ESSENTIAL SURGERY

PROBLEMS, DIAGNOSIS AND MANAGEMENT

CHRIS NUTT
3MBChB
1994-95
UNIVERSITY OF DUNDEE.

ESSENTIAL SURGERY

PROBLEMS, DIAGNOSIS AND MANAGEMENT

H. George Burkitt

BDSc Hons (Queensland) FRACDS MMed Sci (Nottingham) MB BChir (Cambridge)
Medical Author, General Medical Practitioner, Newcastle, NSW, Australia

Clive R.G. Quick

FDS FRCS (England) MS (London)
Consultant General and Vascular Surgeon, Hinchingbrooke Hospital, Huntingdon, and Addenbrooke's Hospital, Cambridge; Associate Lecturer and Examiner in Surgery for MB BChir, University of Cambridge, UK

Dennis Gatt

FRCS (Edinburgh) FRCS (England)
Consultant General, Vascular and Thoracic Surgeon, St Luke's Hospital, G'Mangia; Lecturer and Examiner in Surgery for MD degree, University of Malta, Malta

Drawings by

Philip J. Deakin

BSc Hons MB ChB (Sheffield)
General Medical Practitioner, Sheffield, UK

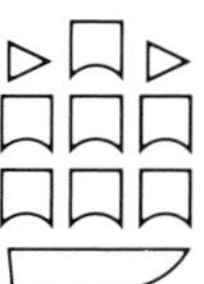

CHURCHILL LIVINGSTONE
EDINBURGH LONDON MELBOURNE AND NEW YORK 1990

CHURCHILL LIVINGSTONE
Medical Division of Longman Group UK Limited

Distributed in the United States of America by Churchill Livingstone Inc., 650 Avenue of the Americas, New York, 10011, and by associated companies, branches and representatives throughout the world.

First published 1990
Reprinted 1990
Reprinted 1991
Reprinted 1992
Reprinted 1993 (twice)
Reprinted 1994

ISBN-0-443-03593-8

British Library Cataloguing in Publication Data
Burkitt, H. George
Essential surgery: problems, diagnosis and management.
1. Medicine. Surgery
I. Title II. Quick, Clive R. G. III. Gatt, Dennis
617

The publisher's policy is to use **paper manufactured from sustainable forests**

Produced by Longman Singapore Publishers (Pte) Ltd
Printed in Singapore

Preface

With so many textbooks of surgery already available, our justification for producing another is that we have taken an entirely new approach to the subject.

This book is written primarily for clinical students. It provides an exposition of the whole field of general surgery and urology suitable for modern clinical courses. It is also a practical manual for junior hospital doctors, up to the level of surgical SHO or junior surgical resident. In addition, this book is designed to be a continuing reference text for doctors in other specialties, including general practice. We hope our book will appeal especially to readers who want to understand surgery rather than merely pass examinations.

There are several major differences between this book and standard surgical textbooks. First, we have tried to explain the pathophysiological basis of surgical diseases and of their management so as to bridge the gap between basic medical sciences and clinical problems. Second, we have adopted a problem-solving rather than a disease-orientated approach to diagnosis and treatment. We believe that understanding how diagnoses are made and why particular treatments are used is more effective and more memorable than rote learning. Third, we have included information about epidemiology, disease prevention and the provision of health care. Fourth, we have extensively used original illustrative material to emphasise important concepts, to avoid unnecessary text and to assist readers in their revision. This includes X-rays, photographs of clinical cases and pathological specimens, anatomical and operative diagrams, tables, flow charts and summaries of the text. Virtually all the clinical photographs and most of the X-rays have been taken from our own practice rather than from commercial libraries, and we have tried to choose typical rather than gross examples of disorders so the student can see how patients commonly present. Fifth, we have included outlines of common surgical operations to enable students and junior doctors to explain operations to patients, to participate intelligently in the operating department, to understand and prevent complications and to perform certain minor operations themselves. Finally, we have included a major section on accident surgery related to the general surgeon.

Surgical practice varies from unit to unit and teaching within each unit tends to reflect local methods. To explain these different but valid approaches to similar problems, we have tried to indicate the principles of how surgical disorders evolve, and the effects of different forms of intervention at various stages. Part I sets the scene by discussing the important pathophysiological processes in clinical terms, and by outlining the principles of cancer management. It also includes an introduction to investigative procedures and the basic principles of operative surgery. These general descriptions are expanded for individual disorders in later chapters.

Junior doctors often find it very difficult to interpret a patient's symptoms and signs to make the correct diagnosis and choose the best treatment option. Abdominal pain, for example, is particularly difficult to sort out. Chapter 6 covers interpretation of non-acute abdominal symptoms, including general aspects of history taking, investigation, diagnosis and management. Chapter 7 deals with clinical aspects of the acute abdomen and acute gastrointestinal haemorrhage, and is based on the pathological processes which produce the physical signs. Chapters 8–31 comprise a systematic and detailed review of surgical disorders. Within this section, Chapters 8–18 cover gastroenterological conditions whilst urological disorders are tackled in Chapters 20–25. Other topics such as breast disease and paediatric surgical disorders are covered in single chapters. The chapter on head and neck problems includes a concise account of dental conditions with which doctors should be familiar.

An important area of concern for the student and junior surgical doctor is the multiplicity of management decisions that must be made. These decisions are faced from moment to moment during assessment, as well as during preoperative and postoperative care. For example, 'Is the patient fit for anaesthesia?', 'Will blood transfusion be necessary?', 'What intravenous fluids are required?', and 'Why is this postoperative patient febrile?' are common surgical questions that must be answered. Throughout the book, we have attempted to view the practical management of patients through the eyes of the trainee. In addition, the whole of Part IV is devoted to specific management problems, and includes chapters on medical problems in surgical patients, complications of surgery, preoperative assessment, postoperative problems, and fluid and nutritional problems.

Teaching surgeons are often unaware of the medical and social aspects of patient care. Yet these are often of vital concern to both doctors in training and their patients. Furthermore, only a small proportion of 'surgical conditions' such as abdominal pain, urinary tract infection or minor injuries ever reach a surgical specialist. Most are managed best outside hospital. Since many doctors will not ultimately work in hospitals, we have tried to relate the community aspects of surgical problems to aetiology, disease prevention, primary care or provision of services.

We cannot pretend that surgery can be taught entirely by a problem-orientated method; at various stages in our text, descriptions of individual diseases have had to be included. Nevertheless, we believe that the benefits of our approach will be apparent and any disadvantages largely overcome by extensive cross-references. We hope readers will enjoy our fresh approach and be stimulated to a greater enjoyment and understanding of the practice of surgery.

H.G.B.
C.R.G.Q.
D.G.

Cambridge, 1990

Acknowledgements

The authors have been honoured by the assistance of many colleagues who provided illustrative material and checked the accuracy of specialist topics. We hope we have done justice to their contributions!

Special thanks are due to Dr Graham Hurst, consultant radiologist at Hinchingbrooke Hospital, Huntingdon, who was responsible for providing the large number of superb radiographs in the book as well as the radiological information in Chapter 2. He was greatly helped in this endeavour by Dr Catherine Hubbard, consultant radiologist at Hinchingbrooke Hospital, and also by many of his radiological colleagues elsewhere who provided valuable radiographs. These include Dr A. Freeman, Dr E.P. Wraight (consultant in nuclear medicine), Professor T. Sherwood, Dr D. Appleton, Dr C. Flower, Dr N. Ashford, Dr R. Coulden, Dr T.D. Hawkins and Dr A.K. Dixon (all of Addenbrooke's Hospital, Cambridge), Dr A. Chalmers (The General Infirmary, Leeds) and Dr L.J. Clark (Queen's Medical Centre, Nottingham).

Dr Alan Stevens, consultant pathologist at the University of Nottingham, reviewed the whole text and gave valuable advice and ideas on pathophysiology. Dr Michael Williams (consultant radiotherapist, Addenbrooke's and Hinchingbrooke Hospitals) provided valuable material for Chapter 4 and reviewed the non-surgical treatment of cancer throughout the book. Dr Paul Wheater of Cambridge provided and photographed the histopathological specimens as well as contributing some fine clinical photographs. Other colleagues who provided clinical illustrations include Mr David Matthews (consultant dental surgeon, Princess Royal R.A.F. Hospital, Ely), Mr W.G. Everett (consultant surgeon, Addenbrooke's Hospital), Dr D. Carr-Locke (consultant gastroenterologist, Leicester Royal Infirmary), Mr M. Owen-Smith (consultant surgeon, Hinchingbrooke Hospital) and Mr Campbell Calder (dental surgeon, Cambridge). To them all, we are greatly indebted.

Black and white photographs of surgical equipment and reproductions of all radiographs and clinical slides were meticulously and painstakingly prepared for publication by Mr Leonard Beard, director of the department of medical photography at Hinchingbrooke Hospital.

Invaluable epidemiological data about cancer in the East Anglian Region was provided by Dr Kingsley Pillars, director of the regional cancer registry in Cambridge, to whom we are grateful.

Many specialist colleagues reviewed our work in their areas of interest and were generous in their criticisms. Any errors that remain are our responsibility, not theirs. Particular thanks go to Mr Andrew Higgins (consultant surgeon and urologist, Hinchingbrooke Hospital), Drs Bill Newsom and Rod Warren (consultant microbiologists, Hinchingbrooke and Addenbrooke's

Hospitals), Dr Howard Smith (consultant anaesthetist, Hinchingbrooke Hospital), Dr Kate Hoggarth (consultant haematologist, Hinchingbrooke Hospital), Dr Michael Williams (consultant radiotherapist, Hinchingbrooke and Addenbrooke's Hospitals), Mr W.G. Everett (consultant surgeon, Addenbrooke's Hospital), Dr Barbara Young (medical registrar), Dr Trevor Wheatley (senior medical registrar), Dr R.J. Dickinson (consultant gastroenterologist, Hinchingbrooke Hospital) and Mr Paul Calvert (consultant orthopaedic and trauma surgeon, St George's Hospital, London). Many other friends, colleagues, junior staff and students willingly contributed time and ideas during the formative stages. To them all, we give our grateful thanks.

As the project neared completion, Dr Jane Hailey, initially as a medical student and later whilst surgical house officer (intern) to C.R.G.Q., spent countless hours reviewing the whole text in meticulous detail, simplifying the language and turning obscurity into clarity. We owe her a great debt of gratitude for this vital work and wish her well in her future writing endeavours.

Finally, our greatest thanks go to our wives who put up with our seemingly endless preoccupation with 'the book' yet always offered their encouragement.

Publisher's note about the authors

The authorship of this book is unusual in that only one of the authors was a consultant surgeon at the time of writing (C.R.G.Q.), while the other two were junior hospital doctors. We believe this has resulted in the radical new and refreshing approach used in this publication.

George Burkitt obtained qualifications in dental surgery and community medicine before studying clinical medicine as a mature student in Cambridge (England). This book was written while he was a senior house officer and represents the book he would like to have had during his training. He has a deep interest in medical education and is co-author of two other popular student texts by the same publisher. These are *Functional Histology* and *Basic Histopathology*, the former written whilst a preclinical medical student in Nottingham and the latter as a clinical student in Cambridge. He has now returned to Australia where he is a family practitioner in Newcastle, NSW.

Clive Quick also trained initially as a dental surgeon but is now a consultant general and vascular surgeon at the teaching hospitals associated with the Clinical School of the University of Cambridge. He has a strong interest in computers as tools of communication. As an associate lecturer in the University, he teaches and examines clinical students in surgery. He is also heavily involved in training junior surgeons which is how he came to know his two co-authors. He is also the organiser of the Cambridge FRCS course and the Cambridge Anastomosis Workshop.

Dennis Gatt is now a consultant general, thoracic and vascular surgeon in his home country of Malta, having become associated with his co-authors whilst undergoing postgraduate surgical training in the Cambridge area. He played a vital role in the conception and planning of the book and also produced the index.

The mechanics of how this book was written were also unconventional. Working from a detailed protocol, the book was written directly onto a word processer by the first two authors working together. Each point was discussed (often heatedly and at length) until it was agreed that the topic was explained as clearly and unambigously as it could be. Editing and formatting were all performed 'on screen' and the whole book was later typeset direct from the computer disks.

The artist, Philip Deakin, first trained in physiology and later in medicine and is now a family doctor in Sheffield. He previously made the drawings for *Functional Histology*, mentioned earlier. For this book, he prepared the drawings from preliminary work by two of the authors, C.R.G.Q. and D.G., using his professional knowledge to achieve unusual accuracy whilst retaining an attractive simplicity and clarity of style.

Contents

PART III: SYMPTOMS, DIAGNOSIS AND MANAGEMENT

PART I
BASIC SURGICAL PRINCIPLES

1 PATHOPHYSIOLOGICAL PROCESSES OF SURGICAL IMPORTANCE

Introduction

Surgical diagnostic method is often taught by comparing a patient's symptoms and signs with standard sets which are known to characterise each disease. But while most disorders match their classical descriptions at certain stages in their evolution, this may not be so at the moment the patient presents for treatment. Perhaps more commonly, patients present before recognisable patterns have developed or else at a late stage, the typical clinical picture having been missed or ignored on the way.

Yet again, the diagnostic process can be confused if all the symptoms and signs expected for a particular diagnosis are not present, or if symptoms and signs are present which seem inconsistent with the working diagnosis.

This chapter, and indeed the whole book, seeks to elucidate a more logical and reliable approach to diagnosis than simple pattern recognition, by attempting to explain symptoms and signs on the basis of the underlying pathophysiology and local anatomy. This chapter provides a review of the main mechanisms of 'surgical' disease against a background of the basic medical sciences.

Fig. 1.1 Principal mechanisms of surgical disease

Trauma
Anatomical abnormalities — congenital or acquired
Disorders of normal function
Inflammation — infection, chemical and immunological mechanisms
Ischaemia and infarction
Metabolic and hormonal disorders
Neoplasia — benign and malignant
Other abnormalities of growth

PRINCIPAL MECHANISMS OF SURGICAL DISEASE

1. Trauma

Tissue trauma, literally injury, in its wider sense includes damage inflicted by any physical means, i.e. mechanical, thermal, chemical, electrical or radiation. Common usage, however, tends to imply blunt or penetrating mechanical injury as caused by accidents in industry or in the home, road traffic accidents, fights, firearms and other missiles. Damage varies according to the nature of the causative agent, and the surface injuries may give no indication of the extent of deep tissue damage as for example, head injuries and bullet wounds.

2. Anatomical abnormalities

Anatomical abnormalities may be developmental in origin, i.e. *congenital*, or else *acquired* as a result of trauma or some other disease process.

Congenital abnormalities of surgical interest range from potentially fatal conditions such as urethral valves and various gut atresias to minor cosmetic deformities. Developmental abnormalities may become manifest at any time from fetal life to old age, although the majority appear at birth or in early childhood. For example, gut atresias may present with grossly excessive amniotic fluid (*polyhydramnios*) during pregnancy, whereas urethral valves may present in the neonatal period as obstructive renal failure. Patent processus vaginalis may result in an inguinal hernia at any stage from birth to early adulthood, while renal abnormalities such as polycystic kidney may present in middle life as an abdominal mass, renal failure or haematuria.

Whilst many congenital abnormalities produce disease by direct *anatomical* effects, other abnormalities may produce disease by more subtle *disruption of function*, the underlying disorder only being revealed on investigation. For example, certain ureteric abnormalities allow urinary reflux from the bladder and predispose to recurrent kidney infections.

Acquired anatomical abnormalities result from *damage* inflicted by a disease, by the body's *response* to a disease or by *treatment* of a disease. For example, obstruction of the bladder outlet may result from benign prostatic hypertrophy, the fibrotic response to gonococcal urethritis or damage inflicted during urethral instrumentation.

3. Disorders of function

A variety of common disorders owe their origin to abnormalities of function. The gastrointestinal tract is particularly susceptible; for example, large bowel malfunction leads to constipation, irritable bowel syndrome and diverticular disease. The modern low-fibre diet is undoubtedly an important cause of these disorders, the colon having evolved on a diet high in fibre.

4. Inflammation

Many surgical disorders result from inflammatory processes, most often the result of infection. Surgical admissions due to infection have markedly decreased since the advent of antibiotics; unfortunately infection remains a common complication of operative surgery. Inflammation may also result from physical irritation, particularly by noxious chemical agents, e.g. gastric acid/pepsin in peptic ulcer disease, pancreatic enzymes in acute pancreatitis. Immunological mechanisms certainly play a part in the inflammatory bowel disorders of ulcerative colitis and Crohn's disease, although whether they constitute cause or effect is not yet known.

5. Ischaemia and infarction

Obliterative atherosclerosis is an enormous cause of morbidity and mortality, particularly in later life. When the disease restricts flow in large distributing arteries to the extent of causing acute or chronic ischaemia, it is often amenable to surgical procedures to improve flow (e.g. aorto-femoral bypass grafting); when atherosclerosis is severe and generalised, however, reconstructive surgery may not be possible and amputation of an ischaemic limb may be the only alternative.

Arterial emboli may also cause acute ischaemia; such emboli usually originate in the heart or atherosclerotic aorta. Surgical embolectomy can often retrieve the occluding material and restore flow in the femoral arteries and occasionally in the superior mesenteric artery.

Atherosclerosis of the carotid bifurcation and other extracranial arteries causes disease in two ways: first, by vascular narrowing or occlusion *inhibiting the blood supply* and, second, by accumulation of platelet thrombi on atherosclerotic ulcers which then *embolise* into the brain causing strokes or transient ischaemic attacks. Either type of disease may require surgical reconstruction.

Chronic venous insufficiency in the lower limb is responsible for the majority of chronic leg ulcers, the elevated hydrostatic venous pressure interfering with nutrition and gas exchange in the superficial tissues of the leg. When a portion of bowel becomes strangulated, the initial mechanism of tissue damage is venous obstruction which eventually progresses to arterial ischaemia and infarction.

6. Metabolic disorders

The lower limb complications of diabetes, particularly the *diabetic foot*, represent an important surgical problem; in addition, diabetes predisposes to atherosclerosis. Diabetes also poses special management problems in the patient undergoing surgery.

Hypersecretion of certain hormones, as in thyrotoxicosis and hyperparathyroidism, may require surgical reduction of glandular tissue. Other metabolic disorders may cause stones in the gall bladder (e.g. haemolytic diseases causing pigment stones) or in the urinary tract (e.g. hypercalciuria and hyperuricaemia causing calcium and uric acid stones respectively).

7. Neoplasia

Malignant tumours are responsible for a large part of the surgical workload. Many surgical referrals are initiated by the fear or suspicion of cancer and many investigations and some operations are performed in the hope of refuting the diagnosis. Some malignant neoplasms are curable by operative surgery but all too often the appearance of distant metastases or subsequent recurrent disease dashes the hope of a cure. In incurable cases, worthwhile surgical palliation may improve the quality of life or even extend life expectancy.

Certain *benign tumours*, such as lipomas, are very common and require surgery mainly for cosmetic reasons. Less commonly, benign tumours are removed either because of obstruction to a hollow viscus or because of surface bleeding. Benign endocrine tumours may have to be removed because of excess hormone secretion, e.g. an insulinoma which causes hypoglycaemia, or a parathyroid adenoma which causes hypercalcaemia. Finally, benign tumours may be indistinguishable clinically from malignant tumours and are therefore removed to obtain a complete histological diagnosis.

8. Other abnormalities of tissue growth

In surgery, the term *cyst* is imprecisely used to describe a mass which appears to contain fluid because of its characteristic fluctuance and transilluminability. In true pathological terms, cysts are epithelium-lined cavities; most represent dilatation of ducts by retained secretion, usually due to obstruction. In some cases there is epithelial hyperplasia, excessive secretion and structural distortion as, for example, in breast cysts. Some cysts arise from ectopic epithelial remnants or as a result of necrosis in the centre of an epithelial mass. Cysts commonly require surgical removal (or drainage) for aesthetic reasons, or to exclude malignancy, e.g. epidermal cysts, epididymal cysts, breast cysts.

Other growth disturbances such as *hyperplasia* and *hypertrophy* give rise to surgical problems, in particular benign prostatic hypertrophy, fibroadenosis of the breast and thyroid goitres.

'The surgical sieve'

The foregoing mechanisms of surgical disease may provide a useful 'first principles' framework or aide memoire upon which to construct a differential diagnosis. This is particularly useful when the symptoms and signs do not immediately point to a diagnosis. This approach is often referred to as the 'surgical sieve'.

ACUTE INFLAMMATION AND ITS OUTCOMES

Acute inflammation is the principal mechanism by which living tissues respond to injury. The purpose of the inflammatory response is to neutralise the injurious agent, to remove damaged or necrotic tissue and to restore the tissue to useful function. The central feature of acute inflammation is the formation of an inflammatory exudate. This has three principal constituents: *serum*, *leucocytes* (predominantly neutrophils) and *fibrinogen*.

Formation of the inflammatory exudate involves three *vascular phenomena* which are collectively responsible for the *'Cardinal signs of Celsus'*, i.e. redness, swelling, heat, pain and loss of function:

- Dilatation of local blood vessels leads to engorgement of the tissues and increased perfusion; clinically this is responsible for local redness, heat and some of the swelling
- Increased capillary permeability results in the passage of serum and plasma proteins (including immunoglobulins and fibrinogen) into the extracellular tissues and this further increases the swelling (oedema). Pain results from swelling and from some of the substances which mediate the inflammatory process, e.g. kinins. The inflammatory exudate serves to irrigate the area, diluting toxins and organisms which are drained away to regional lymph nodes. Fibrinogen polymerises to form fibrin in the damaged tissue which inhibits bacterial spread
- Leucocytes migrate into the area of injured tissues where the neutrophils and macrophages (both tissue-fixed and those derived from blood monocytes)

commence phagocytosis of tissue debris. Macrophages are long-lived but neutrophils die after a burst of lysosomal activity, releasing *endogenous pyrogens* which are at least partly responsible for the fever often associated with acute inflammation

The possible outcomes of the acute inflammatory process are summarised in Figure 1.2.

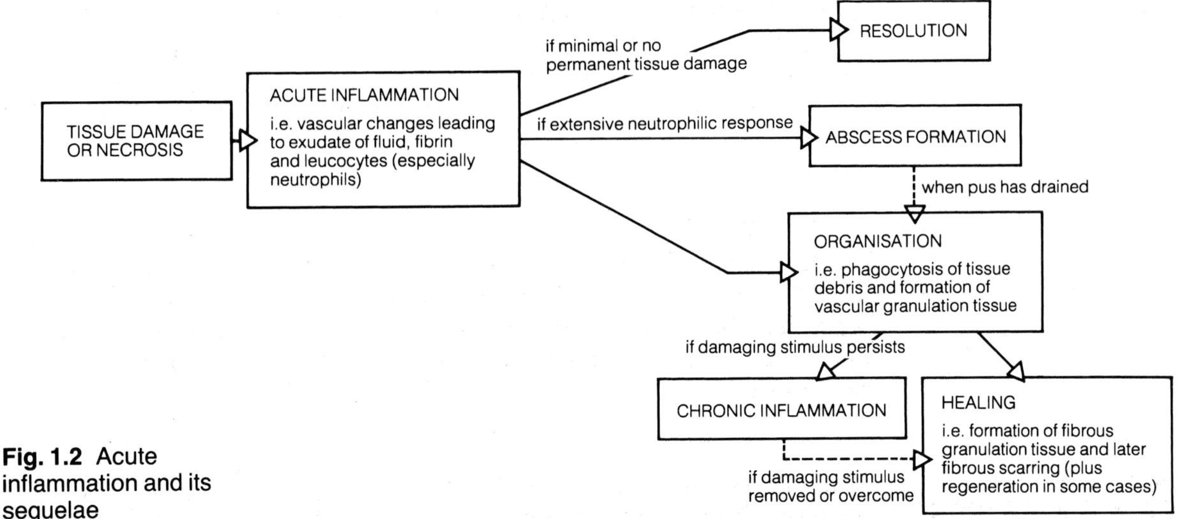

Fig. 1.2 Acute inflammation and its sequelae

1. Resolution

If tissue damage is minimal and there is no actual tissue necrosis, then the acute inflammatory response settles. The tissue returns to normal with no evidence of scarring. A good example is the resolution of sunburn or transient peptic gastritis.

2. Abscess formation

An *abscess* is a collection of pus (dead and dying neutrophils plus proteinaceous exudate) walled off by a zone of acute inflammation. Acute abscess formation occurs particularly in response to certain micro-organisms which attract neutrophils and yet are resistant to phagocytosis or lysosomal destruction. Abscess formation also occurs in response to highly localised tissue necrosis and to some organic foreign bodies (e.g. wood splinters, linen suture material). In such cases, however, infection may also be involved. The main *pyogenic organisms* of surgical importance are *Staphylococcus aureus*, some streptococci (particularly *Streptococcus pyogenes* and *Pneumococci*), *Escherichia coli* and related gram-negative bacilli ('coliforms'), and *Bacteroides*.

In general, without treatment, abscesses tend to 'point' spontaneously to the nearest epithelial surface (e.g. skin, gut, bronchus), eventually discharging their contents; provided the injurious agent is thereby eliminated, drainage leads to healing. If an abscess is far from a surface (e.g. deep in the breast), it progressively enlarges, causing much tissue destruction. Sometimes local defence mechanisms are overwhelmed, leading to runaway local infection.

Even with small and well localised abscesses, showers of bacteria enter the general circulation but are mopped up by the phagocytic cells of the liver and spleen before they can proliferate (*bacteraemia*). This process is responsible for a *swinging pyrexia* which is highly characteristic of an abscess; the site may not be clinically apparent if the abscess is very deep-seated (e.g. subphrenic or pelvic abscess) and the patient may be otherwise well. A typical temperature chart is shown in Figure 1.3. In the presence of an abscess, the number of neutrophils in the bloodstream rises dramatically as they are released in greater numbers from the bone marrow; thus, a marked *neutrophil leucocytosis* (i.e. white cell count greater than 15×10^9/l with more than 80% neutrophils) is usually indicative of a pyogenic infection. Severe infection may result in *septicaemia*, in which case bacteria multiply in large numbers in the general circulation, producing rapid clinical deterioration.

If spontaneous drainage does not eliminate the injurious agent, the neutrophilic response persists and pus continues to be formed, resulting in a *chronic abscess*. This may be manifest only by its secondary effect (i.e. a swinging pyrexia) or, alternatively, as a continuously discharging sinus or an abscess at the surface which cyclically forms, discharges and then heals. From the foregoing, it follows that the essential principle of management of any abscess is to establish drainage, usually by incision or aspiration. Any residual necrotic or foreign material must be eliminated by curettage or excision. Indeed, before the antibiotic era, abscesses were a major cause of hospital admission and the principle of drainage was well known, most hospitals having a separate 'septic' ward for such patients.

Antibiotics are often misused in the treatment of abscesses. Once an abscess has fully formed, antibiotics will seldom effect a cure because the pus and foreign or necrotic material remains and antibiotics cannot gain ready access to the bacteria within the pus; nevertheless, antibiotics may halt expansion or even sterilise the pus, the residual sterile abscess sometimes being known as an *antibioma*. If appropriate antibiotics are given early enough, organisms can be eliminated before they produce an abscess. For example, staphylococcal breast infections are common during lactation and if untreated often lead to formation of a breast abscess; this formerly common surgical problem is now rare because of timely antibiotic treatment by the general practitioner. Likewise, in surgical operations where there is known to be a particular risk of infection, the use of prophylactic antibiotics will dramatically reduce the incidence of postoperative abscess formation.

3. Organisation and repair

The most common sequel to acute inflammation is *organisation* in which dead tissue is removed by phagocytosis, the defect being filled by vascular connec-

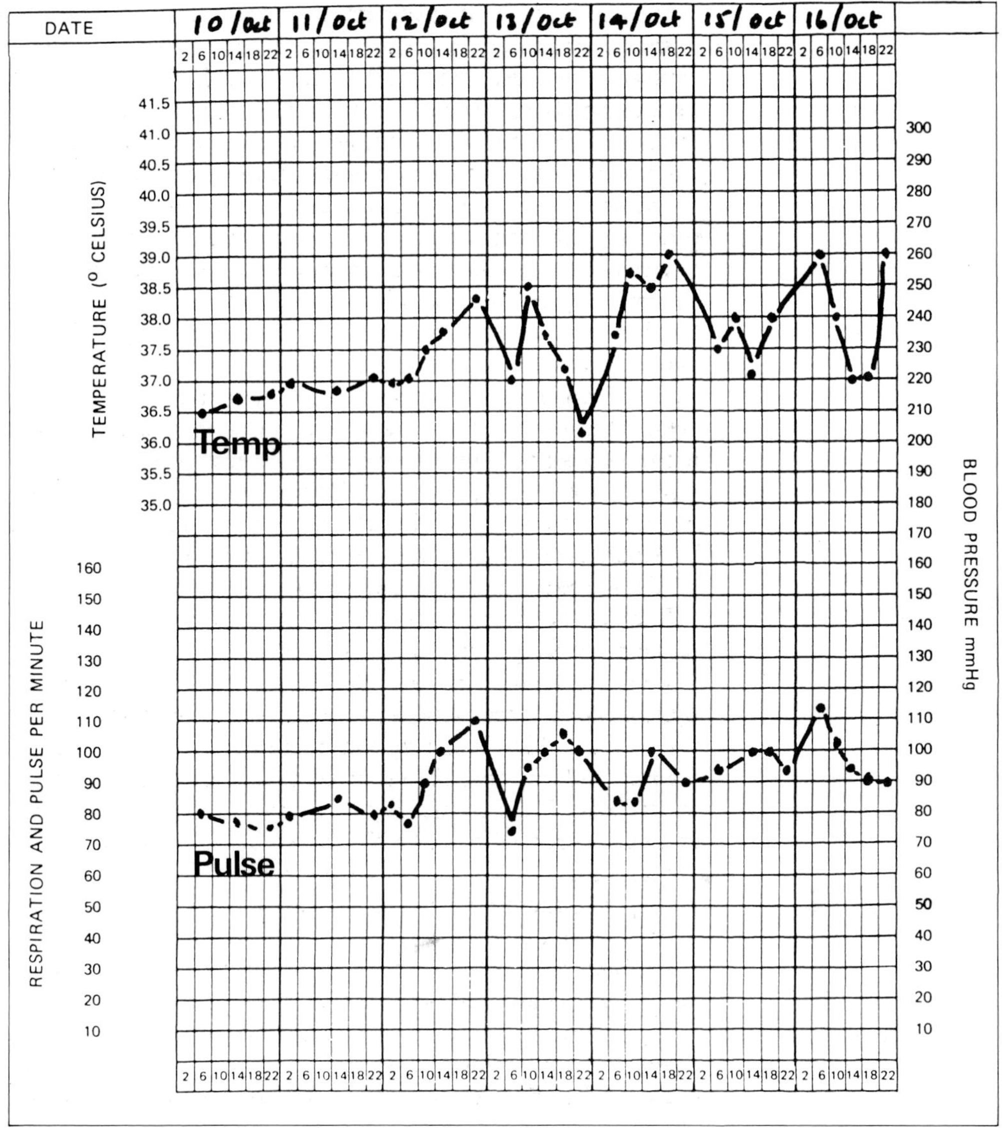

Fig. 1.3 Temperature chart showing swinging pyrexia

tive tissue known as *granulation tissue*. The granulation tissue is gradually 'repaired' by a *fibrous scar*. In some cases the original tissue may regenerate.

The simplest example of organisation and repair is healing of an uncomplicated skin incision. In such cases, there is no necrotic tissue and the margins of the wound are brought into apposition by sutures. An acute inflammatory response develops in the immediate vicinity of the incision and, by the third day, granulation tissue bridges the dermal defect. In the meantime, proliferation of the surface epithelium rapidly restores the epidermis. Fibroblasts invade the granulation tissue, laying down collagen so that the repair is strong enough to permit suture removal after 5–10 days. At this stage the scar is still red but as the blood vessels gradually regress it turns into a pale linear scar. This process is known as *healing by primary intention.*

If the edges of a wound cannot be apposed because of tissue loss, the healing process has to make good the deficiency. The defect is initially filled with blood clot which becomes invaded by vascular granulation tissue from the healthy wound base. At the surface, the inflammatory exudate solidifies, forming a protective scab. Fibrin in the clot contracts, helping to draw the wound edges together, thus reducing the size of the defect. Fibroblasts invade the granulation tissue and collagen is laid down in the extracellular spaces; fibroblast contraction further shrinks the wound defect. Over the succeeding weeks and months, the blood vessels regress and more collagen is formed, leaving a relatively avascular scar; gradual contraction of the collagen (cicatrisation) ensures that the final scar is much smaller than the original defect. The overlying epidermal defect is gradually bridged by epithelial proliferation from the wound margins. The epithelial cells slide over each other on the surface of the granulation tissue and beneath the edges of the scab which is thus eventually shed. This whole process is known as *healing by secondary intention.*

The rate and success of wound healing may be compromised by a variety of local factors including infection, poor or damaged blood supply, and systemic factors such as malnutrition.

4. Chronic inflammation

In certain circumstances, an injurious agent persists over a long period causing continuing tissue destruction. At the same time the body attempts to deal with both the original and the continuing tissue damage by the process of acute inflammation, organisation and repair. In such cases, the damaged area may exhibit several pathological processes concurrently, i.e. tissue necrosis, an inflammatory response, granulation tissue formation and fibrous scarring, the whole process being known as *chronic inflammation*. Histologically this is characterised by a predominance of macrophages (sometimes forming giant cells) which are responsible for phagocytosis of necrotic debris. Lymphocytes and plasma cells are also present, indicating the involvement of immunological mechanisms in chronic inflammation.

Chronic inflammation represents a tenuous balance between a persistent injurious agent and the body's reparative responses. Healing only takes place if the injurious agent is removed and will then occur in the usual manner but with much greater scarring.

A wide range of agents can lead to chronic inflammation and the clinical pattern of disease can be subdivided into three broad categories: *chronic abscesses, chronic ulcers* and the *specific granulomatous infections and inflammations.*

a. Chronic abscesses

As described earlier, a chronic abscess may arise if the injurious agent associated with an acute abscess is not eliminated by spontaneous discharge of the pus or surgical drainage. In this case pus continues to be formed and the abscess

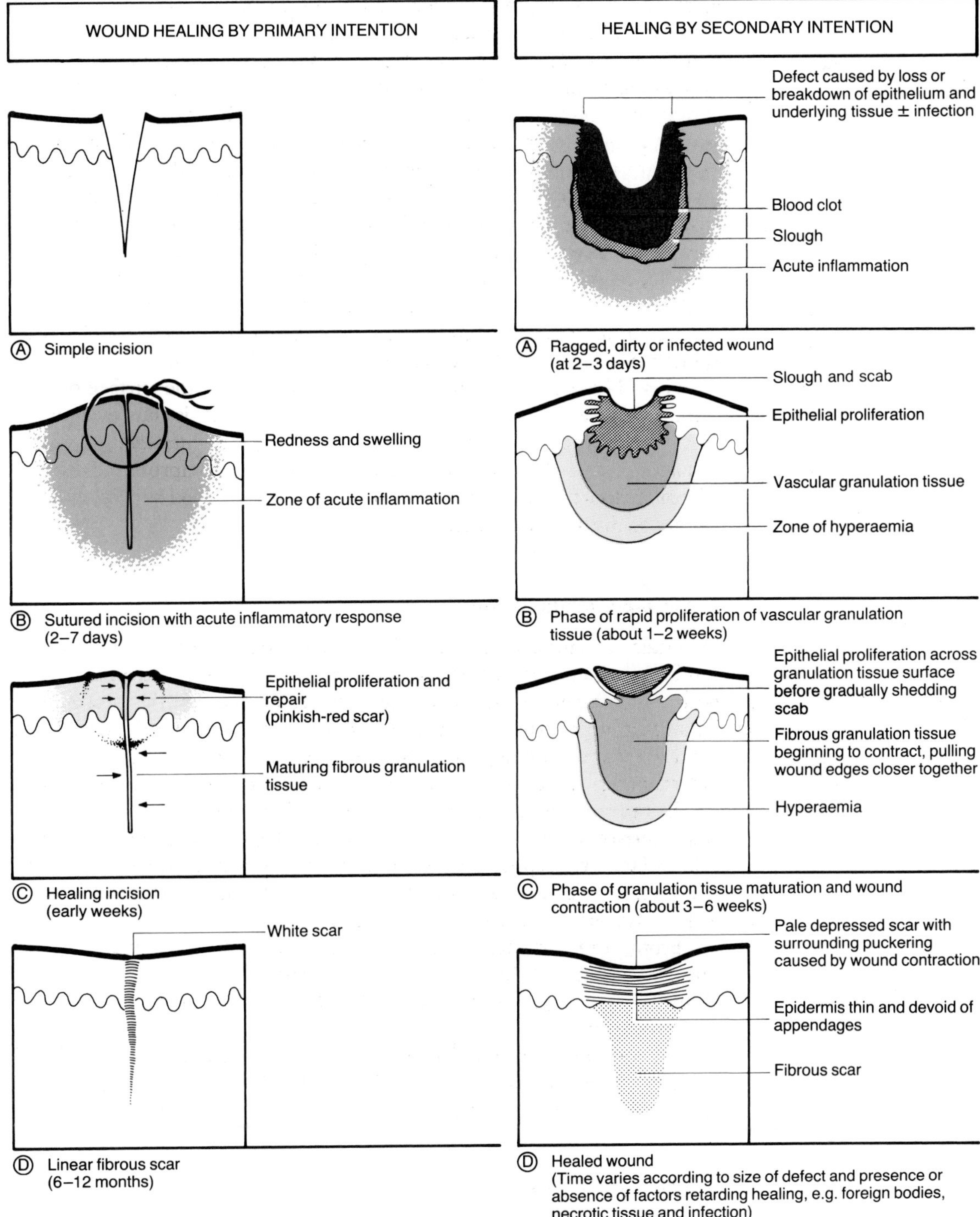

Fig. 1.4 Wound healing by primary and secondary intention

discharges continuously via a sinus or else 'points' and discharges periodically, the sinus healing over between times. The wall of the chronic abscess is formed of fibrous scar and granulation tissue as a result of attempted healing at the periphery.

In modern surgical practice, *infected foreign bodies* are probably the most common cause of chronic abscess formation; such foreign bodies may have been deliberately implanted but have become infected (e.g. deep sutures after inguinal hernia repair, prosthetic hip joint) or have become embedded during an accident (e.g. glass fragments). In addition, dead tissue of any sort can act in the same way as a foreign body, forming a nidus for infection. In this context, hairs becoming deeply implanted in the skin of the natal cleft may cause a pilonidal sinus or abscess. Similarly, an infected dead tooth or root with an associated 'gum boil' is also a manifestation of a chronic abscess (see Figure 1.5). Likewise, chronic osteomyelitis is associated with remnants of dead bone

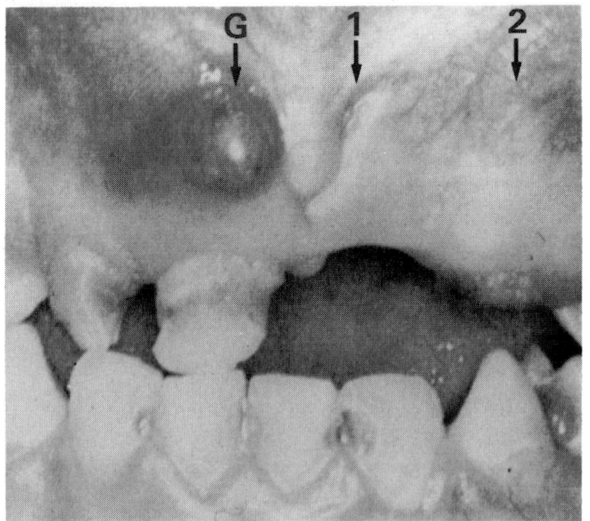

Fig. 1.5 'Gum boil'
Grossly neglected mouth showing widespread dental caries. There is an inflammatory swelling on the buccal aspect of the alveolus **G** caused by a chronic apical dental abscess on the upper right central incisor. Note the left central incisor **1** is missing and the left lateral incisor **2** has fractured at gum level because of caries

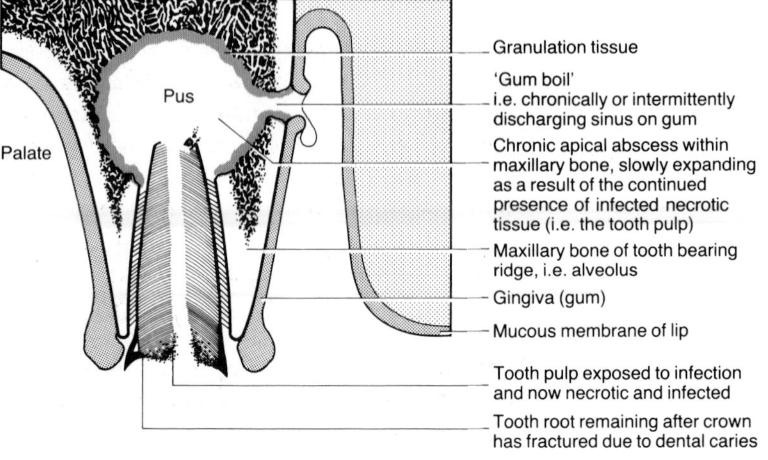

Saggital section through 'gum boil' of upper incisor tooth

known as sequestra. In the foot, diabetes may be complicated by deep infections resulting in necrosis of tendon and bone, leading to chronic abscesses and ulcers. Finally, a chronic abscess can arise without a foreign body if the abscess is so deep and well circumscribed as to prevent spontaneous drainage; the best example is a subphrenic abscess.

b. Chronic ulcers

An ulcer is defined as a persistent defect in an epithelial or mucosal surface. With the exception of malignant ulcers, ulceration usually results from a combination of low-grade traumatic or chemical injury to both epithelium and underlying connective tissue plus some impairment of the reparative response. For example, elderly and debilitated patients are susceptible to pressure sores ('bed sores') which develop over bony prominences such as sacrum and heels. In such cases, the patient does not regularly shift position to relieve the pressure of body weight because of immobility and diminished protective pain response. Tissue necrosis results and subsequent healing is impaired by recurrent pressure ischaemia, poor tissue perfusion (from cardiac or peripheral vascular disease) and malnutrition.

Another common example is the chronic leg ulcer in chronic venous insufficiency; this fails to heal because of local ischaemia induced by the high venous pressure, the problem often being exacerbated by secondary infection.

A chronic peptic ulcer results from persistent acid-pepsin attack upon the gastric or duodenal mucosa, the lesion persisting because the reparative response is just insufficient to tip the balance in favour of repair. The lesion is often initiated and then exacerbated by alcohol, aspirin or other drugs. On the other hand, healing can be assisted by neutralising the acid with antacids, by blocking acid production with H_2 receptor antagonists or by enhancing local protective factors with drugs such as sucralfate.

In summary, a chronic ulcer represents a tenuous, unresolved balance between persistent injurious factors and inadequate reparative responses. The principle of management is therefore to diminish or remove the damaging factors and to promote the healing response.

c. The specific granulomatous infections and inflammations

Certain micro-organisms such as *Mycobacterium tuberculosis, Mycobacterium leprae* and *Treponema pallidum* (causing tuberculosis, leprosy and syphilis respectively) excite a minimal acute inflammatory response and produce almost from the outset a chronic inflammatory response. The lesions are characterised by macrophage accumulation forming *granulomas*, the diseases thus being known as the *specific granulomatous infections*.

Certain extremely fine particulate materials, such as talc and beryllium, produce a similar granulomatous reaction known as *foreign body granuloma*. Talc was traditionally used as a lubricant powder in surgical gloves and sometimes resulted in a diffuse and intense granulomatous peritoneal reaction after laparotomy, causing widespread bowel adhesions. Talc has now been abandoned and replaced by starch, although the present trend is to use gloves without powder.

The tuberculous *cold abscess*, represents a pus-like accumulation of liquefied caseous material containing mycobacteria. In contrast to the pyogenic abscess, the lesion is cold to the touch since there is no associated acute inflammatory vascular response. Tuberculous abscesses are now rare in developed countries but were once common. Cervical lymph node tuberculosis ('scrofula') often produced a 'collar-stud' abscess i.e. a superficial fluctuant abscess communicating via a small fascial defect with a deep (and often larger) lymph node abscess. Tuberculosis of the thoraco-lumbar spine, in addition to local destruction, may track down under the inguinal ligament within the psoas sheath to present as a 'psoas abscess' in the groin.

INFECTION

Clinically significant infection arises when the size of the inoculum or virulence of an organism is sufficient to overcome resistance from protective surface phenomena, non-specific tissue defences and any specific immune responses. Consequently, the virulence of an organism depends on its adherence, invasiveness and its ability to produce toxins. Tissue invasion may be enhanced by production of enzymes (e.g. hyaluronidase and streptokinase), avoidance of phagocytosis (e.g. encapsulation or spore formation), resistance to lysosomal destruction or the ability to kill phagocytes. Toxins may be secreted by the organism (*exotoxins*) or released upon the death of the organism (*endotoxins*); in either case the toxin may produce local tissue damage (e.g. gas gangrene) or systemic effects (e.g. tetanus, septic shock and disseminated intravascular coagulopathy).

Infections may be *community-acquired* (e.g. pneumococcal lobar pneumonia in a fit young adult) or *hospital-acquired*. The latter are known as *nosocomial* infections, and may be with a primary pathogen or post-surgical.

In *post-surgical* infections, organisms gain entry to the tissues through an *abnormal opening*, i.e. surface damage (such as a surgical or traumatic wound) or a perforated viscus. Alternatively, physiological *protective mechanisms* may be disrupted, allowing infection to gain ascendancy; neutropenia predisposes to infection, and bronchopneumonia is liable to develop in a smoker following immobility or anaesthesia.

Furthermore, the surgical patient's *general resistance* may be impaired by malnutrition, malignancy, steroid therapy or other immunosuppressive drugs. In many cases, the infecting organisms are part of the patient's normal skin, gut or respiratory tract flora or are normally present in the external environment. Constantly present is the risk of hospital-acquired infection with a primary pathogen, the infecting organisms arising from 'carriers' among staff, by cross-infection from other infected patients or from contaminated equipment or furnishings.

BACTERIA OF PARTICULAR SURGICAL IMPORTANCE

STAPHYLOCOCCI

Pathophysiology

Staphylococci are gram-positive organisms of which the main pathogenic species is *Staph. aureus*. This typically produces pustules, boils, breast abscesses, wound infections and osteomyelitis. *Staph. epidermidis* (formerly S. albus) is a universal skin commensal which rarely produces significant clinical infection or merits antibiotic therapy, with the exception of infections of prosthetic implants and intravenous cannula sites. In contrast, *Staph. aureus* is a much less widespread commensal, but still about 30% of the general population are nasal carriers and 10% carry it on the perineal skin.

Part of the virulence of *Staph. aureus* is due to its production of *coagulase* which promotes clotting of plasma, thereby erecting a barrier to neutrophil activity. Staphylococci have cell walls which are resistant to adverse conditions such as drying, thus allowing the organism to persist for long periods under dry conditions such as in ward dust.

Antibiotic sensitivity

In the early antibiotic era, most Staphylococci were sensitive to the common antibiotics, including penicillin. More than 85% of strains are now resistant in both general practice and hospital. This is largely due to their ability to produce *penicillinase*. Most *Staph. aureus* strains remain sensitive to a reasonable range of commonly used antibiotics, e.g. *flucloxacillin* (a penicillinase-resistant penicillin), *erythromycin* and some of the *cephalosporins*; gentamicin is also useful against *Staph. aureus*.

A new and potentially devastating problem is the emergence of strains of *Staph. aureus* resistant to methicillin, flucloxacillin and virtually all other antibiotics except the relatively toxic and expensive drug vancomycin; such strains are known by the term *methicillin resistant Staph. aureus* (MRSA). Infections with this organism have appeared sporadically and then spread to cause serious and often fatal infections elsewhere. Radical measures have to be taken to prevent spread of epidemic proportions. Ward areas at greatest risk of MRSA infection are burns units, intensive care units, cardiothoracic surgical wards, neonatal units, orthopaedic wards and geriatric wards.

STREPTOCOCCI

Streptococci are gram-positive organisms which were first described in relation to infected surgical wounds by Billroth in 1874. They are divided into *aerobic* and *anaerobic* groups and, mainly for historical reasons, the aerobes are classified by their ability to haemolyse blood agar culture plates. Alpha organisms produce a narrow band of haemolysis, beta organisms produce a broad band of haemolysis and the gamma group are non-haemolytic. The beta group is subdivided into Lancefield groups or species, labelled A-O; the main human pathogens are in Lancefield group A (*Strep. pyogenes*) and group F.

Aerobic streptococci

a. Alpha streptococci

This group includes the *viridans streptococci* which are oral commensal organisms of low virulence and the most common organism involved in infective endocarditis. The group also includes the pneumococcus (*Strep. pneumoniae*), which causes lobar pneumonia in fit subjects. The pneumococcus also causes bronchopneumonia in susceptible surgical patients and is also associated with chronic bronchitis.

b. Beta streptococci, Lancefield group A (Strep. pyogenes)

These are the main human pathogens. *Strep. pyogenes* is carried in the upper respiratory tract in about 10% of children but not by adults. It is surgically important as the main cause of cellulitis and, less commonly nowadays, erysipelas. *Strep. pyogenes* is also the common cause of sore throat as well as post-streptococcal syndromes such as rheumatic fever, which predisposes to valvular damage and subsequent infective endocarditis.

Cellulitis is a local spreading infection involving the dermis and hypodermis, facilitated by the production of hyaluronidase and streptokinase; *Strep. pyogenes* is the usual cause. In the case of limb infections, organisms draining via lymphatics towards regional lymph nodes may produce perilymphatic inflammation causing painful red streaks along the limb, i.e. *lymphangitis*. The regional nodes react vigorously, becoming enlarged, painful and tender, a condition described as *lymphadenitis*. This also occurs in staphylococcal infections.

c. Strep. faecalis

This group of non-haemolytic aerobic organisms is commonly referred to as the *enterococci*. They form part of the normal bowel flora, but may cause infection where bowel has been opened or where there is faecal contamination of the urinary or genital tracts. Biliary infection is rare and the most common infections are of the urinary tract. *Strep. faecalis* may also cause infective endocarditis.

d. Beta streptococci, Lancefield group F

Strep. milleri is increasing in importance and now forms the commonest single isolate from abscesses in the appendix area, the liver, lung and brain.

Anaerobic streptococci

The anaerobic streptococci include *peptococci* and *peptostreptococci* — bowel commensals which form part of the mixed flora in many intraperitoneal abscesses and diabetic foot ulcers.

Antibiotic sensitivities

Most streptococci are sensitive to *benzyl penicillin* (which must be given parenterally) and oral *penicillin V* (phenoxymethyl penicillin). They are also sensitive to *ampicillin/amoxycillin*. Enterococci (*Strep. faecalis*) are most sensitive to ampicillin/amoxycillin. Streptococci are also usually sensitive to *erythromycin* but are always resistant to the cephalosporins. Development of resistant strains of *Strep. faecalis* is becoming a problem; in some laboratories, 50% of them are resistant to all antibiotics except vancomycin and gentamicin.

ENTEROBACTERIACEAE

Pathophysiology

The Enterobacteriaceae are a large family of gram-negative bacilli (i.e. rods) which usually make up about 1% of the normal intestinal flora (see Figure 1.6); these organisms are commonly referred to as 'coliforms'. The organisms can be cultured under aerobic conditions and, like other members of the bowel flora, grow in bile-salt containing media such as McConkey's agar; this helps in their identification.

Infections of surgical importance are usually opportunistic in nature, the bacteria almost always arising from the patient's own gut. Infection results from direct contamination from opened gut, perineal spread (to nearby wounds or urinary tract) or haematogenous spread. *E. coli* is the most common pathogen of the Enterobacteriaceae and is responsible for many surgical infections, usually in synergy with other bacteria (Kelly's synergy); *E. coli* rarely cause infection alone. *E. coli* is involved particularly in urinary tract infections (about 80% of all UTIs) and gram-negative septicaemia. *E. coli* bronchopneumonia occasionally occurs in debilitated, immunosuppressed or seriously ill patients. *Klebsiella*, *Enterobacter* and *Serratia* are being found more often in surgical gut-related infections. *Proteus* is a common cause of urinary tract infections but occasionally causes other surgical infections, usually originating from the urinary tract.

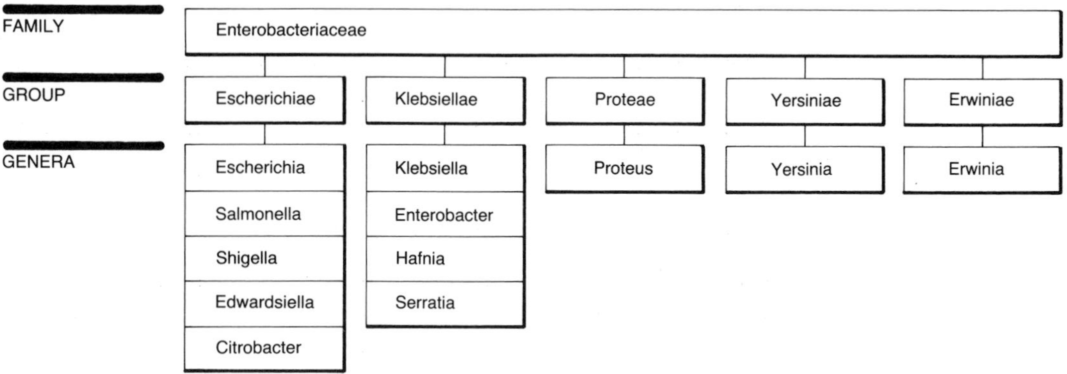

Fig. 1.6 Bacteria of the family Enterobacteriaceae

Antibiotic sensitivities

The coliforms are largely sensitive to *ampicillin* (and amoxycillin), *gentamicin* and the *cephalosporins*, these antibiotics being commonly employed both for prophylaxis in gut and for biliary tract surgery and management of related local and systemic infections. The organisms are also usually sensitive to *co-trimox-*

azole or *trimethoprim* alone, which are often used to treat urinary tract infections. Resistant strains are much more frequent within hospitals than in the community, particularly in respect of urinary tract infection.

'Non surgical' enterobacteriaceae

Other members of the Enterobacteriaceae family produce primary gut infections, although these rarely enter the province of the surgeon; for example, *Salmonella typhi* causes typhoid, *Shigella* causes bacillary dysentery. Rarely, Salmonella is incriminated in acute appendicitis. An increasingly important, often unrecognised variety of *acute haemorrhagic colitis* is caused by *E. coli 0157*; this is clinically indistinguishable from acute ulcerative colitis and should therefore be sought bacteriologically. *Yersinia* sometimes produces an acute inflammation of the ileum which may simulate the clinical picture of acute appendicitis and at laparotomy appear similar to Crohn's disease of the terminal ileum.

PSEUDOMONAS

Pathophysiology

Of these aerobic gram-negative rods, the main pathogen is *Pseudomonas aeruginosa*, an organism of higher virulence than *E. coli*, but an uncommon cause of surgical infection. It tends to cause infections in debilitated, hospitalised patients. It is a normal commensal of the human gut in about 10% of the population. The organism is resistant to many antibiotics and therefore tends to proliferate when other flora have been suppressed by broad-spectrum antibiotic therapy. Like *Klebsiella* and *Enterobacter*, it poses an institutional problem by being able to survive many chemical disinfectants and antiseptics. *Pseudomonas*, however, is killed by the organic iodine compound povidone iodine, hot water and drying.

Pseudomonas may be responsible for fatal septicaemia (especially in terminally ill patients) and pneumonia, particularly in ventilated patients or those with a tracheostomy. Long-standing wounds such as compound fractures and chronic leg ulcers may become infected by *Pseudomonas*, which can be recognised by characteristic blue-green pigmentation of the discharge. The organism is also found in patients with indwelling urinary catheters, although in such cases it is not always clinically significant. *Pseudomonas* is an important pathogen in burn infections found in up to 30% of cases and is often responsible for fatal septicaemia when burns are extensive. Finally, Pseudomonas is an important complication of ophthalmic surgery and may lead to loss of the infected eye.

Antibiotic sensitivity

Because of widespread antibiotic resistance, treatment of pseudomonal infections requires *combination therapy*, usually with an *aminoglycoside* (gentamicin or tobramycin) and a *new-generation cephalosporin* or *penicillin* (ceftazidime or azlocillin). The recently introduced antibiotic, *ciprofloxacin*, is powerful alone against *Pseudomonas*. Despite these, infection tends to persist or recur because of local or systemic predisposing factors which may be difficult or impossible to eliminate (e.g. dead bone in a compound fracture). Local treatment of infected wounds with acetic acid or antibiotic solutions (e.g. polymyxin) may be appropriate in some cases.

BACTEROIDES

Pathophysiology

Bacteroides and related organisms (e.g. *Fusobacterium*) are gram-negative, non-sporing anaerobic bacilli which make up the greatest proportion of normal gastrointestinal flora, outnumbering *E. coli* and its related facultative anaerobes. A small group of these, *B. fragilis*, which make up less than 1% of gut anaerobes, are surgically important. In combination with other gut commensals, *B. fragilis* mainly produces pyogenic infections secondary to faecal contamination of the peritoneal cavity; occasionally they cause septicaemia in debilitated patients. Because of their culture requirements, involving carbon dioxide and incubation for at least 48 hours, identification of these organisms as pathogens was neglected until the early 1970s. Indeed *Bacteroides* was probably responsible for many so-called 'sterile' intra-abdominal abscesses in the past. The importance of *B. fragilis* as a cause of surgical infection is probably still underestimated.

Antibiotic sensitivity

Bacteroides and the other gram-negative anaerobes are highly sensitive to *metronidazole*, which can be given orally, intravenously or rectally, the last giving blood levels equivalent to that achieved by intravenous administration. Metronidazole suppositories are now routinely given for prophylaxis before operation for appendicectomy and large bowel surgery, where they have dramatically reduced the incidence of postoperative peritoneal infections. Bacteroides are also sensitive to the combination of *amoxycillin and clavulanic acid* (Augmentin), *erythromycin* and *cefoxitin*, among others.

CLOSTRIDIA

Clostridia are gram-positive rods which are widely distributed in the soil and as intestinal commensals. They form spores which can survive for long periods, being resistant to drying, heat and antiseptics. Clostridia are obligate anaerobes and thus only proliferate in the absence of oxygen; they are responsible for much of the putrefaction and decay of animal material in nature. The main clostridial disorders of surgical interest are gas gangrene, tetanus and pseudomembranous colitis, the pathological effects resulting from powerful exotoxins produced by the organisms.

Gas gangrene

Gas gangrene results when *Clostridium perfringens* (formerly called *Cl. welchii*) and other anaerobes (e.g. *Bacteroide*s and *anaerobic Streptococci*) proliferate in necrotic tissue, secreting powerful toxins. These rapidly spread and destroy surrounding tissues, at the same time generating gas which gives rise to the characteristic clinical feature of crepitus ('crackling') on palpation and the typical X-ray appearance, shown in Figure 1.7. Deep traumatic wounds involving

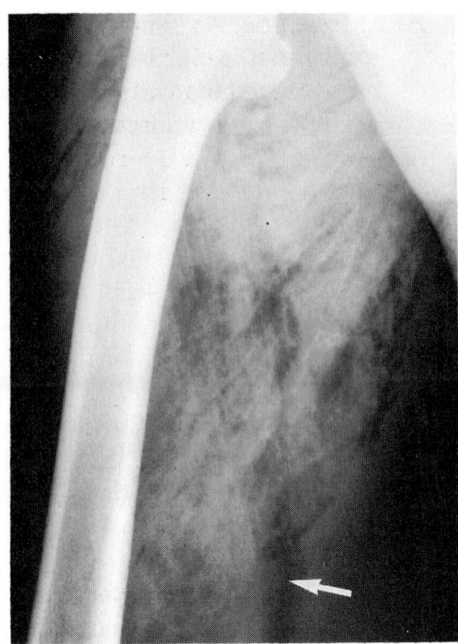

Fig. 1.7 Gas gangrene

Gas gangrene involving all the muscles of the right thigh in a 46-year-old man who sustained extensive contaminated lacerations of the medial thigh (arrowed) in a road traffic accident. Gas gangrene developed because necrotic muscle was not excised early and completely. Note the widespread streaks of radiolucent gas bubbles tracking along the muscle planes. This patient died of toxaemia despite antibiotics, surgery and hyperbaric oxygen therapy

muscle and wounds contaminated with soil, clothes or faeces are most susceptible, the condition being particularly common in battle wounds; indeed gas gangrene was responsible for vast numbers of deaths during the First World War.

In modern surgical practice, the highest risk of gas gangrene is in *lower limb amputations* performed for ischaemia and in high-velocity *gun shot wounds*. The area of muscle necrosis may at first be small, gas gangrene being recognised by blackening of the overlying skin spreading at an alarming rate. Within hours the underlying necrosis rages along the muscle planes and when the skin breaks down, a thin, foul-smelling purulent exudate leaks from the wound. *Toxins* are absorbed into the general circulation causing rapid clinical deterioration and death within 24 to 48 hours unless the process can be halted by timely and vigorous intervention.

The organism is extremely sensitive to *benzyl penicillin* or *mezlocillin* and one of these should be given prophylactically by injection immediately after a traumatic injury to muscle, or an hour or so before amputation of an ischaemic limb. Prevention of clostridial infection in contaminated wounds requires meticulous surgical excision of all necrotic tissue, followed by packing of the wound rather than suturing.

Treatment of established gas gangrene is urgent and must proceed vigorously if there is to be any hope of survival. Treatment is threefold: penicillin, excision of necrotic tissue and hyperbaric oxygen therapy. Massive doses of penicillin are given intravenously to kill organisms in viable and vascularised tissue. Emergency surgery is performed to remove all necrotic tissue. This involves carving back the necrotic muscle to healthy bleeding tissue; the affected muscle is recognised by its brick-red colour and failure to contract on cutting. Hyperbaric oxygen therapy is used to raise the oxygen tension in the necrotic tissues, thereby inhibiting growth of the organisms. The patient is placed in a high pressure chamber with pure oxygen at about three atmospheres pressure for several hours daily. Administration of a multivalent gas gangrene antitoxin may be of some value. However, gas gangrene may continue to spread despite these measures, necessitating further heroic surgical intervention. Even with all this intensive treatment, the prognosis for established gas gangrene remains bleak.

Tetanus

Tetanus is caused by *Clostridium tetani* which infects dirty wounds in a similar manner to gas gangrene; the size of the entry wound may be minute, perhaps caused by a rose thorn or splinter. The organism produces an *exotoxin*, which has little local effect but even in minute quantities has powerful neuromuscular effects, causing widespread muscular spasm. The first signs are often acute muscle spasms, neck stiffness or trismus ('lockjaw'). Untreated, these progress to *opisthotonus* (arching of the back due to extensor spasm), generalised convulsions and eventual death from exhaustion and respiratory failure several days later.

Tetanus is now rare in developed countries because of widespread immunisation during childhood with tetanus toxoid followed by boosters at 5–10 year intervals; booster doses should usually be given after penetrating injuries, however trivial, when patients attend accident and emergency departments. The annual incidence in developed countries is about one in a million; tetanus is now most common following trivial gardening injuries in the elderly, who are least likely to have been properly immunised. If there is doubt about satisfactory immunisation of a patient with a major contaminated injury, *benzyl penicillin* is given prophylactically as well as passive immunisation with *human gamma globulin* collected from people with high titres. Treatment of established tetanus usually requires artificial ventilation with drug paralysis, in addition to the usual antibiotics and passive immunisation. Mortality remains high, especially in the elderly.

Tetanus is still a massive global problem and is particularly common in the neonate as a result of infection of the umbilical stump; the problem is exacerbated by the widespread practice in underdeveloped countries of applying cow dung as a dressing!

Pseudomembranous colitis

Pseudomembranous colitis is the most serious form of antibiotic-associated colitis (see Chapter 16) and is caused by overgrowth of *Clostridium difficile*. The organism has only become identifiable recently because of the difficulty of growing it in culture (hence its name); it requires an atmosphere containing 10% carbon dioxide and special nutritional ingredients to thrive. Infection results in the formation of a thick fibrinous 'membrane' on the large intestinal mucosa, within which the organism proliferates. Its toxin causes a profound watery, sometimes bloody diarrhoea, leading to dehydration and loss of electrolytes.

Fig. 1.8 Summary — main organisms of surgical importance and their antibiotic sensitivities

Organism	Typical infections caused	Antibiotic sensitivities
STAPHYLOCOCCUS *Staph. aureus*	Pustules, boils, abscesses, wound infections, osteomyelitis	flucloxacillin erythromycin cephalosporins gentamicin vancomycin
Staph.epidermidis (albus)	Intravenous cannulae, prosthetic implants	
STREPTOCOCCUS *a. alpha streptococci* *Strep. viridans*	Infective endocarditis	benzyl penicillin penicillin V erythromycin
Strep. pneumoniae	pneumonia	
b. Strep. pyogenes	Cellulitis and lymphangitis	
c. Strep. faecalis (enterococci)	Cause urinary infections and contribute to abscesses associated with bowel surgery	ampicillin and amoxycillin
d. Strep. milleri	Abscesses of appendix, liver lung, brain, etc	
e. Anaerobic streptococci	Contribute to intraperitoneal abscesses associated with bowel surgery; contribute to infection in diabetic penetrating foot ulcers	benzyl penicillin penicillin V ampicillin/amoxycillin metronidazole gentamicin
ENTEROBACTERIA *E. coli, Klebsiella, Proteus, Serratia, Enterobacter*	Urinary tract infections, gram-negative septicaemia, bronchopneumonias in debilitated patients	ampicillin cephalosporins gentamicin co–trimoxazole (or trimethoprim alone) ciprofloxacin
PSEUDOMONAS *Ps. aeruginosa*	Urinary tract infections, pneumonias and septicaemias in ventilated patients, burn infections and septicaemia	gentamicin or tobramycin ciprofloxacin azlocillin, piperacillin ceftazidime
BACTEROIDES *B. fragilis*	Intraperitoneal abscesses associated with bowel surgery, genital tract infections, oral sepsis, brain abscesses	metronidazole (also Augmentin, erythromycin cefoxitin, etc)
CLOSTRIDIA *Cl. perfringens*	gas gangrene	benzyl penicillin
Cl. tetani	tetanus	benzyl penicillin
Cl. difficile	pseudomembranous colitis	metronidazole or vancomycin (orally)

Although uncommon, the condition may develop after even a single dose of almost any antibiotic (except aminoglycosides) but is most often associated with prophylaxis or treatment associated with bowel surgery. Clindamycin and lincomycin were most commonly implicated and are now rarely used. Cephalosporins are now the most common cause. Diagnosis can be made by sigmoidoscopy and biopsy in the 50% of patients with left-sided colonic involvement. The best method of diagnosis is detection of the toxin in the stool; this can be performed rapidly with a latex agglutination test. *Cl. difficile* can also be cultured from the stool. Although the organism is sensitive to penicillin, this fails to penetrate the pseudomembrane. *Oral metronidazole* is effective in most patients, but *oral vancomycin*, which is not absorbed from the gastrointestinal tract, may be used if this is ineffective.

NEOPLASIA

Neoplasms have the characteristic of uncontrolled growth which persists after removal of the initiating stimulus. Most neoplasms can readily be defined as *benign or malignant* according to histological pattern. In most cases, the tendency to invasion or metastasis associated with malignancy can be recognised, although this may occasionally be difficult. For example, the distinction between leiomyoma and leiomyosarcoma may only be made on behaviour of the tumour in the long term. Neoplasms may also be difficult to distinguish clinically from other *tumour-like disorders* such as hyperplasia (e.g. parathyroid adenoma from parathyroid hyperplasia) and hamartomata (e.g. liver secondaries from haemangiomas of the liver).

BENIGN NEOPLASMS

Benign tumours are typically well demarcated and often encapsulated, with a histological appearance reminiscent of the tissue of origin. Benign tumours present to the surgeon in a variety of ways, as summarised in Figure 1.9.

Fig. 1.9 Principal modes of presentation of benign tumours

1. Lesion suspected by the patient to be malignant, e.g. breast lump, oral ulcer
2. Overt bleeding or occult blood loss causing anaemia, e.g. bowel polyps
3. Local obstructive effects. e.g. leiomyoma of small intestine
4. Pressure causing pain or dysfunction, e.g. neurofibroma
5. Unacceptable cosmetic appearance, e.g. subcutaneous lipomas
6. Production of excessive amounts of hormone by endocrine neoplasms, e.g. parathyroid adenoma, insulinoma, phaeochromocytoma

MALIGNANT NEOPLASMS

Malignant tumours are typically non-encapsulated with a poorly-defined, irregular outline due to local invasion. Histologically, both cells and their nucleii tend to be widely variable in shape and size, and the extent of this pleomorphism tends to correlate with the degree of malignancy and the clinical behaviour of the tumour. In anaplastic tumours, there is such loss of differentiation that little similarity with the parent tissue remains.

Carcinogenesis — multiple primary lesions and recurrences

Most cancers are probably caused by a combination of environmental factors and factors intrinsic to the patient. It has been estimated mathematically that about two-thirds of cancers can be attributed in some way to external factors, such as radiation, virus infections and carcinogens in air, food and water. Many such factors are as yet undiscovered but cigarette smoking is now well recognised to be the commonest carcinogen for lung, bladder, and head and neck cancer. When cancer develops, it is likely that the whole of that organ or tissue has been affected in the same way by the carcinogen. Consequently, new primary tumours, as distinct from local recurrences, may develop later; clear distinction between these is often impossible. Certain tissues, particularly those of the bladder, breast, skin, head and neck and possibly large bowel, are at particular risk of new primary carcinomas, and prolonged surveillance is required after an initial tumour has been treated.

Growth and spread of malignant tumours

Malignant tumours spread by *local infiltration* and by *distant metastasis* via lymphatics, the bloodstream and across coelomic cavities. There are two conflicting theories about the significance of regional lymph node involvement in carcinoma. Both views recognise that lymph node involvement implies a worse prognosis. Halsted believed that lymph nodes have an important function in halting spread, at least for a time, and that radical surgery therefore offers the possibility of a cure. The alternative view, expressed by Fisher, is that lymph node metastases indicate failure of the host defences and are therefore a manifestation of systemic metastasis and a contraindication to radical surgery. In the case of breast cancer, Fisher's view has been proved correct and the trend towards ever more radical surgery has been reversed. In more than 50% of large bowel cancers, Halsted's view is probably correct and therefore radical surgery remains the treatment of choice. In the rest, haematogenous spread, often occult, probably occurs at an early stage, rendering the disease incurable by surgery.

Target organs particularly involved in bloodstream spread are the liver, lungs, bone and brain. Haematogenous metastases are usually multifocal and are therefore beyond cure, except in certain cases of testicular tumour and some paediatric malignancies. Occasionally such metastases appear to be solitary and cures may sometimes been effected by partial hepatectomy or pulmonary lobectomy. Multiple metastases often respond temporarily to palliative chemotherapy, radiotherapy or hormone manipulation (e.g. carcinomas of breast, uterus, kidney and prostate). Sarcomas, which are relatively uncommon, usually metastasise early via the bloodstream.

The connective tissue stroma of some malignant tumours may undergo fibrous hyperplasia, which accounts for some of the characteristic clinical features of cancer; these include hardness to palpation, intestinal obstruction by annular carcinomas of the large bowel and retraction of skin overlying breast cancer. On the other hand, in highly aggressive tumours, the connective tissue stroma may be inadequate for nutritional support, leading to necrosis and patchy haemorrhage within the tumour. This often presents as a sudden onset of pain and a mass.

Fig. 1.10 Principal modes of presentation of malignant tumours

The primary lesion

a. Palpable or visible mass, e.g. breast or thyroid cancer

b. Obstruction or other disruption of function of a hollow viscus, e.g. bowel obstruction by colorectal carcinoma, stridor in bronchial carcinoma

c. Overt bleeding, e.g. bladder or left-sided large bowel cancer

d. Occult blood loss causing anaemia, e.g. carcinoma of caecum or stomach

e. Obstructive jaundice, e.g. carcinoma of head of pancreas or extrahepatic bile ducts

f. Skin lesion, often ulcerated, e.g. basal and squamous cell carcinomas, malignant melanoma, breast cancer

g. Nerve invasion, e.g. facial nerve palsy from parotid carcinoma, recurrent laryngeal palsy from anaplastic carcinoma of thyroid

Note: pain is not a common presenting feature of primary malignancy except in the pancreas, lung and nasopharynx; pain is more often associated with metastatic disease

Metastatic deposits

a. Enlarged lymph nodes (nodes tend to be hard, matted and non-tender)

b. Hepatomegaly, e.g. stomach, large bowel and pancreatic carcinomas

c. Obstructive jaundice (usually due to lymph node mass in the porta hepatis compressing the bile ducts, but sometimes extensive liver deposits), e.g. stomach, large bowel and pancreatic carcinomas

d. Abnormal masses distant from the primary lesion, e.g. abdomen, pelvis and skin

e. Bone invasion causing bone pain or pathological fractures, e.g. prostatic and breast cancers

f. Malignant effusions, e.g. pleural effusion in breast cancer, ascites with peritoneal deposits from intra-abdominal malignancies

g. Pulmonary metastases — usually asymptomatic and found on chest X-ray

h. Brain metastases — behaviour or personality changes, headache, fits, paresis, ataxias etc

i. Nerve invasion — backache and abdominal pain in abdominal lymph node metastases

Generalised systemic manifestations (uncommon except for cachexia)

a. Malignant cachexia

b. Fever — characteristic of lymphomas and renal adenocarcinoma but also occurs when there is extensive tumour necrosis

c. Migrating thrombophlebitis and chronic disseminated intravascular coagulation (DIC)

d. Peripheral neuropathies, myopathies and rare autoimmune neuromuscular phenomena, e.g. myasthenic syndrome

e. Other rare autoimmune phenomena e.g. haemolysis

f. Ectopic hormone production, e.g. ADH, ACTH, PTH and gonadotrophins (all rare in malignancies seen in general surgery)

g. Production of fetal and embryonic proteins, e.g. carcinoembryonic antigen (CEA) produced by testicular tumours, colorectal and pancreatic carcinomas; alpha-fetoprotein (AFP) produced by testicular teratomas and hepatomas — may be useful for diagnosis, monitoring treatment and long-term follow up

h. Production of enzymes, e.g. acid phosphatase by extensive carcinoma of prostate — may provide useful diagnostic blood tests

SYSTEMIC RESPONSES TO SURGERY AND TRAUMA

Introduction

In addition to inflammatory and reparative responses at the site of tissue damage, there are a variety of systemic responses, mainly hormonally mediated, which compensate for starvation, provide additional energy and building blocks for tissue repair, and conserve sodium ions and water. Circulating adrenaline and noradrenaline from sympathetic nerve endings and the adrenal medulla play a central role in the systemic response. In addition, increased secretion of adrenocorticotropic hormone (ACTH), glucocorticoids (cortisol), glucagon and growth hormone all contribute to the general catabolic response whilst increased aldosterone and antidiuretic hormone (ADH) production mediate the fluid and electrolyte changes.

Factors responsible for systemic responses to severe injury or major surgery

a. Fall in intravascular volume

This is one of the major factors invoking the systemic response and results from the following:

- Loss of fluid by haemorrhage or burns
- Interstitial sequestration of fluid as oedema both in damaged tissues, and more generally, as a result of the systemic hormonal response
- Restriction of oral intake during the perioperative period

A fall in intravascular volume stimulates sympathetic activity, maintaining blood pressure by increasing cardiac output and peripheral resistance. Thus a mild tachycardia is commonly seen in postoperative patients. Catecholamines also have profound metabolic effects, increasing the metabolism of carbohydrates, proteins and lipids. This explains why many postoperative patients have a mild fever. Decreased renal perfusion activates the renin-angiotensin-aldosterone system, thus increasing renal sodium and water reabsorption. A centrally mediated increase in ADH secretion promotes further water conservation.

b. Reduction in cardiac output and peripheral perfusion

Circulatory efficiency may be impaired by hypovolaemia or myocardial depression from anaesthetics and other drugs. Less commonly, major events, such as septicaemic shock, pulmonary embolism or myocardial infarction, cause cardiovascular collapse.

c. Pain

Pain causes increased catecholamine and ACTH secretion.

d. Stress

Psychological stress associated with injury, severe illness or elective surgery has a similar effect to that of pain on sympathetic function and hypothalamic activity.

e. Infection

Exotoxins and endotoxins initiate intense systemic responses.

f. Inflammation

Products of tissue damage and inflammation may cause systemic effects themselves or via release of catecholamines and other hormones.

g. Excess heat loss

This can occur in long operations and after extensive burns; it imposes great demands upon energy resources. Small babies are particularly vulnerable. Heat loss is counteracted by raising the ambient temperature.

h. Starvation

Even in uncomplicated elective surgery, patients are routinely starved for 6–12 hours before operation and often do not start eating for 12–24 hours after operation. After major gastrointestinal surgery, food may be witheld for several days, or much longer in the event of serious infective complications, anastomotic breakdown or fistula formation. Furthermore, patients with gastrointestinal tumours, malabsorption syndromes or inflammatory bowel disease may already be in a state of chronic starvation even before operation.

Effects of starvation

During starvation, without illness or trauma, blood glucose is maintained by decreased insulin secretion and increased glucagon secretion. Other hormone levels remain normal. Initially, enhanced glycogenolysis maintains blood glucose but liver glycogen is exhausted within 24 hours. Gluconeogenesis in the liver and kidneys is enhanced, utilising amino acids from protein breakdown and glycerol from lipolysis as substrates. Most of the glucose thus produced is utilised by the brain; most other tissues are able to metabolise fatty acids and ketones from adipose tissue. After several weeks, the brain also adapts to using ketones. Overall energy demands fall during starvation and energy is obtained mainly at the expense of body fats. Protein is conserved until a late stage in uncomplicated starvation; this is not the case in severe trauma or surgery.

SURGICAL CATABOLISM

In most elective surgery, many of the factors mentioned above can be avoided by accurate fluid replacement, adequate analgesia, reduction of psychological stress, prevention of infection, and the use of careful operative technique to minimise tissue trauma. The result will be minimal systemic upset with rapid recovery.

On the other hand, in severe trauma and extensive operative surgery, particularly if complicated by major sepsis, the above factors will inevitably cause intense catabolism and drastic changes in fluid and electrolyte balance. Increased sympathetic activity and circulating catecholamines are the key factors in the response to major systemic insults, producing the following metabolic results:

- There is enhanced hepatic glycogenolysis and gluconeogenesis
- Reduced insulin secretion and inhibition of its tissue effects block cellular utilisation of glucose
- Stimulation of glucagon secretion further enhances glycogenolysis and gluconeogenesis
- Catecholamines and glucagon stimulate lipolysis in adipose tissue releasing fatty acids; these provide the major energy source for peripheral tissues
- Breakdown of muscle protein releases amino acids, the main substrate for gluconeogenesis and the raw material for wound healing
- Increased pituitary ACTH release induces a massive rise in circulating glucocorticoids; cortisol levels can increase tenfold immediately after surgery, remaining elevated for days or weeks. Glucocorticoids also enhance gluconeogenesis and promote catabolism of muscle protein and liberation of amino acids
- There is increased secretion of growth hormone and thyroid hormones, both of which inhibit insulin effects and promote catabolism

Effects on carbohydrate metabolism

The overall effect of all these hormonal actions is a rise in blood glucose levels, often resulting in *hyperglycaemia* and a *pseudodiabetic state*; blood glucose levels may reach 20 mmol/l and glucose may appear in the urine. This is in marked contrast to simple fasting, in which glucose levels are normal or slightly depressed.

Effects on body proteins and nitrogen metabolism

In the normal healthy adult, protein turnover results in the daily excretion of 12–20 g of urinary nitrogen which is made good by dietary intake, thus maintaining *nitrogen balance*. In a hypercatabolic state, nitrogen losses can increase three or fourfold. Most importantly, the metabolic environment prevents utilisation of any food or intravenous nutrition. There is therefore an enormous and inevitable daily destruction of skeletal muscle. This state of *negative nitrogen balance* contrasts markedly with starvation, in which body protein is preserved.

Effects on lipid stores and metabolism

The effects of major body insult upon lipid metabolism are little different from simple starvation; most of the energy requirements are met from fat stores. Surgical catabolism only reverses as the patient recovers from the illness and therefore parenteral nutrition has almost no effect; nevertheless, it is often used in the hope of having some benefit. It is worth emphasising that minimising surgical trauma and preventing perioperative complications may well make the difference between recovery and death in the elderly or debilitated patient.

Fluid and electrolyte changes in major surgery and trauma

Major trauma, surgery and illness result in retention of sodium and water, mediated via increased secretion of aldosterone and ADH.

a. Aldosterone secretion

This occurs in response to a fall in renal perfusion and glomerular filtration rate, which tend to accompany significant haemodynamic disturbances. Renin is released from the juxtaglomerular apparatus of the kidney, catalysing the conversion of angiotensin I to angiotensin II in the lungs. The latter has a powerful pressor effect on the peripheral vasculature, counteracting hypotension as well as stimulating aldosterone release from the adrenal cortex. Aldosterone promotes active reabsorption of sodium ions from the distal convoluted tubules of the kidney; this is accompanied by the passive reabsorption of water. Sodium reabsorption is linked to secretion of potassium and hydrogen ions. There is therefore a small volume of acidic urine, which has a low sodium concentration and a raised potassium concentration. Loss of hydrogen ions causes a degree of metabolic alkalosis.

b. ADH secretion

This is stimulated by a rise in serum osmolality, mediated by osmoreceptors in the hypothalamus. After major trauma or surgery, however, additional factors operate: there is a reduction in circulating volume, and stress and pain promote further ADH release via other hypothalamic pathways. ADH acts on the renal collecting tubules, rendering them permeable to water, which is then reabsorbed along a concentration gradient into the vasa recta of the renal medulla.

It is important to recognise the phase of *relative oliguria* and *sodium retention* that occurs after major injury or surgery; this has an important bearing on fluid management. Like surgical catabolism, described earlier, these effects are resistent to external manipulation but resolve with recovery of the patient.

SHOCK

PATHO-PHYSIOLOGY

Shock is defined as an acute change in cardiovascular function of sufficient magnitude to compromise tissue perfusion. Cellular hypoxia and disruption of normal metabolic function, if untreated, rapidly proceed to irreversible organ damage and death. Shock may be encountered anywhere from the acute emergency through to the postoperative period. Treatment depends upon quick and accurate diagnosis.

Shock may be produced in four main ways:

- Sudden loss of fluid from the intravascular compartment (*hypovolaemic shock*)
- Failure of cardiac output (*cardiogenic shock*)
- Severe systemic infection (*septic shock*)
- Severe type I immune reaction (*anaphylactic shock*)

A fifth type of shock, *neurogenic shock*, is represented by the vasovagal attack or 'faint', caused by sudden pain or fear. In this case, there is sudden, autonomically mediated bradycardia and splanchnic dilatation, causing transient hypotension and loss of consciousness. Being transient and spontaneously reversible, this condition does not meet the definition given above and will not be considered further.

1. Hypovolaemic shock

The main causes of hypovolaemic shock are:

- 'Revealed' haemorrhage, e.g. deep skin laceration, large haematemesis from a peptic ulcer, severe blood loss from a wound drain
- 'Concealed' haemorrhage, e.g. intra-abdominal bleeding from ruptured spleen or aortic aneurysm, haemorrhage from a duodenal ulcer into small intestine, intramuscular blood loss from multiple fractures
- Extensive burns, resulting in massive loss of serum into blisters or from surface weeping
- Severe vomiting or diarrhoea, or fluid loss from a small bowel fistula
- Excessive urinary loss, e.g. diabetic keto-acidosis, diuretic phase of acute tubular necrosis, powerful diuretics
- Sequestration of fluid in the bowel due to obstruction
- Massive loss of fluid into the tissues, as occurs in septic shock, or into the peritoneal cavity, in acute pancreatitis or generalised peritonitis

2. Cardiogenic shock

Cardiogenic shock results from any form of 'pump failure', most commonly acute myocardial infarction or an acute ventricular dysrhythmia. The condition can also be caused by valve prolapse from a ruptured papillary muscle. A large pulmonary embolus may also cause cardiogenic shock by obstructing blood flow through the lungs, causing secondary cardiac failure.

3. Septic (septicaemic) shock

Systemic infection with gram-negative organisms typically causes cardiovascular collapse or septic shock. Bacterial endotoxins activate complement and vasoactive amines in peripheral tissue. This results in the opening of arteriovenous shunts, widespread peripheral vasodilatation and greatly increased capillary permeability. The increase in vascular capacity causes relative hypovolaemia and there is massive fluid leakage into the tissues.

4. Anaphylactic shock

Anaphylactic shock is a generalised form of type I hypersensitivity reaction, occurring in response to an antigen to which the patient has previously become sensitised. The antigen binds with antibody attached to the surface of mast cells, triggering degranulation and release of histamine and other vasoactive amines. These cause extensive capillary dilatation and increased permeability, as in septic shock. The systemic effects are compounded by intense bronchoconstriction, which effectively halts ventilation.

In surgical practice, anaphylactic shock usually results from drug administration, particularly via the intravenous route, penicillins being the most common culprit. Anaphylactic reactions may also occur after intravenous injections of radiological contrast media. Insect bites (wasps, bees and hornets) are also an important cause and may be seen in the accident and emergency department.

CLINICAL FEATURES OF SHOCK

The essential feature of any type of shock is a precipitate *fall in arterial blood pressure*. Beyond this, septic shock presents a quite different clinical picture from the other types and is discussed below. In all other types of shock, the immediate homeostatic response is intense sympathetic activity and catecholamine release. The heart rate increases dramatically in a vain attempt to increase cardiac output. There is intense cutaneous vasoconstriction in an attempt to restore intravascular volume by increasing peripheral resistance. Sudomotor activity causes profuse sweating. The hypoxic tissues revert to anaerobic respiration, producing lactic acid sufficient to cause a metabolic acidosis, and the respiratory rate rises in an attempt at compensation. The clinical picture is a cold, white, clammy patient with a rapid thready pulse and increased respiratory rate.

In *septic shock*, there is an endotoxin-mediated peripheral vasodilatation unresponsive to circulating catecholamines. The patient's skin is hot and flushed and cardiac output is increased to fill the dilated periphery. The pulse is typically 'bounding' in quality. Temperature, however, may be normal or even subnormal.

Without treatment, the circulation cannot support the main organ systems. Cerebral hypoxia soon causes confusion, and eventually, coma. Inadequate renal perfusion causes a dramatic fall in urinary output (oliguria) which, if not rapidly corrected, leads to acute tubular necrosis. If shock persists, reduced coronary flow and heart failure cause death. In septic shock, organ damage is exacerbated by endotoxins and deterioration is inexorable unless the source of infection can be rapidly eliminated.

PRINCIPLES OF MANAGEMENT OF SHOCK

Whatever the cause, the aim is to restore tissue perfusion and oxygenation by resuscitative measures while the diagnosis is being made and the specific treatment begun.

Administration of oxygen

A mask delivering 100% oxygen should be immediately secured. The comatose patient must be intubated and positive-pressure ventilation commenced.

Restoration of tissue perfusion

An intravenous infusion must be set up immediately. Unless cardiogenic shock is considered likely, the circulating volume must be rapidly expanded. Plasma or plasma substitutes are preferred; being osmotically active, they draw fluid from the extracellular tissues into the circulatory compartment.

Assessment and monitoring

This involves the following procedures:

- Basic observations of temperature, pulse, blood pressure, respiratory rate and level of consciousness, monitored at frequent intervals; bounding pulse and flushed extremities will suggest the diagnosis of septicaemic shock
- A quick but thorough general examination is performed to search for evidence of infection or concealed haemorrhage, particularly within the abdomen. Elevated jugular venous pressure suggests cardiac failure due to myocardial infarction, a cardiac murmur suggests valvular prolapse, and an expiratory wheeze is suggestive of anaphylaxis or cardiac failure
- An ECG is performed for evidence of myocardial infarction or pulmonary embolism. Note that the ECG changes typical of pulmonary embolism are only seen in massive embolism
- A central venous line is inserted to monitor central pressure and the response to fluid administration

- A urinary catheter is inserted to monitor hourly urinary output
- Venous blood is taken for measurement of haemoglobin, haematocrit, urea and electrolytes and cross-matching of blood; an arterial sample is taken for estimation of blood gas and acid-base status; blood cultures are taken if septic shock is suspected

SPECIFIC TREATMENTS FOR SHOCK

Hypovolaemic shock

Fluid replacement should be equivalent to the estimated fluid loss but adjusted according to the effect on central venous pressure and urine output. Where possible, fluids of similar composition to the fluids lost should be used: whole blood for haemorrhage, plasma after major burns.

Cardiogenic shock

The management of cardiogenic shock is best reviewed in a medical textbook; the management of pulmonary embolism is discussed in Chapter 33. Fluid overload is a significant hazard in cardiogenic shock and must be avoided.

Septic shock

Septicaemia leading to septic shock usually emanates from a specific focus of infection. The source may be obvious but, if not, a careful search must be made bearing in mind the common sites. In surgical practice, septic shock is most commonly seen either as a result of faecal peritonitis following large bowel perforation or as a postoperative complication. In the latter case, intraperitoneal sepsis is the prime suspect but bladder or chest infection or an otherwise 'silent' infection of a central venous cannula are often the cause. Debilitated patients, uncontrolled diabetics and infants are particularly vulnerable to sudden septicaemia; in such cases the source of infection may never be found.

The damaging effects of poor organ perfusion in septic shock are increased by endotoxic tissue damage. Treatment of septic shock is urgent and involves resuscitation, administration of appropriate antibiotics and the tracing and elimination of the source of infection.

Blood cultures must always be taken and intravenous antibiotics administered on a 'best guess' basis. Experience has shown that a broad spectrum combination of gentamicin, benzyl penicillin and metronidazole is one of the most effective regimes and can be modified later if resistant organisms are isolated.

In the meantime, intravenous plasma or plasma expanders are given to correct relative hypovolaemia, the volumes being adjusted according to central venous pressure and urine output. Such volume expansion helps to sustain cardiac output and tissue perfusion. Corticosteroids (e.g. intravenous hydrocortisone 200 mg) are usually given because they are known to stabilise cell membranes; however, objective evidence of their effectiveness in septic shock is lacking.

If the diagnosis of septic shock is correct, such resuscitative measures should produce dramatic improvement in the patient's condition within one to two hours. By that time, the patient should be ready for immediate operation if an abscess or bowel perforation appears to be the cause. A suspect central venous cannula should have been removed and the tip sent for bacteriological examination; specimens of sputum, urine, etc should also be examined. It cannot be emphasised too strongly that the source of infection must be urgently eliminated if the patient is to have any chance of recovery.

Disseminated intravascular coagulation

Another major problem in septic shock is the generalised activation of the clotting cascade causing disseminated intravascular coagulation (DIC). This exhausts the supply of platelets and clotting factors (*consumption coagulopathy*) and becomes manifest as spontaneous bleeding or bruising and uncontrollable haemorrhage from any operation site. Diagnosis is made by finding high levels of *fibrin degradation products* (FDPs) in the serum. Treatment includes intravenous heparin to arrest the coagulation process and infusion of necessary clotting factors, e.g. fresh frozen plasma.

Anaphylactic shock

Anaphylactic shock requires urgent treatment. Adrenaline, 1 ml of 1 in 1000 solution, is given subcutaneously, causing generalised vasoconstriction and increased cardiac output. Hydrocortisone 200–500 mg and an antihistamine such as chlorpheniramine 10 mg are given intravenously, the former stabilising the mast cells and the latter blocking histamine receptors which mediate much of the peripheral vascular response. Intravenous fluids are needed to treat the hypovolaemia.

Because of the risk of anaphylactic shock, a doctor should always administer the first dose of any intravenous agent, including radiological contrast agents and radioisotopes, and a doctor should always be available whenever parenteral drugs (including vaccinations) are being administered. The doctor is legally responsible for ensuring that resuscitation drugs and equipment are immediately available and must check this beforehand, particularly if working in an unfamiliar ward or department.

Fig. 1.11
Summary — shock

	Hypovolaemic	**Cardiogenic**	**Septic**	**Anaphylactic**
Blood pressure	▼▼	▼▼	▼	▼▼
Pulse rate	▲▲ thready	▲? thready	▲? bounding	▲▲ thready
Peripheral vaso-constriction (skin white and clammy)	YES	YES	NO — skin hot and red, peripheral *dilatation.*	YES
Urine output	▼▼	▼▼	▼▼	▼▼
Main treatments	Fluid replacement	Supportive, i.e. treat complications such as pulmonary oedema. Beware of fluid overload	i.v. antibiotics, plasma expander, ? corticosteroids	s.c. adrenaline, i.v. hydrocortisone, antihistamines

2 INTRODUCTION TO INVESTIGATIVE PROCEDURES

This chapter gives an overview of investigative procedures commonly used in surgery. The basis for each method of investigation is described, together with its main indications and shortcomings.

Apart from their use in diagnostic imaging, ultrasound and CT scanning can also be used to guide a needle to obtain tissue for histology. Other diagnostic techniques, such as endoscopy, have therapeutic applications which can be employed at the same time as the diagnostic manoeuvre. An example is the removal of colonic polyps using a wire snare during colonoscopy.

CONVENTIONAL RADIOGRAPHY

Introduction

The various tissues and constituents of the body absorb X-rays by amounts related to the cube of the atomic number of their elements. This results in differential penetration of X-rays through the body and consequent differential exposure of the silver salts in the X-ray film. A radiograph is therefore a 'shadow' picture.

On a plain radiograph, gas and fat absorb few X-rays and appear as *radiolucent* (dark) areas. Bone and other calcified tissues absorb most of the X-rays; they are thus poorly penetrated and appear as *radiopaque* (white) film images. Most urinary tract stones, some gallstones and all heavily calcified atheromatous deposits are also radiopaque. Many X-ray investigations, known as *contrast studies*, obtain their diagnostic information by imaging structures outlined with highly absorptive fluid contrast media, either as positive or negative images.

Certain *foreign bodies* in wounds, such as metal and most glass fragments, are radiopaque, but wood and plastic fragments are completely radiolucent and invisible to X-rays. Gauze swabs used in operating theatres are radiolucent, but have a radiopaque strand woven into them to enable them to be located radiographically if inadvertently left inside a wound.

It is an important principle of radiology to keep irradiation of patients and observers to the minimum. This is achieved by the following methods:

- Improved design of X-ray equipment minimises radiation dose while preserving diagnostic detail; X-ray *scatter* is reduced, and unwanted types of radiation are removed by filters

- Physical barriers to X-rays are provided in all radiology suites to protect the staff. These include barium plaster in walls, lead-glass windows and lead-rubber aprons
- Workers involved in taking X-rays should keep as far as possible from the beam direction during exposure because the inverse square law determines the fall-off of radiation with distance
- All involved in radiography wear X-ray sensitive *film badges* which are regularly monitored for excess radiation

PRINCIPLES OF RADIOGRAPHY

There are several important factors in the production of a useful radiographic image:

- X-ray *power* and *exposure time* are chosen to give a diagnostically useful film exposure, with a range of film densities appropriate to the anatomical area. For example, thoracic spine views require a larger dose than lung fields
- Different *projections (views)* produce different images of the same subject. Since the X-ray tube is effectively a point source which produces a diverging beam (see Figure 2.1), the subject is magnified. This size distortion least affects the side of the patient closest to the source, which is thus more clearly shown on the films. The projection has important consequences for interpretation and should be recorded on the film. The side nearest the tube is written first; for example a chest film might be labelled P.A. (postero-anterior) or A.P. (antero-posterior)

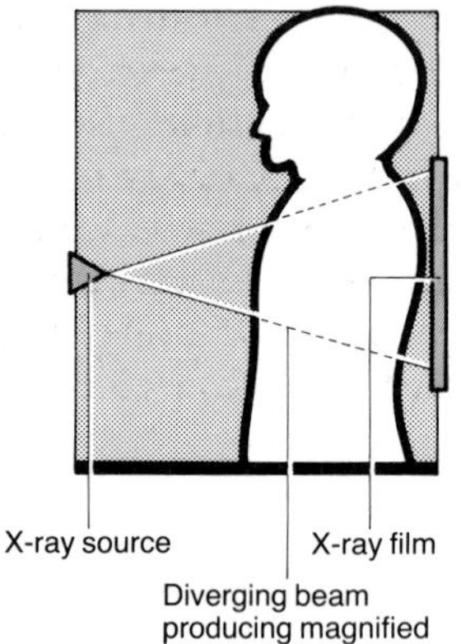

Fig. 2.1 Radiological projection

- Patient *position* during exposure (i.e. supine, prone, oblique or erect) affects the image, because of the effect of gravity upon organs and other body contents such as gas or fluid. Most films are taken with a vertical X-ray beam, but a horizontal beam is sometimes necessary to demonstrate fluid levels in a cavity or in bowel, or free gas under the diaphragm

Tomography

Some body structures, which would otherwise be obscured by overlying or underlying tissues on conventional X-rays, can be distinguished by the use of tomography. In tomography, the X-ray tube and film are moved in opposite

Fig. 2.2 Principle of tomography

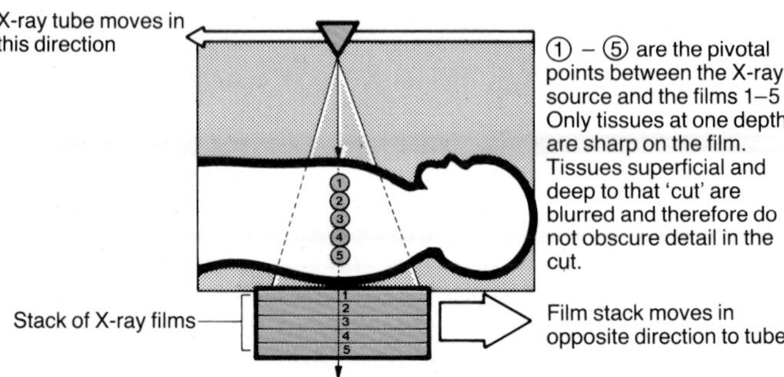

directions during exposure, with the pivotal point between the two centred on the structure under investigation (see Figure 2.2). A transverse slice at the chosen depth is thus defined clearly on the film, and anything superficial or deep to it is blurred into obscurity (e.g. soft tissue, bowel gas, faeces or bones). The technique is particularly useful for demonstrating renal masses during urography and for pulmonary masses. By using a stack of films, one exposure can give a set of 'cuts' at predetermined distances from the surface. Computerised tomography is a development of this principle and for many applications has superceded conventional tomography (see later).

Contrast radiography

When plain radiography is inadequate to study the area of interest, contrast media can often be used to opacify it. Contrast media work in two ways: they outline anatomical structures directly or are concentrated physiologically in the organ they are designed to show.

Direct contrast studies can be made in a variety of ways: contrast material can be swallowed, instilled into body orifices, sinuses or fistulae, or injected into blood vessels or hollow viscera. Commonly-used studies are barium enemas for examining the colon and arteriograms for examining the arterial system.

Indirect contrast studies are made by introducing agents into the body which are concentrated in the organs under investigation. Examples are urography (intravenous injection of contrast which is excreted in the urine) and cholecystography (ingestion of contrast which is excreted in bile concentrated in the gall bladder).

Contrast materials

Barium sulphate is the most satisfactory agent for outlining the gastrointestinal tract. It is insoluble in water and is not absorbed. An aqueous suspension is non-irritant and very radiodense.

Water-soluble *iodinated benzoic acid derivatives* can be injected into vessels and opacify the circulating blood. There is also almost immediate excretion of the contrast through the kidneys into the urine. Thus, two different functions can be achieved: direct opacification of veins or arteries (venography or arteriography), and indirect demonstration of kidneys, collecting systems and bladder. Similar iodine-containing agents given orally are concentrated in the bile, opacifying the gall bladder and biliary tree.

Most water-soluble contrast media have a high osmotic pressure and are therefore irritant (particularly when used for venography) and toxic; this applies particularly at the extremes of age and in diabetic nephropathy. Recently, new agents with an osmotic pressure similar to that of plasma have appeared. These are safer but the price is several times higher.

Finally, care should be taken to ensure that the patient is not sensitive to the contrast medium, as this may produce an anaphylactoid reaction. Resuscitation equipment and drugs should always be on hand when contrast media are injected.

PLAIN ABDOMINAL RADIOGRAPHY

Principles

Most abdominal films are taken with the patient supine and the X-ray beam vertical. Gut is visible when there is gas in it. Normal *small bowel* is less than 3 cm in width and tends to occupy the centre of the abdomen in the supine position; when dilated, it can be recognised by the transverse folds (*plicae circulares*) which completely cross the lumen (see Figure 2.3b). The colon usually lies peripherally in the abdomen and is recognised by its *haustrations*. These are folds that only partly traverse the lumen. Normal colon is less than 6 cm in diameter and is often seen to contain lumps of faeces which have a mottled radiopaque appearance.

Free gas in the peritoneal cavity may be diagnostic of *bowel perforation* and is therefore an important finding. In a supine patient, free gas usually collects in the right upper quadrant. It can be diagnosed when both the inside and outside of the bowel wall are outlined by radiolucent shadows. A chest or upper abdominal X-ray taken with a horizontal beam and the patient erect, will usually (but not always) reveal a radiolucent gas layer under the diaphragm. This can be very small (and easily missed) but may be obvious. The best method of showing free peritoneal gas is to place the patient in the *right-side raised lateral decubitus position* (i.e. lying on the left side), for a period of 10 minutes. A horizontal beam abdominal X-ray is then taken across the table. As little as 2 ml of gas may then be demonstrable above the lateral border of the liver (see Figure 2.3c)

The kidneys may be outlined on a plain abdominal X-ray by a radiolucent border of perinephric fat. However, overlapping bowel gas and faeces often obscure the renal outlines. Also, in a post-nephrectomy patient, the former 'renal outline' may still be visible on a plain film! Small urinary tract stones

Fig. 2.3 Plain abdominal X-rays

(a) Normal supine abdominal X-ray. There is gas in most parts of the colon (transverse colon **T** and sigmoid colon **S**) and some small bowel loops **SB** in the pelvis. Radiopaque lumps of faecal matter **F** are seen in the caecum and ascending colon. A normal pro-peritoneal fat line is present on the left **P**; this would be lost if there was retroperitoneal inflammation. **(b)** Erect abdominal X-ray in a 15-year-old boy with distal small bowel obstruction due to gangrenous appendicitis. There are many dilated small bowel loops and multiple fluid levels (arrowed). The large bowel is collapsed due to absorption of bowel gas beyond the obstruction. **(c)** Right side raised lateral decubitus X-ray (the X-ray beam was horizontal). This 78-year-old woman presented with a sudden onset of severe abdominal pain caused by a perforated duodenal ulcer. Free intraperitoneal gas **G** is seen 'floating' over the liver **L** and beneath the diaphragm **D**. **(d)** A plain abdominal film and an intravenous urogram (IVU) of the same patient showing urinary tract stones. In the plain film (left), several calcified opacities (arrowed) are seen. From the IVU, in which the pelvicalyceal systems and ureters contain contrast material, it can be seen that the three stones **A** lie within the lower right ureter and stone **B** lies within the calyces of the left lower pole of the kidney. Two other opacities on the right side **C** are seen to lie outside the urinary tract, probably representing calcified lymph nodes in the small bowel mesentery

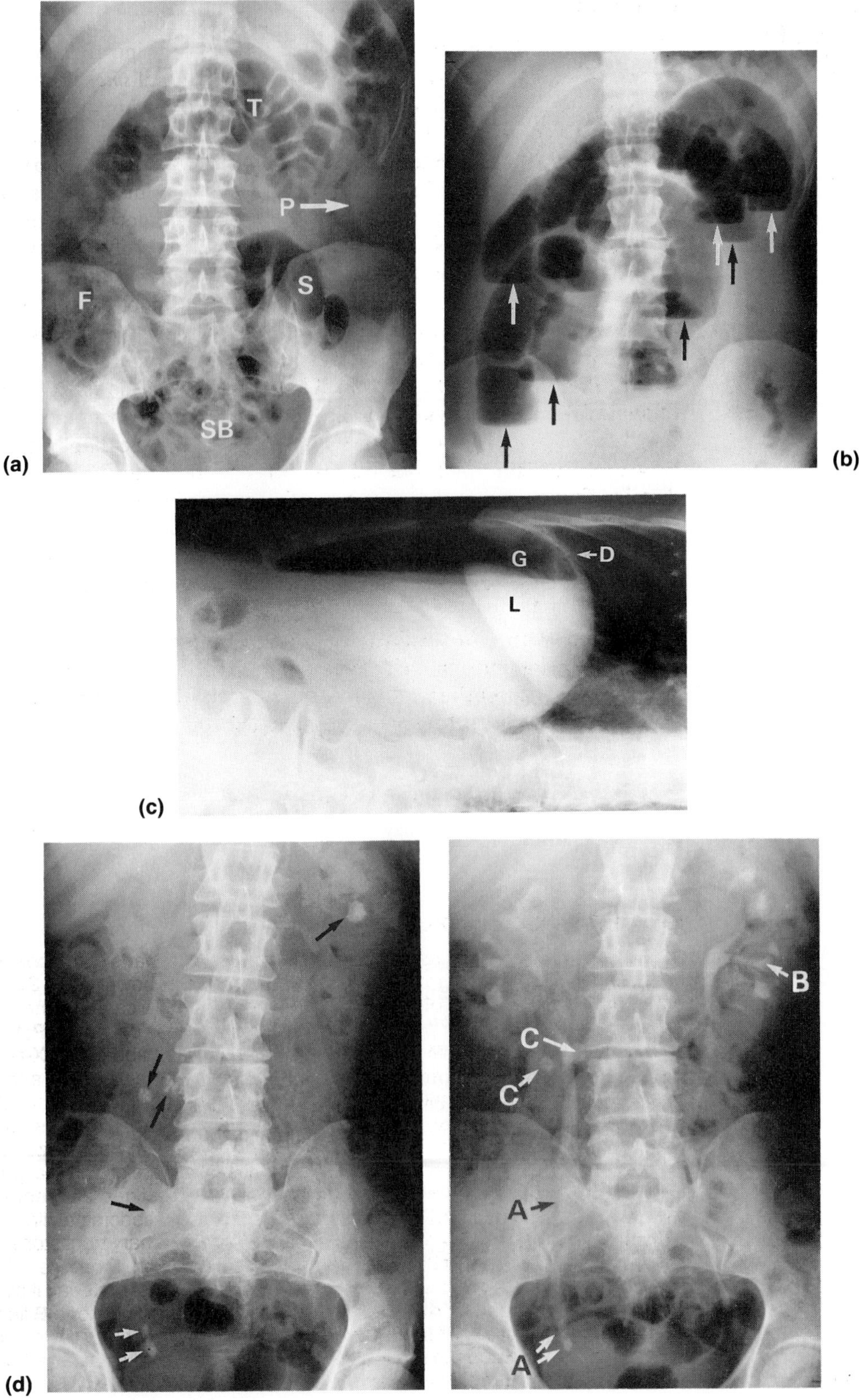
T
P
F
S
SB
(a)
(b)
G
D
L
(c)
B
C
C
A
A
(d)

are easily obscured by overlying bowel gas or faeces, and laxatives are usually given prior to urography to minimise this. The liver may be visible on plain radiographs but its size cannot be accurately estimated.

When examining an abdominal X-ray, the important features to look for are:

- Calcification in areas prone to stone formation, e.g. kidney, ureters, bladder, or biliary tree (see Figure 2.3d)
- Dilated gut (stomach, small bowel or large bowel)
- Free intraperitoneal gas indicating bowel perforation. Note the importance of the patient position when the film was taken
- Gas in abnormal places (e.g. biliary tree or urinary tract) suggesting a fistula into the bowel
- Non-biological objects, e.g. foreign bodies, surgical tubes or pieces of metal
- Pathological calcification, e.g. aortic aneurysm, pancreas, adrenals or uterine fibroids

The limitations of plain abdominal radiography are summarised in Figure 2.4

Fig. 2.4 The limitations of plain abdominal radiography

1. Intraperitoneal structures are not visualised unless they contain gas, displace gas-filled bowel or indent structural fat
2. Non-calcified stones (90% of gallstones, 10% urinary tract stones) are not visible
3. Bowel gas and faeces easily obscure stones
4. Phleboliths, calcified abdominal lymph nodes and costal cartilages readily mimic stones
5. Liver and spleen size cannot be estimated accurately
6. Free intraperitoneal gas may be missed on a supine film (need a horizontal beam film)

BOWEL CONTRAST RADIOLOGY

Techniques

Any part of the gastrointestinal tract can be demonstrated using contrast techniques. For examining the upper gastrointestinal tract, barium suspension is given orally (*barium swallow* for oesophagus and *barium meal* for stomach and duodenum). Progress of the contrast is observed by X-ray *fluoroscopy*. In screening, a technique known as *image intensification* is used to show a moving image on a television screen. The X-ray beam activates a sensing device which converts the output into a video signal. This enables the radiologist to select representative views as *spot films* to record the examination. One minute of screening gives the patient a dose of X-rays equivalent to one film.

Screening is also useful to study rapid gastrointestinal motility, as in swallowing. The images are recorded on video or cine film and studied later in slow-motion.

The large bowel is examined by means of contrast given rectally (*barium enema*). It must be remembered that the rectum is not well shown on this

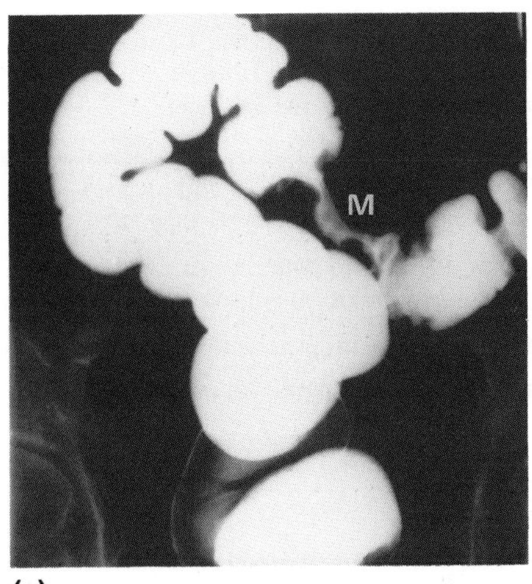

(a)

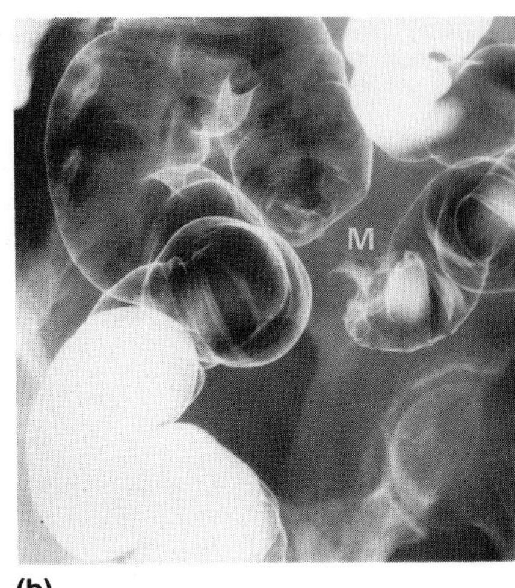

(b)

Fig. 2.5 Single and double contrast barium enemas

Typical annular carcinoma of the proximal sigmoid colon in a woman of 72; **(a)** Single contrast barium enema showing the malignant stricture **M**. Note all mucosal detail in the colon is obscured by barium. **(b)** Double contrast barium enema of the same patient also showing the stricture, but mucosal detail is outlined with a thin coating of barium. The bowel has been inflated with air

examination; a prior sigmoidoscopy should be performed if low lesions are not to be disastrously missed.

For small bowel examination, a barium meal may be 'followed through' distally, but some radiologists prefer to instill contrast into the proximal jejunum through a tube; this is known by the confusing term of *small bowel enema*.

In the early days of barium examinations, a *single contrast* technique was used. Barium was given alone and radiographs taken. However, the dense column of barium obscured much of the finer detail. Most barium studies nowadays use a *double contrast* method. Following the barium, air or carbon dioxide is used to distend the bowel, and this separates the barium-coated bowel walls and acts as a second radiolucent contrast agent (see Figure 2.5b). An anti-cholinergic agent such as hyoscine butylbromide (Buscopan) is often given at the same time to relax the bowel wall muscle and abolish spasm, thereby further improving the image.

Figure 2.5 illustrates various examples of radiological abnormalities on gastrointestinal contrast studies.

Preparation of the patient for bowel contrast studies

For upper gastrointestinal contrast studies, patients should be fasted over-night, except for water. Smoking should be avoided to minimise bowel gas. For small bowel studies, laxatives are sometimes given the day before to empty the colon. This may hasten transit of contrast through the small bowel.

For a barium enema, prior bowel preparation is performed with laxatives and sometimes bowel washouts, so that artefacts are removed (faecal lumps look very similar to polyps) and small mucosal defects are not obscured. Thorough preparation of the colon is vital if important pathology is not to be missed. If a barium enema reveals inadequate preparation, further efforts should be made to clear the colon and the examination repeated.

Some radiologists prefer not to perform barium enema examination for several days after high rectal biopsies, believing there is a risk of perforation.

Fig. 2.6 The limitations of barium contrast studies

1. It is often impossible to distinguish between different types of pathological lesion, e.g. between malignant and inflammatory colonic stenosis, and between malignant and peptic ulcer of the stomach
2. Fine mucosal detail is not shown, e.g. gastric lesions such as inflammation, shallow ulceration or early cancer, or angiodysplasias of the colon. In acute gastrointestinal bleeding, barium meal may miss the bleeding lesion
3. Small bowel is difficult to examine in detail because of contrast dilution by bowel contents, and loops of bowel overlying each other
4. Obstructed gut cannot be satisfactorily demonstrated
5. Barium may turn incomplete colonic obstruction into complete obstruction
6. Major abnormalities may be concealed because of tissue overlap

Complications of barium contrast studies

Barium should be avoided for contrast examinations if substantial peritoneal spillage seems likely, as, for example, when there is a possible perforation or anastomotic leak. In these cases, *water-soluble contrast medium* is best given initially, and if no leak is seen, barium is then substituted. This is because water-soluble materials are less radiopaque and less effective at coating the bowel wall, and therefore show less surface detail than barium. For the same reasons, barium may reveal a tiny leak from the bowel which is invisible with water-soluble contrast.

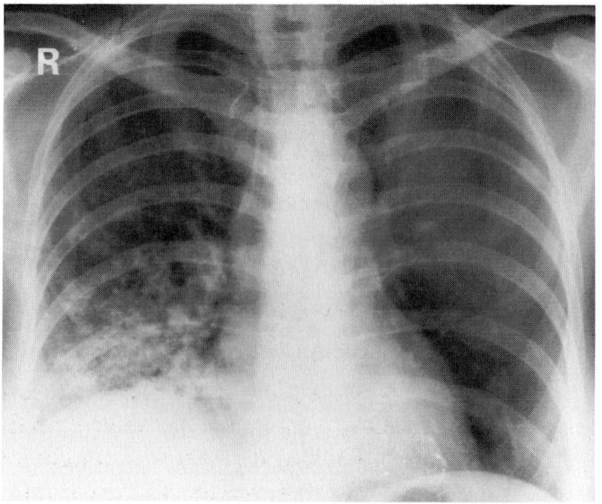

Fig. 2.7 Inhalational pneumonia after barium meal

Right lower lobe consolidation resulting from aspiration of stomach contents, including barium. The patient had undergone a laparotomy several days previously and an abdominal mass was discovered. There was still some (unrecognised) adynamic bowel obstruction (paralytic ileus). This barium follow-through examination was attempted too early and the patient aspirated after vomiting

Constrast studies should be used with caution in patients with bowel obstruction. Barium should not be given by mouth to patients with suspected large bowel obstruction because if it cannot pass through, it solidifies within the bowel and will turn an incomplete obstruction into a complete one. A barium follow-through is sometimes indicated in suspected small bowel obstruction, but there is a risk that contrast material may be vomited and aspirated into the bronchial tree, causing aspiration pneumonitis (see Figure 2.7).

BILIARY CONTRAST RADIOLOGY

Cholecystography

Modified iodinated benzoic acid derivatives given orally are excreted by the liver in the bile, rather than by the kidneys. This weakly opacifies the bile ducts and gall bladder. The contrast medium, however, is concentrated by the normal gall bladder, rendering it more opaque and visible on X-ray. This *concentrating function* is often retained when stones are present. If so, stones will often show as *filling defects* because they are usually radiolucent with respect to opacified bile. If the gall bladder is obstructed by a stone, it will not opacify; if the wall is diseased,its power of concentration is lost and it is unlikely to opacify on cholecystography — this is known as a *non-opacifying gall bladder*. Oral cholecystography is of no value in obstructive jaundice because contrast material is not excreted in sufficient concentration to register an image.

Twelve hours after ingestion of contrast, the cholecystogram films are taken. Lipid prepared from egg yolk is then given (*fatty meal*) which stimulates cholecystokinin-pancreozymin (CCK-PZ) release. This causes contraction of a (healthy) gall bladder which can be demonstrated by a further X-ray. Loss of contractility suggests that the gall bladder has been damaged by inflammation.

Intravenous cholangiography

Iodinated compounds similar to those used for cholecystography can be given intravenously. They are excreted in higher concentration by the liver, thereby allowing imaging of the extra-hepatic biliary system. Intravenous cholangiography has largely fallen from favour because the contrast material is relatively toxic (frequently causing nausea and vomiting) and the image is often of poor quality. Moreover, in the patient with obstructive jaundice, excretion of contrast deteriorates progressively in line with liver function. The technique has now been supplanted by methods allowing direct injection of contrast into the biliary tree (see next sections).

Percutaneous transhepatic cholangiography (PTC or 'perc')

This technique is used mainly for diagnosing the cause of obstructive jaundice and is often an alternative to endoscopic retrograde cholangiography. Using a method similar to percutaneous liver biopsy, dilated intrahepatic ducts can be punctured directly with a long fine (22 G) 'Chiba' needle and injected with contrast. The needle is inserted into the liver under fluoroscopy, using a right lateral or an anterior approach, and contrast is slowly injected as the needle is withdrawn. With a little luck, the end of the needle penetrates a duct and contrast is seen to fill it on X-ray screening. Further contrast is then injected in this position to outline the biliary tree. This test is most useful when there is extrahepatic duct obstruction, when it can show the position and configuration of the obstruction.

Since the jaundiced patient may well have a serious clotting defect, a *clotting screen* should be performed beforehand, including prothrombin time and platelet count.

Endoscopic retrograde cholangio-pancreatography

This investigation is described later in the chapter in the section on endoscopy; its use in obstructive jaundice is described in more detail in Chapter 7.

Operative cholangiography and choledochoscopy

It is now routine to perform cholangiography during operation for cholecystectomy. This is to demonstrate the size and number of stones in the bile ducts which are causing symptoms or, more often, to exclude asymptomatic stones. To perform an operative cholangiogram, a fine plastic cannula is introduced into the common bile duct through a small hole cut in the side of the cystic duct. Water-soluble contrast material is injected in two or three stages to outline the duct system and X-rays are taken at each stage. If stones are demonstrated, the common bile duct is usually opened by a longitudinal incision and explored.

Any stones found in the common bile duct are removed. Many surgeons then inspect the inside of the bile ducts during the operation, using a sterile *choledochoscope*. This can be either an L-shaped rigid instrument which has attachments for removing stones, or a flexible fibre-optic instrument used only for inspection. Choledochoscopy can markedly reduce the incidence of residual stones after exploration of the common bile duct.

T-tube cholangiography

Following exploration of the common bile duct for stones, a T-tube is often left in-situ to drain the duct. The transverse limb of the tube lies in the duct and the long limb drains to the exterior. About a week after operation, contrast can be injected along the T-tube to outline the biliary tree and confirm drainage into the duodenum. Abnormalities such as residual stones, bile leakage and duct stenosis will also be demonstrable.

Fig. 2.8 Some techniques for demonstrating the biliary system

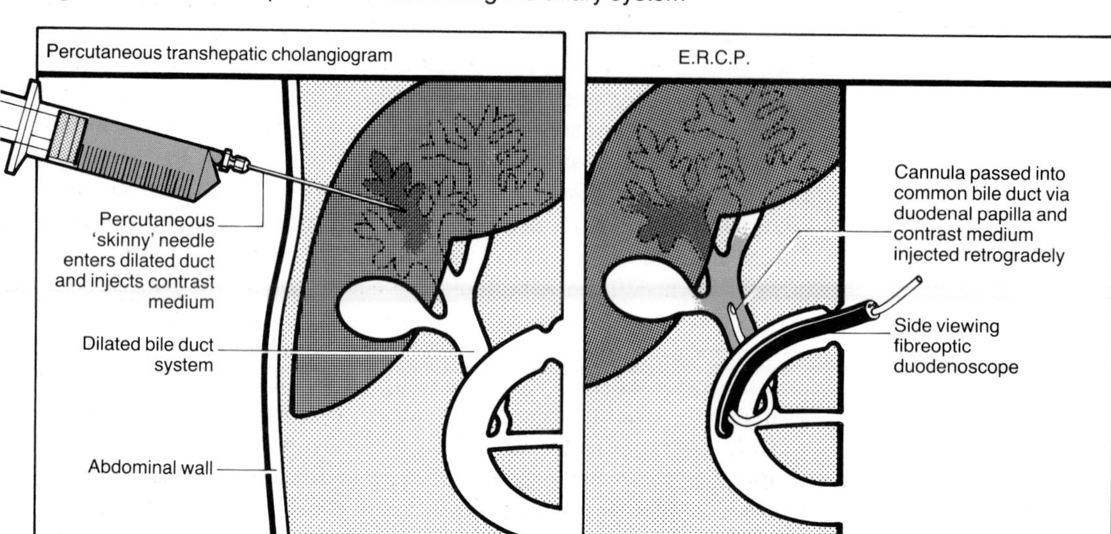

UROGRAPHY

Principles

Urography is a radiological technique for examining the kidneys and urinary collecting systems. It uses intravenous contrast medium which is concentrated and excreted by the kidneys. Laxatives are given beforehand to remove faeces and bowel gas. A plain abdominal *control film* is taken prior to contrast injection, so that any opacities can be compared with films taken after contrast. This helps to identify whether an opacity is a stone or an artefact.

The urinary tract is examined sequentially from kidneys to bladder on films taken at intervals after injection. The renal parenchyma opacifies almost immediately. Contrast then flows successively into the renal pelvis, ureters and bladder. The kidneys can be shown in greater detail by *tomography*. This is especially important when looking for renal masses and is used routinely when investigating adults with haematuria.

Special precautions

Intravenous contrast is potentially nephrotoxic in patients with impaired renal function; patients with diabetic nephropathy are at particular risk.

Conditions which might be associated with renal parenchymal disease should always be specified on the X-ray request form to help the radiologist plan the safest investigation. The important disorders are:

- Diabetes mellitus
- Renal failure (include results of renal function tests on the form)
- Multiple myeloma
- Heart failure

ARTERIOGRAPHY AND VENOGRAPHY

General principles

The veins or arteries of a particular anatomical region can be opacified by intravenous or intra-arterial injection of an appropriate contrast medium. This is known as *angiography*. A catheter is often inserted into a vessel some distance from the target site and manipulated into the correct position. The favourite entry points to the arterial system are the femoral vessels in the groin or, less commonly, the brachial vessels at the elbow.

In *lower limb arteriography*, the abdominal aorta and distal vessels are usually examined via a catheter in a femoral artery (femoral aortography). Occasionally the aorta has to be punctured directly (as when both femoral pulses are absent); this is known as translumbar aortography and is non-selective because the distal vessels are demonstrated by rapid injection and distal 'flush' of contrast. The aorta is punctured from the left lumbar area with the patient lying prone.

Lower limb *venography (phlebography)* is used for two main purposes: to demonstrate whether there is an acute *deep vein thrombosis* in a patient with a swollen or suddenly painful leg, or to investigate suspected *deep venous insufficiency*. Venography for deep venous insufficiency shows the patency of deep veins and any abnormal communications with superficial veins (incompetent perforating veins). A vein is usually cannulated in the foot to inject the contrast and a tourniquet applied around the ankle to direct it into the deep veins.

The results of *clotting studies* should be known prior to vascular radiology to anticipate possible haemorrhagic complications from the vessel puncture site.

Once the vascular catheter is in-situ, water-soluble contrast is injected directly into the artery or vein and images are recorded on rapid-sequence films or a video recorder. Thus obstructions due to thrombosis, atheroma or embolism can be demonstrated. The contrast material is similar to that used for intravenous urography and therefore carries similar hazards. In addition, there is the risk of complication from the arterial or venous cannulation. These include trauma to the vessel, causing bleeding or thrombosis, and loss of part of the catheter into the vessel lumen.

Electronic recording techniques

It is now possible to record X-ray images electronically in *digital* form, as opposed to the *analogue* form of conventional radiographic film. These digital images can be processed to optimise the available information; this includes subtracting background detail (thus removing bony images, for example), enhancing the contrast between tissues, magnifying areas of special interest and abstracting the best parts from a series of images. At present, this process is mainly used in angiography, where it is known as *Digital Subtraction Angiography or Digital Vascular Imaging*.

Background subtraction in real time can produce satisfactory vascular images with much lower concentrations of contrast; indeed, when high resolution pictures are not needed, as in screening for arterial disease or checking the patency of arterial grafts, satisfactory results can be obtained by injecting contrast *intravenously* (via a central venous line) and imaging the arteries when the contrast reaches them.

These electronic techniques are gradually being improved and will undoubtedly be introduced into other areas of radiology. Ultimately a 'film-less' X-ray department will be the norm, with images displayed on terminals dispersed around the hospital.

ULTRASOUND

Medical ultrasound was developed from sonar used for detection of submarines in the Second World War. However, the technology remained an official secret until the 1960s. Since then, the principle has found many applications, ranging from identifying shoals of fish to non-invasive imaging of body organs.

Medical ultrasound was pioneered in obstetrics, where it has become an important part of prenatal assessment. As the technology and electronics have improved the resolution and discrimination, surgical applications have become ever wider. An important advance has been *grey scale ultrasound*, which enables a whole range of tissue echogenicities to be displayed on the screen.

Interpreting ultrasound depends very much on the dynamic picture the radiologist sees during the examination, rather than what is recorded on the static films. The film record may mean little to anyone but the radiologist who performed the study!

PRINCIPLES OF MEDICAL ULTRASOUND

Ultrasound is non-invasive, painless and almost certainly safe. An ultrasound probe containing the transducer is applied to the skin over the area of interest while the image is displayed on a screen. The probe must be 'coupled' to the skin with jelly to exclude an air interface. The probe is then moved in different directions and at different angles to best display the organ and any abnormality. 'Spot' films are taken to record the examination.

The transducer, which has a piezo-electric crystal, both transmits and receives the ultrasound. A one microsecond pulse of ultrasound is emitted every millisecond, and the transducer then 'listens' for reflected ultrasound echoes over the next 999 microseconds. A fan-shaped image, representing a slice through the body, is generated electronically, with reflections showing as bright spots on a dark screen. The brightness of each spot is proportional to the sound reflectivity of the tissue interfaces. The moving image is displayed on a television screen as the examination proceeds and is thus desribed as *real time ultrasound*.

The length and breadth of organs or lesions displayed on the screen can be accurately determined by measuring the image. Furthermore, the volume of some structures such as the urinary bladder or the left ventricle can be estimated. This can give useful functional information: for example, the volume of residual urine in the bladder in chronic retention, or the completeness of left ventricular emptying in cardiac failure.

Bone, stones and other calcified tissues cause an abrupt and marked change in acoustic impedance, resulting in virtually complete reflection of ultrasound. Thus the surface of hard tissue, such as gallstones, is revealed by its echogenicity, and also by the fan-shaped *acoustic shadow* it casts. A similar, though lesser change in acoustic impedance occurs at gas/soft tissue interfaces, such as the bowel wall.

Minimal patient preparation is needed for ultrasound examination. For biliary ultrasound, the patient should be fasted to minimise gas shadows. For examining the pelvis, the bladder should be full of urine. This provides a fluid-filled, non-reflective 'window' for the ultrasound to reach the pelvic organs.

APPLICATIONS OF ULTRASOUND IN GENERAL SURGERY

Ultrasound has already largely replaced cholecystography for diagnosing gall bladder disease and, for many purposes, replaces intravenous urography.

Ultrasound is useful for:

- Distinguishing *solid* from *cystic* lesions, e.g. a thyroid cyst from a solid nodule, a renal or pancreatic cyst from a solid tumour
- Assessing palpable *abdominal masses* in the upper abdomen or pelvis. (Mid-abdominal masses are not well seen because they are usually obscured by bowel gas)

- Detecting *abnormal tissues* in a homogeneous organ, e.g liver metastases or renal adenocarcinoma
- Obtaining information about the nature of lesions from the way the echo *texture* contrasts with normal (e.g. liver secondaries from normal liver)
- Detecting *movement*, such as pulsation of an aneurysm, cardiac movement and fetal movements
- Detecting upper urinary tract dilatation *(hydronephrosis)*
- *Measuring* physical dimensions, e.g. the diameter of an abdominal aortic aneurysm or a dilated bile duct, the volume of residual urine in the bladder after micturition
- Detecting *stones* in the gall bladder or urinary bladder
- Guiding *percutaneous interventional procedures* for tissue sampling, e.g. aspiration or biopsy of liver metastases, pancreatic tumours or retroperitoneal masses

Fig. 2.9 Limiting factors in diagnostic ultrasound

1. Bone completely reflects ultrasound and obscures any tissues beyond it. Ultrasound is therefore no use for examining the brain and spinal cord

2. Bowel gas partly reflects ultrasound which may prejudice the examination. Starving the patient and giving laxatives may help

3. A thick layer of fat scatters ultrasound. It may not therefore be the first choice for investigating the gall bladder in obese patients

Doppler-shifted ultrasound

Ultrasound can be used for detecting and studying blood flow by applying the Doppler principle. Using a special probe placed on the skin, a beam of ultrasound is directed at an artery. Ultrasound is reflected from the red cells, which cause a frequency shift related to their velocity. The reflected ultrasound is used to generate a simple audible signal (for detecting blood flow) or else is electronically processed to reveal information about the nature of flow. The pitch of the simple audio signal is related to blood velocity and provides some qualitative assessment about whether flow is normal or abnormal.

The applications of Doppler-shifted ultrasound are:

- Measuring systolic blood pressure when it is low. This includes brachial pressure in shock or in infants, and ankle systolic pressure in lower limb ischaemia. For this purpose, an inexpensive portable Doppler instrument is used to detect flow (an electronic stethoscope) beyond a sphygmomanometer cuff placed around the arm or ankle
- Detecting the fetal heart rate
- Studying flow dynamics and estimating volume flow. Complex and expensive apparatus is required for this. The main application is occlusive carotid artery disease

COMPUTERISED TOMOGRAPHY (CT SCANNING)

GENERAL PRINCIPLES

Computerised tomography involves X-raying a series of thin transverse 'slices' of the patient's head or body. A precise fan-shaped beam of X-rays is repeatedly pulsed from successive angles around the circumference of each slice and the transmitted radiation electronically recorded on the other side. Each element of the beam is attenuated according to the density of the tissue it traverses. These numerous radiation counts are analysed by a computer, which builds up a picture of the tissue densities in the slice by solving many simultaneous equations. Each picture element is called a *pixcel* and each volume element is known as a *voxcel*. The images are displayed on a screen where they can be electronically edited and then recorded on film.

APPLICATIONS OF CT SCANNING

Pathological anatomy can be studied in great detail by computerised tomography and a vast new array of information can now be obtained to aid surgical diagnosis. Indeed, the accuracy of this information often could not be rivalled by exploratory operation; this is particularly so in brain injury after trauma. Management of serious head injuries has been transformed by head scanning, which enables timely and appropriate surgical intervention and avoids unnecessary exploratory operations.

Good CT images can be obtained in obese patients because fat separates the organs; this is the opposite of conventional radiography. Water-soluble contrast is often given before CT scanning to enhance the image in certain areas. Contrast may be given by mouth or by enema to enable gut to be recognised, or injected to show the aorta, the kidneys or the brain (if the blood-brain barrier is damaged).

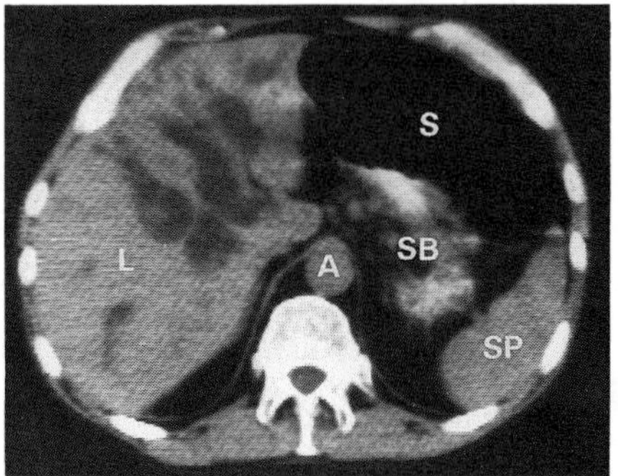

Fig. 2.10 CT scan

This CT scan image of the upper abdomen is from a 68-year-old woman who presented with a change in bowel habit and a palpable liver. By convention, the image is presented as if it were being viewed from the patient's feet, i.e. the left of the image is the patient's right. The liver **L** is seen to contain multiple large radiolucent lesions which represent metastases. The stomach **S** is filled with air. The spleen **SP**, aorta **A** and ribs and vertebrae are easily seen. The small bowel **SB** contains contrast material but is poorly displayed

The main indications for CT scanning are:

- Investigating areas difficult to examine by standard radiology or ultrasound. Examples include the retroperitoneal area and pancreas (deep inside the body), the lungs and mediastinum, and the brain and spinal cord (encased in bone)
- Investigating abdominal pathology when ultrasound has proved unsatisfactory
- Planning radiotherapy or chemotherapy, e.g. for staging lymphomas (replaces staging laparotomy), assessing intrathoracic tumours

- Planning surgery, e.g. establishing the extent of local invasion of oesophageal carcinoma, identifying the upper level of an aortic aneurysm
- Assessing solid organ damage in abdominal or thoracic trauma
- Guiding needles during biopsy of masses, drainage of fluid collections or obtaining aspiration cytology specimens

INTERVENTIONAL RADIOLOGY

Many of the conventional X-ray, ultrasound and CT techniques already described have been adapted to obtain biopsy material and to allow less invasive therapeutic manoeuvres than were formerly required. Many of these techniques have revolutionised treatment, for example of obstructive jaundice, and have established the radiologist as a front-line clinician. This is a rapidly expanding field of radiology, with a growing list of techniques. Some of the main surgical applications are described below.

TISSUE SAMPLING

Fine needle aspiration cytology

A fine needle (22 gauge) can be safely passed through most organs or gut to aspirate small fragments of tissue from a suspicious lesion. The depth and direction of the needle can now be accurately guided by ultrasound or CT to ensure a representative sample is taken. For example, pancreatic masses can be reached by transfixing bowel lying in front of the pancreas; this causes remarkably few side effects.

Needle biopsy

This is similar in concept to fine needle aspiration, except that a larger biopsy needle (14 or 18 gauge) is employed. This method is frequently used for sampling liver nodules or for taking renal biopsies in diffuse renal disease.

DILATATION TECHNIQUES

Percutaneous transluminal angioplasty

This technique, also known as *Gruntzig dilatation*, has rapidly become established as an alternative to surgery for overcoming certain arterial stenoses. In general, short stenoses are most suitable for this approach. The method is particularly useful for lower limb arterial disease (particularly of the iliac arteries) and for renal and even coronary arterial stenoses.

Angioplasty is usually performed under local anaesthesia (see Figure 26.16 later). A needle is first inserted into an accessible artery (usually femoral or brachial) and a flexible guide-wire and catheter passed through the stenosis. A special catheter, with a rigid plastic inflatable balloon at its end, is exchanged for the first catheter and then manipulated into position across the arterial stenosis. Positioning is guided by X-ray fluoroscopy and injections of contrast. Arterial pressure above and below the stenosis is measured via the catheter.

The balloon is then inflated to three or four atmospheres pressure to dilate the stenosis. Arterial pressures are measured as before. If dilatation has been successful, the pressure differential across the stenosis should have been eliminated.

Balloon dilatation of gastrointestinal strictures

Large balloon catheters similar to Gruntzig catheters can be used to dilate oesophageal strictures secondary to oesophagitis. They are sometimes used in achalasia or benign rectal strictures.

THROMBOLYTIC THERAPY

An artery that is freshly occluded by thrombosis and causing ischaemia can be recanalised by intravenous infusion of *streptokinase* or *urokinase*. However, systemic thrombolytic therapy is dangerous because it can cause serious bleeding and may provoke allergic reactions. However, if the tip of a catheter can be manoeuvred, under radiological control, to lie within the clot, small amounts of thrombolytic agents can be infused locally to achieve a high concentration where it is needed, but not in the systemic circulation; the clot may thus be safely dissolved. Unfortunately, the technique will not remove mature embolic material.

The same technique can be used for pulmonary emboli although the indications and efficacy are not yet well established.

OBTAINING ACCESS

Radiological access to the upper urinary tract

The renal pelvis can be reached percutaneously and punctured with a needle guided by ultrasound or CT scanning. The tract can be dilated to allow tubes of various sizes and types to be inserted. This access can be used to remove stones from the renal pelvis, to drain the kidney in distal urinary obstruction and to conduct sophisticated pressure and flow measurements in suspected pelviureteric junction obstruction. Gaining access to the kidney in this way is known as *percutaneous nephrostomy*.

Insertion of stent tubes

In obstructive jaundice caused by malignant compression of bile ducts, drainage of bile may be restored by placing a stent tube across the narrowed area under radiological control. The technique involves percutaneous needling of a dilated intrahepatic duct and passing a guide-wire through the stenosis. After dilatation of the tract (which can be traumatic and painful), the stent is then passed over the guide-wire to lie across the stenosis. This method is being superceded by endoscopic stenting.

EMBOLISATION

Highly vascular lesions, which would be difficult or impossible to treat by surgery alone, can have their arterial supply reduced or obliterated by embolisation. The main supplying artery is identified by selective arteriography and a catheter manoeuvred into it, close to the lesion. A small quantity of occlusive material is injected along the catheter to arrest in the artery where it narrows. The usual materials for embolisation are *gelatin foam, lyophilised human dura mater or minute steel coils*. The process is repeated for all the feeding vessels.

Embolisation is useful to reduce the vascularity of a lesion prior to otherwise difficult surgery (e.g. carotid body tumour) or to treat lesions not amenable to surgery (e.g. hepatic metastases or extensive arteriovenous malformations).

RADIOISOTOPE SCANNING

GENERAL PRINCIPLES

Radioisotope scanning is the diagnostic application of *nuclear medicine* techniques to identify sites of abnormal physiology, e.g the presence of pus, abnormal phagocytic activity, areas of excessive bone turnover. Isotope scanning, however, gives poor anatomical detail. Suitable tracer agents combine a substance physiologically taken up in the target tissue and a *radioactive label*. The usual label is ^{99m}Technetium.

The tracer is concentrated in a specific type of tissue (such as thyroid gland) or tissues with similar physiological or pathological activity (such as reticuloendothelial cells or areas of inflammation, respectively).

In the early days of nuclear medicine, tracer was detected using a rectilinear scanner which tracked back and forth over the patient for an hour or more to build up the image. Nowadays, a gamma camera, consisting of multiple detector units, simultaneously collects and counts the level of radioactivity across the area of interest. This produces a complete image in one exposure (see Figure 2.11). Several views are taken from different directions (usually anterior, posterior and oblique), and this provides more diagnostic information than a single view.

Some pathophysiological functions can be investigated by *dynamic imaging*. For this, isotope detection continues for a period and the changing level of radioactivity is recorded by computer for later analysis. Examples of this include estimating renal blood flow and studying renal clearance.

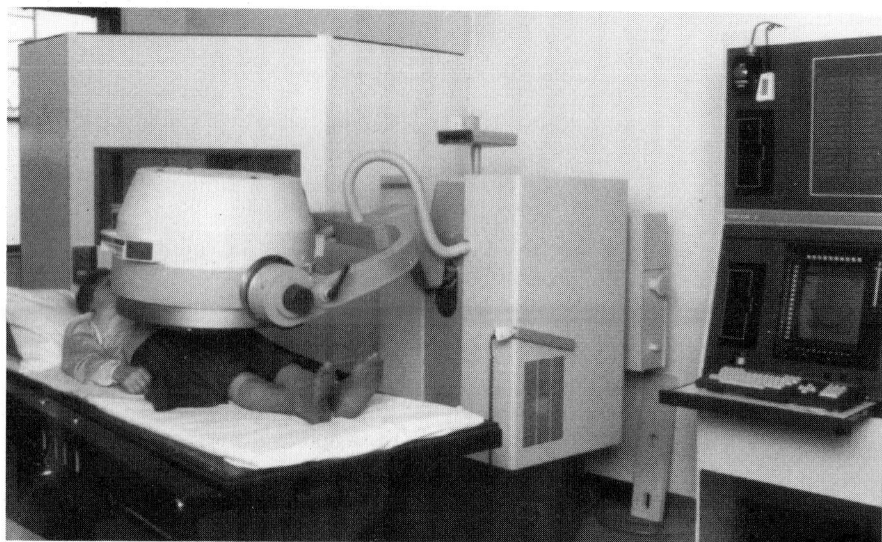

Fig. 2.11 Isotope scanning using a gamma camera

APPLICATIONS OF NUCLEAR MEDICINE SCANNING

Liver and spleen scans

a. Reticuloendothelial imaging ('liver scanning')

Technetium-labelled sulphur colloid is the usual tracer agent. This is taken up by reticuloendothelial cells in the liver (Kupffer cells) and spleen, and demonstrates the general morphology of the parenchyma. Areas of increased phagocytic activity are revealed by abnormal uptake of tracer.

Liver and spleen scanning may be indicated in the following circumstances:

- Unexplained abnormalities of liver function tests
- Parenchymal liver disease
- Suspected liver metastases
- Splenic function is in doubt
- Secondary spleens need to be located

b. Hepatobiliary imaging ('HIDA scanning')

Technetium-labelled imido-diacetic acid (IDA) derivatives are concentrated by the hepatocytes and excreted into the bile even in the presence of jaundice. This provides a useful means of testing the patency of the biliary tree, including the gall bladder.

Hepatobiliary imaging is mainly used for the following purposes:

- Demonstrating cystic duct obstruction in suspected acute cholecystitis
- Demonstrating the presence of bile duct obstruction (confirming obstructive jaundice) and its site. This investigation is being superceded by other investigations described earlier, particularly ultrasound and ERCP

c. Hepatoma imaging

More than 90% of primary liver tumours (hepatomas) preferentially take up *gallium*, whereas this is true for less than 50% of liver metastases. If liver tumour nodules are present but do not take up the tracer, then they can be diagnosed as metastases. The tracer agent, ^{67}Ga citrate, is also taken up by granulation tissue and was formerly used for detecting occult abscesses.

Bone scanning

Phosphate-based agents (phosphates or diphosphonates) labelled with technetium are usually used for bone scanning. These have replaced the former fluoride tracers. The tracer is taken up by areas of increased bone deposition and resorption, indicating sites of bone growth and repair. These include *growth plates, secondary tumours, foci of bone infection* and *active arthritis.*

The tracer agent is injected intravenously and becomes distributed in all body fluids. The highest concentration in sites of osteogenesis is about six hours later, and the patient is then scanned. The tracer is also taken up in areas of *dystrophic calcification* and thus may sometimes reveal an unsuspected carcinoma of breast, an old myocardial infarction or a uterine fibroid.

The main indications for bone scanning are:

- Suspected bone metastases (e.g. staging breast carcinoma) or investigation of bone pain
- Biochemical abnormalities suggesting bone disease (e.g. hypercalcaemia or raised serum alkaline phosphatase)
- Suspected occult (stress) fractures of bone
- Suspected osteomyelitis

Renal scans

Renal scanning is an important method of investigating the urinary tract. It can obtain information not available from any other source, it is quick and simple to perform and it allows the function of each kidney to be assessed independently. There are two main varieties of renal scan which use different isotopes: DTPA (diethylene tetramine pentacetic acid) is excreted in the urine like urographic contrast, whereas DMSA (dimercaptosuccinic acid) remains in cortical tissue.

Both DMSA and DTPA can give an estimate of excretory activity; this is useful in investigating unilateral renal parenchymal disease. A further application of DTPA scanning is to follow up children with reflux nephropathy. The isotope is injected and allowed to accumulate in the bladder. The child then voids urine while being scanned and any vesico-ureteric reflux is shown.

DTPA and DMSA are used to estimate differential renal function. This is useful for investigating renal artery stenosis, and also the function of transplanted kidneys. DMSA is also used to image the renal parenchyma and is useful for demonstrating renal scars or tumours.

Scanning for gastrointestinal bleeding

Scanning of the patient's own isotopically-labelled red cells may help to locate a source of gastrointestinal bleeding. This is useful in patients with recurrent acute haemorrhage, or in acute bleeding where the source cannot be identified by endoscopy or contrast radiology.

A quantity of the patient's blood is taken, labelled with technetium and reinjected. The abdomen is scanned at intervals over the next 24 hours for 'hot spots' indicating fresh gastrointestinal haemorrhage. If the rate of bleeding is more than about 1 ml per minute, the scan will usually reveal concentration of activity in one part of the gut. Unfortunately, slower blood loss is not usually detectable by this method. Scanning reveals the general area of

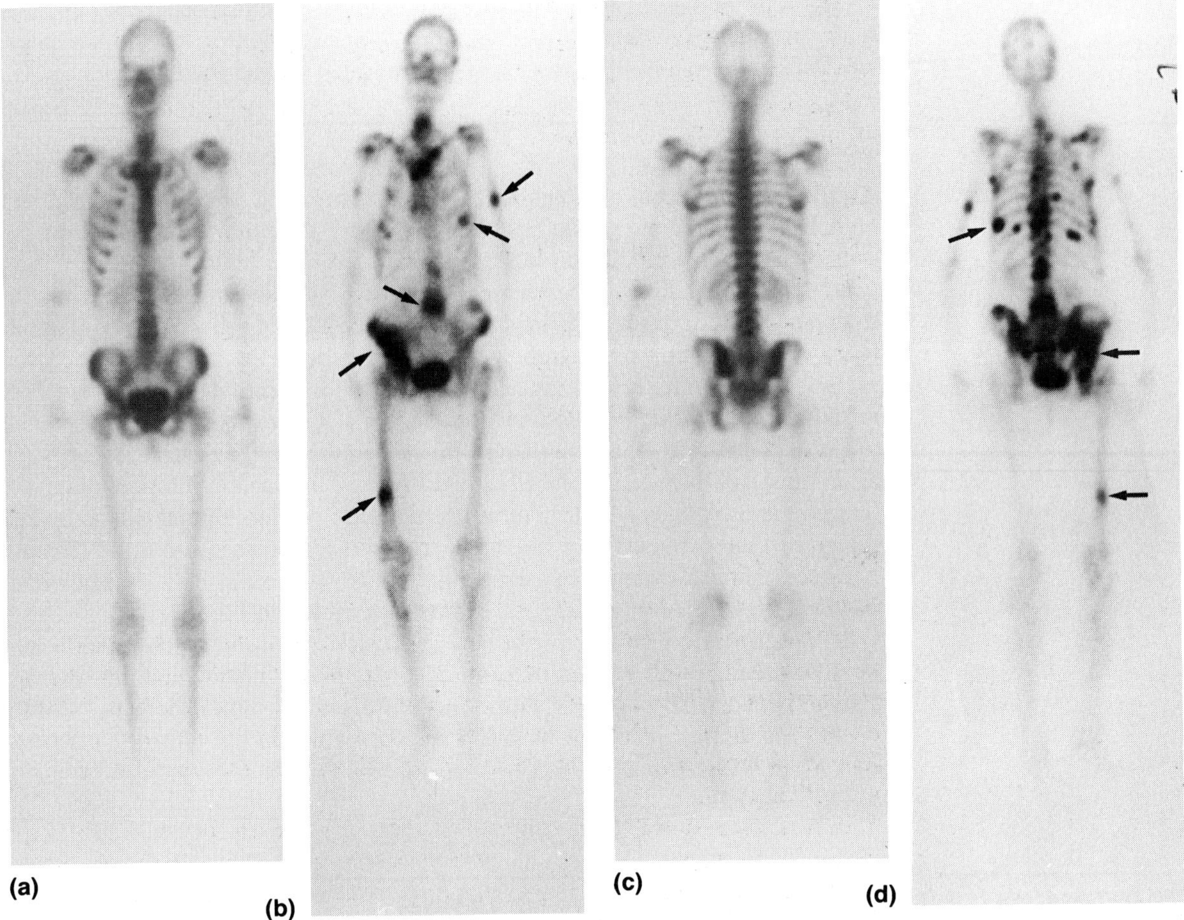

Fig. 2.12 Isotope bone scans of the whole body

(a) Anterior view of normal bone scan. **(b)** Anterior view of bone scan in a patient with multiple bony metastases (arrowed) from breast cancer. **(c)** Posterior view of normal bone scan. **(d)** Posterior view of bone scan in the same patient as in (b)

haemorrhage rather than the precise location, and therefore enables the surgical search to be focussed, for example, on the distal stomach and duodenum, or the right side of the colon. Isotope scanning has the advantage of detecting an accumulation of blood over a period, whereas the alternative investigation of selective angiography, although equally sensitive, requires active bleeding at the moment of injection.

Abscess scanning

When an abscess or other infected focus is suspected but cannot be localised, the patient's own white blood cells may be labelled with ^{111}Indium, reinjected and scanned. Typical indications for this are patients with a high swinging pyrexia after operation, or patients with a septicaemia of unknown origin. The process is expensive because it requires a cell separator. It gives high specificity and sensitivity, but there is a small proportion of false negative tests, where a hidden abscess is not revealed by the scan.

Lung scanning

The most important application of lung scanning is detecting pulmonary emboli. The principle is that pulmonary emboli obliterate patchy areas of the pulmonary arterial circulation but do not interfere with lung ventilation. Often, a *perfusion scan* alone is performed. For this, technetium-labelled albumin microspheres are injected intravenously. These lodge in the pulmonary capillaries after traversing the chambers of the right side of the heart. For improved accuracy, a separate *ventilation scan* may be performed first. The two together are known as *ventilation/perfusion scanning* or *V/Q scanning*.

For a ventilation scan, the patient inhales a gaseous radioactive tracer, such as a 'mist' of technetium-labelled DTPA or ^{133}Xenon, and the lungs are imaged from front and back. The ventilation and perfusion scans are compared for areas that are ventilated but not perfused (embolism), and areas that are perfused but not ventilated (consolidation or collapse). This is known as *ventilation/perfusion mismatch*. An example is shown in Figure 33.8.

If a right-to-left shunt is present, perfusion scanning is contraindicated because the microspheres can pass into the systemic circulation and may damage critical organs. Right-to-left shunts occur in cardiac septal defects, arterio-venous malformations of the lung and sometimes within pulmonary metastases.

MAGNETIC RESONANCE IMAGING (MRI)

GENERAL PRINCIPLES

Magnetic resonance imaging (MRI), also known as nuclear magnetic resonance, is a newly developed technique with rapidly expanding diagnostic applications.

MRI involves applying a powerful magnetic field to the body which causes the protons of all hydrogen nuclei to become aligned. These are then excited by pulses of radio waves at a frequency which causes them to resonate and emit radio signals; these are recorded electronically. Sophisticated computation then produces images which, uniquely, can be viewed in any plane, transverse, longitudinal or at any obliquity.

Lipids have a particularly high hydrogen content and are therefore clearly seen on MRI. Not surprisingly, the main applications of MRI so far have been in examining the brain and spinal cord. Atheroma can also be demonstrated. An exciting new application of MRI is in the study of blood flow and cardiac function. The direction and velocity of blood flow can be determined without need for contrast injection, and volume flow in particular vessels can be calculated. These techniques will undoubtedly play an increasing part in cardiac and arterial surgery in the future.

(a) 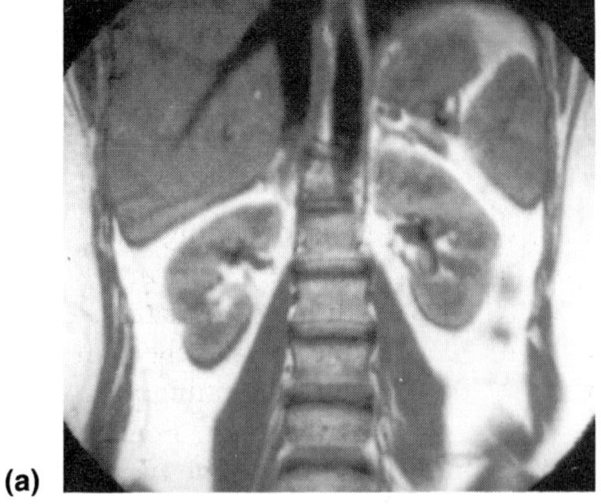

(b) 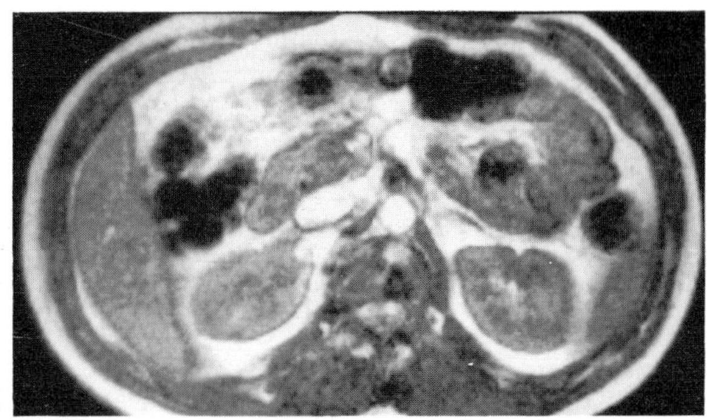

Fig. 2.13 MRI images

Longitudinal and transverse magnetic resonance images of the abdomen. Note the normal kidneys, liver and spleen. These images have both been generated from the same scan information. Any other oblique plane could also be generated if required

ENDOSCOPY

PRINCIPLES

Strictly speaking, endoscopy applies to any method of looking into the body through an instrument, either via an orifice such as the nose or mouth, or via an artificially created opening (e.g. peritoneoscopy or arthroscopy). Endoscopy, using simple tubular instruments, has been in use for many years and most of these methods are still in regular use, e.g. rigid sigmoidoscopy and oesophagoscopy. The term *endoscopy*, however, is now often used to mean endoscopy using flexible fibre-optic instruments.

Developments in fibre-optics first led to a major improvement in illumination for conventional endoscopes, and later to the creation of flexible endoscopes, which greatly extend the range and sophistication of endoscopic techniques.

Fibre-optic illumination

Rigid endoscopes and the early flexible instruments were illuminated by tiny incandescent bulbs which were prone to failure. The amount of light they could emit was limited by their production of waste heat. These have now largely been replaced, for both rigid and flexible endoscopes, by *fibre-optic light guides*.

Fibre-optic light guides are used to channel light from a powerful, fan-cooled light source remote from the patient, to the distal end of an endoscope. The light guides are made up of thousands of glass fibres, each with total internal reflection so that very little light is lost in transmission but no heat is transmitted. A powerful and cool light beam can thus emerge from the distal end of even the longest endoscope.

Fibre-optic image transmission

The second development, crucial in the design of flexible endoscopes, was the manufacture of *coherent viewing bundles*. In these bundles, the orientation of fibres at the distal end exactly matches that at the proximal viewing end. Each fibre thus transmits a tiny part of the distal scene to the viewing end. Here it can be inspected or photographed with a still or video camera. The view is not altered by angulation of the flexible conduit between the ends. The distal end of most flexible endoscopes allows a viewing angle of over 100°, and the lenses give a remarkable depth of focus. The image is so clear that accurate diagnosis can often be made on inspection alone.

Structure of flexible endoscopes

Flexible endoscopes all include a mechanism to steer the distal end in four directions, a coherent viewing bundle, one or two fibre-optic light guides, a suction channel, a channel for inflating the hollow viscus being inspected and a lens washing channel (see Figure 2.14). The suction channel is also used to pass slender flexible operating tools such as tiny forceps for taking biopsies.

APPLICATIONS OF FLEXIBLE ENDOSCOPY

Flexible endoscopes were first used to inspect the stomach in the late 1960s and the range of available instruments has progressively expanded ever since. There are now instruments available to inspect and cannulate the duodenal papilla, to examine all or part of the large bowel, to inspect the interior of the bile ducts at operation and to examine the bladder interior using only a local anaesthetic, as well as many others.

Narrow fibre-optic *bronchoscopes* can be passed under simple local anaesthesia. They are used to inspect bronchi for disease and can be used to aspirate mucus plugs which cause postoperative lobar collapse — important in general surgery. Further applications will undoubtedly appear as endoscopes become smaller and more sophisticated.

Gastroscopy

Oesophago-gastro-duodenoscopy, also known as *OGD* or *gastroscopy*, involves-inspection of the upper gastrointestinal mucosa using a steerable, flexible fibre-optic endoscope. It is usually carried out under intravenous sedation and hospital admission is not usually required. Gastroscopy enables the whole area prone to peptic ulcer disease to be directly and comprehensively examined.

Gastrointestinal contrast radiology suffers from the following disadvantages compared with fibreoscopy:

- Structural abnormalities (such as chronic ulcers) are only seen as two-dimensional images which give little information about the surface
- Shallow mucosal abnormalities like superficial ulceration or vascular malformations are easily missed

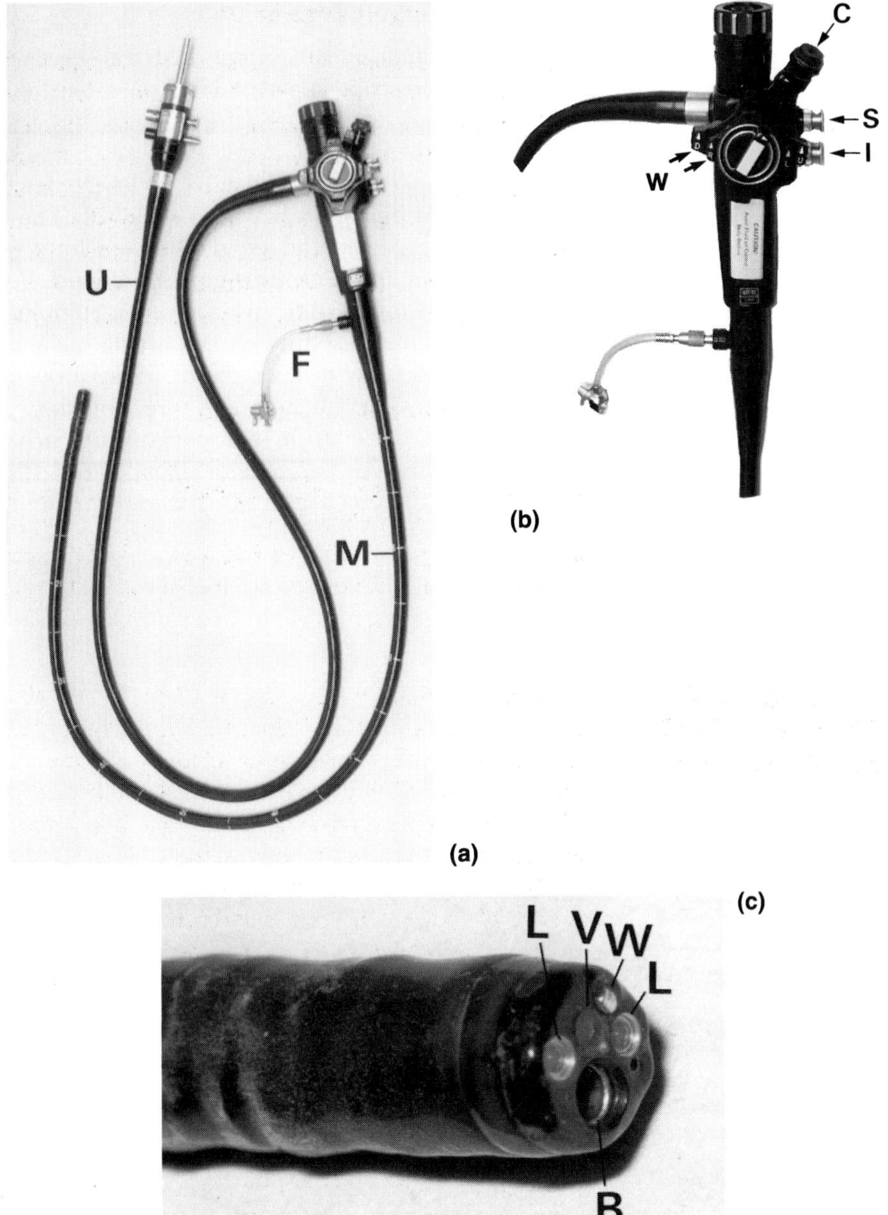

Fig. 2.14 Flexible fibre-optic gastroscope

(a) This end-viewing gastroscope is composed of a flexible main shaft **M** which is 1 metre long and marked at 10-cm intervals; the distal 10-cm can be flexed in 4 directions to steer the instrument and obtain the best view. There is also an umbilical cord **U** which is plugged into the control box and carries air to inflate the viscus, water to wash the viewing lens and suction to aspirate fluid from the lumen. There is a flush tube **F**, through which fluid can be injected to wash the bowel wall. The steering controls are better seen in photograph **(b)**. These consist of two concentric wheels **W** labelled respectively D & U (down and up) and L & R (left and right). There is a channel **C** to pass instruments, buttons to control suction **S** and air inflation and lens washing **I**. **(c)** shows the tip of the instrument in detail. The two light guides are marked **L**, **V** is the lens at the end of the viewing bundle, **W** is the exit of inflation air and lens washing water and **B** is the channel for passage of instruments and for suction

- Fibrosis and anatomical distortions from previous disease or surgery seriously interfere with recognition of what is abnormal
- Abnormal areas such as ulcers can be biopsied at endoscopy. Benign ulcers and early malignancies may be indistinguishable on radiology
- Tracing the source of acute upper GI haemorrhage is often impossible radiologically. Fibreoscopy can often identify the exact site of the lesion and the rate of haemorrhage

Treatment of oesophageal strictures

Endoscopic methods are often used for dilating benign oesophageal strictures. The endoscope is passed until the stricture is visible and then a flexible wire is passed through it into the stomach. The endoscope is removed, leaving the wire in-situ. Plastic *(Celestin)* or metal *(Eder-Puestow)* dilators of increasing size are then passed over the wire, which guides them through the stricture, until sufficient dilatation has been achieved. The technique is relatively safe, can easily be repeated and avoids the need for a general anaesthetic, which is necessary when a rigid oesophagoscope is used. Perforation of the oesophagus is a risk but is fortunately an uncommon complication (see Figure 2.15).

For dysphagia caused by an inoperable malignant stricture, a tube can be placed endoscopically to keep the oesophagus open. This involves first dilating the stricture, as for a benign stricture, and then pushing a flanged and reinforced latex tube down the oesophagus until it lies across the stricture. This technique, known as *pulsion intubation*, avoids an operation and may provide worthwhile palliation for an obstructing tumour.

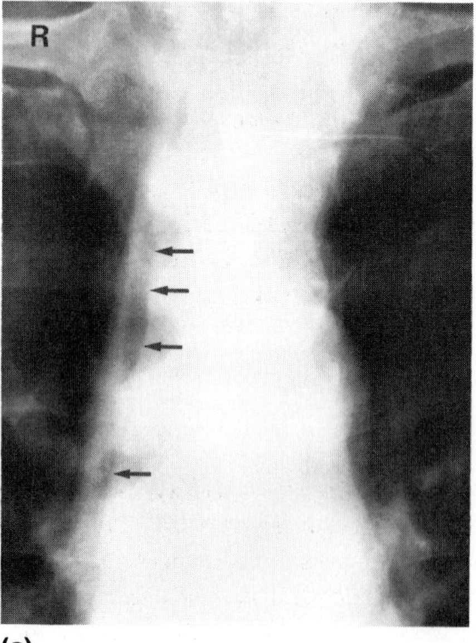

(a)

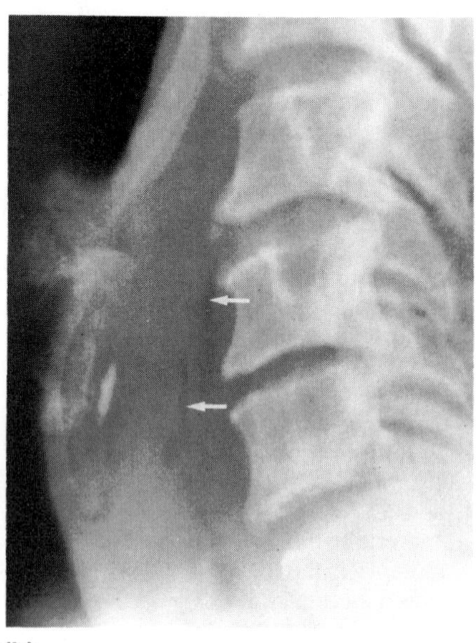

(b)

Fig. 2.15 Pneumomediastinum following perforation of an oesophageal tumour during endoscopy

This 56-year-old man was being investigated for difficulty in swallowing but after the examination, he complained of chest pain. Crepitus was found in the neck and was due to surgical emphysema. This results from oesophageal air leaking out of the perforation and tracking up the mediastinum into the neck. **(a)** Part of PA chest X-ray showing radiolucent line of gas (arrowed) in the right side of the mediastinum beneath the parietal pleura. **(b)** Lateral view of the neck in the same patient showing gas (arrowed) tracking up the prevertebral area behind swollen prevertebral soft tissues

Duodenoscopy

A special side-viewing duodenoscope is used to inspect the duodenal papilla, allowing insertion of a cannula. This allows injection of contrast material into the common bile duct and the pancreatic duct. The technique is known as ERCP *(endoscopic retrograde cholangio-pancreatography)* and has now become an important part of gastroenterological investigation. It is often used to image the biliary duct system in preference to percutaneous transhepatic cholangiography. Bile duct stones can often be removed endoscopically by slitting the sphincter at the lower end *(sphincterotomy)* and retrieving them with a balloon catheter or a Dormia basket. This may avoid the need for a hazardous operation.

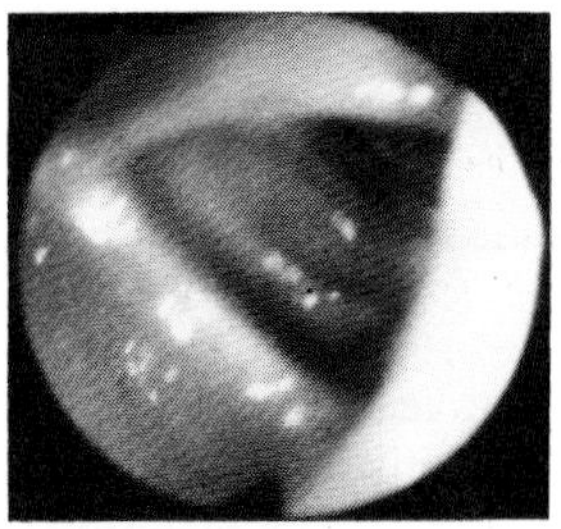

Fig. 2.16 Colonoscopic view of normal transverse colon

The transverse colon is typically triangular in cross section when seen colonoscopically; the taenia form the apices. Note how the image is made up of a series of dots, each transmitted by a single optical fibre

Large bowel endoscopy (colonoscopy)

Flexible endoscopes of different lengths are available for large bowel examination. The shortest, the *fibre-optic sigmoidoscope*, is about 60 cm long. It is simple to use and allows examination of the rectum, sigmoid and descending colon. Longer colonoscopes enable inspection of the entire large bowel including the caecum. Polyps can be removed by wire snares and diathermy, and other suspicious lesions can be biopsied. In follow up of long-standing ulcerative colitis, multiple biopsies can be taken at intervals from all around the colon, thus enabling early detection of dysplasia.

Urological endoscopy

Endoscopic urology is becoming a progressively larger part of urological surgery.

Cystourethroscopy (cystoscopy), using rigid instruments, is an important diagnostic and therapeutic tool for disease of the urethra, prostate and bladder. Transurethral resection of the prostate has virtually eliminated the need for open retropubic prostatectomy, and most early bladder tumours can be treated endoscopically.

A similar but longer instrument, the *ureteroscope*, can now be used for retrieving stones from the lower half of the ureter.

More recently, endoscopic methods of percutaneous stone removal from the renal pelvis have become possible. This involves creating a channel from the skin into the renal pelvis and dilating it until an endoscope can be passed. When the stone is seen, various instruments can be used to fragment it and effect removal.

Peritoneoscopy

Peritoneoscopy or *laparoscopy* is widely used by gynaecologists for diagnosing pelvic disorders and for sterilisation. It involves inflating the abdomen with carbon dioxide and passing a rigid peritoneoscope into the peritoneal cavity through a small subumbilical incision. Some general surgeons use the technique to obtain liver biopsies under direct vision and others are testing its value in diagnosing appendicitis.

METHODS OF OBTAINING TISSUE FOR DIAGNOSIS

BIOPSY

If major surgery or other therapy is being contemplated for a suspected malignant lesion, an accurate *tissue diagnosis* should be made if possible.

Skin lesions can be biopsied by incision under local anaesthetic. Rectal lesions can be biopsied using forceps through a rigid sigmoidoscope, while gastric and colonic lesions can be biopsied endoscopically. Breast lumps can be sampled using percutaneous needle biopsy (or aspiration cytology).

Enlarged lymph nodes can often be diagnosed by removing one completely for histological examination (excision biopsy). This often requires general anaesthesia, particularly for lumps in the neck.

Biopsy guided by ultrasound or CT scanning

Abdominal masses such as liver metastases or pancreatic lesions can now be biopsied accurately with the aid of ultrasound or CT scanning. The lesion is first imaged and then a biopsy needle guided to it. Guided biopsy techniques have greatly assisted surgical diagnosis and have saved many patients from unnecessary exploratory laparotomy when inoperable tumour has been confirmed.

CYTOLOGY

Special staining techniques for malignant cells can be applied to material obtained by fine needle aspiration. Cytological diagnosis requires special skills but often permits accurate diagnosis (e.g. of malignancy), which renders further, more invasive investigations unnecessary. A negative cytological result, however, must usually be disregarded because it may be due to sampling error.

Cytological diagnosis may be useful for the following:

- Examining fluid aspirated from cystic lesions such as from the breast
- Examining ascitic fluid obtained from the abdomen by *paracentesis*, or pleural effusions from the chest by aspiration
- Examining cells aspirated from solid masses such as in the pancreas, the breast or thyroid

3 PRINCIPLES OF OPERATIVE SURGERY

Introduction

This chapter outlines the essential principles of operative surgery and minor surgical techniques. These should be understood not just by surgeons but by all doctors, so as to give them an appreciation of the scope of surgery, to enable them to provide adequate explanation to patients before and after surgery, and to help them participate intelligently at operations. Furthermore, most doctors are required at one time or another to perform minor operations, casualty procedures and invasive investigations which require a knowledge of surgical technique.

Various suffixes derived from Greek and Latin are used in the description of certain surgical techniques; these are summarised in Figure 3.1.

Fig. 3.1 Surgical terminology

–oscopy = examination of a hollow viscus, body cavity or deep structure employing an instrument specifically designed for the purpose, e.g. gastroscopy, colonoscopy, laparoscopy, arthroscopy, bronchoscopy; the general term is endoscopy.

–ectomy = removal of an organ, e.g. gastrectomy, orchidectomy (i.e. removal of testis)

–orrhaphy = repair of tissues, e.g. herniorrhaphy

–ostomy = fashioning an artificial communication between a hollow viscus and the skin, e.g. tracheostomy, colostomy, ileostomy; the term may also apply to artificial openings between different viscera, e.g. gastrojejunostomy, choledocho-duodenostomy (i.e. anastomosis of duodenum to common bile duct)

–otomy = cutting open, e.g. laparotomy, arteriotomy, fasciotomy, thoracotomy

–plasty = reconstruction, e.g pyloroplasty, mammoplasty, arthroplasty

–pexy = relocation and securing in position, e.g. orchidopexy (for undescended testis), rectopexy (for rectal prolapse)

ANAESTHESIA

GENERAL PRINCIPLES

Some form of anaesthesia is required for almost every surgical procedure, with the aim of preventing pain in all cases, minimising stress for the patient in most, and providing special conditions for some operations, e.g. muscular relaxation in abdominal surgery. The choice of anaesthetic techniques includes *topical (surface) anaesthesia, local anaesthetic infiltration or nerve block, regional anaes-*

thesia and *general anaesthesia*. Methods other than general anaesthesia may be supplemented with *intravenous sedation* (e.g. with benzodiazepines) if the patient is anxious. Intravenous sedation with such drugs produces relaxation, relieves anxiety and has a marked amnesic effect; the patient is able to cooperate yet maintains protective reflexes. Intravenous sedation with benzodiazepines does not provide pain relief, which must be achieved by other means such as local anaesthesia or intravenous analgesics.

A combination of local or regional anaesthetic (for pain relief) with a light general anaesthetic can minimise postoperative respiratory and cardiovascular

Fig. 3.2 Choice of anaesthetic technique

1. Local anaesthesia
— in general for cooperative, calm and rational patients when no autonomic discomfort is anticipated
— minor operations, e.g. excision of small skin lesions or dental operations
— minor but painful procedures, e.g. insertion of chest drain
— unavailability of general anaesthetic expertise, e.g. in undeveloped countries
— patients unfit for general anaesthesia, e.g. cardiac and respiratory cripples
— ambulatory ('day case') surgery
— patient unwillingness to undergo general anaesthesia
— use of combined local anaesthetic and vasoconstrictor to provide a relatively bloodless operative field (note: this must never be used in the extreme peripheries, e.g. digits, penis, nose)

2. Regional nerve block
— minor surgery requiring wide field of anaesthesia, e.g. femoral nerve block for varicose vein surgery, pudendal block for forceps delivery
— when it is undesirable to inject into the operation site, e.g. drainage of an abscess
— to avoid tissue distortion from local infiltration in delicate surgery
— short-lived, wide-field ambulatory anaesthesia for reduction of forearm fractures, hand surgery (Bier's intravenous regional anaesthesia)

3. Epidural and spinal anaesthesia
— lower limb surgery e.g. amputations
— lower abdominal, groin and pelvic surgery e.g. caesarean sections, inguinal hernia repair, prostate, bladder and urethral surgery

4. Intravenous sedation or intravenous analgesia alone
— short-lived uncomfortable procedures where local anaesthesia is impractical, e.g. gastrointestinal endoscopy, musculoskeletal manipulation

5. Intravenous sedation combined with local anaesthesia
— unpleasant procedures without autonomic side effects, e.g. wisdom tooth extraction, toe-nail operations, vasectomy

6. Local anaesthesia with light general anaesthesia
— caudal epidural anaesthesia for operations in the perineal area, e.g. haemorrhoidectomy, circumcision

7. General anaesthesia
— where all of the above are unsuitable or difficult to achieve
— severe patient apprehension or patient preference for general anaesthesia for uncomfortable or unpleasant procedures
— major or prolonged operations
— abdominal and thoracic operations requiring muscle relaxation
— where it is necessary to secure the airway by intubation

depression, reducing postoperative morbidity (e.g. caudal anaesthesia in perineal operations). Local or regional anaesthesia can also be used at the end of an operation to provide postoperative pain relief; for example, intercostal nerve blocks after an abdominal operation will allow more comfortable breathing and coughing, reducing the likelihood of respiratory complications. The main factors influencing choice of anaesthesia are summarised in Figure 3.2.

Careful selection of appropriate drug combinations for each case and close liaison between surgical and anaesthetic staff before, during and after operation greatly enhance postoperative recovery. The use of a 'high dependency' recovery area where at-risk patients can be intensively nursed and monitored postoperatively, also plays an important part.

PRINCIPLES OF ASEPSIS AND INFECTION CONTROL

Introduction

The main organisms involved in surgical infections have already been described in Chapter 1. The chief sources of infection are the patients themselves (particularly their bowel flora), less commonly the hospital environment, food or cross infection from other patients and, rarely, bacteria carried by theatre personnel. Very rare sources of infection are contaminated surgical instruments or equipment, dressings and parenteral drugs and fluids.

The risk of postoperative infection depends on the extent of bacterial contamination of the wound at operation. Bacteria may enter a wound by five possible routes:

- Airborne bacteria-laden particles
- Direct innoculation from instruments and operators
- From the patient's skin
- From the flora of the patient's internal viscera, especially the large bowel
- Via the blood stream

Modern operating theatre design and aseptic procedures, if correctly observed, minimise wound contamination but infections still occur. Their results can be devastating, especially in relation to artificial prostheses, bowel anastomoses, skin grafts and bone. Furthermore, some patients are particularly vulnerable to infection, notably neonates, the immunosuppressed, the debilitated and the malnourished. Treatment of established infection is no substitute for prevention.

The introduction in the 1970s of perioperative prophylactic antibiotics has revolutionised the scope and outcome of certain types of operative surgery in a manner comparable to the surgical revolution of the late 19th century heralded by Lister's techniques of antisepsis.

METHODS OF INFECTION CONTROL

1. The operating environment

Modern *operating theatre design* plays a major role in the control of airborne wound contamination. This is important mainly for staphylococci carried on airborne skin scales.

The main factors influencing infection rate are:

- Concentration of organisms in the air
- Size of bacteria-laden particles
- Duration of exposure of the open wound

The last one can be minimised by avoiding unnecessarily long procedures but the first two are mainly influenced by theatre design and air supply. Operating theatre complexes are laid out so as to minimise introduction of infection from elsewhere in the hospital via air, personnel or patients. Air is drawn from the relatively clean external environment, filtered and supplied to the operating theatres at a slightly higher pressure than outside to ensure constant outward flow. Air turnover is the most important factor; the aim is to ensure 3–15 air changes per hour which 'scrubs out' the theatre air by dilution. Standard air delivery systems aim to achieve a constant flow of clean air towards the operating table which is then exhausted from the theatre. Despite this, convection currents allow some recirculation of air, which may have been contaminated, into the operation site.

The crucial importance of infection in joint replacement surgery has led to the development of sophisticated *ultra-clean air delivery systems*. These have been shown to reduce postoperative infection two to fourfold but the cost of such measures makes them difficult to justify for general surgery. Enclosure of the patient in a sterile tent in which the surgeons wear space-type suits can reduce infection rates by a further 5–7.5% but such measures are probably not warranted except in specialised joint replacement units. A simpler isolation system, known as the *Trexler system*, encloses the patient in a plastic chamber filled with clean air; the theatre staff operate via gloves sealed into the walls of the chamber.

2. Minimising infection from operating theatre personnel

Studies of bacterial types in wound infections have shown that a modest proportion of wound infections are derived from theatre personnel. Bacteria reach the wound via the air or by direct innoculation. About 30% of healthy people carry *Staph. aureus* in the nose but pathogenic organisms may also be present in the axillae and perineal area, the latter probably the most important source. In addition, minor skin abrasions are usually infected, as are skin pustules and boils; thus personnel with such lesions should not enter the operating theatre.

Airborne, personnel-derived infection is reduced by changing from potentially contaminated day clothes to clean theatre clothes and shoes which should not then be worn outside the theatre complex. Trouser cuffs should be elasticated or tucked into boots. Some studies suggest that females should wear trousers instead of dresses, in order to reduce 'perineal fallout'. *Facemasks* are worn to deflect bacteria-containing droplets in expired air, but their effectiveness falls over a relatively short period, especially if they become wet. With the exception of nasal *Staph. aureus* (particularly important in infection of prostheses), bacteria derived from the head do not generally cause wound infection. The efficacy of wearing masks, and even hair coverings, is unknown.

Sterile gloves and gowns are worn by surgeons and staff directly involved in the operation to prevent direct innoculation of bacteria. Gloves are impermeable to bacteria but hands and forearms are washed before gloving and gowning with antiseptics which persist on the skin. This minimises bacterial contamination if a glove is punctured or the sleeve of the gown becomes wet. *Thorough washing* with soap and water removes extraneous contaminants but not resident flora, the numbers of which can be considerably reduced by using detergent solutions containing antiseptics such as *chlorhexidine* and *povidone-iodine*; disinfection is further improved by a final *alcohol rinse*. These are most effective if they are not rinsed off but merely dried with a sterile towel. The traditional ritual of scrubbing with a brush for three minutes is actually less effective than washing the hands thoroughly because it causes microtrauma to the hands and brings more bacteria to the surface.

Despite the wearing of gloves and gown, the less the wound is handled the better. This principle particularly applies when aseptic conditions are less than ideal. On the ward, minor procedures such as bladder catheterisation or insertion of a chest drain should be performed using a *no-touch technique*.

3. Minimising infection from the patient's skin

The patient's skin, especially the perineal area, is the source of up to half of all wound infections. These can be minimised by the following measures:

- *Shaving the skin* — body hair was once thought to be an important source of wound contamination but shaving produces numerous small abrasions which then become infected with skin commensals. Hair removal should therefore be restricted to clipping away just enough hair to provide adequate skin access; if shaving is required, it should be done on the ward just before the patient is sent to theatre rather than the day before. Ideally, it should be done in theatre

- *Painting the skin with antiseptic solutions* — povidone-iodine or chlorhexidine in alcoholic solution is applied to a wide area around the proposed operation site ('skin prep'); this is now done only when the patient is on the operating table, but in the past patients were subjected to a series of applications of antiseptics such as gentian violet for several days beforehand!

- *Draping the patient* — the standard procedure is to place sterile cotton drapes over all but the immediate field of operation to isolate the area. However, if the drapes become soaked with blood or other body fluids, bacteria may be drawn through by capillary action. Therefore, impermeable sterile paper sheets known as *ventiles* are usually placed beforehand beneath the drapes. For high risk surgery, e.g. joint replacements, plastic or impermeable paper drapes with adhesive borders may be used in addition

- *Investing the skin* at the operation site with a thin film of adherent clear plastic — the skin incision is then made through the plastic film so that little bare skin is exposed. This method has proved counter-productive because bacteria multiply beneath the film

4. Reducing infection from internal viscera

The large bowel teems with potentially pathogenic bacteria and the peritoneal cavity is inevitably contaminated in any operation at which the large bowel is opened. Therefore, wherever possible the large bowel should be mechanically cleansed prior to operation. Pathogenic bacteria are also found in obstructed small bowel. The same applies to the stomach and small bowel of patients on H_2 receptor blocking drugs (see Chapter 9) where the normal bactericidal effect of gastric acid is lost.

5. Sterilisation of instruments and other supplies

In modern surgical practice, infection from instruments, swabs, equipment and intravenous fluids has been virtually eliminated by their being supplied in sterile packs from a central sterile supplies department (CSSD). Re-usable instruments and drapes are sterilised by *high pressure steam autoclaving* according to strict regulations. Most disposable items are purchased in pre-sterilised, sealed packs. Sterilisation in small autoclaves near the operating theatre should only be performed if instruments in short supply are required for successive operations.

Fig. 3.3 Time and temperature requirements for sterilisation by different methods

	TEMP	TIME
Steam autoclave		
Unwrapped instruments and bowls	126° C	10 mins
Instrument sets, dressings and rubber	134° C	3 mins
Ethylene oxide gas		
Heat sensitive materials — plastics, endoscopes electrical equipment	55° C	2–24 hrs
Liquid glutaraldehyde		
Cystoscopes and other urological equipment, plastics and heat sensitive equipment required urgently	Room temp	10 mins

6. Surgical technique

Surgical technique plays an important part in minimising the risk of operative infection. Non-vital tissue and collections of fluid and blood are particularly vulnerable to colonisation by infecting organisms, which may enter via the bloodstream even if direct contamination has been avoided by aseptic technique. Tissue damage in the course of surgery should be kept to the minimum by careful handling and retraction and by avoiding unnecessary diathermy coagulation. Haematoma formation is minimised by careful attention to haemostasis and placement of drains into potential sites of fluid collection; *closed-drainage* or *suction-drainage systems* reduce the risk of organisms tracking back into the wound from the ward environment.

Faecal contamination is associated with a high risk of infection and great care is taken in operations where the bowel is opened or has perforated. After large bowel anastomoses, a drain is usually placed in the vicinity to minimise the danger of general peritoneal contamination should the anastomosis leak.

Management of drains in the postoperative period

Abdominal drains provide a potential route for infection to enter the abdomen even though the intra-abdominal pressure nearly always exceeds the external pressure. The risk can be minimised by ensuring the drain opens into a sterile environment such as a drainage bag *(closed drainage)* and by removing the drain as soon as its task is completed. Decisions about removal of drains should rest with the operating surgeon who will undoubtedly have personal preferences.

The general principles of drain management are as follows:

- Suction drains help to collapse down spaces left in the tissues at operation as well as to drain blood and inflammatory exudate. These drains are mainly used after extensive excisional surgery where a large enclosed raw surface remains, e.g. after mastectomy or excision of the rectum. The drain is usually only retained for 24 hours after operation unless drainage persists for a longer period
- Non-suction drains (e.g. large bore silicone or rubber tubes, or corrugated drains) are mainly used for bowel and biliary anastomoses and in abscess drainage. In this case, the drain is left in place for about five days. Some surgeons prefer to withdraw the drain in stages so that the deep part of the drainage tract can collapse progressively, reducing the risk of leaving a deep pool of fluid

7. Prophylactic antibiotics

Despite the best aseptic techniques, some operations carry a high risk of postoperative wound infection and septicaemia; this can be dramatically reduced by the prophylactic use of antibiotics. The antibiotics chosen should be *bactericidal* rather than bacteriostatic and should be matched to the anticipated organisms in the area of the operation. The relative risk of postoperative infection in different types of operation is summarised in Figure 3.4.

As a general principle, prophylactic antibiotics are indicated if the anticipated risk of infection exceeds 10%, i.e. all emergency abdominal surgery, all elective colonic operations and upper gastrointestinal operations for malignancy. Prophylactic antibiotics are also used by some surgeons for operations in the 5–10% risk category, e.g. cholecystectomy. In addition, prophylactic antibiotics are indicated for low-risk cases such as artificial implants where the consequences of infection are catastrophic. Prophylactic antibiotics can reduce postoperative infection in high risk cases by 75%, and in lower risk cases, may almost entirely eliminate the risk.

Fig. 3.4 Relative risk of infection in surgical wounds

1. Clean operations, i.e. no preoperative infection and gastrointestinal, respiratory and urinary tracts not opened (e.g. inguinal herniorrhaphy, breast lump excision, ligation of varicose veins) — risk is 2–5%

2. Clean operations with gastrointestinal, respiratory or urinary tracts being opened but with minimal contamination (e.g. elective cholecystectomy, elective peptic ulcer surgery, transurethral resection of prostate, excision of minimally inflamed appendix) — risk is less than 10%

3. Operations where tissues inevitably become contaminated but without pre-existing infection e.g. elective large bowel operations, fresh traumatic skin wounds — risk is about 20%

4. Operations in the presence of infection, e.g. abscesses within the body cavities, bowel perforations, delayed operations on traumatic wounds — risk is greater than 30%

5. Emergency colonic surgery (bowel unprepared), i.e. perforation or obstruction — risk greater than 50%

In the vast majority of wound-related infections, the organisms are introduced during the operation and become established during the next 24 hours. Thus, if prophylactic antibiotics are to be effective, high blood levels must be achieved during the operation, when contamination occurs. To achieve the latter, the first dose of antibiotic should be given either an hour before operation or at induction of anaesthetic; antibiotics should not be given any earlier as this may encourage proliferation of resistant organisms. A single preoperative dose of antibiotic is probably sufficient, provided it is rapidly bactericidal and the inoculum of bacteria is small. However, many surgeons prefer to give two additional doses postoperatively. Longer courses of prophylactic antibiotics are not beneficial and may encourage resistant strains of organisms to emerge.

In general, intravenous antibiotics provide the most predictable blood levels; peak tissue levels are achieved within one hour of injection. Metronidazole administered rectally gives equally reliable blood and tissue levels although these are not reached until 2–4 hours after administration. Oral metronidazole is usually inappropriate because of unreliable absorption and enforced perioperative starvation.

a. Operations involving bowel and biliary system

Patients having these operations are at risk mainly from a mixture of gram-negative bacilli (Enterobacteriaceae family and *Pseudomonas*), faecal anaerobes (*Bacteroides fragilis*) and *Staph. aureus*. The most commonly used prophylactic antibiotic regimens are:

- For biliary surgery — a cephalosporin alone (e.g. cefotaxime or ceftizoxime)
- For colonic and other bowel surgery — either a combination of a cephalosporin (as for biliary surgery) and metronidazole, or a combination of

gentamicin, benzyl penicillin and metronidazole. Mezlocillin alone should no longer be used because 10–20% of *E. coli* are now resistant

- For appendicectomy — rectal metronidazole alone, given two hours pre-operatively. This has proved as effective as any other regimen

The choice of antibiotics for prophylaxis must be kept under review because organisms change their sensitivities. An important consideration in this regard is that aminoglycosides such as gentamicin do not alter the gut flora because their concentration in the lumen is low; this is in contrast to the cephalosporins and ampicillin. In consequence, there is a rising tide of *beta-lactam resistant* gut organisms, which are insensitive to the cephalosporins and ampicillin but not to the aminoglycosides. If resistant staphylococci become more troublesome, vancomycin may become necessary for prophylaxis.

b. Operations involving implantation of prostheses

Vascular grafts and joint replacements are at particular risk from *Staph. aureus* infection. *Staph. epidermidis (albus)* may also be implicated and, very rarely, coliforms. Flucloxacillin is the agent of first choice for prophylaxis but gentamicin may be added for extra protection. Cephalosporins are often used but their efficacy against staphylococci is less than flucloxacillin or gentamicin.

c. Operations where ischaemic or necrotic muscle may remain

Lower limb amputations for arterial insufficiency and major traumatic injuries involving muscle are susceptible to gas gangrene and tetanus. Clostridia are highly sensitive to benzyl penicillin and metronidazole, one of which should be given as early as possible after major trauma and before major amputations for ischaemia.

8. Prevention of cross-infection

Cross-infection is the term used to describe infection derived from other patients in the nearby hospital environment, and it is rare. It should be distinguished from colonisation with other patients' bacteria, which is common. Cross-infection is mainly spread via food, staff, medical equipment or ward furnishings. Outside the operating theatre, whenever there is patient contact which might result in infection, the same principles of asepsis should be applied, although the achievable level of aseptic technique is lower. Doctors are probably the worst offenders as regards transfer of infection, e.g. by removing dressings to inspect wounds in the open ward, by failing to wash hands between patients, and by careless aseptic technique when performing ward procedures such as bladder catheterisation.

A patient with an infection which is potentially dangerous to other patients should be isolated and barrier-nursed in a single room. These infections include Lancefield group A streptococci, open tuberculosis and infective diarrhoeas. Infection with multiply-resistant strains of staphylococcus requires a patient to be transferred to an isolation unit or, if the patient is in intensive care, the unit should be closed to new admissions.

ESSENTIAL SURGICAL TECHNIQUES

INCISION TECHNIQUE

Choice of incision

The purpose of most skin incisions is to gain access to underlying tissues or body cavities, and the first consideration when planning a surgical incision must be to achieve good access. Furthermore, the incision should be placed in a position which will allow it to be extended if necessary. Despite patients' impressions, the length of an incision (and the number of sutures required for closure!) has little bearing on the rate of healing; the success of an operation should not be put at risk by 'key-hole' surgery.

Secondary considerations in the choice of incision are as follows:

- Orientation of skin tension lines *(Langer's lines)* and skin creases — wherever possible, incisions should be made parallel to these lines (e.g. a 'collar' incision for thyroid operations) as this causes minimal distortion, gives a better cosmetic result and is less likely to break down
- Strength and healing potential of the tissues — the nature and distribution of muscle and fascia, particularly in different parts of the abdominal wall, influences the strength of the repair. For example, a vertical lower midline incision situated where the abdominal wall consists only of fascia, may be more prone to subsequent incisional herniation than a paramedian vertical incision a few centimetres lateral to the midline; here the rectus abdominis muscle imparts extra strength to the wound
- The anatomy of underlying structures, particularly nerves — if possible, the incision line should run parallel to, but some distance away from the expected course of underlying structures, reducing the risk of damage. For example, to gain access to the submandibular gland, the incision is made parallel and 2 cm below the lower border of the mandible to avoid the mandibular branch of the facial nerve
- Cosmetic considerations — wherever possible, incisions should be placed in the least conspicuous position, such as in a skin crease or where it will later be concealed by clothing, e.g. a transverse suprapubic *(pfannanstiel)* incision below the 'bikini' line for operations on the bladder, uterus or ovary

Handling of deeper tissues

The skin consists not only of thin epidermis and the dense, somewhat thicker dermis, but also includes the underlying fatty hypodermis which may be as much as 10 cm thick in an obese individual.

Once the skin incision has been made, the scalpel is mainly reserved for incising fascia and other fibrous structures like breast tissue. Anatomical detail is exposed and displayed by a combination of blunt and sharp dissection. The purpose of dissection is to protect structures which might be damaged by bold incisions, and to preserve blood supply and venous drainage. *Blunt dissection* involves teasing or stripping tissues apart using the fingers, swabs or blunt instruments, following natural tissue planes. *Sharp dissection*, with scissors and forceps, is used where tissues have to be cut and also to display small structures. Some surgeons generally prefer sharp to blunt dissection, believing it causes less tissue trauma.

PRINCIPLES OF HAEMOSTASIS

Bleeding is an inevitable part of surgery. Blood loss should be minimised because the loss has to be made up later, and because bleeding obscures the operative field and hampers operative technique. Excessive bleeding can be averted by judicious dissection, controlling bleeding as the operation proceeds, and by minimising the area of raw tissue exposed at the operation site by accurately siting the incision and by avoiding opening unnecessary tissue planes.

Clipping and ligation

Ligation is obligatory when large vessels are divided and desirable for vessels larger than about 1 mm calibre (see Figure 3.5). If the end of a bleeding vessel cannot be grasped by the haemostat forceps, a suture can be used to encircle the vessel and its surrounding tissues, a technique often described as 'under-running'. It is particularly useful for a bleeding vessel in the base of a peptic ulcer.

Fig. 3.5 Techniques of haemostasis

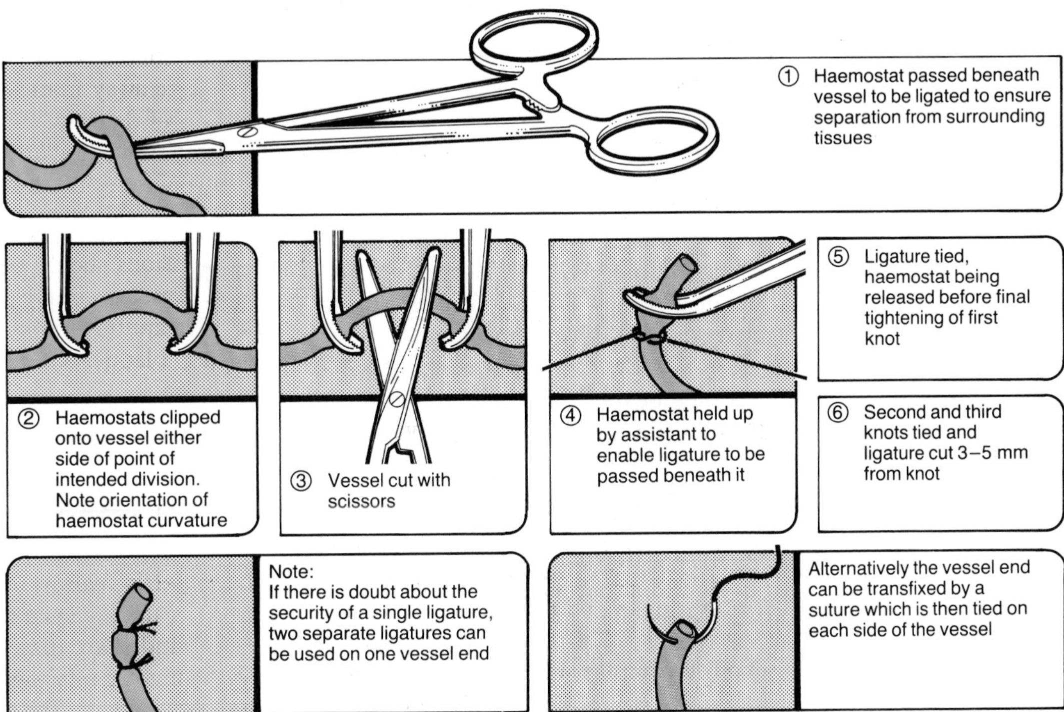

Diathermy

Diathermy achieves haemostasis by local intravascular coagulation using a particular electrical waveform. However, enough heat is also produced to burn the tissues, which may be needlessly damaged by careless use, particularly near the skin. Diathermy is ineffective for large vessels which should be ligated. There are three main variants of diathermy, illustrated in Figure 3.6.

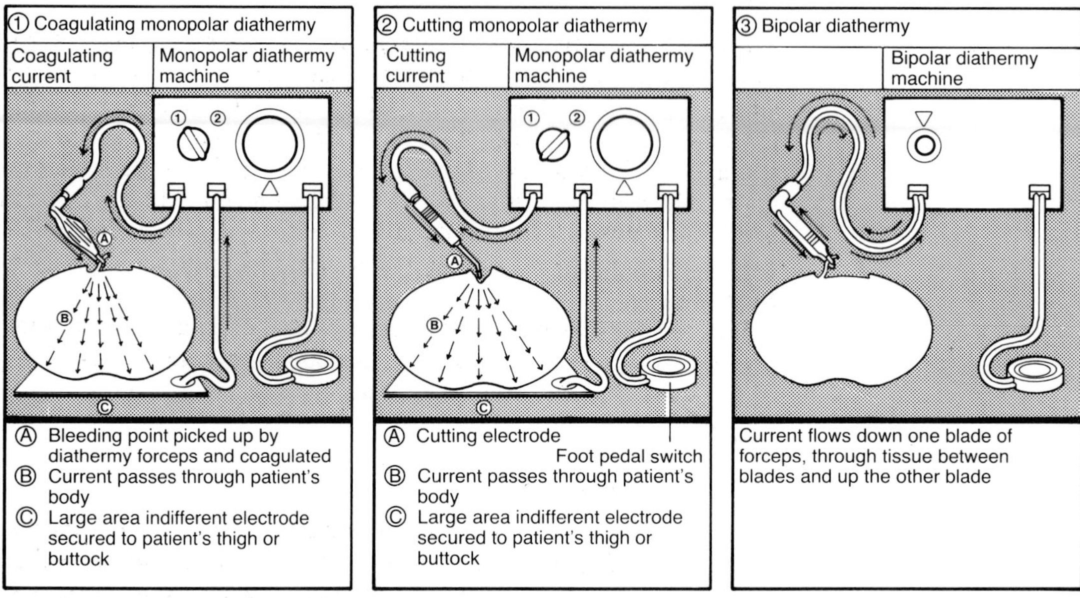

Fig. 3.6 Three modes of diathermy

Monopolar diathermy is the most widely used for routine haemostasis but there is wide dispersion of the coagulating and heating effects, making it unsuitable for use near nerves and other delicate structures. Since the current passes through the patient's body, there is a risk of coagulating vessels en passant (e.g. diathermy used in circumcision may cause penile thrombosis), as well as provoking arrhythmias in patients with cardiac pacemakers. Monopolar diathermy may also result in skin burns at the indifferent electrode plate if it becomes wet during operation.

Bipolar diathermy is mainly used for fine surgery and requires accurate grasping of the bleeding vessel. Its main advantages are minimal tissue damage at the point of coagulation, and its safety in relation to nearby nerves, vascular structures and cardiac pacemakers.

Cutting diathermy is mainly used for dividing large masses of muscle (e.g. during thoracotomy or access to the hip joint), and cutting vascular tissues (e.g. breast). The intention is to coagulate the numerous small blood vessels as the tissue is cut; unfortunately this is not always effective.

Tourniquet and exsanguination

This technique is used in surgery of the limbs and digits where a bloodless field is particularly desirable. For the whole limb, a pneumatic tourniquet is placed proximally around the limb. The limb is exsanguinated by elevation and spiral application of a rubber bandage (Esmark) from the periphery; the tourniquet is then inflated. Upper limb tourniquets must not be left inflated for more than 30 minutes and lower limb tourniquets for more than one hour to avoid the risk of necrosis.

Pressure

Pressure is a useful means of controlling bleeding until platelet aggregation, reactive vasoconstriction and blood coagulation take over. It can be used for emergency control of severe arterial or venous bleeding but is equally useful for controlling diffuse small-vessel bleeding from a large raw area, e.g. liver bed after cholecystectomy. Pressure is usually applied with gauze swabs which must be kept in position for at least 10 minutes. For intractible bleeding which is not amenable to ligature, diathermy or suture, various resorbable packing materials can be left in position to encourage haemostasis, allowing the wound to be closed.

When a raw cavity has been created beneath the skin, external pressure dressings are a useful method of controlling postoperative oozing and minimising haematoma formation, e.g. after breast lump excision.

Hypotensive anaesthesia

This method of anaesthesia is sometimes employed when marked diffuse bleeding is anticipated, e.g. prostatectomy, or where a bloodless field is desirable for fine dissection but where a tourniquet is impossible, e.g. parotid surgery. The anaesthetist achieves controlled hypotension by the judicious infusion of drugs such as nitroprusside.

SUTURING, SURGICAL REPAIR AND IMPLANTS

Types of suture material

Numerous types of suture are available (see Figure 3.7), the most important distinction being between *absorbable* and *non-absorbable* materials. This clear-

Fig. 3.7 Suture materials and their characteristics (typical brand names in brackets)

Absorbable:

Plain catgut — natural monofilament
Chromic catgut — natural monofilament
Polyglycolic acid — synthetic braided (Dexon)
Polyglactin — synthetic braided (Vicryl)
Polydioxanone — synthetic monofilament (PDS)

Non-absorbable:

Silk — natural braided
Linen — natural braided
Stainless steel wire — monofilament or braided
Nylon — synthetic, usually monofilament (Ethilon)
Polyester — synthetic braided (Ticron, and others)
Polypropylene — synthetic monofilament (Prolene)
Polytetrafluoroethylene (PTFE) — synthetic 'expanded/teased' monofilament (Goretex)

cut difference has been blurred by the advent of slowly absorbed sutures, e.g. polydioxanone (PDS). The groups can be subdivided into *natural* and *synthetic* materials and further subdivided into *monofilament* and *polyfilament* (braided) materials. The choice of suture material depends upon the task at hand, the handling qualities and personal preference.

a. Absorbable versus non-absorbable materials

The strength of absorbable sutures declines at a predictable rate for each type of material, although the suture material remains in the wound for a much longer period.

In increasing duration of useful strength, the main absorbable materials are:

- Plain catgut and chromic catgut — last three and five days respectively
- Polyglycolic acid (Dexon) and polyglactin (Vicryl) — both lasting about 10 days
- Polydioxanone (PDS) — retains its strength for at least 14 days

The strength of catgut declines even more quickly in the presence of infection but this is not true of the synthetic absorbable sutures.

The eventual elimination of such materials from the body overcomes the problem of a permanent foreign body which can harbour infection. Absorbable sutures are often used in the skin to avoid the need for removal; typical applications are minor skin operations, surgery in children, circumcisions and vasectomies. Absorbable skin sutures generally give a poorer cosmetic result because of the inflammatory response they provoke.

Non-absorbable sutures retain their strength indefinitely. They are used where the repair will take a long time to reach full strength (e.g. abdominal wall closure) or will be inherently weak (e.g. incisional and inguinal hernia repairs). Non-absorbable sutures are also widely used for skin closure; synthetic monofilament sutures give the best cosmetic results and are most easily and painlessly removed.

b. Natural versus synthetic materials

Catgut has been used as a suture and ligature material since before Roman times, being originally derived from musical instrument strings. It consists of collagen and is actually made from the dried small bowel submucosa of sheep. Catgut is still the most widely used material, and modern manufacturing techniques have ensured a high and consistent quality. Silk and linen also have a long and distinguished history but their use is declining. Many surgeons believe that silk has the best handling and knotting properties of any material, but it provokes a strong inflammatory response exceeded only by linen. Silk is mainly used for skin sutures, where its softness means there are no sharp ends to prick the nearby skin. This is particularly important for operations involving the mouth and the perineum. Linen thread is now relatively unpopular, being used mainly for ligation of blood vessels. In general, natural materials are about half the price of the synthetics, a factor of importance in underdeveloped countries.

The main advantages of synthetic suture materials are that they provoke little or no inflammatory reaction and that they can be designed to meet specific requirements of absorbability, duration of strength and handling.

c. *Monofilament versus polyfilament sutures*

Monofilament materials have an extremely smooth surface and can be pulled through the tissues with minimal friction; this makes them easier to insert and remove than polyfilament braided materials. On the other hand, monofilament materials are stiff, springy and more difficult to knot. Braided materials have the best handling qualities, but their interstices provide a haven for bacteria. When used at a surface (e.g. skin or bowel wall) they tend to act as a 'wick', drawing infected material in. This problem is partly overcome by the application of surface coatings.

d. *Wire sutures*

Metal wire sutures have now been displaced by the non-absorbable synthetics. Stainless steel wire is, however, extensively used in orthopaedic surgery for bone fixation. It is virtually inert, its main disadvantage being breakage due to metal fatigue.

Gauge of suture material

The gauge of suture chosen for a particular task depends largely on practical experience. This takes into account the following factors:

- Strength of repair required
- Number of sutures to be placed — the greater the number, the finer can be the gauge
- Type of suture material being used — for a given gauge, the various materials have different strengths; catgut is the weakest
- Cosmetic requirements — multiple fine sutures give a better result than fewer heavier sutures

The traditional method of describing suture gauge is confusing for the newcomer and derives from the time when sutures were much thicker than those used today. The finest suture then was designated gauge 1, with gauge 2 and upwards applying to heavier sutures. As finer and finer sutures came into use, the scale had to be taken progressively backwards from 1, i.e. gauges 0, 00 (i.e. 2/0), 000 (3/0) and so on. Nowadays, the finest suture is 10/0 which is used for extremely delicate surgery such as in the eye. A more rational metric gauge, based on suture diameter, is in use but the traditional gauge is still more widely used. A simple guide to the use of different gauges is outlined in Figure 3.8.

Fig. 3.8 Guide to suture gauges for common procedures

skin
face 5/0 or 6/0
hands and limbs 3/0 or 4/0
elsewhere 2/0 or 3/0

abdominal wall
two strands of gauge 0 ('loop nylon'), gauge 1 or gauge 2

gut anastomoses
2/0 or 3/0

arterial anastomoses
2/0 down to 7/0 according to size of vessel

microsurgery (e.g. eyes, microvascular, nerve repair)
7/0 down to as fine as 10/0

Types of suture needle

A vast range of needles have been designed to accomodate both the stringent requirements of microsurgery and the various different demands of general and specialist surgery. Characteristics of needles and the broad indications for their use are summarised in Figure 3.9 and illustrated in Figure 3.10.

Fig. 3.9 Types of suture needle

1. Method of use

Hand-held needles — routine use for skin suturing; sometimes used for abdominal wall closure

Instrument-held needles — necessary for deeper access and fine control

2. Shape of needle

Straight — skin suturing

Curved — half-circle used for most purposes, quarter-circle for microvascular anastomoses, three-quarter circle for hand closure of abdominal wall

3. Length of needle

Range from 2–60 mm — according to depth of penetration and delicacy of surgery

4. Tissue penetration characteristics

Round bodied with smooth pointed tip — most soft tissues, e.g. gut, fat, muscle

Trocar point (semi-cutting) — moderately tough tissues, e.g. atherosclerotic arteries, fascia

Cutting needles — tough tissues, e.g. skin, breast tissue

5. Means of attachment of suture to needle

Needles with an eye requiring suture material to be threaded by hand — mainly used in the Third World so that needles can be re-used

'Atraumatic' needles with suture material already attached (swaged into the end) — there is no double thickness of suture material to cause extra drag and trauma as it is pulled through the tissues, and the suture material does not detach from the needle during use

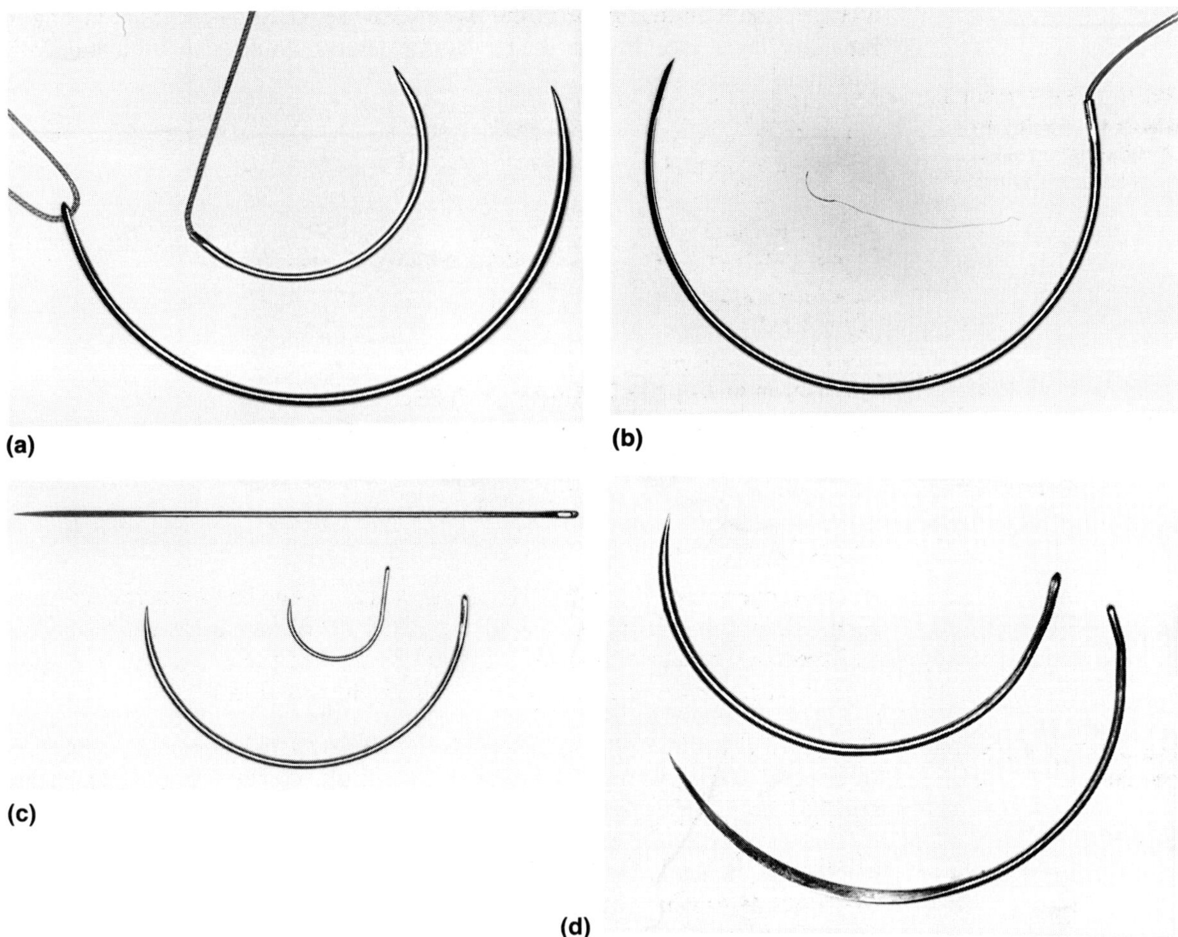

Fig. 3.10 Various types of surgical needle

(a) Two half-circle round-bodied needles, the larger with a threaded 'eye', and the smaller with the suture material swaged into it ('atraumatic' needle). Note the braided nature of the suture material. **(b)** The largest and smallest needles in common use. The larger needle is a $\frac{5}{8}$ circle needle with a semi-cutting point, used in the hand for abdominal wall closure. Note the two strands of nylon swaged into the end. The smaller needle is used in ophthalmic surgery and has 10/0 suture material. **(c)** Three shapes of needle. The straight needle has a cutting point and is used for skin suturing. The J-shaped needle is used mainly for femoral hernia repairs, and the large half-circle needle is for abdominal wall closure. **(d)** Two large needles showing the difference between round-bodied and cutting ends

Methods of skin suturing

The objective of skin suturing is to approximate the cut edges so they will heal rapidly, leaving a minimal scar. Edges to be apposed should have been cut in a clean line and at right angles to the skin surface; ragged or angled edges should be trimmed. The cut edges should be able to be brought neatly together and without tension, otherwise the wound may break down or the scar slowly stretch, giving an ugly result. To achieve this, it may be necessary to insert a layer of subcutaneous sutures or even mobilise the skin by undercutting in the fatty layer (see Figure 3.11). Undue laxity should also be avoided by trimming excess skin.

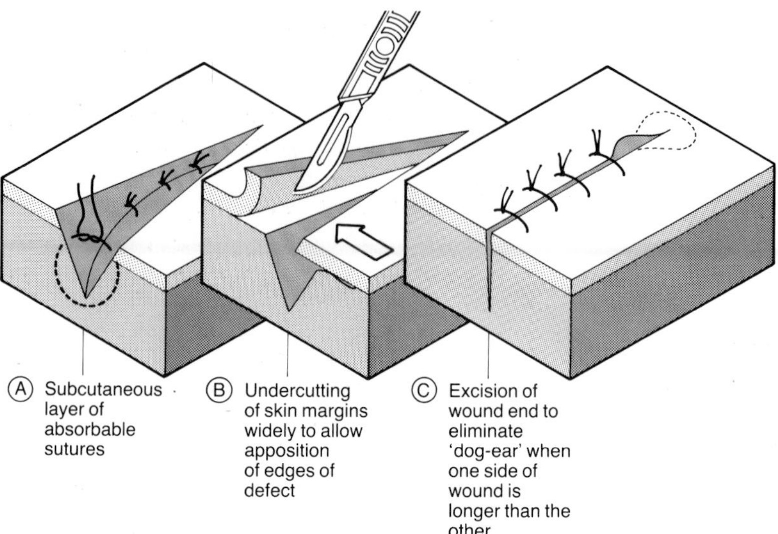

Fig. 3.11 Methods of approximating skin edges before suturing

There are many techniques of skin closure, the choice being governed by the nature and site of the operation and by the surgeon's personal preference. In general, facial wounds are closed with multiple fine sutures which are removed after four or five days. Subcuticular sutures are used for longer wounds in cosmetically sensitive areas, provided the risk of infection is low. Elsewhere, the choice is between interrupted and continuous suture techniques. Interrupted sutures are indicated if there is a particular risk of infection, in which case some of the sutures can be removed early to facilitate drainage. The commonly used methods of skin suturing are illustrated in Figure 3.12.

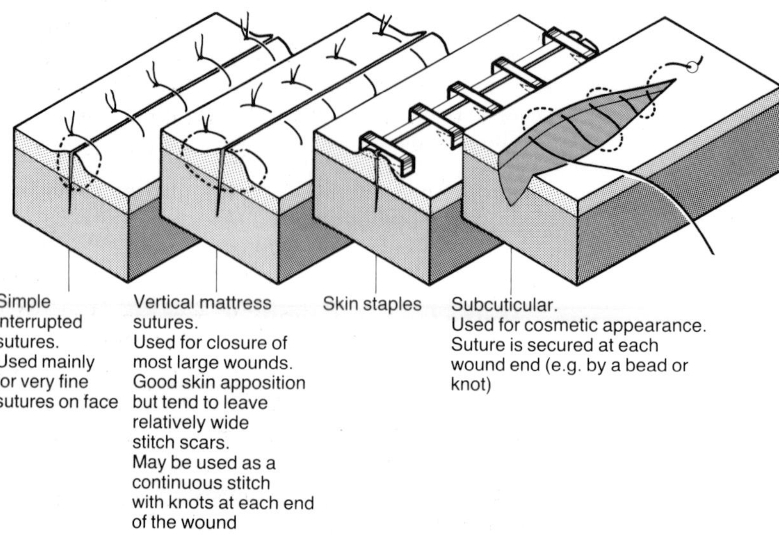

Fig. 3.12 Commonly used skin closure techniques

Clips and staples

Stainless steel clips (e.g. Michel clips) have been used for several decades for closing skin wounds and are popular for neck incisions after thyroidectomy. As the clips do not penetrate skin yet give good edge apposition, the cosmetic result is excellent. Staples are a recent development in surgery and various instruments are used for skin closure and bowel surgery. The skin closure devices are similar in concept to ordinary paper staplers, the staples being held in a magazine and applied singly instead of sutures. More complex devices, which apply multiple staples simultaneously, are available for bowel anastomoses and closure of tubular viscera. Some of these devices have revolutionised surgical practice, e.g. resection of low rectal carcinomas. When used in the internal viscera, the staples remain in place indefinitely.

POSTOPERATIVE WOUND MANAGEMENT

Once a wound has been closed, the doctor has three main responsibilities: choosing the dressing, monitoring the progress of healing and deciding when to remove the sutures.

The purposes of dressings are as follows:

- To protect the wound from bacterial contamination and interference
- To absorb or contain any superficial bleeding or inflammatory exudate
- To prevent the wound from drying out
- To prevent sutures catching on clothing or other objects
- To conceal the wound from the patient
- To apply pressure to the wound if haematoma formation is likely

Types of wound dressing

For small surgical wounds, a dressing is often unnecessary, the linear crust of inflammatory exudate performing this task admirably. In most other cases, pre-packed adhesive dressings are used, incorporating an absorbent pad with non-stick film in contact with the wound surface. While convenient, these dressings tend to conceal accumulations of blood, inflammatory exudate or infected discharge. Wound inspection requires painful removal of the dressing which can be an opportunity for infection to enter. The recently developed transparent plastic film type of dressing neatly overcomes this problem.

Paraffin gauze (tulle gras) is used mainly for covering raw areas (e.g. skin-graft donor sites) as it tends not to stick to the underlying surface and damage the delicate new epithelium when it is removed. *Gamgee* describes thick cotton-wool dressings enveloped by a thin layer of gauze; these are variously used for padding sites vulnerable to trauma (e.g. amputation stumps), as pads beneath pressure bandages or as absorbent dressings for leaking wounds. *Dry dressings* are wads of dressing material (e.g. gauze), usually taped or bandaged in place; such dressings need regular replacement and may be prevented from sticking by first placing a piece of non-adherent dressing material (e.g. Melolin) against the wound.

Removal of dressings and sutures

Provided the dressing remains clean and dry and the patient afebrile and generally well, there is no need to inspect the wound until the time of suture removal. If wound complications are suspected, the dressing should be removed and the wound checked and redressed as appropriate. If infection is apparent, a wound swab should be taken for culture and sensitivity; spreading cellulitis requires antibiotic therapy, whilst localised abscess formation requires suture removal and probing to effect drainage.

Skin sutures should be removed as soon as the wound is strong enough to remain intact without support. In the abdomen, this takes about seven days (longer in the case of steroid therapy or infection) but in the face and neck healing is more rapid and is less influenced by functional stresses. Here, sutures can be safely removed after 4–5 days, giving a better cosmetic result.

SURGERY INVOLVING INFECTED TISSUES

Management of abscesses

The first pinciple of management of an abscess is to *establish drainage* of the pus. When an abscess is 'pointing' to the surface, this involves a skin incision at the site of maximum fluctuance, followed by blunt probing with sinus forceps or a finger to ensure that all loculi are drained; necrotic material is removed at the same time.

Small abscesses only need a dry dressing, the cavity filling in rapidly from beneath. Larger and deeper abscesses need a method of keeping the skin opening patent until the cavity has filled with granulation tissue. A corrugated drain, which is gradually withdrawn ('shortened') over a few days, will achieve this or else the cavity may be packed with ribbon gauze soaked in antiseptic solution, e.g EUSOL (Edinburgh University Solution Of Lime) or povidone-iodine; these packs are usually changed daily or every other day.

Management of infected surgical wounds

Grossly infected surgical wounds must be opened up, to ensure free drainage, and cleaned. Any necrotic tissue is excised leaving only healthy tissue, and the wound packed daily thereafter with antiseptic-soaked gauze. The wound is usually allowed to heal by secondary intention (see Chapter 1), although a large wound can be sutured later when infection is no longer a problem. In the case of deep, slowly healing wounds, a *silicone foam dressing* can be poured into the wound where it sets to form a sponge. This can be removed, washed and replaced as required and can largely be managed by the patient alone until a new, smaller foam dressing is needed.

Management of dirty or contaminated wounds

Major soft tissue injury results in crushing and tearing of tissues, leaving devascularised areas and deep impregnation with soil, road grit or fragments of clothing. If such a wound is merely sutured, pyogenic infection is certain, and there is a serious risk of gas gangrene.

The principles of managing these wounds were first established during the First World War, as follows:

- Thorough cleansing of the wound of all foreign material (debridement)
- Excision of all non-viable tissue
- Loose open packing of the wound with cotton gauze without suturing
- Inspection of the wound under anaesthesia two to three days later, drainage of any new abscesses and removal of any residual non-viable tissue
- Suturing of the wound when it looks clean, but avoiding tension; this is known as *delayed primary closure*

MINOR OPERATIVE PROCEDURES

Many skin lesions are amenable to simple excision or biopsy, often under local anaesthesia. These may be performed in general practice or in dermatological or surgical outpatient departments. A strict aseptic technique must be employed.

LOCAL ANAESTHESIA

The usual method is by infiltration of local anaesthetic (e.g. lignocaine 1% or 2%) into the skin surrounding the lesion. Between 1 and 10 ml of solution is usually required. A vasoconstrictor (e.g. adrenaline 1 in 200 000) may be incorporated to reduce vascularity in the operative field, but this must never

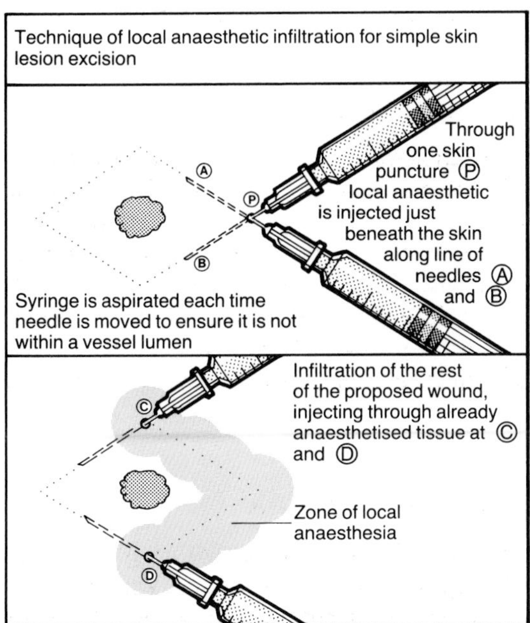

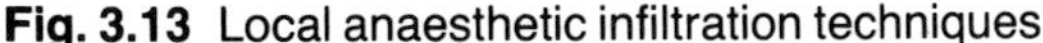

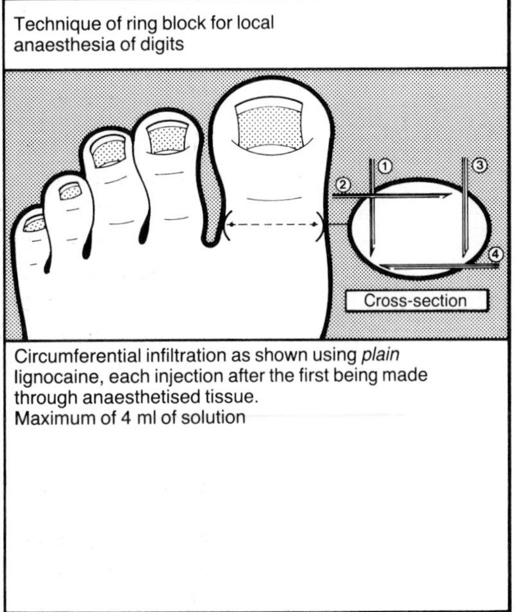

Fig. 3.13 Local anaesthetic infiltration techniques

be used on the extreme peripheries, e.g. fingers, toes, penis or nose, because of the high risk of ischaemic necrosis. The injecting needle should be as fine as possible and inserted into the skin as few times as possible to avoid causing unnecessary pain. Before each injection, aspiration should be attempted to ensure that the solution is not injected into a blood vessel. Intravascular injection of local anaesthetic may cause systemic toxicity. The method of local anaesthetic infiltration is illustrated in Figure 3.13.

BIOPSY TECHNIQUES

Excision biopsy

The technique of excision biopsy illustrated in Figure 3.14 is appropriate for most small lesions not considered to be malignant. The lesion is removed in a fusiform piece of normal skin, the long axis being orientated along skin creases and tension lines. The specimen should include a millimetre or two of normal skin on either side of the lesion and should include the full depth of the skin down to the subcutaneous fat.

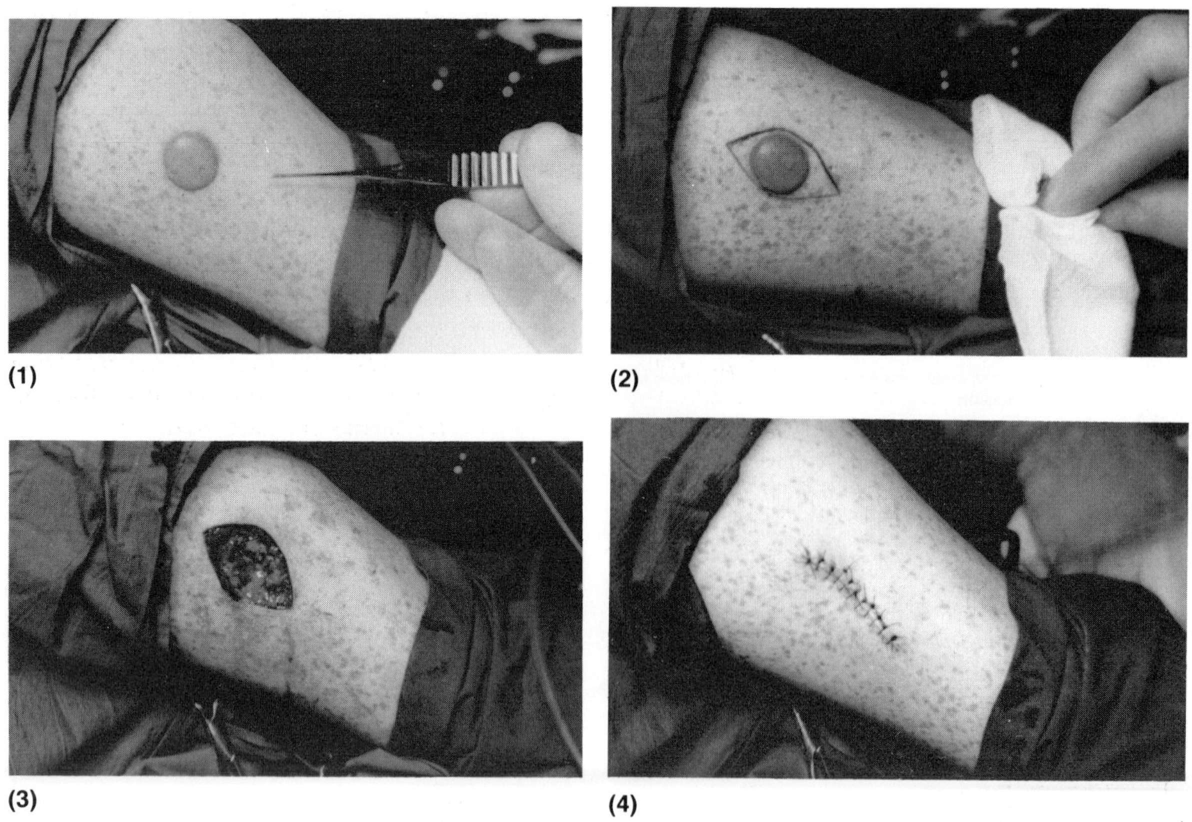

Fig. 3.14 Excision biopsy technique

(1) (2) (3) (4)

Incision biopsy

Incision biopsy is a technique of obtaining a tissue sample from a lesion too large or anatomically unsuitable for excision biopsy, e.g. a skin rash or a suspected malignant tumour. Major surgical procedures or radiotherapy should

Fig. 3.15

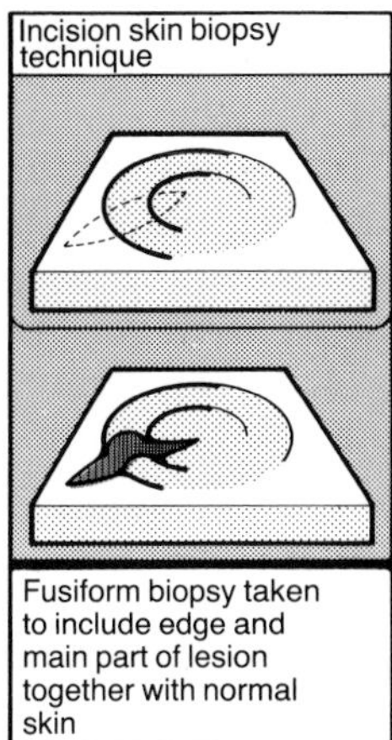

Fig. 3.16

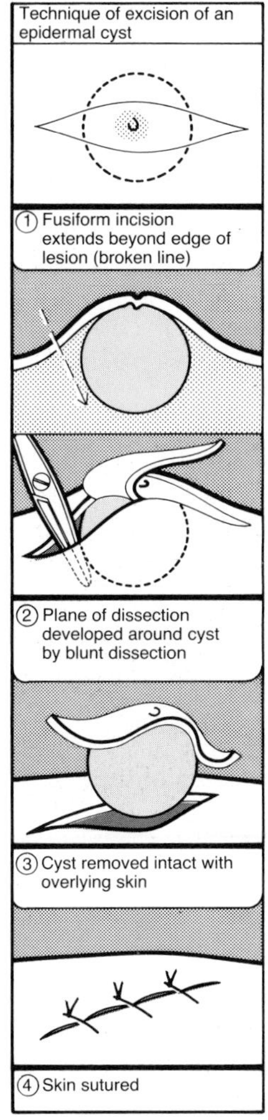

not be performed without histological confirmation of the diagnosis. The objective is to obtain a representative sample of the full depth of the lesion, including an area of the margin and adjoining normal tissue (see Figure 3.15).

Destruction of lesions by diathermy, electrocautery, or cryocautery and curettage

These techniques are used for small lesions where there is no clinical suspicion of malignancy and a histological diagnosis is not required, the lesion being destroyed in the process of removal. Local infiltration of anaesthetic is usually necessary.

Removal of cysts

A cyst is a fluid-filled lesion, lined by epithelium and usually encapsulated by a condensation of surrounding fibrous connective tissue. The aim of treatment is to remove the whole epithelial lining because any remnant will lead to recurrence. The technique of removal is outlined in Figure 3.16. Ideally, the cyst is dissected out intact without puncturing the cavity. If this occurs, the cyst collapses, making it difficult to identify and remove the epithelial lining.

Marsupialisation

This technique is usually employed in the treatment of cysts or other fluid-filled lesions which are too large, inaccessible or technically impossible to remove. It is rarely appropriate for skin lesions but is often used for large salivary retention cysts in the floor of the mouth, cysts in the jaw and pancreatic pseudocysts. The technique is illustrated in Figure 3.17. The surgeon removes a disc from the wall of the cavity and sutures the lining to the overlying epithelium around the cut edge. This leaves a pouch, which slowly fills from below once the pressure of the cyst contents has been removed.

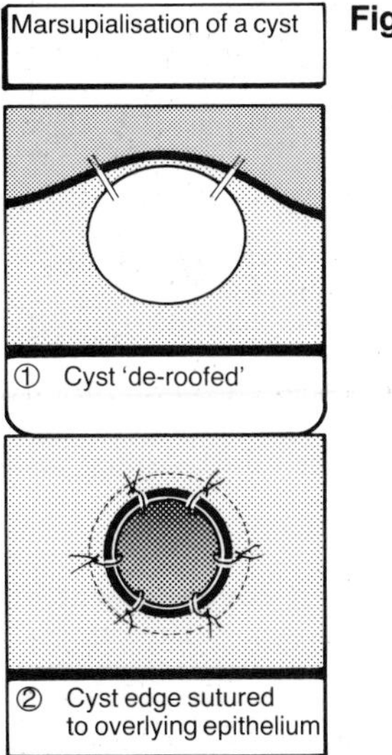

Fig. 3.17

PRINCIPLES OF PLASTIC SURGERY

The discipline of plastic surgery was born during the First World War in response to the appalling disfigurement caused by blast injuries and burns. Since then, specialised techniques of skin reconstruction have progressed further, especially in the field of microvascular reconstructive surgery. The scope of modern plastic surgery is outlined in Figure 3.18. There is a considerable degree of overlap and collaboration between the field of plastic surgery and other surgical specialties, especially ear nose and throat, maxillofacial and orthopaedic surgery.

Fig. 3.18 The scope of plastic surgery

Reconstruction after mutilating surgery or trauma
Correction of congenital defects, e.g. cleft palate
Management of facial soft tissue trauma
Management of burns
Replantation surgery, e.g. digits and limbs, nerve and tendon repairs
Cosmetic surgery, e.g. scar removal, breast remodelling, 'face-lifts', eyelid surgery, nasal reshaping
Surgery for obesity, e.g.liposuction, apronectomy (for pendulous abdomen)

TISSUE TRANSFER TECHNIQUES

Obtaining satisfactory skin cover is one of the major problems in plastic surgery and, until recently, other tissues such as fat and muscle could not be satisfactorily transferred. Free transplantation of full thickness skin or any other tissue without revascularisation is usually unsuccessful.

Tissue transfer can be achieved in four main ways:

- Split skin (Thiersch) grafting
- Skin advancement or flap transposition
- Pedicle grafting
- One stage free tissue transfer

Split skin (Thiersch) grafting

This involves transplantation of a very thin layer of skin consisting of little more than epidermis. It is commonly employed in burns and after wide excision of skin lesions, provided there is a base of healthy tissue. The donor site heals very rapidly since small islands of epithelium are left behind (see Figure 3.19).

Skin advancement or flap transposition

This involves wide undercutting of nearby skin and, if necessary, raising strategically placed skin flaps; this may provide sufficient mobility to close a moderate sized defect.

Pedicle grafting

In pedicle grafting, a flap of skin is raised and formed into a tube while remaining attached at both ends to its site of origin. After about three weeks, one end of the tube is divided (the 'donor end') and transposed to the recipient site. After another three weeks, when a new blood supply from the recipient site will have become established, the other end of the tube is divided and the flap opened out, shaped and sutured at the recipient site, to restore the defect.

The early *random flaps*, devised by Gillies, were limited in scope because the blood supply prevented construction of a flap which was longer than its width. Their principal use was in the head and neck but they have been largely superceded by 'free tissue transfer'. *Axial flaps* were devised in the 1960s; with this technique, which is suitable for sites such as the forehead and groin, a long flap can be raised with its blood supply and transposed to provide full thickness cover in the vicinity. In the 1970s, *musculocutaneous flaps* were devised, enabling transfer of a long flap of muscle and overlying skin to make good a substantial tissue loss, e.g latissimus dorsi flap after mastectomy.

One stage, free tissue transfer

In free tissue transfer, an appropriate piece of tissue is first dissected out, complete with at least one main artery and vein. The whole graft is then relocated to the recipient site where the vessels are connected to a suitable local

Fig. 3.19 Methods of skin grafting

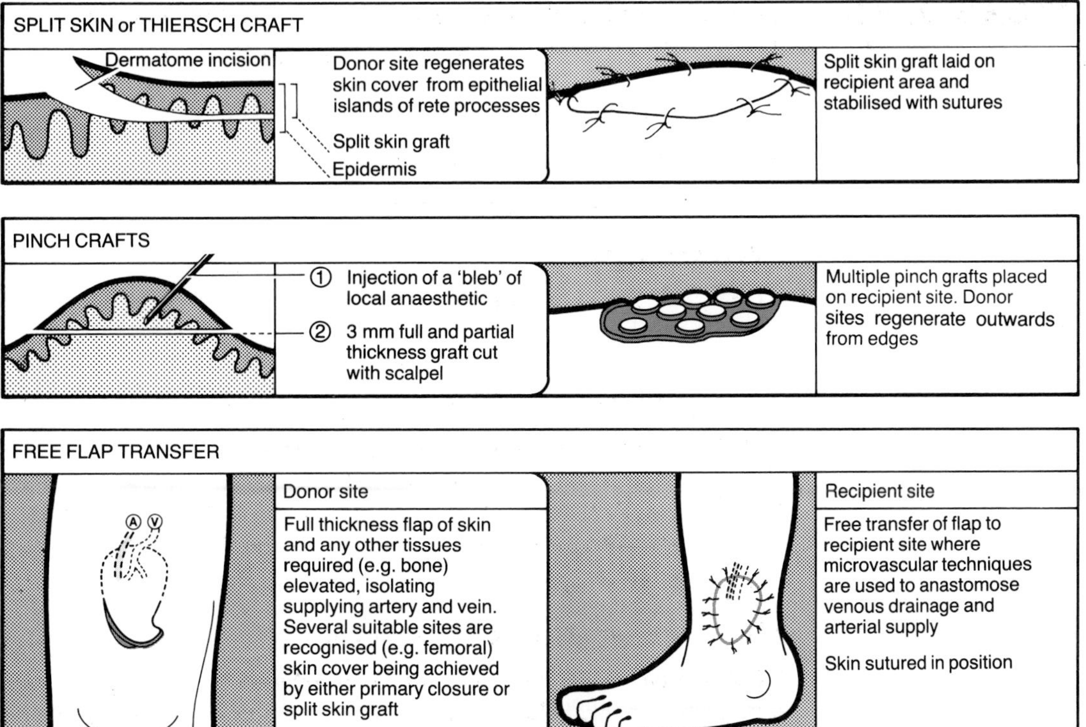

artery and vein by microvascular surgery. The donor site can often be primarily closed or else is covered with a split skin graft. The needs of this technique have led to new investigations into surgical anatomy aimed at discovering areas of the body which can be removed and transplanted. Examples are the *radial forearm flap* which supplies bone, muscle and skin, and the big toe which has been used to replace a lost thumb.

PRINCIPLES OF TRANSPLANTATION SURGERY

Introduction

Transplantation of tissue from one individual to another has always offered the tantalising prospect of recovery of function; indeed John Hunter transplanted teeth from one individual to another as long ago as the 18th century.

In order to transplant organs, special surgical techniques have to be developed but the major obstacle in most cases remains the problem of *graft rejection*. Pig heart valves can be treated to prevent rejection, and have been successfully transplanted to humans for over 20 years. Transplantation of the human cornea, kidney and bone marrow are now accepted as routine, although by no means free of rejection and other complications. Promising results are also being obtained with heart, combined heart-lung, liver and pancreatic transplants, although these are still to some extent experimental.

Grafts between members of the same species are known as *homografts* but since individuals are genetically different (except for identical twins), the term *allograft* is used to describe human transplants. Grafts from another species (e.g. pig heart valves) are known as *heterografts*.

TRANSPLANT IMMUNOLOGY

Major histocompatibility complex

Most tissue cells have at their surface a number of different glycoproteins which, if transplanted from one individual to another, excite a rejection response by the recipient's immune system. These *histocompatibility antigens* are recognised by the recipient's lymphocytes as they circulate through the graft; the response includes both cell-mediated and humoral mechanisms. The end result is destruction of the transplanted cells.

Each individual has a large number of histocompatibility antigens but only one group is responsible for major graft rejection problems. These *major histocompatibility antigens* are coded for by a set of genes known as the *major histocompatibility complex (MHC)*. In humans, the MHC is located on a segment of the short arm of chromosome number 6. Because it was first discovered in leucocytes, it is also rather confusingly known as the *HLA complex* (Human Lymphocyte Antigen system A). Within the human major histocompatibility complex, four *loci* have been identified as responsible for the important transplant antigens. These *loci* are known as A, B, C and D. Since chromosomes function in pairs, any two individuals may thus differ in respect of eight HLA antigen systems.

The normal biological function of the HLA system is recognition and destruction of cells which become altered by viral incorporation or neoplasia.

Certain HLA types are associated with particular autoimmune disorders, most notably ankylosing spondylitis and coeliac disease, although their aetiology is unknown.

Tissue typing

The greater the mismatch in HLA antigens between donor and recipient, the greater is the likely rejection response. HLA typing of individuals is used to match the donor and recipient as closely as possible. It is performed serologically, using specific antisera or, more recently, using *monoclonal antibodies*. HLA matched siblings have the best chance of graft survival, but there is still some rejection due to minor histocompatibility antigens. Results are less good for grafts from HLA matched individuals who are not related because they possess different alleles at each HLA locus. ABO blood group compatibility is an obvious prerequisite for organ transplantation.

Immunosuppression

With all major organ transplants, the recipient's immune response must be suppressed even if there is full HLA compatibility, otherwise the graft will not survive. Therapy must be continued indefinitely, although after the first year doses may be reduced because rejection is often less aggressive. Drugs are employed in various combinations, the most common agents being *prednisolone, azathioprine, cyclophosphamide* and *actinomycin D*. Lymphocyte proliferation, antibody production and inflammation are all suppressed by therapy and complications include poor healing, peptic ulceration, vulnerability to infection, bone marrow suppression and development of malignancy (especially lymphomas).

A new drug, *cyclosporine A*, is showing great promise. It suppresses only the cell-mediated response, thus preserving humoral antibacterial protection. This drug also appears to confer some immunological tolerance to the graft, allowing gradual withdrawal of immune suppression after about 12 months. The main disadvantage of the drug is its toxic effect upon the renal tubules.

Graft rejection

Serious graft rejection may occur at any time after transplantation. The main clinical problems are:

a. Hyperacute rejection

This occurs within minutes or hours of transplantation and results from the actions of preformed antibodies, either due to previous transplantation, blood transfusions or ABO incompatibility.

b. Acute rejection

This cell-mediated response usually occurs after about two weeks in unsuppressed, first-time grafts; *accelerated rejection* is a similar but earlier phenomenon occurring in patients already sensitised by previous graft attempts.

c. Chronic rejection

This may occur months to years after transplantation and is mediated by humoral responses which become resistant to long-term immunosuppression.

PRACTICAL PROBLEMS OF TRANSPLANTATION

Source of organs for transplantation

Most tissues for transplantation are derived from cadavers, the organ being removed from the body as soon as possible after death has been diagnosed. Young, previously well subjects dying unexpectedly from head injuries or intracranial vascular catastrophes are the main source of major organs. Most victims have been resuscitated from the outset, circulation and respiration being maintained by artificial means.

In the case of renal transplants, relatives may volunteer one of their own kidneys. Results from first degree relatives are better than those obtained from unrelated donors. The risk to the donor is the small possibility of losing the remaining kidney, apart from the minimal risk of operative and anaesthetic complications. The donor's remaining kidney hypertrophies over succeeding months, restoring renal reserve to near normal.

'Brain death'

A set of criteria has evolved to form the legal definition of death for transplantation donors. The criteria allow withdrawal of life support measures at an appropriate time, usually after discussion with relatives. Once these criteria have been satisfied, the subject becomes eligible for organ donation. The legal criteria for brain death in the UK are summarised in Figure 3.20; similar criteria are used in other countries.

Fig. 3.20 Legal criteria for diagnosis of brain death (UK)

1. There must be a positive diagnosis of severe structural brain damage
2. The condition causing brain damage must be irreversible
3. There must be complete loss of brain stem function — evidenced by fixed pupils, no spontaneous eye movements or response to caloric testing, absent corneal, eyelash and blink reflexes, absent laryngeal and cough reflexes, and no response to deep painful stimuli (note: some tendon reflexes may be retained despite brain death)
4. On removal of ventilatory support, there must be no spontaneous respiratory activity
5. Any possible effects of hypothermia and drugs (e.g. muscle relaxants, respiratory depressants, alcohol) must be excluded

Clinical criteria alone are sufficient to make the diagnosis of brain death in the UK. EEG, cerebral blood flow and other neurophysiological tests are not required. Clinical examination must be performed by two doctors independent of the transplant team and must be repeated on at least two occasions more than 12 hours apart

Consent

Consent to organ donation is the second major ethical dilemma. The doctor is faced with a conflict between duty to his own dying patient and his wider responsibility to potential organ recipients. The law requires that the relatives agree and that there should be no known objection by the potential donor. The matter is simplified if the potential donor carries a donor cord or has left other written instructions, but the bereaved relatives must always be approached. The trauma many doctors face in informing relatives of the death is compounded by having to request organ donation at the same time. This is a limiting factor in the number of organs available for transplantation. With current public awareness and opinion, the bereaved often gain comfort from the knowledge that something has been salvaged from the tragedy. Doctors should be aware that a request for organ donation may be silently appreciated by the donor's relatives.

Organ preservation and transport

Because of geographical and organisational limitations, the organ must usually be removed from the donor some hours before transplantation. The period between organ removal and cooling by fluid perfusion is known as *warm ischaemia* and should be reduced to a minimum. For kidneys, normal function will usually recover if warm ischaemia does not exceed 40 minutes.

Two methods are used for preserving organs between donation and transplantation:

- Hypothermia — the organ is flushed with ice-cold, osmotically inactive solution; it is then kept on ice, allowing satisfactory storage for up to 24 hours
- Continuous pulsatile perfusion with special plasma or albumin solutions — this enables organs to be stored for up to three days; the equipment is portable and can be used during transportation

SPECIFIC ORGAN TRANSPLANTS

Kidneys

Kidney transplantation is the longest established and most successful of major organ transplants. The main indications are end-stage chronic renal failure requiring regular dialysis, and renal disorders such as polycystic kidneys causing intractable hypertension. Donors should be young (under 55) and healthy with no disorder likely to impair renal function.

The kidney is transplanted into an extraperitoneal location in the iliac fossa, the renal vessels being anastomosed to the iliac artery and vein. The ureter is implanted into the bladder through a mural tunnel to prevent reflux. The non-functioning kidneys are usually left in-situ unless infected or causing unmanageable hypertension.

It is now legal to remove organs from 'heart-beating' brain-dead donors. Because of this, results have improved dramatically and the survival rate of transplanted kidneys is as high as 85% at one year. This falls by 5–10% each year thereafter. The quality of life is markedly improved over that of chronic dialysis; in particular the general feeling of malaise and tiredness usually disappears. Signs of rejection are oliguria, proteinuria and pain and tenderness of the transplanted kidney.

Heart and lung transplants

Cardiac transplantation, in certain specialised units, has become almost a standard treatment for patients with terminal cardiomyopathies and young patients with end-stage ischaemic heart disease. A reliable operative technique has now been established involving suturing of the donor ventricles to the recipient's own atria. Rejection is no more likely than with kidney transplantation, but monitoring for early rejection requires regular cardiac catheterisation and endocardial biopsy. These procedures, coupled with the need for immediate re-transplantation in the event of irreversible rejection, demand massive investment in personnel and hospital facilities. The shortage of donors and the costs involved mean that cardiac transplantation therapy will probably never be available to all those that could benefit.

Combined heart and lung transplants have recently been performed for patients with lung damage secondary to major cardiac disease. This procedure is still experimental, but holds promise for the future.

Liver transplants

The indications for liver transplantation are terminal non-malignant parenchymal liver disease in otherwise fit young patients, and young children with congenital biliary atresia. Cholangiocarcinoma, hepatocellular carcinoma and multiple liver secondaries are no longer indications for liver transplantation, as malignancy inevitably recurs. The problems of rejection are less than for kidney transplantation but there are formidable technical problems, which are complicated by the effects of pre-existing liver failure in the recipient. Biliary tract anastomoses are prone to ischaemic breakdown causing catastrophic biliary peritonitis. Blood loss is often in excess of 30 units, due to the multiple and inaccessible vascular anastomoses, the clotting abnormalities secondary to liver failure, and the extreme abdominal vascularity resulting from portal hypertension.

Pancreas transplants

Pancreas transplantation offers a tantalising hope of cure for diabetes but results so far are extremely disappointing. Attempts at transplanting the entire pancreas or the pancreatic tail have been largely unsuccessful. Apart from rejection, there is the problem of disposing of the pancreatic exocrine secretions. Problems of pancreatic rejection in combined pancreas and kidney transplants for diabetic angiopathy seem to be less troublesome because the latter organ somehow 'absorbs' the immune rejection response.

A different approach is the transplantation of pancreatic endocrine islets alone, these being extracted from pancreatic segments after treatment with collagenases. The islets are then injected into the hepatic portal vein. The need for several donor organs to provide for one recipient and the overwhelming immunological response to islet cell transplantation are, at present, insurmountable problems.

PRINCIPLES OF BLOOD TRANSFUSION

Introduction

Transfusion of blood and to a lesser extent blood products has revolutionised the management of major trauma. It has also facilitated extraordinary advances in major surgery which involve heavy blood loss such as arterial reconstruction, open heart surgery and organ transplantation. Nevertheless, blood transfusion is not without risk, for example from transfusion reactions and transmission of infection. The problem of infection has been tragically highlighted by the development of AIDS in haemophiliacs and other patients after unwitting transfusion of infected blood. Thus, the decision to transfuse blood products must be based on clear indications and only after considering alternatives where appropriate, such as gelatin infusion for hypovolaemia or iron therapy for anaemia.

The technique of *auto-transfusion*, by which the patient's own blood is collected and stored before operation, is applicable to elective surgery but is

Fig. 3.21 Types of transfusion and indications for their use

Whole blood — substantial haemorrhage, e.g trauma, major surgery, bleeding peptic ulcer

Packed red cells — for raising haemoglobin where circulating volume is adequate, especially if there is a risk of circulatory overload, e.g chronic anaemia with cardiac failure

Plasma (now called 4.5% human albumin) — replacement of plasma, e.g. burns, crush injuries

Fresh frozen plasma (FFP), separated from fresh blood and then frozen, conserving all clotting properties — used to replace clotting factors exhausted during major haemorrhage (due to a combination of consumption of clotting factors by attempted haemostasis and poor clotting ability of stored blood). Transfusion of FFP should be considered whenever bleeding is continuing and a clotting screen is abnormal. Also used in patients short of clotting factors for other reasons, e.g. liver disease or on anticoagulants. (Note: FFP must be blood group compatible)

Platelet concentrates — for platelet exhaustion during major haemorrhage and in thrombocytopenia

Cryoprecipitate and other specific clotting factor concentrates — for various specific coagulation deficiencies, e.g. haemophilia

Fibrinogen — treatment of disseminated intravascular coagulation

20% human albumin — hypoalbuminaemia, e.g. severe malnutrition, catabolism, liver disease

Plasma substitutes. These are solutions of macromolecules with similar colloid osmotic pressure and viscosity characteristics to plasma, e.g. gelatin solutions ('Haemaccel', 'Gelofusin') which have now largely replaced dextrans ('Dextran-70') — used for initial restoration of circulating volume in haemorrhage or burns while awaiting compatible blood or plasma; also used to maintain volume, blood pressure and renal perfusion intraoperatively where blood transfusion is not indicated.

not yet widely used. In cases of acute massive intra-abdominal blood loss which is uncontaminated by bowel contents, e.g. multiple trauma or liver transplantation, a 'cell saver' can be used. Blood is collected at operation by suction and the cells are washed, resuspended in physiological solution and transfused. By this method, losses of over 100 units have been recycled.

The immediate advantage of transfusing stored blood for replacing blood loss is that it remains within the vascular compartment; nevertheless, the oxygen carrying capacity of this blood is low for the first 24 hours or so as a result of the storage process. Furthermore, white cells and platelets in the transfused blood are virtually inactive and the clotting properties are greatly diminished. The types of transfusion currently available and the general indications for their use are summarised in Figure 3.21.

PRACTICAL ASPECTS OF BLOOD TRANSFUSION

Blood grouping and compatibility testing (cross-matching)

Transfusion of incompatible blood in respect of the major blood group antigens (ABO factor) is potentially fatal. Transfusion practice, developed to minimise this risk, involves two main steps. First, the patient's ABO and Rhesus groups are established and second, each unit of group-compatible donor blood intended for this transfusion is matched directly against the patient's serum to ensure complete compatibility. In the process, minor incompatibility factors may be discovered and require more extensive cross-matching procedures. Fortunately the donor blood is compatible at first attempt at cross-match in about 99% of cases.

In an emergency, group-compatible blood can be given without specific cross-matching. After the transfusion of many units of blood (e.g. massive haemorrhage from liver trauma), the patient's own antibodies are so depleted that further group-compatible blood is usually given without cross-matching. In an emergency (e.g. obstetric haemorrhage at home) where group-compatible blood is not available, then group O, Rh negative blood *(universal donor)* can be given with comparative safety, but there is a long-term risk of antibodies developing, making future cross-matching difficult.

In elective surgery, patients usually fall into one of three categories i.e. *transfusion not anticipated* (e.g. hernia repair), *transfusion possible but unlikely* (e.g. cholecystectomy), and *transfusion probable* (e.g. major arterial reconstruction). For patients in the second category, a blood sample should be sent in advance for ABO and Rhesus grouping, and the serum retained in the laboratory for compatibility testing later if required *('group and save serum')*. For patients in the third category, an appropriate number of units of blood is requested to be available for transfusion at the time of operation. In this case, the blood group is established on receipt of the request and the blood is *cross-matched* a day or so preoperatively. If blood is transfused and a further transfusion is required more than two days later, a new sample of blood is required for cross-matching since antibodies may have developed in the meantime.

To guard against the disaster of the wrong blood being given to the wrong patient, scrupulous attention must be paid to correct and complete labelling of blood samples sent for grouping and cross-matching. Immediately before transfusion, the label of the supplied blood must be checked with the identity and blood group of the patient.

Storage and useful life of blood

Blood and blood products have exacting requirements if their quality is to be preserved. Maintenance of blood quality is essentially the responsibility of the supplying laboratory; the value of blood and blood products is easily diminished if they are handled inappropriately thereafter.

Blood is stored chilled between 2 and 4° C, when it has a shelf-life of about five weeks. With recent developments in preservative solutions (e.g. CPD-A) there is little deterioration of red cell quality during storage but pH changes occur and clotting factors diminish. Blood must not normally be frozen, although expensive techniques for freezing of patients' own blood for later autotransfusion have been developed for patients with rare blood groups or unusual antibodies and, recently, for preventing blood-borne viral infections.

To ensure vitality, blood should not be removed from the laboratory or theatre refrigerator until immediately before use. If blood has been out of the refrigerator for more than 30 minutes and has not been transfused, it should be returned to the laboratory unused. Indeed, all unused blood should be returned to the laboratory as soon as it becomes apparent that it will not be required, as it may still be suitable for another patient. Empty used blood packs are routinely kept on the ward for 24 hours so that they can be returned to the laboratory for further testing in the event of a transfusion reaction.

Volume and rate of transfusion

The volume of blood required and the rate of transfusion depends on the age of the patient, the indications for transfusion and the patient's general and cardiovascular condition.

a. Haemorrhage

Whole blood (or plasma or plasma substitutes if blood is not available) should be transfused as fast as necessary to maintain adequate blood pressure (i.e. systolic above 100 mm Hg), and a positive central venous pressure. If rapid transfusion is required, an inflatable bag surrounding the blood pack is used to increase the pressure. If many units are to be given, or the blood is for neonates or small children, it should be warmed by passing it through a special blood warming device.

b. Anaemia

Surgery should not generally be performed on a patient whose haemoglobin is less than 10 g/dl. Ideally, preoperative transfusion should be given at least two days beforehand. This maximises the effect of the blood and permits stabilisation of fluid balance. One unit of blood (450 ml blood + 63 ml preservative/anticoagulant solution) will raise the haemoglobin concentration by approximately 1 g/dl in an adult. If a large amount of blood is required to treat anaemia, it is preferable to use packed cells and to transfuse in two stages, waiting 48 hours before the second transfusion. If whole blood is given, each unit should be transfused over about four hours and diuretics may be needed after every two units to avoid circulatory overload.

RISKS AND COMPLICATIONS OF BLOOD TRANSFUSION

Febrile reactions

Fever during blood transfusion is common and is usually due to pyrogens in the transfused blood. If the fever is less than 38°C then the transfusion should be allowed to continue. If the fever is higher, or there are systemic symptoms (e.g. chills or rigors), then the transfusion should be stopped immediately and the blood returned to the laboratory for testing.

Haemolytic reactions

Massive haemolysis will occur if there is major ABO incompatibility. A lesser degree of haemolysis is associated with incompatibility in minor determinants. Almost all haemolytic reactions are caused by human error in transfusing incompatible blood. The clinical features of a haemolytic reaction are summarised in Figure 3.22. Diagnosis is confirmed by finding haemoglobinaemia, haemoglobinuria and a positive Coomb's test, and by demonstrating an antibody on repeat crossmatching. The transfusion must be halted immediately and the patient resuscitated. Oliguria is treated by osmotic diuresis (e.g. mannitol), aided by a loop diuretic if appropriate.

Fig. 3.22 Clinical features of a haemolytic transfusion reaction

1. Rapidly developing pyrexia at onset of transfusion
2. Dyspnoea, constrictive feeling in chest, intense headache
3. Severe loin pain
4. Hypotension
5. Acute oliguric renal failure with haemoglobinuria (due to obstruction of tubules with haemoglobin, hypotension causing acute tubular necrosis)
6. Jaundice (developing hours or days later)
7. Disseminated intravascular coagulation with spontaneous bruising and haemorrhage (e.g. cerebral, gastrointestinal)

Allergic reactions

Allergic reactions to transfusion are occasionally seen and manifest as fever, pruritus (itching), skin rashes, wheals or angioneurotic oedema (periorbital, facial and laryngeal swelling). These tend to appear either towards the end of transfusion or else some time later. Transfusions still in progress should be discontinued and symptoms treated with antihistamines.

Infection

Infection may arise from three sources: the donor, the process of blood preparation and storage, and the giving set or cannula site.

Hepatitis (either type B or 'non-A non-B'), cytomegalovirus and syphilis are well recognised complications of blood transfusion, especially in countries where blood donors are paid. It is now standard practice for all blood to be tested for these agents before being accepted by blood banks. Discovery of the AIDS virus (HIV) and its transmission via transfusion of blood products, has led to the adoption of new test methods so that all blood is as far as possible free from known transmissible agents. Factor VIII concentrates for haemophiliacs are now all heat treated before release.

Blood may be contaminated by bacteria during preparation; these may proliferate if storage conditions are inadequate or blood is left unchilled before transfusion. Giving sets may become contaminated unless strict aseptic technique is maintained during the setting-up or changing of any component of transfusion equipment. Finally, peripheral intravenous cannulae or central venous lines may become infected by opportunistic skin commensals (e.g. *Staph. epidermidis*) or contaminating pathogens (e.g. *Staph. aureus*, *E. coli*) causing local infection (see Figure 3.23), bacteraemia or even septicaemia. Cannula sites should be inspected daily and changed every two days.

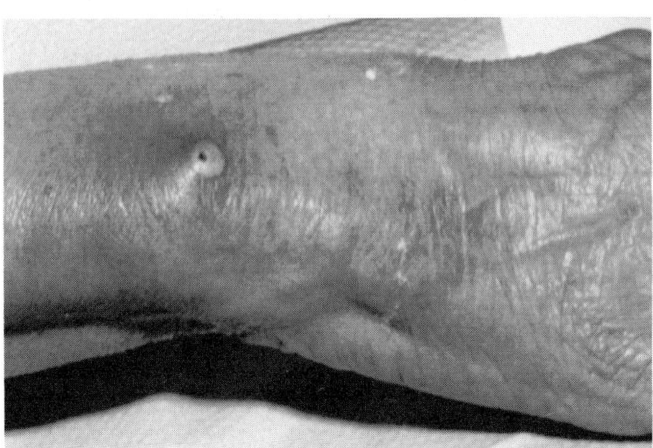

Fig. 3.23 Infected cannula site at the wrist

Fluid overload

Fluid overload is rarely a problem in healthy adults but may easily develop if the cardiovascular system is already compromised, if large volumes are given or when transfusing babies and small children.

Special problems of large transfusions

The problems of large transfusions are summarised in Figure 3.24.

Fig. 3.24 Special problems of large transfusions

1. Hypothermia — avoided by warming the blood during administration.
2. Cardiac arhythmias induced by large quantities of cold blood — risk reduced by warming
3. Adult respiratory distress syndrome (probably due to multiple microemboli by platelet and leucocyte aggregates) — minimised by the use of a blood filter
4. Air embolism (if blood administered from glass bottles which require ventilation, especially if pressure used for rapid transfusions) — avoided by using a closed system and collapsible blood packs; these are now universal in developed countries
5. Hyperkalaemia (potassium leaks out of ageing erythrocytes) — avoided by using blood as fresh as possible
6. Citrate intoxication (citrate is the standard anticoagulant) — prevented by intermittent calcium gluconate infusion during large transfusions
7. Haemorrhage (caused by loss and consumption of clotting factors during haemorrhage which are not replaced by transfused blood) — treated with fresh frozen plasma and platelet concentrates (ideally overcome by use of fresh blood just donated)

4 PRINCIPLES OF CANCER MANAGEMENT

Introduction

Patients with malignant disease form a major part of the surgical workload, and are responsible for as much as 40% of general surgical bed usage. Cancer patients impose disproportionate demands on services, since operations are more extensive and the patients are generally older, slower to recover and more prone to complications. At the same time, the total number of patients with malignant disease is rising because of increasing life expectancy. In the younger age groups, surgical workload from cancer is also expanding because of earlier detection, increased technical sophistication and increasing patient expectation.

Fig. 4.1 Incidence of common solid tumours as a proportion of all malignancies (UK 1985)

Lung	16%
Colorectal	15%
Breast	13%
Prostate	10%
Stomach	7%
Head and neck	6%
Bladder	4%
Pancreas	3%

Two broad considerations determine the approach to treatment in any cancer patient. The first is whether an attempt should be made to achieve a *cure* or whether only *palliation* is appropriate; the approach depends on the nature of the tumour, the extent of local spread and whether distant metastases are present. The second consideration is the prognosis. This takes into account the extent of disease, the likely natural history of the tumour type and the patient's age and constitution. Systems of *staging* have been devised for each tumour type, many based on the *TNM system* which scores characteristics of the **T**umour, the extent of regional lymph **N**ode involvement and presence of **M**etastases. Staging is used in planning treatment, as a guide to prognosis and as a standardised descriptive tool in comparing efficacy of treatment in different patients.

Unfortunately, measures of outcome of cancer treatment are relatively inaccurate, success of any particular treatment often being described in terms of patient survival after a given number of years. *Five year survival* is often used as the yardstick of success in cancer therapy and in many cases can be taken to imply cure. Nevertheless, some tumours, particularly breast cancer, may recur in a disseminated form as long as 30 years after apparently successful eradication. Conversely, testicular teratoma and seminoma almost never recur after the patient has survived five years.

Treatment options

The main treatment options for malignant disease are *surgical excision, radiotherapy, cytotoxic chemotherapy and hormone manipulation*, two or more often being used in combination. For a small proportion of patients, disease is so advanced or the patient so unfit at the time of first presentation that active treatment is inappropriate and *terminal care* is the only reasonable option. In many other patients, the disease will progress despite treatment and patients will eventually require terminal care. This must be accorded as great a priority as active treatment.

Most cancer treatments involve unpleasant *side-effects* which may easily be overlooked by both doctor and patient in their enthusiasm for treatment. Thus it is essential that the benefits and disadvantages are carefully considered in every case and where possible the patient should be involved in making decisions. There are few circumstances where a diagnosis of cancer should be concealed from a patient because suspicion and fear of the unknown often causes more distress than a frank explanation of the diagnosis and its ramifications.

EARLY DETECTION OF CANCER

As a general principle, the earlier in its natural history that a malignancy is diagnosed and treated, the better the prognosis. The ideal is to detect cancer before invasion has actually occurred, i.e. during the 'in-situ' stage. Where this applies, health education plays an important part in alerting the public to early symptoms and warning signs. In the case of breast and testicular tumours, this should be extended to include regular self-examination.

Screening

Screening is defined as the examination of an asymptomatic population at risk of a particular disease, with the objective of diagnosis at a very early stage, to maximise the cure rate. There are two essential prerequisites before any screening programme is introduced. First, it must have been demonstrated that early diagnosis and treatment either improves the cure rate or decreases the side effects of treatment. Second, the high cost of screening vast numbers of healthy individuals must be justified by the yield. Screening for pulmonary tuberculosis by mass miniature X-rays was highly successful in the 1950s and 1960s but was eventually abandoned in the 1970s when the number of new cases discovered fell to such a low level that the cost could no longer be justified.

Screening for cancer of the uterine cervix was widely introduced in the late 1970s and has proved successful, despite the reluctance of many women at greatest risk to be screened. As regards screening for breast cancer by radiography (*mammography*), there has been conflicting evidence about whether it improves prognosis. Recently, however, it has been demonstrated that survival can be prolonged and perhaps lives saved by early detection. Improved radiological techniques enable even earlier breast cancer, and sometimes carcinoma-in-situ, to be diagnosed. Mass breast cancer screening programmes are likely to be implemented in most developed countries over the next few years. These will be monitored by computer call and recall systems which should overcome some of the obvious inadequacies of some of the current cervical screening programmes.

SURGERY FOR CANCER

PRINCIPLES

The ideal result of cancer surgery is the complete eradication of the malignant disease. Nearly a third of cancer patients, mainly those with primary disease only, can be cured in this way.

Where metastases appear confined to local lymph nodes, these nodes are usually excised along with the primary tumour or at a second operation. Even in the presence of metastases, surgical excision of the primary lesion is often required to relieve the local effects of the tumour, e.g. bleeding, pain or bowel obstruction, although palliative surgery is not often indicated in advanced breast or lung cancer. Surgery may be required in advanced disease as a palliative measure to deal with specific distressing symptoms (e.g. severe haemorrhage from a bladder tumour) or some emergency problem (e.g. acute bowel obstruction).

Sometimes surgery is used to *debulk* a tumour; this is combined with chemotherapy, either in an attempt to improve the efficacy of chemotherapy (as in ovarian carcinoma), or to avoid leaving unstable tissue behind in abdominal lymph nodes (as in testicular teratoma).

RADIOTHERAPY

PRINCIPLES

The value of ionising radiation in treating malignant tumours was recognised soon after the discovery of X-rays in 1895. *Orthovoltage* X-rays (up to 250 kV) were the basis of conventional radiotherapy until the development of *megavoltage* irradiation in the late 1950s. Cobalt-60 machines and the later generation of linear accelerators provide photon beams of an energy exceeding 1×10^6 V. The radiation dose is concentrated deep to the skin, thus avoiding the former severe skin reactions. Absorption of radiation by the target tissue results in the appearance of highly reactive free radicals which damage DNA and result in cell death at subsequent mitosis. Malignant tumours can thus be destroyed with minimal damage to surrounding normal tissues, provided that radiotherapy is given in *multiple dosage fractions* to allow recovery of normal tissues between treatments.

The larger the volume of tumour, the greater the dosage of irradiation required for its destruction. Since the dose is limited by the tolerance of normal tissues, radiotherapy is more effective for small lesions. If cure, as opposed to palliation, is the aim, accurate staging and tumour localisation is needed. This will help to establish whether radiotherapy is the appropriate treatment, and will ensure that the whole tumour can be included in the field of irradiation. CT scanning has greatly improved radiotherapy planning for lesions deep within the body, such as bladder or head and neck cancer.

Radiation can be directed to a tumour in three ways:

- *External beam irradiation* — this is the method most commonly employed for both skin and deeply located tumours. For deep lesions, modern megavoltage irradiation spares the skin and superficial tissues from the reactions that formerly beset the use of conventional X-ray treatment
- *Implantation radiotherapy* — this involves placing the radiation source within the tissue to be irradiated. Radioactive iridium wires or caesium needles can be implanted in the oral cavity, perineum, skin, or sometimes breast, giving high-dose local irradiation. Implantation is usually performed under general anaesthesia. For cancer of the uterus and cervix, the radioactive source is placed in the uterine or vaginal cavity rather than implanted in the tissues
- *Systemic therapy* — radioactive iodine given by mouth is a well established treatment for non-neoplastic thyrotoxicosis in older patients, but can also be used for treating well differentiated thyroid tumours provided they have a high uptake of iodine. Similarly, radioactive phosphorus is used systemically for treating polycythaemia rubra vera. Attempts are being made to direct radioisotopes precisely to cancer cells by attaching them to tumour-specific monoclonal antibodies, thus realising the dream of a 'magic bullet'; alas this technique is still in the experimental stage

MAJOR APPLICATIONS OF RADIOTHERAPY

Radiotherapy has three major applications in cancer treatment as a primary cure, as adjuvant treatment or palliation. The objective should be clearly defined before treatment is begun.

1. Primary curative radiotherapy

This application, also known as *radical radiotherapy*, is widely used for basal cell and squamous cell carcinomas of the skin. It is also used for certain tumours which are technically difficult to remove or where surgery would be particularly mutilating, as in the head, neck and larynx. Radiotherapy can be directed at the primary lesion and regional lymph nodes if appropriate, and rates of cure are comparable to those achieved by surgical excision. For example, in head and neck cancers without distant metastases, cure rates of 50–90% are being achieved with radiotherapy alone; similar results can be obtained in carcinoma of the cervix. Radiotherapy is the standard treatment for Hodgkin's disease, giving excellent results. Radiotherapy can also achieve cure in a high proportion of patients with seminoma and metastases in para-aortic lymph nodes.

2. Adjuvant radiotherapy

The principle underlying *adjuvant therapy*, whether radiological or chemical, is that clinically undetectable micrometastases are often present in tissue surrounding a primary lesion and in regional nodes. These are believed to be responsible for subsequent local and regional recurrence after a primary lesion has apparently been completely removed. Adjuvant radiotherapy is applied after surgery to local tissue and regional nodes to try to eliminate micrometastases. Adjuvant radiotherapy is most widely employed for carcinoma of the breast after removal of the primary lesion by simple lumpectomy or mastectomy. This avoids the need for radical lymph node clearance and more mutilating operations. Survival rates are comparable to those achieved after more extensive surgery.

3. Palliative radiotherapy

Radiotherapy is particularly effective in controlling metastatic deposits in bone and brain. The pain of bone metastases can often be completely relieved by radiotherapy, as can some of the neurological manifestations of brain secondaries. Radiotherapy is also valuable in providing symptomatic relief in advanced disease. In ulcerating breast cancer, radiotherapy can shrink the

Fig. 4.2 Reactions and complications of radiotherapy

Non-specific tiredness and lassitude — very common and settles spontaneously

Nausea, vomiting and anorexia — mainly occur in wide field abdominal irradiation. Controlled with antiemetics and rest

Skin reactions — rare with modern megavoltage radiotherapy, except when treating skin cancer when moist breakdown of skin is inevitable; this takes three to four weeks to heal. Occasional mild redness and soreness occurs when irradiation involves axilla, groin or perineum

Progressive endarteritis obliterans — causes dense fibrosis and impairs blood supply. Progresses for years after treatment. Particularly serious effects on the gastrointestinal tract, causing strictures and obstruction. (The next two complications in this list are probably also caused by endarteritis obliterans)

Slow or incomplete healing after subsequent surgery — may cause failure of skin and bone grafts, breakdown of intestinal anastomoses and, occasionally, formation of internal fistulae

Intestinal damage — radiotherapy absorbed by the colon during treatment of cervical cancer may result in 'radiation colitis' causing troublesome rectal bleeding; small bowel may be damaged in the same way but tends to form strictures. Radiotherapy for bladder cancer tends to leave a friable bladder mucosa susceptible to bleeding

Atrophy and fibrosis of salivary glands — head and neck radiotherapy may result in *xerostomia* (dryness of the mouth) and atrophy of mucous membranes. Xerostomia (which may partly recover) causes dysphagia and accelerated dental caries. In such cases, special dental care and prophylactic fluoride therapy is indicated.

Osteoradionecrosis — a feared complication of the former low voltage radiotherapy but now rare. Necrosis of bone occurs in the vicinity of the irradiated lesion, e.g. ribs after radiotherapy for breast cancer (see Figure 4.3)

primary lesion, controlling exudation and bleeding and permitting healing of overlying skin. Similarly, the distressing symptoms of cough, haemoptysis and pleuritic pain from advanced lung cancer can be eased by palliative radiotherapy. Symptoms associated with local tumour recurrence can often be controlled, e.g. haematuria from advanced bladder cancer or pain from rectal carcinoma. In abdominal malignancy, the main factor limiting the use of radiotherapy is concurrent radiation injury to normal bowel which can cause stricture formation, obstruction and continual bleeding, often years later.

The dosage and number of fractions of radiotherapy employed in palliative treatment is much less than are used for curative treatment in order to minimise side effects. Indeed palliative radiotherapy can only be justified if therapeutic benefits are likely to ensue.

COMPLICATIONS OF RADIOTHERAPY

Despite the precise use of high energy radiotherapy, side effects and complications still occur; the main ones are outlined in Figure 4.2.

CHEMOTHERAPY

PRINCIPLES

Success with chemotherapeutic agents in curing many haematological and childhood malignancies has encouraged the use of similar drugs against solid tumours, hitherto treated by surgery or radiotherapy.

Drugs destroy tumour cells in a variety of different ways, capitalising on their increased mitotic and metabolic rates. The main types of chemotherapeutic agent are as follows:

- *Antimetabolites* — analogues of normal cellular nutrients, e.g. methotrexate substitutes for folinic acid
- *Alkylating agents* — bind to DNA, e.g. nitrogen mustards
- *Drugs which crosslink DNA*, e.g. cisplatin
- *Drugs which disrupt the mitotic spindle*, e.g. vinca alkaloids

These cytotoxic mechanisms also operate upon normal tissues, though usually to a lesser extent, and are responsible for many of the side effects. For many tumours, the best results are obtained by combinations of cytotoxic drugs. The drug combinations are chosen so their toxic effects impinge upon different organ systems; this means that each drug can be given in full tumour-toxic dose without excessive damage to normal tissues. The most effective drug combinations and doses for each tumour type have been established mainly by empirical trials (and some good luck!). Drugs are usually given intra-

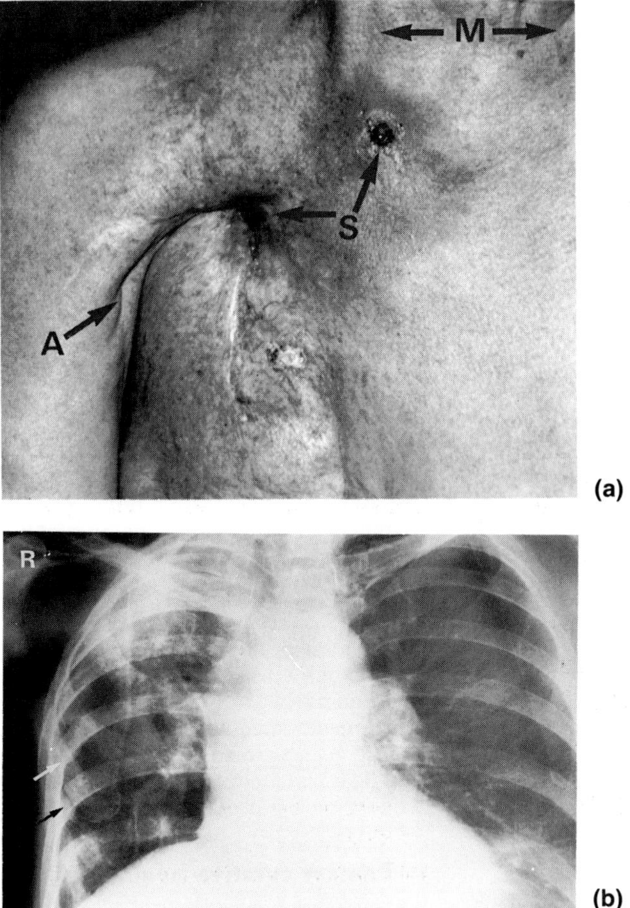

Fig. 4.3 Osteoradionecrosis after breast irradiation

A 75-year-old woman who had a radical mastectomy and low-voltage irradiation for carcinoma of the right breast 40 years ago. She presented with two discharging skin sinuses just below the clavicle. **(a)** Gross deformity of chest wall caused by excision of pectoral muscles (axilla **A**, sternomastoids **M**). Note sinus openings **S** leading down to sequestra, and widespread telangiectasia, a late result of radiotherapy. **(b)** Chest X-ray showing osteoradionecrosis of the ribs and scapula on the right side. There is typical patchy osteoporosis and osteosclerosis. Several healing pathological fractures are also evident (arrowed). Irradiation has induced lung fibrosis and pulmonary contraction resulting in a shift of the mediastinum towards the right

venously, in a series of four to six short courses separated by three to four weeks to allow recovery of normal tissues.

Experience has revealed a wide spectrum of sensitivities of different malignant tumours to cytotoxic therapy, ranging between total destruction and no therapeutic value. The sensitivities of different tumour types are summarised in Figure 4.4.

Fig. 4.4 Tumour sensitivity to cytotoxic chemotherapy

1. Highly sensitive tumours — reasonable prospect of cure

Hodgkin's disease
High-grade lymphomas
Testicular tumours
Choriocarcinoma
Childhood leukaemias
Wilms' tumour (nephroblastoma)
Ewing's sarcoma
Osteogenic sarcoma (lung metastases)

2. Moderately sensitive tumours — palliation is the main objective

Breast cancer
Ovarian malignancies
Small cell (oat-cell) carcinoma of lung
Multiple myeloma
Acute and chronic leukaemias in adults
Low-grade lymphomas

3. Relatively insensitive tumours — cytotoxic therapy only indicated in special circumstances or with techniques of regional infusion

Carcinoma of lung other than small cell type
Colorectal cancer
Squamous carcinomas, especially in the head and neck
Carcinoma of uterus and cervix
Melanoma
Hepatoma
Osteogenic sarcoma (primary lesions)
Renal adenocarcinoma
Bladder carcinoma

MAJOR APPLICATIONS OF CHEMOTHERAPY

1. Primary curative treatment

This is mainly indicated for highly sensitive *germ cell tumours*, high-grade *lymphomas* and *solid tumours of childhood*. Chemotherapy may be used alone after obtaining a biopsy diagnosis (e.g. Hodgkin's disease), it may follow removal of the primary tumour (e.g. teratoma, Wilms' tumour), or chemotherapy may be used first and be followed by resection of any residual tumour to achieve complete remission (e.g. abdominal para-aortic nodes in testicular teratoma).

2. Adjuvant chemotherapy

This involves chemotherapy after treatment of the primary lesion in an attempt to destroy already disseminated but undetectable micrometastases. Adjuvant chemotherapy is sometimes used for breast cancer where axillary lymph nodes are involved; in such cases, widespread metastases would be almost certain to appear later. Unfortunately, the treatment has proved unacceptably toxic and improves survival by no more than 5%.

3. General palliative treatment

This is the rationale for the use of chemotherapy for disseminated malignancy in highly sensitive and moderately sensitive tumours. Cure is rarely achieved but quality of life may be greatly improved and, in some cases, life may be prolonged.

4. Palliation of distressing local symptoms

Cytotoxic therapy may sometimes be indicated for relatively insensitive tumours if local tumour effects are so distressing that even a small reduction in tumour mass might relieve them, e.g. breast cancer causing lymphatic obstruction. The objective is not to prolong life but to improve its quality.

5. Direct administration of cytotoxic agents to the tumour

In isolated primary or secondary tumours in the liver or kidneys, it is sometimes possible to cannulate the arterial supply of the lesion and administer the cytotoxic agent directly. This may successfully shrink the tumour. For superficial bladder tumours which are too extensive for local surgical treatment, a chemotherapeutic agent may be instilled into the bladder.

SIDE EFFECTS OF CHEMOTHERAPY

Chemotherapy is not only toxic to tumour cells but also to normal body cells, especially those with rapid rates of turnover, e.g. bone marrow and gastrointestinal epithelium. Toxic effects are summarised in Figure 4.5. Side effects are common and often so severe that they greatly diminish the quality of the patient's remaining life. This must be balanced against the expected benefits of therapy; advantages and disadvantages must be clearly defined and discussed with the patient. Patients should never be subjected to chemotherapy on the basis that 'it might do some good'. In such cases it is more likely to do harm and may even prove fatal!

While chemotherapy offers significant benefit and a chance of cure in certain well defined malignancies, less than 10% of cancer patients can benefit from present chemotherapeutic agents. To save unwarranted suffering, therapy must be reserved for these patients.

Fig. 4.5 Toxic effects of chemotherapy

Bone marrow suppression — causes anaemia, thrombocytopenia and leucopenia (potentially fatal)

Immunosuppression — causes diminished resistance to opportunistic infections

Non-specific CNS toxicity — causes nausea and vomiting (tends to occur one hour or more after chemotherapy)

Disruption of gastrointestinal epithelial turnover — causes diarrhoea and oral ulceration

Toxicity to hair follicles — causes hair loss (recovers two to six months after treatment)

Gonadal injury — loss of libido, sterility and possible mutagenesis

Long-term risk of inducing other malignancies — 20 to 30 times the normal risk

Rapid tumour destruction on a massive scale — leads to release of purines and pyrimidines (only a problem in leukaemias and lymphomas). These cause hyperuricaemia, presenting as obstructive uropathy and renal failure. Can be prevented by giving prophylactic allopurinol

HORMONAL MANIPULATION

PRINCIPLES

The growth of certain tumours, notably carcinoma of the prostate and some breast cancers, is partially dependent on sex hormones. Removal of the gonads or use of drugs which block or antagonise the appropriate hormone may have a valuable inhibitory effect on tumour growth.

Surgical removal of the testes *(orchidectomy)* is now the preferred treatment for metastatic carcinoma of the prostate, although *stilboestrol*, a form of oestrogen, was widely used in the past. Stilboestrol has fallen from favour because of greatly increased risk of thromboembolic disease, fluid retention and cardiac failure. *Luteinising hormone releasing hormone* (LHRH) is a new agent used for prostatic cancer, given by monthly injection. It acts by driving testosterone release to the point of exhaustion, thereby lowering blood levels after a preliminary rise. *Cyproterone acetate*, a drug which blocks testosterone at cellular level, shows promise in the treatment of disseminated prostatic carcinoma. The drug blocks testosterone both from testes and adrenals, and may therefore be more efficacious than other methods already described.

In metastatic breast cancer, particularly with bony metastases, *oophorectomy* brings relief from pain in about 50% of cases. A recent development is the oral drug *tamoxifen*, an anti-oestrogen, which can give effective palliation in all forms of recurrent or metastatic breast cancer. It is usually worth a trial of treatment, particularly as the drug has minimal side effects. Paradoxically, tamoxifen, given as an adjunct to primary surgical treatment, has been shown to prolong survival in breast cancer most effectively in patients over the age of 60, i.e. after the menopause. In former days, *adrenalectomy* was sometimes performed following relapse after oophorectomy, the aim being to eliminate all traces of sex hormone production. Occasionally, the drug *aminoglutethimide* is given to perform a 'medical adrenalectomy', although tamoxifen seems to have removed the need for adrenalectomy because it also opposes oestrogen of adrenal origin.

TERMINAL CARE

GENERAL PRINCIPLES

Despite all efforts to save them, many patients with malignant tumours eventually die from progression of the primary tumour or widespread metastases. The management of terminal disease should be given as much attention as preceding attempts at cure. Indeed, high technology medicine can be indicted for concentrating on the primary disorder while failing to perceive and treat the patient as a whole being. This means reserving active treatments for conditions where their efficacy has been clearly established; there should be no ethical dilemma in witholding treatment when there are no sound indications for it. It is as much the doctor's duty to 'do no harm' as to try to do some good.

Most patients with disseminated malignancy deteriorate insidiously until they reach a terminal phase when it becomes obvious that death will occur soon.

As various organ systems begin to fail, symptoms develop unpredictably and patient care becomes highly demanding of the doctor's skills. Diagnostic tests should be kept to a minimum because most are unpleasant and may remove the patient from familiar surroundings for little real benefit. The doctor must rely more on 'old-fashioned' clinical skills and be prepared to act on them. Most of all, the doctor must not lose sight of the purpose of treatment, which is to ensure the best possible quality of life, even at the expense of duration.

Drugs should be used in ways that achieve the optimum therapeutic effect, despite possible longer-term adverse effects; for example, dependency on opiate analgesics is irrelevant in a dying patient in pain. The correct dose is the one which relieves the pain, even if it seems enormous by the usual standards. It must, however, be remembered that distress may not be due to pain alone, and attention to simple matters like constipation can relieve much suffering.

The principles of terminal care are summarised in Figure 4.6. These should not be imposed, but rather offered after discussion with the patient and the caring relatives. A flexible approach must always be maintained. If handled well, terminal care can bring great rewards to both patient and doctor.

Fig. 4.6 Principles of terminal care

1. Assess prognosis and the most likely sequence of terminal events
2. Discuss prognosis and life expectancy with the patient and close relatives (but avoid precise predictions of survival time or terminal events)
3. Arrange regular consultations by the patient's general practitioner, who ideally should be personally available to be called at any time
4. Ensure immediate availability of hospital medical care and advice in the event of sudden deterioration or onset of new symptoms, i.e. 'open door' policy.
5. Identify future nursing requirements and make contingency plans, e.g. home aids (commodes, incontinence devices, etc), community nursing care, hospice or hospital relief
6. Anticipate the development of symptoms and initiate treatment before problems get out of hand
7. Pay particular attention to prevention and early treatment of pain, diarrhoea and constipation, and nausea and vomiting, by the use of appropriate drugs
8. Continually review drug therapy, titrating doses against new and changing symptoms to minimise side effects

The most common problems of the dying cancer patient and suitable measures for their relief are as follows:

- *Pain* — seek the cause of pain, much of which can be relieved by simple nursing measures. For the pain of malignant disease, give regular opiate analgesics in high enough dose and sufficient frequency to prevent pain from 'breaking through' or becoming established. Slow release morphine tablets given eight-hourly are often effective and their effect can be enhanced by chlorpromazine tablets and oral prednisolone. This treatment often raises 'mood' and relieves anorexia. Morphine can also be made up as an elixir in water or in an antiemetic syrup, but this needs to be given at shorter intervals, e.g. 4-hourly. Mixtures containing several ingredients (e.g. Brompton cocktail, which contains alcohol, cocaine, chloroform water, etc) are best avoided as accurate titration of the dose of each component is impossible

- *Constipation* — regular laxatives or enemas
- *Nausea* — often relieved by anti-emetics such as metoclopramide, domperidone and prochlorperazine (which can be given as suppositories)
- *Intestinal obstruction and vomiting* — difficult to palliate but powerful anti-emetics and 'little and often' by mouth are helpful measures
- *Dysphagia* — liquidised food, presented as attractively as possible
- *Oral ulceration* — helped by metronidazole gel
- *Mouth care* — careful attention to oral hygiene prevents oral infection (e.g. candidiasis) and acute parotitis
- *Cough and dyspnoea* — eased by morphine and codeine
- *Insomnia* — use benzodiazepines or chlorpromazine

PART II
PRINCIPLES OF ACCIDENT SURGERY

5 ACCIDENTS, HEAD INJURIES AND BURNS

Introduction

Trauma patients constitute up to 20% of general surgical admissions in the average district general hospital, the percentage depending to some extent on local policy as to which department is responsible for head injuries. In most centres, head injuries are the responsibility of either general surgeons or orthopaedic surgeons; in regional neurosurgical centres, all head injuries are usually admitted directly to the neurosurgeons.

This chapter discusses the principles of management of multiple injuries, head injuries, injuries to the chest and abdomen, soft tissue injuries and finally burns.

PRELIMINARY MANAGEMENT OF SERIOUS INJURIES

TRIAGE

The accident and emergency department (A & E) will usually be given prior warning by the ambulance service when seriously injured patients are on the way to the hospital. This gives casualty staff time to alert the surgical and anaesthetic teams who should be standing by when the patient arrives. The resuscitation room and essential equipment are made ready for immediate use, e.g. infusion sets run through, drugs laid out. Successful management of life-threatening injuries depends on good organisation. One doctor must take overall responsibility and coordinate the activities of the different specialties involved; this is of paramount importance in the case of the multiply injured.

For *major disasters* such as train or air crashes, where many casualties can be expected, each receiving hospital should have a detailed and rehearsed *major disaster plan*. This should clearly demarcate the responsibilities of each individual. One of the most important tasks is sorting patients on arrival into management priority groups, a process known as *triage*.

The usual triage categories are:

- Require immediate surgery
- Require surgery but can wait
- Minor injury
- Dead

Prevention of secondary injuries

Most trauma deaths result from either head injuries alone or multiple injuries which also involve the chest, abdomen and limbs. The management priorities for the multiply injured patient are summarised in Figure 5.1. Initial *assessment* is carried out at the same time as appropriate *resuscitation*, according to urgency. There is now good evidence that the sequence of resuscitation and elective ventilation, followed by stabilisation of long bone fractures, provides the best conditions for assessment of head, chest and abdominal injuries.

Any unconscious patient may have an *unstable vertebral injury* and subsequent spinal cord injury may occur unless the patient is nursed and moved with extreme care. Unconscious trauma patients should always have X-rays of the cervical spine performed. Conscious patients with suspected cervical spinal injury should be moved with extreme caution. Passive movements of the neck should never be attempted; it is safer to allow the patient to perform active movements unaided, which will be restricted by spasm or pain if there is a significant injury.

Fig. 5.1 Management priorities for the patient with multiple injuries

1. Resuscitation and support of cardiovascular and respiratory function

A. Ensure a clear **AIRWAY**
— remove any oropharyngeal obstructions, e.g. teeth, dentures or blood
— intubate trachea if necessary especially if the patient is unconscious or has multiple jaw fractures

B. Ensure that the patient is **BREATHING** adequately to maintain oxygenation
— ventilate if necessary, e.g. for flail chest or serious head injuries
— seal open chest wounds which are allowing air into the pleural cavity in order to limit mediastinal 'flap' movement with each breath
— relieve tension pneumothorax, drain haemothorax

C. Maintain the **CIRCULATION**
— ensure adequate circulating volume by controlling haemorrhage and replacing lost fluids by intravenous infusion
— relieve cardiac tamponade by long needle aspiration
— apply external cardiac massage in the case of cardiac arrest
— catheterise the bladder to monitor urine production and provide a guide to renal perfusion

2. Treat life threatening injuries

— relieve rising intracranial pressure, e.g. surgical decompression of extradural haemorrhage
— perform thoracotomy for major heart and great vessel injuries
— perform laparotomy for gastrointestinal perforation or splenic rupture
— repair major peripheral vascular injuries, e.g. penetrating groin injury

3. Treat major fractures and dislocations including spinal injuries

4. Treat less serious injuries

— perform wound toilet of soft tissue injuries, suturing or packing as appropriate
— reduce fractures and dislocations
— repair tendon and peripheral nerve injuries

INITIAL ASSESSMENT OF THE SERIOUSLY INJURED PATIENT

Despite the urgency of the situation, assessment of the trauma patient must be performed in a *systematic* manner, i.e. history, examination and special tests.

1. History

A history is obtained from the patient if possible, and from ambulance personnel and other witnesses. The history should include the following details:

- Time of the accident
- Nature and speed of impact
- Conscious level of patient when discovered and subsequent changes in conscious level
- An estimate of blood loss at scene of accident
- Details of drugs, fluids and other treatments administered at scene of accident
- Previous state of health including past medical history, drug history and drug allergies
- Details of prior food, alcohol or drug intake

2. Examination

A rapid preliminary examination is performed as soon as the patient arrives. The main observations are:

- State of consciousness
- Signs of distress, i.e. difficulty in breathing, obvious pain
- Appearance of the skin for evidence of pallor and cyanosis
- Vital signs, i.e. pulse rate, blood pressure, respiratory pattern
- The presence of gross injuries
- Ability to move all limbs

From this, immediate *management priorities* can be identified and resuscitation measures implemented. Once this has been done, a detailed 'head to toe' examination is then performed for signs of serious head, spine, chest, abdominal, pelvic and limb injuries; the particular observations are summarised in Figure 5.2 and details of the individual systems are described later. The examination findings must be carefully recorded in the patient's notes, not least for medicolegal purposes.

X-rays and other investigations

In most seriously injured patients, the chest and cervical spine are X-rayed in the resuscitation room using portable equipment. The diagnostic quality of the films must be good enough to exclude major chest, mediastinal and lung

Fig. 5.2 Special points to note in systematic examination of the seriously injured patient

Head and neck — lacerations, depressed vault fractures, facial and jaw fractures, pupil size and responsiveness, range of neck movements (if in doubt do not perform passive movements before X-rays are available)

Chest (front and back) — penetrating injuries, bruising and skin imprinting, pattern and rate of respiration, symmetry of chest movement, gross mediastinal shift, pattern of air entry throughout the lung fields, crepitus (subcutaneous air)

Abdomen — external injuries as for chest, distension by gas or fluid, abdominal girth, tenderness, presence of palpable or percussible bladder, pelvic fractures, bleeding from urethral meatus

Limbs — neurovascular status of each limb, lacerations, deformities, soft tissue swelling, fractures and dislocations

injuries, and also to provide a baseline for comparison should the patient subsequently deteriorate. Cervical spine X-rays often fail to include C1, C7 and T1 and must be interpreted with caution and, if necessary, repeated later.

Portable skull X-rays should only be performed if this will affect immediate management because the diagnostic quality tends to be inadequate. All other X-rays are performed later, preferably in the radiology department, once the patient has been stabilised.

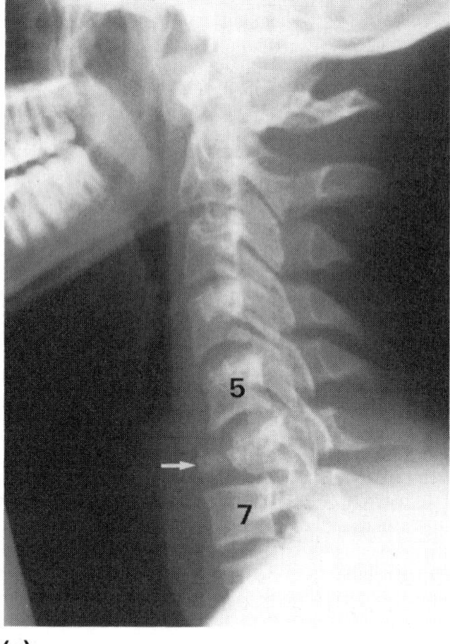

(a)

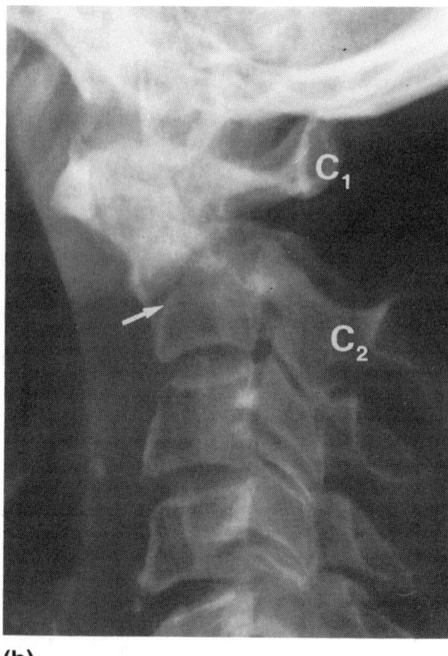

(b)

Fig. 5.3 Cervical spine fractures

(a) Lateral cervical spine X-ray of a 17-year-old boy admitted semi-conscious after coming off his motor-cycle and landing head-first in a ditch. On examination he was not moving his lower limbs or hands although there was some movement at the shoulders. The X-ray shows a burst fracture of the body of C6 (arrowed) with fragments in the spinal canal; there is also some posterior subluxation of C5.
(b) Left lateral cervical spine X-ray from another unconscious young patient showing a fracture (arrowed) of the body of C2 and severe anterior subluxation of C1

Initial blood tests should include haemoglobin, and blood grouping and cross-matching. In a desperate emergency, universal donor blood (group O, Rh negative) can be transfused without grouping or cross-matching, although plasma substitutes or plasma will usually suffice until blood becomes available. Plasma electrolytes and glucose are usually measured, and arterial blood gases are estimated if there is any suggestion of respiratory failure.

Any further investigations are guided by the nature of the injury, as detailed below.

HEAD INJURIES

Introduction

Head injuries cause approximately 5000 deaths per annum in the UK, representing about 0.8% of all deaths. As illustrated in Figure 5.4, however, deaths represent only a small part of the workload caused by head injuries.

Fig. 5.4

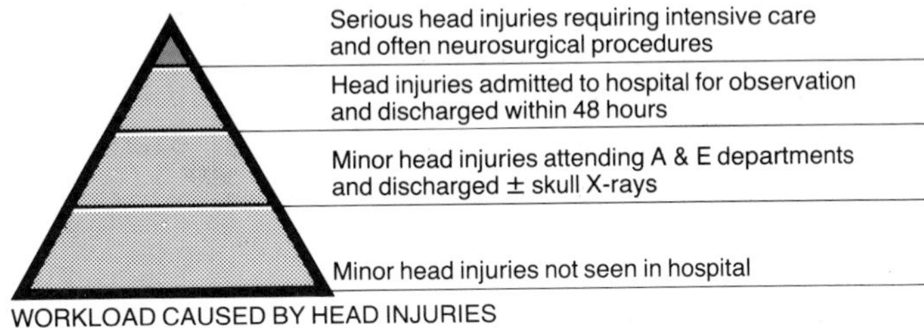

One of the problems in providing trauma services is the vast number of head injury patients. Less than half will require hospital admission and of these only a small proportion will require specialist neurosurgical investigation and care. Most of those with serious injuries are readily identifiable, but a small proportion of the remaining patients will deteriorate later. The problem is to recognise those at risk without investigating and admitting every single case.

PATHO-PHYSIOLOGY OF TRAUMATIC BRAIN INJURY

Traumatic brain injuries are divided into *primary brain injury*, i.e. the immediate result of the trauma, and *secondary brain injury*, which develops later as a result of complications. Treatment cannot reverse the primary brain injury but can sustain the patient during the natural recovery period. Secondary brain injury, however, is largely preventable by appropriate intervention and prophylactic measures; indeed, the death rate from head injury could be halved by implementation of well recognised management protocols.

In general, the younger the patient the better the prognosis. Young children can sustain remarkably severe injuries and yet recover full function because of the plasticity of the developing nervous system. With increasing age, the brain shrinks in relation to the cranial vault, allowing greater movement under impact. Consequently there is a greater chance of tearing intracranial vessels causing haemorrhage.

Primary brain injury

Minor primary brain injury, known as *concussion*, results in disruption of brain function without detectable structural damage. Clinically, concussion presents as transient loss of consciousness, followed by a short period of diminished consciousness and minor cognitive disturbances such as brief memory loss. With more serious injury, there is *cerebral contusion* or sometimes *laceration*, the site and extent of the injury depending on the nature of the damaging force (see Figure 5.5).

Brain injury is more likely in the presence of a skull fracture, but skull fracture of itself does not indicate brain injury. With overt brain injury, there is usually a period of coma, followed by a degree of cognitive disturbance related to the extent of brain damage.

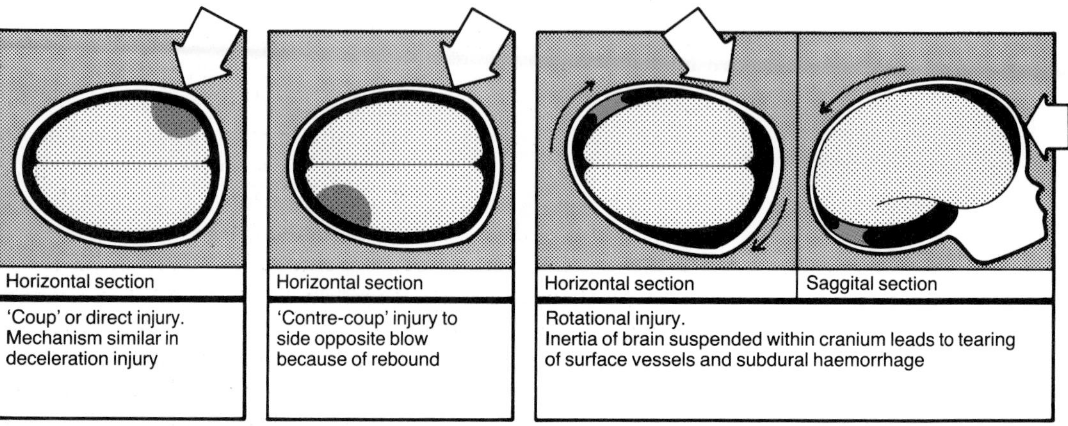

Fig. 5.5 Mechanisms of brain injury

Secondary brain injury

Secondary brain injury may be caused by intracranial bleeding, cerebral hypoxia and infection. These are discussed in detail below:

INTRACRANIAL BLEEDING

Post-traumatic intracranial bleeding may be *extradural*, *subdural* or *intracerebral* (subarachnoid haemorrhage is rarely a feature of trauma). Local brain compression causes focal neurological effects as well as a general rise in intracranial pressure. This may cause temporal lobe herniation under the tentorium cerebelli or 'coning' of the brain stem through the foramen magnum, or both.

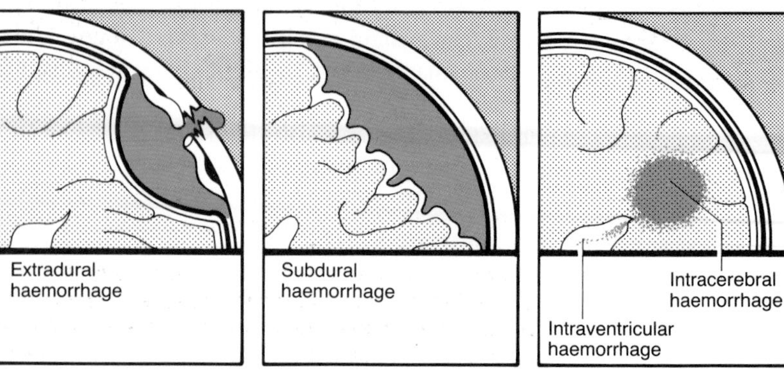

Fig. 5.6 Types of post-traumatic intracranial bleeding

An acute rise in intracranial pressure manifests as:

- Falling pulse rate
- Rising blood pressure
- Deteriorating level of consciousness
- Central respiratory depression

1. Extradural haemorrhage

Extradural haemorrhage is usually caused by disruption of a *meningeal artery*, particularly the middle meningeal and its branches. Haematoma rapidly accumulates between the skull vault and the tough dura mater; the extent of lateral spread is limited by the dural attachments. The haematoma bulges into the underlying brain substance, causing *local compression* and a general *rise in intracranial pressure*. This may be accompanied by focal neurological signs, as well as the signs of acutely raised intracranial pressure.

Extradural haematomas are most commonly seen in children, adolescents and young adults and are most likely to occur when there is a skull fracture in the temporal region. An extradural haematoma can, however, occur without a fracture. In either case, the patient may be unconscious from the outset, or else may have apparently recovered from the initial injury and appear lucid before suddenly deteriorating. Unless the haematoma is evacuated urgently, death is likely to ensue. Extradural haematomas nearly always present within 24 hours of trauma.

(a)

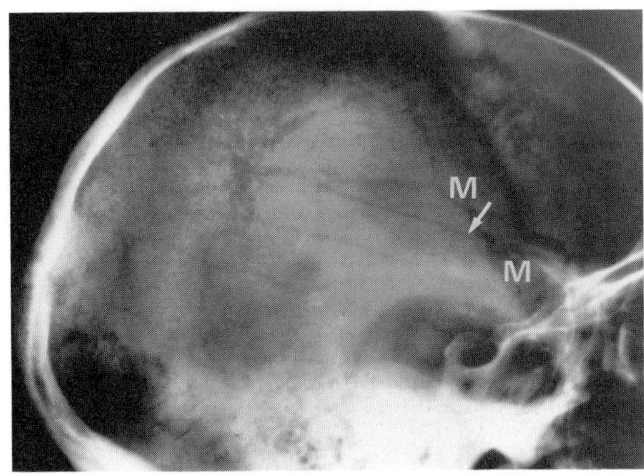

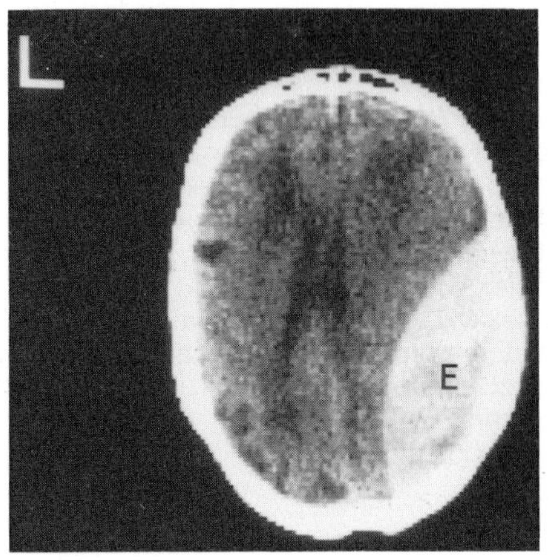

(b)

Fig. 5.7 Temporo-parietal fracture with extradural haematoma

A 20-year-old man admitted fully conscious after being knocked off a bicycle but who deteriorated rapidly two hours later. **(a)** Lateral skull X-ray showing a linear fracture of the right temporo-parietal bones (arrowed) crossing the course of the anterior branch of the middle meningeal artery **M** on the temporal bone. **(b)** CT scan showing a right extradural haemorrhage **E**. The extradural haematoma has a characteristic convex outline because bleeding is under high pressure and the haematoma is confined by the dura mater. Note that CT scanning is of little value in showing skull fractures

2. Subdural haemorrhage

Subdural haemorrhage is usually caused by the tearing of *veins*, with blood leaking slowly into the large potential space between dura mater and arachnoid mater. The haematoma tends to spread laterally over a wide area. In contrast to extradural haemorrhage, there is usually underlying *primary brain contusion*. Subdural haematomas commonly occur in more than one site, which may be on the same side or both sides.

In an acute subdural haemorrhage, there is usually clinical evidence of significant brain injury at the outset, with subsequent deterioration. A lucid interval is rare. Acute subdural haemorrhage is more common in older adults because of increased brain mobility. Evacuation of the clot may halt deterioration but recovery is usually incomplete; most elderly patients die from this condition even when expeditiously treated.

Chronic subdural haematoma

Subdural haematomas may develop gradually in the elderly, following trivial, often unrecalled, head injury. A chronic subdural haematoma may become manifest weeks or months later as non-specific neurological deterioration, headache or coma. Most patients do not present with a head injury, the diagnosis being made on investigation of neurological symptoms.

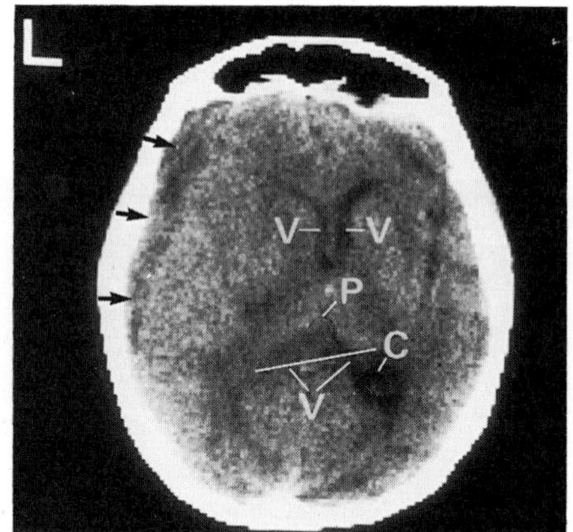

Fig. 5.8 Subdural haematoma

This 78-year-old woman developed increasing confusion for one month following a minor fall when she hit her head on a stone window ledge. This horizontal 'slice' was taken at the level of the top of the pinna and passing through the frontal sinuses. It shows a subdural haematoma (arrowed) in the left fronto-parietal area and shift of the calcified pineal **P** to the right. Note the normal ventricles **V** and calcified choroid plexuses **C**. Unlike the extradural haematoma seen in Figure 5.7, the subdural haemorrhage is radiolucent because the long-standing clot has liquefied

3. Intracerebral haemorrhage

Haemorrhage into the brain is caused by primary brain injury; continuing haemorrhage produces an expanding, space-occupying lesion which causes secondary brain damage. The haemorrhage may be within the brain substance itself (*intracerebral haemorrhage*) or extend into the ventricles (*intraventricular haemorrhage*). An intracerebral haematoma which is discrete may be amenable to evacuation, minimising secondary brain damage.

CEREBRAL HYPOXIA

Oxygen deprivation to the brain after head injury is a major and preventable cause of secondary brain injury. Damage is caused both by cellular hypoxia and by raised intracranial pressure due to cerebral oedema. The most common cause is *inadequate pulmonary oxygenation* due to airway obstruction, chest injury, inhalational pneumonitis, shock lung or central respiratory depression. Hypotension reduces cerebral perfusion, which may also contribute to cerebral hypoxia.

INFECTION

Meningeal infection may cause secondary brain injury, organisms entering via compound skull fractures. Fractures underlying *scalp lacerations* are clearly compound fractures, but others may be deceptive; for example, *fractures of the base of the skull* may communicate with the sphenoid or ethmoid sinuses, the nasal cavity or the external auditory canal. Similarly, fractures of the frontal bone often involve the frontal sinuses. Fractures of this type are thus always considered to be compound. Infection usually becomes evident several days after injury and can largely be prevented by using prophylactic antibiotics for all compound fractures. The antibiotic must cross the blood-brain barrier. Current practice is to use ampicillin and flucloxacillin for a minimum of one week; sulphadimidine is now used less commonly.

SKULL FRACTURES

Importance of skull fractures

A skull fracture indicates that a severe impact has taken place. It is not suprising, therefore, that patients with fractures are more likely to have suffered primary brain damage than those without. Most important, however, is the fact that patients with skull fractures are 30 times more likely to suffer secondary brain damage by the mechanisms described above. Patients with skull fractures therefore merit hospital admission for close observation, even if fully conscious.

Depressed fractures are usually associated with some primary injury to the underlying brain but, paradoxically, the process of fracture may have absorbed some of the energy of impact and protected the brain.

Most skull fractures can only be reliably diagnosed by skull X-ray. It is easy to X-ray every patient who presents with a head injury, however trivial, but such a policy is expensive and time-consuming. To identify those at particular risk of a skull fracture, the criteria shown in Figure 5.9 have been established.

Fig. 5.9 Criteria for skull X-ray after recent head injury (based on guidelines of the working party on head injuries, Royal College of Surgeons of England, July 1986)

1. Loss of consciousness or amnesia at any stage
2. Any neurological symptoms or signs
3. Cerebrospinal fluid or blood emanating from the nose or ear
4. Suspected penetrating injury or marked scalp bruising or swelling (simple scalp laceration alone is not a criterion for skull X-ray)
5. Alcohol intoxication (since this makes neurological assessment difficult)
6. Difficulty in assessing the patient, e.g. young children, epileptics

Fig. 5.10 Clinical signs of a fracture of the skull base

Anterior fossa fractures

Periorbital haematoma — usually bilateral and limited by the margins of the orbicularis oculi

Subconjunctival haemorrhage — the blood tracks from behind forward and therefore no posterior limit can be seen (unlike the localised subconjunctival haematoma which results from direct trauma)

CSF rhinorrhoea — clear fluid running from the nose

Middle fossa fractures, i.e. involving petrous temporal bone

CSF otorrhoea — clear fluid running from the ear

Bruising behind the ear over the mastoid area (Battle's sign)

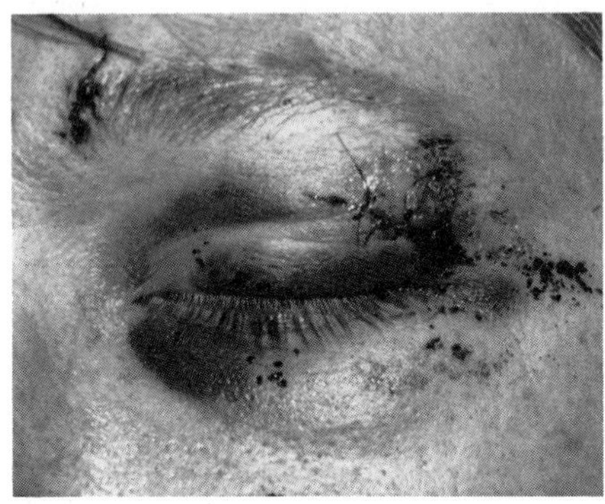

(a)

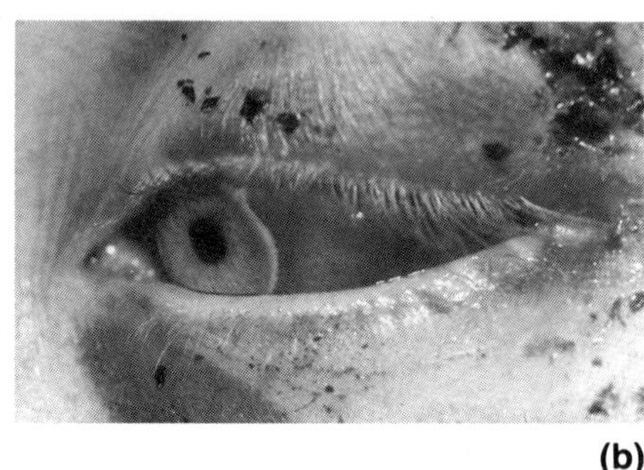

(b)

Fig. 5.11 Periorbital and subconjunctival haematoma following a head injury

This 14-year-old boy fell off his bicycle and momentarily lost consciousness. **(a)** periorbital haematoma; this might have been caused by local haemorrhage from the laceration in his eyebrow but **(b)** shows a subconjunctival haematoma with no posterior limit, indicating a fracture of the orbital wall, in this case the petrous temporal bone of the base of the skull

Types of skull fracture

a. Linear fractures

These mainly involve the skull vault, often with little external sign of injury, although there may be some overlying scalp bruising or swelling. If there is a deep scalp laceration or a history of penetrating injury, the scalp should be deeply probed with a gloved finger, which may reveal a small bony defect or step. Linear fractures rarely exhibit displacement unless there are multiple fracture lines.

b. Depressed fractures

These fractures are usually caused by blunt injuries and the overlying scalp is usually lacerated or severely bruised; such fractures rarely produce serious brain injury unless they are depressed more than 1 cm; this is regarded as an indication for elevation.

c. Fractures of the base of skull

These usually involve the anterior or middle cranial fossae. The characteristic clinical features are summarised in Figure 5.10.

X-rays used for diagnosis of skull fractures

A standard set of three X-ray films is normally all that is required to diagnose a skull fracture. These are *lateral skull, AP skull* and *Towne's view* (see Figure 5.12). The X-rays should be examined not only for presence of a fracture but also for pineal shift and fluid levels in the sphenoid and frontal sinuses. Fluid levels indicate a basal skull fracture. For suspected facial and orbital fractures, an *occipito-mental* view is the standard investigation.

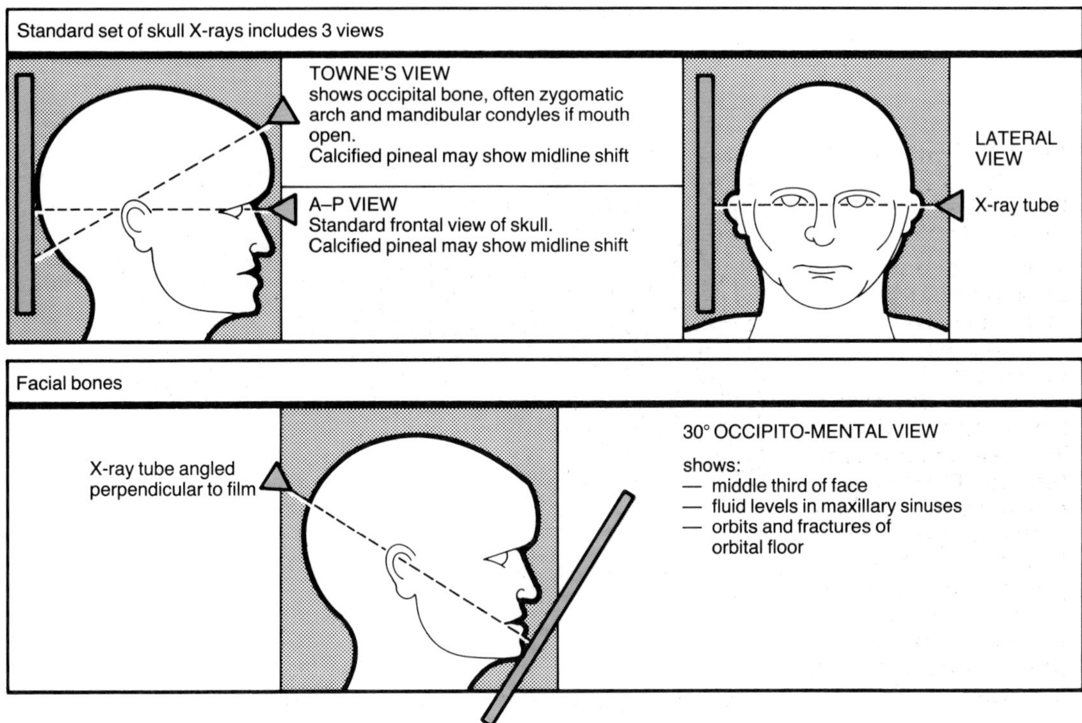

Fig. 5.12

ASSESSING ACTUAL (OR POTENTIAL) BRAIN DAMAGE

History

The history is of great value in deciding whether minor head injuries need skull X-rays or admission to hospital for observation. The most important factors which indicate brain injury and a risk of future complications are a history of *unconsciousness*, and *amnesia* for events around the time of the accident. Amnesia for events prior to the accident (*retrograde amnesia*) may be more significant than for events after it. The duration of unconsciousness and amnesia are proportional to the severity of brain injury. Witnesses should be questioned

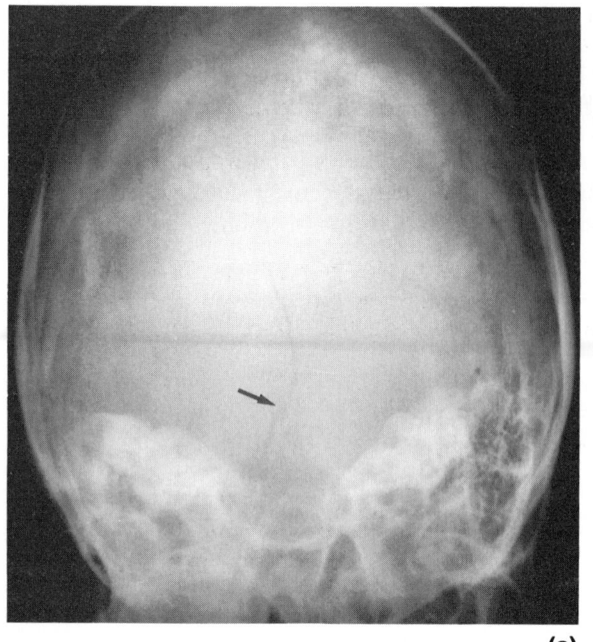

(a)

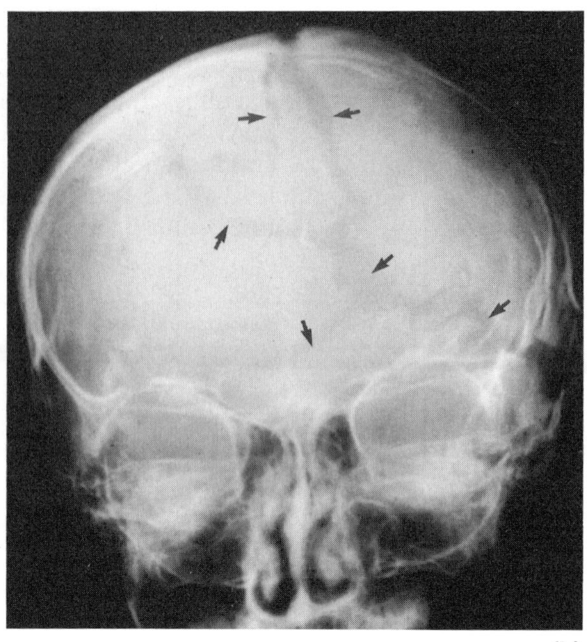

(b)

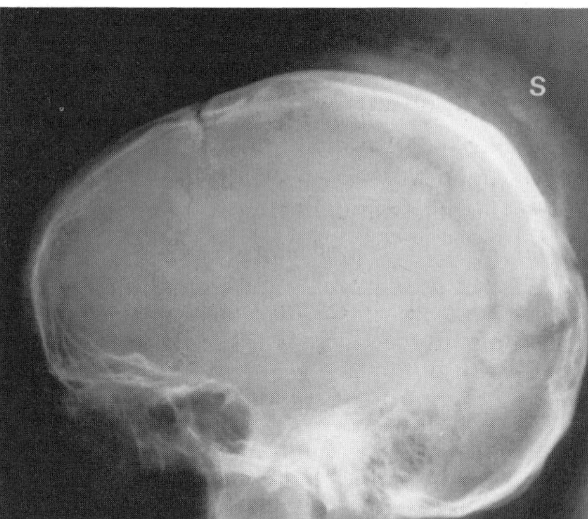

(c)

Fig. 5.13 Standard skull X-ray views

(a) Towne's view from a fully conscious 30-year-old man showing a linear fracture in the parietal bone just lateral to the midline (arrowed). **(b)** and **(c)** AP and lateral views from an unconscious 24-year-old woman. There were deep scalp lacerations and the X-rays show extensive fractures (arrowed) in parietal, occipital and squamous temporal bones. Because of the lacerations, these fractures were *compound*. In (c), note the gross swelling of the overlying scalp soft tissues **S** and the radiolucent air trapped in the lacerations

Fig. 5.14 Glasgow coma scale (worst total score is 3, best total score is 14)

Eye opening	**Score**
spontaneous	4
to speech	3
to pain	2
none	1
Verbal response	
oriented	5
confused	4
inappropriate words	3
incomprehensible sounds	2
none	1
Motor response	
obeys commands	5
localises pain	4
flexion to pain	3
extension to pain	2
none	1

as to whether or not the patient was 'knocked out'. In practice however, the evidence is often equivocal. Careful questioning of the patient about events leading up to the accident will usually reveal the duration of retrograde amnesia; *post-grade amnesia* is more difficult to assess because cerebral function tends to recover gradually.

Examination

In addition to general examination, a systematic neurological examination must be performed in every case of head injury, however trivial. Particular attention should be paid to level of consciousness, limb movements and responses and pupillary responses.

a. Level of consciousness

The level of consciousness is the most important single observation in head injury patients. However, subjective clinical judgement is prone to error and lacks reproducibility. Level of consciousness can be categorised simply and reproducibly using the *Glasgow Coma Scale* (Figure 5.14), and this is now in widespread use. In the majority of minor head injuries, the patient is fully conscious by the time of assessment. If there is any depression of conscious level, the patient must be admitted for observation. The extent to which brain injury is responsible for depression of consciousness is difficult to assess if the patient is *intoxicated* with alcohol or other drugs; any such patient with a history of head injury must be admitted to hospital.

Aggressive behaviour in patients smelling of alcohol must not be assumed to result from intoxication (i.e. removal of social inhibition), because such behaviour also commonly arises from brain injury or hypoxia. A thorough examination must be performed with this in mind before employing sedation to quieten a disruptive patient. Comatose patients or those with multiple injuries are often hypoxic. This causes cerebral swelling, thereby further depressing consciousness and damaging the brain. Accurate assessment of brain injury can therefore only be performed in a fully oxygenated patient.

b. Limb movements and responses

In the fully conscious patient, tone, power and coordination are readily assessed in the standard manner. If a subtle abnormality is suspected, the patient should be asked to close his eyes and hold his arms outstretched, palms upwards, for one minute. Pronation or downward drift on one side is indicative of brain injury. For the semi-conscious or unconscious patient, the pattern of limb response to painful stimuli (e.g. pressure on nailbed, earlobe or sternum) provides a useful indication of the conscious level.

c. Pupillary responses

Normal pupillary size and light responses require the integrity of both the second and third cranial nerves. *Pupillary asymmetry* is fairly common in a population, even without injury and if a patient has asymmetry after an accident, it is sensible to find out whether this existed before the trauma. Otherwise, unilateral change in pupil diameter or response is usually caused by *third nerve* involvement, except in the uncommon case of injuries to the *optic tract* or *occipital cortex*.

Pupillary changes are a sensitive indicator of developing intracranial bleeding. Pressure on one side of the brain results in the medial edge of the temporal lobe being pushed through the tentorial hiatus. This compresses the third nerve on the same side in its long intracranial course. The result is *pupillary dilatation* and *loss of the constrictor response to light* on the same side as the lesion.

Unilateral pupillary dilatation may sometimes be associated with injury to the eye itself, but in this case, there is usually a *hyphaema* (bleeding into the anterior chamber) or other obvious eye injury. *Bilateral pupillary dilatation* and loss of the light reflex is an indication of *brain stem injury* i.e. 'coning'.

MANAGEMENT OF MINOR HEAD INJURIES

For most patients presenting with head injury, only two management decisions have to be made: whether to *perform skull X-rays* and whether to *admit to hospital* for observation. Suggested criteria for skull X-rays are shown earlier in Figure 5.9 and for hospital admission in Figure 5.15.

The purpose of admission after minor head injury is to monitor the patient's condition for about 24 hours, during which period the majority of complications, particularly intracranial bleeding, will become apparent. Those who do not need admission should spend the first night with a responsible adult who can return the patient to hospital in the unlikely event of deterioration. A printed sheet with details of warning symptoms and signs should always be given to the accompanying adult.

Fig. 5.15 Criteria for hospital admission after head injury (based on the report of the working party on head injuries, Royal College of Surgeons of England, July 1986)

Confusion or any other depression of conscious level at the time of examination (note: a short period of unconsciousness or amnesia by itself is not a criterion for admission)

Severe headache or vomiting

Any neurological abnormality

Skull fracture

Difficulty in assessing the patient, e.g. alcohol intake, children, epileptics

Poor social circumstances or person living alone

Head injury observations

The essential observations for head injury patients admitted to hospital are shown in Figure 5.16. These are sufficiently sensitive to provide early warning of developing complications. Observations are performed by the nursing staff, the frequency depending on the state of the patient. If there is a skull fracture or any suggestion of confusion, disorientation, alcohol effects or reduced consciousness, observations should be made at 30 minute intervals, at least overnight, but otherwise at hourly intervals. Observations are recorded on a special head injury chart so that deterioration will be immediately obvious and can be reported to the medical staff at once.

Patients with minor uncomplicated head injuries who are fully alert can be safely allowed to go home after 24 hours even if there is a simple skull fracture. Patients should be advised to rest at home for about a week as some cognitive functions such as power of concentration may not completely recover for some days ('*post-concussion syndrome*').

Fig. 5.16 Essential observations for head injury patients

Observation	Sign of neurological deterioration
Pulse rate	Falling pulse rate
Blood pressure	Rising blood pressure
Respiratory pattern and rate	Irregularity, slowing or reduced depth of breathing
Conscious level (Glasgow coma scale)	Falling score
Pupil size and reaction	Dilatation, loss of light reaction or developing asymmetry

MANAGEMENT OF MORE SEVERE HEAD INJURIES

Initial management

Any patient who is unconscious, has focal neurological signs, or whose conscious level is moderately depressed (Glasgow coma score 10 or less) must be considered to have a serious head injury. The patient is resuscitated and a decision made as to whether CT scan and neurosurgical consultation should be sought. The criteria for these are listed in Figure 5.17. Unfortunately, as many district general hospitals (DGHs) do not yet have CT scanning facilities, the patient may require transfer to a regional centre. This must not be done until the patient is fully resuscitated. If the patient is deteriorating rapidly and an extradural haemorrhage is suspected, *burr holes* must be made immediately in the temporal region if the patient's life is to be saved; this emergency procedure should fall within the competence of any general surgeon.

Fig. 5.17 Head injuries: criteria for CT scan and/or consultation with a neurosurgical unit (based on the guidelines of the working party on head injuries, Royal College of Surgeons of England, July 1986)

Fractured skull in combination with any of the following:
- Confusion or other depression of conscious level
- Focal neurological signs
- Fits or seizures

Confusion or other neurological disturbance persisting for more than 12 hours, even if there is no skull fracture

Coma continuing after resuscitation

Suspected compound fracture of the vault or base of the skull

Depressed skull fracture

Deterioration of conscious level or other neurological signs

The management of intracerebral haemorrhage and other major head injury complications is highly specialised. Some patients, however, who have serious primary brain injury but no special neurosurgical requirements, will be returned to the district hospital after CT scan and will therefore remain under the care of general surgeons. Many such patients will have other serious injuries and are ideally nursed and monitored in an intensive care unit with the assistance of anaesthetic staff.

Continuing care

The continuing care of the patient with stable serious brain injury will involve some or all of the following procedures:

- *Intensive monitoring* of vital signs and neurological status
- *Endotracheal intubation* and *artificial ventilation* if hypoxaemic
- *Nasogastric aspiration* of stomach contents, to prevent inhalation, is required for all unconscious patients
- *Monitoring of fluid and electrolyte balance* (hyponatraemia and hypoproteinaemia exacerbate cerebral oedema)
- *Measures to temporarily control raised intracranial pressure* e.g. intravenous *mannitol* (for its osmotic effect in reducing cerebral oedema), or *controlled hyperventilation* (reducing pCO_2 causes cerebral vasoconstriction, reduced cerebral oedema and hence reduced intracranial pressure)

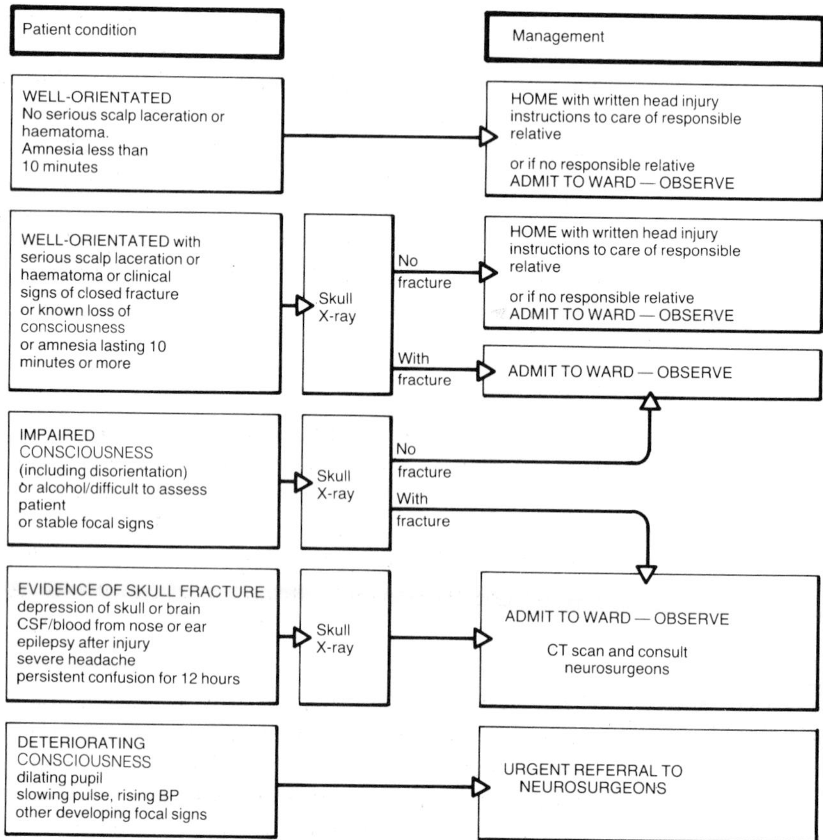

Fig. 5.18 Management protocol for head injury patients

Long-term recovery of intellectual function after serious brain injury is slow and cannot be hastened, although physiotherapy and occupational therapy can aid physical recovery. Patients may easily languish in the community and should therefore be encouraged to join self help groups.

MAXILLOFACIAL INJURIES

GENERAL PRINCIPLES

Fractures of the facial skeleton are common, particularly after sporting injuries, road accidents and fights. The main fractures involve the mandible, the middle third of the face, the nasal bones, the orbit and the zygoma. Facial fractures rarely pose urgent management problems except for major *middle third fractures* (in which the upper jaw becomes detached from the base of the skull), and multiple *mandibular fractures*; both may result in upper airway obstruction, and these patients require endotracheal intubation to safeguard the airway. Facial fractures are generally managed by maxillofacial surgeons, who may not be available in smaller hospitals. In most cases, delaying treatment for a few days does not affect the patient adversely.

Examination for facial fractures

If there is any facial injury, the contour of the facial bones must be carefully palpated before oedema develops as this can obscure underlying bony deformities. As the extraocular muscles may be disrupted by orbital wall fractures, the full range of *eye movements* must be formally examined and the patient questioned about *diplopia* in all positions. The patient should be asked 'if the teeth bite together normally' and the *dental occlusion* examined. Abnormalities of occlusion are a common sign of a jaw fracture, which might otherwise be missed. Similarly, the full range of *mandibular movements* should be checked to exclude fractures or dislocations involving the mandibular condyles.

Radiology

X-rays of the facial bones should be taken if fractures are suspected, the particular view being determined by the bones under suspicion. Interpretation of facial radiographs can be difficult for the non-specialist but most fractures can be identified if the main bony contours are carefully traced and compared with the opposite side. Opacities or fluid levels in the maxillary sinuses usually represent haematoma. This commonly follows fractures of the bones surrounding the maxillary sinuses, e.g. zygoma or orbital floor.

MANDIBULAR FRACTURES

The common sites of mandibular fractures are shown in Figure 5.19. A fracture on one side is often accompanied by a fracture on the other side which is in a different position because of the effects of oblique trauma. Fracture lines tend to occur through points of weakness e.g. mental foramina, unerupted third molar teeth or condylar necks. Most undisplaced mandibular fractures require no active intervention but displaced fractures require fixation. This can be achieved by wiring the lower teeth to the upper teeth or by direct bone wiring. Any fracture passing through a tooth socket defines the fracture as 'compound' and prophylactic antibiotics should therefore be used.

Fig. 5.19

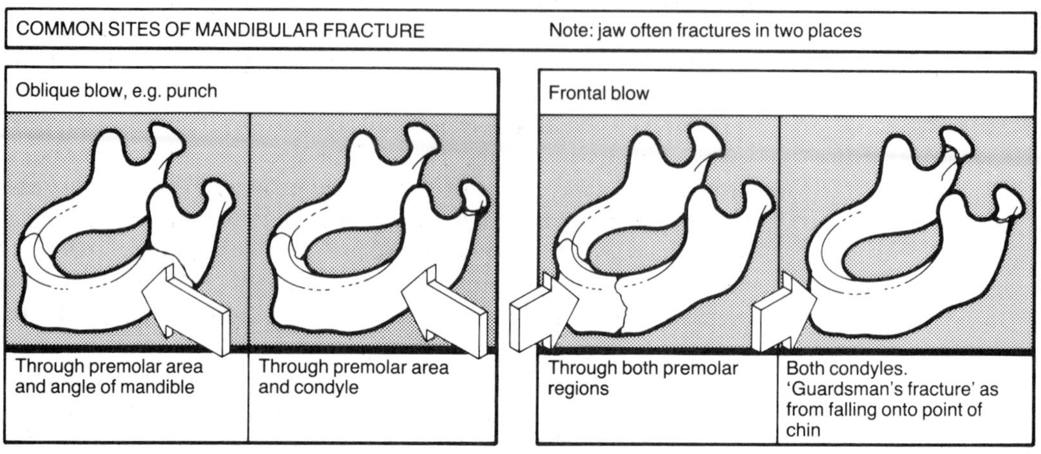

Fig. 5.20 Common sites of mandibular fractures

Oral pantomograph (OPG) showing mandible fractured in two places. Oblique fracture lines can be seen running down from between the left first and second premolars and from the medial root of the right first molar. The fractures have been immobilised by interdental wiring, visible on the teeth in both jaws

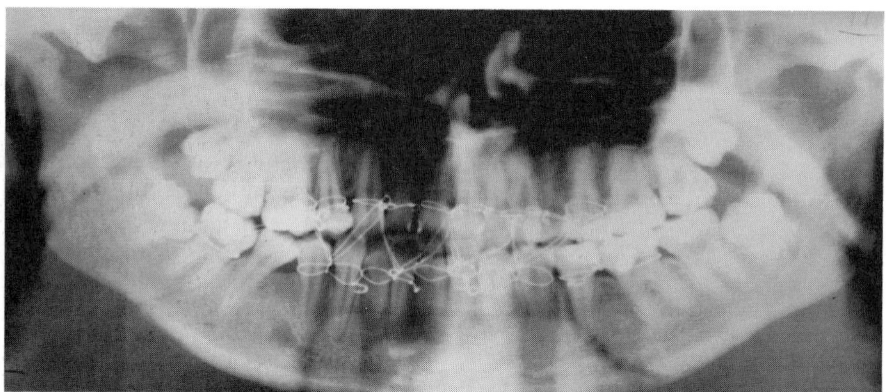

MIDDLE THIRD FRACTURES

Fractures of the middle third of the facial skeleton range from detachment of the palate and dental arch to complete separation of the maxillary complex from the base of the skull. Diagnosis is based on clinical assessment. One of the simplest tests is to grasp the upper teeth or jaw between the fingers and attempt to move it independently of the skull! Treatment may involve disimpaction, and usually requires some sophisticated external fixation to the skull.

FRACTURES OF THE NASAL BONES

Trauma to the nose is extremely common and often results in nasal bone fracture. Less often, fracture dislocations of the septum occur which may interfere with the nasal airways. Diagnosis is made on clinical grounds, the main features being flattening or lateral displacement of the nasal bridge.

Bleeding from the nose often indicates a nasal fracture. Reduction is usually performed several days later by an ENT surgeon.

FRACTURES OF THE ORBIT AND ZYGOMA

Depressed fractures of the zygoma

The most common fracture in relation to the orbit is a depressed fracture of the zygoma resulting from a blow to the cheek. The fracture line usually passes through the *infraorbital foramen* and causes a palpable step in the inferior orbital margin. With any significant degree of depression, the infraorbital nerve becomes compressed, causing paraesthesia or numbness in its area of sensory innervation, i.e. the upper lip, upper teeth and buccal mucosa.

Diagnosis may be suspected by flattening of the cheek contour; this is best seen from above and behind the patient. Overlying oedema may obscure a depressed fracture, and these patients warrant radiological examination. An associated fracture of the lateral orbital wall may produce enough bleeding for it to track forward under the conjunctiva. This subconjunctival haemorrhage has no visible posterior limit, and is the characteristic sign of an orbital wall fracture.

Treatment is indicated if there is inferior orbital nerve compression or a cosmetically unacceptable deformity. Reduction is usually accomplished via a temporal approach, an elevator being slid down under the root of the zygoma, deep to the temporalis fascia.

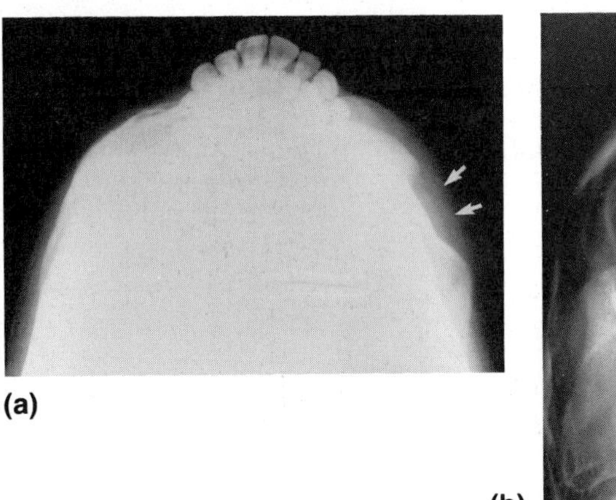

(a)

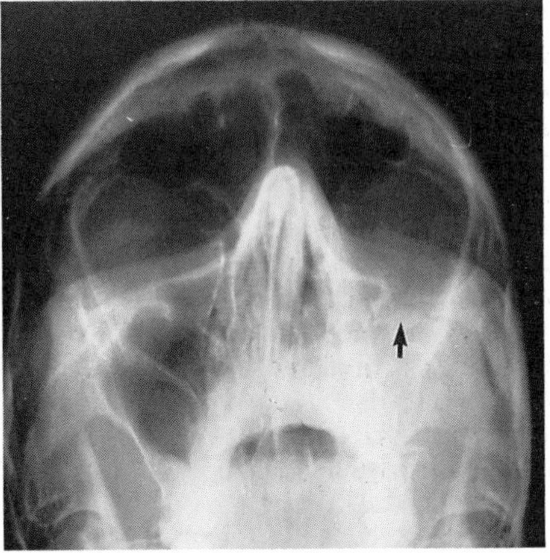

(b)

Fig. 5.21 Depressed zygomatic fractures

(a) Submento-vertical projection of a 43-year-old man who had been punched on the left cheek. This film shows a depressed fracture of the zygomatic arch (arrowed). **(b)** 30° occipito-mental radiograph after a similar injury in a different patient. This patient had a depressed tripod fracture of the zygoma manifest by discontinuity of the lower orbital margin (arrowed). Note that since the roof of the maxilla is involved, the maxillary sinus (antrum) typically fills with blood and is rendered radiopaque

Blow-out fractures of the orbit

A direct frontal blow to the orbit from an object about the size of a squash ball may act like a plunger, causing a 'blow-out' fracture of the orbital wall, without damaging the orbital margin. The blow-out most commonly involves the floor of the orbit where the bony walls are thinnest. This causes herniation of peribulbar fat into the maxillary sinus and disrupts the function of the extraocular muscles, causing *diplopia* and *restricted upward gaze*. Hence the importance of testing eye movements in any patient with a facial injury. Diagnosis is suggested by the finding of an antral opacity (haematoma) on occipitomental X-ray, but tomography of the orbit is required if the bony defect needs to be demonstrated. Treatment involves exploration of the orbital floor and may require a bone graft or silicone implant.

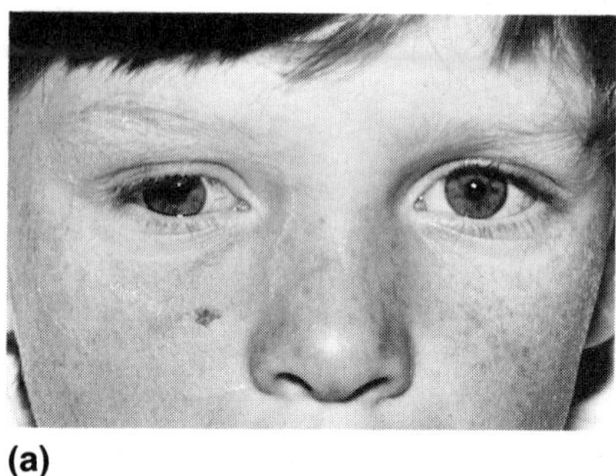

(a)

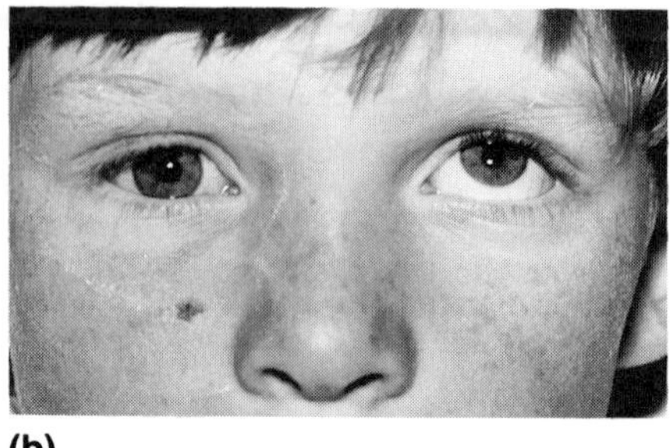

(b)

Fig. 5.22 Blow-out fracture of orbital floor

This 12-year-old boy was punched in the right eye, causing a blow-out fracture of the orbital floor. Note failure of upward gaze on the right in (b) due to trapping of the extraocular muscles in the fractured orbital floor

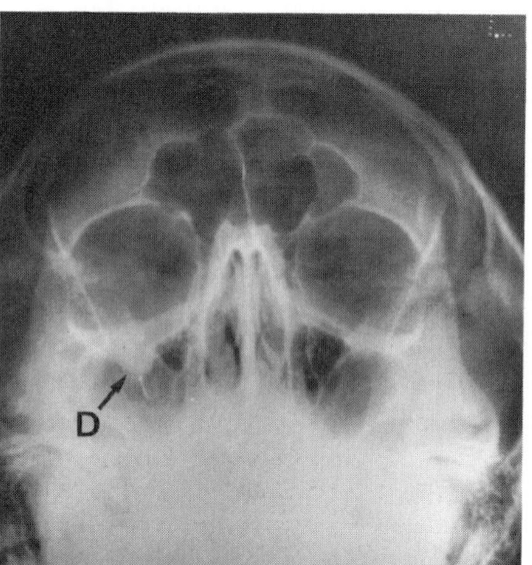

Fig. 5.23 Blow-out fracture of orbital floor

This 30-year-old man was hit in the right eye by a squash ball, causing a *blow-out fracture* of the orbital floor by hydraulic pressure. Orbital fat and extraocular muscles have been forced into the maxillary antrum and held there by the fractured bone edges. This causes the characteristic *hanging drop sign* **D**. Upward gaze is restricted resulting in vertical diplopia

INJURIES TO THE TEETH

Fractures and avulsions of the anterior teeth are common and may require immediate treatment in the accident and emergency department. Correct first-aid treatment may preserve teeth which would otherwise be lost.

Fractures involving the loss of more than a third of the crown should be seen urgently by a dental surgeon as the pulp may be exposed or endangered. Partially avulsed teeth need to be pushed back into position. This can usually be done with the fingers, after local anaesthetic infiltration. Urgent dental referral for tooth splintage is then required.

If a tooth is completely avulsed, it can often be successfully reimplanted by a dentist if the tooth has been carefully cleaned and wrapped in a sterile, saline-soaked swab. Absent or broken teeth in the unconscious patient should alert the examining doctor to the possibility of inhalation or impaction of tooth material in the lips or pharynx. Chest X-ray and examination of the perioral soft tissues should therefore be performed in such cases.

CHEST INJURIES

GENERAL PRINCIPLES

Chest injuries are a common cause of death in the patient with multiple injuries, although the number of deaths has fallen dramatically since the introduction of compulsory wearing of seat belts. Seat belts, however, often cause typical sash pattern bruising obliquely across the chest, and minor rib and sternal fractures.

Serious chest injuries, particularly tearing injuries of the mediastinal contents e.g. aorta, bronchi and oesophagus, may be present even without evidence of external injury. Diagnosis of serious chest injuries goes hand in hand with urgent resuscitative measures. Clinical signs may provide clues to the nature of the injury but the various diagnostic possibilities must all be considered or they may be missed. Good quality chest X-rays are mandatory and will usually clinch the diagnosis.

The types of chest injury, their clinical features and treatment are summarised in Figure 5.24. The main mechanisms of chest injury are penetrating trauma, blunt impact and crush injuries, deceleration injuries and rupture of the diaphragm by abdominal compression. Fewer than 10% of chest injuries require thoracic surgery but early recognition of these patients may save their lives.

Fig. 5.24 Types of chest injury and their management

NATURE OF THE INJURY	CLINICAL FEATURES	TREATMENT
Rib fractures	Localised pain on respiration or coughing; tenderness over fractures; usually visible on chest X–ray	Analgesia, physiotherapy, prophylactic antibiotics in chronic bronchitics.
Flail chest, i.e. multiple rib fractures producing a loose segment	Respiratory embarrassment, 'paradoxical' indrawing of the flail segment on inspiration	Intercostal block anaesthesia; endotracheal intubation and ventilation if hypoxic
Pneumothorax, i.e. air in pleural cavity causing lung collapse	Unilateral signs: loss of chest movement and breath sounds, percussion note resonant; sometimes chest wall emphysema; confirmed by chest X–ray	Intercostal drain with underwater seal
Sucking chest wound, i.e. open pneumothorax with mediastinum 'flapping' from side to side with each respiration	Gross respiratory embarrassment, audible sucking of air through chest wound	Seal chest wound with impermeable dressing; intercostal drainage

Fig. 5.24 Types of chest injury and their management (continued from previous page)

NATURE OF THE INJURY	CLINICAL FEATURES	TREATMENT
Tension pneumothorax, i.e. expanding pneumothorax causing progressive mediastinal shift to the opposite side and tracheal deviation	Signs of pneumothorax with disproportionate and increasing respiratory distress and hypoxaemia	Urgent chest drain
Lung contusion	Deteriorating respiratory function; opacification of affected lung field on chest X–ray	Oxygenation, physiotherapy, artificial ventilation in severe cases
Rupture of bronchus (uncommon)	Respiratory distress, surgical emphysema in the neck; suggested by air in mediastinum on chest X–ray (see Figure 2.15) and confirmed by bronchoscopy	Operation by thoracic surgeon
Rupture of oesophagus (very rare)	May have surgical emphysema in the neck and pneumomediastinum on chest X–ray but diagnosis often missed until mediastinitis or empyema develop	Surgical repair if recognised early but surgical drainage and diversion for a late presentation
Haemothorax, i.e. blood in the pleural cavity usually from a chest wall injury	Dull percussion note, breath sounds absent, tachycardia and hypotension due to blood loss	Urgent intercostal drain, even before chest X–ray (in sixth intercostal space in posterior axillary line), blood transfusion, thoracotomy if bleeding excessive. The usual cause is a ruptured intercostal or internal mammary artery
Cardiac tamponade, i.e. bleeding into pericardial cavity (usually penetrating trauma)	Hypotension, inaudible heart sounds, distended neck veins with systolic waves; enlarged, rounded heart shadow on chest X–ray	Long needle aspiration via epigastric approach; operation if tamponade recurs
Cardiac contusion	May have dysrhythmia or ECG changes similar to myocardial infarction	Conservative management
Rupture of aorta — fatal unless false aneurysm develops in mediastinum (usually results from deceleration injury)	Back pain, hypotension; systolic murmur or signs of tamponade in some cases; characteristic widening of mediastinum on chest X–ray; diagnosis confirmed by arteriography	Urgent thoracotomy and dacron graft
Rupture of diaphragm — linear split usually in left diaphragm with herniation of gut into chest (penetrating or abdominal crush injury)	Respiratory distress, bowel sounds heard in the chest; diagnosis by chest X–ray and confirmed by barium meal	Repair of diaphragm usually via an abdominal approach

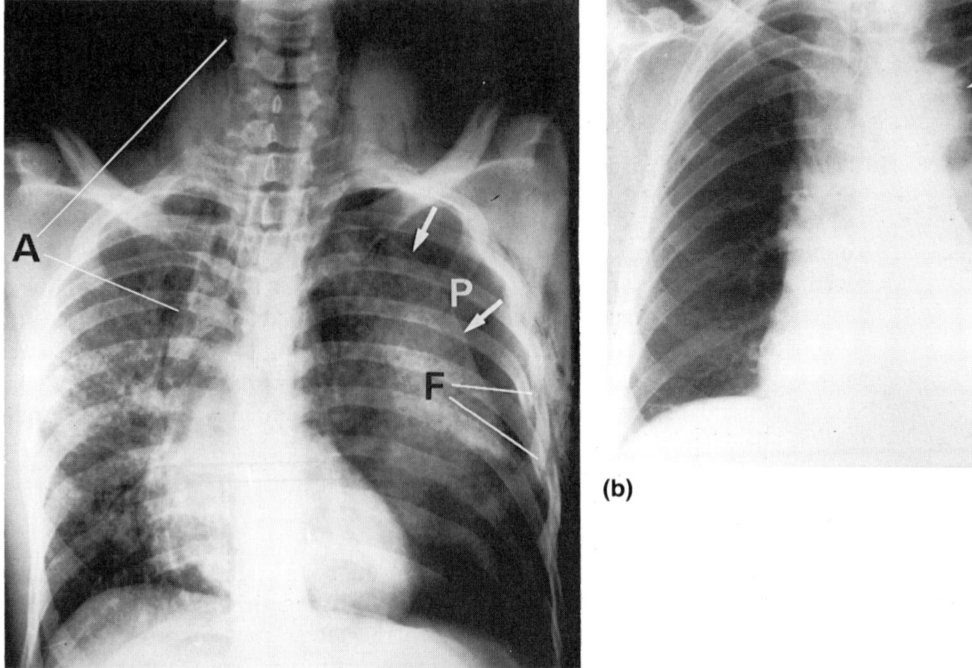

Fig. 5.25 Serious chest injuries

(a) A 20-year-old driver of a car involved in a head-on road traffic accident. He was not wearing a seat belt and his chest hit the steering wheel with great force. The chest X-ray shows multiple rib fractures **F** on the left side, associated with a flail segment which moved paradoxically on breathing. A left pneumothorax **P** is also shown, the lung border being clearly visible (arrowed). Mediastinal shift towards the right strongly suggests a tension pneumothorax; the lung would not be expected to collapse completely because of extensive contusion. Lung contusion on both sides is manifest by the patchy shadowing. There is also a pneumo-mediastinum **A** with air from ruptured alveoli tracking alongside the airways to the mediastinum and thence up into the soft tissues of the neck causing surgical emphysema. **(b)** This chest X-ray was taken following a crushing central chest injury. The patient was well, but the X-ray shows the aortic knuckle has a double shadow **A** and is wider than normal. CT scanning confirmed this was due to a ruptured aortic arch, the blood being contained only by a thin layer of adventitia

ABDOMINAL INJURIES

Compared with head and chest injuries, abdominal injuries are relatively uncommon and mortality is low if management is prompt and appropriate. One of the problems in the management of abdominal injuries is making the diagnosis. Especially after closed injuries, there may be considerable delay between the injury and the development of overt signs of intra-abdominal bleeding or perforation of a hollow viscus. In civilian life, the principle cause of death is uncontrollable bleeding, particularly from bursting injuries of the liver and spleen.

Penetrating abdominal wounds

Penetrating wounds usually result from stabbing or gunshot. The severity of bullet injuries depends to a large extent on the *velocity* of the missile. The essential difference between high- and low-velocity bullet wounds is the *extent and depth of damage*. High-velocity (i.e. rifle) bullet wounds injure widely and deeply. In low-velocity missile wounds (e.g. hand-gun bullets or shrapnel) damage is confined to the tissues in the wound track. The size of the skin wound, however, is no guide to the extent of injury, or to the size of the weapon because of the elastic recoil of skin after injury. For this reason, virtually all penetrating abdominal wounds should be assumed to have breached the peritoneum and caused visceral damage. Buttock wounds may breach the pelvic peritoneum and should be treated in the same way as abdominal wounds.

As a general principle, all penetrating wounds should be explored under general anaesthesia.

Closed abdominal injuries

Closed abdominal injuries usually occur during road traffic accidents, falls and kicking injuries from sportsmen or horses. The *spleen* is the most vulnerable organ, especially in left-sided injuries to the lower chest or upper abdomen (see Figure 5.26). *Liver* injury requires greater impact, usually from the front

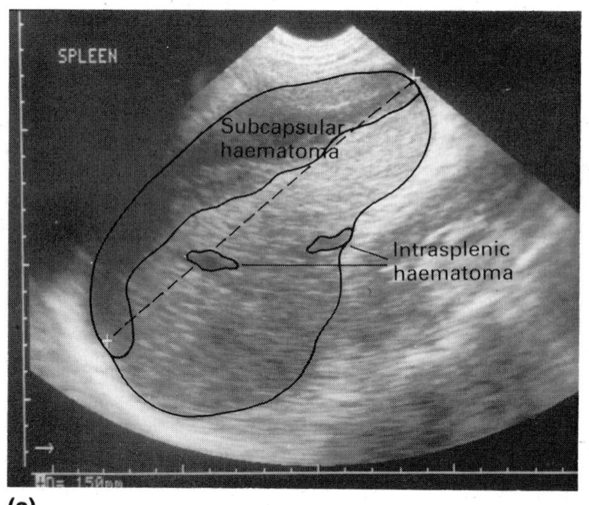

(a)

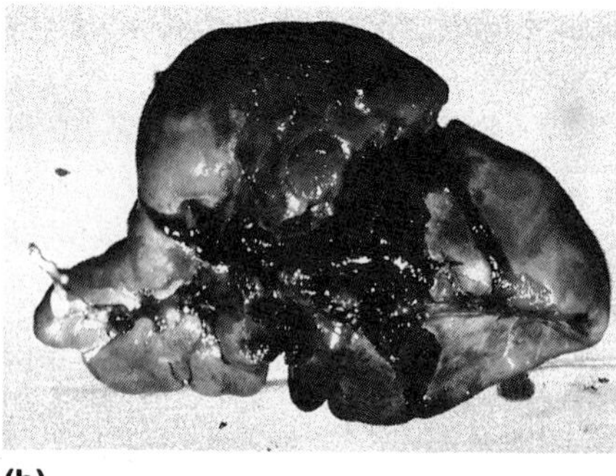

(b)

Fig. 5.26 Ruptured spleen

(a) This 67-year-old woman sustained fractures of the left lower ribs in a fall. She was discharged from hospital the following day but presented again 6 weeks later with abdominal swelling, tenderness and anaemia. This ultrasound scan shows a large subcapsular splenic haematoma, which had presumably developed slowly over the intervening period. She rapidly recovered after splenectomy. **(b)** This 15-year-old girl fell off her pony which then trod on the left side of her chest. She was admitted to hospital with bruising over the lower ribs and a tachycardia. Photograph of the operative specimen; at laparotomy, her spleen was found to be split completely in half and was removed

or right side. *Pancreatic* injuries are uncommon and usually result from a massive central abdominal impact, the pancreas being transected by pressure against the vertebral bodies. The *kidneys* are vulnerable in punches or kicks to the loins.

The *gut* tends to be damaged by deceleration or crushing injuries, tearing in areas where freely mobile bowel is attached to the retroperitoneum, e.g. either end of the transverse colon, duodenojejunal flexure, ileocaecal area. A full *bladder*, commonly found in accidents after heavy drinking, may rupture into the peritoneal cavity after abdominal impact. The bladder and *urethra* are also liable to tearing in displaced pelvic fractures. The clinical features and investigation of closed abdominal injuries are shown in Figure 5.27.

Fig. 5.27 Clinical features of closed intra-abdominal injury

1. History

Substantial trauma to the abdomen
Abdominal pain after trauma
Haematuria following trauma to back or loin

2. Physical signs

Skin bruising immediately after injury — suggests impact of sufficient force to cause internal damage

Imprinting of cloth pattern on skin — implies skin compressed against vertebral bodies

Unexplained hypotension — suggests concealed haemorrhage into the abdominal cavity

Abdominal distension, i.e. increasing abdominal girth — from accumulating blood, urine or gas in the peritoneal cavity

Increasing abdominal tenderness, guarding and rigidity (difficult to assess in the presence of abdominal wall bruising) — may indicate gut perforation or intra-abdominal bleeding

Lateral lower rib fractures — may be associated with injury to spleen, liver or kidney

Pelvic fractures, especially 'butterfly' fractures of all four pubic rami — often associated with bladder or urethral injury, especially in males

Blood at the urethral meatus and inability to pass urine — implies rupture of the urethra, usually at the pelvic diaphragm (urethral catheterisation must not be performed)

3. Investigation options

Chest and plain abdominal X-rays (supine and erect or decubitus views) in all cases may show free intraperitoneal gas, rib and pelvic fractures, retroperitoneal fluid obscuring psoas shadow

Peritoneal lavage (instillation of 500–1000 ml normal saline via peritoneal dialysis catheter which is then allowed to run out) — blood staining indicates intra-abdominal injury but a negative result does not exclude serious injury

Ultrasound (or CT) scanning — particularly useful in investigation of solid organs i.e. spleen, liver, kidneys (see Figure 5.26)

Intravenous urography — investigation of haematuria

Urethrography — investigation of suspected urethral rupture

PRINCIPLES OF MANAGEMENT OF ABDOMINAL INJURIES

If laparotomy is not indicated at the outset, patients with abdominal trauma should be admitted to hospital and closely observed. Nursing observations such as pulse, blood pressure and abdominal girth are made at half-hourly to hourly intervals and the patient should be re-examined regularly by a doctor for signs of visceral injury. Significant injuries will almost always become manifest within 24 hours.

Solid organs

Splenic rupture is treated by urgent splenectomy. In contrast, isolated liver injury may be treated by surgical repair or local resection if the injury is small, but is best treated conservatively if there is major injury. This is because surgery may be incapable of controlling bleeding from torn hepatic vessels deep within its substance, particularly from the hepatic veins which directly enter the inferior vena cava. In conservative management, large volume blood transfusions are given until abdominal tamponade stops the bleeding. If a major liver injury is encountered at surgical exploration of the abdomen, it should be packed with gauze and the abdomen closed. The packs can usually be removed safely about 48 hours later.

Pancreatic transection is treated by surgically removing the distal half and oversewing the stump. A crushing pancreatic injury may have to be treated with just drainage. Renal injuries are usually managed conservatively unless nephrectomy is required for uncontrollable bleeding.

Bowel

Injuries to the small bowel are dealt with by simple suture or if the vascular supply is impaired, by resection and reanastomosis. Large bowel injuries on the right side are treated by resection and anastomosis to small bowel. Localised injuries to the rest of the colon, without substantial intra-abdominal faecal contamination, can usually be resected and joined end-to-end. Extensive injuries with contamination require exteriorisation of the damaged ends, the proximal end as a colostomy and the distal end as a mucous fistula (see Chapter 15).

High-velocity injuries wreak havoc upon the gut, causing extensive devascularisation and multiple perforations; all necrotic or ischaemic tissue must be excised. The immediate danger is fatal peritonitis from gross contamination. Exteriorisation of bowel ends is mandatory.

Lower urinary tract

Intraperitoneal rupture of the bladder is treated by laparotomy and suturing of the bladder, a urethral catheter being left in-situ for about a week until the defect is healed. Extraperitoneal bladder rupture is treated conservatively with prolonged urethral catheterisation. Urethral tears in which the lumen is partly intact (as shown on urethrography) can be treated by catheterisation. Complete urethral avulsion injuries are treated by suprapubic catheterisation and formal repair after local inflammation has settled. Alternatively, an attempt can be made to 'rail-road' a catheter through the disrupted urethra at operation, by passing instruments down the urethra from the bladder and up the urethra from below.

SOFT TISSUE INJURIES

Soft tissue injuries are responsible for many visits to A & E departments. The vast majority are minor injuries which can be dealt with on the spot by the casualty officer. Only a small proportion of patients require hospital admission and many of these have other injuries, particularly fractures or head injuries. Injuries range from minor cuts to deep, contused and dirty wounds. Any wound may contain a *foreign body* which will retard healing and may result in infection. An unrecognised foreign body may also result in litigation!

MANAGEMENT OF SOFT TISSUE INJURIES

The detailed management of any particular injury depends on its site, the tissues involved, the extent of contamination and the possibility of a foreign body. In every case, the danger of *tetanus* must be considered and tetanus toxoid administered if immunisation is inadequate. Deep, soil-contaminated wounds (however small) in an unimmunised patient warrant prophylactic penicillin.

The majority of wounds can be cleaned and sutured immediately but contused or grossly contaminated wounds require debridement and excision of dead tissue. They should either be closed by *delayed primary suture* several days later or, less commonly, allowed to heal by *secondary intention* (see Chapter 3).

Foreign bodies

The history of the injury will provide clues as to the likelihood of a foreign body being present. The main foreign bodies are road dirt and gravel, wood splinters, glass and metal fragments. Radiology will show metal and usually glass. The radiopacity of glass, however, depends on its lead content and a negative X-ray does not exclude its presence.

As a general principle, foreign bodies should be removed, especially if they are organic or likely to be contaminated. Glass and metal fragments are often small, multiple and deeply imbedded. They may be difficult or impossible to locate and extricate despite X-ray diagnosis. In this case, it is inappropriate to embark on extensive exploratory surgery. Rather, the fragments should be left in-situ where they rarely cause much problem; superficial fragments usually work their way to the surface and are shed spontaneously. If such foreign bodies are known to be present, the patient must be informed and this fact recorded in the notes to safeguard against future legal action.

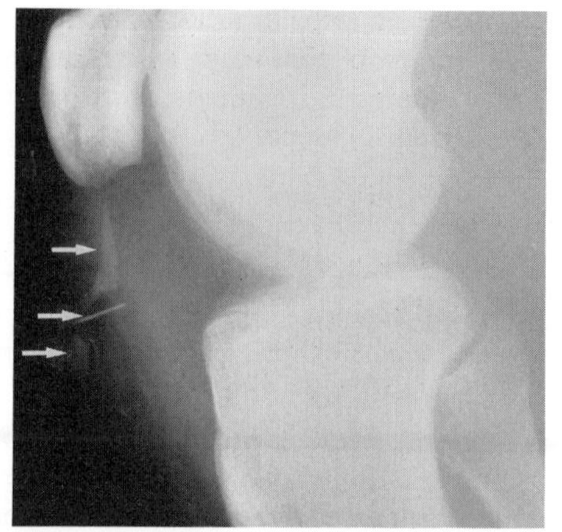

(a)

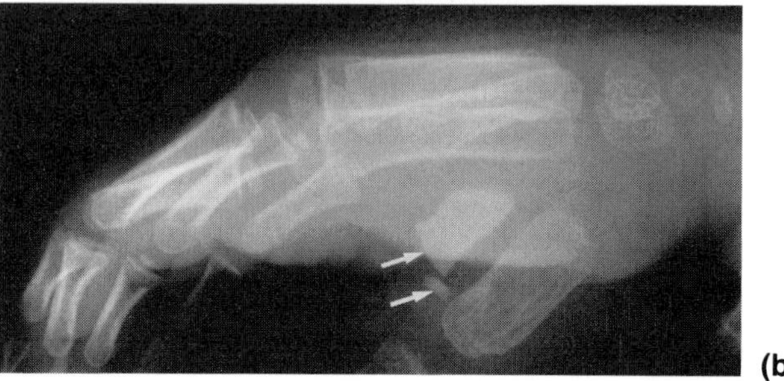

(b)

Fig. 5.28 Glass in soft tissue wounds

(a) A 19-year-old woman with lacerations near the knee after falling onto a broken glass. Note several fragments of glass (arrowed) in the infrapatellar soft tissues. **(b)** Fragments of glass (arrowed) in the palm of a 12-year-old boy after falling through a glass door. In both these cases, the fragments were missed by casualty officers because X-rays were not requested despite a history of glass injury!

Facial lacerations

Facial lacerations heal well. Provided they are cleaned meticulously, they can invariably be primarily sutured; because of the excellent blood supply, infection is rarely a problem. Even ragged skin edges do not become devitalised and trimming is therefore rarely necessary. The main consideration is the cosmetic outcome and therefore great care should be taken with suturing technique, employing general anaesthesia if necessary. Complex lacerations, especially on children and women, should be sutured by a plastic surgeon.

Scalp lacerations

Apart from the possibility of brain injury or skull fracture, the main considerations in dealing with scalp lacerations are haemostasis and whether the aponeurotic layer has been breached. Assessment and proper exploration are difficult without shaving the wound edges; large lacerations should be dealt with under general anaesthesia.

If the aponeurosis is breached, this layer must be sutured separately to prevent formation of a *subaponeurotic haematoma* which is vulnerable to infection. The major scalp vessels lie in the superficial fascia between the dermis and aponeurosis. Dense collagenous bands traverse the superficial fascia and may inhibit vascular contraction and spontaneous arrest of bleeding; these vessels should be individually ligated or sutured. The extent of blood loss from scalp lacerations is easily underestimated and may well be sufficient to cause shock.

Lacerations to the limbs and hands

The main considerations with this type of injury are as follows:

- The possibility of associated nerve, tendon or vascular injury — this necessitates careful assessment of sensation, movement, peripheral pulses and tissue perfusion (i.e. warmth, colour, capillary refilling after blanching)
- Tissue viability — this is particularly important in the case of crush injuries and flap lacerations, especially of the shin
- Risk of infection — the fingers and hands are vulnerable to infection in the *pulp spaces* and *deep palmar spaces*. Such wounds require meticulous exploration, cleansing and antibiotic prophylaxis against staphylococci and streptococci (e.g. flucloxacillin plus ampicillin or amoxycillin). *Gas gangrene* must be considered in the case of large contaminated and contused wounds involving muscle. Dead tissue should be thoroughly excised, benzyl penicillin given prophylactically, and delayed primary closure undertaken. Injuries from *bites* (especially by dogs or humans) and *bones* (usually in meat workers) almost invariably become infected unless antibiotic prophylaxis is given (e.g. flucloxacillin plus ampicillin or amoxycillin)

PRINCIPLES OF RE-PLANTATION SURGERY

Complete amputation of digits is common, especially in industrial accidents, but sometimes whole limbs are severed. With clean-cut injuries, it is possible to reattach the amputated part using microsurgical techniques to join the vessels and nerves. This cannot be done in crush or avulsion injuries or in grossly contaminated wounds. Even in ideal cases, recovery is slow and usually incomplete, necessitating many months away from work. Therefore, replantation should never be undertaken without careful evaluation of the real benefits. In digital amputation, the greatest disability results from loss of the thumb. There is no place for replantation of a single finger, even the index finger, because the remaining fingers rapidly adapt to the loss.

The indications for replantation are as follows (there must be no major crushing or degloving injury):

- Loss of whole upper limb or hand
- Loss of thumb alone
- Loss of all digits (replant thumb and one or two fingers)
- Loss of all fingers (replant one or possibly two fingers)

At the scene of the injury, the severed digit should be washed and placed in a plastic bag which is then immersed in ice. In this way it can be successfully preserved for up to 12 hours.

BURNS

Burns and scalds are common injuries, resulting in 12 000 hospital admissions annually in England and Wales. Many times this number are treated on an outpatient basis. Two-thirds of burns occur in the home, the rest largely occurring in industrial accidents. The vast majority are preventable. Young children and the elderly are at greatest risk of sustaining burns and also suffer disproportionate mortality from them. Among the most common burns are those involving toddlers who pull containers of hot fluid down over themselves from cookers and tables. These result in scalds to the outstretched arm, face, neck and front of the chest (see Figure 5.29).

PATHO-PHYSIOLOGY OF BURNS

Fig. 5.29

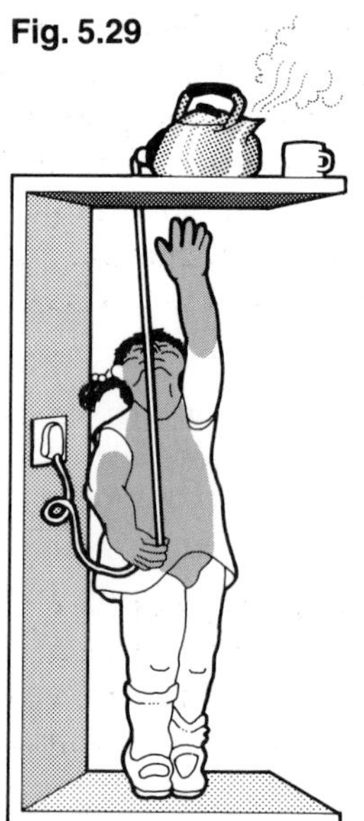

Typical pattern of burns in young children.
The child pulls a teapot or cup of hot liquid from a table or when being held by a seated adult.
The area shaded pink is typically burned

1. Thermal burns

For thermal burns of the skin, the depth of tissue destruction is an important determinant of outcome. Skin burns are divided into partial or full thickness. *Partial thickness burns* are those in which epidermal elements are spared, allowing spontaneous healing without skin grafting. In deep partial thickness burns, the only epithelial remnants may be hair follicles and sweat glands which extend into the hypodermis; thus with deep burns, the regeneration is slower.

Full thickness burns are those in which all epidermis has been destroyed. Skin grafting is usually necessary because epithelialisation from the margins is slow and prone to complications, particularly infection, fibrotic scarring and contractures. The extent of damage caused by a thermal burn is not only related to the temperature of the burning agent but also to the duration of contact. Water at a temperature of only 45°C, if applied for long enough, will cause full thickness burns (scalds). This is often the mechanism of tragic burns in childhood.

Loss of the epidermis removes the barrier to evaporation of body water, and evaporation is exacerbated by exudation of protein-rich inflammatory fluid. Large volumes of fluid can be lost, but the amount depends on the area and not the depth of the burn. In large burns, vasoactive amines from the inflammatory response are released into the general circulation. These cause a generalised increase in capillary permeability, increasing the volume of plasma lost from the circulation. Burns involving 15% or more of the body surface in adults and 10% in children result in hypovolaemia sufficient to cause shock.

Extensive epidermal loss and the presence of necrotic tissue place the patient at particular risk of *infection*. The main organisms are Strep. pyogenes during the first week and Pseudomonas aeruginosa thereafter. Pseudomonas septicaemia is responsible for considerable mortality, even in this antibiotic era.

2. Electrical burns

Electrical burns are caused by the conversion of electrical energy into heat, and the severity of burning is proportional to the electrical resistance of the tissue through which the current is transmitted. Bone offers the highest resistance. If current passes through a limb, the bones become heated and nearby structures such as muscle and blood vessels suffer greatly. Consequently, the extent of damage is often much greater than is immediately apparent. Deep tissue necrosis may not become clinically apparent until some days after an electrical burn.

3. Inhalational injuries

Respiratory and systemic damage from inhalation of hot air, smoke and toxic gases (e.g. carbon monoxide or cyanides from burning upholstery) is a major cause of death and complications even when skin burns are slight. The heat of inhaled gases is often sufficient to cause inflammatory oedema of the oral, nasal and laryngeal mucosa or even serious burns. In addition, noxious gases injure the lung parenchyma, resulting in pulmonary oedema, atelectasis and secondary pneumonias.

ASSESSMENT OF THE BURNED PATIENT

The history should include information about the source of the burn, the temperature and the duration of contact, and whether there was any inhalation of noxious gases. The percentage of skin area burned must be estimated accurately for purposes of fluid replacement. The usual method is the '*rule of nines*' and is illustrated in Figure 5.30. Another method is to compare the burned area with the patient's palm, which is equivalent to about 1% of total body area. The depth of burn is often difficult to assess at the time of presentation. Signs of partial thickness burns are skin redness with blanching to finger pressure and normal pinprick sensation; charred skin or thrombosed skin vessels invariably indicates a full thickness burn.

Fig. 5.30

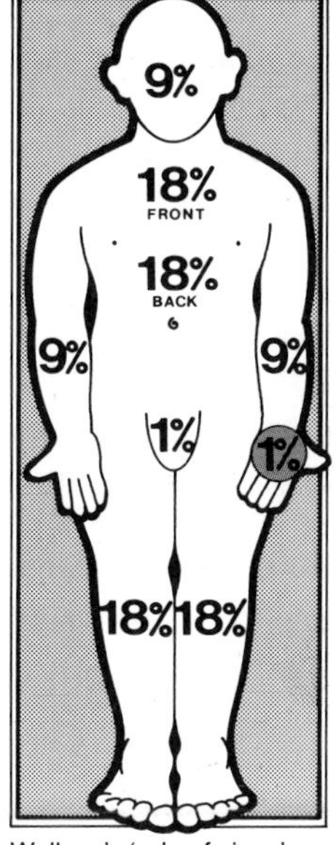

Wallace's 'rule of nines' for estimating percentage of skin surface area burned. A useful alternative estimate is that the area of the patient's own palm is approximately 1% of total skin area

PRINCIPLES OF MANAGEMENT

One of the first management decisions is whether the patient requires hospital admission. The criteria are summarised in Figure 5.31. Patients with extensive burns, i.e. involving more than 30% of body surface, should generally be transferred to a specialist burns unit as soon as initial treatment has been carried out.

Fig. 5.31 Criteria for hospital admission after burns

Adults with burns involving 15% or more of total skin area, and children with 10% or more
Full thickness burns
Circumferential burns on the limbs
Suspicion of inhalation of hot gases or smoke
Burns to face, hands, feet or perineum (difficult to manage at home)
Electrical burns

Outpatient management of minor burns

The main objective is to prevent dehydration and infection of the burn site. Any blisters are punctured and a non-stick antiseptic dressing applied. Tulle gras (paraffin gauze) impregnated with chlorhexidine or povidone-iodine may be used or alternatively *silver sulphadiazine* cream (e.g. Flamazine). Either dressing is then covered by a thick absorbent layer of gauze and wool or gamgee. Burns on the fingers and hands are best managed with a liberal coating of silver sulphadiazine cream, the hand then being enclosed in a plastic bag. The patient should be reviewed at least every second day and skin slough excised as it separates. Partial thickness burns re-epithelialise within 14–21 days. If this does not occur, they are full thickness burns and will require skin grafting.

Application of the dressing gives considerable relief from pain but even minor burns are extremely painful and require prescription of suitable analgesia.

MANAGEMENT OF EXTENSIVE BURNS

The main aspects of early management of serious burn victims are fluid replacement, assessment and treatment of respiratory problems and local management of the burns.

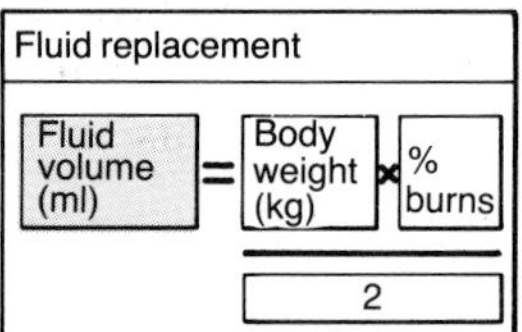

Example

Fluid replacement regimen in first 36 hours for 70 kg man with 20% burns

Fluid volume = 70 × 20 / 2 = 700 ml

Theoretical fluid loss

Rate of i.v. infusion

1st 700 ml given i.v. | 2nd 700 ml | 3rd 700 ml | 4th 700 ml | 5th 700 ml | 6th 700 ml

0 12 24 36

Hours elapsed since burns sustained

Fig. 5.32 Serious burns – a method for estimating fluid requirements over the first 36 hours (after Muir and Barcley)

Fluid management

As previously described, adults with 15% body involvement and children with 10% lose sufficient fluid to be at risk of hypovolaemic shock. Most fluid is lost in the first 12 hours but substantial fluid loss continues for at least another 36 hours. Since much of the fluid lost is essentially plasma, the mainstay of fluid replacement is 4.5% human albumin (formerly known as PPF), while the remainder is isotonic electrolyte solutions, e.g. Hartmann's solution.

Fluid requirements should be calculated by reference to a well-tried formula, such as that of Muir and Barcley, shown in Figure 5.32. With this formula, the anticipated fluid loss in each of the three 4-hour periods immediately following the burn is half the product of the percentage area of the burn and the body weight in kilogrammes; by way of example, for a 20% burn in a 70 kg patient, 700 ml fluid replacement is a reasonable estimate for each of the first three 4-hour periods. After the first 12 hours, this volume is again administered in each of the next two 6-hour periods and then over the following 12-hour period. Fluid balance must also be monitored according to pulse, blood pressure and urine output. For the last, catheterisation is usually necessary in the extensively burned patient.

Management of inhalational injuries

If there is a history of possible smoke or gas inhalation, the patient must be carefully examined for evidence of soot or skin burning around the mouth, nostrils and throat. These usually indicate serious inhalation injury. Investigations include chest X-ray, blood gas and carbon monoxide estimations and fibre-optic bronchoscopy.

Treatment involves administration of humidified air by mask and antibiotics to prevent chest infection; a course of high dose steroids may help to limit inflammatory pulmonary damage. The development of pulmonary oedema and hypoxia may signal the need for endotracheal intubation and artificial ventilation.

Local management of the burn

The principles of local management of extensive partial thickness burns are the same as for minor burns. Full thickness burns will require *skin grafting* at some stage. Fingers, eyelids and genitalia nearly always require primary grafting so on after injury. In specialist centres, smaller burns are excised and grafted at the outset before infection can develop. Otherwise grafting is usually delayed for two weeks or so and then performed, often in several stages, provided the wounds are clear of infection.

Full thickness *circumferential burns* of the limbs and thorax begin to contract early and may restrict blood flow and respiratory movements; should these signs develop, a procedure known as *escharotomy* is performed, involving incision of the eschar longitudinally down to bleeding tissue.

Long-term problems

Even after grafting, full thickness burns across joint flexures, including the neck, may undergo such severe fibrotic contraction that movement is seriously limited. This difficult problem may require multiple plastic operations.

PART III
SYMPTOMS, DIAGNOSIS AND MANAGEMENT

6 NON-ACUTE ABDOMINAL PAIN AND OTHER ABDOMINAL SYMPTOMS

Introduction

Diagnosis and management of abdominal complaints form an important part of the surgical outpatient workload, although the proportion of abdominal problems varies from one centre to another depending on the availability of a medical gastroenterology service. Only a proportion of patients with abdominal complaints eventually need hospital admission or operation, the remainder being investigated and treated as outpatients. Figure 6.1 shows a typical case mix in a general surgical outpatient clinic.

Fig. 6.1 Types of case referred to general surgical outpatient clinics (Note: the conditions in bold type are discussed in this chapter)

Breast disorders	15%
Varicose veins	15%
Minor skin lesions	15%
Suspected lower limb ischaemia	15%
Hernia/scrotal/preputial disorders	10%
Vasectomy	7%
Haemorrhoids/other anal complaints	**7%**
Abdominal pain including gallstones and peptic ulcer	**7%**
Change in bowel habit	**3%**
Head and neck including thyroid and salivary glands	3%
Minor surgical conditions in children including phimosis, inguinal hernia and undescended testis	3%

The diagnoses which emerge from outpatient referrals are quite different from emergency diagnoses. Nevertheless, the clinician must remain alert for unfamiliar presentations of common acute disorders, e.g. an appendix mass.

The principal presenting symptoms of non-acute abdominal disorders are abdominal pain, difficulty in swallowing (dysphagia), loss of appetite (anorexia), weight loss, nausea and vomiting, changes in bowel habit, and anal or perianal symptoms. In addition, patients are often referred to the surgeon after the discovery of an abdominal mass, obstructive jaundice or an iron deficiency anaemia caused by chronic blood loss. The history provides the most important clues to diagnosis and should therefore be taken accurately and with great care.

This chapter provides a problem-solving approach to interpreting non-acute abdominal symptoms and signs. The following chapter then deals with acute abdominal problems. Chapters 8–18 then describe the important clinical entities, and their diagnosis and management from a more disease-oriented perspective.

Although examination of the groin and (male) genitalia are essential parts of a complete abdominal examination, problems in these areas are usually identifiable as such from the history; for this reason, they are considered separately in Chapter 19. Similarly, urinary tract disorders usually present with symptoms which are obviously urological; these problems are discussed in Chapters 20–25. Abdominal pain or an abdominal mass may, however, be the only clinical feature of a urinary tract lesion (e.g. renal adenocarcinoma in adults, urinary tract infection in children). Thus, the possibility of a urinary tract disorder must be remembered when formulating a differential diagnosis.

Fig. 6.2 Main presenting features of non–acute abdominal disorders

Abdominal pain
Difficulty in swallowing (dysphagia)
Weight loss, anorexia and associated symptoms
Change in bowel habit, including rectal bleeding
Anal and perianal symptoms
Iron deficiency anaemia
Obstructive jaundice
Abdominal mass or distension

PAIN

Nature of the pain

Pain is described by patients in many different ways, although each pathological entity tends to have its own pain characteristics. The pattern will only come to light if a meticulous history has been compiled. Pain is, however, a highly subjective phenomenon and the history will be coloured by the patient's own perception of the pain and its possible significance. Patients often use vague terms such as 'indigestion' and 'dyspepsia' to describe upper abdominal pain or discomfort associated with food, and what the patient actually means must be clarified in each case. These terms should have little place in medical terminology. The key points to be covered in taking a history of abdominal pain are summarised in Figure 6.3.

The *site of origin* of the pain suggests the anatomical structures most likely to be involved. These are shown in Figure 6.4. The *distribution* and *radiation* of the pain provide further clues. Pain that extends through to the back suggests involvement of retroperitoneal structures, e.g. pancreas (carcinoma or chronic pancreatitis) or abdominal aorta (aneurysm). Gall bladder pain tends to radiate from the right hypochondrium around to the back on the right side. Renal pain tends to radiate from the loin down towards the groin and occasionally to the genitalia.

Diseases causing non-acute abdominal pain

The following conditions cause non-acute abdominal pain; each has certain characteristic features:

- *Gallstones and gall bladder dysfunction* — long-standing grumbling ('nagging') pain, often with short-lived, more severe episodes. Usually located in the right upper quadrant, less often in the epigastrium. May radiate to the back

Fig. 6.3 Assessing abdominal pain from the history

Location of pain — e.g. central, epigastric, right or left subcostal (hypochondrial), in right or left iliac fossa, suprapubic, 'lower abdominal', or loin pain. Is pain well or poorly localised (i.e. is parietal peritoneum with its somatic innervation involved)? Is there any radiation of the pain?

Severity and character of pain — e.g. discomfort, moderate or severe pain? What descriptive words are used by the patient: 'sharp', 'blunt', 'burning', 'crushing', 'deep', 'gnawing', 'boreing', 'bloating', 'knife-like', 'stabbing'? How much does the pain affect normal living? Could the pain be physiological (e.g. pre-defecation colic or dysmenorrhoea) or pathological? Are there any changes in the character of the pain with time?

Variation of pain severity with time — e.g. constant, intermittent, 'colicky' (i.e. coming in waves), background pain with exacerbations, episodic

Duration of pain — i.e. when did the pain really begin?

Periodicity — e.g. weekly, monthly, hourly. Daytime or night-time? Any periods free from pain? Any previous similar episodes or attacks?

Exacerbating and relieving factors — e.g. improved or made worse by food, posture or drugs?

Associated symptoms — e.g. vomiting, change in bowel habit

on the right. Often precipitated by rich or fatty foods and may be associated with vomiting

- *Peptic ulcer disease* — typically intermittent 'boreing' epigastric pain (although retrosternal 'burning' pain in peptic oesophagitis) which recurs several times a year and lasts for days or weeks at a time. The association with food varies according to the site of the disease: duodenal ulcer pain tends to be relieved by bland food and recurs three to four hours afterwards, typically in the early hours of the morning, whereas the pain of gastric ulcer and oesophagitis tends to be aggravated by food, especially if acidic or spicy. Peptic pain is generally relieved by antacids and virtually always by H2 antagonist drugs, e.g. cimetidine

Fig. 6.4 Anatomical significance of the site of abdominal pain

Right upper quadrant	Biliary tract, liver
Epigastric	Usually foregut structures, i.e. stomach, duodenum, lower oesophagus, biliary tract, pancreas (cardiac pain can also present in the epigastrium)
Left upper quadrant	Rarely directly related to anatomical structures, occasionally spleen or stomach
Central	Midgut structures, i.e. small and large bowel or pancreas (deep pain radiating to the back)
Right iliac fossa	Caecum and appendix (when parietal peritoneum is involved), ovary, right kidney and ureter, mesenteric adenitis
Suprapubic	Bladder, uterus and adnexae
Left iliac fossa	Sigmoid colon, left kidney and ureter
Loins	Kidneys and ureters

- *Chronic pancreatitis and carcinoma of pancreas* — typically severe 'gnawing', persistent, poorly localised central pain which usually radiates through to the back. The pain is often associated with anorexia and weight loss. The pain may be relieved by leaning forwards. Early carcinoma of the pancreas, however, is often painless

- *Irritable bowel syndrome, constipation, diverticular disease and Crohn's disease* — these conditions may all produce partial obstruction of the bowel which is manifest by episodes of colicky pain. This is poorly localised, often 'bloating' pain of highly variable intensity and is often associated with transient disturbances of bowel function; passage of flatus or stool often temporarily relieves the symptoms

- *Renal outflow obstruction by stone, tumour or fibrosis* — 'dull', poorly defined, fairly constant loin pain which may be accompanied by typical urinary tract symptoms e.g. haematuria and dysuria. Often aggravated acutely by a high fluid intake

- *Gynaecological conditions, particularly chronic pelvic inflammatory disease and ovarian tumours* — these may reach the surgeon because of poorly defined lower abdominal pain. Gynaecological history is important and pelvic examination may reveal the cause

- *Non-surgical* (i.e. 'medical') disorders causing abdominal pain include liver congestion in heart failure (common), splenic infarcts or diabetes (both uncommon but important), porphyria or tertiary syphilis (very rare). Patients with various psychological disturbances sometimes present with abdominal pain for which no organic cause can be found despite extensive investigation. Unnecessary operations may be performed on these patients (*Munchausen syndrome*)

Note: non-acute abdominal pain in children is uncommon; the main organic causes are constipation, grumbling appendicitis and sometimes hydronephrosis. The 'periodic syndrome' is characterised by recurrent episodes of poorly defined and inconsistent abdominal pain, sufficiently severe for the child to avoid school. There are no other consistent features; psychological and environmental factors are the usual underlying cause.

Approach to the investigation of non-acute abdominal pain

A differential diagnosis must first be made on clinical grounds. The choice (and order) of numerous possible investigations should be efficient and economical. Their aim should be to support or eliminate the most probable (and common) diagnoses. Rarer diagnoses will need further investigation.

The following example shows the diagnostic pathway in a patient presenting with chronic epigastric pain:

i. Once the main complaint has been stated, a preliminary differential diagnosis forms in the clinician's mind, even before a detailed history is taken. Acid-peptic disorder of oesophagus, stomach or duodenum or, alternatively, gall bladder disease are statistically the most likely. Irritable bowel syndrome, and angina pectoris are less likely.

ii. A detailed history and direct questioning strengthens the possibility of certain diagnoses and diminishes the likelihood of others; rarer conditions such as chronic pancreatitis might now enter the differential diagnosis.

iii. Physical examination may add further weight to one diagnosis over another. The clinician will be particularly seeking signs of anaemia, jaundice, tenderness or a mass.

iv. A narrower and weighted set of diagnostic probabilities will by now have evolved which will form the basis for planning special investigations.

v. If the most likely diagnosis is acid-peptic disorder, either gastroscopy or barium meal examination will be considered, although if the symptoms are mild, a diagnostic trial of antacid therapy might be more appropriate. A full blood count is performed if anaemia is suspected and, if confirmed, specimens of faeces are tested for occult blood. If biliary tract disease seems most likely, cholecystography or ultrasound of the upper right quadrant is performed.

vi. By this stage, investigation will usually have confirmed or eliminated the most likely diagnoses. If no diagnosis has been confirmed, alternative diagnoses are considered, probably at a subsequent visit, by further history taking and examination. Symptoms and physical signs may have persisted unchanged, they may have changed or may even have resolved completely during the period of investigation. Changed symptoms may suggest new diagnostic possibilities and new lines of investigation. If the symptoms have decreased, a less serious disorder such as irritable bowel syndrome might become the working diagnosis and a trial of treatment initiated. Further investigation will depend on the patient's response to either treatment or reassurance.

DYSPHAGIA

Clinical presentation

Dysphagia is the term used to describe difficulty in swallowing. The most common symptom is inability to swallow solid food, which the patient will describe as 'becoming stuck' or 'held up' before either passing on into the stomach or being regurgitated. The patient usually reports that particular types of food are more difficult than others; fibrous foods, such as meat, usually cause the most trouble. The patient can usually indicate a precise level for the perceived obstruction. The true level of obstruction is usually some way below that point.

Dysphagia is almost always caused by disease in or adjacent to the *oesophagus*, but occasionally the lesion is in the *pharynx* or *stomach*. Oesophageal narrowing usually causes symptoms only when the lumen is unable to expand beyond a diameter of 11 mm — the narrower the lumen, the more severe the symptoms. In many of the pathological conditions causing dysphagia, the lumen becomes progressively constricted and indistensible. Initially only fibrous solids cause difficulty but later the problem extends to all solids and even later to fluids. Because narrowing is an insidious process, patients often compensate to a suprising degree (e.g. by liquidising all food) and may only present when they have difficulty in swallowing fluids or even their own saliva. By this time there is usually marked weight loss.

The common causes of dysphagia are outlined in Figure 6.5. *Pain on swallowing* (usually provoked by both food and drink, particularly if hot) is a distinctive symptom which is highly suspicious of carcinoma.

Fig. 6.5 Causes of dysphagia

Obstruction arising in the oesophageal wall

Peptic oesophagitis or fibrous stricture (often associated with hiatus hernia) — common

Carcinoma of oesophagus or cardia of the stomach — common

Pharyngeal pouch — extremely rare

Oesophageal web (Plummer–Vinson syndrome) — extremely rare

Leiomyoma of the oesophageal muscle — extremely rare

Disorders of muscle function

Achalasia — uncommon

Pseudobulbar palsy — rare

External compression of the oesophagus

Sub-carinal lymph node secondaries from carcinoma of the bronchus — common

Left atrial dilatation in mitral stenosis — rare

Dysphagia lusoria (compression from abnormal great vessels) — very rare

Achalasia is a major exception to the usual pattern of dysphagia, in that swallowing of fluids tends to cause more difficulty than swallowing solids. In achalasia, there is idiopathic destruction of the parasympathetic ganglia in *Auerbach's* (submucosal) *plexus*, which results in functional narrowing of the lower oesophagus and peristaltic failure throughout its length. Thus the oesophagus becomes markedly distended and dilated, solids settling towards the lower end, with fluids spilling over into the airways, causing *spluttering dysphagia*. This overspill tends also to occur when the patient is lying flat at night. Achalasia often presents with chronic chest infection rather than dysphagia.

Bolus obstruction is an acute form of dysphagia, where a lump of food sticks at a narrow part, completely obstructing the oesophagus.

Approach to investigation of dysphagia

Dysphagia, particularly of recent onset, must be regarded seriously and fully investigated. A plain *chest X-ray* should be taken to exclude bronchial carcinoma; occasionally an oesophageal fluid level behind the heart may be seen due to an oesophageal stricture from hiatus hernia or achalasia. The next investigation is usually a *barium swallow and meal*, although some clinicians prefer *fibreoptic endoscopy* (oesophago-gastro-duodenoscopy or OGD). When a lesion has been demonstrated radiologically, endoscopy allows direct inspection and biopsy to confirm (or change) the diagnosis. In disorders of function, swallowing of barium-soaked bread or a cinematographic record of a barium swallow may be helpful in reaching a diagnosis.

WEIGHT LOSS, ANOREXIA AND ASSOCIATED SYMPTOMS

Marked weight loss (*cachexia*), and loss of appetite (*anorexia*) are frequently manifestations of serious, insidious, often malignant abdominal disorders. They may be associated with a variety of other symptoms such as malaise, bloating, nausea, sporadic vomiting and regurgitation. Such symptoms may have been unnoticed or have been dismissed as trivial by the patient and are only elicited by direct questioning.

The diseases which cause these symptoms may be grouped into three broad categories:

- Intra-abdominal malignancies, e.g. carcinoma of stomach or pancreas, metastatic disease in the liver or peritoneum (arising particularly from stomach, large bowel, ovary, breast or bronchus), bowel lymphomas
- 'Medical' conditions, e.g. alcoholism and cirrhosis, viral diseases (e.g. hepatitis or infectious mononucleosis), diabetes, thyrotoxicosis, malabsorption, renal failure
- Psychiatric disorders, e.g. depression, anorexia nervosa

Approach to investigation of weight loss, anorexia and associated symptoms

In many patients, there may be other clinical clues to the main diagnosis or line of investigation, e.g. pain, signs of anaemia or jaundice, or a palpable abdominal mass. More difficult are those cases where the symptoms occur alone. In this situation, basic screening investigations (full blood count and ESR, urea and electrolytes, liver function tests and urinalysis) begin to differentiate 'medical' conditions from 'surgical' ones. If these screening tests fail to produce a lead, abdominal ultrasound or CT scanning may be indicated to exclude an occult intra-abdominal malignancy.

If investigations still reveal no cause, a psychological cause should be seriously considered. Before such a diagnosis can be accepted, there must be positive evidence of psychiatric disturbance. In practice, by this stage, previously concealed psychiatric features often become apparent.

CHANGE IN BOWEL HABIT, RECTAL BLEEDING AND RELATED SYMPTOMS

Normal bowel habit varies widely between different individuals in both frequency of defecation and consistency of stool. For the individual, transient changes in bowel habit are usually insignificanct but persistent change often leads to the patient seeking medical advice. Departure from the norm may have several different aspects, occuring in various combinations.

1. Frequency of defaecation and stool consistency

Chronic constipation or diarrhoea mark the extremes of change, although some patients develop an erratic pattern of bowel action. All may signify serious disease and deserve investigation. The index of suspicion is further raised if there is rectal bleeding or tenesmus. Waking from sleep to evacuate the bowels should be treated seriously, especially if it occurs frequently.

Stool consistency varies according to diet, but the stool is usually 'formed'. Persistently unformed stools, i.e. 'looseness', is only abnormal if it represents a change from the patient's usual habit.

a. Constipation

Constipation arises for three main reasons:

- There may be incomplete bowel obstruction. This may be caused by faecal impaction, an obstructing carcinoma or stricture in the bowel wall, or occasionally an extrinsic lesion such as ovarian cancer
- Constipation may be caused by loss of peristalsis, e.g. due to drugs such as codeine or iron, diverticular disease, chronic laxative abuse and inactivity
- Inadequate fibre intake may decrease faecal volume and prolong intestinal transit time

b. Diarrhoea

Chronic diarrhoea is most often caused by irritation or inflammation of the small or large bowel. The inflammatory bowel diseases (ulcerative colitis and Crohn's disease) are important diagnoses. Chronic parasitic infestations of the large bowel with amoeba or giardia are easily overlooked, but in such patients there is often a history of foreign travel. Less commonly, a *blind loop* of small bowel remaining after bypass surgery becomes colonised with gut flora, causing chronic inflammation (*blind loop syndrome*).

Bile salts irritate the bowel. Therefore if the enterohepatic circulation is disrupted, e.g. after distal small bowel resection, defective reabsorption of bile salts may cause diarrhoea. A less common cause of diarrhoea is the increased volume of bowel contents in malabsorption syndromes. Finally, when no physical cause can be found, concealed laxative abuse or an anxiety state should be considered.

c. Erratic bowel habit

Some patients develop an erratic bowel habit with bouts of constipation interspersed with episodes of frequency and looseness of stool. The most common cause is irritable bowel syndrome, which can be attributed to large bowel spasm followed by excessive peristalsis. In diverticular disease, constipation and 'rabbit-pellet' faeces are the dominant characteristics but there may be episodic diarrhoea, often during periods of inflammation. This may be caused by intermittent release of partially obstructed faeces. Incomplete bowel obstruction, as may occur in carcinoma of the left colon, Crohn's disease or faecal impaction, may cause *spurious diarrhoea*. This occurs when proximal liquefied stool overflows past the obstruction.

Fig. 6.6 Differential diagnosis of change in bowel habit

Carcinoma of colon, rectum or anus
Diverticular disease
Irritable bowel syndrome
Crohn's disease in small or large bowel
Ulcerative colitis
Drug effects, e.g. codeine phosphate, iron, laxative abuse
Change in fibre content of diet
Parasitic infestations, e.g. giardiasis
Bacterial infection or overgrowth
Malabsorption syndromes
Thyrotoxicosis

Note: in many cases, no cause is found

2. Nature of the stool

Stools are normally brown due to the presence of *stercobilinogen*, a breakdown product of bile. In biliary obstruction, stools therefore become pale and are often described as 'putty coloured'. This is usually associated with obvious jaundice. Stools may also be pale when they contain excess fat, as occurs in various malabsorption syndromes. In coeliac disease (*gluten enteropathy*) the stool is often loose and offensive, and this is known as *steatorrhoea*. In malabsorption, the stools tend to float due to the excessive fat content and the patient has difficulty flushing them away.

Undigested food in the stool indicates failure of digestion and absorption. This can be normal when the diet is extremely high in fibre. It may, however, indicate malabsorption or a 'short-circuit' in the bowel due to previous bowel resection or a fistula between bowel loops.

3. Presence of frank blood, altered blood or mucus in the stool

a. Frank rectal bleeding

When a patient has seen blood in the stool, a careful history should be taken of colour, i.e. fresh or altered blood, and also the relationship of the blood to the stool. Blood alone may be passed, or it may appear before or after the stool. There may be blood mixed in with the stool or coating it.

Bright red blood usually indicates a lesion in the rectum or anus. When blood is clearly separate from the stool it suggests an anal lesion, most commonly haemorrhoids but occasionally proctitis or a carcinoma. If the blood is on the surface of the stool it suggests a lesion further proximal in the rectum or descending colon such as a polyp or carcinoma.

When blood is mixed with the stool, it usually indicates even more proximal disease. This is usually in the left side of the colon or occasionally the transverse colon. Carcinoma or inflammatory ulceration are often the cause. In such cases the blood, being 'older', is darker. When the blood originates further proximally in the gastrointestinal tract, e.g. peptic ulcer or caecal cancer, it is so altered by 'digestion' that it may not be recognised as blood by the patient. The stool is typically shiny black or plum-coloured. In rapid bleeding from stomach or duodenum, the stools become fluid and are described as 'tarry'.

This is known as *melaena* and has a characteristic foul odour. Patients on iron therapy will have greenish-black, formed stools which should not be mistaken for altered blood.

b. Occult faecal blood loss

A persistent trickle of blood from the gastrointestinal tract may not alter the appearance of the stool. This 'occult' blood may only be detectable in the laboratory. Despite the small daily quantities involved, this insidious blood loss can cause serious iron deficiency anaemia.

c. Rectal passage of mucus or pus

Mucus ('slime') or pus may be passed alone or with the stool. Patients rarely volunteer this information, but will report it when asked. Villous adenomas typically secrete copious mucus, but this may also occur with frank carcinoma of the rectum. Mucus and pus may be noted in the inflammatory bowel diseases and occasionally in diverticular disease. An anal leak of mucus may be a feature of haemorrhoids and causes itching (pruritus ani). A patient will sometimes report passing a mass of purulent material. This usually represents spontaneous discharge of a perianal or pararectal abscess, and will often have been preceded by anal or perineal pain.

4. Tenesmus

Tenesmus is an unpleasant sensation of incomplete evacuation of the rectum. The sensation causes the patient to attempt defaecation (often with straining) at frequent intervals. The most common cause is an abnormal mass in the rectum or anal canal. This may be a carcinoma, polyp or thrombosed haemorrhoid. Occasionally a prostatic carcinoma invades around the lower rectum producing tenesmus. Despite extensive investigation, no cause is found for tenesmus in some cases. The cause could be psychosomatic but an organic lesion may become apparent later.

Approach to investigation of change in bowel habit

The first step in investigation is *sigmoidoscopy* (rectoscopy). This permits direct visual examination and biopsy of the mucosa up to the rectosigmoid junction; most large bowel lesions responsible for altered bowel habit occur in this region. In the case of chronic diarrhoea, stool specimens should be examined for ova and parasites and cultured for *Shigella* and *Salmonella* species.

Further investigation will be based on the differential diagnosis assembled during clinical examination, but barium enema X-rays will be indicated in the majority of cases. Note that low rectal lesions cannot be reliably demonstrated on barium enema and preliminary sigmoidoscopy is mandatory. If Crohn's disease is suspected, barium studies of the small bowel may also be required.

Flexible fibreoptic endoscopes of different lengths are used to examine the colon above the rectosigmoid junction. The shortest, the *fibreoptic sigmoido-*

scope, requires minimal bowel preparation and can be used in the outpatient clinic. An excellent view can be obtained as far as the splenic flexure, allowing examination of the area in which 70% of large bowel cancers occur. The longer instruments, *colonoscopes*, require prior bowel clearance with laxatives. They tend to be reserved for detailed inspection and biopsy of lesions already demonstrated or suspected on barium enema. Since colonoscopy is a time consuming and rather unpleasant procedure, patients usually require intravenous sedation and analgesia, and sometimes general anaesthesia. Therefore colonoscopy patients are usually admitted to hospital for the procedure, if only for the day.

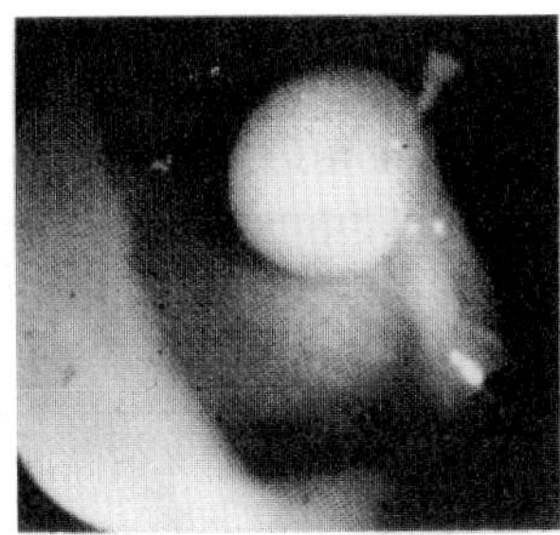

Fig. 6.7 Colonoscopic appearance of a polyp in sigmoid colon

This 1-cm polyp was found to be the cause of rectal bleeding. It was easily removed with a snare soon after this photograph was taken.

ANAL AND PERIANAL SYMPTOMS

Anal symptoms generate a large number of surgical outpatient referrals. Symptoms include bleeding and discharge, pain and itching, local swelling, and a sensation of 'something coming down'. They cause distress out of proportion to their pathological importance. The most common diagnoses are haemorrhoids, anal fissures and local abscesses, although the occasional infiltrating anal carcinoma or low rectal carcinoma or polyp must not be overlooked.

1. Anal bleeding

This is an extremely common symptom. It is well tolerated by patients who usually believe that 'piles' (haemorrhoids) are responsible. Patients often present when the bleeding becomes excessive or when new, different symptoms develop. The characteristic feature of anal bleeding is fresh blood separate from the stool which may only be seen 'on the paper'. Fresh bleeding, however, may arise from malignancy in the rectum, sigmoid colon or anal canal and must be treated seriously. All patients require at least sigmoidoscopy, and patients over 40 require barium enema examination to exclude large bowel cancer, whether or not a benign anal cause, such as haemorrhoids, has been found.

2. Anal pain and discomfort

The principal causes of anal pain and discomfort are anal fissure and haemorrhoids. Haemorrhoids cause anal discomfort rather than severe pain, unless they become strangulated or thrombosed, at which time they present as an acute problem.

Intermittent severe perianal pain following defecation usually indicates a fissure-in-ano. This is a longitudinal tear in the posterior anal mucosa ending externally in a characteristic 'sentinel pile', a small skin tag visible at the posterior anal margin. An anal fissure is often initiated by unaccustomed constipation.

A perianal abscess may be responsible for anal pain even before the abscess is clinically detectable, and the rare intersphincteric abscess may elude detection for weeks. Anal carcinoma is usually painless but may present with haemorrhoid-like pain. The difference is obvious on rectal examination.

3. Perianal itching and irritation

The most common cause of these symptoms is inadequate hygiene resulting in local skin irritation, often exacerbated by scratching or application of various topical medications. The discharge associated with haemorrhoids, fistulae or tumours tends to keep the perianal skin moist, predisposing to low-grade fungal and bacterial infections. The longer such symptoms persist, the more difficult they are to eradicate and in fastidious patients a 'fixation' can develop. In children, threadworm is a common cause of perianal itching; the itching is usually worse at night.

4. 'Something coming down'

Haemorrhoids, skin tags (the residuum of past haemorrhoids) and occasionally mucosal or rectal prolapse cause this symptom. It is exacerbated by defecation. Many patients tolerate the condition for some time before seeking medical advice and may routinely push the lumps back manually after defecation, presenting only when this becomes impossible. A low rectal pedunculated polyp may occasionally come through the anus and be confused with prolapsed haemorrhoids. Perianal warts are occasionally mistaken for lumps arising in the anus itself.

5. Perianal discharge

A perianal discharge results from leakage of pus, inflammatory exudate or mucus from the anus or anal area. Pus may arise from a pilonidal sinus in the natal cleft or from a fistula-in-ano. Inflammatory exudate and excess mucus may be produced by haemorrhoids, ano-rectal mucosal inflammation (*proctitis*), a villous adenoma or an ulcerating carcinoma.

Approach to investigation of anal and perianal symptoms

Proctoscopy is mandatory and should be conducted after inspection and digital rectal examination. If these examinations are impossible due to pain, a young patient can usually be assumed to have a fissure. In an older person, carcinoma of the anus must be excluded by examination under anaesthesia. Haemorrhoids appear as bulging blueish masses beneath the anal mucosa. They all arise above the squamo-columnar junction or dentate line ('internal piles') but may later extend beneath the perianal skin ('external piles') or prolapse through the anus.

A typical anal fistula appears as an inflammatory 'nipple' near the anal margin; often it exudes a discharge. A pilonidal sinus arises in the natal cleft and usually presents as a swelling with one or more associated sinuses, often with hairs protruding. In proctitis, the rectal mucosa is granular and reddened when seen on proctoscopy, and often bleeds to the touch (friability). An anal or low rectal carcinoma is a discrete ulcerated lesion with an indurated (firm, woody) base and a thickened margin. Diagnosis is confirmed by histological examination of a biopsy taken with special forceps.

The lymphatic drainage of the anal canal below the dentate line is to the inguinal lymph nodes and these should always be examined when an anal lesion is found.

IRON DEFICIENCY ANAEMIA

A common reason for surgical referral is persistent or severe anaemia believed to be caused by chronic blood loss. The patient may have presented initially with symptoms of chronic anaemia, namely lethargy, generalised weakness, breathlessness or even angina. Just as often, the anaemia has been recognised during general examination or on routine blood count.

Chronic anaemia has many causes. Iron deficiency is the commonest and is the only one with a cause likely to be amenable to surgical treatment. In blood films, iron deficiency anaemia is characterised by hypochromic, microcytic red

Fig. 6.8 Conditions causing chronic occult blood loss

Lesions in the gastrointestinal tract

Ulcerating tumours or polyps of the following (in order of frequency): caecum, stomach, the rest of the large bowel, and (rarely) connective tissue tumours of small bowel, e.g. leiomyosarcoma

Chronic peptic ulceration, i.e. hiatus hernia with reflux oesophagitis, gastric and duodenal ulcers, stomal ulceration following gastric surgery. All may be induced or aggravated by ingestion of aspirin and other non-steroidal anti-inflammatory drugs. These drugs can also cause chronic gastric haemorrhage from superficial erosions

Other 'ulcerating' lesions of the bowel, e.g. haemorrhoids, angiodysplasias of colon or small bowel

Chronic parasitic infestations, e.g. hookworm (extremely common in some underdeveloped countries)

Lesions in the urinary tract

Transitional cell carcinoma of bladder, pelvicalyceal systems or ureters

Renal adenocarcinoma (commonly causes haematuria but rarely iron deficiency anaemia)

Chronic parasitic infestations, e.g. schistosomiasis (common in underdeveloped countries)

Lesions in the female genital tract

Heavy menstrual loss (menorrhagia is an extremely common but easily overlooked cause)

Carcinoma of uterus or cervix (usually presents as abnormal vaginal bleeding rather than anaemia)

blood cells. Serum iron level is low and iron binding capacity (*transferrin*) elevated. Iron deficiency anaemia can be caused by chronic low grade blood loss (which is often occult), inadequate dietary iron intake or absorption, or a combination of both. In some patients, the pattern of iron deficiency may be complicated by a coexisting anaemia of another cause, particularly the 'anaemia of chronic illness'. For example, an elderly patient with rheumatoid arthritis may have a chronic normochromic, normocytic anaemia due to chronic disease, as well as an iron deficiency anaemia caused by gastric bleeding secondary to non-steroidal anti-inflammatory drugs.

Approach to investigation of anaemia

Investigation of a patient with suspected iron deficiency anaemia has five main components:

- History — seeking sources of blood loss from the various tracts and excluding inadequate dietary iron intake. Previous gastrectomy resulting in diminished acid output, may prevent adequate iron absorption
- Physical examination — seeking an abdominal mass or signs of a 'medical' cause
- Confirmation of iron deficiency anaemia and exclusion of common 'medical' causes of anaemia such as rheumatoid disease or chronic leukaemias — analysis of blood film, ESR, serum iron and iron binding capacity. When there is a 'mixed' anaemia, measurement of iron stores on a marrow biopsy is the definitive method of diagnosing iron deficiency
- Testing of specimens of urine and stool for occult blood (at least three stool specimens should be tested)
- Pursuing clues that suggest the origin of bleeding by using special investigations such as contrast radiography and endoscopy. When occult blood is found in the faeces, double contrast barium enema is usually performed first. If negative, it is followed by a barium meal or gastroscopy (enema precedes meal to avoid carry-over of contrast). If these are negative or unsatisfactory, it may be appropriate to repeat one or all of them before proceeding to colonoscopy (particularly looking for angiodysplasias) and small bowel contrast radiography. In the case of occult haematuria, the minimum investigation is cysto-urethroscopy and intravenous urography
- Occasionally, gastrointestinal bleeding continues, even though all investigations appear normal. The next step is often to repeat the appropriate investigations. If they are still negative and if bleeding becomes acute, radioisotope scanning, using the patient's own radiolabelled red cells may show the general area of bleeding, as labelled blood leaks into the lumen and accumulates there. Selective mesenteric angiography may be more precise, but the patient must be actively bleeding at the time of the examination. If bleeding is slower, but serious enough to merit operation, the whole small bowel may be examined by operative endoscopy. The small bowel is opened and a colonoscope threaded along its full length, transilluminating the bowel in the process. Only by this means can angiodysplasias be located.

OBSTRUCTIVE JAUNDICE

Patients with jaundice usually reach the surgeon after a provisional diagnosis of obstructive jaundice has been made. There is often evidence that the obstruction involves the bile ducts.

The normal enterohepatic circulation

The *haem* component of spent red cells is normally broken down to *bilirubin* (mainly in the spleen and bone marrow) and then transported to the liver bound to albumin. In the liver, bilirubin is conjugated making it water soluble, and it is then excreted in bile; the level of *conjugated bilirubin* in the blood is normally very low. Bacterial action in the bowel converts the conjugated bilirubin to urobilinogen. Some of this is oxidised to stercobilin which imparts the brown colour to normal faeces. Some urobilinogen however is reabsorbed, passing to the liver in the portal blood. It is then re-excreted in the bile. The entire process is called an *enterohepatic circulation* (see Figure 6.9). A small amount of urobilinogen escapes into the systemic circulation and is excreted in the urine.

Bile acids (salts) are synthesised in the liver from cholesterol-based precursors. Excreted in the bile to the duodenum, they facilitate lipid digestion and absorption in the small intestine. In the distal ileum, 95% of the bile acids are reabsorbed, returning to the liver in the portal vein, only to be re-excreted in the bile. Thus the enterohepatic circulation involves both bilirubin and bile acids.

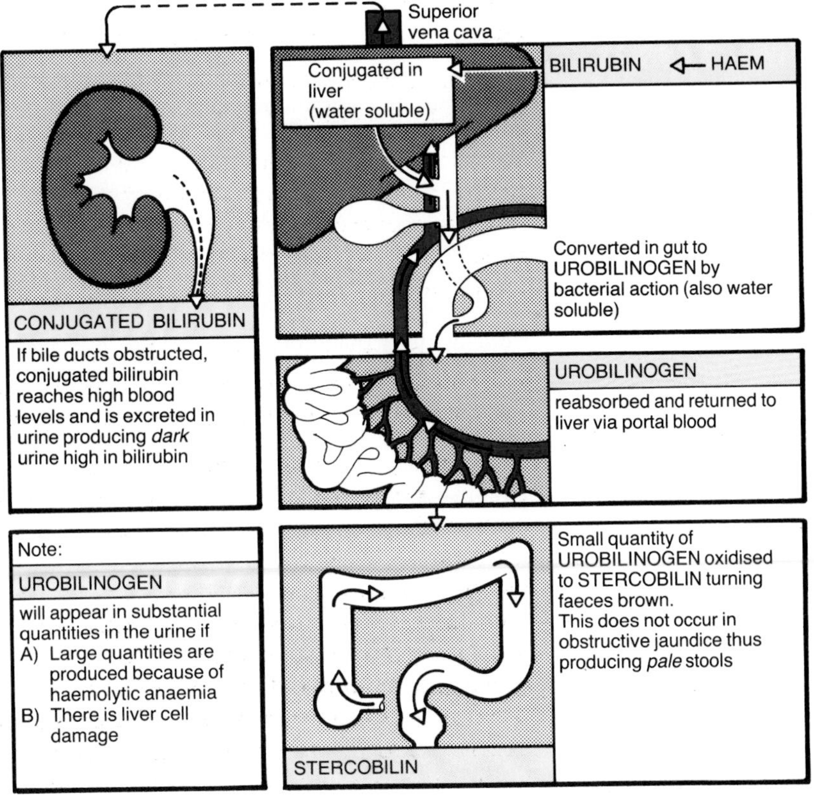

Fig. 6.9 Dynamics of bilirubin in obstructive jaundice

Pathophysiology of obstructive jaundice

If biliary outflow becomes obstructed, conjugated bilirubin is dammed-back in the liver, where it enters the blood stream and causes an insidious rise in serum bilirubin. Once the serum bilirubin level exceeds about 30 μmol/l, jaundice should be clinically detectable. Above 60 μmol/l, jaundice is obvious. Conjugated bilirubin, being soluble, is excreted in the urine, turning it dark. The presence of bilirubin in the urine, and an indication of its concentration, is easily established by ward dipstick testing. Significant quantities usually mean biliary obstruction.

With the diminished or absent excretion of bile into the gut in obstructive jaundice, there are changes in the faeces. There is less stercobilin to darken the stool, and there is less bile acid, which results in defective fat absorption. The two combine to give the stool a characteristic 'putty' colour.

Malabsorption of vitamin K is a particular consequence of poor dietary fat absorption and leads to decreased hepatic synthesis of clotting factors, notably prothrombin. Clotting impairment is not so great as to cause spontaneous haemorrhage or bruising, but there is a significant risk of haemorrhage at surgery or during liver biopsy. The biliary obstruction also dams back bile acids. These become more concentrated in the blood and are deposited in the skin, often causing intense itching.

Biochemically, obstructive jaundice is manifest by an elevated level of serum bilirubin, which is predominantly in the conjugated form. There is marked elevation of serum alkaline phosphatase (liver isoenzyme) which is derived from bile canaliculi, but the transaminases, derived from hepatocytes, are usually

Fig. 6.10 Conditions causing obstructive jaundice

Stones in the common bile duct (very common) — suggested by the presence of pain or a history of pain typical of gall stones. Jaundice may be progressive (if a stone is firmly impacted), fluctuant without ever disappearing altogether (if a stone alternately impacts and disimpacts), or intermittent (if multiple stones successively impact then pass through the lower end of the common bile duct)

Carcinoma of the head of the pancreas (common) — typically painless jaundice which is persistent or progressive. The gall bladder may be palpable (Courvoisier's law, see Figure 6.11)

Periampullary tumours i.e. of ampulla, bile duct or duodenum (uncommon) — clinical features similar to carcinoma of head of pancreas

Benign strictures of the common bile duct may be due to surgical damage or previous stone (uncommon) — clinical features similar to carcinoma of head of pancreas

Other malignant tumours may cause bile duct obstruction above the ampulla, e.g. secondaries in the porta hepatis (fairly common), cholangiocarcinoma (uncommon), carcinoma of the gall bladder (rare)

Intrahepatic bile duct obstruction, e.g. by cholangiocarcinoma, liver secondaries, cirrhosis, sclerosing cholangitis (all rare)

Intrahepatic cholestasis is diagnosed when jaundice is obstructive but the duct system is normal. Idiosyncrasy to certain drugs interferes with bile excretion from hepatocytes, presumably by affecting membrane transport. These drugs include chlorpromazine, oral contraceptives and chlorpropamide. Hepatic lymphoma is another classic, but rare, cause of intrahepatic cholestasis

only mildly elevated. When the biliary obstruction is from an intrahepatic cause (e.g. cholangiocarcinoma obstructing only one duct) there may be a mixed biochemical picture with evidence of hepatocyte damage as well as duct obstruction.

History and examination in patients with obstructive jaundice

History taking should enquire about episodes of pain suggestive of gall stone disease, episodes of obstructive jaundice which resolved spontaneously, or biliary tract surgery. Attacks of recurrent pancreatitis also suggest gall stone disease. A history of anorexia, weight loss and non-specific upper gastrointestinal disturbances is common in carcinoma of the pancreas, especially likely in the elderly. Inflammatory bowel disease predisposes to sclerosing cholangitis although this is very rare.

Several special points are important when examining the jaundiced patient. Early jaundice is a subtle physical sign and will be missed unless the patient is examined in a good light, preferably daylight. Jaundice is first detectable in the conjunctivae and soon afterwards in the smooth skin of the abdominal wall. In some cases of obstructive jaundice, the patient develops generalised itching (pruritus), and scratch marks may be apparent. The general stigmata of liver disease such as spider naevi and liver 'flap' are only found when jaundice is caused by primary liver disease rather than extrinsic obstruction.

The abdomen should be examined particularly for ascites, an enlarged liver or spleen, abnormal masses or a palpable gall bladder. An enlarged liver may be caused by primary or secondary malignancy. Splenomegaly with hepatomegaly is an important sign of chronic parenchymal liver disease, usually cirrhosis, and indicates portal hypertension. Ascites, in a patient with obstructive jaundice, is almost always due to disseminated intra-abdominal malignancy. *Courvoisiers 'law'* (Figure 6.11) states that obstructive jaundice in the presence of a palpable gall bladder is not due to stone (and is therefore likely to be caused by tumour). The argument is that gall stones cause chronic inflammation and fibrosis of the gall bladder, thus preventing its distension. (More likely, intermittent stone obstruction leads to muscular hypertrophy of

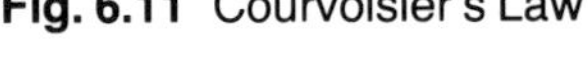

Fig. 6.11 Courvoisier's Law

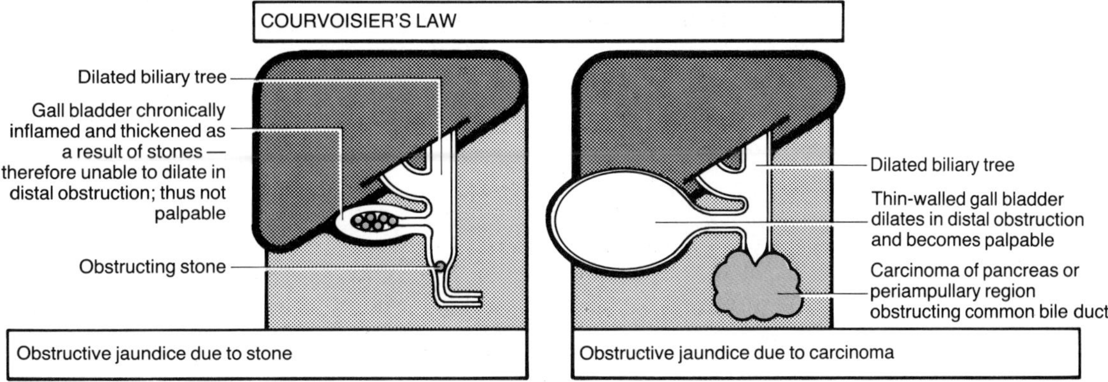

the gall bladder which prevents distension). In malignancy, progressive obstruction occurs over a short period, and the gall bladder distends easily.

At rectal examination, particular attention is paid to the colour of the stool, a pale stool being characteristic of obstructive jaundice. The urine should also be inspected in obstructive jaundice. It is dark yellow or orange from the presence of conjugated bilirubin, and froths when shaken due to the detergent effect of bile acids.

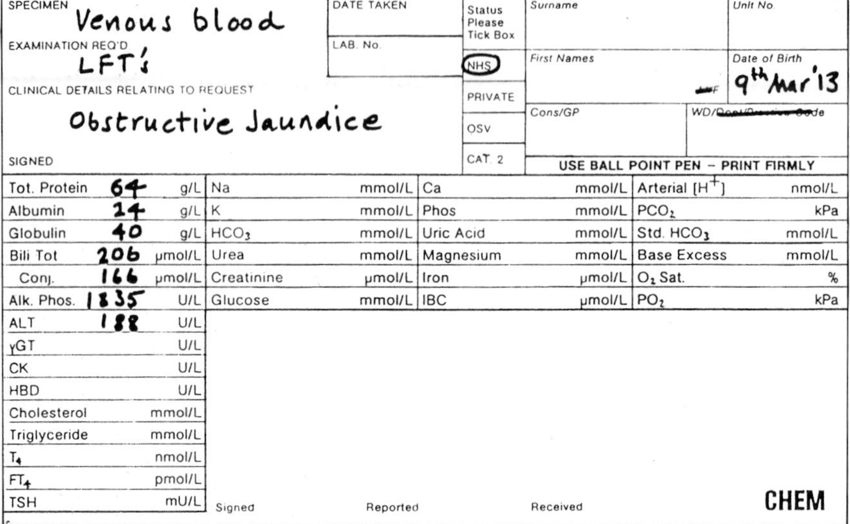

SPECIMEN Venous blood
EXAMINATION REQ'D LFT's
CLINICAL DETAILS RELATING TO REQUEST Obstructive Jaundice
SIGNED
DATE TAKEN
LAB. No.
Status Please Tick Box: NHS (circled) / PRIVATE / OSV / CAT. 2
Surname
Unit No.
First Names
Date of Birth 9th Mar '13
Cons/GP
WD/
USE BALL POINT PEN – PRINT FIRMLY

Tot. Protein 64	g/L	Na	mmol/L	Ca	mmol/L	Arterial [H⁺]	nmol/L
Albumin 24	g/L	K	mmol/L	Phos	mmol/L	PCO_2	kPa
Globulin 40	g/L	HCO_3	mmol/L	Uric Acid	mmol/L	Std. HCO_3	mmol/L
Bili Tot 206	µmol/L	Urea	mmol/L	Magnesium	mmol/L	Base Excess	mmol/L
Conj. 166	µmol/L	Creatinine	µmol/L	Iron	µmol/L	O_2 Sat.	%
Alk. Phos. 1835	U/L	Glucose	mmol/L	IBC	µmol/L	PO_2	kPa
ALT 188	U/L						
γGT	U/L						
CK	U/L						
HBD	U/L						
Cholesterol	mmol/L						
Triglyceride	mmol/L						
T_4	nmol/L						
FT_4	pmol/L						
TSH	mU/L	Signed		Reported		Received	CHEM

Fig. 6.12 Typical liver function test result in obstructive jaundice

Approach to investigation of jaundice

Jaundice is usually investigated step by step as follows:

- Exclude hepatitis B by screening for the surface antigen of the virus (HBsAg). Other antigen and antibody tests may be carried out if suspicion of infective hepatitis is high
- Confirm that the jaundice is obstructive by means of liver function tests. Obstructive jaundice is characterised by a predominance of conjugated bilirubin and a high alkaline phosphatase level (liver isoenzyme); transaminase levels are only moderately elevated
- Hepatobiliary ultrasound is the simplest means of demonstrating dilated intrahepatic ducts, liver secondaries, a dilated extrahepatic biliary system or gall bladder abnormalities including stones. Ultrasound may also reveal the cause of obstructive jaundice to be a tumour in the head of the pancreas or enlarged lymph nodes in the porta hepatis. CT scanning may be the next stage if the findings are equivocal. It is particularly useful for demonstrating tumours
- If ultrasound demonstrates dilated ducts, endoscopic retrograde cholangiopancreatography (ERCP) is the investigation of choice if it is available.

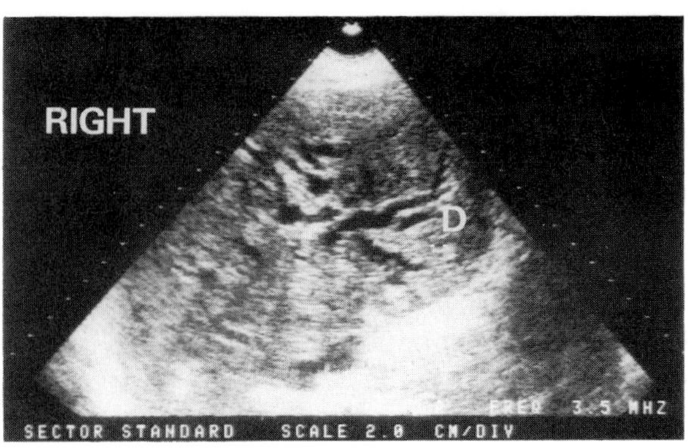

Fig. 6.13 Ultrasound showing dilated intrahepatic ducts

An ultrasound scan in an 80-year-old man with obstructive jaundice. This transverse section through the liver shows the characteristic *double-barrel shotgun* sign, **D**, with two parallel tubular structures representing major branches of the bile duct and portal vein. Normally, the portal vein is four times wider than the corresponding bile duct. Here they are the same diameter

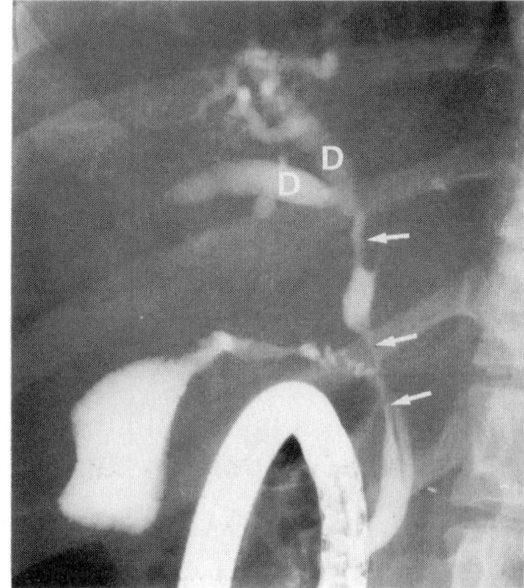

Fig. 6.14 Malignant lymph nodes in the porta hepatis causing obstructive jaundice

This woman of 54 presented with obstructive jaundice. Ultrasound showed no gallstones. This endoscopic retrograde cholangiogram (ERC) shows extrinsic compression of the common bile duct over much of its length (arrowed), and dilatation of the intrahepatic bile ducts **D**. At laparotomy, the compression was found to be due to malignant lymph nodes in the porta hepatis but no primary carcinoma was found. The primary was probably a tiny lesion in the stomach or pancreas

Alternatively, percutaneous 'skinny needle' transhepatic cholangiography can be performed. Both tests show the site and often the nature of an obstruction, although the latter test is more invasive. If bile ducts are not dilated, liver biopsy or biopsy of demonstrated secondaries (with ultrasound or CT guidance) may be performed. Because clotting is frequently abnormal, clotting must be checked before any invasive procedure. Abnormalities are corrected by giving daily vitamin K injections and giving fresh frozen plasma preoperatively if a clotting defect remains

- Despite the above, a firm diagnosis cannot always be made and laparotomy may be the only method of making the diagnosis. It provides an opportunity for treatment at the same time. Alternatively, laparoscopy may also be used to visualise the liver directly and to obtain biopsy specimens, but its use in general surgery is in its infancy

Principles of management of obstructive jaundice

The primary aim of treatment is to relieve the obstruction to the biliary tract. Obstructed bile is commonly infected and a fulminant cholangitis can develop at any time. Back-pressure interferes with other liver functions, such as synthesis of albumin and clotting factors. Eventually structural liver damage ensues.

Three categories of obstruction may be defined according to surgical treatment options:

a. Removable obstructions

These include bile duct stones and strictures, as well as small tumours of the lower bile ducts and periampullary region.

Bile duct stones can be removed by surgical exploration of the duct, at which time the gall bladder is usually removed. The number, size and position of stones may have been identified preoperatively by ERCP or percutaneous transhepatic cholangiography. Alternatively, stones can be identified by cholangiography performed during the operation (peroperative cholangiography). Operative choledochoscopy allows a visual check of completeness of stone removal.

Less commonly, stones may be removed by dividing the ampullary sphincter via a duodenal endoscope. This is the treatment of choice in the acute situation (particularly if acute cholangitis is present), in patients who have already had a cholecystectomy, or in a debilitated elderly where laparotomy is specially hazardous.

Small tumours in the periampullary region may be amenable to complete excision, thereby relieving biliary obstruction. Often a complete cure is achieved.

Fig. 6.15 Some remediable causes of obstructive jaundice

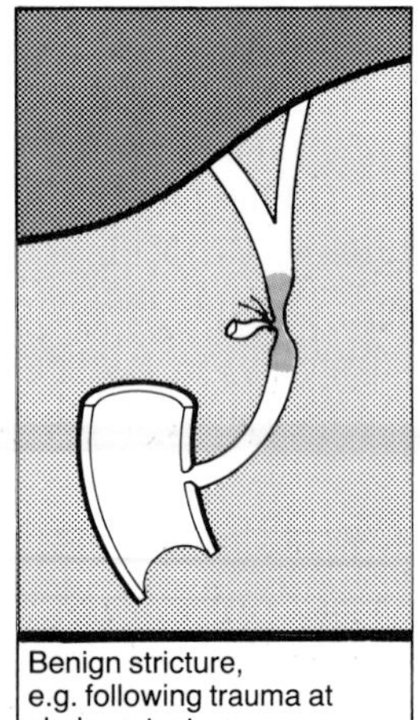

Benign stricture, e.g. following trauma at cholecystectomy

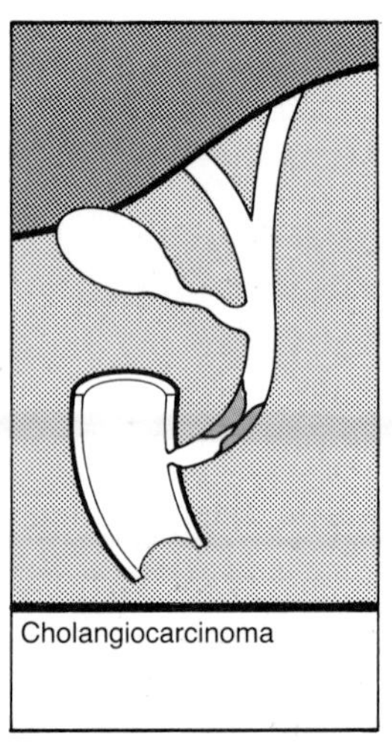

Cholangiocarcinoma

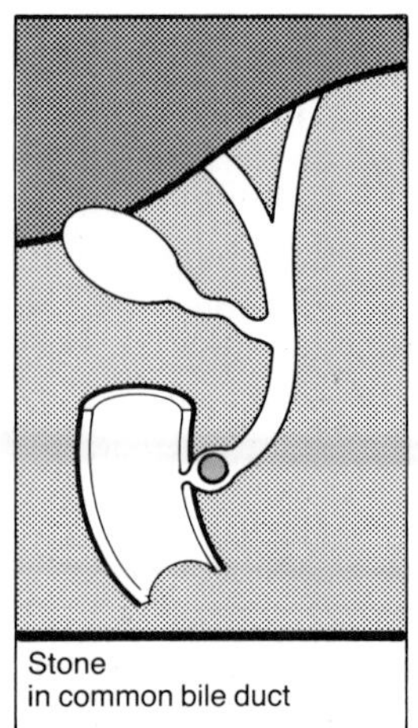

Stone in common bile duct

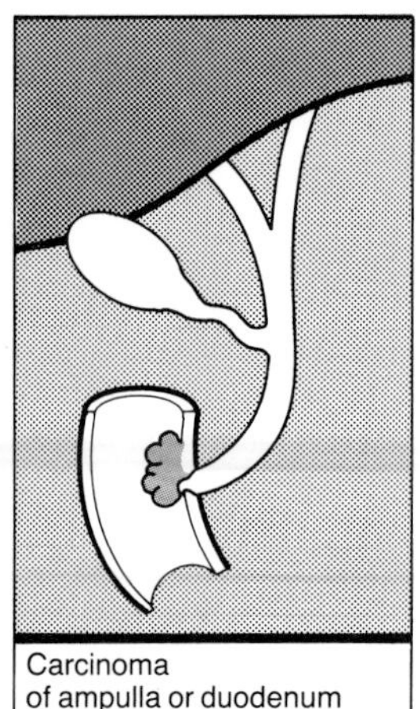

Carcinoma of ampulla or duodenum

b. Obstruction due to extensive tumour

This commonly results from carcinoma of the head of the pancreas, less often from secondaries in porta hepatis lymph nodes and rarely, from carcinoma of the gall bladder. A similar problem sometimes results from bile duct strictures following surgery. Provided the obstruction is below the bifurcation of the common bile duct, various operations can bypass the obstruction by joining the small bowel to the gall bladder or bile duct proximal to the obstruction. The most commonly performed operation of this type is the *triple bypass* for carcinoma of the head of the pancreas (see Chapter 12).

Inoperable tumours can usually be intubated to provide internal biliary drainage. This may be done by the percutaneous transhepatic route or endoscopically. The tubes are known as *Stents*, being named after the inventor of earlier devices of this kind. With the recent development of large bore duodenal endoscopes, per-oral placement of Stents up to 4 mm in diameter has become possible, and is now the preferred method.

All these techniques merely overcome the problem of obstructive jaundice and have no influence on the course of the disease. Eventually, the patient succumbs to some other manifestation of the malignancy, often within a few months.

c. Terminal disease

By the time obstructive jaundice has developed, some patients have reached a terminal stage of their malignancy. In these cases, interference is unjustified and the aim should be to relieve distress and allow a dignified death. Some patients experience severe itching. This may be lessened by drugs such as antihistamines and cholestyramine. Oral cholestyramine binds bile salts in the gut, removing them from the circulating pool. Unfortunately, this can only occur if bile reaches the gut; this rarely occurs in terminal patients. Chlorpromazine often gives relief from itching.

Special risks of surgery in the jaundiced patient

The jaundiced patient is at greater risk from peroperative and postoperative surgical complications as follows:

- Obstructed bile is nearly always infected by aerobic and anaerobic gut organisms and instrumentation may precipitate ascending cholangitis. This can easily lead to peritoneal contamination and wound infection or septicaemia and death. The ideal preventative measure is preoperative drainage of bile into the gut by endoscopic sphincterotomy or intubation, but this may not be practicable. Prophylactic antibiotics (e.g. ceftizoxime and metronidazole) should be used

- Biliary obstruction leads to diminished fat absorption and therefore of vitamin K, the substrate for prothrombin synthesis. This result is defective clotting. Intramuscular vitamin K for several days pre-operatively will usually improve the prothrombin time sufficiently to permit operation. If not, fresh frozen plasma is given peroperatively

- There is usually some degree of hepatic impairment due to biliary back-pressure. This disrupts hepatic metabolism of drugs and results in defective synthesis of clotting factors, even if vitamin K has been given
- Endotoxins reaching the liver from the gut are not detoxified. These predispose to renal failure, particularly if renal perfusion is impaired; this is known as the *hepatorenal syndrome*. Renal function can be protected by ensuring that the patient does not become dehydrated during the preoperative period of oral fluid restriction. Intravenous fluids are given preoperatively overnight and a diuresis is stimulated during operation with an osmotic diuretic such as mannitol
- Paradoxically, considering the clotting deficiency, postoperative deep vein thrombosis is particularly common in the jaundiced patient. Prophylactic measures should be taken to reduce this risk, e.g. low dose subcutaneous heparin
- Patients with chronic parenchymal liver disease withstand the stresses of major abdominal surgery and anaesthesia poorly

Fig. 6.16 Special precautions to be taken when operating on patients with obstructive juandice

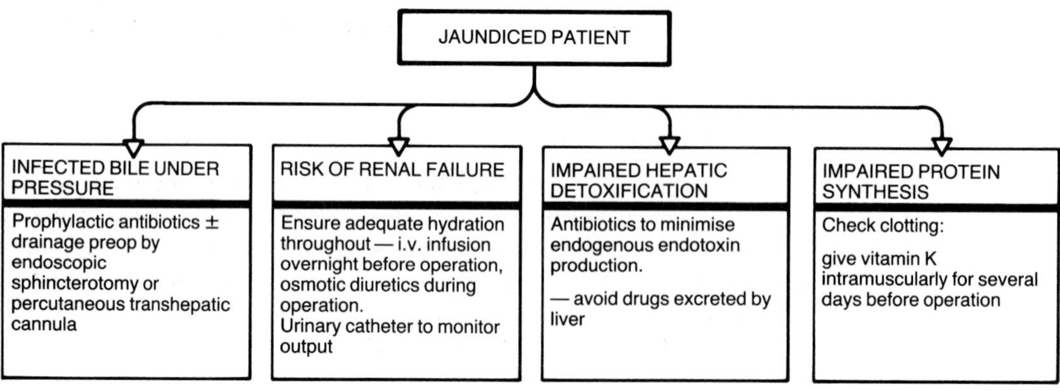

ABDOMINAL MASS OR DISTENSION

An abdominal mass is sometimes discovered by the patient himself but more often by a doctor. If a definite mass is palpable, the likely diagnosis is a malignant tumour, although benign cysts, inflammatory masses, aneurysms or atypical hernias may be responsible. Occasionally masses are due to a 'medical' cause e.g. hepato-splenomegaly of chronic lymphocytic leukaemia. Commonly, one of the 'five F's' — fetus, faeces, flatus, fat or fluid — may masquerade as a 'surgical' mass. The first is a common cause of embarrassment!

An abdominal mass may be discovered without related abdominal symptoms, but usually the patient has presented with anaemia, jaundice or an abdominal symptom. A careful history will often reveal useful clues as to the cause.

Clinical assessment of an abdominal mass

The location of the mass, its relations and mobility, and its physical characteristics, such as size, shape and consistency, give valuable information about the organ of origin and the likely pathology. Incisional, umbilical and sometimes Spigelian hernias may present as localised swellings, but they reduce or disappear when the patient is supine. Unless this diagnosis is considered, it may be overlooked. An incarcerated (irreducible but not obstructed) hernia is more appropriately considered a true 'mass'.

a. Mass in the right hypochondrium

A right hypochondrial mass is usually of hepatic origin. If so, it will be continuous with the main bulk of the liver both to palpation and percussion. It will also descend on inspiration. When the liver is diffusely enlarged the inferior margin is regular and well defined and the consistency is usually normal. When infiltrated with tumour, the palpable liver margin may be hard and irregular, but more often the liver appears diffusely enlarged. Rarely, *Riedel's lobe*, a congenitally enlarged part of the right lobe, is mistaken for a pathological mass. The expanding liver usually remains in contact with the anterior abdominal wall and is consequently dull to percussion. Less commonly, a right hypochondrial mass is a diseased gall bladder. The mass is continuous with the liver above but may be recognisable by its typical pear-shaped rounded outline. When a liver or gall bladder mass is suspected, signs of liver disease should be sought.

b. Epigastric mass

A mass in the epigastrium is usually due to a tumour of the stomach or transverse colon, or sometimes omental secondaries from ovarian carcinoma. Such masses are usually hard and irregular, and are mobile or fixed according to the degree of invasion. Occasionally an epigastric mass may represent isolated enlargement of the left lobe of the liver, or massive para-aortic lymph nodes due to lymphoma or testicular secondaries.

c. Mass in the left hypochondrium

Tumours of the stomach and splenic flexure of the colon may present as a mass in the left hypochondrium. Tumour can usually be distinguished clinically from an enlarged spleen which has a discrete 'edge' and lies more posteriorly. The spleen also has a band of overlying resonance due to gas in bowel superficial to it. It is easier to palpate a spleen if the patient rolls partially onto his right side; the examiner then puts his left hand behind the patient's lower left ribs pulling the spleen towards the examining hand. Note that a normal sized spleen is rarely palpable by any means.

d. Mass in the loin or flank

A mass in either loin or flank is most likely to be of renal origin and can best be felt by bimanual palpation. This involves pushing the mass forward from behind with the left hand so that it can be palpated anteriorly. Furthermore, since the kidneys lie just beneath the diaphragm, a renal mass will descend with inspiration. Very rarely, hernias occur in the lumbar region; they are usually reducible and bowel sounds may be heard on auscultation.

e. Mass in the left iliac fossa

Masses in the left iliac fossa usually arise from the sigmoid colon. A hard faecal mass simulates a tumour but it can often be indented like putty. A sigmoid mass is usually due to tumour or peridiverticular inflammation. Ovarian masses and sometimes eccentric bladder lesions may be palpable in either iliac fossa. Such lesions however, continue down into the pelvis and may be pushed up onto the abdominal examining hand by digital pressure in the rectum or vagina. A rectal examination is mandatory in a thorough abdominal examination.

Hernias in the groin are common and may be chronically irreducible. Occasionally, an interstitial (Spigelian) hernia develops above the groin in the iliac fossa. This presents a somewhat confusing picture on examination by virtue of its site and because the peritoneal sac herniates between the muscle layers of the abdominal wall.

f. Suprapubic mass

Suprapubic masses usually arise from pelvic organs such as bladder or uterus and its adnexae. A palpable bladder is most commonly due to chronic urinary retention. A distended bladder is dull to percussion and disappears on catheterisation. Bladder enlargement is usually symmetrical and may extend above the umbilicus. The margins may be difficult to define accurately because of the bladder's soft consistency. Only massive bladder tumours are palpable and there are accompanying urinary tract symptoms. Sometimes, large bladder stones are palpable abdominally.

The uterus, enlarged by pregnancy or fibroids, may be palpable abdominally. A bimanual technique involves digital examination of the vagina at the same time as palpation of the lower abdomen with the other hand. Ovarian tumours, particularly cysts, may become enormous and extend well up into the abdomen; again, vaginal examination helps to distinguish the origin.

g. Mass in the right iliac fossa

The right iliac fossa is a common site for an asymptomatic mass. It may be due to unresolved inflammation of the appendix which becomes surrounded by a mass of omentum and/or small bowel, giving rise to an 'appendix mass'; there is usually a recent history of right iliac fossa pain and fever. A carcinoma of the caecum may become very large without causing symptoms of obstruction because the caecum is large and distensible. Thus, a caecal carcinoma may present as an asymptomatic right iliac fossa mass; iron deficiency anaemia is usually apparent by this stage.

h. Central abdominal mass

A central abdominal mass may originate in large or small bowel or from retroperitoneal structures, i.e. lymph nodes, pancreas or connective tissues. Retroperitoneal masses are only palpable if they are large. One of the most common central abdominal masses is an aneurysm of the abdominal aorta. Aneurysms usually arise just above the aortic bifurcation (at the umbilical level) which explains their central location. The characteristic feature of an aneurysm is its expansile pulsation; other solid masses may transmit pulsation from large vessels nearby, but these masses are not expansile.

Several different types of hernia may present near the centre of the abdomen. Most common is an *incisional hernia* which protrudes through part or the whole of an abdominal wall incision. This may occur at any time postoperatively, from days to years later. It usually results from poor closure technique or post-operative infection. *Paraumbilical hernias*, common in the obese, occur centrally and diagnosis is usually straightforward. *Divarication of the recti* represents a form of hernia, the recti being splayed apart (often as a result of pregnancy), leaving the lower anterior abdominal wall devoid of muscular support; this condition is easily recognised and rarely requires treatment.

i. Rectal mass

An abdominal or pelvic mass may be palpable solely on rectal (or vaginal) examination. The mass may be a rectal tumour, or a tumour of the sigmoid colon lying in the pelvic cavity; the latter is unlikely to be visible on sigmoidoscopy. Sometimes, secondary deposits from an impalpable tumour in the upper abdomen may seed the pelvic cavity. This may produce a palpable pelvic lump or even a solid mass filling the pelvic cavity. The latter condition is known as a *frozen pelvis*.

Diffuse abdominal distension

Diffuse distension of the abdomen is a separate problem from a solid but discrete abdominal mass.

Widespread peritoneal involvement with tumour secondaries, particularly if there is also an accumulation of fluid (ascites), may cause abdominal distension. It is often difficult to recognise on abdominal examination. This should be suspected if the patient has other symptoms suggestive of malignancy like anorexia and marked weight loss. Ultrasound or CT scanning will usually reveal this.

Gas within the bowel is a common cause for long-standing and often intermittent abdominal distension. It usually occurs in healthy young adults, particularly women, in association with irritable bowel syndrome or air swallowing during hyperventilation. Women of reproductive age often complain of abdominal distension in the premenstrual phase, which may be due to fluid retention. A detailed history and examination will usually diagnose these problems and avoid the need for further investigation.

Abdominal wall and intraperitoneal fat may give the impression of diffuse abdominal distension, especially if the patient has a lumbar lordosis. In the middle-aged and elderly, more sinister conditions should be excluded before fat is blamed.

Gross faecal loading may also be responsible for diffuse abdominal distension. This is often seen in children with abdominal pain, and sometimes in young adults with irritable bowel syndrome. Asymptomatic chronic constipation is very common in the elderly but can also be a symptom of incomplete bowel obstruction due to diverticular disease or tumour. A faecal mass palpable through the thin abdominal wall of an elderly patient can give the impression of a sinister mass. This commonly leads to fruitless but unavoidable investigations.

Ascites

Ascites is defined as the accumulation of fluid within the abdominal cavity and has many causes, both malignant and non-malignant.

Sometimes, in ovarian or colonic tumours, the peritoneum is seeded with tumour deposits, resulting in secretion of a protein-rich fluid containing malignant cells. This *malignant ascites* may reach a volume of several litres. The peritoneum may be peppered with thousands of minute seedlings without a palpable mass, or there may be several large masses hidden by the ascitic fluid. A rare cause of ascites is massive obstruction of abdominal lymphatic drainage.

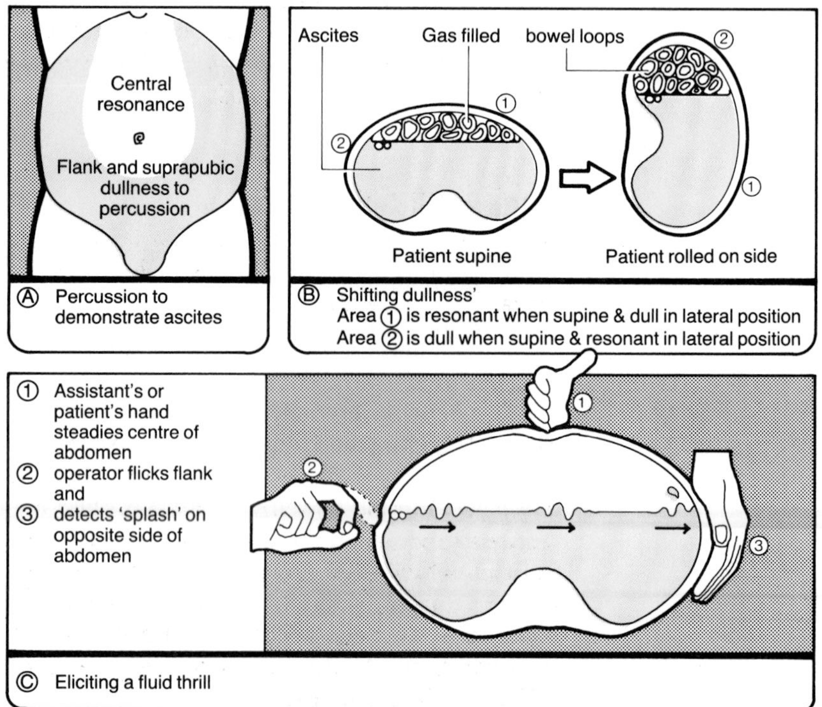

Fig. 6.17 Clinical signs of ascites

This is usually caused by malignant involvement of para-aortic lymph nodes with lymphoma or metastatic testicular tumour. *Chylous ascites*, in which the ascitic fluid is milky white is an occasional cause and is due to the presence of chylomicrons originating from mesenteric lymphatics.

Ascites may also be caused by gross congestive cardiac failure, severe hypoalbuminaemia or portal venous obstruction, the last occurring in cirrhosis and occasionally with liver metastases. Tuberculosis can occasionally present as ascites; this form of tuberculosis is characterised by multiple tiny peritoneal tubercles, clinically indistinguishable from tumour secondaries. Tuberculosis must be considered in this situation, and biopsies taken, because the condition is usually curable, unlike its malignant counterpart.

Ascites can usually be recognised only when the volume exceeds two litres, but even then it is easily overlooked. Dullness to percussion in the flanks and suprapubic region with central resonance is suspicious of ascites and should be followed by an attempt to elicit a fluid thrill or 'shifting dullness' (Figure 6.17).

Approach to investigation of an abdominal mass or distension

a. History and examination

A thorough history will probably provide clues to the specific organ system involved. A history of intra-abdominal malignancy, even many years previously, should be regarded with grave suspicion. The disease may have recurred or a new primary developed. This is especially common in large bowel cancer.

General examination should seek systemic signs of disease, e.g. cachexia, anaemia and jaundice, or signs of malignant dissemination, e.g. supraclavicular lymphadenopathy in suspected stomach cancer. Abdominal and pelvic examination must be thorough.

b. Laboratory tests

Blood, urine and stool investigations will be performed as suggested by the history and examination, e.g. full blood count, liver function tests, dipstick urinalysis and faecal occult bloods.

c. Radiology

Plain abdominal and chest X-rays should be performed if malignancy is suspected. Ultrasound scanning is useful in demonstrating the size and origin of a mass. It is also the first choice if pathology is suspected in the liver, biliary tree, pancreas, aorta or pelvic organs, or to confirm ascites. CT scanning is most valuable in defining masses, particularly in the retroperitoneal area, e.g. pancreas, aorta, kidneys. Ultrasound or CT scanning can be used to direct a biopsy needle precisely to the abnormality, a process which may avoid the need for laparotomy. Finally, contrast studies, e.g. barium meal, barium enema or IVU, may be indicated.

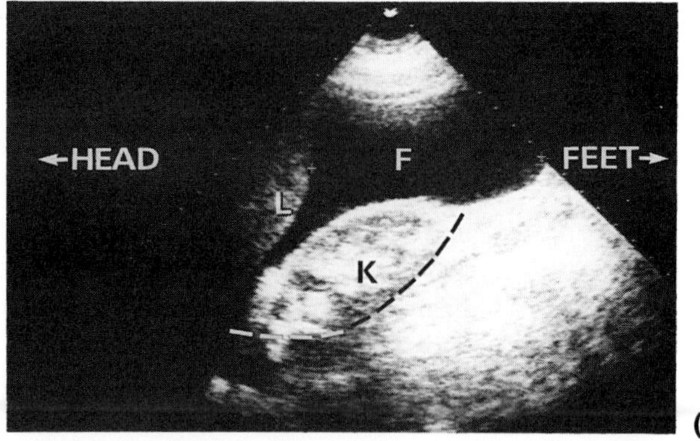

(a)

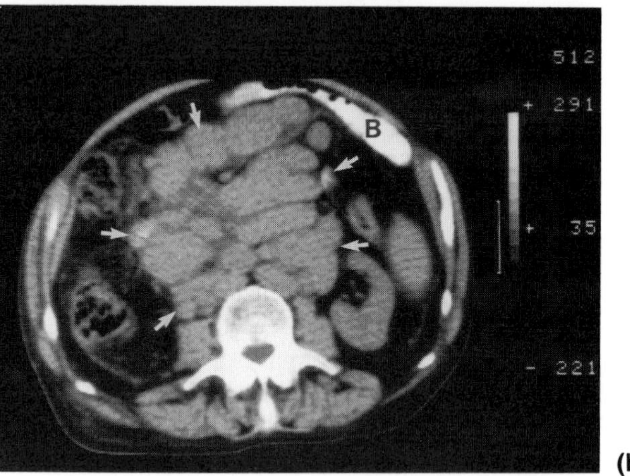

(b)

Fig. 6.18 (a) Ultrasound showing ascites

This 60-year-old man presented with weight loss and abdominal distension. This ultrasound examination in longitudinal section shows free fluid **F** within the peritoneal cavity; note the lack of internal reflections characteristic of clear fluid. The liver **L** and right kidney **K** are also shown. The renal image is enhanced because it lies behind the fluid.

(b) Retroperitoneal mass of lymph nodes due to lymphoma

This CT scan was taken to assess the 'stage' of a known lymphoma. This 40-year-old woman with lymphoma presented with a large rubbery lymph node mass in her neck and was also found to have a large central abdominal mass. Abdominal CT scanning showed an enormous mass of lymph nodes (arrowed). Small bowel **B** is seen anteriorly, enhanced by orally administered contrast material

d. Endoscopy

Endoscopic techniques such as gastroscopy or colonoscopy, enable direct examination and biopsy of many gastrointestinal lesions. ERCP may be used to inject contrast material into the biliary and pancreatic duct systems if appropriate. Laparoscopy, widely used in gynaecology, is gradually being introduced in general surgery for direct inspection and biopsy, particularly of liver nodules. Laparoscopy may avoid the need for formal laparotomy.

e. Other methods of tissue diagnosis

A tissue diagnosis should be obtained even if disseminated malignancy seems obvious. It can influence palliative and supportive treatment and occasionally, an apparently hopeless case proves on histology to be treatable or even curable. Examples are tuberculosis or a germ cell tumour, such as teratoma. Techniques of obtaining tissue for histology include excision biopsy of enlarged cervical lymph nodes, percutaneous biopsy of liver or an intra-abdominal mass (which may be guided by ultrasound or CT). *Paracentesis* (i.e. needle aspiration of ascitic fluid) is a safe and simple way of obtaining a specimen for cytology and microbiology. Finally, direct biopsy of tumour at operation usually provides the definitive diagnosis.

f. Examination under anaesthesia and exploratory laparotomy

Examination under anaesthesia (EUA) is often necessary, especially in patients with a suspected pelvic mass. General anaesthesia with a muscle relaxant, allows thorough abdominal palpation and bimanual examination of the pelvis via rectum and vagina. Without anaesthesia, this may not be possible because of tenderness or abdominal wall muscle tone. Cystoscopy and sigmoidoscopy are often performed at the same time. Diagnostic laparotomy, formerly often necessary, is fortunately now required only when less invasive procedures have failed to provide a diagnosis, or when treatment is required urgently to relieve symptoms such as bowel obstruction.

7 THE ACUTE ABDOMEN AND ACUTE GASTROINTESTINAL HAEMORRHAGE

Introduction

The term *acute abdomen* is widely understood but is difficult to define precisely. Typically, the symptoms are of acute onset and strongly suggest an abdominal cause; abdominal pain is almost always a prominent feature. The illness is of such severity that admission to hospital appears necessary with operative surgery a likely outcome. Many of the disorders causing an 'acute abdomen' are serious and potentially life-threatening unless treated promptly. On the other hand, simple and relatively trivial conditions such as constipation can produce acute and severe symptoms. These lesser diagnoses may only become apparent after a period of observation or after special investigations.

Fig. 7.1 Common causes of acute abdominal emergencies in adults

Non-specific abdominal pain which resolves without operation

Acute appendicitis

Acute biliary tract disorders — biliary colic, cholecystitis, ascending cholangitis

Acute pancreatitis

Acute manifestations of peptic ulcer disease — severe exacerbations of pain, haemorrhage, perforation, pyloric stenosis

Acute diverticular disease — acute inflammation, abscess, haemorrhage, perforation, large bowel obstruction

Strangulated hernias, and other small bowel obstructions, e.g. bands or adhesions

Colorectal carcinoma — large bowel obstruction, perforation, fistula

Constipation

Sigmoid volvulus

Urinary tract infections

Ureteric colic

Acute urinary retention

Leaking or ruptured abdominal aortic aneurysm

Mesenteric arterial occlusion causing bowel ischaemia

Abdominal trauma causing bleeding or perforation

Gynaecological emergencies — ruptured ectopic pregnancy, torsion or bleeding of ovarian cyst, acute salpingitis

Fig. 7.2 Composition of acute general surgical admissions in a typical district general hospital

Non-specific abdominal pain, resolving without surgery 25%

Acute appendicitis 12%

Acute abdomen due to other causes 12%

Head injuries 20%

Abscesses 10%

Arterial emergencies 5%

Urological emergencies 5%

Hernia/scrotal emergencies 5%

Gastrointestinal haemorrhage 3%

Soft tissue wounds 2%

Burns 1%

By the time of hospital admission, a patient with an 'acute abdomen' may well have been managed conservatively at home for a day or two, during which time the symptoms have either failed to settle or become progressively worse.

Major gastrointestinal haemorrhage, revealed by vomiting of blood (*haematemesis*) or rectal bleeding, is also a common reason for acute surgical referral. Many of these patients are initially referred to a physician, especially if the presumptive diagnosis is a bleeding peptic ulcer.

The common abdominal causes for emergency admission are summarised in Figure 7.1. The list is not meant to be exhaustive and excludes obscure medical causes like acute intermittent porphyria or tabes dorsalis, and conditions mainly confined to infants and children (see Chapter 31).

Acute surgical emergencies constitute about half of all general surgical admissions, as shown in Figure 7.2. Approximately half of the acute surgical admissions are for abdominal symptoms, mainly pain, and half of those resolve without operation. Most of the rest undergo emergency surgery and many of the remainder require surgical procedures later.

In managing the acute abdomen, the goal is to make a definitive diagnosis before proceeding to an operation. This is often impossible in the emergency situation, and the crucial consideration then is whether an urgent operation is required.

Firstly, the basic pathophysiological phenomenon responsible for the patient's clinical state should be identified. Is the clinical picture suggestive of obstruction, bowel strangulation, peritonitis, intra-abdominal abscess or acute bowel ischaemia, or is it obviously gastrointestinal haemorrhage? More than one of these phenomena may occur at once, for example strangulation is usually associated with signs of obstruction. Once the phenomenon has been diagnosed, a set of probabilities as to the underlying cause can be put together from the clinical evidence.

Each of the basic pathophysiological phenomena is described in detail below.

BOWEL OBSTRUCTION

Pathophysiology and clinical features

Any part of the gastrointestinal tract may become obstructed and present as an acute abdomen. The possible causes are many and varied, as outlined in Figure 7.3, but only a few of them account for most cases of obstruction.

Obstruction leads to proximal dilatation of the bowel and disrupts peristalsis. The presentation depends on the level of obstruction (i.e. stomach, proximal or distal small bowel or large bowel), and on the completeness of obstruction. The most acute presentation is upper small bowel obstruction. This is because of obstruction to the large volume of pancreatic and biliary secretion. In contrast, distal large bowel obstruction is often much more chronic.

Obstruction of the bowel eventually leads to vomiting. The more proximal the obstruction, the earlier it develops. Vomiting occurs, even if nothing is taken by mouth, because saliva and other gastrointestinal secretions continue to be produced and enter the stomach. At least 10 litres of fluid are secreted into the gastrointestinal tract each day. The nature of the vomitus gives important clues to the level of obstruction. For example, semi-digested food eaten a day or two previously strongly suggests gastric outlet obstruction, particularly if there is no bile present. Copious vomiting of bile-stained fluid suggests upper small bowel obstruction. If vomitus is thicker and foul-smelling (*faeculent*), a more distal obstruction is likely.

Fig. 7.3(a) Mechanical causes of bowel obstruction

Adhesions or bands resulting from previous surgery or intraperitoneal infection

Bowel strangulation, e.g strangulated hernias, obstructing fibrous bands, volvulus

Tumours, e.g. gastric carcinoma near the pylorus, colonic carcinoma, small bowel tumours

Inflammatory strictures, e.g. diverticular disease, Crohn's disease

Bolus obstruction, e.g. impacted faeces (common), foreign bodies or solitary gallstone (rare), phytobezoar i.e. a mass of impacted vegetable matter such as orange pith (very rare except after partial gastrectomy)

Intussusception, i.e. a segment of bowel becoming telescoped into the segment distal to it — usually initiated by a mass in the bowel wall which is dragged along by peristalsis; rare in adults but common in children

(a)

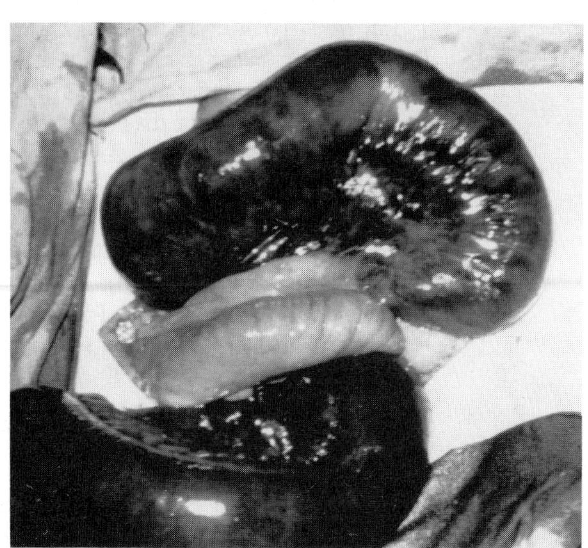

(b)

(b) Necrotic bowel after strangulation

This photograph, taken at operation for bowel obstruction, shows a dilated necrotic loop of small bowel which has strangulated by passing through a congenital defect in the sigmoid mesocolon. The bowel was on the point of perforation

Proximal distension of the bowel by fluid and swallowed air causes pain. The general area of the pain gives a clue to the embryological origin of the affected bowel: upper, middle or lower abdominal pain originates in foregut, midgut or hindgut respectively. In obstruction, pain is not usually the most prominent symptom; it is of variable intensity, often quite mild, and usually colicky as peristalsis tries to overcome the obstruction. In large bowel obstruction, symptoms develop more gradually because of the large capacity of the colon and caecum and their absorptive activity. If the ileo-caecal valve remains competent (as in about half the cases), the thin-walled caecum progressively distends with swallowed air, and will eventually rupture. The ileo-caecal valve becomes incompetent in about half of large bowel obstructions, and this allows the small bowel to distend, thereby delaying the onset of symptoms.

Distal to the obstruction, bowel gas is absorbed and propulsion of bowel contents is arrested. The resulting *absolute constipation*, i.e. neither faeces nor flatus is passed rectally, is pathognomonic of bowel obstruction.

If the bowel is only partially obstructed, the clinical features are less clearly defined. Vomiting may be intermittent and bowel habit erratic. Chronic incomplete obstruction leads to gradual hypertrophy of the muscle of the bowel wall proximally. Peristaltic activity in this hypertrophic muscle is responsible for the bouts of colicky pain which are more prominent than in complete obstruction. The pain is often accompanied by *visible peristalsis*, which is the hallmark of incomplete obstruction.

Physical examination

Vomiting, diminished fluid intake and sequestration of fluid in the small bowel commonly lead to dehydration. This is manifest clinically by extreme dryness of the mouth and characteristic loss of skin turgor and elasticity. Gas-filled loops of bowel produce abdominal distension; the more distal the obstruction, the greater the distension. Episodes of visible peristalsis may be observed in thin patients in whom the obstruction is incomplete and of long duration. General examination may reveal signs of anaemia or lymphadenopathy attributable to the primary disorder.

The most striking feature on abdominal palpation is the lack of tenderness; the exception is when strangulation has occurred. Obstruction with tenderness must be diagnosed as strangulation, necessitating urgent operation. An obstructing abdominal mass may be palpable if large. The groin must always be examined for hernias. An obstructed femoral hernia rarely causes local symptoms but instead produces symptoms and signs of small bowel obstruction. A strangulated femoral hernia is often no bigger than a large grape and is rarely red or tender; consequently, it is easily missed if not specifically sought.

On percussion, the centre of the abdomen tends to be resonant and the periphery dull, because bowel gas tends to rise to the most elevated point; this may be difficult to distinguish from ascites.

Bowel sounds in obstruction are traditionally described as being loud and frequent, high-pitched and tinkling; nevertheless, in practice, obstructed bowel sounds may or may not be increased. They have an echoing, cavernous quality or can sound like the gentle lapping of water against a boat. This is due to fluid sloshing about in distended, gas-filled loops of bowel.

Investigation of suspected bowel obstruction

The most useful investigation is plain abdominal X-ray. This is usually performed in both erect and supine positions, although the need for an erect film is doubted by some clinicians. Bowel proximal to the obstruction is distended by gas. Distally, bowel gas is absent, but some rectal gas may be seen if a digital examination has been done. The pattern and distribution of gas will often indicate the approximate site of obstruction, as illustrated in Figure 7.4. Fluid levels may be seen in small bowel obstruction on an erect film.

In obstruction of the large bowel at any point distal to the caecum, the caecum and ascending colon take the brunt of the distension, being less muscular. When the radiological diameter of the caecum reaches 12 cm, it is considered to be in imminent danger of rupture, and therefore needs urgent operation. In large bowel obstruction of less acute onset, a barium enema is helpful to demonstrate the site and nature of the obstruction.

Adynamic bowel obstruction

Temporary disruption of normal peristaltic activity without mechanical blockage causes adynamic bowel obstruction. Most commonly, it arises after abdominal surgery in which the bowel has been handled. Small bowel is particularly susceptible and the condition is known as *ileus* or *paralytic ileus*. Normal post-operative ileus should not persist for more than about four days. It is one of the reasons why fluids and solids must be introduced gradually after abdominal surgery. Persisting postoperative ileus is usually due to a complication of surgery such as anastomotic leakage or intra-abdominal infection, which has local noxious effects upon the bowel wall.

Occasionally, electrolyte disturbances like hypokalaemia or anti-Parkinsonian drugs are responsible for adynamic obstruction. The condition is common in patients in intensive care. A form of adynamic obstruction peculiar to the large bowel is called *pseudo-obstruction*, and is caused by a wide range of apparently unrelated conditions. These include retroperitoneal inflammation or haemorrhage, certain drugs, pregnancy, multiple trauma and prolonged recumbency.

Physical signs are similar to those of mechanical obstruction with the exception that bowel sounds are not of the obstructed type or may be inaudible.

Principles of management of intestinal obstruction

Once intestinal obstruction has been recognised and the approximate level of obstruction identified, management proceeds as follows:

- Oral intake is discontinued and intravenous fluids given, the volume and type of fluid depending on the state of hydration and serum electrolyte estimations. After prolonged vomiting, patients may be seriously depleted of fluid and electrolytes
- If the patient is vomiting or there is marked small bowel dilatation, a naso-gastric tube is passed and gastric contents aspirated. This will control nausea

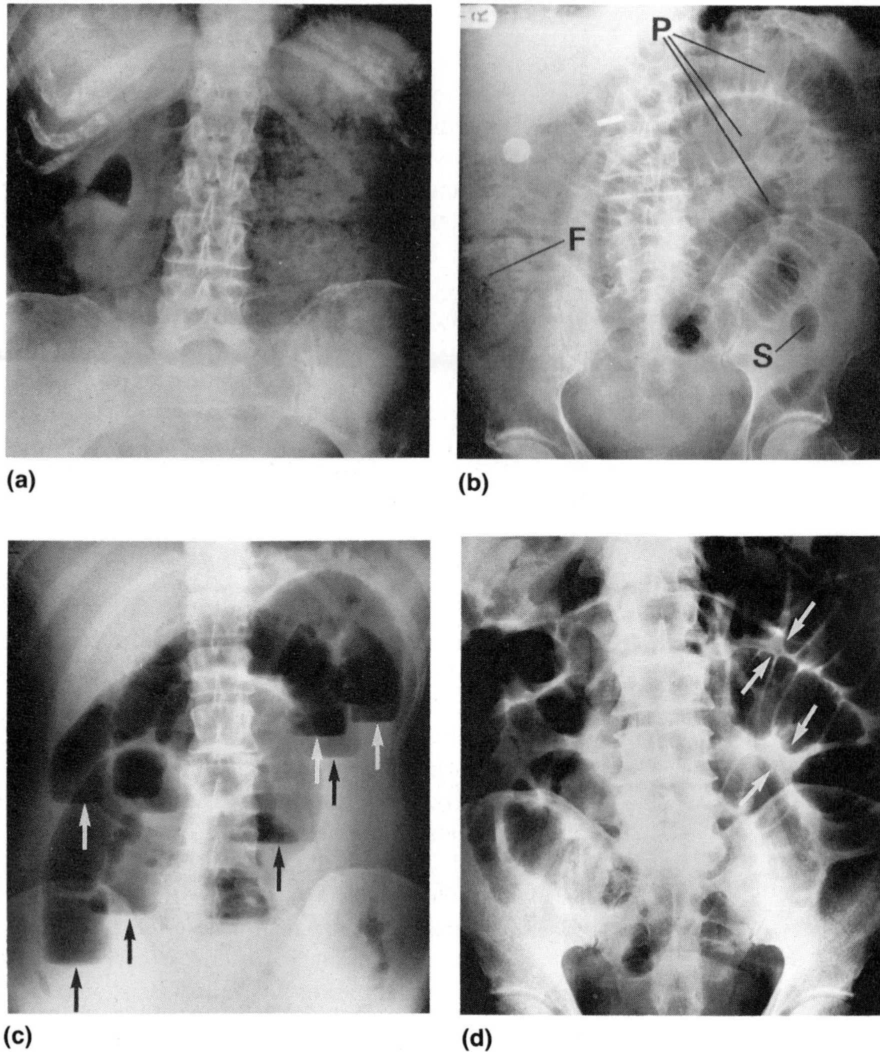

Fig. 7.4 Radiological appearances of obstructed bowel

(a) Plain abdominal film showing gastric outlet obstruction. The stomach is grossly distended with food, giving a typical mottled appearance over the whole left side of the abdomen. Bowel gas distal to the obstruction has been absorbed or expelled and so the rest of the abdomen is relatively gas free. **(b)** Supine abdominal film showing mid small bowel obstruction. Dilated small bowel fills the upper left quadrant and centre of the abdomen, and can be identified by the plica circulares **P** which extend across the whole width of the lumen. Distal small bowel is collapsed and is not seen on this film. The large bowel is also collapsed distal to the obstruction, with only a small amount of gas seen in the sigmoid colon **S**; there is faecal loading of the ascending colon **F**. Note also the metallic tip of the nasogastric tube and the incidental radiopaque gallstone. **(c)** Erect film from the same patient as in (b), showing multiple loops of dilated small bowel and multiple fluid levels (arrowed). **(d)** Supine abdominal X-ray in a middle-aged man with several days of small bowel obstruction due to adhesions. The abdomen is filled with grossly dilated small bowel loops. In addition, the small bowel wall is thickened, as shown by the apparent space between loops of bowel (arrowed); this is a characteristic feature of

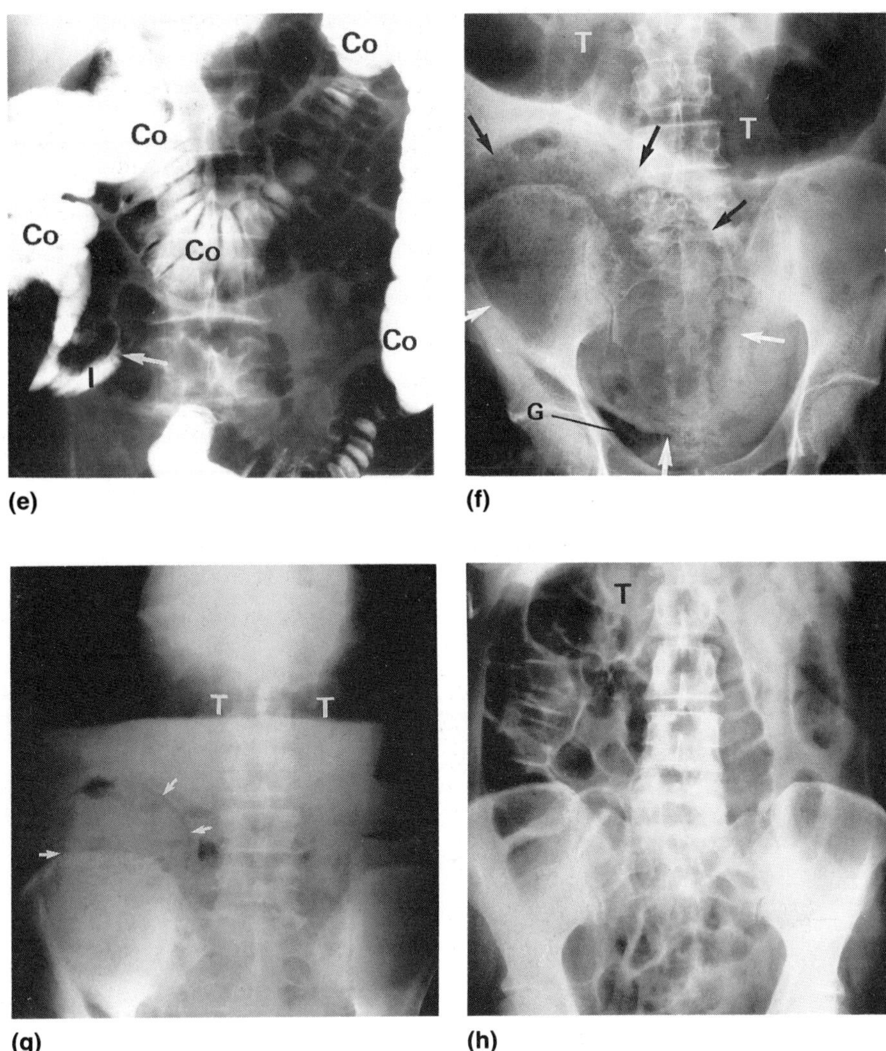

prolonged obstruction **(e)** 'Instant' barium enema on the same patient as (d), showing contrast filling the normal colon **Co** and distal ileum **I** which abruptly terminates at the obstruction (arrowed). **(f)** Supine film showing gross caecal dilatation (outline arrowed) with loss of haustration. It can be deduced that the colon is obstructed near the splenic flexure because the transverse colon **T** is also dilated with gas whilst there is complete absence of colonic gas down the left side of the abdomen in the position of the descending and sigmoid colon. Gross caecal dilatation occurs in large bowel obstruction when the ileo-caecal valve remains competent. In this patient, the caecum has perforated, as shown by the presence of gas **G** in the extra-peritoneal tissues. **(g)** Erect film of the same patient as in (f) showing gas in the caecal wall (arrowed); this indicates necrosis. Note also the long fluid-level in the transverse colon **T**. This patient was an elderly man with an obstructing carcinoma at the splenic flexure. **(h)** Plain supine abdominal X-ray of another elderly man, also with an obstructing carcinoma at the splenic flexure. In this patient, the ileocaecal valve has become incompetent. Note the dilated transverse colon **T** and the multiple dilated loops of small bowel in the centre of the abdomen

and vomiting, remove swallowed air, and reduce gaseous distension. Most important, it will minimise the risk of inhalation of gastric contents, particularly during induction of general anaesthesia

- Uncomplicated cases of obstruction due to adhesions will usually resolve with conservative measures. Those that do not will require operation
- Large bowel obstruction due to faecal impaction can be relieved by enemas or manual removal of faeces
- Adynamic bowel obstruction in most cases eventually resolves with conservative measures and removal of any precipitating cause
- Operation may be required to relieve the obstruction. Provided strangulation can be excluded and the caecum is not dangerously distended, operation can safely be deferred for a day or two. This gives time for the patient to be stabilised and for any other desirable investigations. During this period of *conservative management*, the obstruction may well settle, particularly if caused by adhesions from previous surgery
- At operation the cause of the obstruction is confirmed and dealt with appropriately

Fig. 7.5

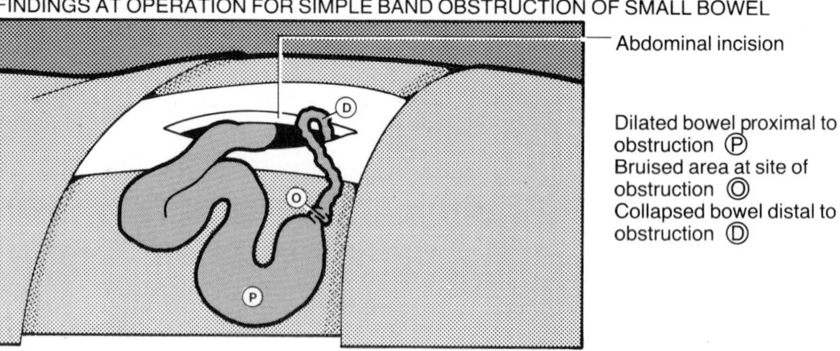

BOWEL STRANGULATION

Pathophysiology and clinical features

Strangulation occurs when a segment of bowel becomes trapped so that its lumen becomes obstructed and its blood supply disrupted. If unrelieved, this progresses to infarction and perforation. Strangulation can occur when there is an external hernia, when loops of bowel become trapped within the abdominal cavity or when there is mass rotation of bowel (*volvulus*).

The process of strangulation begins with partial obstruction of the bowel due to external pressure or twisting. This leads to oedema of the bowel wall which aggravates the obstruction and prevents venous return. The closed loop of bowel becomes progressively dilated by gas from fermentation. The combination of gas pressure and venous back-pressure inhibit arterial inflow, causing ischaemia and then infarction.

Strangulation most commonly occurs when small bowel is caught within a hernia (inguinal, femoral, umbilical or incisional). The bowel undergoes necrosis and soon perforates within the hernial sac; initially this may be contained, but generalised peritonitis usually ensues. Clinically, the patient develops symptoms and signs of small bowel obstruction. A newly irreducible hernia can usually be found and this is likely to be tender and inflamed. However, a strangulated femoral hernia is a trap for the unwary. As indicated earlier, these are often deceptively small and non-tender and will be missed unless the groins are carefully examined.

Bowel may also become strangulated within the abdominal cavity if a loop becomes trapped by fibrous bands or adhesions, or passes through an omental or mesenteric defect. Similarly, strangulation occurs if a large loop of bowel becomes twisted several times on its mesentery, a condition known as volvulus. The sigmoid colon is particularly susceptible to volvulus in chronic constipation, and in countries where the staple diet is extremely high in fibre. Small bowel volvulus is rare. Intra-abdominal strangulation exhibits the usual symptoms and signs of bowel obstruction but is accompanied by abdominal tenderness which is not a feature of uncomplicated bowel obstruction. The tenderness is probably due to distension of the closed loop. When compared with uncomplicated obstruction, patients with strangulation are systemically more unwell, with a tachycardia and a leucocytosis.

Fig. 7.6 Clinical features of bowel obstruction and strangulation

SYMPTOMS

Vomiting — time of onset and nature of the vomitus suggests the level of obstruction

Abdominal pain — usually colicky in character, often mild in uncomplicated obstruction and more severe in strangulation

Absolute constipation (i.e. no flatus or faeces passed rectally) — pathognomonic of complete obstruction (but not present in partial obstruction)

PHYSICAL SIGNS

Dehydration — caused by vomiting, lack of fluid intake and fluid sequestration

Abdominal distension — due to gas-filled loops of bowel. The more distal the obstruction, the greater the distension

Visible peristalsis — uncommon finding, usually in a very thin patient with prolonged distal obstruction

Central resonance to percussion with dullness in the flanks — gas within dilated bowel loops rising to the uppermost point in the abdomen

Abdominal tenderness — important feature distinguishing bowel strangulation from uncomplicated obstruction

Abnormal bowel sounds — exaggerated, lapping, sloshing, perhaps high-pitched or tinkling. Bowel sounds are absent in adynamic obstruction

Principles of management of suspected bowel strangulation

When strangulation is diagnosed, or even suspected, operation must be performed urgently to try to prevent infarction and perforation. The patient is otherwise managed as for uncomplicated obstruction. Specific investigations are limited to plain abdominal X-ray in which a single dilated, gas-filled strangulated loop may be prominent. There are no other investigations to help diagnose bowel strangulation, which is a clinical diagnosis.

PERITONITIS

Pathophysiology and clinical features

Peritonitis is defined as inflammation of the peritoneal cavity. This includes the serosal covering of the bowel and mesentery, the omentum and the lining of the abdominal cavity. At the outset, peritoneal inflammation is often localised and the affected area contained by a wrapping of omentum, adjacent bowel and fibrinous adhesions. This may, however, be insufficient to prevent spread, resulting in generalised peritonitis. Sudden perforation of any viscus almost invariably leads to life-threatening generalised peritonitis.

Fig. 7.7 Causes of peritonitis

Localised peritonitis

Transmural inflammation of the bowel, e.g. appendicitis, Crohn's disease, diverticulitis

Transmural inflammation of other viscera, e.g cholecystitis, salpingitis

Generalised peritonitis

Irritation of the peritoneum by noxious materials, e.g. bile, stomach or small bowel contents (due to perforation), enzyme-containing exudates of acute pancreatitis

Spreading intraperitoneal infection, e.g. rupture of intra-abdominal abscess or faecal contamination due to bowel perforation, trauma, surgical spillage or anastomotic leak

Localised peritonitis occurs in the vicinity of any primary intra-abdominal inflammatory process. Appendicitis is a typical example. Once the parietal peritoneum becomes involved, pain becomes localised to the affected area and is exacerbated by movement of the abdominal musculature. The area is tender to palpation and there is contraction of the overlying abdominal wall muscles when examination is attempted. This sign is known as *guarding*. If the palpating hand is quickly removed, the sudden movement of the peritoneum causes intense pain which is described as *rebound tenderness*. However, this test is unkind and its diagnostic value overstated. Rebound tenderness is better elicited by gentle percussion. Rectal examination should always be performed as anterior tenderness can be a sign of pelvic peritonitis. Localised peritonitis is usually accompanied by mild systemic 'toxicity', i.e. low-grade fever, malaise, tachycardia and leucocytosis.

With *generalised peritonitis*, the patient is seriously ill. There is massive exudation of inflammatory fluid into the peritoneal cavity causing hypovolaemia. This is often compounded by toxaemia from absorbed products, or septicaemia if infection is present. The severity of the systemic illness depends on the cause of the peritonitis, being most severe when there is widespread contamination by faeces, pus or infected bile. Peritonitis is less severe when infection is absent (e.g. perforated duodenal ulcer in its early stages).

On examination, the abdomen is rigid and tender and bowel sounds are absent because of peristaltic paralysis. Rectal examination provides a means of direct palpation of the pelvic peritoneum and will usually reveal anterior tenderness. This is a most important sign which if present, is strong evidence of pelvic peritonitis.

There is no specific investigation which will confirm the diagnosis but plain abdominal X-ray may provide additional clues as to the cause. It is unkind and unnecessary, however, to subject a patient to abdominal X-rays if a decision has already been taken to perform an emergency laparotomy.

Intra-abdominal haemorrhage

Blood may enter the abdominal cavity from a variety of sources, including ruptured ectopic pregnancy, leaking aortic aneurysm or blunt trauma, especially to the liver and spleen. Blood in the abdominal cavity causes moderate peritoneal irritation and symptoms similar to peritonitis, but often muted. Distinguishing between the two is usually not difficult because the history and other symptoms and signs give enough clues. Intraperitoneal bleeding may be confirmed by *peritoneal lavage* which involves instillation of saline via a peritoneal cannula; retrieval of blood-stained fluid is diagnostic.

Principles of management of peritonitis

Local peritonitis is treated according to the diagnosis. For example, appendicitis requires urgent appendicectomy whilst acute diverticulitis and salpingitis are usually managed with antibiotics.

With generalised peritonitis, the patient is at risk of death from toxaemia or septic shock. As soon as the diagnosis is made, high doses of antibiotics are given intravenously. With the exception of acute pancreatitis, generalised peritonitis requires urgent laparotomy to discover the cause and to clear the contaminating material (*peritoneal toilet*).

INTRA-ABDOMINAL ABSCESS

Pathophysiology and clinical features

There are two common causes of intra-abdominal abscess. The first occurs after bowel perforation, when omentum and adjacent gut attempt to wall off the defect. The second is a complication of bowel surgery where there has been localised faecal contamination or an anastomotic leak. Appendiceal perforation may cause a local abscess or one which tracks down into the pelvis. Diverticular disease often causes a pericolic abscess, particularly in the recto-sigmoid area or pelvis. Less commonly, perforation of a colonic tumour results in a pericolic abscess. Gall bladder perforation is rare and occasionally results in a right-sided subphrenic abscess. Finally, perforation of an ulcer in the posterior wall of the stomach may produce a lesser sac abscess.

With intra-abdominal abscess, abdominal pain is usually continuous rather than colicky and tends to increase inexorably. Local bowel irritation may cause diarrhoea or adynamic obstruction. A swinging pyrexia is an important sign which points to the diagnosis. There is usually a marked leucocytosis. The patient is otherwise relatively well, except the patient with a postoperative abscess, where there is a degree of toxaemia or even septicaemia. There may be a palpable abdominal inflammatory mass which most commonly originates with appendicitis or acute diverticular disease. Rectal examination may reveal a hot, tender mass (*a pelvic abscess*), displacing the rectum backwards. Such a patient will usually have complained of diarrhoea, due to inflammation in the vicinity of the rectum.

Ultrasound of the abdomen and pelvis is most useful in demonstrating the site and size of an abscess; drainage may be possible under ultrasound control. CT scanning may also be useful. When an abscess is suspected but cannot be demonstrated, radioisotope scanning, using the patient's own white cells labelled with indium, may be helpful (see Figure 7.8)

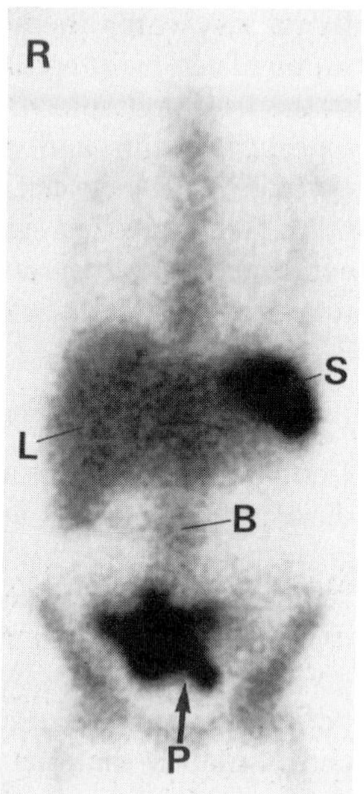

Fig. 7.8 Radioisotope scan showing large pelvic abscess

Radionuclide scan of a 47-year-old woman who presented with lower abdominal tenderness and a swinging pyrexia. The patient's own leucocytes were labelled with radioactive indium and reinjected. This scan shows a large pelvic abscess **P**, shown later to be due to diverticular perforation. Note also the normal radioisotope uptake by the spleen **S**, liver **L** and bone marrow **B**, which is a normal feature of such scans

Principles of management of an intra-abdominal abscess

There is no benefit in attempting to drain a pelvic abscess or to treat the patient with antibiotics if the patient is otherwise well, because the abscess will usually drain spontaneously into the rectum in time. Discharge of the abscess is recognised when the patient passes pus and blood per rectum; this is followed by resolution of the fever and healing.

Small subphrenic abscesses may also resolve without intervention but larger subphrenic abscesses can usually be drained percutaneously under ultrasound control. With these exceptions, intra-abdominal abscesses require laparotomy to effect drainage and deal with the source. Antibiotics should not be used, except in patients with systemic toxicity or septicaemia.

PERFORATION OF AN ABDOMINAL VISCUS

Pathophysiology and clinical features

Disease in any hollow abdominal viscus may be complicated by perforation into the peritoneal cavity. The common sites of perforation are stomach and duodenum (from peptic ulcer), sigmoid colon (from diverticular disease) and the appendix (from appendicitis). The symptoms and signs of a perforated viscus depend on the nature of its contents, the volume of spillage and the effectiveness of the local defences.

A small perforation may be immediately walled off by omentum and nearby bowel, but a local abscess will then develop. In this case, symptoms and signs are often grumbling and rather non-specific at first but subsequently develop into those of an intra-abdominal abscess. A typical example of this is appendicitis in adults. A small diverticular perforation without faecal spillage may cause localised peritonitis, which may even resolve spontaneously. At the opposite extreme, a large colonic perforation causes sudden overwhelming faecal peritonitis, which is often fatal despite treatment. A perforated peptic ulcer causes marked abdominal signs of peritonitis but little systemic upset. This is because the fluid spilled is usually sterile.

Perforation is essentially a clinical diagnosis but can usually be confirmed by the presence of free gas in the peritoneal cavity on plain abdominal X-ray. This can usually be seen as a radiolucent line beneath one or both hemidiaphragms on an erect chest film (see Figure 7.9) or on a lateral decubitus film of the abdomen. Radiology does not always demonstrate free gas when there is a perforation; if X-rays fail to support the clinical diagnosis, action should be taken on the clinical diagnosis. In the case of perforated appendicitis, free gas is very rarely seen.

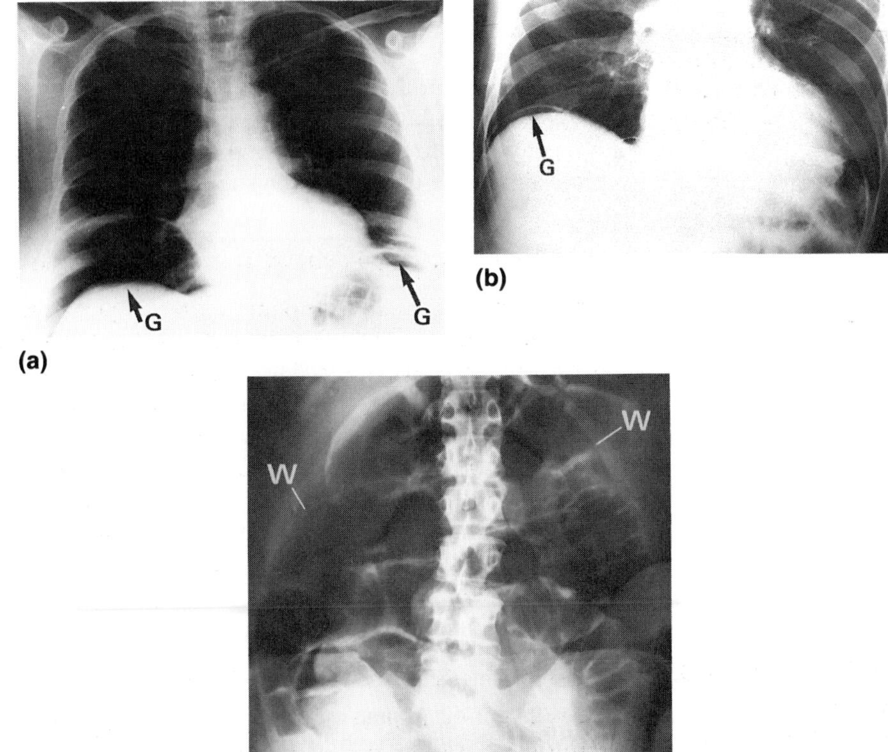

Fig. 7.9 Free perforation of an abdominal viscus

(a) Erect chest X-ray from a man of 60 with a perforated sigmoid diverticulum who presented with a sudden onset of severe abdominal pain. The film shows large radiolucent gas shadows **G** under each hemidiaphragm. Fortunately in this case, no faeces entered the peritoneum and the patient did not suffer shock or peritonitis.
(b) Similar view to (a) from a different patient, showing a smaller pneumoperitoneum **G** beneath the right hemidiaphragm.
(c) Supine abdominal X-ray showing free gas in the peritoneal cavity. This can be diagnosed because the outer wall of bowel **W** is clearly visible due to the presence of gas within and without

Principles of management of perforation

Perforation is a surgical emergency. Most cases require urgent laparotomy to repair the defect or resect the segment of diseased bowel. A temporary colostomy is often required in large bowel perforations because healing may be impaired if there has been peritoneal contamination. Occasionally, conservative management is appropriate, e.g. a perforated peptic ulcer in a debilitated patient.

ACUTE BOWEL ISCHAEMIA

Pathophysiology and clinical features

Occlusion of the superior mesenteric artery may lead to acute midgut ischaemia (i.e. of jejunum, ileum and right colon). This causes massive infarction and later, fatal perforation. There are two fairly distinct types of acute superior mesenteric occlusion. The first is embolism, which originates from left atrial thrombus in atrial fibrillation or from left ventricular wall thrombus after recent myocardial infarction. Secondly, thrombosis of the artery may occur. This is usually a terminal event in gross low output cardiac failure; thrombosis takes place more readily if the mesenteric vessels are already atherosclerotic. The particular vulnerability of the superior mesenteric artery is poorly understood as is the sparing of the coeliac and inferior mesenteric territories. It probably relates to the nature of the collateral blood supply.

Acute bowel ischaemia can be a difficult diagnosis to make because of the lack of specific clinical features and diagnostic tests. The severity of abdominal symptoms and signs often gives no clue to the catastrophe within. There may be diffuse tenderness, abdominal distension and absent bowel sounds. Typically, there is a disproportionate degree of cardiovascular collapse or shock. Diagnosis depends therefore on clinical suspicion. In the late stages, gas may appear within the bowel wall and be visible on plain abdominal X-ray; by this time surgery is unlikely to be successful.

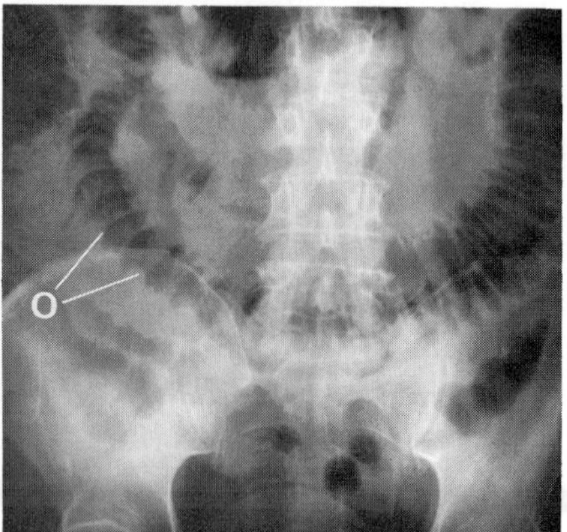

Fig. 7.10 Intestinal ischaemia

This 68-year-old woman with atrial fibrillation presented with collapse but only moderate abdominal pain. The patient had embolised her superior mesenteric artery *(acute SMA occlusion)* which supplies the primitive mid-gut. The whole of her small bowel and the right half of her colon was necrotic but the left half of the colon was intact. This film shows the typical gross thickening of small bowel folds **O** caused by swelling from oedema and intramural haemorrhage

Principles of management of intestinal ischaemia

If intestinal ischaemia is suspected, laparotomy must be performed urgently. It is sometimes possible to restore the mesenteric arterial supply by embolectomy or vascular bypass before the bowel becomes necrotic. If the infarcted segment is not too extensive and the rest of the bowel looks healthy, resection gives a reasonable chance of recovery and an adequate amount of bowel to sustain nutrition. In nearly half the cases, however, the extent of necrosis is so great that resection is unrealistic and the patient should be allowed to die with as little interference as possible.

Fig. 7.11 Summary — special points to note in examining a patient with an acute abdomen

General examination

— general demeanour, alertness and state of consciousness

— posture and movement

— state of hydration, skin colour (anaemia or cyanosis), perfusion and sweating

— temperature

— pulse (rate, character and regularity), blood pressure

— respiratory pattern and rate, breath sounds on auscultation

Abdominal examination

Inspection

— distension, visible peristalsis, previous operation scars, obvious hernias, abdominal movement with respiration

— always inspect the loins and back

Palpation and percussion

— tenderness, guarding, rigidity, rebound, pain on percussion

— free fluid, succussion splash

— hernias and their reducibility, external genitalia

— abdominal masses (including full bladder)

— abnormal pulsation (aneurysm)

Auscultation

— bowel sounds, mesenteric arterial bruits

Rectal examination (and vaginal examination if appropriate)

— inspection of anal margin

— peritoneal tenderness (unilateral tenderness may be uterine tube)

— lesions in the bowel wall, pelvic lesions

— stool colour and consistency, bleeding

— prostate size and consistency

MAJOR GASTROINTESTINAL HAEMORRHAGE

Pathophysiology and clinical features

Major gastrointestinal haemorrhage presents either as vomiting of blood or passage of frank or altered blood rectally. Vomited blood (*haematemesis*) may be fresh or partly digested. In the latter case, it is dark in colour and may have the typical appearance of 'coffee grounds'. Haematemesis usually indicates bleeding from the oesophagus or stomach but may indicate bleeding from the duodenum. Blood emanating beyond the duodenum will usually be passed rectally. The extent to which it is altered by digestion and the degree of mixing with the stool are useful indicators of its level of origin (described in Chapter 6). Upper gastrointestinal bleeding is often manifest by *melaena*. This is the passage of loose, black, tarry stools with a characteristic foul smell. The main causes of major gastrointestinal haemorrhage are summarised in Figure 7.12.

Fig. 7.12 Causes of major gastrointestinal haemorrhage

Chronic gastric and duodenal ulcers, acute gastric erosions and stress ulcers (very common) — haematemesis and/or melaena

Diverticular disease (common) — fresh rectal bleeding

Oesophageal varices (uncommon) — haematemesis and/or melaena

Mallory–Weiss oesophageal tears (uncommon) — haematemesis

Colonic or small bowel angiodysplasias (uncommon) — fresh or altered blood per rectum

Fulminant inflammatory bowel disease (uncommon) — bloody diarrhoea

Malignant small bowel tumours (rare) — altered blood per rectum

Principles of management of severe gastrointestinal haemorrhage

Any patient presenting with severe gastrointestinal haemorrhage is at risk of death from hypovolaemic shock. The volume of blood vomited or passed per rectum is unreliable as a measure of true blood loss because a great deal may still remain in the gut. It is therefore essential during resuscitation to adjust the rate and volume of intravenous fluid replacement (whether plasma expanders or blood) against the responses of pulse rate, blood pressure, central venous pressure and hourly urine output.

Once the patient is stable, further details of the history can be taken, including any relevant previous history of peptic ulceration and gastric surgery, diverticular disease or cirrhosis. Abdominal examination is usually unremarkable but general examination may show signs of chronic liver disease suggesting possible oesophageal varices. Rectal examination may reveal melaena stool or altered blood, and this can be helpful if the history of haematemesis is not substantiated e.g. 'coffee-ground' vomit not seen by a doctor.

After the initial haemorrhage precipitating admission to hospital, most patients stop bleeding with conservative management. All such patients should be assessed early by a surgical team, even if admitted under the care of a gastroenterologist or physician. This is because of the very real danger of rebleeding which may be catastrophic. The same surgical team should ideally remain responsible for that patient until recovery. This continuity of surgical care ensures that a decision to operate can be made without procrastination, if conservative management shows signs of failing.

The nature and timing of investigation for gastrointestinal haemorrhage depends on the rate of bleeding and where it seems to be coming from. If the patient is in a stable state and an upper gastrointestinal lesion seems likely, gastroscopy should be performed as soon as practicable, certainly within 24 hours. More distal bleeding is usually not investigated initially but managed conservatively, the site and nature of the lesion being investigated later as appropriate.

If bleeding persists, an operation will be needed. The source of bleeding may be difficult or impossible to find at laparotomy, therefore, any help that can be obtained from prior investigation is well worthwhile. Even in the most acute case of upper gastrointestinal haemorrhage, gastroscopy can usually be performed on the operating table before operation. The common causes, namely duodenal or gastric ulcer, should be easily identifiable by gastroscopy, but these could be found at operation without this assistance; the real value of gastroscopy is the ability to diagnose unusual sources of bleeding, most of which present particular operative problems. Thus, oesophageal ulceration or a Mallory–Weiss tear may be discovered, and the surgeon can avoid operating on unsuspected variceal haemorrhage. Nevertheless, when blood loss is extremely rapid, a laparotomy must be performed immediately to staunch the flow.

If bleeding is less rapid but recurrent or persistent, it is even more important to know the source before operation. In addition to gastroscopy, investigation may include colonoscopy, radioisotope scanning using the patient's own labelled red cells or highly selective arteriography (see Figure 7.13). As a last resort, a colonoscope can be used to examine the whole colon and small bowel for bleeding sites; in suspected small bowel bleeding, the colonoscope is inserted

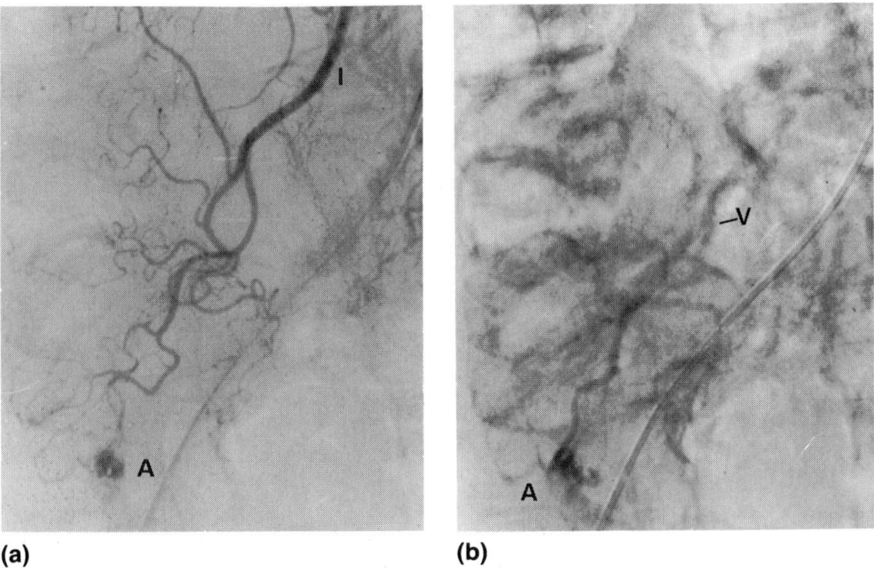

Fig. 7.13 Angiogram showing angiodysplasia of caecum

This man of 70 had been admitted to hospital on 12 occasions for rectal bleeding and chronic anaemia and had received 55 units of blood transfusion in all. On the last admission, this superior mesenteric arteriogram was performed, revealing the source of blood loss. **(a)** Subtraction film showing the arterial phase; the ileo-colic artery **I** feeds a knot of abnormal blood vessels, an angiodysplasia **A** at the lower pole of the caecum, which had been bleeding. **(b)** Subtraction film of the venous phase; the angiodysplasia **A** is still visible and there is early filling of a large draining vein **V**. These appearances are typical of angiodysplasia, and this is the most common site of occurrence

through an incision in the bowel wall at laparotomy. This may be the only means of diagnosing angiodysplasia.

Fig. 7.14 Summary — investigation of the acute abdomen

BLOOD TESTS

Haemoglobin — may be normal immediately after an acute bleed; low haemoglobin concentration may represent chronic anaemia due to occult blood loss rather than acute haemorrhage

White blood count — leucocytosis is non-specific and rarely of much diagnostic value

Serum amylase — whenever pancreatitis cannot be excluded

Urea and electrolytes — indicated in vomiting and diarrhoea, dehydration, poor urine output, diuretic therapy, urinary tract disease, known or suspected renal failure, pancreatitis and septicaemia

Glucose — for diabetics or those with glycosuria (beware of hyperglycaemia due to acute stress and steroid therapy)

Blood group and cross match — for anaemic patients, major haemorrhage or when major surgery is contemplated

Liver function tests and calcium estimation — for pancreatitis and acute biliary disease

Clotting studies — for acute pancreatitis and septicaemia (*disseminated intravascular coagulation*), severe bleeding (*consumption coagulopathy*) or those with a history of bleeding disorders

URINE TESTS

Ward ('stick') testing — for blood, protein, bile, glucose

Microscopy — for red and white blood cells, organisms

Culture and sensitivity — suspected urinary tract infections

Strain urine for stones — in ureteric colic

RADIOLOGY

Chest X-ray

— cardiovascular disease or abnormality e.g. hypertension, cardiac failure

— chest disease

— suspected visceral perforation (gas under diaphragm)

Plain abdominal X-rays (supine plus erect or decubitus)

— gut (gas pattern and dilatation, fluid levels, gas in the wall, faeces and faecoliths)

— urinary tract (kidney size and position, calculi)

— biliary tract (gallstones, gas in biliary tree in gallstone ileus)

— aortic calcification (aneurysm)

— psoas shadows (obscured by retroperitoneal inflammation or haemorrhage)

Contrast radiology

— 'instant' barium enema in colonic obstruction or acute colitis

— emergency intravenous urography in ureteric colic

8 GALLSTONE DISEASES AND RELATED DISORDERS

Introduction

Gallstones and related disorders account for all but a small proportion of biliary tract disease. The remainder, cholangiocarcinoma and sclerosing cholangitis, are discussed in Chapter 12. Gallstone disease is also known as *cholelithiasis*. When stones are present in the bile ducts, this is known as *choledocholithiasis*.

Most gall stone related disease presents with pain, typically located in the epigastrium or right hypochondrium. The character of the pain varies with the diagnosis; in most cases, it is neither acute nor particularly severe, but rather chronic or intermittent and often rather poorly defined. For this reason, gall stone disease tends to be investigated from the outpatient clinic. Less commonly, gallstone disease presents as jaundice caused by a stone passing into and obstructing the common bile duct.

Non-acute upper abdominal pain is a common cause of surgical referral, accounting for up to 7% of outpatient referrals in a typical District General Hospital. Of these, about half will be diagnosed as having gall stone disease. Furthermore, about 25% of adult elective laparotomies in district general hospitals are performed for gall bladder disease. As gall bladder surgery is fraught with potentially serious complications, there is considerable scope for the development of effective preventive measures, safer surgical techniques and better non-surgical methods of managing gallstone disease.

Fig. 8.1 Surgical anatomy of the gall bladder, biliary tract and pancreas

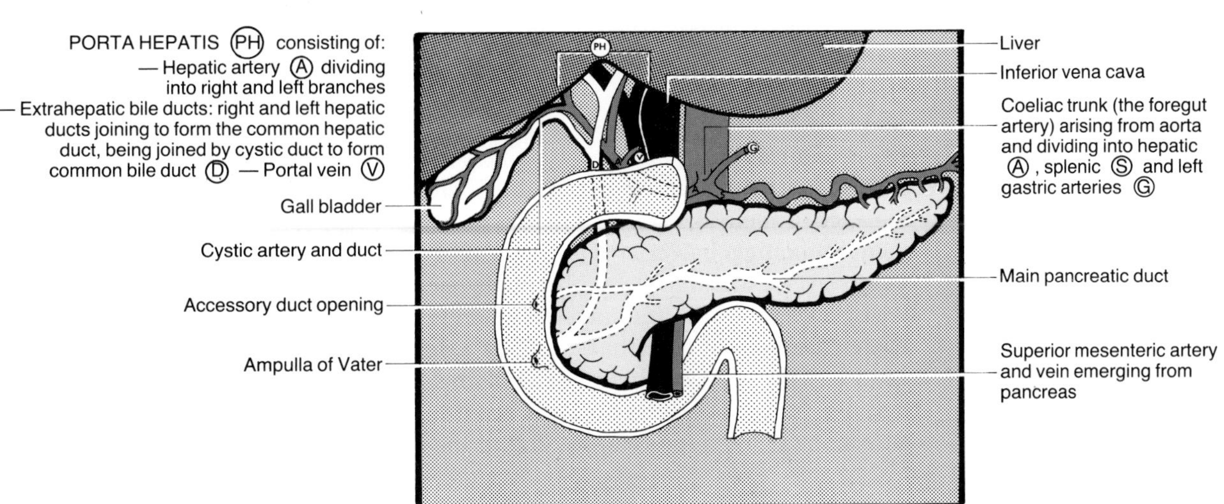

STRUCTURE AND FUNCTION OF THE BILIARY SYSTEM

Bile collects in the canaliculi between hepatocytes and drains via collecting ducts in the portal triads into a system of ducts within the liver. These increase in diameter until they become the *right* and *left hepatic ducts* which fuse to form the *common hepatic duct*; 3–4 cm outside the liver, this is joined by the *cystic duct* to become the *common bile duct*. The common bile duct is 4–5 cm long and passes down behind the duodenum near the head of the pancreas to drain via the *ampulla of Vater* into the second part of the duodenum. Reflux of duodenal contents is prevented by the *sphincter of Oddi*. In most cases, the *main pancreatic duct* joins the common bile duct at the ampulla, although it may enter the duodenum independently.

The *gall bladder* is a muscular sac lined by a single, highly folded layer of tall columnar epithelial cells. The lining epithelium is supported by loose connective tissue which contains numerous blood vessels and lymphatics. Mucus-secreting glands are found at the neck of the gall bladder but are absent from the body and fundus. The gall bladder lies in a depression in the under surface of the right hepatic lobe, and is covered by the same peritoneal covering as the liver. The common bile duct is a fibromuscular tube lined by a simple, tall columnar epithelium. It is normally up to 0.6 cm in diameter.

Bile is continuously made by the liver and passes down the biliary tract into the gall bladder where it is stored. Bile is concentrated by as much as ten times in the gall bladder by active mucosal reabsorption of water. Lipid-rich food passing from stomach to duodenum promotes secretion of the hormone *cholecystokinin-pancreozymin* (CCK) by endocrine cells of the duodenal mucosa. This hormone stimulates contraction of the gall bladder, forcing bile into the duodenum. Bile acts as an emulsifying agent and facilitates hydrolysis of dietary lipids by pancreatic lipases. If bile fails to reach the duodenum because of biliary tract obstruction, lipids are neither digested nor absorbed, resulting in the passage of loose foul-smelling fatty stools (steatorrhoea). Furthermore, the fat-soluble vitamins (A, D, E and K) are not absorbed, the lack of vitamin K soon leading to inadequate prothrombin synthesis and hence defective clotting; this may pose problems if surgery is necessary in a patient with obstructive jaundice.

PATHOGENESIS OF GALLSTONE DISEASE

Gallstone composition

In developed countries, most gall stones contain a predominance of *cholesterol* mixed with some *bile pigment* (calcium bilirubinate) and other *calcium salts*. A small proportion are virtually 'pure' cholesterol stones ('cholesterol solitaire'). In Asia, most gall stones are composed of bile pigment alone. The composition and pathogenesis of the various types of gall stone are summarised in Figure 8.2.

The physical structure of mixed gall stones gives an insight into the time sequence of their formation. There is usually a small core of organic material, often containing bacteria. The main part of the stone is made up of concentric layers, which suggests that the stone does not form in a single episode, but by a series of discrete precipitation events. Furthermore, there are often several 'families' of gall stones, each of a different size, found in the same gall bladder. This suggests that each family began at a different time, presumably due to a transient change in local conditions. All families then build up by lamination at the same rate, leading to the variety of different sizes. Radioisotope dating studies have shown that the average gall stone is 11 years old when it is removed!

The full story of how the common cholesterol-predominant (or mixed) stones are formed has not yet been elucidated, but several clues are available. The main factors are changes in concentration of the different constituents of bile, biliary stasis and infection. It is likely that several subtle abnormalities combine to encourage precipitation of bile constituents.

Bile salts and lecithin are responsible for maintaining cholesterol in a stable micelle formation. The normal micellar structure of bile supports a greater concentration of cholesterol than could normally be held in solution, and it is therefore inherently unstable. An excess of cholesterol in relation to bile salts and lecithin is probably one of the main factors. This is supported by the observation that patients whose terminal ileum has been resected or who have chronic distal ileal disease, have a three-fold risk of developing cholesterol-rich stones. The terminal ileum is the main site for reabsorption of bile salts. When this is removed or diseased, reabsorption falls off, leading to loss of bile salts via the gut and a consequent reduction in the bile salt pool. Bile salts are thus insufficient to maintain the micellar structure of cholesterol suspension.

Precipitation is enhanced by biliary stasis. This occurs if the gall bladder becomes obstructed or contractility becomes defective. It is not known whether

Fig. 8.2 Composition and pathogenesis of gallstones

CHEMICAL COMPOSITION	PATHOGENESIS	MORPHOLOGY
1. Mixed stones *(75–90% of all stones)* Cholesterol is the predominant constituent. Heterogenous mixture of cholesterol, bile pigments and calcium salts in a 'core' and laminated structure	Combination of: • Abnormalities of bile constituents • Bile stasis • Infection	Multiple stones, several generations of different sizes often found together. Stones may be hard and facetted (where they have developed in contact) or irregular 'mulberry' shaped and softer. Colour ranges from near white through yellow and green to black. Most are radiolucent but 10% are radiopaque.
2. Cholesterol stones *(up to 10% of all stones)*	As for mixed stones	Large, smooth, egg– or barrel–shaped and usually solitary ('cholesterol solitaire') Yellowish. Up to 4 cm diameter and may fill the gall bladder. Radiolucent
3. Pigment stones Calcium bilirubinate (uncommon in developed countries, common in Asia)	Excess bilirubin excretion due to haemolytic disorders, e.g. haemolytic anaemias, malaria, leukaemias	Multiple, jet black, shiny 'jack' stones; 0.5-1cm diameter. Usually of uniform size and often friable
4. Calcium carbonate stones (rare)	Excess calcium excretion in bile	Greyish facetted stones. Radiopaque

obstruction of the gall bladder outlet is a primary event in the formation of stones, but it is believed to play a part in their continued accretion. Obstruction could be caused by dysfunction of the spiral valve in the cystic duct, by reflux of duodenal contents (which may be infected) or by small stones already formed. The muscular gall bladder wall is damaged by long-standing inflammation or infection, which interferes with its ability to empty.

The role of inflammation and infection

The relative roles of inflammation and infection in gall stone formation are still in doubt, but probably both play a part. Abnormalities of bile composition may cause chemical inflammation of the gall bladder, resulting in inflammatory exudation and perhaps accumulation of inflammatory debris. Infection probably plays a part in the pathogenesis of gall stones. Bacteria usually form the organic nidus upon which gall stones are built: they enter the gall bladder intermittently by reflux from the duodenum or via the blood stream. This process is probably normal in itself but becomes pathological if the bacteria are not flushed out — as when the gall bladder does not adequately empty. Once stones are formed, episodic bacterial ingress could be responsible for periods of precipitation during which layers of the laminated structure are built up. Indeed, some gall stones continue to harbour bacteria so the process becomes self-perpetuating; in support of this is the fact that faecal organisms can be cultured from at least 25% of cholecystectomy specimens.

The role of chronic obstruction

Transient obstruction of the gall bladder by stone may cause episodes of acute pain (*biliary colic*). If the obstruction persists, the gall bladder becomes chemically inflamed causing *acute cholecystitis*. If obstruction does not resolve by itself and the contents do not become infected, the gall bladder becomes distended with mucus; this is known as a *mucocoele*, and is often palpable and tender. If however, the contents become infected, an abscess develops within the gall bladder. This is known as an *empyema of the gall bladder*.

The majority of gall bladders removed for chronic pain show a range of histological features much more in keeping with a *chronic obstructive aetiology* than an infective one. These features include intact but often atrophic mucosa, submucosal and subserosal fibrosis, hypertrophy of the muscular wall, and mucosal diverticula extending into the muscular layer (known as *Rokitansky–Aschoff sinuses*). Evidence of active or previous infection is uncommon. Inflammatory infiltrates are mainly associated with traumatic gallstone erosion of the mucosa or intrusion of inspissated bile into the gall bladder wall, particularly around the mucosal diverticula. In some cases the gall bladder is so grossly scarred, distorted or contracted that its absorptive and contractile functions must have been completely destroyed.

Other pathological mechanisms

In nearly 20% of patients with gall bladder disease, no stone can be demonstrated during investigation or at operation. In some of these cases, a stone

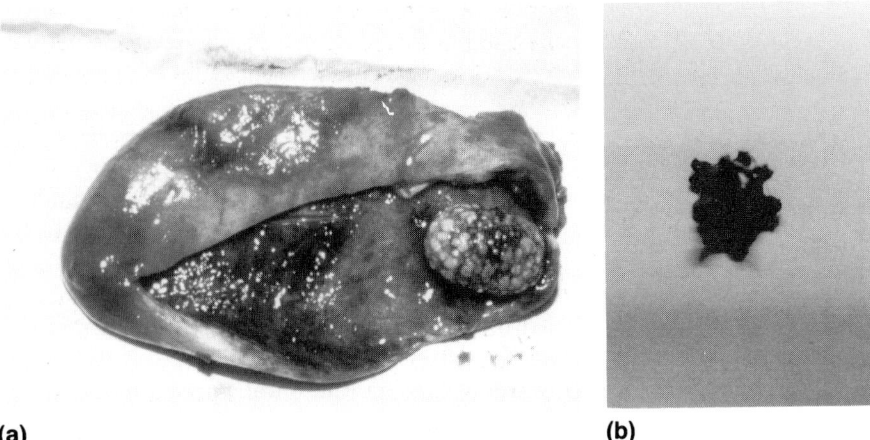

(a) (b)

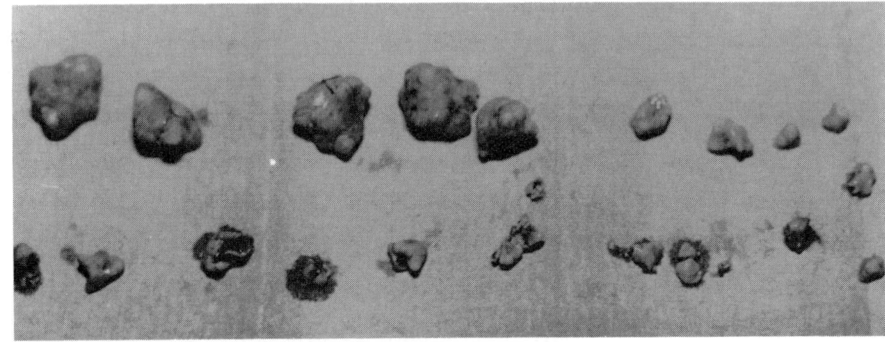

(c)

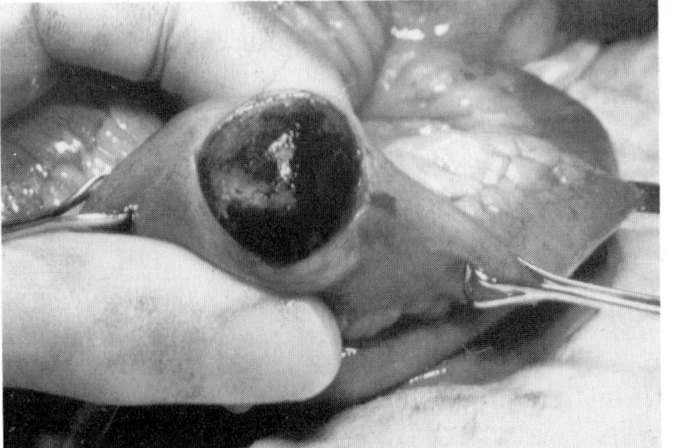

(d)

Fig. 8.3 Types of gallstones

(a) Thick-walled chronically inflamed gall bladder which was found to be obstructed at its neck by a single stone. Note the stone is an aggregate of many smaller stones.
(b) 'Jack-stone' type of gallstone. This single non-obstructing gallstone was found in a mildly inflamed gall bladder.
(c) These families of stones were all from one gall bladder and presumably originated at different times.
(d) Cholesterol 'solitaire' which had caused gallstone ileus by obstructing the terminal ileum. The photograph shows it being removed from the distal ileum at operation

may have passed out of the duct system into the bowel. In other cases, chronic inflammation occurs independently of stones, the so-called '*cholecystitis sans stones*'; again, chronic obstruction may be the aetiology. Finally, the terms 'biliary dyskinesia' and 'cystic duct syndrome' have been adopted by some people to explain the situation where patients have typical symptoms of gall bladder disease but essentially normal investigations. The idea is that the cystic duct is too narrow to allow normal biliary drainage. Confirming this diagnosis is difficult because there are no reliable tests, and only a proportion of patients suspected of this are cured by cholecystectomy. The resected specimen is found to be normal both macroscopically and histologically.

Epidemiology of gallstones

In developed countries, at least 10% of the adult population probably have gall stones although most remain asymptomatic. Gall stones are rare before adulthood and increase in prevalence with age. Women are affected four times as often as men and it appears that pregnancy, obesity and diabetes are important predisposing factors. The typical patient is said to be a Fair Fat Fertile Female of Forty, but many gall stone patients do not fit this description! Gallstone disease is rare in the rural communities of undeveloped countries but is increasing with urbanisation. Western style processed foods, high in fats and refined carbohydrates but poor in fibre, may be responsible. Their contribution to gall bladder disease would be compatible with the theory that changes in the composition of bile are the most important factors in stone pathogenesis.

INVESTIGATION OF SUSPECTED GALLSTONES

When gall stone disease is suspected, investigation has the following objectives:

- Exclude haematological, liver function and other systemic abnormalities
- Establish whether gall stones are present in the gall bladder or common duct
- Evaluate gall bladder function (i.e. ability to concentrate bile and to contract)
- Assess integrity of the bile duct system and the pancreatic duct (if there is any suggestion of obstruction)

Blood tests for haematological and liver abnormalities

In many straightforward cases, no blood tests are necessary except perhaps to exclude anaemia in susceptible groups such as women of child-bearing age. *Haemolytic disorders* such as hereditary spherocytosis, thalassaemia and sickle cell trait should be considered as they may predispose to pigment stones. Liver function tests will be indicated if there is any suggestion of jaundice or other liver abnormality. Finally, blood cultures to exclude septicaemia may be appropriate in seriously ill patients.

Investigation of gall bladder pathology

Investigation for gall bladder disease aims to demonstrate the presence of stones and some aspects of gall bladder function. Both ultrasound and oral cholecystography have a place in investigation.

a. Ultrasound

Ultrasound is now reliable for identifying stones in the gall bladder and in estimating gall bladder wall thickness (caused by inflammation or fibrosis). Unfortunately, ultrasound is unreliable for identifying duct stones, particularly at the lower end; it does, however, provide a simple and accurate means of demonstrating *duct dilatation*, which might indicate distal duct obstruction. Ultrasound also has the great advantage of being suitable for the seriously ill or jaundiced patient.

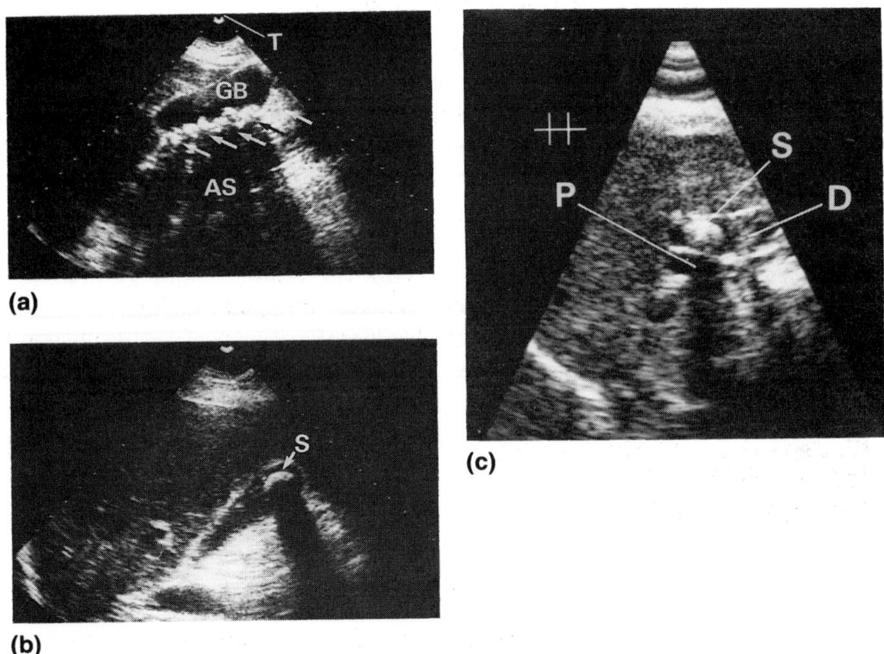

Fig. 8.4 Biliary ultrasound scans

(a) Longitudinal scan of gall bladder in a 46-year-old woman who complains of intermittent attacks of right upper quadrant pain. The scan shows the outline of the gall bladder **GB** and a layer of gallstones (arrowed) along its posterior wall. The stones each cast a clear acoustic shadow **AS** beyond them. Note that these shadows can be projected back to the transducer **T**. **(b)** Longitudinal scan of the gall bladder in a 37-year-old woman showing a single large stone **S** in the fundus. Note that only the anterior surface of the stone is seen (as an arc) because all sound waves are reflected from it, casting a dense acoustic shadow beyond.
(c) Longitudinal scan of the common bile duct in a 66-year-old woman who had transient right upper quadrant pain and jaundice. The scan shows a stone **S** in the upper part of the common bile duct. The duct **D** can be recognised by its relationship to the portal vein **P**. Note that ultrasound is a poor method of demonstrating stones at the lower end of the common bile duct because the image tends to be obscured by overlying duodenal gas

b. Oral cholecystography

Oral cholecystography provides a different perspective by showing gall bladder function, and only incidentally revealing stones. It involves ingestion of contrast medium which is absorbed, excreted by the liver and then radiographically demonstrated in the extrahepatic biliary system. At the outset, a plain radiograph of the biliary area (*control film*) is taken; this may demonstrate stones, although only about 10% of all stones are radiopaque. It may occasionally show *calcification* in the pancreas (indicating previous pancreatitis), or a gall bladder outlined by calcification ('porcelain gall bladder').

Immediately after the plain radiograph, the contrast medium is given by mouth. Twelve hours later, further films are taken. The standard position is *prone*, but various other projections are used if necessary.

If the concentrating function of the gall bladder is normal, the gall bladder will be visible as a radiopaque viscus in which negative shadows of stones may be seen as *filling defects* (see Figure 8.5). If the gall bladder fails to opacify, this implies that the gall bladder is either obstructed by a stone blocking the gall bladder neck or is unable to concentrate bile because of inflammatory damage to the wall. This condition is sometimes called a 'non-functioning gall bladder'. Oral fatty liquid or chocolate (*fatty meal*) is usually given to cause release of cholecystokinin into the blood stream. The normal gall bladder contracts and this is visible radiologically. Failure to contract suggests inflammatory damage to the gall bladder.

Oral cholecystography is of little value in jaundice, hepatic failure, intestinal malabsorption and vomiting. The investigation is rarely indicated in acute gall bladder disease because the gall bladder is usually obstructed, and in any case, a negative result would not influence management.

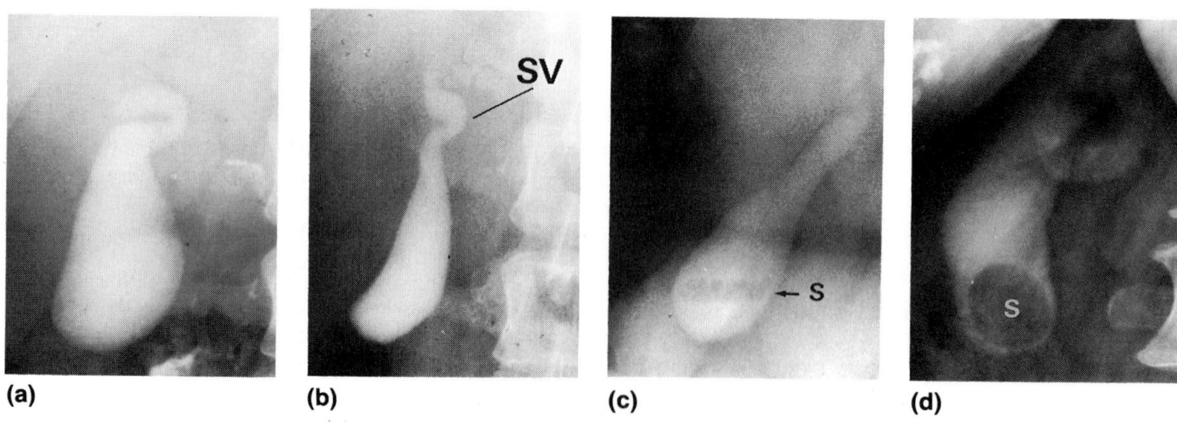

Fig. 8.5 Oral cholecystography

(a) Normal oral cholecystogram. This film was taken, as usual, in the prone position 12 hours after the patient swallowed contrast. There is good opacification of the gall bladder and cystic duct and there are no filling defects within. **(b)** A second view of the same patient taken after a fatty meal. The gall bladder has contracted vigorously and contrast can now be seen in the 'spiral valve' **SV** of the cystic duct. **(c)** Oral cholecystogram in a 33-year-old woman complaining of attacks of epigastric pain for several years following her third pregnancy. This film was taken in the erect position. The gall bladder opacifies well and a horizontal layer of radiolucent stones **S** can be seen. **(d)** Oral cholecystogram in a woman of 72 who complained of grumbling upper abdominal pain. The gall bladder opacifies well and a single large gallstone **S** is seen occupying the fundus. This type of stone is usually known as a *cholesterol solitaire*. It can ulcerate through into the duodenum and obstruct the distal ileum, causing *gallstone ileus* (see Figures 8.3d and 8.9)

Investigation of the biliary duct system

a. The non-jaundiced patient

Patients with gall stones but no history of obstructive jaundice do not require preoperative investigation for duct stones. This is performed routinely by *peroperative cholangiography* at cholecystectomy. The bile duct system is outlined by passing a cannula through the cystic duct into the common bile duct and injecting radiopaque contrast material (see Figure 8.11). This fills the biliary tree and should flow into the duodenum. X-rays or fluoroscopic imaging are then used to demonstrate the duct morphology and any abnormalities such as duct dilatation, filling defects caused by stone or distortion of the tapering lower end of the common duct, as well as obstruction of flow into the duodenum. If cholangiography shows a stone or stones, the duct is explored as described later.

A different problem is the patient with a history of *transient jaundice* possibly attributable to stones. Most cases will only have peroperative cholangiography at cholecystectomy, but some surgeons endeavour to make a firm preoperative diagnosis. This permits better planning of the operation but represents an extra procedure. Oral cholecystography is unreliable for the duct system, and intravenous cholangiography is out of favour because of poor definition and unpleasant side effects like nausea or even anaphylaxis. A better alternative is endoscopic retrograde cholangio-pancreatography (ERCP), described in Chapter 2.

b. The jaundiced patient

When obstructive jaundice has been diagnosed, it is important to distinguish between stone and tumour in order to plan appropriate management. Cholecystography and intravenous cholangiography are no use in the presence of jaundice because contrast is not excreted.

Ultrasound is usually the initial investigation. This shows the extent of dilatation of both intra- and extrahepatic ducts and may even show a stone lodged at the lower end of the duct. If stones are demonstrated in the gall bladder, this adds weight to the idea that stones are blocking the duct rather than tumour, but both can coexist. The ultrasound scan will usually demonstrate a carcinoma of the pancreatic head or enlarged lymph nodes in the porta hepatis; either may cause extrahepatic biliary obstruction.

Ultrasound may make the diagnosis, but if more detailed information is required, biliary tract morphology can be outlined by direct injection of contrast. There are two methods: *endoscopic retrograde cannulation* of the ampulla of Vater (ERCP), and *percutaneous transhepatic cholangiography*. ERCP is a more useful and less invasive investigation; it avoids needle injection into the liver and also allows the ampullary region to be inspected for tumour. Furthermore, the pancreatic duct may be outlined if required. If stones are found in the common bile duct, it is often possible to perform immediate *endoscopic sphincterotomy*, releasing the stone, thus diagnosing and relieving the jaundice in one procedure. This may be life-saving for the patient with ascending cholangitis and is the treatment of choice for the patient who is a poor risk for laparotomy.

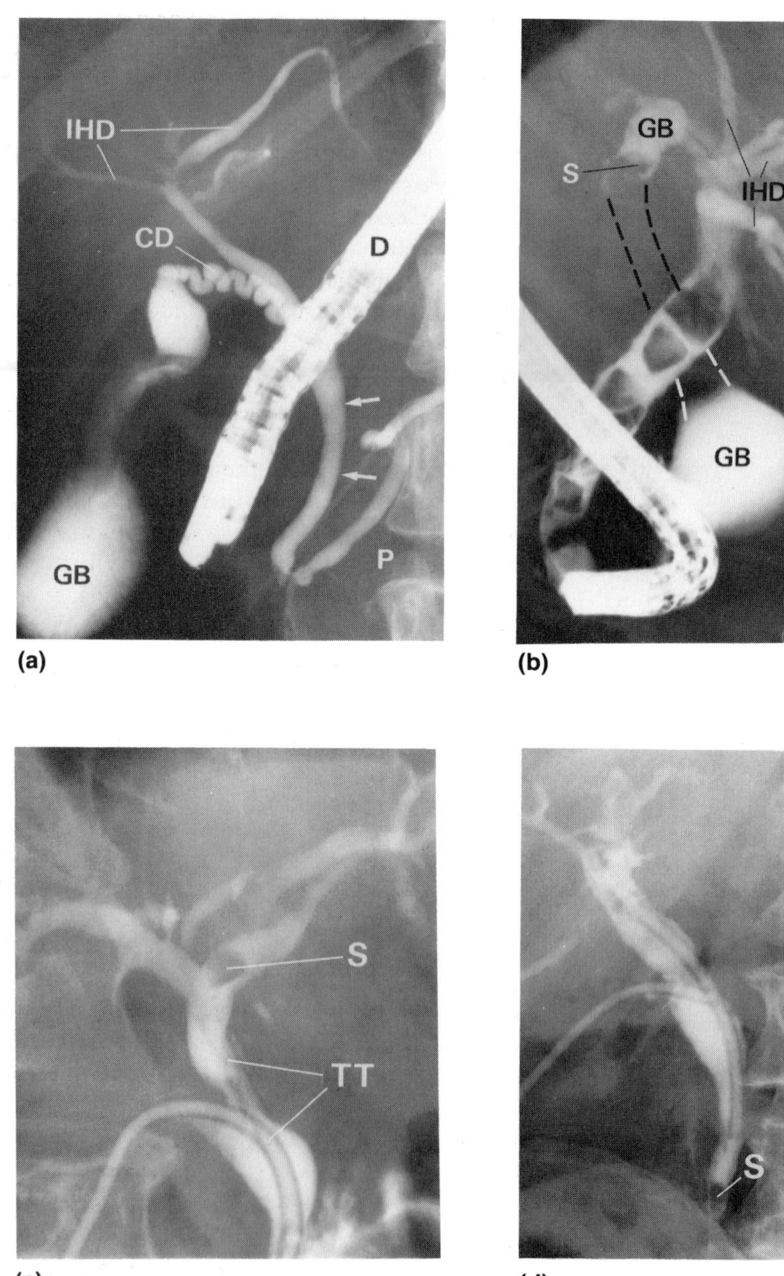

Fig. 8.6 Investigation of the biliary duct system

(a) Normal ERCP showing duodenoscope **D** in the second part of the duodenum. Contrast has been injected first into the pancreatic duct **P** and then into the common bile duct (arrowed). Note also the cystic duct **CD**, gall bladder **GB** and intrahepatic bile ducts **IHD**. **(b)** Endoscopic retrograde cholangiogram in a woman of 77 who presented with mild epigastric pain and obstructive jaundice. The film shows multiple large stones in the common bile duct, represented by filling defects. The common bile duct is moderately dilated, but the intrahepatic ducts **IHD** are not. The fundus and neck of the gall bladder **GB** are shown, but the body is empty of contrast (dotted lines). There is a stone **S** near the neck of the gall bladder. **(c)** and **(d)** Postoperative *T-tube cholangiogram* films taken (routinely) 7 days after a cholecystectomy and removal of stones from the common bile duct. The films show the T-tube **TT** in situ. In (c), a stone **S** can be seen in the left hepatic duct, and in (d), another stone **S** can be seen at the lower end of the common bile duct. Both stones were successfully retrieved percutaneously 6 weeks later. The T-tube was removed and steerable grasping forceps passed into the biliary system through the skin defect. Each stone was then grasped and drawn to the surface along the track.

Percutaneous cholangiography is used if ERCP is unavailable or unsuccessful. It involves inserting a fine (22 gauge) needle through the skin into one of the dilated intrahepatic ducts, under radiological control. Contrast medium is then injected in an antegrade direction. An obstructing stone produces a characteristic rounded filling defect, as opposed to the tapering stricture typical of tumour (see Figure 8.6).

CLINICAL PRESENTATIONS OF GALL STONE DISEASE

The names attached to the various clinical syndromes associated with gall stones are somewhat confusing and at best imprecise. This is partly because more than one pathological process may occur at once; hence the true diagnosis can often be made only in the histology laboratory.

Most commonly, gall stones cause chronic, low-grade symptoms, probably due to a combination of obstruction and inflammation. This condition does not have a generally agreed clinical name, being variously known as '*gall stones*', *chronic cholecystitis* or *flatulent dyspepsia*. 'Chronic low-grade obstructive gall bladder disease' is probably as good a descriptive term as any and is used throughout this text; 'chronic obstructive cholecystopathy' would be more elegant and is perhaps more accurate.

Severe pain occurs if the gall bladder becomes acutely obstructed, even transiently. This is known as *biliary colic*. Acute inflammation of the gall bladder is known as *acute cholecystitis*. It may be complicated by mucocoele of the gall bladder, abscess formation (empyema), free perforation or, rarely, by fistula formation or gall stone ileus. Finally, gall stones probably predispose to carcinoma in the very long term. The spectrum of clinical disorders associated with gall stones is summarised in Figure 8.7.

CHRONIC LOW-GRADE OBSTRUCTIVE GALL BLADDER DISEASE

Clinical features

Intermittent cystic duct obstruction by stone is probably the most common reason for symptoms from gall stones. Typically, patients are female and fall into two groups: the young or middle-aged, often overweight woman, where there is likely to be little histological evidence of inflammation in the gall bladder, and the elderly woman in whom the gall bladder is grossly thickened, chronically inflamed and shrunken. In either case, there is often a long history of almost daily pain, which is poorly localised in the right upper quadrant or epigastrium. It is often accompanied by nausea or even vomiting. The pain is exacerbated by large or fatty meals and may radiate around towards the back. The symptoms are often rather vague and ill-defined; this probably explains why patients often delay consulting a doctor. However, not all patients with these symptoms have gall stones or any gall bladder pathology!

Examination rarely reveals more than mild upper abdominal tenderness. Differential diagnosis includes peptic ulcer disease, urinary tract infection, chronic constipation or irritable bowel syndrome.

Management

If a patient has upper abdominal symptoms and demonstrable gall stones, this does not prove the one is caused by the other. Asymptomatic gall stones are a common enough incidental finding, and it sometimes takes fine clinical judgement to decide whether cholecystectomy is likely to cure the symptoms.

When symptoms are characteristic of gall bladder disease, no other special investigations are required. When the symptoms are less clear-cut, a more

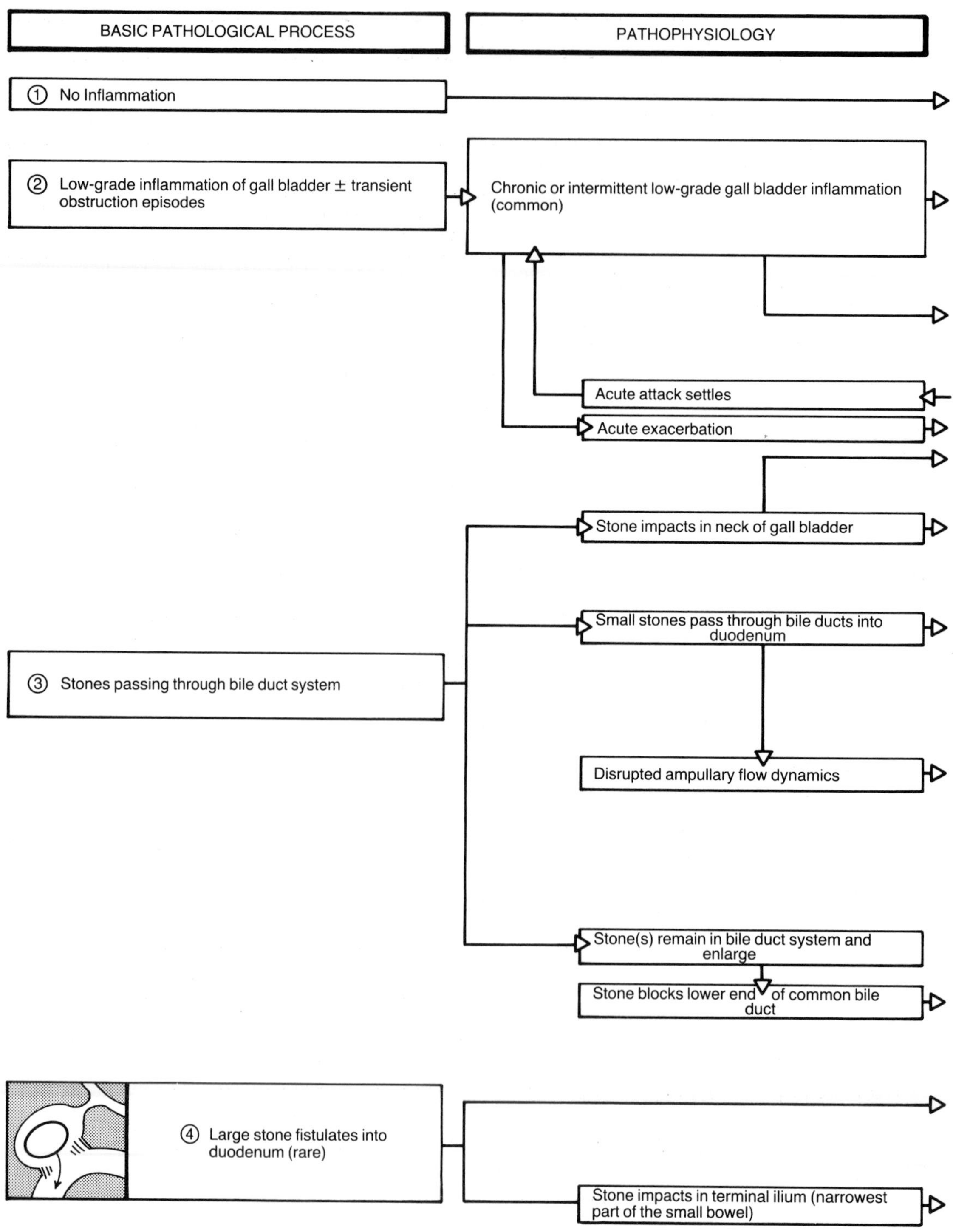

Fig. 8.7 Clinical consequences of gallstones

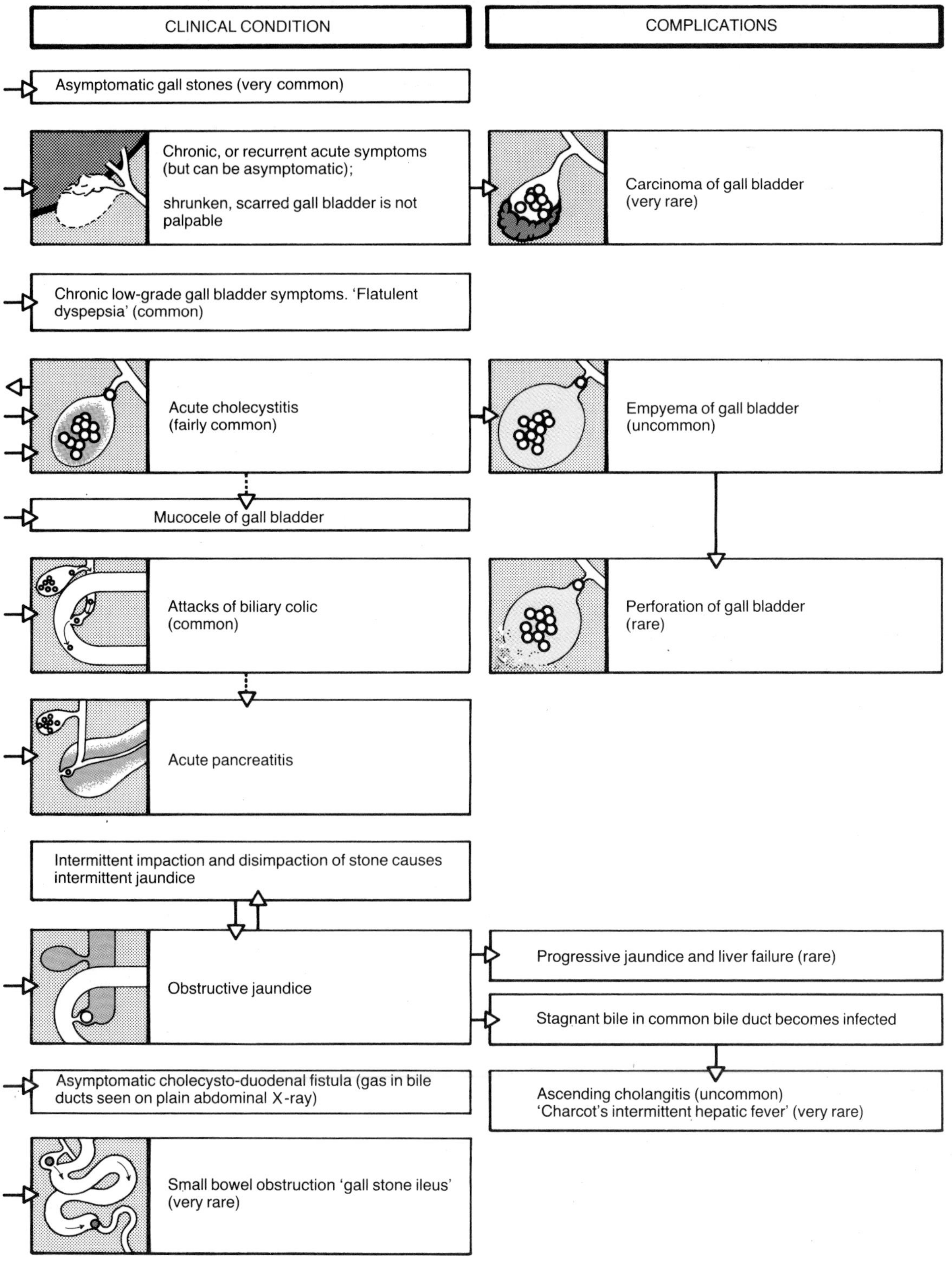
CLINICAL CONDITION
COMPLICATIONS
Asymptomatic gall stones (very common)
Chronic, or recurrent acute symptoms (but can be asymptomatic);
shrunken, scarred gall bladder is not palpable
Carcinoma of gall bladder (very rare)
Chronic low-grade gall bladder symptoms. 'Flatulent dyspepsia' (common)
Acute cholecystitis (fairly common)
Empyema of gall bladder (uncommon)
Mucocele of gall bladder
Attacks of biliary colic (common)
Perforation of gall bladder (rare)
Acute pancreatitis
Intermittent impaction and disimpaction of stone causes intermittent jaundice
Obstructive jaundice
Progressive jaundice and liver failure (rare)
Stagnant bile in common bile duct becomes infected
Asymptomatic cholecysto-duodenal fistula (gas in bile ducts seen on plain abdominal X-ray)
Ascending cholangitis (uncommon)
'Charcot's intermittent hepatic fever' (very rare)
Small bowel obstruction 'gall stone ileus' (very rare)

extensive search is necessary, perhaps including upper gastrointestinal endoscopy, serum amylase and ECG.

Cholecystectomy is the definitive treatment for chronic low-grade obstructive gall bladder disease. Patients are frequently put on a low fat diet initially or while awaiting operation; this often relieves symptoms, presumably by removing a stimulus to gall bladder contraction; it also facilitates weight loss, if appropriate.

In younger patients, cholecystectomy is usually straightforward. The gall bladder is usually found to contain stones or thick dark biliary sludge and its wall is often thin, although it may be inflamed. Occasionally a *mucocoele* is found.

In the elderly, the operation is often much more difficult; the gall bladder is usually grossly inflamed, thickened and scarred and has to be patiently dissected out of the liver bed. Great care has to be taken to avoid damaging the bile ducts. The gall bladder often contains several stones and is filled with pus. A culture swab should be taken from within the gall bladder at operation as any postoperative infective complications are likely to involve the same organisms.

CARCINOMA OF THE GALL BLADDER

Chronic irritation by stone over a long period is believed to predispose to *adenocarcinoma of the gall bladder*. This condition is rare and only found in the elderly. The presenting symptoms are similar to chronic inflammatory gall bladder disease. Jaundice may develop if the tumour obstructs the bile ducts. Carcinoma of the gall bladder is usually an unexpected finding at cholecystectomy for stones and is usually incurable at the time of detection. The possibility of malignant transformation is one argument in favour of removing a chronically inflamed gall bladder, even if symptoms are not severe.

BILIARY COLIC

Clinical features

Biliary colic describes the symptom complex arising from sudden and complete obstruction of the cystic duct by stone. The pain produced is severe, typically rising to a plateau over a few minutes, then continuing unrelentingly. The patient writhes in agony until the pain resolves spontaneously after several hours or after opiate analgesia. A bout of vomiting often heralds the end of the attack. There is commonly a history of previous similar episodes. On examination, there are few positive findings. There is no fever but there may be some local tenderness due to gall bladder distension. If the attack does not settle within 24 hours, acute cholecystitis is a more likely diagnosis.

Management

Most cases of biliary colic can safely be managed at home if the diagnosis is recognised. Pain relief usually requires only one injection of an opiate and the attack then passes. Severe attacks of biliary colic usually lead to emergency hospital admission, since the differential diagnosis includes other conditions which may require urgent operation. A presumptive diagnosis can be made on clinical grounds, but ultrasound is useful in making a definitive diagnosis.

Ultrasound examination should be performed as soon as possible, since early diagnosis may save several unnecessary days in hospital. Immediate cholecystectomy is preferred by some surgeons, but most still perform the operation electively at a later date.

If a mucocoele of the gall bladder is found, the attack is likely to persist and cholecystectomy becomes necessary during the current admission.

ACUTE CHOLECYSTITIS

Pathophysiology and clinical features

Several factors contribute in varying degrees to acute inflammation in an obstructed gall bladder. These include physical and chemical irritation, and probably less important, bacterial infection. The clinical result is acute cholecystitis which often presents as a surgical emergency. In contrast to biliary colic, the patient is often systemically unwell with fever and tachycardia. On examination there is tenderness in the right upper quadrant, more marked on inspiration, and an inflammatory gall bladder mass may be palpable. The term 'Murphy's sign' is often misused in this context: it was originally used to describe tenderness at the tip of the 9th rib. The clinical course of acute cholecystitis is more prolonged than biliary colic, usually lasting several days before settling.

Management

As with biliary colic, a presumptive diagnosis may be made on clinical grounds, but it is worthwhile obtaining an early definitive diagnosis. Ultrasound may support the diagnosis by revealing stones and a thickened gall bladder wall. A more positive diagnosis can be made by nuclear medicine scanning: radiolabelled HIDA is excreted in bile and normally outlines the gall bladder and bile duct system. An obstructed gall bladder fails to take up the isotope and is not demonstrated (see Figure 8.8).

As previously described, most patients with acute cholecystitis have a chemical inflammation, which therefore does not require antibiotics. Oral intake should be restricted to fluids and an intravenous infusion set up if necessary. If gall bladder infection is present, symptoms and signs are more marked and antibiotics should then be given.

The patient with acute cholecystitis will need a cholecystectomy at some stage. Early cholecystectomy, performed within a few days of the onset of the attack, is becoming more popular. The procedure is safe, convenient for the patient and efficient in terms of hospital bed usage. The alternative policy of conservative management is to discharge the patient after resolution of the acute attack and readmit for elective cholecystectomy after about 6 weeks, by which time the inflammation has usually settled. However, in the meantime, there is a risk of a further acute attack or some other manifestation of gall stone disease like acute pancreatitis. Even if delayed cholecystectomy is preferred, the acute attack may not settle necessitating cholecystectomy on the same admission.

When laparotomy is performed during the acute illness, the gall bladder is found to be obstructed and tense. The serosal surface is oedematous and inflamed with petechial haemorrhages or even purulent exudate and there are

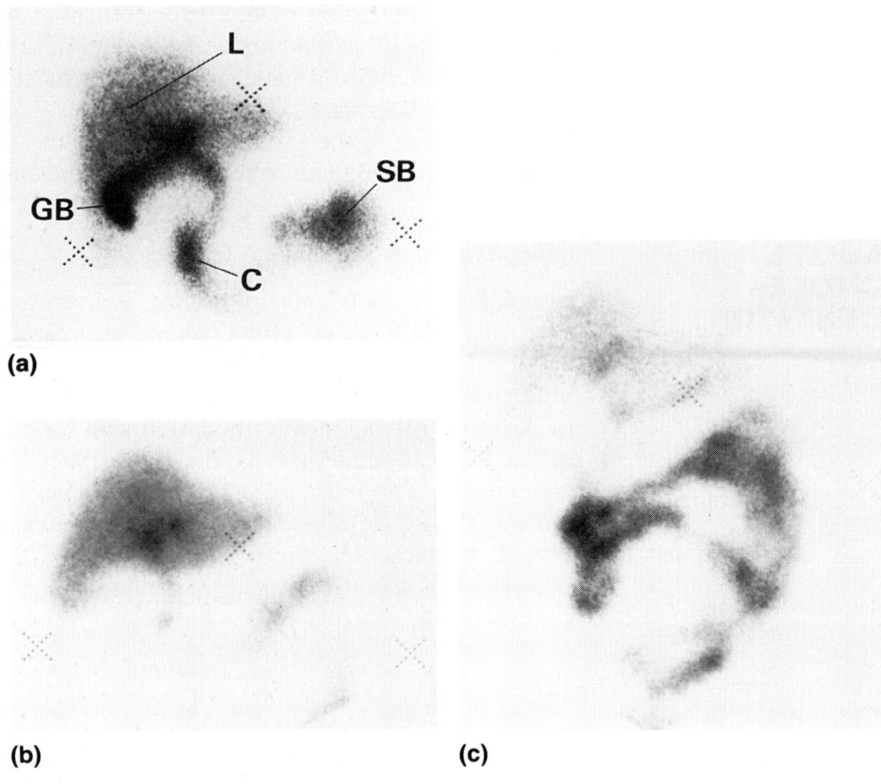

Fig. 8.8 HIDA scanning for acute cholecystitis

(a) Normal HIDA scan. This scan was taken 30 minutes after ingestion of the radioisotope. Radioactivity has been detected in the liver **L**, gall bladder **GB**, common bile duct **C** and small bowel **SB**, demonstrating patency of the whole biliary system. **(b)** HIDA scan in a patient with symptoms and signs suggesting acute cholecystitis. This scan at 30 minutes shows contrast in the liver and a little in the common bile duct and small bowel; there is none in the gall bladder. **(c)** HIDA scan of the same patient taken at 60 minutes. The isotope has now virtually cleared from the liver and is seen in small bowel. There is still no filling of the gall bladder, which must therefore be obstructed, confirming the diagnosis of acute cholecystitis

fibrinous adhesions to nearby structures. The gall bladder neck or cystic duct is blocked by an impacted stone, and the gall bladder is found to contain further stones or sludge mixed with inflammatory exudate. Gut organisms can be cultured from the contents in about 70% of cases.

Empyema of the gall bladder

In a more extreme clinical variant, the gall bladder becomes distended with pus. The condition, known as an empyema, is an abscess of the gall bladder. A swinging pyrexia is often found, as with abscesses elsewhere. Sometimes part of the gall bladder wall becomes necrotic, leading to perforation. This is usually walled off by adjacent omentum resulting in localised abscess formation and a palpable gall bladder mass. Occasionally perforation leads to a subphrenic abscess or generalised peritonitis. Gangrenous cholecystitis and perforation is rare because the gall bladder has a rich blood supply from its hepatic bed as well as from the cystic artery. These patients require surgery without delay.

GALLSTONE ILEUS

This uncommon complication of chronic cholecystitis results from the gall bladder becoming adherent to the adjacent duodenum and a stone ulcerating through the wall to form a *cholecysto-duodenal fistula*. The fistula decompresses the obstructed gall bladder and allows stones to pass into the bowel and gas to enter the biliary tree. As such, the condition is usually harmless and unsuspected. It may be diagnosed on plain abdominal X-ray by the presence of gas outlining the biliary tree. Sometimes it is discovered at operation.

Occasionally, a solitary cholesterol stone passing into the bowel is so large that, after traversing the small bowel, it impacts in the narrow distal ileum causing *gallstone ileus*. This occurs in the elderly and presents as an unexplained gradual onset of small bowel obstruction. Unfortunately, the diagnosis is often difficult to make, and the delay is detrimental to the patient. Diagnosis can be confidently made if gas is recognised in the biliary tree on a plain abdominal X-ray of an elderly patient with distal small bowel obstruction.

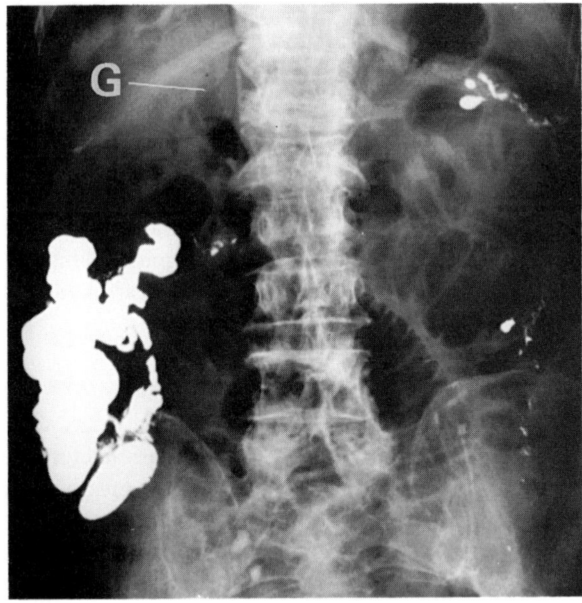

Fig. 8.9 Gallstone ileus
This 78-year-old woman presented with a gradual onset of small bowel obstruction. A large cholesterol solitaire stone had ulcerated from gall bladder into duodenum, travelled down the small bowel and finally impacted in the distal ileum causing complete obstruction. This plain supine abdominal X-ray shows residual barium from a barium enema performed 2 weeks previously. There is widespread small bowel dilatation. The diagnostic feature is the presence of gas **G** in the biliary tree (in this case, the common bile duct and cystic duct)

BILE DUCT STONES

Pathophysiology

Bile duct stones have nearly always originated in the gall bladder, and passed through the cystic duct. Most stones are small enough to pass out of the biliary system into the duodenum, but may cause biliary colic or mild jaundice during transit. This explains many of the symptoms of recurrent gallstone disease.

Stones in the bile duct system are usually small initially, progressively enlarging in situ. This is evident from the frequent finding of multiple faceted gall stones fitting neatly together, which have obviously formed within the bile duct. The common bile duct is narrowest at its lower end, and stones too large to pass out tend to lodge at this point. A stone here either becomes impacted, causing *progressive jaundice* or acts as a ball-valve which causes *intermittent jaundice*. Obstruction results in gradual dilatation of the biliary tree; if dilatation is long standing it does not regress even after removal of the obstruction and may lead to stagnation of bile and further stone formation. Note that the gall bladder rarely distends in this condition even when the common bile duct is completely obstructed. This is because of the inflammatory fibrosis caused by gall stones (Courvoisier's law — see Chapter 6).

Clinical presentations of stones in the biliary tract

a. Obstructive jaundice

Stones in the common bile duct are, as stated earlier, a common cause of obstructive jaundice and must be considered in the differential diagnosis; details are given in Chapter 6.

b. Asymptomatic duct stones

Any patient with gall stones may have duct stones. Therefore, at cholecystectomy, it is standard practice to investigate the biliary tree by peroperative cholangiography and to remove any stones by exploration of the common bile duct (see earlier). This avoids the need for a subsequent procedure.

c. Acute pancreatitis

Stones near the ampulla of Vater may interfere with drainage of pancreatic enzymes into the duodenum. This induces bile reflux into the main pancreatic duct causing acute pancreatitis (see Chapter 13).

d. Ascending cholangitis

Bile stasis in the common duct, which occurs with chronic obstruction and dilatation, predisposes to bacterial infection. The infection then extends proximally to involve the intrahepatic duct system. The condition is known as ascending cholangitis and is characterised by intermittent attacks of pain, swinging pyrexia and jaundice. This triad is also referred to as *Charcot's intermittent hepatic fever*, and is often accompanied by marked weight loss. Ascending cholangitis is a serious condition and may culminate in life-threatening *acute suppurative cholangitis*. The bile duct must be drained urgently, either by surgical operation or by endoscopic sphincterotomy.

Ascending cholangitis more commonly develops as a late complication of biliary tract surgery, particularly bypass operations.

MANAGEMENT OF GALLSTONE DISEASE

Non-surgical treatment

Whatever the clinical manifestation of gall stone related disease, most cases are treated surgically. A small proportion however, are suitable for oral drug therapy. *Chenodeoxycholic acid* and related drugs increase the bile salt pool and inhibit hepatic cholesterol secretion. When administered over a long period, they cause slow dissolution of cholesterol stones. Unfortunately, these drugs have several disadvantages apart from their very slow action. Only cholesterol-predominant stones can be dissolved and even if this treatment is successful, there is a high rate of stone recurrence; there are frequent side-effects such as severe diarrhoea and hepatic damage. Thus, drug therapy should be restricted to young patients with small radiolucent stones in a gall bladder which concentrates contrast and contracts in response to a fatty meal.

Fig. 8.10 Incisions for biliary surgery

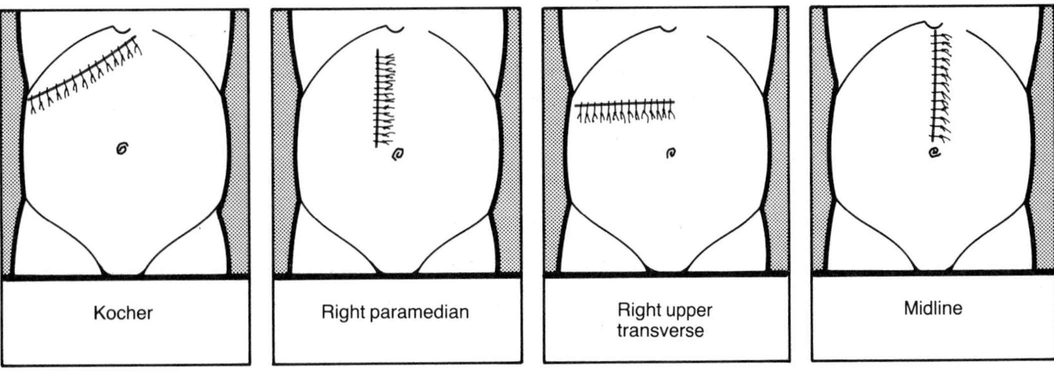

Fig. 8.11 Principal steps in cholecystectomy

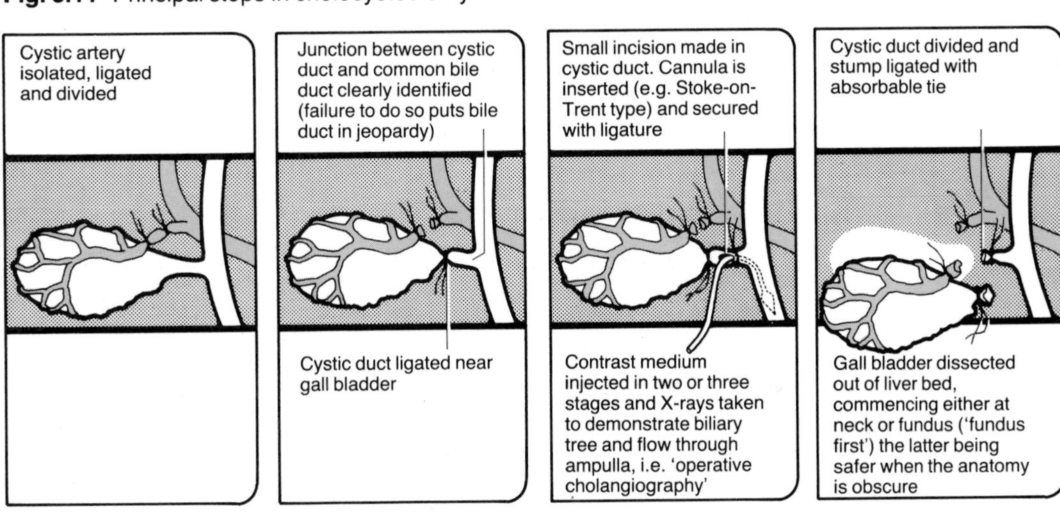

(b)

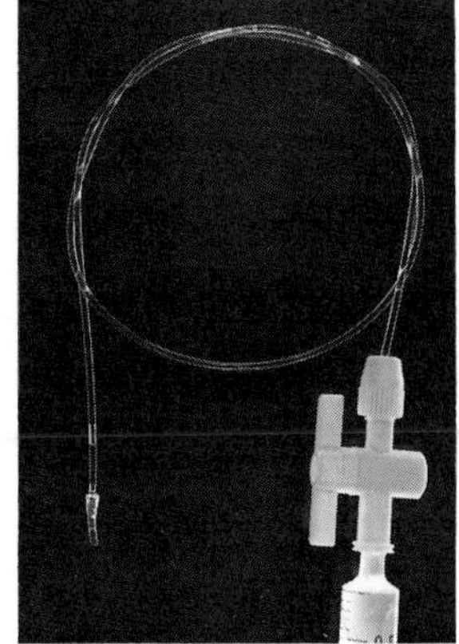

Cannula for peroperative cholangiography

Surgical management

There are two main indications for cholecystectomy:

- Symptomatic gall bladder disease
- Asymptomatic gall stones, if there is a reasonable likelihood of future symptoms or complications

Common duct exploration is added to cholecystectomy if there are stones in the duct system. A jaundiced patient is at particular risk during surgery because of infection, hepatic impairment, defective clotting, acute renal failure and venous thrombosis.

Cholecystectomy

The main incisions for biliary surgery are illustrated in Figure 8.10 and the main steps in cholecystectomy are shown in Figure 8.11. These should be familiar to students and junior surgical staff if they are to assist at operation as well as appreciate the potential for operative complications.

Exploration of the common bile duct

The common duct is opened through a longitudinal incision. Stones are retrieved, often with some difficulty, by a combination of manipulation, irrigation, grasping with stone forceps and use of a balloon catheter. *Choledochoscopy* is increasingly being used to check for residual stones and to remove difficult stones. The flexible fibreoptic choledochoscope gives good visibility and manoeuvrability but, unlike its rigid counterpart, lacks the range of instrumentation for retrieving stones. After exploration, a latex T-tube is usually inserted to drain bile to the exterior, with the transverse limb placed within the common bile duct. The main purpose of a T-tube is to provide access to the biliary tree for a further cholangiogram about a week postoperatively (*T-tube cholangiography*). This is to ensure that no stones remain. If no stones are found on surgical exploration, or if the surgeon is satisfied that no stones remain, the common bile duct can be closed without T-tube drainage.

Procedures to facilitate bile duct drainage

When the common bile duct is grossly dilated and contains multiple stones, it may be difficult to ensure complete stone clearance at exploration. This is because fragments of stone adhere to the wall. Furthermore, such a duct is usually stretched and baggy and remains so postoperatively, predisposing to stasis and further stone formation. It is therefore a useful precaution to make an anastomosis between the bile duct and adjacent duodenum known as a *choledocho-duodenostomy*. This ensures biliary drainage even if stones or debris have been left behind. The anastomosis should be wide or it will predispose to ascending cholangitis.

An alternative operation, *transduodenal sphincteroplasty*, involves opening the second part of the duodenum and splitting the sphincter of Oddi by a large longitudinal incision. The mucosal edges are then sutured in apposition, to minimise stricture formation. This operation may also be used to remove a firmly impacted stone from the lower end of the common duct. After any operation in which bile ducts are opened, an abdominal drain should be placed nearby to minimise the hazards of any biliary leakage.

With the widespread availability of ERCP and endoscopic sphincterotomy, stones in the common duct can often be retrieved without an open operation. This technique represents a real advance in the management of duct stones. *Endoscopic sphincterotomy* may be employed in the following circumstances:

- Urgent drainage of the bile duct in obstructive jaundice which is complicated by cholangitis. Definitive surgery can thus be deferred until the risks of infection have been overcome
- Retrieval of stones missed at operation. This avoids a difficult and hazardous operation to explore or re-explore the duct
- Removal of duct stones in patients unfit for operation

Complications of biliary surgery

a. The retained stone

Despite considerable care, stones occasionally remain in the duct system after operation and are revealed by postoperative T-tube cholangiography. Until recently there were only two courses of remedial action. The first, attempting to flush the stone into the duodenum by irrigating the T-tube with heparin, saline or bile acids, was rarely successful. The second choice was a further laparotomy. Reoperation is technically difficult and carries a greatly increased risk of morbidity and mortality.

It is now possible, however, to retrieve such stones percutaneously by means of steerable grasping forceps or a Dormia basket, provided a large T-tube has been used. The T-tube is left in-situ for at least six weeks and then removed, to leave a 'mature' fistulous track through which instruments can be passed. The most satisfactory option for retained stones, however, is endoscopic sphincterotomy.

Retained stones sometimes make themselves known many years later, when, having enlarged, they cause obstructive jaundice. This possibility should always be considered if a patient with previous biliary tract surgery develops obstructive jaundice.

b. Biliary peritonitis

Bile leaking into the peritoneal cavity is irritant and causes a chemical peritonitis. If the bile is infected, it causes generalised peritonitis and septicaemia with a high risk of fatality. Bile tends to leak through suture lines because of its detergent action. Therefore, whenever the duct system has been opened, a drain should be left in the vicinity for at least five days. Small leaks after biliary operations usually settle spontaneously but if biliary peritonitis develops, the area must be re-explored urgently and drained under intravenous antibiotic cover.

c. Bile duct damage

The bile ducts can easily be damaged at cholecystectomy or common duct exploration unless their anatomy, which is commonly aberrant, is carefully displayed. The most serious error is unrecognised transection or ligation of the common duct. This presents as a major biliary leak or increasing jaundice; urgent re-exploration is mandatory. Lesser degrees of bile duct damage from crushing or a careless suture line will heal, but result in a fibrotic stricture. This presents much later with obstruction. Regardless of how the bile ducts are damaged, complex reconstructive surgery is usually required, although endoscopic placement of a Stent promises the chance of rescuing some strictured ducts without operation.

d. Haemorrhage

The cystic and hepatic arteries and the vascular liver bed are vulnerable to operative trauma and bleed profusely. Removing a grossly inflamed or fibrotic gall bladder is particularly hazardous. Manoeuvres to control haemorrhage may damage other structures, passing unnoticed at the time; this is a common cause of bile duct trauma.

e. Complications of pre-existing jaundice

This is discussed under 'Obstructive jaundice' in Chapter 6.

f. Ascending cholangitis and other infections

Ascending cholangitis can be a late complication of biliary surgery where there is an anastomosis between bile ducts and gut. Reflux of intestinal contents and organisms takes place continually in such cases, but active infection only occurs when bile stagnates in the duct system due to inadequate drainage. Ascending cholangitis may also occur early after common duct exploration for jaundice, since bile in this situation is nearly always infected. Prophylactic antibiotics should always be used when operating on jaundiced patients to minimise this complication.

Another early complication of biliary surgery is a *subphrenic abscess*. This must be considered if the patient develops an unexplained swinging fever a few days after operation. Diagnosis may be elusive and is best made by ultrasound. Treatment is by percutaneous needle drainage under ultrasound guidance or occasionally by open operation.

9 PEPTIC ULCERATION AND RELATED DISORDERS

Introduction

Peptic ulcer disease encompasses disorders of the oesophagus, stomach and duodenum. All have the common aetiology of mucosal inflammation caused, to a greater or lesser extent, by gastric acid-pepsin secretions. The conditions also share the symptom of epigastric pain. Together with gallstone disease, peptic disorders are the commonest cause of organic upper abdominal pain.

With the advent of highly effective pharmacological agents, and more reliable diagnostic and treatment monitoring techniques such as fibreoptic endoscopy, the use of surgery in peptic ulcer disease has declined by over 70% in the last 20 years. Most patients with suspected peptic ulcer disease are treated by general practitioners; the rest are largely managed by physicians. Only a minority present to surgeons because of failed medical treatment or emergency complications such as perforation, haemorrhage or pyloric stenosis. Nevertheless, because of the diagnostic difficulties posed by upper abdominal symptoms, surgeons still manage many patients who turn out to have peptic disorders.

PATHO-PHYSIOLOGY OF PEPTIC ULCERATION

Inflammation caused by the combined effect of gastric acid and pepsin upon the mucosa of the upper gastrointestinal tract is the cause of all peptic disorders. Normally, a dynamic balance is maintained between the inherent protective characteristics of the mucosa and the irritant effects of acid-pepsin secretions. This delicate balance may be disrupted by excessive acid-pepsin secretion, diminution of mucosal resistance or a combination of both. In some cases, the mucosal surface may be eroded by the action of some external agent, e.g. non-steroidal anti-inflammatory drugs (NSAIDs). Whatever the aetiology, the possible pathological outcomes are similar, as summarised in Figure 9.1. If, at any stage, the balance of resistance over attack is restored, the disease is halted, and the tissue repaired. This explains the chronic and remittent nature of peptic ulcer disease.

When the protective mucosal surface is breached, the delicate underlying connective tissue is exposed to acid-pepsin attack, exciting an acute inflammatory response. If the protective balance is restored at this early stage, the inflammation will resolve and the epithelium regenerate. Little if any residual scarring will result. If, however, the healing balance is not restored, continued acid-pepsin attack on the unprotected submucosa leads to an *acute peptic ulcer*. This tends to become progressively larger and deeper.

From here, there are several possible outcomes. Sometimes the ulcerative process continues virtually unchecked through the full thickness of the gut wall.

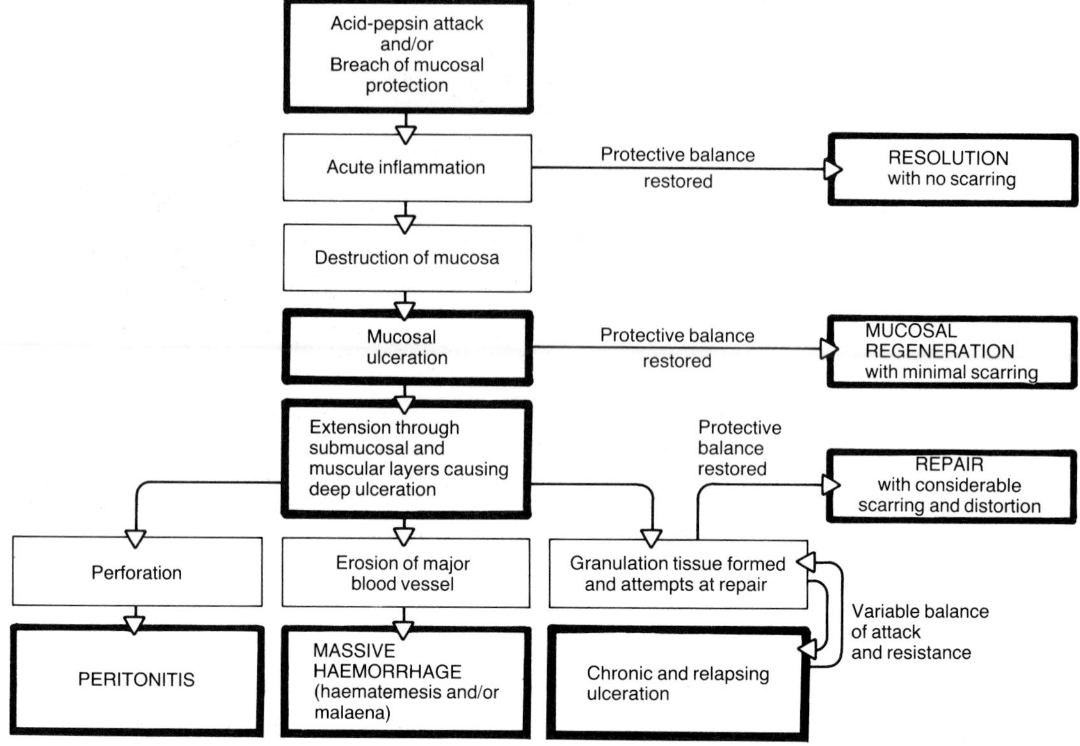

Fig. 9.1 Pathogenesis of peptic ulceration and its possible outcomes

The ulcer perforates and gut contents escape into the peritoneal cavity, resulting in peritonitis. More often, the layer of necrotic slough and acutely inflamed underlying tissue in the ulcer base temporarily resist acid-pepsin attack. This allows granulation tissue to form, which initiates the process of fibrous repair. If for example, acid reducing drugs are used, the ulcer may heal, leaving a small scar with normal overlying mucosa. Usually, however, a tenuous balance is established between resistance and attack, matched by an unstable equilibrium between the rate of repair and the rate of tissue destruction. A *chronic peptic ulcer* then results which may persist for many years, its size and symptoms varying as mucosal resistance and exacerbating factors fluctuate.

If local or systemic factors change and swing the balance in favour of repair, the lesion may heal completely. Internally, the healed ulcer site is usually puckered by scar contraction in the muscular wall. Externally, the serosa is thickened and may adhere to adjacent structures. If scarring occurs in a narrow part of the tract, i.e. the lower oesophagus or pyloric region, the lumen may become even narrower, and subsequent acute mucosal inflammation and swelling may then precipitate obstruction. If healing does not occur at all, a chronic ulcer may slowly enlarge and deepen. This may eventually erode into a large blood vessel causing major haemorrhage (see Figure 9.2), or perforate into the peritoneal cavity.

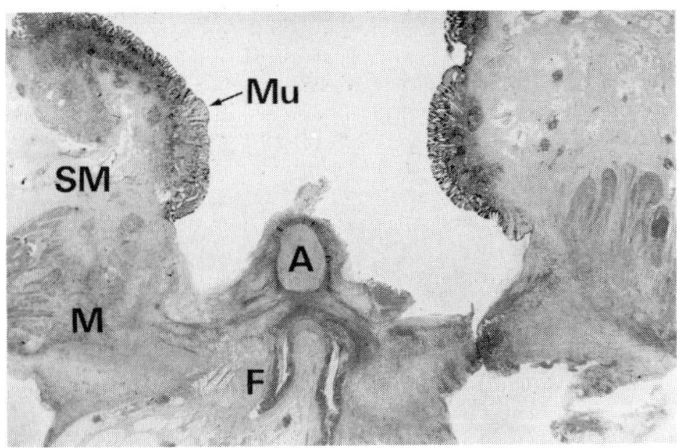

Fig. 9.2 Bleeding gastric ulcer — histopathology

This micrograph shows a chronic gastric ulcer from a patient who died of massive haemorrhage. The inflammatory process has completely destroyed the mucosa **Mu**, submucosa **SM** and muscular wall **M**, leaving only an old fibrous scar **F** in the base of the ulcer which prevented perforation. The scar contains the large artery **A**, erosion of which caused the fatal haemorrhage

EPIDEMIOLOGY AND AETIOLOGY OF PEPTIC ULCER DISEASE

The size of the problem

Chronic peptic disease is very common in developed countries, affecting around 10% of the population at some time in their lives. In contrast, peptic ulceration is quite rare in undeveloped rural communities. This may implicate stress as a cause of the disease. In many sufferers, symptoms are trivial or sporadic and settle either spontaneously or with the help of antacids. Medical advice may never be sought.

Sites of peptic ulceration

Ninety-eight percent of all chronic peptic ulcers occur in either the duodenum or stomach, and sometimes both at the same time. The most common sites are in the first part of the duodenum (duodenal bulb) or the gastric antrum, particularly along the lesser curve.

Peptic inflammation and superficial ulceration may also involve the lower oesophagus and it is almost always secondary to acid-pepsin reflux, which is often associated with hiatus hernia. A chronic peptic ulcer may also develop at the lower end of the oesophagus when reflux is severe and of long standing. Gastric-type mucosa, probably ectopic or possibly metaplastic in origin, may be present in the distal oesophagus and become subject to ulceration; this is known as *Barrett's ulcer*. A chronic *stomal ulcer* may also appear at the margin of a surgically-created communication between stomach and intestine (gastroenterostomy).

In the rare *Zollinger-Ellison syndrome*, a gastrin-secreting tumour, usually of pancreatic origin, causes severe and widespread peptic ulceration. The ulcers commonly extend into the second part of the duodenum or even further distally.

Gastric	Duodenal
Common in later middle age and increasing in frequency with age	Common in middle age (peak 30–50 years)
Slight male preponderance	Males 7 : 1 female
Excess in blood group A	Excess in blood group O
Most common in lower socio–economic groups (at least until recently)	More common in higher socio–economic groups (at least until recently)
Acid–pepsin secretion tends to be normal or low	Acid–pepsin secretion tends to be abnormally high
Probably caused by inadequate resistance to acid–pepsin attack	Probably caused by excess acid–pepsin production

Fig. 9.3 Comparative epidemiology and aetiology of chronic gastric and duodenal ulceration

Aetiological factors in peptic disease

Despite extensive research, the precise aetiology of peptic ulcers is unknown. There are fascinating differences in epidemiology between gastric and duodenal ulcers as outlined in Figure 9.3. These suggest that the two conditions are different pathological entities. In both conditions, acid-pepsin secretion is a prerequisite, hence the expression 'no acid, no ulcer'. Ulceration occasionally occurs in both stomach and duodenum; in this situation, gastric ulceration is considered to be a secondary phenomenon.

a. Acid-pepsin production

In patients with *gastric ulcers*, measured acid secretion is either normal or low, and the essential problem seems to be diminished resistance to acid-pepsin attack. In *duodenal ulceration*, however, the fundamental abnormality appears to be excessive production of acid-pepsin by the stomach, both basal (i.e. overnight) and stimulated. Indeed, such patients tend to have an abnormally large parietal cell mass.

The cause of excess acid-pepsin production in duodenal ulceration is mysterious. The APUD endocrine cells of the gastric antrum secrete gastrin in response to gastric distension and protein ingestion, and this is an important factor in controlling acid-pepsin secretion. However, resting gastrin levels are not elevated in duodenal ulcer patients, although there appears to be an exaggerated gastrin response to food intake.

b. Mucosal resistance

The mechanism which normally prevents autodigestion of the gastric and duodenal mucosa is poorly understood, and by the same token, it is not known why gastric ulcer patients have diminished resistance to acid-pepsin attack. The most important factors are believed to be the integrity of intercellular junctions and the protection afforded by gastric mucus. With increasing age, there is reduced turnover of surface cells and generalised mild mucosal atrophy, which might explain why the incidence of gastric ulcers rises with age.

c. Other mucosal irritants

Alcohol, aspirin and other NSAIDs are all known to induce acute mucosal inflammation *(acute gastritis)*. In a susceptible individual, the inflammation may persist, resulting in chronic ulceration. Indeed, in elderly patients presenting with upper gastrointestinal bleeding or perforation, NSAIDs prescribed for arthritic disorders are commonly and increasingly being identified as the initiating cause of the peptic ulceration. Ulceration may occur after only a few tablets have been taken or at any stage during a long period of medication. The risk of NSAID-induced ulceration increases steeply in later life. Prolonged heavy alcohol intake is also a recognised risk factor.

Reflux of pancreatic digestive enzymes back through the pylorus may also play a part, and is probably caused by defective pyloric closure. Another possible factor is antral stasis (perhaps also caused by abnormal pyloric function), leading to increased gastrin secretion. The area of the junction between parietal and antral cells on the lesser curvature of the stomach has been noted to be particularly vulnerable to ulceration, although the reason is not understood.

d. Smoking

Cigarette smoking is twice as common in patients with chronic peptic ulcer disease as in the general population, but any role of smoking in ulcer pathogenesis is uncertain. Cessation of smoking, however, greatly assists in healing of peptic ulcers.

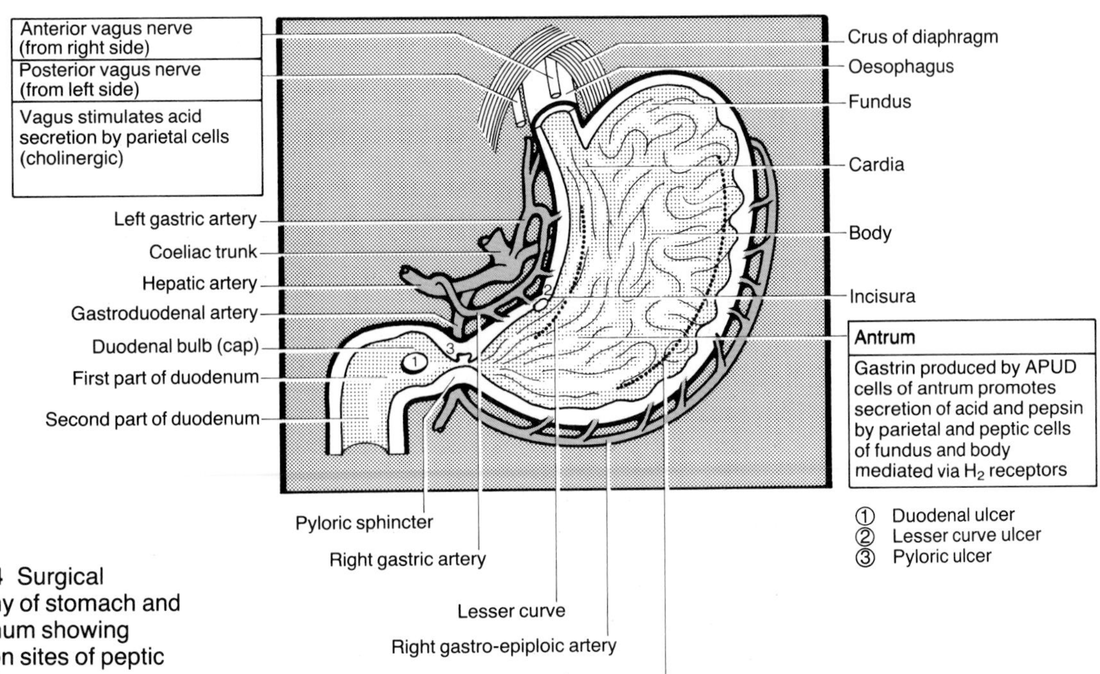

Fig. 9.4 Surgical anatomy of stomach and duodenum showing common sites of peptic ulceration

e. Infection

Evidence is emerging for the involvement of a bacterium, *Campylobacter pylori* (formerly known as C. pyloridis), in the causation, or at least initiation, of some peptic ulcer disease. These spiral-shaped organisms appear to be able to penetrate protective surface mucus and accumulate in the region of intercellular junctions. There they may excite inflammation or compromise normal protective intercellular adhesions. Should this infective aetiology be proven, antibiotic therapy may revolutionise management of peptic ulcer disease in the future.

INVESTIGATION OF SUSPECTED PEPTIC ULCER DISEASE

The diagnosis of peptic disorders relies on contrast radiography and fibre-optic endoscopy, the latter having revolutionised diagnosis and management since its introduction in the late 1960s.

Contrast radiology

Contrast radiography of the upper gastrointestinal tract involves the patient swallowing barium suspension *(barium meal)*. Its passage is followed through the upper GI tract by fluoroscopic imaging, with films being exposed to record points of special diagnostic importance. During the investigation, the patient is tilted and rolled in various directions to demonstrate the whole region of interest. Effervescent tablets are given to produce gaseous distension of the stomach and duodenum and spread the contrast in a thin, even layer over the mucosal surface. This *double contrast technique* is now routine and improves the imaging of mucosal detail, particularly when the duodenum is relaxed by intravenous anti-cholinergic drugs such as hyoscine butylbromide.

Endoscopy

Oesophago-gastro-duodenoscopy, also known as OGD or gastroscopy, involves visual examination of the mucosa using a steerable, flexible fibre-optic endoscope. Gastroscopy enables direct and comprehensive examination of the whole area of the upper GI tract prone to peptic ulcer disease.

In peptic ulcer disease, fibreoscopy has definite advantages over contrast radiography, which by its nature can only demonstrate substantial structural abnormalities, and then only as two-dimensional images. Shallow mucosal abnormalities, like superficial ulceration or vascular malformations which are invisible on barium meal, can be inspected directly and diagnosed from their endoscopic appearance. Distortion resulting from previous disease or surgery often interferes with radiological interpretation. This too can usually be overcome by endoscopic inspection.

Benign peptic ulceration can be reliably distinguished from malignancy if endoscopic biopsies are taken from several places around the ulcer edge. In acute upper gastrointestinal haemorrhage, fibreoscopy can identify the site of the bleeding more reliably than contrast radiology. This is particularly useful if another lesion, such as oesophageal varices, is present but is not the source of bleeding. Gastroscopy also demonstrates whether the lesion is actively bleeding at the time of examination.

Tests of gastric secretory function

Tests of gastric acid secretion are used in severe ulceration where hypergastrinaemia is suspected, or in recurrent ulceration after surgery. They are also used experimentally to test the efficacy of new types of surgical vagotomy (see later).

Pentagastrin test

The pentagastrin test is the standard investigation. Gastric secretions are collected via a nasogastric tube, and the rate of acid secretion determined at specified intervals. Unstimulated or basal secretions are first collected, followed by an intravenous injection of pentagastrin (a synthetic gastrin analogue) to stimulate maximal acid output. The rates of basal and stimulated secretion at hourly intervals are then calculated and plotted against time.

When surgery was used more often, the pentagastrin test was a regular part of the assessment of duodenal ulcer patients. It helped to decide who might benefit from surgery. Patients with a normal or elevated basal rate of acid secretion but with an exaggerated response to pentagastrin were thought likely to respond best to an operation. In this respect, the test may still be appropriate in investigating patients with recurrent ulceration.

If basal acid secretion is grossly elevated and uninfluenced by pentagastrin, a diagnosis of autonomous gastrinoma (Zollinger–Ellison syndrome) must be suspected. This can be confirmed by measuring serum gastrin levels, using a radioimmunoassay.

Insulin test

This test, used to investigate vagal integrity, is based on the fact that hypoglycaemia induces vagally-mediated gastrin secretion. The test is similar to the pentagastrin test, with insulin substituted for pentagastrin. The insulin test is mainly used in post-vagotomy patients with recurrent ulceration; a positive result means that the vagus nerves have been incompletely divided.

PRESENTING FEATURES OF PEPTIC ULCER DISEASE

The various ways in which peptic inflammation affects the oesophagus, stomach and duodenum are summarised in Figure 9.5.

Epigastric pain (usually described as ‘boring’, ‘gnawing’ or ‘burning’) is the principle presenting symptom and is common to peptic disorders whatever the site. Pain is often accompanied by other forms of discomfort, often described by the patient as ‘indigestion’ or ‘dyspepsia’. A more specific description may suggest particular diagnostic entities. Retrosternal pain (‘heartburn’) suggests reflux oesophagitis, whereas bitter regurgitation (‘waterbrash’) is characteristic of both oesophageal reflux and duodenal ulceration. Nausea or vomiting, anorexia (loss of appetite) and abdominal fullness or bloating are common in gastric ulcer and pyloric stenosis, but may also occur in a variety of other upper gastrointestinal disorders, e.g. gallstone disease, irritable bowel syndrome.

The relationship of symptoms to food intake may help to distinguish gastric from duodenal ulceration; gastric ulcer pain is typically exacerbated by food and duodenal ulcer pain relieved by it.

Fig. 9.5 Clinical consequences of peptic ulcer disease in different anatomical sites

PATHOLOGICAL PROCESS	CLINICAL LESION	SYMPTOMS
Oesophagus		
Transient acid reflux	Mild reversible acute inflammation, i.e. transient oesophagitis	Burning retrosternal pain (i.e. 'heartburn')
Recurrent acid reflux or failure of oesophagus to expel acid by peristalsis (often found in hiatus hernia)	Episodes of acute inflammation, i.e. reflux oesophagitis — probably reversible with no scarring. Chronic low–grade blood loss	Recurrent epigastric and retrosternal pain Chronic iron deficiency anaemia may occur
Persistent severe reflux	Continuous severe inflammation with superficial ulceration. May lead to chronic ulceration and/or stricture	Severe retrosternal pain, dysphagia, and sometimes recurrent small haematemeses
Stomach		
Acute gastric irritation e.g. by NSAIDs or alcohol	Acute (reversible) mucosal inflammation, i.e. acute gastritis or erosive/haemorrhagic gastritis	Epigastric pain,vomiting, acute upper GI bleeding
Long–standing diminished resistance to acid–pepsin attack, with or without extrinsic irritation	Chronic or recurrent gastric ulceration	Epigastric pain — characteristically exacerbated by food (especially if acid or spicy), anorexia and weight loss
Duodenum		
Episodic acid–pepsin attack	Acute (reversible) mucosal inflammation, i.e. duodenitis	Episodic epigastric pain
Persistent acid–pepsin attack	Duodenal ulceration (may involve pyloric canal)	Epigastric pain — typically relieved by food and occurring several hours after food, especially at night
Chronic duodenal ulceration with scarring of pyloric region	Pyloric stenosis	Intermittent vomiting, anorexia, feeling of fullness.
Pre–existing pyloric stenosis with superadded acute inflammation and mucosal swelling	Complete pyloric obstruction	Severe vomiting, dehydration, shock, gross electrolyte disturbance (hypochloraemic alkalosis)
The following features apply to both stomach and duodenum:		
Periodic loss of protective equilibrium	Recurrent ulceration	Intermittent symptomatic episodes
Erosion of a major vessel in ulcer floor	Severe haemorrhage	Massive haematemesis or melaena
Unchecked ulceration	Perforation and peritonitis	Acute severe abdominal pain and shock

Peptic disorders are by nature protracted, with exacerbations and remissions over weeks or months. Symptoms tend to follow the disease activity, and may wax and wane over many years.

Iron deficiency anaemia is a common finding in patients with chronic peptic ulcers. Asymptomatic peptic ulceration should always be suspected if there is no obvious cause for anaemia.

NON-ACUTE CLINICAL PRESENTATIONS OF PEPTIC ULCER DISEASE

PEPTIC DISORDERS OF THE OESOPHAGUS

Reflux of gastric contents initiates all peptic disorders of the oesophagus. These range from mild reversible inflammation, through moderate acute inflammation with superficial ulceration *(reflux oesophagitis)*, to severe persistent inflammation. The latter may lead to *fibrotic scarring and stenosis* (see Figure 9.6) and sometimes *chronic peptic ulceration*. In many patients, reflux is associated with hiatus hernia but in the remainder, the mechanism of the damaging reflux is poorly understood.

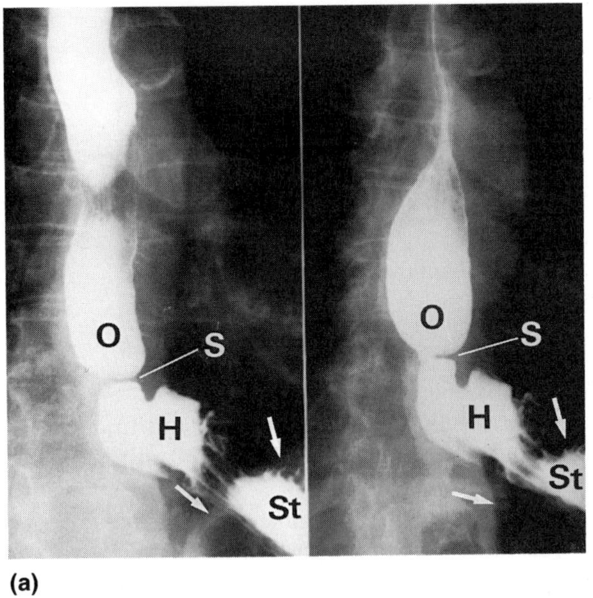

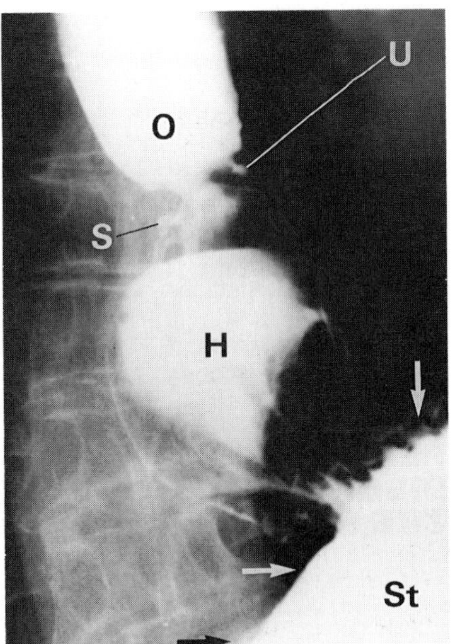

Fig. 9.6 Peptic stricture of the oesophagus

(a) Two views from a barium swallow in a 60-year-old woman who complained of burning retrosternal pain when lying flat (present for several years), and recent onset of pain and difficulty when swallowing solid foods. The X-rays show the lower end of the oesophagus **O** and stomach **St**, part of which lies above the level of the diaphragm (position arrowed), forming a sliding hiatus hernia **H**. There is a tight stenosis in the last two cm of the oesophagus due to a peptic stricture **S**. **(b)** At greater magnification, barium can be seen filling the crater of a chronic peptic ulcer **U** immediately above the stricture

Barium meal examination is of limited value except in demonstrating strictures, hiatus hernia or the existence of gross reflux.

On endoscopy, reflux oesophagitis is characterised by mucosal reddening and, in more severe cases, by typical linear superficial ulceration (see Figure 9.7). Peptic strictures only occur in the last few centimetres of the distal oesophagus and are recognised if the lumen is found to be too narrow to allow the endoscope to pass. The stricture usually lies just above the oesophago-gastric junction, which, because of inflammatory shortening of the oesophagus, often lies well above the diaphragm. The normal oesophago-gastric junction, as seen on endoscopy, is about 40 centimetres from the incisor teeth. The mucosa near the stricture varies in the amount of inflammation and ulceration. Carcinoma must be excluded by biopsies because the appearance of a carcinoma may not be characteristic. Occasionally, a deep chronic ulcer occurs in the lower oesophagus; this looks and behaves like a gastric or duodenal ulcer. When squamous oesophageal epithelium is repeatedly damaged by reflux, it may be replaced by ectopic or metaplastic gastric columnar epithelium. This is known as Barrett's oesophagus and there is some evidence that it predisposes to malignant change. If found, it should be biopsied to exclude dysplasia.

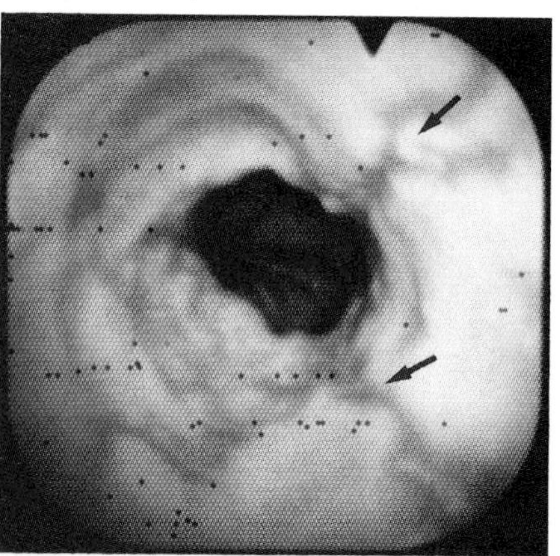

Fig. 9.7 Reflux oesophagitis

Gastroscopic view of the lower end of the oesophagus in a woman of 62 with a long history of reflux. Note the linear ulceration (arrowed) and the irregular fibrotic cardia caused by recurrent ulceration and attempts at healing. Further scarring may cause stricture formation. The small black dots represent broken glass fibres in the gastroscope

PEPTIC DISORDERS OF THE STOMACH

Peptic disorders of the stomach range from mild inflammation *(gastritis)* to *chronic gastric ulcers*, and most often occur in the antral region and along the lesser curve beyond the incisura.

Chronic gastric ulcers must be distinguished from malignant ulcers. The position may help recognise a benign ulcer but carcinoma has no predilection for any part of the stomach. Malignancy can only be excluded by histological examination of the whole ulcer in a resection specimen, or of multiple representative biopsies taken from around the ulcer circumference. In most cases, carcinoma probably arises de novo, but occasionaly, a benign ulcer may undergo malignant transformation. For this reason, operation should be considered for any gastric ulcer which fails to heal after conservative treatment.

Gastritis

Gastritis can only be proved by endoscopy and appears as widespread reddening of the mucosa. The inflamed mucosa is often awash with bile, and sometimes referred to as 'biliary gastritis', on the assumption that it is caused by the irritant effect of biliary and pancreatic secretions. Acute gastritis, often caused by alcohol (chronic alcoholism or single alcoholic binges) or aspirin ingestion, can cause symptoms of sufficient severity to warrant gastroscopy. The mucosa often exhibits patchy shallow ulceration (erosive gastritis) and is friable and easily traumatised, causing bleeding. Acute gastritis is sometimes so severe as to cause severe and diffuse mucosal bleeding (haemorrhagic gastritis) which may present as major upper gastrointestinal haemorrhage.

Chronic gastric ulceration

Chronic gastric ulcers vary greatly in size but the majority are small (less than 2 cm in diameter). Giant ulcers (up to 10 cm) are occasionally seen in the elderly; if posteriorly situated, they may erode through the stomach wall, obliterating the lesser sac, and adhere to the surface of the pancreas. In such cases, the ulcer base or floor is composed of pancreatic tissue.

Benign gastric ulcers are typically regular in outline, with a base consisting of white fibrinous slough. The ulcer gives the impression of having been punched out of the gastric wall, and there is no heaping-up of the mucosal margin as is seen in malignant ulcers. The surrounding mucosa is surprisingly normal, although there may be radiating folds due to fibrotic contractures. The typical endoscopic appearance of a gastric ulcer is shown in Figure 9.8 and the barium meal appearance in Figure 9.9.

Peptic disorders of the stomach typically cause severe, often disabling, epigastric pain which tends to be exacerbated by food, especially if acidic or

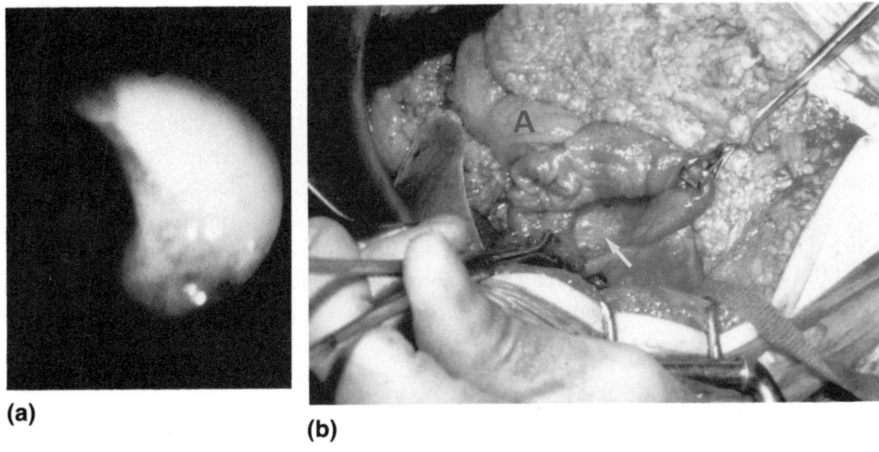

(a) (b)

Fig. 9.8 Peptic ulcers

(a) Large lesser curve gastric ulcer as seen through a gastroscope. The large white area in the upper part is fibrous tissue exposed in the ulcer base. Little more detail can be seen in this photograph, emphasising that information from endoscopy depends on the dynamics of the investigation. **(b)** Photograph taken at emergency laparotomy for bleeding duodenal ulcer. The gastric antrum is seen at **A**; the pylorus has been opened longitudinally and a deep chronic posterior ulcer crater is identified (arrowed). A bleeding artery in the ulcer crater was under-run with sutures to arrest the haemorrhage

spicy. The pain may be so severe that patients lose weight and develop a fear of food. Symptoms tend to persist for weeks or months, fluctuating in intensity and then disappearing completely only to recur weeks or months later. Symptoms are a poor guide to disease activity or response to treatment; both can only be monitored by repeated gastroscopy. A rare complication of peptic disease is perforation of a gastric ulcer into the transverse colon. The resulting gastro-colic fistula causes true faecal vomiting.

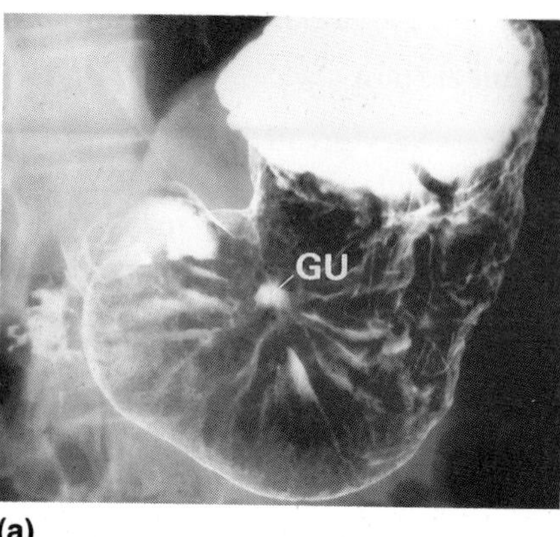

(a)

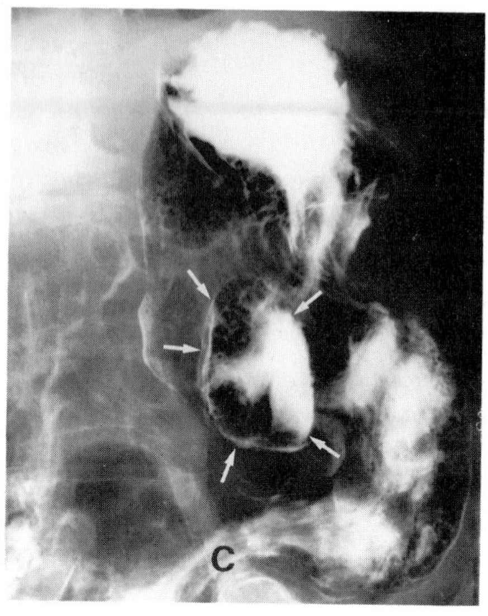

(b)

Fig. 9.9 Chronic gastric ulcer

(a) Double contrast barium meal in a 54-year-old man with a 6-month history of epigastric pain after meals. A gastric ulcer crater **GU** containing barium is seen on the lesser curve. Abnormal folds of gastric mucosa radiate out from the ulcer. Endoscopy and biopsy is indicated to exclude malignancy.
(b) Barium meal in an 88-year-old woman who suffered a haematemesis. The patient had been taking non-steroidal anti-inflammatory drugs for several months. The X-ray shows a *giant gastric ulcer* (outline arrowed) on the lesser curve, partly filled with barium

Stress ulcers

Acute 'stress' ulcers are single or multiple small discrete superficial lesions that may develop rapidly in seriously ill patients. They tend to occur after severe burns or trauma, major surgery, major head injuries or intracranial surgery, or during severe infections, uraemia or terminal illness. Stress ulcers typically present with haemorrhage which is sometimes catastrophic, and occasionally with perforation. There is minimal mucosal inflammation around the ulcers and their aetiology is not primarily peptic. Nonetheless, the risk of this life-threatening complication can be minimised in vulnerable patients by the routine use of parenteral H_2 blocking drugs to control acid secretion.

PEPTIC DISORDERS OF THE DUODENUM

Duodenitis

Duodenitis, a non-ulcerative form of duodenal inflammation, has a similar endoscopic appearance to gastritis. It is commonly discovered in patients suspected of having duodenal ulceration, and probably represents a mild form of peptic disease.

Chronic duodenal ulceration

Chronic duodenal ulcers almost exclusively occur in the pyloric channel and the first part of the duodenum. The latter area is known endoscopically as the 'duodenal bulb' and radiologically as the 'duodenal cap'. On endoscopy, duodenal ulcers have a range of appearances similar to chronic gastric ulcers. There is usually a single ulcer but two or more ulcers at one time are common. Malignancy is very rare in the duodenal bulb, so biopsy is seldom necessary. The radiological characteristics of duodenal ulcers are shown in Figure 9.10.

Duodenal ulcer symptoms follow the same general pattern as for gastric ulcer but with important exceptions. The pain tends to appear several hours after a meal ('hunger pain'), and is relieved by eating. A typical history includes episodic early morning waking (often around 2 a.m.) with epigastric pain; this pain is relieved by drinking milk and eating bland foods. Consequently, patients gain weight from the increased intake of food and milk. This is in contrast to

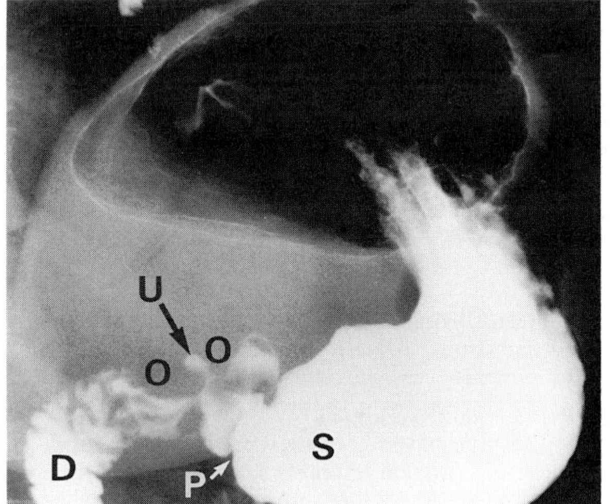

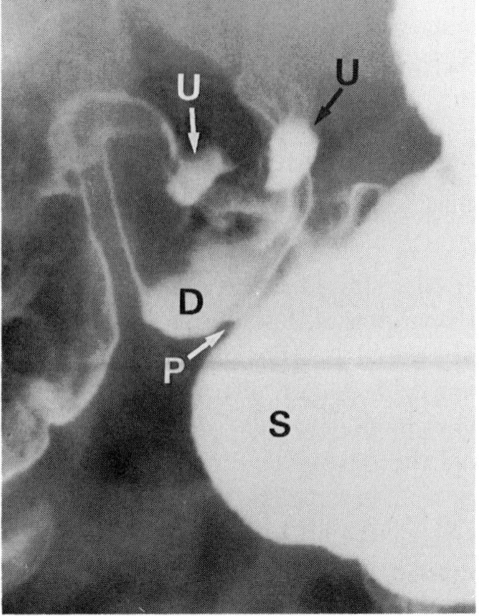

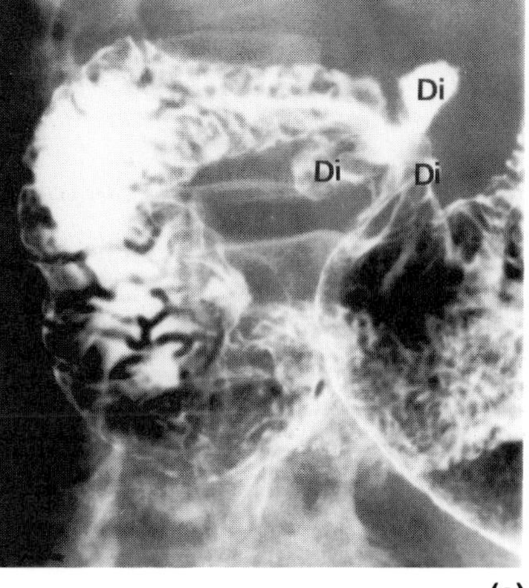

Fig. 9.10 Chronic duodenal ulceration

Barium meal examinations; stomach marked **S**, duodenum **D** and pylorus **P** in each X-ray. **(a)** A 35-year-old man complaining of epigastric pain at night and before meals. The X-ray shows a deep chronic duodenal ulcer **U** with contrast filling the ulcer crater; on either side are large areas free of contrast **O** caused by a ring of oedematous duodenal mucosa surrounding the ulcer. **(b)** Two contrast-filled duodenal ulcers **U** in a 50-year-old male who smoked heavily. Note the otherwise normal duodenal appearance. **(c)** 'Trefoil' deformity of duodenal cap. This appearance is produced by long-standing duodenal ulceration leading to marked scarring and contraction of the first part of the duodenum resulting in the formation of three pseudo-diverticula **Di** which may or may not contain active ulceration. Endoscopy is required to establish whether there is active disease

the weight loss often associated with gastric ulcer. Symptoms in duodenal ulcer are more useful as a guide to disease activity and the response to treatment than in gastric ulcer; this removes the need for regular gastroscopic follow-up in most cases of duodenal ulcer.

MANAGEMENT OF CHRONIC PEPTIC ULCER DISEASE

Both the nature and the management of peptic ulcer disease have undergone extraordinary changes over the past four decades. The aim of treatment has always been to heal the ulcer with the minimum harm or inconvenience to the patient and the lowest risk of recurrence. Several decades ago, medical management was relatively ineffective and was largely confined to antacid drugs, bland diets and bed-rest. The only definitive treatment was major surgery and it was therefore widely employed. Partial gastrectomy offered the best cure rate and was thus the most common operation despite its mortality of 2–10% and its serious long-term complications. Surgery was deferred as long as possible in the hope of spontaneous remission, and patients often had to 'earn' their operations by years of suffering!

The principles of modern management of peptic disorders are summarised in Figure 9.11.

Fig. 9.11 Principles of management of peptic disorders

Control predisposing or aggravating causes:
modify diet, reduce alcohol intake, cease smoking, avoid irritant drugs (aspirin and other NSAIDs), avoid stress, reduce oesophageal reflux by losing weight and attention to posture

Diminish irritant effects of acid-pepsin and promote ulcer healing:
antacid drugs, alginate preparations, liquorice derivatives, bismuth preparations, pirenzepine, prostaglandins, sucralfate

Reduce acid secretion:
H_2 receptor blocking drugs (cimetidine, ranitidine or famotidine), surgical vagotomy (trunkal or highly selective)

Surgical removal of intractable ulcers and gastrin-secreting tissue:
partial gastrectomy

Correct secondary anatomical problems:
dilatation of oesophageal strictures, operations for pyloric stenosis

Control of predisposing or aggravating causes

The history may reveal adverse factors which can be easily removed. These are summarised in part of Figure 9.11. Radical dietary modification is unnecessary; patients should merely be advised to avoid food which they find aggravates the symptoms. Spicy or acidic foods are often blamed.

Aspirin and other NSAIDs should be avoided, although this is often difficult in patients with painful arthritic disorders; the detrimental effect of these drugs is greatest in the elderly, the main sufferers from arthritis. The ulcerogenic effect of these drugs is directly proportional to their effectiveness and relates to their anti-prostaglandin activity; it is thus largely a systemic effect rather than a local irritant effect. There is therefore little to be gained from changing drugs within the group or by using them in enteric-coated or suppository form.

If NSAIDs cannot be avoided in patients with a predisposition to peptic ulceration, concurrent use of cytoprotective drugs such as sucralfate may be indicated. Patients with oesophageal reflux, especially if associated with hiatus hernia, can minimise the damage by simple mechanical measures such as losing weight, elevating the head end of the bed and avoiding stooping.

Control of irritant effects of acid-pepsin and promotion of ulcer healing

An array of proprietary antacid preparations is available over the counter and on prescription. When used assiduously, they promote ulcer healing as effectively as any other drug, although perhaps more slowly. The main active ingredients are few. Sodium bicarbonate offers rapid but temporary relief of symptoms, while magnesium trisilicate or aluminium hydroxide promote ulcer healing. Bismuth compounds are claimed to be effective in duodenal ulceration but have been implicated in causing encephalopathy.

Alginate preparations form a foamy layer on the surface of gastric contents, coating the upper stomach and lower oesophagus and protecting it from oesophageal reflux. The liquorice derivative carbenoxolone is used to heal gastric ulcers but tends to cause marked fluid and sodium retention; it should be avoided in the elderly.

Reduction of acid secretion

Acid secretion by the gastric mucosa is controlled by two mechanisms:

- Direct cholinergic stimulation of parietal cells mediated via the vagus nerve. This is under reflex control originating in the cerebral cortex e.g. the sight and taste of food
- Gastrin, which is secreted by APUD cells in the gastric antrum, promotes acid secretion via histamine, which is released from mast cells in the vicinity of the parietal cells. The histamine receptors on the parietal cells are distinct from those elsewhere in the body and are designated as type 2 (H_2) receptors; these receptors are not blocked by standard 'antihistamine' drugs such as chlorpheniramine. Gastrin secretion is partly controlled by the vagus and partly by local (vagally-independent) reflexes initiated by gastric distension and the presence of food or alcohol in the stomach

From this, two practical methods have been found to reduce acid secretion, drugs which selectively block H_2 receptors and surgical division of the vagus nerve.

H_2 receptor blockade

H_2 receptor blocking drugs were developed in the 1970s and have revolutionised the management of peptic disorders. *Cimetidine* was alone in the market for several years but has more recently been joined by *ranitidine*, which has a few minor advantages. Several newer drugs of this type are in various stages of development. H_2 receptor antagonists are highly effective in reducing gastric acid secretion. Symptomatic response is rapid, usually within a day or two, and healing follows within a few weeks. The drugs have remarkably few side-effects and are normally prescribed for six to eight weeks in active disease. Long-term use in lower doses (usually once in the evening) prevents ulcer recurrence in susceptible patients. H_2 receptor blockade is indicated for both gastric and duodenal ulcers but efficacy is probably greater for the latter.

Vagotomy

Vagotomy (an operation first described by Dragstedt in 1938) has gradually superceded partial gastrectomy as the surgical treatment of choice for chronic duodenal ulcer. The various vagotomy operations are illustrated in Figure 9.12. The simplest and most widely used method involves dividing the anterior and posterior vagal trunks close to the abdominal oesophagus just below the diaphragm (*trunkal vagotomy*). The operation is highly effective in reducing gastric acid secretion and promoting ulcer healing but paralyses gastric motility and restricts pyloric emptying. A surgical *drainage procedure*, such as *pyloroplasty or gastro-jejunostomy*, is therefore a necessary part of the operation (Figure 9.12).

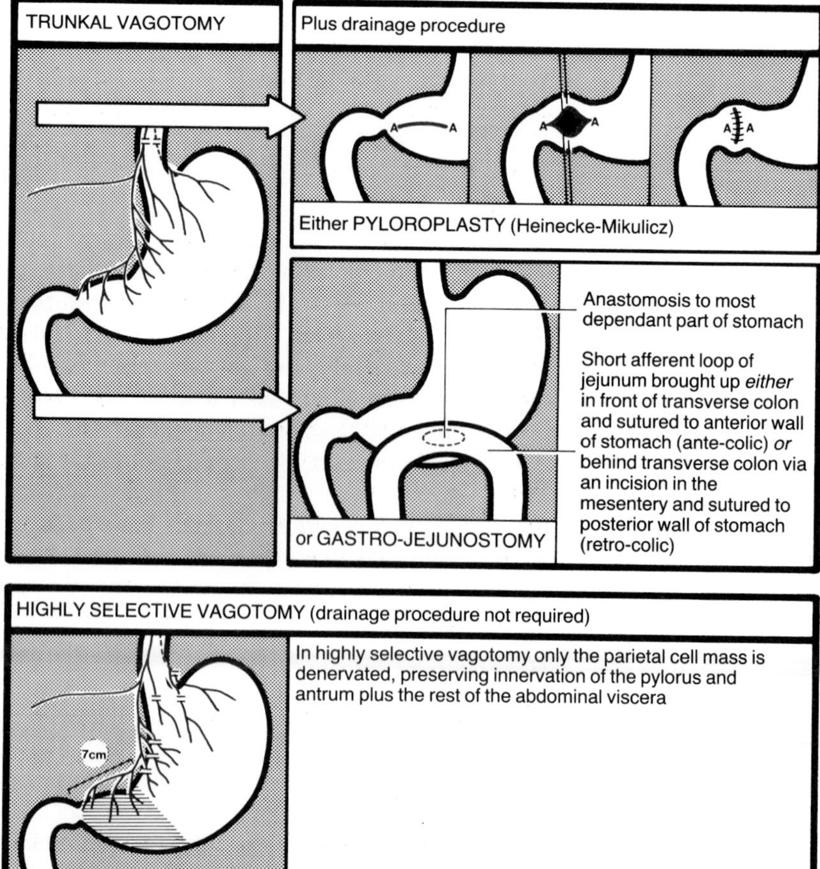

Fig. 9.12 The vagotomies and gastric drainage procedures

The operation of trunkal vagotomy plus drainage has few serious side-effects although most patients experience epigastric fullness after meals. Major metabolic disturbances and malabsorption are rare. A few patients experience *dumping syndromes*, discussed below, or severe diarrhoea. Trials of more selective operations led to the popular *highly selective vagotomy* which preserves the pyloric vagal branches and avoids the need for a gastric drainage procedure. The ulcer recurrence rate is slightly higher than for trunkal vagotomy but side-effects are fewer. All surgical treatments for duodenal ulcer have been eclipsed by the introduction of the H_2 receptor antagonists; only about a tenth of the number of operations performed two decades ago for duodenal ulcer take place nowadays.

The vagotomies are mainly employed for chronic duodenal ulceration, where acid production is excessive. Vagotomy is less commonly used for chronic gastric ulcers, where acid production is probably normal or low; for these, partial gastrectomy remains the operation of choice.

Surgical removal of intractable ulcers and gastrin secreting tissue

Partial gastrectomy is used mainly in patients in whom medical management has failed to heal a gastric ulcer or to prevent repeated recurrence. Patients on long-term NSAIDs have particular problems with recurrent ulceration. Partial gastrectomy has the dual role of removing the ulcer (and preventing possible malignancy) as well as removing the gastrin-secreting mucosa. This greatly reduces acid production. The standard operation for chronic gastric ulcer is known as the *Billroth I* type of gastrectomy (Billroth, 1881) and involves removal of half to two-thirds of the distal part of the stomach. The gastric remnant is then anastomosed to the first part of the duodenum (see Figure 9.13).

As described above, vagotomy is the usual surgical treatment for chronic duodenal ulcers. However, if it fails to prevent recurrence and the patient has exceptionally high levels of acid secretion, partial gastrectomy may be indicated. In this case, the usual technique, known as a *Polya-type gastrectomy*, involves resection of the distal two-thirds of the stomach. The anastomosis is then made to the side of a loop of proximal jejunum. The cut end of the duodenum (duodenal stump) is closed and the ulcer left in situ to heal (see Figure 9.13). Numerous variations have been described over the years, and many still carry their authors' names, e.g. Polya (1911), Finsterer (1909), Billroth II (1881), Hofmeister (1908), Balfour (1934).

Most surgeons have their own personal techniques of partial gastrectomy, often incorporating elements from various sources. Consequently, the use of eponymous titles to describe particular operations has become somewhat confused.

The main variable elements of a Polya-type partial gastrectomy are as follows:

- The extent of gastric resection — often determined by acid output (measured or assumed)
- The relationship of the anastomosis to the transverse colon — this is made either behind the transverse colon via an incision in the mesocolon (retrocolic) or in front of the transverse colon (antecolic)

- The type of stoma — either the whole width of the cut end of the gastric remnant is anastomosed to the jejunum or part of the cut end is closed, which narrows the stoma and provides a 'valve' to direct duodenal contents away from the stomach

Partial gastrectomy and trunkal vagotomy may be combined for duodenal ulceration *(vagotomy and antrectomy)*. In this operation, only the gastric antrum is removed, i.e. the gastrin secreting tissue. The operation is more successful in preventing recurrence than the vagotomies and is thus more popular in the litigation-conscious USA. It is a more extensive operation than vagotomy, and the risks and side-effects include those of both gastrectomy and vagotomy.

In general, partial gastrectomy is highly effective in relieving symptoms and preventing recurrence of peptic disease, but side-effects may be a problem.

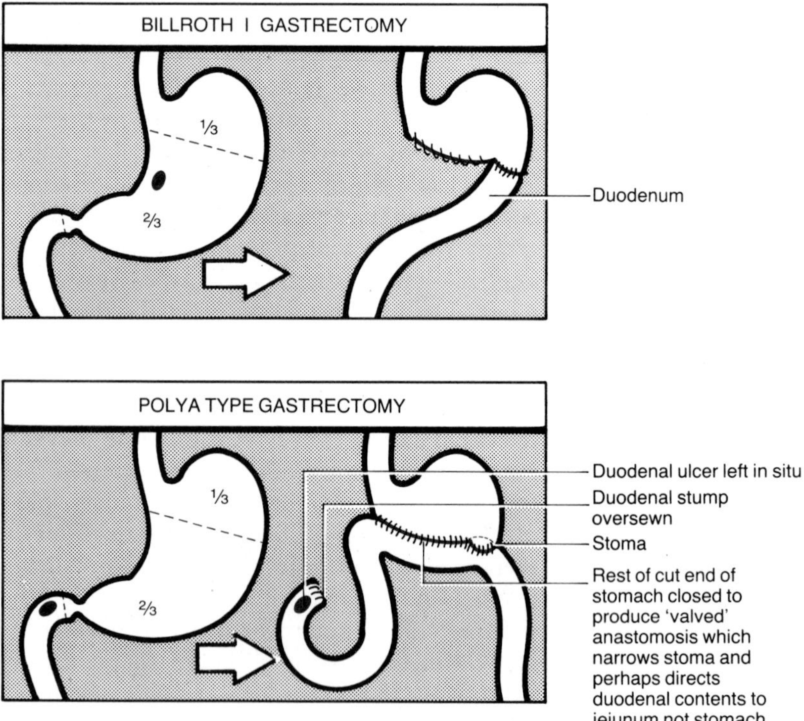

Fig. 9.13 Common types of partial gastrectomy

Complications and side-effects of partial gastrectomy

Partial gastrectomy is a major operative procedure, yet recovery tends to be surprisingly straightforward. A small proportion of patients develop serious complications such as duodenal stump leakage and anastomotic breakdown. However, the main complications of partial gastrectomy occur in the long-term and may not become manifest for years (Figure 9.14).

Fig. 9.14 Side–effects of partial gastrectomy

Inability to eat normal sized meals due to reduced gastric capacity — very common but tends to improve over first few months

'Dumping' due to rapid emptying of stomach contents — common but most patients adapt with time

Episodic bilious vomiting due to reflux of bile into stomach via the anastomosis — fairly common but variable in severity and persistence

'Blind-loop syndrome' due to bacterial overgrowth in a blind-ended loop (Polya type gastrectomy) — causes diarrhoea and malabsorption

Tendency to bolus obstruction of the gastric outlet stoma

Tendency to 'intestinal hurry' and diarrhoea — fairly common but usually only of minor inconvenience

Weight loss due to a combination of above factors and malabsorption — especially common in women

Vitamin B_{12} deficiency due to loss of gastric intrinsic factor; may present as macrocytic anaemia or subacute combined degeneration of the spinal cord — potentially catastrophic, occurring many years after operation and preventable by regular vitamin B_{12} (hydroxycobalamin) injections

Iron deficiency anaemia due to reduced iron absorption — common but easily prevented by taking iron tablets, e.g. once weekly

Recurrent ulceration of gastric remnant or stomal margin — approximately 1% of cases

Osteomalacia due to malabsorption of both calcium and vitamin D — rare

Malignant change in gastric remnant possibly due to bacterial production of carcinogens — rare

'Dumping' syndromes

Two physiological disturbances are responsible for the symptoms described as 'dumping':

- *Early Dumping* — after partial gastrectomy, food passes rapidly into the small bowel. The contents produce an osmotic gradient which draws a large volume of fluid into the bowel from the blood stream. The result is *transient hypovolaemia*, causing faintness, sweating, pallor, tachycardia and sometimes hypotension. Early dumping occurs soon after eating, but is rarely severe. The patient may need to lie down for a short while after meals
- *Late Dumping* — the 'dumping' of a lage bolus of carbohydrate-rich food into the small bowel provokes a steep rise in blood glucose concentration. An exaggerated insulin response follows, leading to *rebound hypoglycaemia* an hour or two later. The symptoms are similar to those of early dumping, but often more severe

Dumping symptoms can be reduced by taking smaller, more frequent meals. Eating dry foods and avoiding fluids with meals will also retard gastric emptying. Late dumping can be further helped by taking small carbohydrate snacks an hour or two after a meal.

Recurrent ulceration after partial gastrectomy is rare and occurs in the gastric remnant or at the stomal margin. The usual reason is that insufficient stomach has been removed leaving behind acid-secreting tissue; occasionally malignant change is responsible. Abnormally high acid production is another cause, sometimes due to Zollinger–Ellison syndrome or hyperparathyroidism.

Correction of secondary anatomical problems

The main anatomical problems secondary to peptic disease are oesophageal stricture and pyloric stenosis. The latter is described later in this chapter.

Oesophageal strictures can usually be eased by periodic dilatation. With the patient sedated intravenously, a guide wire is inserted across the stricture endoscopically, and then metal or plastic dilators are inserted over it. Of course this must be coupled with the usual medical management to promote ulcer healing. Occasionally reflux continues to cause damage and stricturing; it may then become necessary to perform major anti-reflux surgery.

EMERGENCY PRESENTATIONS OF PEPTIC ULCER DISEASE

The emergency presentations of peptic ulcer disease are acute haemorrhage, perforation and pyloric stenosis. Peptic ulcer disease was responsible for much major emergency abdominal surgery until the early 1970s. Since then there has been a remarkable reduction in emergency presentations of peptic ulcer; emergency surgery for peptic ulcer is now a rarity. This change was well under way before the introduction of effective modern drug therapy, and can probably be attributed to the progressive improvement in living standards following World War II.

HAEMORRHAGE FROM A PEPTIC ULCER

Acute bleeding from a peptic ulcer presents with haematemesis or melaena or both (see Chapter 7). Patients with major upper gastrointestinal haemorrhage are usually admitted under the care of a physician who is responsible for initial management.

The principles of management are as follows:

- Resuscitation, including blood transfusion
- Monitoring of vital signs, central venous pressure and serial haemoglobin estimations, looking for signs of continued bleeding or rebleeding
- Intravenous H_2 receptor antagonists (although value unproven in acute haemorrhage)
- Endoscopic diagnosis of site and severity of the bleeding lesion
- Surgical team should be alerted even if operation is not anticipated
- Urgent operation is required if there is continued or recurrent bleeding, the patient is elderly, or an actively bleeding vessel is seen at endoscopy

The standard operation for a bleeding duodenal ulcer is first to open the duodenum and arrest the haemorrhage by 'underrunning' the ulcer with deep sutures, and then to perform a vagotomy and pyloroplasty. Rebleeding is uncommon after this procedure. For a bleeding gastric ulcer, the standard operation is a Billroth I partial gastrectomy, but lesser operations may be used in certain cases, e.g. a patient too ill to withstand a larger operation.

PERFORATION OF A PEPTIC ULCER

Perforation of a gastric or duodenal ulcer into the peritoneal cavity causes peritonitis. Until about 20 years ago, these perforations were a common cause of an acute abdomen, but the incidence has fallen in parallel with the general decline in peptic ulcer disease. Nowadays, perforations of peptic ulcers occur most commonly in elderly patients who are taking NSAID drugs for arthritic conditions. Occasionally, a younger patient presents with a perforated duodenal ulcer without an obvious predisposing cause.

Duodenal ulcer perforations are two or three times more common than gastric ulcer perforations. They typically occur on the anterior surface of the duodenal bulb just beyond the pylorus. There is often a short history of NSAID ingestion, but a long history of taking such drugs does not rule them out as an aetiological factor. About half the patients with a peptic ulcer perforation have had recent ulcer symptoms, however, the other half give no history of indigestion.

Gastric ulcer perforations are uncommon and occur only in the elderly. About a third of these are due to perforation of a gastric carcinoma but present in the same way as a perforated peptic ulcer. This explains why the standard surgical treatment for gastric perforation includes excision of the ulcer. Oesophageal peptic ulcers occur much less commonly and perforate even more rarely.

Clinical presentation of perforated peptic ulcer

Perforation of a gastric or duodenal ulcer usually presents as a sudden onset of epigastric abdominal pain, rapidly spreading to the whole abdomen. The pain is continuous and is aggravated by moving about. Paradoxically, there may be vomiting of brownish or even blood-stained fluid. On examination, the patient is in obvious pain but not shocked or toxic.

There is generalised involuntary abdominal guarding, which in younger patients is so tense as to be described as 'board-like' rigidity. There is also generalised abdominal tenderness, but this may only be detectable on firm palpation because of muscle spasm of the abdominal wall. After several hours, abdominal wall rigidity tends to relax although tenderness remains. In older patients, rigidity is less marked because of a lack of muscle bulk. Peptic ulcer perforation initially causes a chemical, as opposed to bacterial peritonitis, unlike more distal bowel perforations. This explains the lack of general toxicity in the early stages. If untreated for more than 24 hours, secondary infection takes place and signs of sepsis appear.

If posterior wall gastric ulcers perforate, they leak gastric contents into the lesser sac, which tends to confine the peritonitis. These patients thus present with more muted symptoms.

Diagnosis of perforated peptic ulcer

Diagnosis of an upper gastrointestinal perforation can usually be made from the symptoms and signs alone. A plain erect radiograph of the upper abdomen will often reveal gas under the diaphragm, confirming the perforation, but not its origin. Radiographic evidence of perforation, however, is not always present. If perforation is suspected but the signs are equivocal, an abdominal radiograph may be taken after the patient has swallowed 25 ml of barium; this may confirm the leakage. Gastroscopy is contraindicated because the stomach must be inflated during this examination, and air and gastric contents would erupt into the peritoneal cavity.

Surgical management of peptic perforation

Emergency surgery is indicated in nearly all cases of upper gastrointestinal perforation. The patient is first resuscitated and a nasogastric tube inserted. Prophylactic antibiotics should be given before operation. The abdomen is opened through an upper midline incision and fluid contaminating the peritoneal cavity is sucked out. Perforated duodenal ulcer is usually obvious as a punched-out hole near the pylorus. An anterior gastric perforation is also obvious, but a posterior gastric ulcer is not visible unless the lesser sac is opened, usually along the greater curve.

In duodenal perforation, the question is whether to simply close the perforation or whether to perform a definitive operation to treat the peptic ulcer at the same time. If the ulcer is simply oversewn, at least 50% of patients will return with an active ulcer; the availability of effective medical treatment has, however, swung the balance in favour of oversewing.

Several other factors influence the choice of operation. A long history of treated peptic ulcer, particularly if there have been previous complications, merits a definitive operation (usually a trunkal vagotomy and pyloroplasty). Similarly, if pyloric stenosis is found at operation or if the ulcer has also been bleeding substantially, a definitive procedure should be performed.

In perforated gastric ulcer, the standard surgical operation is a Billroth I gastrectomy, including the whole ulcer in the resection. This ensures that a malignant ulcer is not unwittingly left behind.

Conservative management

If an elderly, unfit patient presents late with a perforated ulcer, many surgeons treat this conservatively. This involves nasogastric aspiration, intravenous infusion and antibiotics. Many of these patients recover satisfactorily, but would have succumbed under major surgery.

PYLORIC STENOSIS

The pyloric canal and the immediate pre-pyloric area are common sites of chronic ulceration. Ulcers in this area are probably aetiologically related more closely to duodenal than gastric ulcers and should be managed accordingly. There may be typical symptoms of chronic duodenal ulcer, or the presentation may be with pyloric stenosis and a minimal history of ulcer pain. Chronic ulceration near the pylorus causes fibrosis which may progress to stricture formation. In the early stages, this leads to partial gastric outlet obstruction. An acute exacerbation of the ulcer leads to mucosal swelling and pyloric sphincter spasm which then precipitates complete luminal obstruction.

Clinical features of pyloric stenosis

These patients rarely give any recent history of peptic ulcer pain but tend to present with a short history (a few weeks at most) of episodic and sometime projectile vomiting. This is unrelated to eating, and the vomitus typically contains foul-smelling semi-digested food eaten a day or more previously. It does not contain bile. Often patients do not seek medical advice until they have become severely dehydrated with gross electrolyte disturbance.

On clinical examination, undernourishment, constipation, weakness and weight loss may dominate the picture. Because the stomach is full of residual fluid and food, shaking the patient's abdomen from side to side produces an audible *succussion splash*. In long-standing cases, gastric peristalsis may be visible, and a dilated stomach full of residual food palpable. On plain abdominal X-ray, it may be possible to see the grossly dilated stomach filled with mottled food material.

Several gastric washouts, using a large-bore oral tube, will be necessary to clear the gastric residue before endoscopy or barium meal is attempted. In any case, the stomach must be clear before surgery.

The differential diagnosis of gastric outflow obstruction includes antral carcinoma, carcinoma of head of pancreas (with or without obstructive jaundice) and rarely, chronic pancreatitis.

Biochemical abnormalities in pyloric stenosis

The biochemical disturbances in these patients are complex, and depend on the volume and composition of fluid lost by vomiting and on the body's compensatory mechanisms. Hydrogen and chloride are the principal ions lost in the vomitus. In response, the kidney conserves hydrogen ions by exchanging them for sodium ions (and some potassium ions), which are necessarily lost in the urine. The kidney also conserves chloride ions by exchanging them for bicarbonate ions. The net result may be a profound depletion of total body sodium (which is not accurately reflected in the plasma sodium level), profound hypochloraemia and profound metabolic alkalosis (*hypochloraemic alkalosis*). The plasma urea level is often high due to dehydration. Finally, the proportion of ionised calcium in the serum may fall as a result of the alkalosis, inducing tetany.

Management of pyloric stenosis

The first management priority in gastric outlet obstruction is resuscitation. Fluid and electrolyte deficiencies are corrected by infusion of physiological saline with added potassium chloride. The volume required often amounts to 10 litres or more. Rehydration will usually return the blood urea level to normal but may unmask an anaemia serious enough to require blood transfusion. Once the patient is stable, operation is considered.

Operative treatment of peptic pyloric stenosis aims to prevent further ulceration and establish gastric drainage. The choice of operation depends of the surgeon's preference but includes trunkal vagotomy with either pyloroplasty or more often, gastro enterostomy, or occasionally, a Polya-type partial gastrectomy.

10 DISORDERS OF THE OESOPHAGUS

Introduction

Diseases of the oesophagus form a small but significant part of the workload of the general surgeon. *Peptic disorders* of the lower oesophagus (often associated with hiatus hernia) and *oesophageal carcinomas* are the main conditions encountered. *Achalasia* and *pharyngeal pouch* are occasionally seen, but *oesophageal web* (as in Plummer Vinson syndrome), and *leiomyoma* are extremely rare. Difficulty in swallowing, dysphagia, is the most common presenting symptom.

Oesophageal varices secondary to cirrhosis usually present as massive haematemesis. Surgical treatment may be required, either as an emergency or later.

CARCINOMA OF THE OESOPHAGUS

Pathology and clinical features

The oesophagus is lined by stratified squamous epithelium and thus the majority of oesophageal malignancies are *squamous carcinomas*. The rest are *adenocarcinomas*, probably derived from ectopic gastric mucosa, and tend to occur in the lower third of the oesophagus. Tumours at the gastro-oesophageal junction often arise at the cardia of the stomach and grow upwards. Both histological forms are usually only moderately differentiated and behave aggressively.

Oesophageal tumours may fungate into the lumen but more often infiltrate diffusely along and around the oesophageal wall. Once through the wall, the tumour invades surrounding mediastinal organs.

Difficulty in swallowing (dysphagia) is the classical symptom, but it tends to develop insidiously. Patients initially have trouble with solids but they tend to compensate (liquidising their food, for example) before seeking medical advice. Later they have trouble swallowing liquids. By the time a patient presents with dysphagia, the tumour is usually inoperable (i.e. incurable). Sometimes, involvement of other mediastinal organs, e.g. recurrent laryngeal nerve invasion or an oesophago-tracheal fistula, produces the first symptoms. Lymphatic spread to mediastinal nodes has often occurred by the time of presentation. Low oesophageal lesions tend also to metastasise to upper abdominal nodes and the liver.

Epidemiology of oesophageal carcinoma

Compared with carcinoma of the colon and stomach, the incidence of oesophageal carcinoma is relatively low. Because the disease is usually advanced

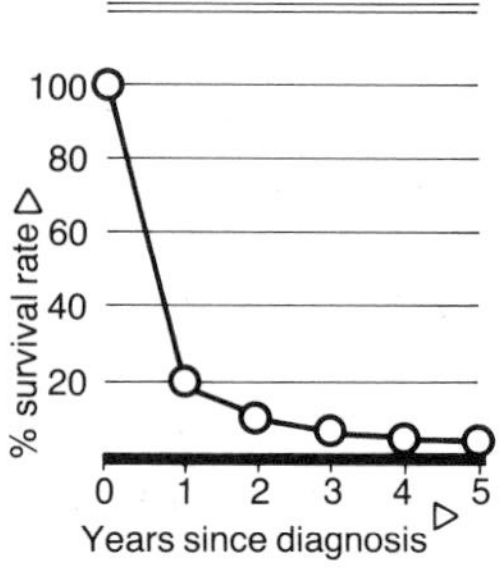

Fig. 10.1 Survival after diagnosis of oesophageal carcinoma

by the time of presentation, the mortality rate is appalling; 75% die within one year of presentation and only 6% survive five years. In the UK, oesophageal carcinoma accounts for 3% of all deaths from cancer, with minimal difference between males and females.

Oesophageal carcinoma is uncommon below the age of 50 years. At least half the tumours occur in the lower third of the oesophagus with only about 15% in the upper third. Heavy alcohol intake is associated with at least a 20 times greater risk of developing the disease; smokers have at least five times the risk of non-smokers. There appears to be no familial predisposition. These figures suggest that chronic local tissue irritation is the principle aetiological factor. This is supported by the fact that people with structural and functional disorders, such as peptic oesophagitis and stricture, achalasia, oesophageal web or pharyngeal pouch, are all at considerably greater risk of the disease. The majority of women who develop upper third lesions have a pre-existing oesophageal web or pharyngeal pouch, both very rare. In addition, areas of exceptionally high incidence have been reported in China and elsewhere in the Far East. There is some evidence that a fungus which grows on food grain may be responsible.

Investigation of suspected oesophageal carcinoma

Dysphagia or pain on swallowing in a middle-aged or elderly patient demands investigation in order to exclude carcinoma. Physical examination is usually unrewarding except in very advanced disease when there may be signs of wasting, hepatomegaly due to secondaries or sometimes hoarseness due to involvement of the recurrent laryngeal nerve.

Barium swallow examination is the investigation of first choice. The typical appearance of carcinoma is an irregular narrowing of the oesophageal lumen as illustrated in Figure 10.2. With early tumours, there may be minimal stricturing or even no visible abnormality. If radiological examination suggests tumour, or is not in agreement with the symptoms, direct inspection is necessary using either a flexible endoscope or a rigid oesophagoscope. Biopsies are taken of any suspicious areas.

Once carcinoma of the oesophagus is diagnosed, it is desirable to establish the extent of local invasion and discover whether metastasis to thoracic lymph nodes or the liver has occurred. CT scanning is the investigation of choice.

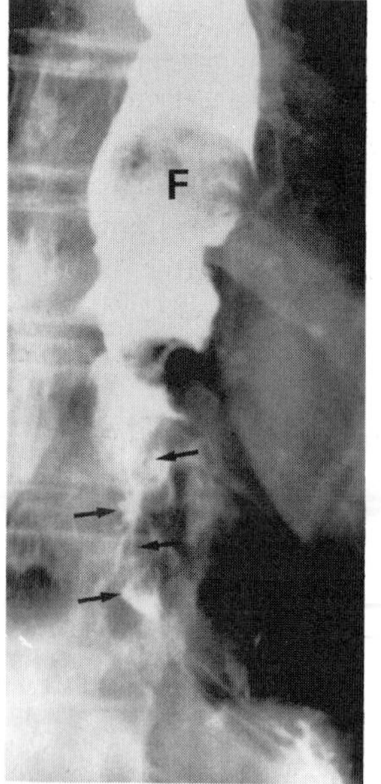

Fig. 10.2 Oesophageal carcinoma

Barium swallow in an elderly man who presented with almost complete dysphagia. The film shows the lower end of the oesophagus which has an irregular narrowing of the lumen (arrowed). This appearance did not alter in several views of the same area and is characteristic of malignancy. Nevertheless, endoscopy is usually performed to obtain histological confirmation by means of biopsies. The oesophagus above is moderately dilated and contains a bolus of food **F** which cannot pass onwards

Management of carcinoma of the oesophagus

The objective of treatment is of course to eliminate the tumour. In practice, this can rarely be achieved because of overt or occult spread. Even if cure is impossible, oesophageal obstruction must be relieved to allow the patient to eat and to prevent the appalling consequence of complete obstruction, i.e. inability to swallow even saliva.

Resection of the tumour is the only possible means of cure and provides good palliation in patients with a reasonable life expectancy. However, intubation of the tumour is preferable if life expectancy is short or the patient is not fit for a major operation.

Radiotherapy has a role in some patients with squamous carcinoma of the oesophagus but adenocarcinoma is insensitive. Intubation of the tumour may be necessary before commencing radiotherapy. Results of radiotherapy are disappointing mainly because of side-effects, for example mucosal swelling, which causes acute obstruction and later fibrosis. Radiotherapy tends to be reserved for palliation.

Surgery

The choice of operation depends on the level of the lesion and the usual approach is via a right thoracotomy. The lesion is resected along with a large margin of apparently normal oesophagus. Because of possible submucosal spread, frozen sections of the cut ends should be examined peroperatively to ensure removal has been complete. Some surgeons advocate excision of the entire oesophagus for the same reason. Continuity is restored by drawing up a portion of bowel, mobilised through a separate abdominal incision. This is known as the *Ivor Lewis operation*. The proximal oesophageal remnant is usually anastomosed to the gastric remnant but if this is impossible, a loop of jejunum is used to make the connection.

If the tumour is high or extensive, or if a sub-total oesophagectomy is the treatment of choice, the anastomosis is fashioned in the neck, wholly outside the mediastinum. An operation which has recently gained popularity is *transhiatal total oesophagectomy*. This avoids a thoracotomy, and the oesophagus is mobilised by blunt dissection from the abdomen and neck. Otherwise, subtotal oesophagectomy is performed through three separate incisions, when it is known as the *McKeown operation*. In some cases, it is necessary to use a *colonic conduit* to replace the excised oesophagus. A section of colon (usually right or left hemicolon) is isolated, retaining its original blood supply, and used to restore continuity.

Oesophagectomy is always a major undertaking and carries the potentially fatal risk of anastomotic breakdown. This may lead to mediastinitis, lung abscess or oesophago-pleural fistula. Patients should be made aware of the risks in relation to the benefits as well as the expected prolonged convalescent period.

Inoperable lesions

If operation is inappropriate, patency can often be restored by inserting a permanent reinforced rubber or plastic tube through the lesion. This may be done at an open operation or more often nowadays, under intravenous sedation using the endoscopic technique of *pulsion intubation*, preceded by dilatation (see Figure 10.3). Such tubes relieve symptoms but require food to be liquidised and must be kept 'clean' by taking fizzy drinks after eating.

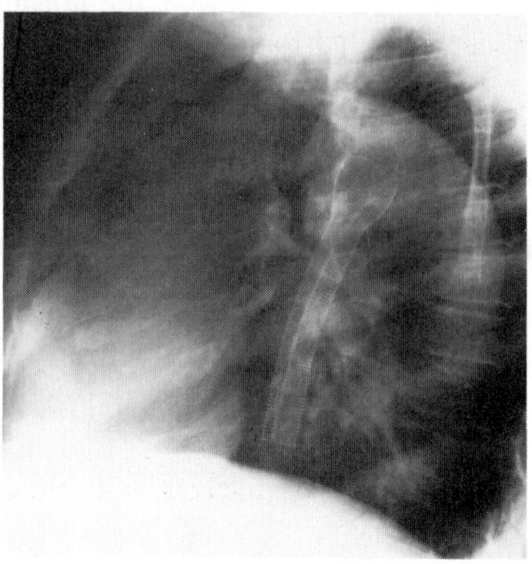

Fig. 10.3 Celestin tube
This 63-year-old man presented with inoperable carcinoma of the middle third of the oesophagus. The malignant stricture was dilated via a flexible gastroscope and a Celestin tube pushed in place to keep the stricture open. This lateral chest X-ray shows the tube in situ

HIATUS HERNIA AND REFLUX OESOPHAGITIS

Pathophysiology

The oesophagus is essentially a tube of smooth muscle conveying food to the stomach by peristalsis. At the lower end of the oesophagus there is a tonically active sphincter mechanism. Its activity coordinates with peristalsis, relaxing to allow food to enter the stomach. Otherwise, the sphincter mechanism prevents reflux of stomach contents into the oesophagus.

After passing through the diaphragm, the oesophagus continues for about two centimetres within the abdomen before joining the stomach. The sphincter mechanism is not completely understood but it probably involves several components: there is a functional (but not anatomical) sphincter of the oesophageal wall immediately above the diaphragm and the smooth muscle at the gastric cardia. This is reinforced by contraction of the diaphragmatic crura, by the acute angle of entry of oesophagus to stomach and by the 'flutter valve' effect of intra-abdominal pressure on the abdominal oesophagus causing collapse of the lumen.

Hiatus hernia occurs when the proximal part of the stomach passes through the diaphragmatic hiatus into the chest; 90% of hiatus hernias are of the *sliding type* in which the gastro-oesophageal junction is drawn up into the chest, and a segment of stomach becomes constricted at the diaphragmatic hiatus. The hernia tends to slide up into the chest with each peristaltic contraction. Such hernias may reach a huge size. In the other 10% of cases, the gastro-oesophageal junction remains below the diaphragm and a bulge of stomach herniates through the hiatus beside the oesophagus. These are described as *para-oesophageal* or *rolling hiatus hernias* and are usually small. In sliding hiatus hernia, the lower oesophageal sphincter mechanism is defective, causing reflux of acid-peptic stomach contents into the oesophagus. This is not a problem with rolling hiatus hernias.

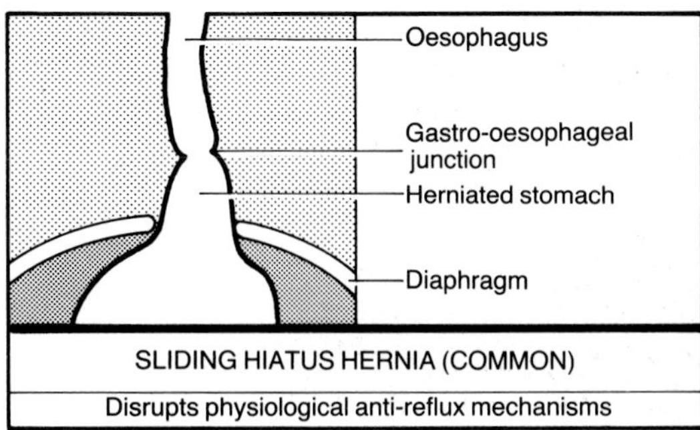

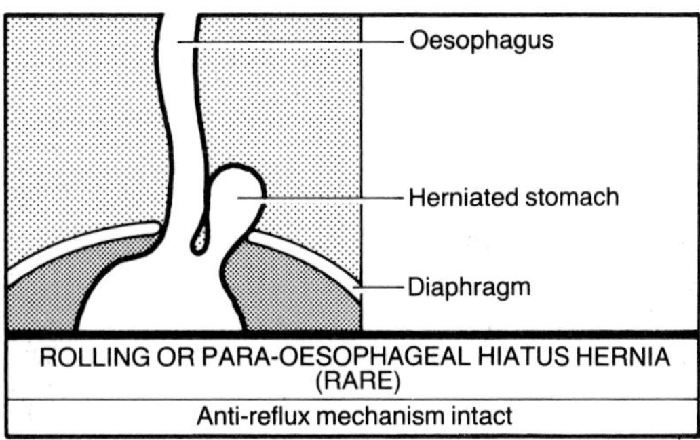

Fig. 10.4 Sliding and rolling hiatus hernias

Hiatus hernia in adults is commonly associated with obesity. Perhaps the pressure of intra-abdominal fat is contributory. Hiatus hernia can also be a congenital abnormality presenting in early infancy.

Clinical features

Hiatus hernia is common, especially in women, and with advancing years. Only a small proportion of patients with a hiatus hernia experience symptoms of acid-peptic reflux. Reflux causes acute inflammation (oesophagitis). This is experienced as burning retrosternal pain, bitter tasting regurgitation, other forms of 'indigestion' and occasionally small haematemeses. Symptoms are typically worse at night when the patient lies flat in bed or during the day with bending forwards.

If reflux is severe and persistent, inflammation becomes chronic; progressive fibrosis of the wall may lead to narrowing (stricture) of the lumen and the symptom of dysphagia. Long-standing oesophageal ulceration predisposes to the development of *Barrett's oesophagus* in which oesophageal epithelium is replaced by ectopic gastric glandular epithelium. The condition is probably premalignant.

Occasionally, oesophageal reflux symptoms are severe and acute, causing chest pain which may easily be mistaken for angina or even myocardial infarction. There is often an element of *oesophageal spasm* which, like angina, is relieved by GTN and similar drugs. This may confuse the diagnosis.

In general, hiatus hernia and reflux can be demonstrated by barium swallow examination (see Figure 10.5) but assessment of mucosal inflammation requires endoscopy and biopsy. The latter is important to exclude carcinoma, especially if dysphagia is experienced.

Management of hiatus hernia and reflux oesophagitis

Most patients can be managed conservatively; surgery is reserved for intractable cases. Treatment is aimed at reducing acid-pepsin activity and preventing reflux.

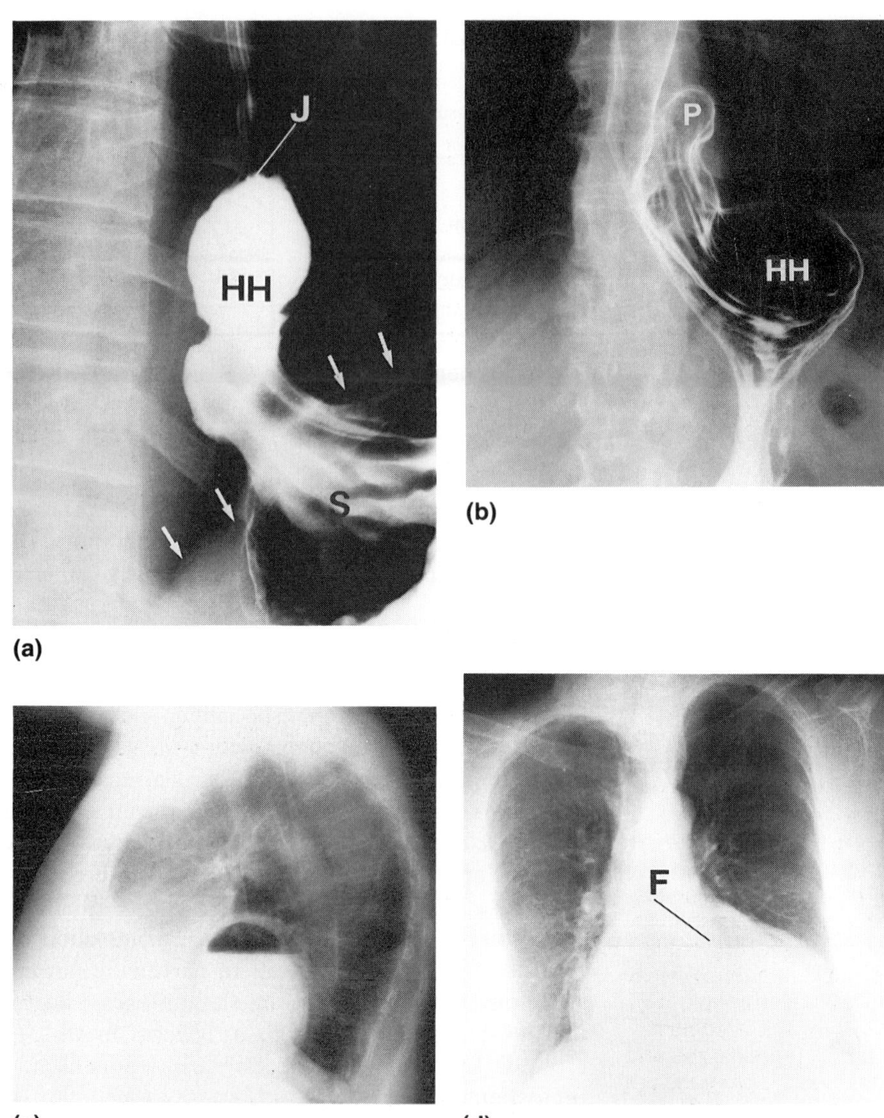

Fig. 10.5 Hiatus hernia

(a) Sliding hiatus hernia in a 63-year-old woman. The hiatus hernia is marked **HH**, the stomach **S**, the oesophago-gastric junction **J** and the position of the diaphragm is arrowed. **(b)** and **(c)** Large incarcerated (irreducible) sliding hiatus hernia in an elderly woman with few symptoms. Note there is also a small para-oesophageal 'rolling' hiatus hernia **P**. The lateral film shows the hernia containing barium and a fluid level. **(d)** Plain chest X-ray of the same patient showing a fluid level **F** strongly suggestive of a hiatus hernia

Reduction of reflux

Reflux can be reduced considerably by taking smaller, more frequent and drier meals, by using blocks to elevate the head of the bed, and by sleeping on more pillows in an upright position. Smoking induces sphincter relaxation and quitting often reduces reflux dramatically. Weight reduction, however, is the most effective long-term measure. *Alginate drugs*, such as 'Gaviscon', available in liquid or chewable tablet form, produce a foamy surface layer on the stomach contents, diminishing reflux. These drugs are most effective if taken soon after food.

Reduction of acid-pepsin production

Reduction of acid-pepsin attack is accomplished as for chronic peptic ulcer disease. *Antacid drugs* and *H_2 receptor antagonists* are the drugs of choice. Drugs and food which irritate the lower oesophagus should be avoided.

Management of strictures

Inflammatory fibrous strictures can be dilated with gum-elastic bougies of progressively increasing size. This was done under general anaesthesia via a rigid oesophagoscope. More commonly now, a guide-wire is positioned across the stricture endoscopically and graded metal or plastic dilators inserted over it to dilate the stricture; only intravenous sedation is required. If, despite suitable conservative treatment of reflux, the stricture recurs causing dysphagia, an anti-reflux operation is usually performed. This allows healing of ulceration and inhibits further stricture formation.

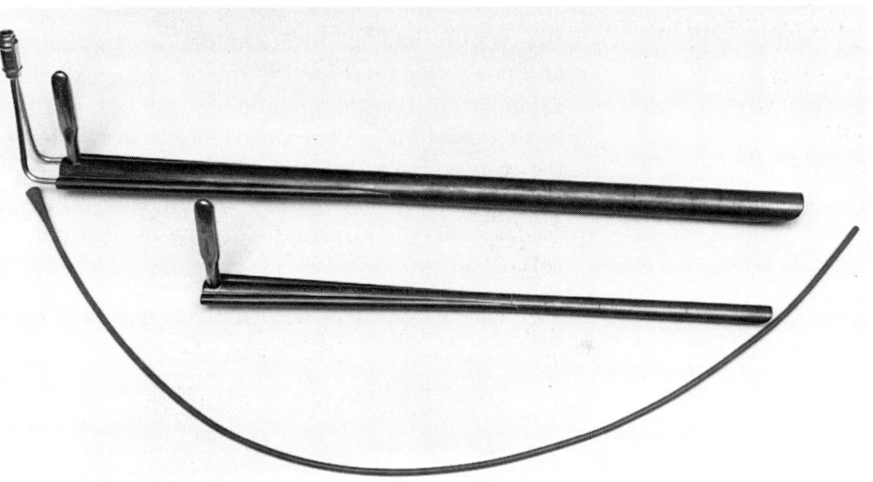

Fig. 10.6 Oesophagoscopes and an oesophageal bougie

This shows two rigid oesophagoscopes, adult and paediatric sizes. Note the 'beaked' distal ends and the markings at 5-cm and 1-cm intervals along the length of each instrument. The fibre-optic guide used to transmit illumination to the distal end is seen at the proximal end of the adult instrument. A small gum-elastic bougie is also shown. These come in sets of graded sizes and are used to progressively dilate oesophageal strictures under direct vision

Surgery for hiatus hernia and reflux oesophagitis

Surgery is reserved for intractable symptoms, recurrent stricture and chronic peptic ulceration, particularly with Barrett's oesophagus. The traditional operations for repair of hiatus hernia, performed via chest or abdomen, have largely been superseded by the *Nissen fundoplication*. This abdominal operation involves wrapping the gastric fundus around the intra-abdominal portion of the oesophagus to create a flutter valve. Recently, the *Angelchik ring device* (filled with liquid silicone) has been introduced; it is placed around the intra-abdominal oesophagus. The operation is very simple but long-term efficacy has not yet been established.

ACHALASIA

Pathophysiology and clinical presentation

Achalasia is an uncommon disorder of oesophageal motility. Normal peristalsis is lost causing uncoordinated relaxation of the lower oesophageal sphincter.

In pathological terms, there is a poorly understood neurological defect involving Auerbach's myenteric (parasympathetic) plexus. The entire oesophagus is affected rather than just the cardia, as the outdated term 'achalasia of the cardia' implies. The condition presents in two main age groups, young adults and the elderly. In the latter, the cause may be a central rather than a local neurological defect. Achalasia, as with any structural abnormality of the oesophagus, predisposes to carcinoma.

Clinically, the cardiac sphincter becomes constricted and the proximal oesophagus dilates with accumulated fluid and solids. Difficulty in swallowing fluids is the usual presenting symptom. Solids tend to sink to the lower end of the dilated oesophagus, whereas fluids spill over into the trachea causing spluttering dysphagia (see Chapter 6). Vomiting and retrosternal pain may occur in more severe cases. The degree of dysphagia tends to be variable, probably depending on the amount of food residue in the oesophagus at any one time.

Investigations

Chest X-ray may show a widened mediastinal shadow of dilated oesophagus and possibly a fluid level in the oesophagus behind the heart. Barium swallow examination reveals dilatation of the oesophagus and a tapering constriction at the lower end. The constriction barely allows the passage of contrast into the stomach (see Figure 10.7). Under fluoroscopic screening, uncoordinated, purposeless peristaltic waves can often be seen; these are described as 'tertiary contractions', contrasting with the normal pattern of primary and secondary contractions.

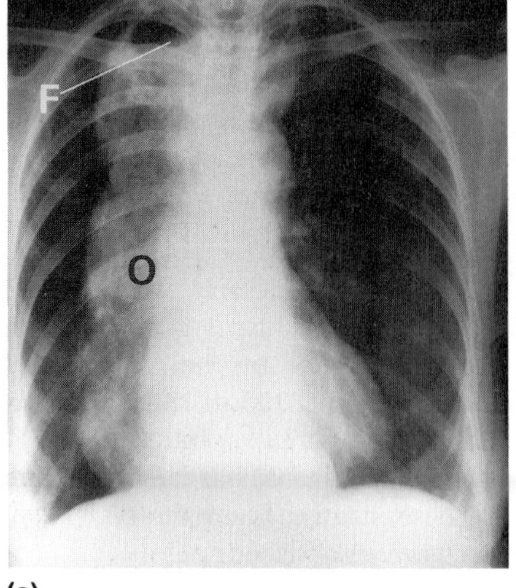

(a)

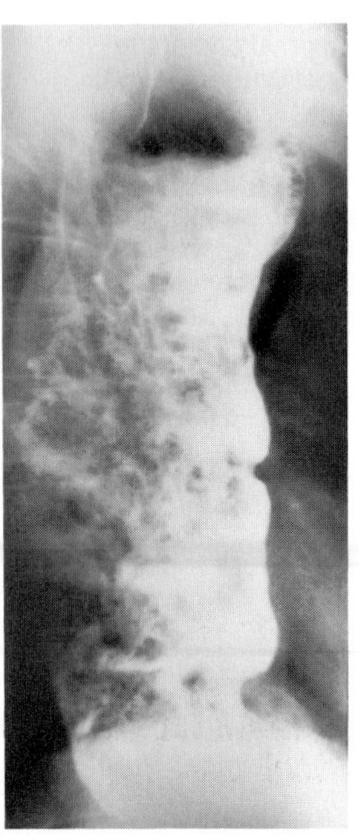
(b)

Fig. 10.7 Achalasia

Late stage achalasia in a 60-year-old man. **(a)** The chest X-ray shows gross mediastinal widening caused by a massively dilated oesophagus **O** filled with food debris. Note the mottled appearance of the oesophagus and the fluid level **F** at its upper end. Note also the absence of a gastric air bubble which is characteristic of achalasia. **(b)** Barium swallow in the same patient. This confirms the findings on the chest X-ray

Management of achalasia

The condition is, by its nature, incurable, and treatment is directed at relief of the distal obstruction. The standard operation is via the abdomen, and involves a longitudinal incision of the lower oesophageal and upper gastric muscle wall until the mucosa bulges through (*Heller's cardiomyotomy*). Recently, balloon dilatation has been introduced as an alternative to operation. Patients with achalasia should be followed up and periodically endoscoped to exclude carcinoma.

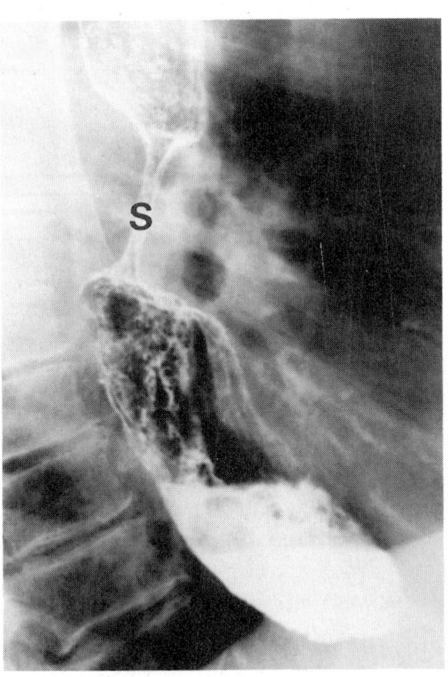

Fig. 10.8 Oesophageal carcinoma secondary to achalasia

Malignant stricture **S** in the middle third of the oesophagus in a 60-year-old woman with achalasia of long standing. She had a Heller's myotomy at the age of 26. Note that surgery does not alter the predisposition to carcinoma

PHARYNGEAL POUCH

Pharyngeal pouch is a rare cause of dysphagia. It arises at the junction of pharynx and oesophagus, and probably results from lack of coordination of the inferior constrictor muscle and cricopharyngeus during swallowing. The result is progressive mucosal outpouching between the two muscles. The condition is best diagnosed by barium swallow and treated by surgical excision from the side of the neck.

OESOPHAGEAL WEB

Circumferential mucosal folds (or webs) may occur in the oesophagus producing annular narrowing of the lumen and causing dysphagia. In the upper oesophagus, they are found in association with severe iron deficiency anaemia, particularly in women. The triad of dysphagia, anaemia and atrophic glossitis is known as *Plummer Vinson syndrome*.

OESOPHAGEAL VARICES

Pathophysiology

Oesophageal varices result from *portal venous hypertension*. The most common cause is cirrhosis of the liver, usually associated with alcohol abuse. Less

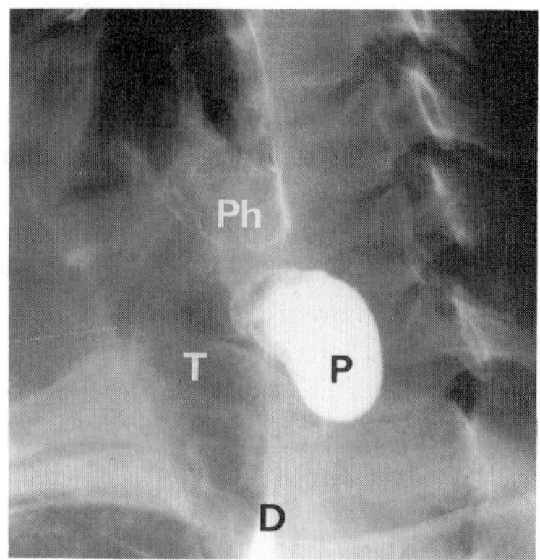

Fig. 10.9 Pharyngeal pouch

Lateral view during barium swallow examination in a 41-year-old man complaining of mild dysphagia; the X-ray shows a contrast-filled pouch **P** extending from the pharynx **Ph**. Note the gas-filled trachea **T** lying anteriorly and the barium-containing oesophagus **D** below

common causes include portal vein thrombosis, hepatic vein thrombosis (*Budd–Chiari syndrome*) and schistosomiasis.

As resistance to flow and pressure in the portal venous system rises, abnormal venous communications develop between the peripheral part of the portal system and the systemic circulation. This is known as *portal-systemic shunting*. Multiple large veins appear in the peritoneal cavity and retroperitoneal area, making operative surgery hazardous. Large submucosal veins also appear at the lower end of the oesophagus and gastric fundus and these are known as *oesophageal varices* (see Figure 10.10). These varices are easily traumatised by food and produce massive gastrointestinal haemorrhage. Up to 40% of cirrhotic patients suffer variceal haemorrhage at some stage.

A further result of portal hypertension is splenic enlargement. This may result in *hypersplenism*, causing anaemia, thrombocytopenia and leucopenia. Patients in late stages of cirrhosis also develop ascites.

If there is massive portal-systemic shunting, either spontaneous or resulting from a surgically created shunt, *portal-systemic encephalopathy* may occur. This is due to toxins such as ammonia passing directly into the systemic circulation without traversing the liver, where they would normally be detoxified.

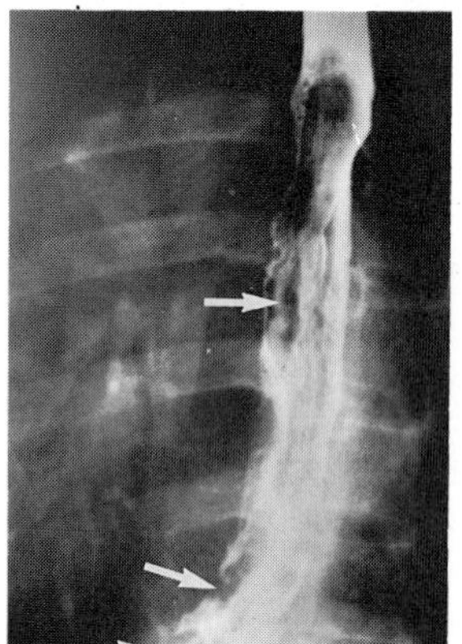

Fig. 10.10 Oesophageal varices

A 51-year-old woman with primary biliary cirrhosis in whom a barium swallow was performed to assess possible complications. Oesophageal varices are represented by ragged filling defects (arrowed) typically extending from the stomach **S** up as far as the level of the aortic arch. The patient subsequently underwent injection sclerotherapy

Management of oesophageal varices

Oesophageal varices do not usually require treatment unless haemorrhage has occurred. However, elective injection sclerotherapy (described below) may be carried out if prophylactic treatment is considered desirable.

Acute variceal haemorrhage

When a patient with known cirrhosis or varices presents with massive upper gastrointestinal haemorrhage, the first priority is resuscitation. Following this, the source of haemorrhage is sought. In fact only about half of these patients will be bleeding from varices. The rest have bleeding duodenal or gastric ulcers. Clearly, management varies according to the diagnosis. It must be remembered, however, that cirrhotic patients often have defective clotting. Clotting studies should be performed and specific corrective factors given.

Balloon tamponade

If bleeding is from varices, an attempt is made to apply tamponade. A special tube is passed through the mouth into the stomach and a balloon inflated. Traction is exerted on the upper end for up to four hours in the hope that haemorrhage will stop. Several varieties of tube are in use: the *Minnesota* and *Sengstaken tubes* have separate intragastric and oesophageal balloons and depend for their action upon physiological arrest of bleeding. The *Linton balloon*, however, has a single large intragastric balloon (200–300 ml), which allows simultaneous endoscopy and injection of varices with sclerosant. This method of treating acute variceal haemorrhage is steadily becoming more popular.

Surgical treatment of variceal haemorrhage is much less commonly performed nowadays. Operations include *transgastric oesophageal stapling*. A circular stapler is passed into the oesophagus via a gastrotomy, a ligature tied around the oesophagus between the staples and the anvil, and the gun fired. This places two rows of staples through the full thickness of the oesophageal wall, disconnecting the longitudinal veins.

Emergency portal-systemic shunting is hardly used now because of the risk of portal-systemic encephalopathy and the unpredictable outcome with regard to haemorrhage. These operations are still sometimes used following recovery from the acute haemorrhage to prevent further haemorrhage, although many doctors now believe that repeated injection sclerotherapy via a flexible endoscope is the best treatment.

All surgical portal-systemic shunts carry a risk of encephalopathy, although newer shunts have been designed to minimise this risk. These operations include *porta-caval shunting*, in which the main portal vein is anastomosed to the inferior vena cava, *meso-caval shunting* in which the superior mesenteric vein is connected to the inferior vena cava via an interposition graft, and *lieno-renal shunting* (the *Warren shunt*) in which the splenic vein is anastomosed to the left renal vein. The last is said to cause the lowest incidence of encephalopathy, but is also the least effective at decompressing the portal venous pressure.

Operative risk has been calculated using *Child's criteria*, as shown in Figure 10.11.

Operative surgery for oesophageal varices has dwindled in recent years because of the effectiveness of injection sclerotherapy. Now that the problem of variceal haemorrhage can be overcome, the mortality in these patients is related to the mortality from the underlying cirrhosis.

Fig. 10.11 Child's criteria for assessing operative risk in portal hypertension

Score points	1	2	3
Encephalopathy	none	minimal	marked
Ascites	none	slight	moderate
Bilirubin (micromoles/L)	<35	36–50	>50
Albumin (g/L)	>35	28–35	<28
Prothrombin ratio	<1.4	1.4–2.0	>2.0

Each criterion is scored and the total added:
Child's grade A (good risk) scores 5–6
grade B (moderate risk) scores 7–9
grade C (bad risk) scores 10–15.

11 TUMOURS OF THE STOMACH AND SMALL INTESTINE

Introduction

Although benign tumours can occur in the stomach, most gastric tumours are malignant. Most of these are adenocarcinomas, while lymphomas, and occasionally carcinoid tumours and sarcomas, make up the remainder.

Tumours of the small bowel are rare. Of the malignant tumours, lymphomas and leiomyosarcomas are much more common than adenocarcinomas. *Peutz–Jehger syndrome* is a rare inherited disorder characterised by multiple benign polyps in the small bowel and perioral pigmentation. It is most commonly seen at student examinations!

CARCINOMA OF STOMACH

Pathology

Gastric carcinomas are almost exclusively adenocarcinomas. They may develop in three morphological forms:

- Fungating tumours — these tend to be polypoid and may grow to a huge size. They have a somewhat better prognosis than the other types
- Malignant ulcers — these lesions probably result from necrosis at the centre of broad-based solid tumours. Malignant ulcers are often larger than peptic ulcers (except for the giant benign ulcer of the elderly), with a heaped-up indurated margin. There is no surrounding mucosal puckering typical of inflammatory scarring
- Infiltrating carcinoma — this form of gastric cancer spreads widely beneath the mucosa and diffusely invades the muscular wall. This causes considerable wall thickening and rigidity, and the whole stomach contracts to a very small capacity. This is known as *linitis plastica* and its appearance is likened to a 'leather bottle'. Linitis plastica affects a slightly younger age group and has a very poor prognosis

Most gastric cancers are moderately well differentiated histologically, with an acinar structure and mucus secreting ability. In linitis plastica, the tumour cells are poorly differentiated with large intracellular mucin droplets which displace the nuclei peripherally. This gives a characteristic *signet ring appearance*. There is often a pronounced fibrotic stromal reaction.

Aetiology and epidemiology of gastric carcinoma

The epidemiology of gastric carcinoma gives tantalising clues as to the cause of the disease, but no single aetiological factor has been established which might

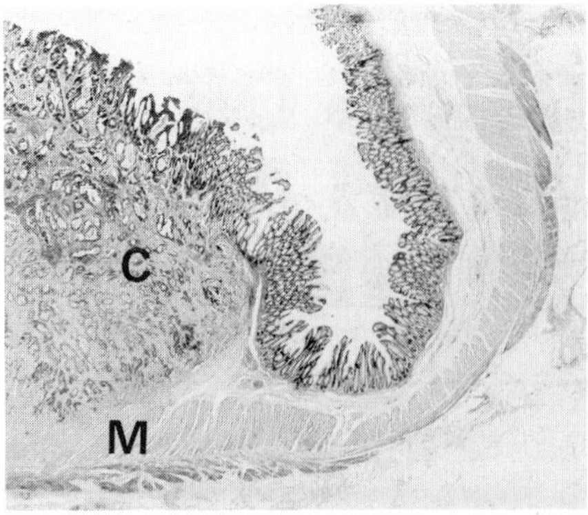

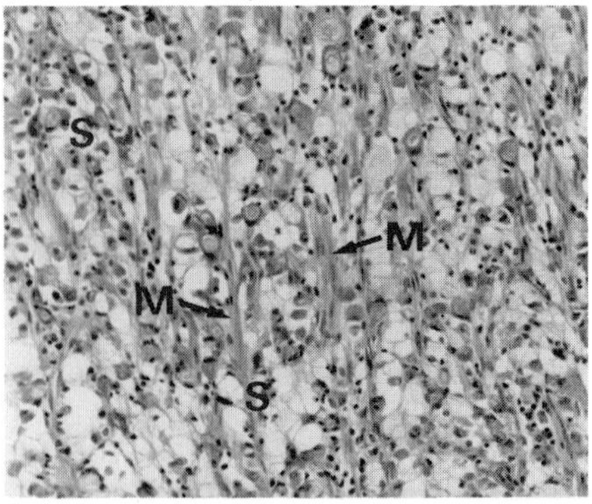

Fig. 11.1 Carcinoma of the stomach — histopathology

(a) Typical moderately differentiated fungating gastric carcinoma **C** invading the muscular wall **M** of the stomach in a 60-year-old man.
(b) High power view of linitis plastica in a 63-year-old woman showing masses of signet ring cells (arrowed) invading between strands of smooth muscle **M**

(a) (b)

be amenable to preventative measures. The incidence of gastric carcinoma is declining worldwide, as shown in Figure 11.2. Nevertheless, gastric carcinoma still ranks fifth as a cause of deaths from cancer in the UK, accounting for about 7% of all cancer deaths.

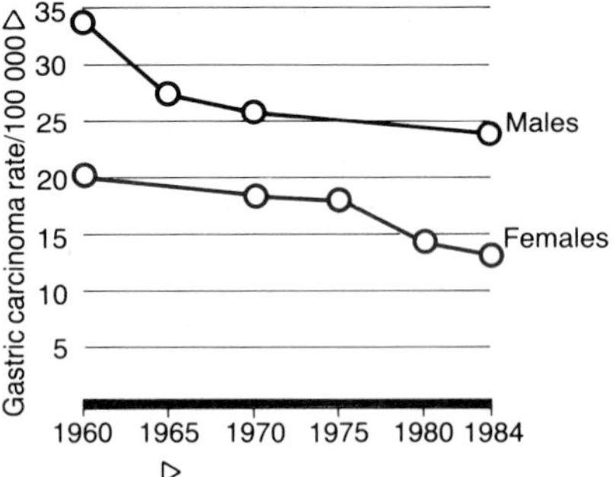

Fig. 11.2 Declining incidence of gastric carcinoma

Cancer of the stomach is rare before the age of 50 and increases in frequency thereafter. Males have one and a half times the risk of females, and the disease is more common in lower socio-economic groups. Constitutional factors play some part, since the close family relatives of those affected have a four-fold risk of developing the disease. A higher incidence has been observed in people with blood group A.

There are significant international differences in the incidence of gastric cancer. It is especially common in Japan, Scandinavia and Chile. The offspring of Japanese immigrants to America, however, appear to have the same risk as other Americans, suggesting that environmental rather than racial factors are responsible for the regional variation. Polycyclic hydrocarbons in smoked fish and meat products, as well as nitrosamines derived from nitrates in food and water, have been implicated in causing gastric carcinoma, but there is no conclusive evidence.

Gastric cancer is seldom seen in its early stages, so little is known of its origins. In patients with overt malignancy, there are often metaplastic and dysplastic changes in the rest of the gastric epithelium. Up to 20% of apparently benign gastric polyps show areas of dysplastic change but polyps are much less common than frank carcinoma. Gastric mucosal atrophy (which occurs in atrophic gastritis, achlorhydria and pernicious anaemia), is a definite predisposing factor. As many as 10% of patients with pernicious anaemia eventually develop cancer.

In most countries, gastric carcinoma in usually incurable by the time of presentation and the five year survival rate is below 10%. In Japan however, screening of high risk groups by endoscopy and barium studies has led to earlier diagnosis, and an improved cure rate.

Clinical features of gastric carcinoma

Since the stomach is so capacious, local symptoms rarely develop until the gastric lesion is extensive and metastasis has occurred. Symptoms tend to be vague and non-specific. They include epigastric discomfort or pain, anorexia and weight loss, or a feeling of fullness after only a small amount of food. Vomiting may occur if the gastric outlet becomes obstructed. Severe weight loss usually indicates advanced disease and may be its only manifestation; indeed, dramatic weight loss in the absence of other symptoms should alert the clinician to possible gastric carcinoma.

Physical examination gives few clues except in advanced cases where cachexia and a craggy epigastric mass make the diagnosis obvious. Anaemia resulting from chronic occult blood loss is common.

Metastatic spread initially involves local lymph nodes in the coeliac axis and periduodenal area. Later the para-aortic and porta hepatis nodes become involved, the latter causing obstructive jaundice. Left supraclavicular (*Virchow's*) nodes may become invaded via the thoracic duct and give rise to a palpable mass (*Troisier's sign*). These nodes are palpable in a small proportion of cases at initial presentation. Hepatic metastasis through haematogenous spread is also a common initial finding. Widespread metastasis to lungs, brain and bone may also occur. Gastric carcinoma sometimes spreads across the peritoneal cavity, particularly to the surface of the ovaries (*Krukenberg tumour*) or the pouch of Douglas. In either case, a mass is often palpable on rectal examination. Direct spread into the transverse colon is not unusual and sometimes results in fistula formation.

Fig. 11.3 Summary — presenting features of gastric carcinoma

Often asymptomatic until a late stage
Marked weight loss
Anorexia
Feeling of abdominal fullness or discomfort, often after only small meals
Epigastric mass
Iron deficiency anaemia
Left supraclavicular mass (secondaries in Virchow's node)
Obstructive jaundice (secondaries in the porta hepatis)
Pelvic mass

Investigation of suspected gastric carcinoma

Barium meal has been for many years the standard investigation for upper gastrointestinal symptoms, but it is often impossible to differentiate between gastric ulcer and carcinoma radiologically. The typical radiological appearances of gastric malignancies are, however, shown in Figure 11.4. Endoscopy and biopsy are essential if there is any doubt of the diagnosis on radiological grounds, and endoscopy alone is now becoming the preferred investigation for suspected carcinoma of stomach. Carcinomas can arise in any part of the stomach, including the lesser curve, whereas benign gastric ulcers are usually found on the lesser curve or prepyloric area. The site of a lesion may therefore be of diagnostic significance. CT scanning may be used to assess the site and extent of metastases before embarking upon surgery. This investigation is useful for showing local spread, lymph node involvement and hepatic metastases.

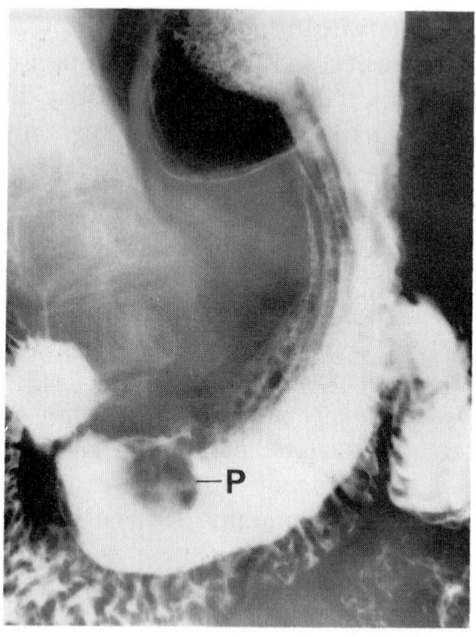

(a)

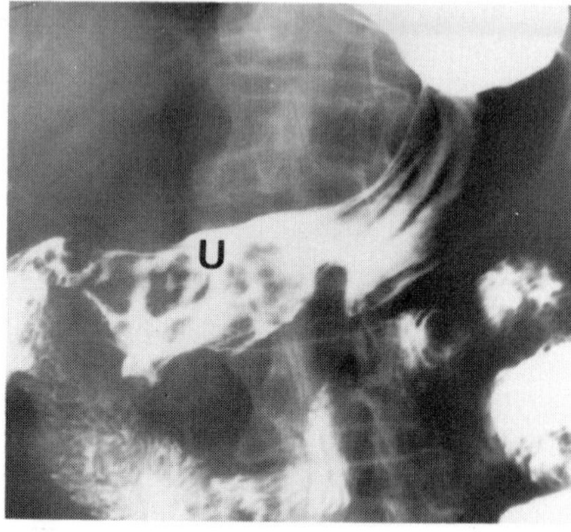

(b)

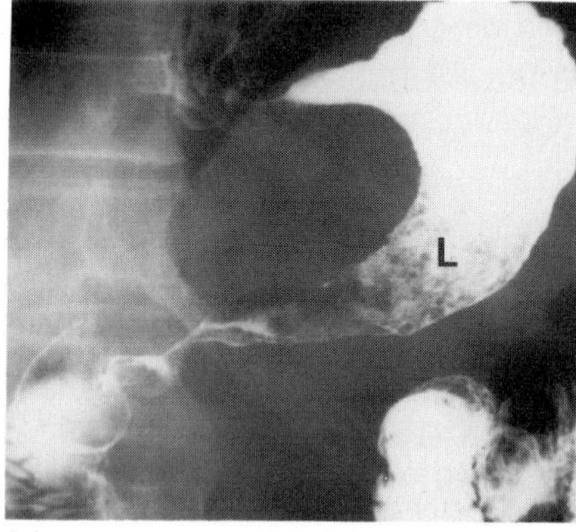

(c)

Fig. 11.4 Barium meals of carcinoma of the stomach

(a) Polypoid carcinoma of stomach **P** discovered during investigation of iron deficiency anaemia in a 60-year-old man. Diagnosis was confirmed by endoscopic biopsy.
(b) Ulcerating carcinoma of stomach **U** in a 55-year-old man presenting with weight loss.
(c) Linitis plastica type of carcinoma of stomach **L**. Note the shrunken appearance of the whole stomach caused by widespread submucosal invasion of tumour. Endoscopic biopsy may not give the correct diagnosis because the mucosa is often intact. This 60-year-old woman presented with anorexia. She had a total gastrectomy but died five months later of widespread metastases

Management of gastric carcinoma

Metastasis in gastric cancer tends to be early and widespread. Therefore, surgery usually offers little prospect of cure even when the tumour is small. The only real hope of cure is when tumours are found at an early stage. This usually happens only fortuitously, for example, when a patient is gastroscoped for dyspepsia and an incidental early cancer is found. Screening for the disease by regular gastroscopy is becoming popular in Japan, where gastric cancer is extremely common. Early detection before symptoms appear and before the tumour becomes invasive allows curative surgery.

Even if the disease has progressed to local lymph nodes, palliative gastrectomy may be indicated to treat local problems such as chronic blood loss or obstruction. In a few cases, this may effect a cure. The usual operation is a radical gastrectomy: excision of the tumour and a wide margin of normal stomach, clearance of lesser curve and coeliac axis lymph nodes, and removal of the greater omentum and the nodes within it. Japanese surgeons have developed more extensive, radical gastrectomies (known as R2 and R3 gastrectomies) which involve clearance of further lymph node fields, including the porta hepatis and splenic nodes, and splenectomy. With such procedures, five year survival rates up to 25% can be achieved and local recurrence is almost eliminated.

The decision to attempt removal of a gastric cancer depends on the general fitness of the patient as well as the stage of the tumour. It is kindest to treat patients with advanced cancer symptomatically, and only perform lesser palliative procedures (such as gastroenterostomy to bypass an obstructing antral carcinoma). Patients with obviously incurable tumours may have very few symptoms and their quality of life may only be diminished by surgery. In other cases, tumour bleeding, necrosis or encroachment on the gastric lumen results in distressing symptoms. These include nausea, anorexia, vomiting (sometimes complete gastric outlet obstruction), or symptoms of anaemia. These symptoms can be greatly relieved by palliative partial gastrectomy. Afterwards, patients survive about 12 months on average, compared with about three months without operation. Unfortunately, radiotherapy and chemotherapy have no proven benefit in control of gastric carcinoma.

GASTRIC POLYPS

Gastric polyps are small benign adenomas of the gastric mucosa, with histological and morphological forms similar to the more common polyps of the large intestine. Polyps may be solitary or multiple, and sessile or pedunculated in form. They rarely grow to more than a few centimetres in diameter and are usually asymptomatic. Most are found only incidentally on radiological or endoscopic examination.

Up to 20% of gastric polyps show histological features of dysplasia but they probably account for only a small proportion of gastric adenocarcinomas.

Treatment is by endoscopic excision biopsy. Regular endoscopy is usually arranged to monitor recurrence or the appearance of new lesions.

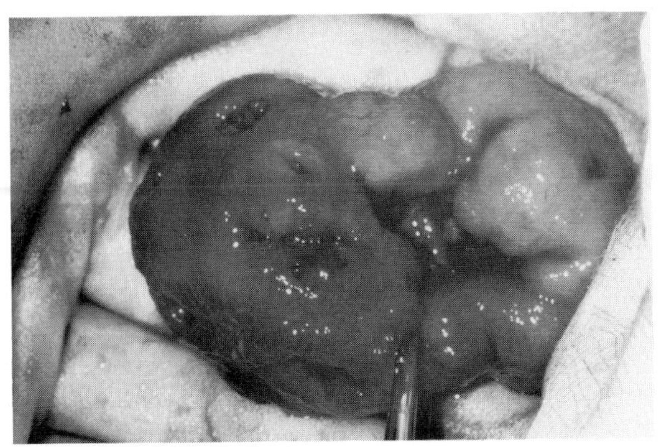

Fig. 11.5 Gastric polyp

This 64-year-old woman presented with recurrent iron deficiency anaemia. A large ulcerated polyp had been seen at endoscopy. Here, the stomach has been opened at laparotomy and the polyp is held up in the surgeon's hand. Deep peptic ulcers can be seen on its surface. Histologically, it proved to be a benign leiomyoma

LEIOMYOMAS

Leiomyomas are benign tumours of smooth muscle and may arise anywhere in the muscular wall of the gastrointestinal tract. They are especially common in the stomach and small bowel. These lesions are usually only a few centi-

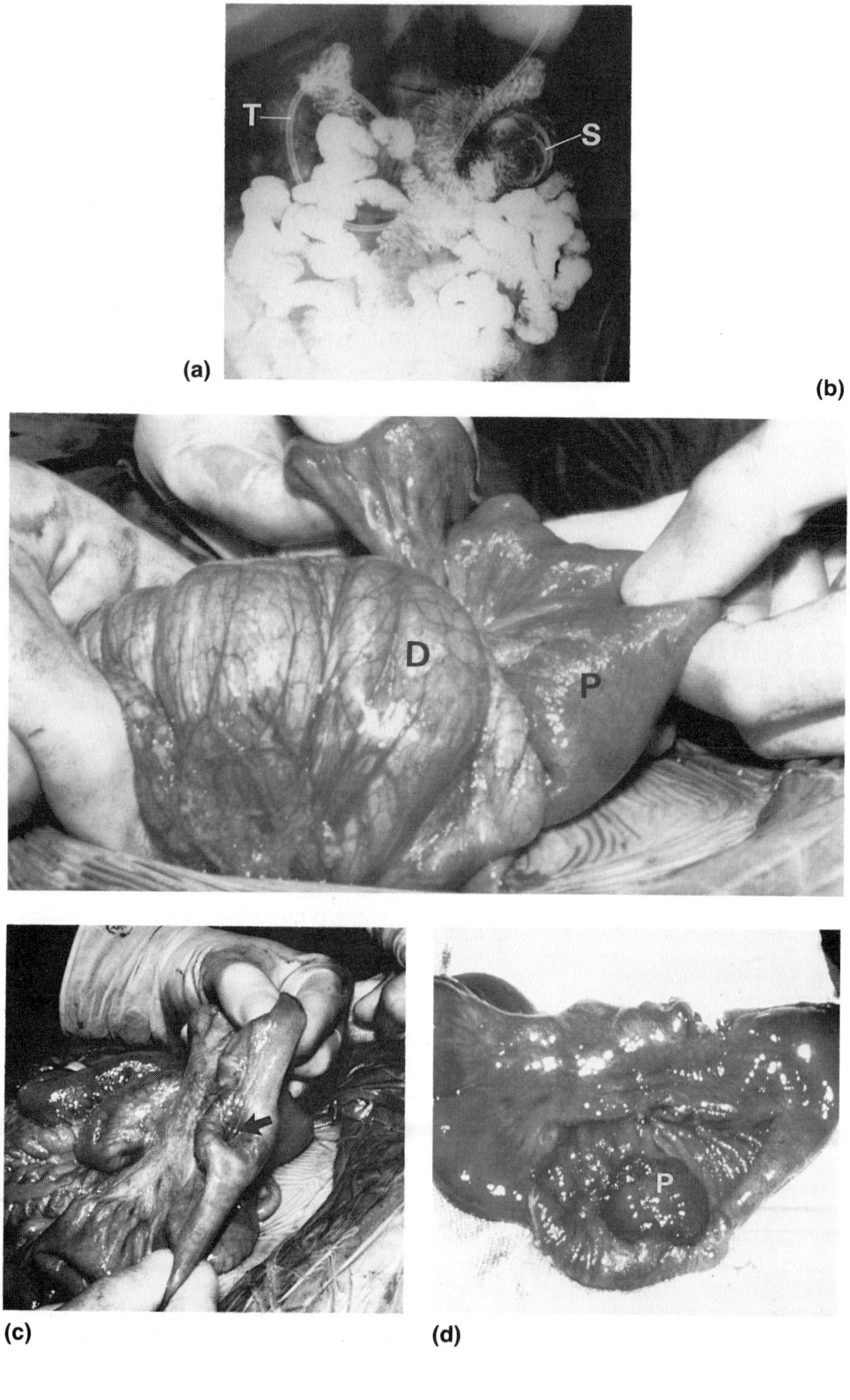

(a)

(b)

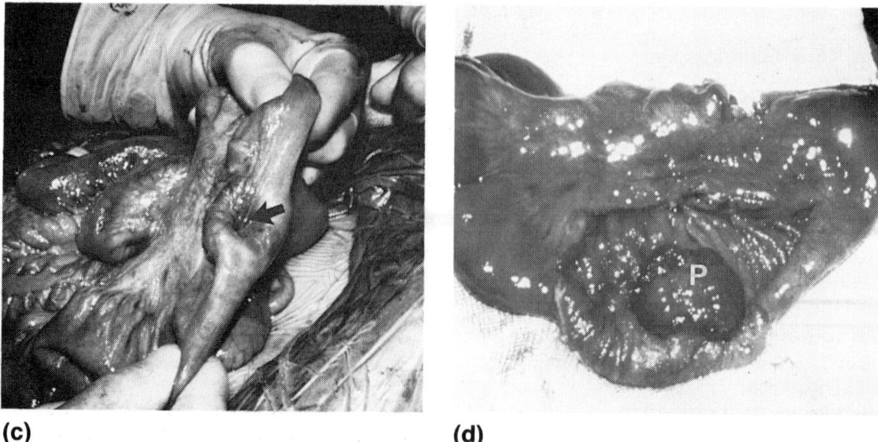

(c) (d)

Fig. 11.6 Intussuscepting tumours of small bowel

(a) This 35-year-old woman suffered several self-limiting episodes of small bowel obstruction. A small bowel barium enema, shown here, was performed during one of these episodes, by placing the tip of a nasojejunal tube **T** just distal to the duodenojejunal flexure and instilling barium. A small bowel intussusception is demonstrated by the 'coiled-spring' sign **S**, due to the presence of barium between the telescoping layers of bowel. At surgery, a leiomyoma was found to be responsible. **(b)–(d)** This 22-year-old man presented with small bowel obstruction. At laparotomy, the obstruction was found to be caused by an ileo-ileal intussusception. In this set of operative photographs (b) shows the proximal ileum **P** had intussuscepted into the distal ileum **D**. When this was reduced (c), an abnormality of the bowel wall could be seen to have formed the apex of the intussuscipiens (arrowed). In (d), a polypoid tumour **P** can be seen on the luminal surface, which proved histologically to be a lymphoma

metres in diameter and are discovered incidentally on endoscopy or barium examinations. Occasionally, larger lesions are found to be the cause of chronic gastrointestinal blood loss or intermittent gastric outlet obstruction. Morphologically, leiomyomas are sessile or pedunculated lesions covered by normal mucosa. This may ulcerate, causing insidious blood loss and anaemia. Major haemorrhage is rare.

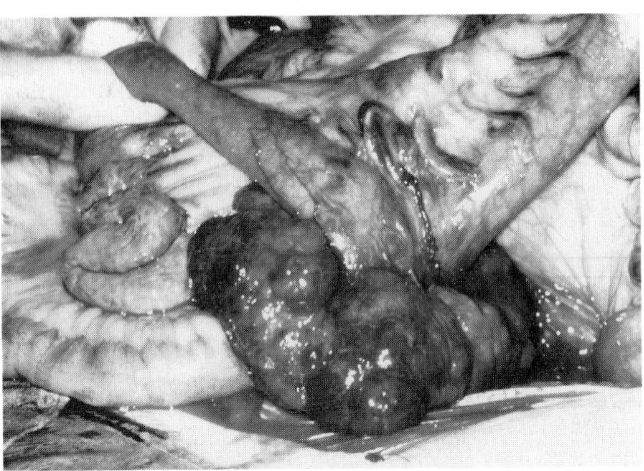

Fig. 11.7 Leiomyosarcoma of the jejunum

This operative specimen shows a large fleshy lesion on the outer surface of the upper jejunum. The patient was a 33-year-old woman who presented with iron deficiency anaemia refractory to oral iron. An abnormality was finally seen on a barium small bowel study after many fruitless investigations. This tumour was histologically well-differentiated and amenable to resection; after 5 years, there has been no recurrence

Leiomyosarcomas, the malignant counterpart of leiomyomas, are rare and present with similar symptoms or as an abdominal mass. Leiomyosarcomas spread locally and tend to metastasise early via the blood stream. Treatment involves resection of the primary lesion plus palliative chemotherapy if metastasis has occurred.

LYMPHOMAS

Pathology and clinical features

Primary lymphomas may arise in the stomach or small bowel. In the stomach, they constitute about 10% of malignancies. The lymphoid tissue of the small bowel may also become secondarily involved in non-Hodgkin's lymphomas.

In the stomach, lymphomas become extensive, either projecting into the lumen as a bulky ulcerating mass or diffusely infiltrating the stomach wall. They closely resemble gastric carcinoma in symptoms and endoscopic appearance, but it is particularly important to make the distinction because the prognosis of treated lymphoma is much better than adenocarcinoma. Biopsy is the only reliable means of diagnosis. In contrast to gastric carcinoma, lymphomas tend to occur in children and young adults.

In the small intestine, lymphomas also produce bulky lesions which may obstruct, ulcerate, bleed or even perforate. Coeliac disease is a strong predisposing factor to primary small bowel lymphoma.

Management

In both stomach and small intestine, investigation involves barium studies and endoscopic biopsy. But only laparotomy can usually distinguish primary lymphomas from secondary lesions. Primary lymphomas are often discrete and amenable to surgical excision. Subsequent radiotherapy or chemotherapy, or both, may be necessary. Treatment gives a five year survival rate of around 50%. Radiotherapy alone can succeed in treating some primary gastric lymphomas, emphasising the importance of a tissue diagnosis before surgery is embarked upon.

CARCINOID TUMOURS

Pathology

Carcinoid tumours probably arise from APUD cells of the gastrointestinal endocrine system. Thus, they can arise anywhere in the gastrointestinal tract or in tissues embryologically derived from it, including the pancreas and biliary system. More than half of carcinoid tumours are found in the appendix, and most of the remainder occur in the small intestine.

Clinical presentation

Appendiceal carcinoid tumours are usually discovered incidentally in appendicectomy specimens, and generally remain small and benign. In contrast, carcinoid tumours elsewhere in the bowel spread locally in the bowel and mesentery, later become disseminated to the liver and other sites. The bowel lesions usually present with symptoms of partial or complete obstruction.

Carcinoid tumours secrete a variety of catecholamines, including *serotonin* (5 hydroxytryptamine or 5HT). When there is a large mass of tumour, usually in the form of liver metastases, enough catecholamines are secreted to produce the *carcinoid syndrome*. This is characterised by an array of clinical phenomena including transient 'hot flushes', hypotension, asthma and diarrhoea. A metabolite of serotonin, *5 hydroxy-indoleacetic acid* (5 HIAA), can be measured in the urine as a diagnostic test.

Management of carcinoid tumours

Treatment involves resection of local bowel lesions only. Metastatic disease progresses very slowly and is not curable by radiotherapy or chemotherapy.

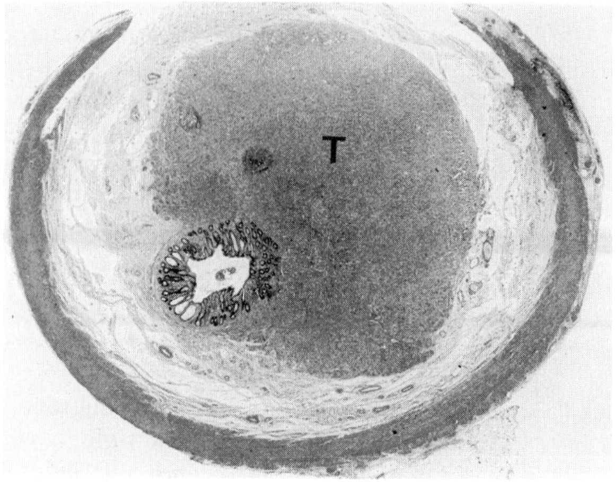

Fig. 11.8 Carcinoid tumour in the appendix — histopathology

Carcinoid tumour **T** found incidentally in the appendix of a 40-year-old man with acute right iliac fossa pain. The appendix was not inflamed but, as is standard practice, it was removed

Radiotherapy is, however, useful for pain caused by massive liver enlargement. The full-blown carcinoid syndrome is rare and may be mitigated by catecholamine blocking drugs.

OTHER TUMOURS OF THE SMALL INTESTINE

In addition to leiomyomas, other small bowel tumours include solitary benign adenomas, lipomas and angiomas. They are usually found incidentally at operation or autopsy, but sometimes present with intussusception or chronic haemorrhage.

Adenocarcinomas do occur in the small intestine (especially in the duodenum) but they are rare compared with their incidence in stomach and large bowel. Adenocarcinomas present with symptoms of obstruction of bowel or periampullary region, bleeding or metastases. Barium examination for chronic symptoms may demonstrate the lesion, but more commonly it is found and resected at laparotomy for acute obstruction, only being categorised later by histological examination. In many patients, spread has already occurred to regional lymph nodes or the liver by the time of presentation.

PEUTZ-JEHGER SYNDROME

Peutz-Jehger syndrome is a rare inherited autosomal dominant disorder in which multiple small benign polypoid lesions develop in the small intestine. These are accompanied by characteristic pigmentation of the lips, gums, hands and feet. The bowel lesions represent hamartomatous malformations of mucosa, submucosa and smooth muscle rather than true adenomas. They may cause chronic intestinal blood loss. Malignant transformation does not occur. This condition should not be confused with familial polyposis coli, which is characterised by multiple adenomatous colonic polyps, which almost invariably undergo malignant change (see Chapter 15).

12 TUMOURS OF THE PANCREAS AND HEPATOBILIARY SYSTEM

Introduction

Carcinoma of the pancreas usually means adenocarcinoma derived from cells of the exocrine pancreas. Much less commonly however, tumours arise from islet cells. These are generally benign and sometimes multiple. Most are insulinomas or glucagonomas, which become apparent by the effects of their excess hormone secretion.

Most pancreatic carcinomas arise in the head of the pancreas, which makes up the bulk of the gland. Intractable abdominal pain and marked weight loss are the most common presenting features, but obstructive jaundice caused by compression of the common bile duct is almost as common. In jaundiced patients, pain may develop at a later stage. Obstructive jaundice is also a common presentation of carcinomas of the biliary tree, ampulla of Vater and duodenum ('periampullary carcinomas'), but these are less common. Sclerosing cholangitis, a rare non-malignant condition, has a similar mode of presentation, and is thus included in this chapter. In contrast, the uncommon carcinoma of the gall bladder does not usually present with jaundice.

Primary liver tumours are rare in developed countries but relatively common in some underdeveloped countries. Secondary liver tumours are common everywhere.

CARCINOMA OF THE PANCREAS

Pathology

Histologically, carcinoma of the pancreas is usually adenocarcinoma arising from cells lining the duct system. About 70% of tumours arise in the head of the gland (the largest part) and the remaining 30% in the body or tail. Histologically, the tumours tend to form a well-differentiated ductular pattern but the sheets of cells may have a more anaplastic appearance. Despite the organised histological pattern, carcinoma of the pancreas is a highly malignant tumour. It metastasises early to local lymph nodes (including nodes in the porta hepatis) and to the liver via the portal vein. By the time pancreatic carcinoma presents, the tumour has already disseminated and the prognosis is poor. Despite all treatment, the five-year survival rate is only 3%.

Carcinoma of the pancreas is a disease of the elderly and is extremely rare under the age of 50 years. Males and females are equally affected. After cancer of the large bowel and stomach, pancreatic carcinoma ranks third in incidence among gastrointestinal carcinomas. It is responsible for about 6500 deaths annually in the UK. Nevertheless, it is a relatively uncommon cancer. Its incidence is only half that of gastric carcinoma, and it represents only about 3% of all malignancies. The aetiology of pancreatic cancer is unknown, although some studies have incriminated excess coffee or alcohol intake. The incidence of pancreatic cancer is increasing steadily in developed countries; thus, factors in the modern environment are probably responsible.

Clinical features

Because the pancreas is so inaccessible to palpation, pancreatic carcinoma rarely presents as a mass. The main presenting symptoms are abdominal pain and obstructive jaundice, and systemic symptoms like weight loss and malaise. At the time of presentation, it is not uncommon to find liver enlargement and abdominal distension due to ascites. Proportions of patients with different clinical features at the time of diagnosis are shown in Figure 12.1.

Fig. 12.1 Presenting features of pancreatic carcinoma

Common presenting features

Substantial weight loss (about 80%)
Abdominal pain (about 60%)
Obstructive jaundice, often without pain (about 50%)
Malignant ascites with hard 'knobbly' liver (about 30%)

Less common presenting features

Gastric outlet obstruction (due to external compression)
Thrombophlebitis migrans
Acute pancreatitis
Gastrointestinal haemorrhage (by erosion of the duodenum)
Pancreatic steatorrhoea (due to pancreatic duct obstruction)
Diabetes mellitus

The pain of pancreatic carcinoma is severe and continuous and typically described as 'deep' and 'gnawing'. It tends to be relieved by leaning forwards in a sitting position. There are often ill-defined dyspeptic symptoms like anorexia, nausea or sporadic vomiting. Weight loss may be dramatic even without liver metastases, and is much more than can be explained by anorexia alone.

Painless jaundice develops insidiously over several weeks, during which time the patient gradually assumes a deep greenish-yellow hue. Suprisingly, pruritis and other distressing symptoms are uncommon. Obstructive jaundice is usually caused by compression of the common bile duct where it lies in contact with the pancreas. Thus, the proximal duct system becomes dilated, including the gall bladder which often becomes palpable (*Courvoisier's law*, see Chapter 6). Bile duct obstruction may also be caused by enlarged lymph nodes in the porta hepatis. Liver metastases alone rarely cause jaundice until a late stage and even then, jaundice is usually mild. Note that carcinoma of the pancreas and other obstructing tumours of the biliary tree typically produce an unremitting and progressively deepening jaundice, whereas the jaundice of gall stone disease tends to fluctuate, and there is usually a typical history of gall bladder pain.

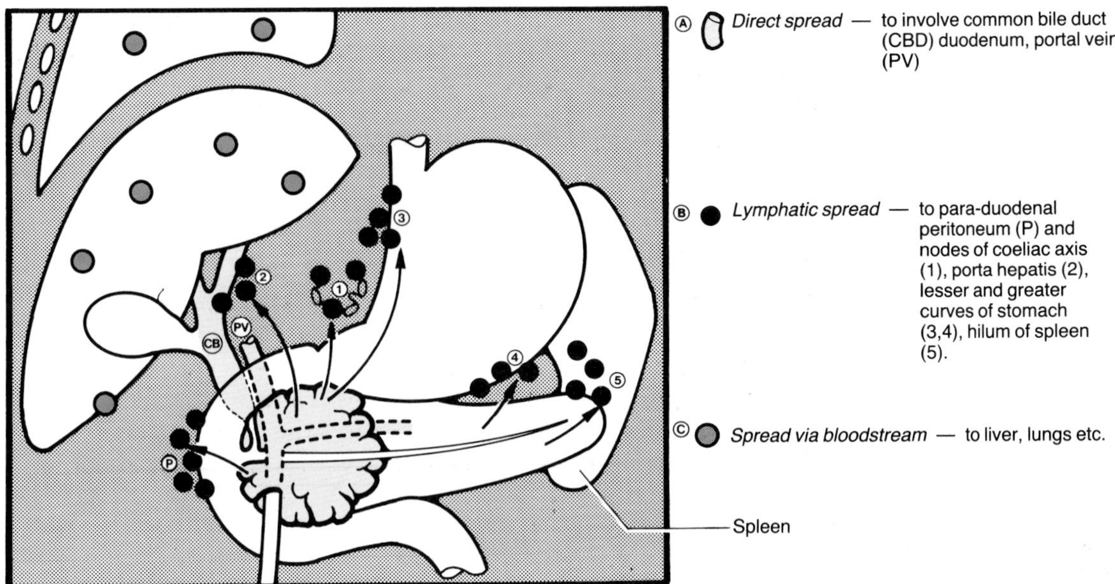

Fig. 12.2 Spread of carcinoma of the pancreas

Approach to investigation

The patient presenting with obstructive jaundice should be investigated as described in Chapter 6. Ultrasound to look for dilated ducts and stones is followed by ERCP or transhepatic percutaneous cholangiography. When pancreatic carcinoma is suspected in the non-jaundiced patient, CT scanning is the most reliable (though not infallible) method of diagnosis and may also demonstrate metastatic deposits in the porta hepatis or liver parenchyma. CT scan will also show the extent of local invasion into the retroperitoneal area and portal vein, providing some indication of whether the lesion might be resectable. If it is not apparent whether a CT- demonstrated pancreatic lesion is benign or malignant, fine-needle aspiration may be performed percutaneously using ultrasound or CT control, and the sample sent for cytological examination.

Management of pancreatic carcinoma

Pancreatic carcinoma is essentially incurable since metastasis occurs at such an early stage. Not only is curative resection impossible, but the tumour is virtually unresponsive to radiotherapy and chemotherapy. Thus, any treatment must be regarded as palliative.

If there is obvious widespread disease, the patient should be allowed to die without surgical interference. Adequate analgesia is essential and if pain is severe, may require percutaneous coeliac ganglion blockade. If obstructive jaundice is the dominant feature, this can be relieved with a bypass operation or by the recent technique of inserting a tubular stent into the compressed bile duct. An endoscopic approach is preferable for this, but a percutaneous transhepatic route may be necessary; various techniques are illustrated in Figure 12.4.

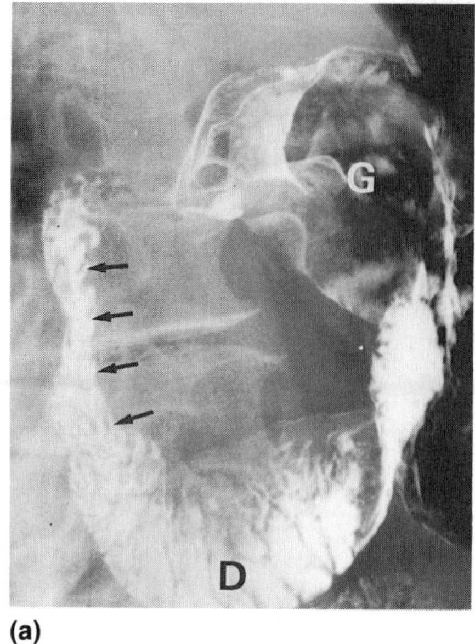

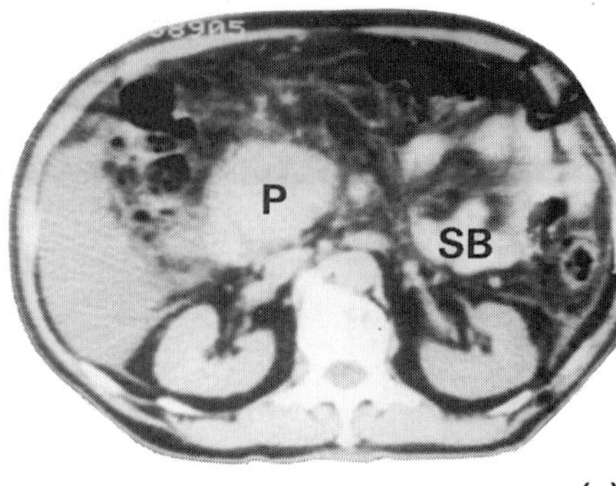

(a) (c)

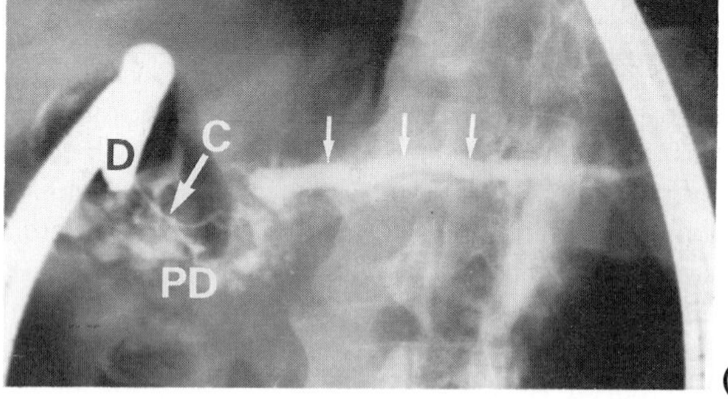

(b)

Fig. 12.3 Carcinoma of the head of the pancreas

(a) This 77-year-old man presented with four weeks of painless obstructive jaundice. This barium meal shows the gastric antrum **G** and duodenum. The duodenal loop **D** is grossly expanded by a large carcinoma of the head of the pancreas. The medial wall of the second part of the duodenum (arrowed) is compressed and distorted by the tumour.
(b) Endoscopic retrograde pancreatogram in a jaundiced patient with carcinoma of the head of the pancreas. The tip of the duodenoscope **D** lies opposite the ampulla of Vater, into which a catheter **C** is passed. The distal pancreatic duct is dilated (arrowed) and the proximal duct **PD** is compressed and distorted by the tumour.
(c) CT scan showing a homogeneous mass lesion in the head of the pancreas **P**. The small bowel **SB** is outlined by dilute contrast medium given orally at the start of the examination. The appearance of the mass is typical of carcinoma. Such lesions are amenable to biopsy using CT guidance to confirm the diagnosis

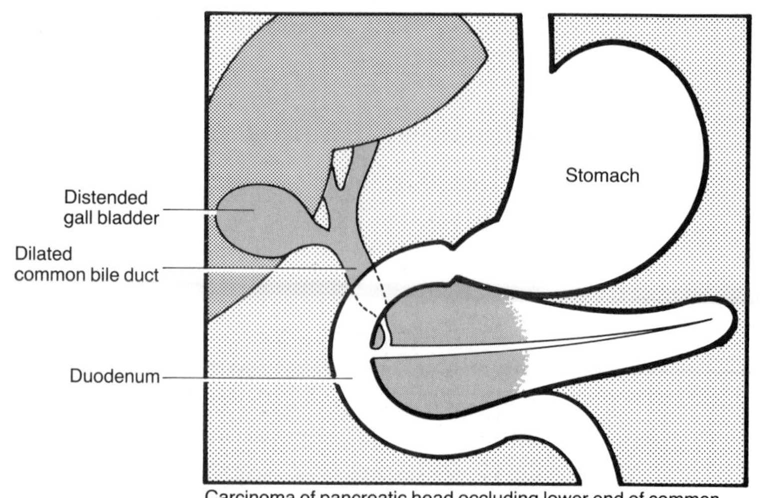

(a)

Carcinoma of pancreatic head occluding lower end of common bile duct and actually, or more often potentially, obstructing the duodenum, i.e. gastric outlet

Fig. 12.4 Palliative procedures for obstructive jaundice (**(b)–(e)** opposite)

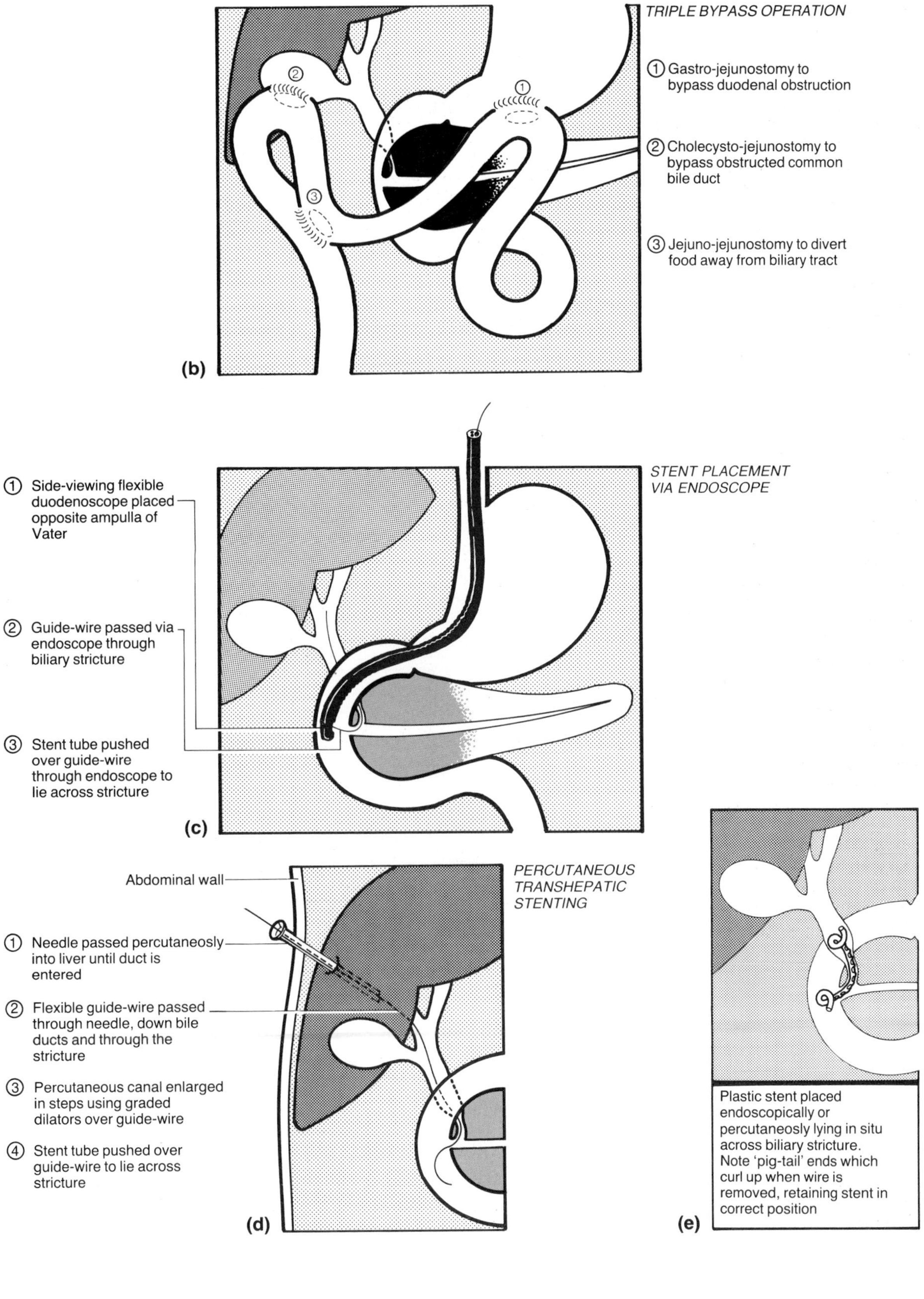

TRIPLE BYPASS OPERATION

① Gastro-jejunostomy to bypass duodenal obstruction

② Cholecysto-jejunostomy to bypass obstructed common bile duct

③ Jejuno-jejunostomy to divert food away from biliary tract

(b)

STENT PLACEMENT VIA ENDOSCOPE

① Side-viewing flexible duodenoscope placed opposite ampulla of Vater

② Guide-wire passed via endoscope through biliary stricture

③ Stent tube pushed over guide-wire through endoscope to lie across stricture

(c)

PERCUTANEOUS TRANSHEPATIC STENTING

Abdominal wall

① Needle passed percutaneosly into liver until duct is entered

② Flexible guide-wire passed through needle, down bile ducts and through the stricture

③ Percutaneous canal enlarged in steps using graded dilators over guide-wire

④ Stent tube pushed over guide-wire to lie across stricture

(d)

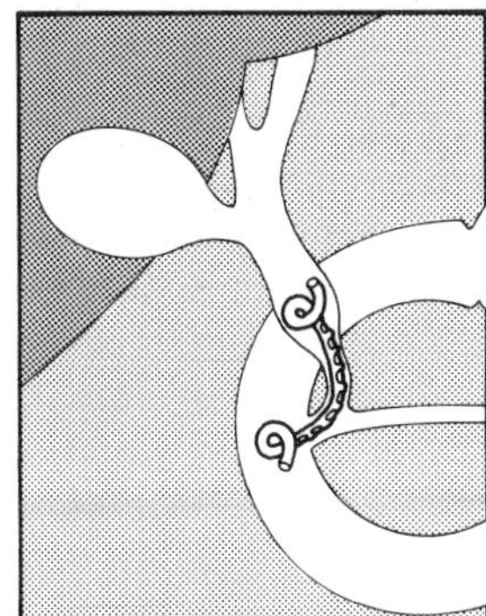

Plastic stent placed endoscopically or percutaneosly lying in situ across biliary stricture. Note 'pig-tail' ends which curl up when wire is removed, retaining stent in correct position

(e)

Whipple's operation (pancreatico-duodenectomy) is rarely indicated for pancreatic carcinoma since it offers virtually no hope of cure or prolonged survival. It is a major undertaking with high operative morbidity and mortality, and is mainly indicated for periampullary lesions (see Figure 12.6).

As mentioned above, intractable pain, which is common in pancreatic carcinoma, can often be dramatically relieved by coeliac ganglion blockade.

BILIARY AND PERI-AMPULLARY TUMOURS

Adenocarcinomas originating from the epithelium lining the biliary duct system are known as *cholangiocarcinomas*. They may develop anywhere in the intra-hepatic or extrahepatic duct system.

Intrahepatic cholangiocarcinomas tend to invade the liver parenchyma, presenting in a similar manner to primary hepatocellular carcinomas. Since most of the biliary system remains patent in these cases, jaundice is rare.

In contrast, extrahepatic cholangiocarcinomas tend to obstruct bile drainage. They present with painless progressive jaundice in the same way as carcinoma of the pancreatic head. Unlike pancreatic cancer, cholangiocarcinomas are slow growing and metastasise late so that complete resection is often possible. Cholangiocarcinomas have a dense fibrous stroma and, rather than producing a focal proliferative lesion, tend to grow along the duct system. The resulting smooth elongated stricture can be demonstrated by ERCP or transhepatic cholangiography.

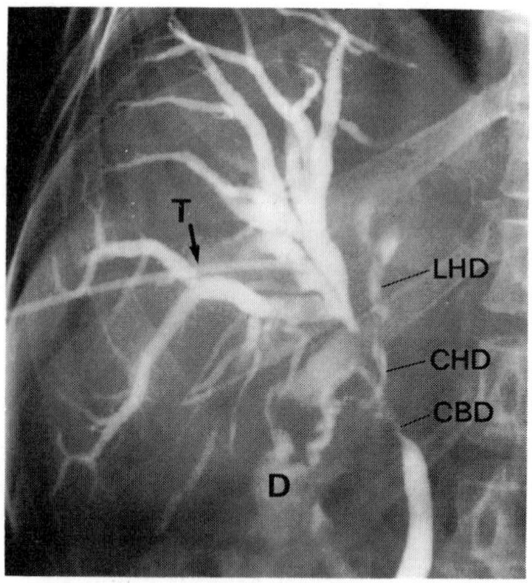

Fig. 12.5 Cholangio-carcinoma

Percutaneous transhepatic cholangiogram in a 66-year-old man with painless progressive jaundice from an inoperable cholangio-carcinoma; the X-ray shows a long stricture of the common bile duct **CBD**, common hepatic duct **CHD** and left hepatic duct **LHD**. Some contrast has flowed through into the duodenum. The cystic duct is obliterated, preventing filling of the gall bladder. A percutaneous drainage tube **T** has been inserted into the right hepatic duct system prior to an attempt to place a stent across the stricture by the same route

Adenocarcinoma sometimes arises at the ampulla of Vater, forming a polypoid lesion which projects into the duodenum and obstructs biliary drainage. Obstructive jaundice is thus a common presentation of periampullary tumours. These tumours are friable and tend to bleed insidiously, giving a positive result on faecal occult blood testing. Diagnosis is made at ERCP, the tumour being visible and accessible to biopsy. Very rarely, adenocarcinoma arises in the duodenal mucosa, causing obstructive jaundice if in the vicinity of the ampulla. Again, the lesion is readily diagnosed at ERCP.

Management of extrahepatic cholangiocarcinoma, ampullary and duodenal carcinoma

Extrahepatic and periampullary lesions are often amenable to curative resection by Whipple's operation. This extensive procedure involves resection of most of the extrahepatic biliary system as well as the whole duodenum, distal stomach and head of the pancreas ('pancreatico-duodenectomy'), as illustrated in Figure 12.6. Operative morbidity and mortality is high due to the difficulty of preventing leakage of exocrine secretions from the pancreatic remnant, the overall extent of the operation, and the complications of jaundice.

Fig. 12.6 Whipple's operation

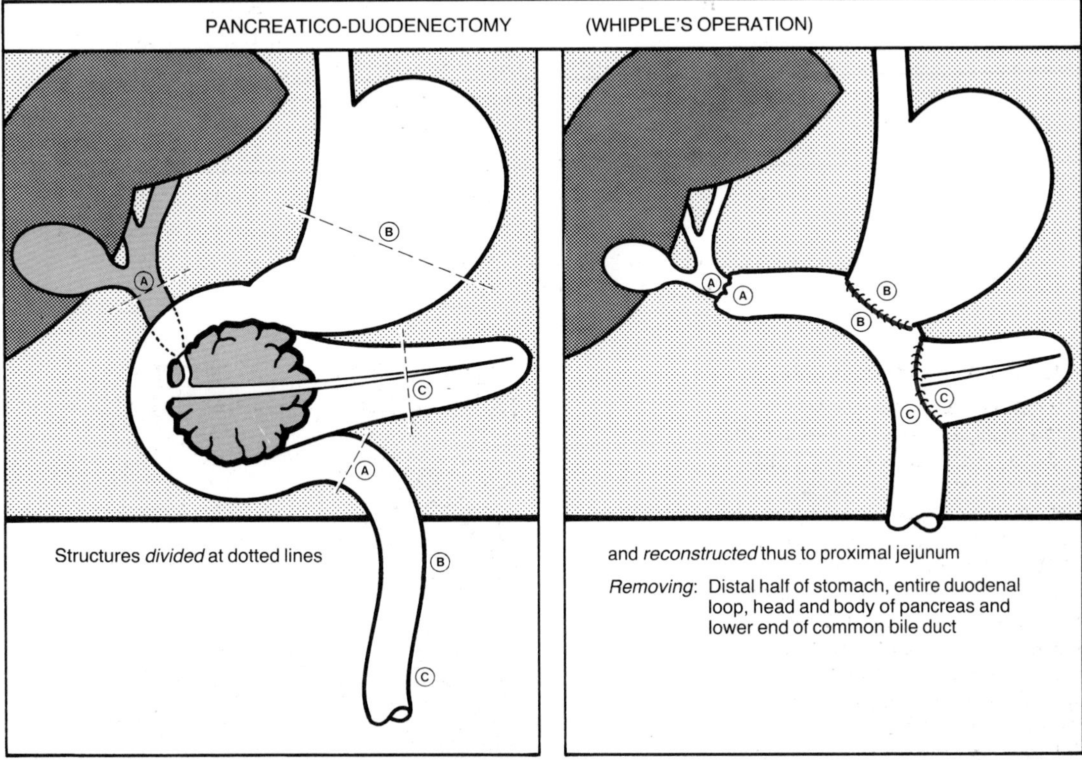

CARCINOMA OF THE GALL BLADDER

Carcinoma of the gall bladder is a disease of old age, and nearly always arises in association with pre-existing stone disease. Chronic inflammation may be the carcinogenic factor. These tumours are often diagnosed incidentally at cholecystectomy being performed for pain attributed to gall stone disease. The tumour tends to invade the liver bed at an early stage making resection impracticable and the prognosis poor. At a late stage, gall bladder carcinomas may invade the biliary system causing obstructive jaundice.

SCLEROSING CHOLANGITIS

Sclerosing cholangitis is a rare condition, probably of autoimmune origin, which results in progressive fibrosis of the biliary system. The luminal narrowing causes insidious and progressive obstructive jaundice and secondary cirrhosis.

The condition may arise sporadically but often occurs in association with long standing ulcerative colitis. Bile duct sclerosis is usually diffuse with a characteristic appearance on ERCP (see Figure 12.7), but occasionally the condition is localised to the extra hepatic biliary system. Here it gives a radiological appearance indistinguishable from cholangiocarcinoma.

In the case of localised obstruction, an indwelling plastic stent may be passed through the stricture, either via the transhepatic percutaneous route or at laparotomy. More extensive intubation procedures have been devised for diffuse disease but life expectancy is only about five to ten years.

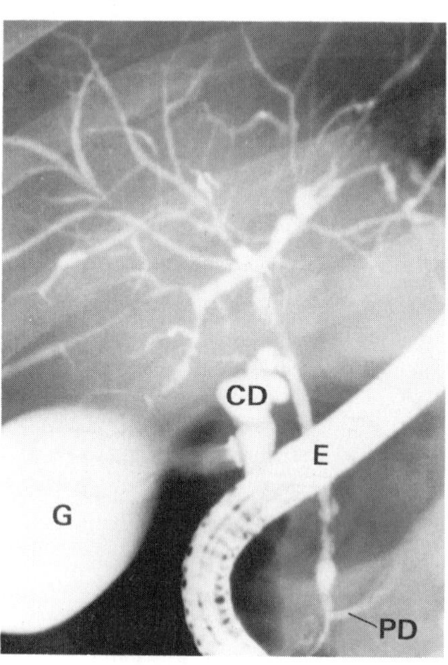

Fig. 12.7 Sclerosing cholangitis

ERCP in a 52-year-old man with long-standing ulcerative colitis who developed painless jaundice. There is widespread irregular narrowing of both the intrahepatic and the extrahepatic bile ducts which is typical of *sclerosing cholangitis*. Note the endoscope **E**, the normal gall bladder **G** and cystic duct **CD** filling with contrast. The proximal part of the pancreatic duct **PD** also contains contrast

ENDOCRINE TUMOURS OF THE PANCREAS

The APUD cells of the islets of Langerhans may give rise to a variety of tumours which cause excess hormone secretion which is responsible for their presenting features. The majority of these tumours are benign.

The most common endocrine tumours of the pancreas are *insulinomas*, derived from beta cells, which cause attacks of hypoglycaemia, particularly when fasting and exercising. The attacks are relieved by oral or intravenous glucose. Ninety per cent of insulinomas are benign and amenable to curative resection. Diagnosis is usually made after metabolic investigation for bizarre 'funny turns'. Once hyperinsulinism has been confirmed, CT scanning or selective pancreatic arteriography, or both, are used to identify the site of the lesion. Alpha cells may give rise to *glucagonomas* which are very rare and present with hyperglycaemia.

The islets of Langerhans (and sometimes APUD cells elsewhere in the gut) also give rise to gastrin-secreting tumours which cause severe and intractable peptic ulceration and diarrhoea. The condition is known as *Zollinger–Ellison syndrome*. Diagnosis is made by demonstrating persistently high serum gastrin levels, and the tumour is localised by CT scanning or selective pancreatic

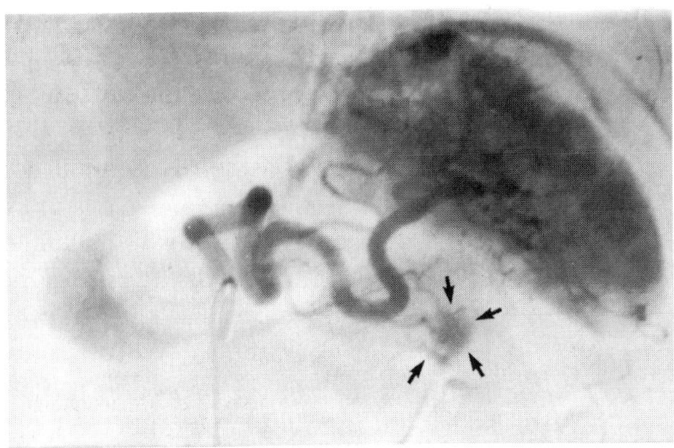

Fig. 12.8 Insulinoma as seen on a selective arteriogram

This 31-year-old woman suffered from bouts of faintness which proved to be caused by intermittent hypoglycaemia. Selective splenic arteriography demonstrated an abnormal mass of blood vessels about 1.5-cm in diameter (arrowed) in the tail of the pancreas and representing an insulinoma. The tail of the pancreas was excised and the patient's symptoms disappeared

angiography. Many of the lesions are too small to be demonstrated by either method and their location can only be established at laparotomy by mobilisation and palpation of the pancreas. Sixty per cent of gastrinomas are classified as malignant but they grow slowly and metastasise late. Thus, excision is often curative. However, some surgeons prefer the operation of total gastrectomy for Zollinger–Ellison syndrome. In cases where the primary tumour cannot be found, this may be the only treatment that can be offered.

Pancreatic APUD cell tumours sometimes form part of a *multiple endocrine neoplasia syndrome* (MEN) of which two types are recognised:
MEN I — islet cell tumours, pituitary adenomas and parathyroid hyperplasia
MEN II — medullary carcinoma of the thyroid, phaechromocytoma and parathyroid adenoma

PRIMARY TUMOURS OF THE LIVER

Primary tumours of the liver are uncommon, the majority being hepatocellular carcinomas derived from hepatocytes. A small minority of primary liver tumours are haemangiomas derived from the vascular system; these benign neoplasms are a separate pathological entity from the common congenital vascular hamartomas of the liver.

Hepatocellular carcinoma

Hepatocellular carcinomas (also known as hepatomas) are malignant, slow-growing tumours which often arise multicentrically throughout the liver. It is of great interest that an aetiological factor can be identified in nearly all cases; these include pre-existing alcoholic cirrhosis, haemochromatosis, chronic active hepatitis and various environmental agents. In 80% of cases, there is some form of pre-existing cirrhosis. Alcoholic cirrhosis is the most common aetiological factor in developed countries; indeed, hepatoma occurs in about 25% of patients with cirrhosis of more than five years standing. The risk in patients with haemochromatosis and chronic active hepatitis is even higher.

Although uncommon in developed countries, hepatocellular carcinoma is one of the most common tumours in certain parts of Africa. A variety of environmental carcinogens have been implicated; these include aflatoxin, a toxin produced by a species of Aspergillus which grows on stored grains and peanuts.

Various parasitic infestations, e.g. shistosomiasis, echinococcus (tape worm) and clonorchis sinensis (liver fluke) also predispose to hepatocellular carcinoma. In developed countries, the peak incidence of hepatocellular carcinoma is between the ages of 40 and 60, but in those underdeveloped countries where the disease is common, the majority of cases occur between 20 and 40 years of age.

The presenting features of hepatocellular carcinoma are anorexia, weight loss, abdominal pain and distension. These are often in association with stigmata of underlying cirrhosis. On examination, a liver mass is usually palpable. Ultrasound (or preferably CT scanning) can be used to establish the size and position of the liver mass and to guide needle biopsy.

By the time it is diagnosed, hepatocellular carcinoma is usually widespread within the liver and the only surgical option would be liver transplantation. Unfortunately, recurrence has proved inevitable after transplantation and the procedure has largely been abandoned for this condition. Isolated lesions are occasionally amenable to segmental resection but again recurrence is likely. Perhaps recurrence is due to the multicentric origin of the tumour, although this does not explain recurrence after transplantation. Embolisation and local administration of cytotoxic drugs via intra-arterial cannulae are sometimes attempted by way of palliation but complication rates are high and the efficacy unproven.

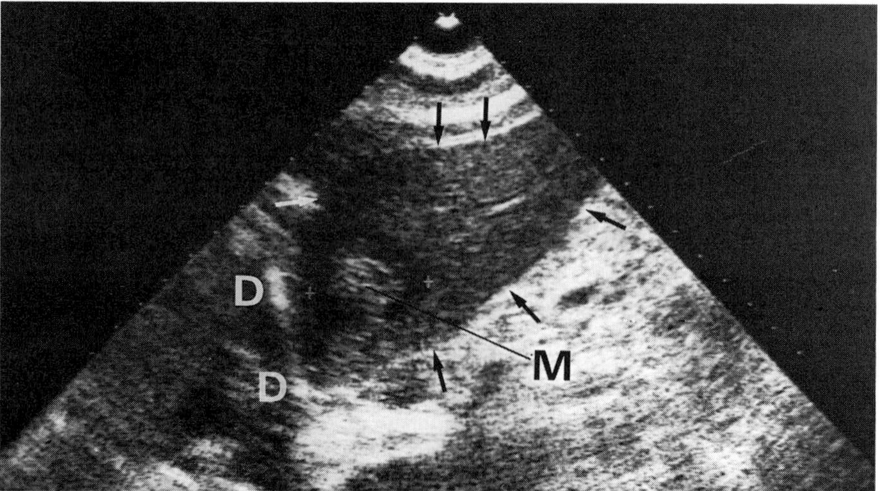

Fig. 12.9 Isolated liver metastasis from carcinoma of colon

Longitudinal ultrasound scan of the left lobe of the liver in a 58-year-old man whose colonic carcinoma appeared to have been completely resected 18 months previously. The scan shows an isolated metastasis **M** 2.6 cm in diameter in the left lobe of the liver. Note that the liver (outline arrowed) is relatively echo-poor whereas the nearby aorta and diaphragm **D** are strongly echogenic. The metastasis is echo-poor but with an echogenic centre. An isolated hepatic metastasis like this can sometimes be resected with some hope of cure

SECONDARY LIVER TUMOURS

Secondary tumours in the liver are extremely common. They arise from a wide variety of primary sources, especially the stomach, pancreas, large bowel, breast and bronchus. Liver metastases are usually asymptomatic but as the liver parenchyma is progressively destroyed, the patient begins to feel unwell with associated anorexia and weight loss. Jaundice is unusual and tends to appear only at a terminal stage of the illness. Jaundice results from a combination of compressive obstruction of the intrahepatic biliary system and gross loss of parenchyma so that bile pigments cannot be excreted. Consequently, the biochemical picture tends to be that of a mixed hepatitic and obstructive pattern.

As a rule, the presence of liver secondaries is indicative of incurable disease. Isolated metastases, however, especially of colonic or renal origin, may be amenable to excision by segmental resection. If liver metastases are responsible for pain, systemic chemotherapy may retard their growth and suppress symptoms. Sometimes large secondaries cause intractable pain which can be controlled by selective angiographic embolisation of the supply vessels.

13 PANCREATITIS

Introduction

Pancreatitis is an inflammatory disorder of the pancreas that is characterised by abdominal pain. Most cases present in an acute form known as *acute pancreatitis*. Attacks range in severity from relatively mild to life threatening. Some patients suffer recurrent acute attacks, and a small proportion appear to suffer a persistent form known as *chronic pancreatitis*.

ACUTE PANCREATITIS

Pathophysiology

Acute pancreatitis is characterised by the sudden onset of diffuse inflammation of the pancreas associated with activation of pancreatic enzymes within the gland. It probably results from some form of obstruction to pancreatic duct flow.

In its most severe form, acute pancreatitis causes haemorrhagic necrosis of the gland and release of lytic enzymes into the peritoneal cavity. A major feature of the resulting chemical peritonitis is lipase attack upon intraperitoneal and retroperitoneal fat. Systemic absorption of enzymes and toxic products through the peritoneum produces a profound toxaemia. This is responsible for the high mortality, in excess of 75%, in cases of *necrotising haemorrhagic pancreatitis*. At autopsy, the peritoneal cavity is filled with a foul, blood-stained inflammatory exudate containing fine lipid droplets. The peritoneal surface is grossly inflamed and semi-digested and all that is left of the pancreas is a necrotic mass. Severe pancreatic damage is accompanied by disruption of islet cell insulin secretion, leading to a diabetic state. In patients who survive severe attacks, diabetes often persists; there may also be chronic pancreatic malabsorption.

Fortunately, in most cases the extent and severity of inflammation is considerably less. The gland becomes swollen and oedematous but not actually necrotic, and peritoneal inflammation is less marked. If laparotomy is inadvertently performed, clear peritoneal fluid can be seen with whitish patches on the great omentum and mesentery, representing areas of fat necrosis. In these patients, the systemic effects are much less profound.

Calcium is sequestered in areas of fat necrosis and tends to cause a fall in the serum calcium level. The presence of damaged or necrotic tissue predisposes to secondary infection by gut bacteria. Infection may lead to suppurative necrosis or frank abscess formation in the pancreas or retroperitoneal area. An accumulation of pancreatic enzymes, inflammatory fluid and necrotic debris in the lesser sac may result in formation of a *pancreatic pseudocyst*.

Epidemiology and aetiology of acute pancreatitis

Acute pancreatitis is relatively uncommon, seen about once in 100 acute general surgical admissions. It now has approximately the same frequency as perforated peptic ulcer. Less than 10% of cases fall into the category of necrotising haemorrhagic pancreatitis.

The main aetiological factors for acute pancreatitis are pre-existing gallstone disease and chronic excess alcohol intake. The former is more common in women and the latter more common in men. Overall, similar numbers of men and women are affected and the majority are over 45 years of age. When younger patients are affected, alcohol is the usual culprit.

Gallstone disease probably causes pancreatitis by disrupting the flow of bile and pancreatic juice through their common pathway into the duodenum. Small stones may pass through the ampulla of Vater causing transient obstruction or larger stones may impact at the lower end of the common bile duct. Alcohol is known to strongly stimulate pancreatic secretion, but it may also obstruct flow by causing ductal oedema and increased tone in the sphincter of Oddi. Bile reflux may then activate pancreatic proteases and lipases within the pancreatic duct system, causing pancreatic damage and acute inflammation.

Acute pancreatitis sometimes develops after a huge meal, perhaps due to massive secretion of pancreatic juice and relative obstruction of the duct. Pancreatitis is more common in hyperparathyroidism and hypercalcaemia, where small pancreatic duct calculi may be the predisposing factor. Hyperlipidaemias also predispose to pancreatitis although the mechanism is obscure. Children rarely suffer from pancreatitis, but a viral illness or hyperlipidaemia is often the causative factor when they do.

Clinical features of acute pancreatitis

Acute pancreatitis presents as an acute abdomen. Pain begins suddenly and is severe and continuous from the outset. Initially it is poorly localised in the upper abdomen and is often described by the patient as 'going through to the back'. As the peritoneal cavity becomes involved over the next few hours, the pain spreads throughout the abdomen, and may be referred to the shoulder tips if the diaphragmatic peritoneum becomes inflamed. Vomiting is an early feature. In the early stages, the patient is restless, constantly changing posture in the search for a comfortable position. Pain is most often relieved by leaning forward in the so-called 'pancreatic position'. With the onset of peritonitis, movement becomes increasingly painful and the patient tends to lie still. The clinical signs depend on the severity of the inflammatory process and the stage to which it has progressed.

a. Severe acute pancreatitis

In a severe attack the patient looks apathetic, grey and shocked and there are typical abdominal signs of generalised peritonitis, i.e. extreme tenderness, guarding and rigidity. In this case, the differential diagnosis includes other major abdominal catastrophes, especially faecal peritonitis from perforated large bowel, and concealed haemorrhage from a leaking aortic aneurysm. Massive bowel infarction due to arterial occlusion may present in this way, but the abdominal signs are often less marked. An important and dangerous complication of severe acute pancreatitis is adult respiratory distress syndrome.

b. Moderate acute pancreatitis

Much more commonly, the attack is less severe, with only moderate systemic features like tachycardia. The abdomen is usually distended and diffusely tender with little guarding. Bowel sounds are absent as a result of inflammatory ileus. Rectal examination is usually normal. The patient may be mildly jaundiced due to periampullary oedema. Differential diagnosis includes acute cholecystitis, biliary colic, perforation of a peptic ulcer or even a small diverticular perforation without faecal spillage.

c. Mild acute pancreatitis

In mild attacks, the patient looks generally well with minimal systemic features and unimpressive abdominal tenderness; nevertheless, there is often considerable pain. The differential diagnosis in this situation includes biliary colic, acute cholecystitis, an acute exacerbation of a peptic ulcer or even a small perforation of a peptic ulcer. Lower lobe pneumonia or an inferior myocardial infarct may sometimes present in this way.

Fig. 13.1 Summary — clinical features of acute pancreatitis

Severe attack
Severe acute abdominal pain
Severe toxaemia and shock
Generalised peritonitis (diffuse abdominal tenderness, guarding, rigidity, absent bowel sounds)
'Shock lung' (ARDS)

Moderate attack
Severe acute abdominal pain
Tachycardia
Abdominal distension, some abdominal tenderness and guarding, absent bowel sounds

Mild attack
Acute abdominal pain
Minimal or rapidly resolving abdominal signs
Minimal systemic illness

Investigation of suspected pancreatitis

Acute pancreatitis must be excluded in any adult presenting with acute abdominal pain, and in any child with peritonitis not readily attributable to appendicitis.

Amylase is one of the enzymes absorbed into the circulation in pancreatitis; *serum amylase* measurement is simple to perform in the laboratory and provides a reliable diagnostic test. A serum amylase level above 1200 i.u./ml is usually regarded as diagnostic of acute pancreatitis. However, any upper abdominal inflammatory condition which impinges on the pancreas (e.g. cholecystitis, perforated peptic ulcer or strangulated bowel) causes a moderate rise in serum amylase, but this rarely reaches 1000 i.u./ml.

Serum amylase levels rise rapidly at the outset of an attack of pancreatitis and levels as high as 10 000 i.u./ml or more may be recorded on admission to hospital. The peak amylase level is no indicator of severity of the pancreatitis or the likelihood of subsequent complications.

Plain X-rays of chest (erect) and abdomen (supine) will usually have been performed during the initial investigation. Abdominal X-ray may show a 'ground-glass' appearance if peritoneal exudate is present. Bowel gas tends to be absent except perhaps for a 'sentinel loop' of dilated adynamic small bowel in the centre of the abdomen. These signs are often absent in pancreatitis and even if present, are not pathognomonic.

Management of acute pancreatitis

Mild attacks

Mild attacks require no further emergency investigation and are managed by conservative measures designed to 'rest' the pancreas and bowel. Oral intake is prohibited and intravenous fluids are given. Recovery from mild attacks is usually rapid. Subsequent management attempts to treat predisposing factors. Gall stones should be sought by ultrasound or later, by cholecystography, and removed endoscopically or surgically; alcohol abuse must be discouraged.

Moderate attacks

Even when pancreatitis is clinically severe, supportive measures are still the mainstay of treatment. In addition to intravenous fluids, a nasogastric tube is passed and the stomach aspirated. This keeps the upper gastrointestinal tract empty of gas and fluid, minimising stimulation of pancreatic secretory activity. It also prevents distension of the adynamic bowel by swallowed air. Antibiotics (e.g. a cephalosporin) are given parenterally as prophylaxis against the development of a pancreatic abscess. Serum amylase is measured daily to chart the progress of the inflammation — as the inflammation begins to resolve, the serum amylase level falls accordingly. If the level remains elevated beyond several days, complications such as pancreatic abscess and pseudocyst may be responsible.

Severe attacks

Patients with severe pancreatitis may die because of profound systemic toxaemia complicated by adult respiratory distress syndrome (ARDS), fluid and electrolyte disturbances and hypocalcaemia. Any patient who is recognised to have severe pancreatitis or anyone with acute pancreatitis, however mild, who shows signs of serious deterioration should be admitted to an intensive care unit without delay, for close monitoring and treatment. Figure 13.2 lists recommended investigations to guide management.

Deteriorating arterial pO_2 heralds ARDS. This is an indication for urgent ventilatory support before the condition becomes established. Fluid balance of the shocked patient is complicated by massive loss of protein-rich fluid into the peritoneal cavity. This needs to be replaced by large amounts of colloid solutions, carefully monitored by measurement of central venous pressure and hourly urine output. Peritoneal lavage is sometimes employed in desperation in an attempt to reduce systemic absorption of enzymes and other toxins, however, the efficacy of this procedure is doubtful.

Fig. 13.2 Recommended daily investigations in severe acute pancreatitis

Haemoglobin estimation and white cell count
Arterial blood gas estimations
Blood sugar
Serum electrolytes and urea
Serum amylase
'Liver function tests' (i.e. bilirubin, alkaline phosphatase, lactate dehydrogenase (LDH), transaminases, serum proteins)
Serum calcium and phosphate

Early indicators of prognosis in acute pancreatitis

The initial clinical picture cannot be relied upon to predict which patients are likely to deteriorate. Only a small proportion of patients eventually suffer necrotising haemorrhagic pancreatitis, but a patient who appears at first to have mild pancreatitis can rapidly deteriorate to death's door without warning. Results of the tests recommended in Figure 13.2, however, are known to provide useful prognostic information. When considered together, the tests enable early and more accurate identification of severe cases. Figure 13.3 lists the main harbingers of serious trouble. If three or more of these factors are present, the patient is assumed to have 'severe pancreatitis' and should be admitted to intensive care immediately.

Fig. 13.3 Criteria for early identification of severe pancreatitis (after RANSOME)

'Severe pancreatitis' is defined by the presence of three or more features within 48 hrs of admission

Age over 55 years
Blood glucose greater than 10 mmol/l (patient not diabetic)
Leucocyte count greater than 15 000 × 10^9/l
LDH greater than 600 i.u./l
Transaminases >100 u/l
Hypocalcaemia (corrected serum Ca < 2.0 mmol/l)
Blood urea >16 mmol/l despite adequate i.u. therapy
Rising haematocrit
Low arterial pO_2 (<8kPa or 60 mmHg)
Metabolic acidosis
Serum albumin <32 g/l

Surgery in acute pancreatitis

As a general rule, surgery plays no part in the early management of acute pancreatitis. Later, biliary tract surgery may be appropriate to remove causative gall stones. Occasionally, acute surgery is appropriate if a stone is impacted at the lower end of the common duct, preventing resolution of an attack of acute pancreatitis. Sometimes, in a last ditch attempt in a desperately ill patient, laparotomy is carried out to perform *peritoneal toilet* and to drain any retroperitoneal collections of pus. At the same time the necrotic pancreas is readily removed. By now it has formed a discrete red-grey mass lying loose within the pancreatic bed and acting as a foreign body.

Fig. 13.4 Summary — principles of management of acute pancreatitis

(Treatments added according to severity of attack)

'Nil by mouth' and intravenous fluids
Nasogastric aspiration
Broad spectrum intravenous antibiotics
Intensive care
— fluid and electrolyte management
— treatment of hypocalcaemia
— ventilatory support
— peritoneal lavage
Laparotomy and peritoneal toilet

Complications of acute pancreatitis

The main complications of acute pancreatitis are pancreatic pseudocyst and abscess formation. Diabetes mellitus, and malabsorption due to loss of pancreatic secretions sometimes occur after severe attacks, but it is suprising how uncommon these are considering the extent of pancreatic damage that occurs.

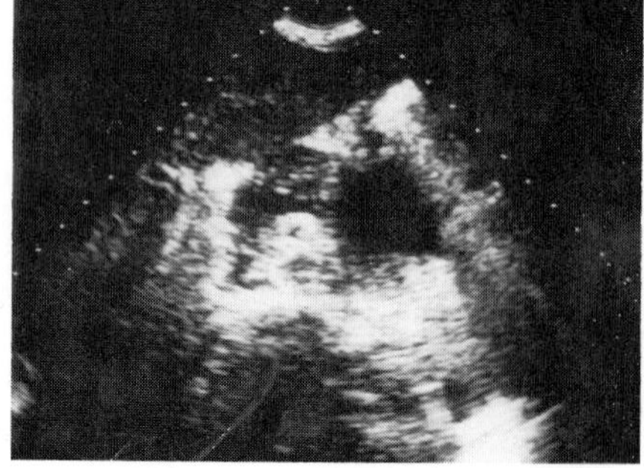

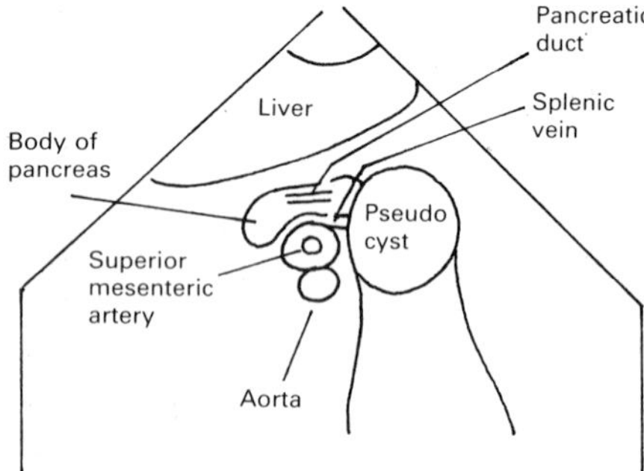

Fig. 13.5 Pancreatic pseudocyst

This 62-year-old man was admitted to hospital with an acute abdomen three weeks before this scan. He was found to have acute pancreatitis due to gallstones. The symptoms and signs of pancreatitis smouldered on and the serum amylase failed to return to normal. This transverse ultrasound scan of his upper abdomen shows the cause of the persistent pancreatitis, a pseudocyst arising from the tail of the pancreas. Anatomical landmarks recognisable on ultrasound are shown in the diagram

a. Pancreatic pseudocyst

A pancreatic pseudocyst is a collection of pancreatic enzymes, inflammatory fluid and necrotic debris in the lesser sac. It is not a true cyst (i.e. there is no epithelial lining) although the surrounding tissues become thickened by the inflammatory response, and effectively encapsulate the fluid. Pseudocysts may occur after only a moderate attack of acute pancreatitis and often reach the size of a football!

Clinically, the acute attack fails to resolve completely; at the end of the first week, the serum amylase remains elevated and normal bowel peristalsis has not returned. An upper abdominal mass may be palpable. If a pseudocyst is suspected, ultrasound is the investigation of choice (see Figure 13.5).

Management usually involves laparotomy, at which the pseudocyst is 'marsupialised' into the bowel, usually the posterior wall of the stomach. This can be performed after two or three weeks, by which time the wall of the pseudocyst has 'matured' enough to hold sutures.

b. Pancreatic abscess

This complication only occurs after a severe attack of pancreatitis and is caused by bacterial invasion of necrotic material. It may occur despite the use of prophylactic antibiotics. The abscess may remain small and confined to the pancreatic bed, or it may spread extensively in the retroperitoneal tissues. Infection complicating necrotising pancreatitis is often lethal. However, a chronic abscess, even if large, tends to be walled-off and produces a less serious illness than might be expected. The clinical picture is similar to that of a pseudocyst (i.e. failure of recovery of an acute attack after about a week) but there is also a swinging pyrexia and tachycardia. Ultrasound is usually performed first but often fails to demonstrate the abscess clearly. CT scanning is usually more revealing. Treatment requires abdominal exploration and surgical drainage of loculated collections of pus and removal of necrotic pancreas.

RECURRENT, RELAPSING AND CHRONIC PANCREATITIS

Some patients suffer recurrent attacks of acute pancreatitis, usually resulting from either alcohol abuse or gall stone disease. The patient is entirely well between attacks. In different patients, the attacks vary in severity, but are rarely extreme. This condition is often described as 'acute relapsing pancreatitis' but is better described as *recurrent acute pancreatitis*.

Chronic pancreatitis

Other patients suffer persistent and severe upper abdominal pain, similar in character to a prolonged attack of acute pancreatitis. This condition is known as *chronic pancreatitis*. These patients do not develop the other clinical features of acute pancreatitis. The pain is so severe and so persistent as to drive some patients to suicide. Carcinoma of the pancreas and chronic pancreatic inflammation should both be considered in patients with this pattern of pain. Inflammatory swelling of the pancreatic head occasionally causes obstructive jaundice but carcinoma in this position is a far more common cause.

Despite the pain, there are usually no abnormal abdominal signs. The serum amylase may be moderately elevated on occasions; the diagnosis of chronic pancreatitis may, however, be missed if raised serum amylase levels are not detected. This may be because tests are not done at an appropriate time or because the patient is unfortunate enough never to have elevated levels. There is a danger that these patients may be dismissed as suffering from psychosomatic pain.

Ultrasound or CT scans may show glandular swelling, sometimes difficult to distinguish from pancreatic carcinoma. If ERCP is performed, the pancreatic duct system may look normal or else may be distorted and irregular in calibre, thus confirming chronic inflammation and fibrosis (see Figure 13.6). Sometimes pancreatic duct stones are demonstrable.

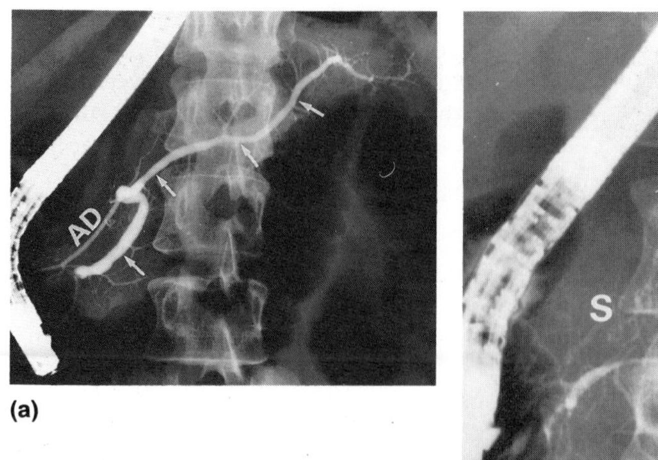

Fig. 13.6 Retrograde pancreatography

These films were both obtained by injecting contrast into the pancreatic duct using a flexible fibreoptic duodenoscope. **(a)** This pancreatogram is normal. The main duct (arrowed) narrows regularly towards the tail of the pancreas and there are no strictures nor dilatations along its length. The accessory pancreatic duct **AD** also fills in this patient. **(b)** This pancreatogram is from a man of 26 with a history of severe upper abdominal pain. There is a long stricture of the main duct **S** (of unknown origin). Typical changes of chronic pancreatitis, i.e. irregularity of the wall with dilatations and poor filling of small ducts, are seen in the duct behind the stricture

Chronic pancreatitis may cause years of misery, perhaps eventually 'burning out' as the gland completely atrophies. It is important to make the diagnosis so that pain can be relieved. In the long term, malabsorption or diabetes may develop.

Pancreatic calcification seen on abdominal X-rays is diagnostic of chronic pancreatitis but is rare, and is sometimes found in asymptomatic patients. It is therefore of little clinical value.

Treatment of chronic pancreatitis is far from satisfactory. Surgery is only useful if structural abnormalities can be found. Surgical procedures include removal of pancreatic duct stones, partial pancreatectomy of the body and tail for duct stenosis, sphincteroplasty of the pancreatic duct opening, or occasionally complete pancreatectomy. If there are multiple duct strictures, the pancreatic duct can be is split along its whole length and a loop of jejunum sutured to the gland to allow unrestricted drainage. Coeliac ganglion blockade provides useful (and usually permanent) pain relief, but does nothing to prevent inflammation.

Occasionally, pancreatitis may pursue a prolonged course with a series of acute relapses and remissions; this condition is known as *chronic relapsing pancreatitis* and is managed in a similar manner to chronic pancreatitis.

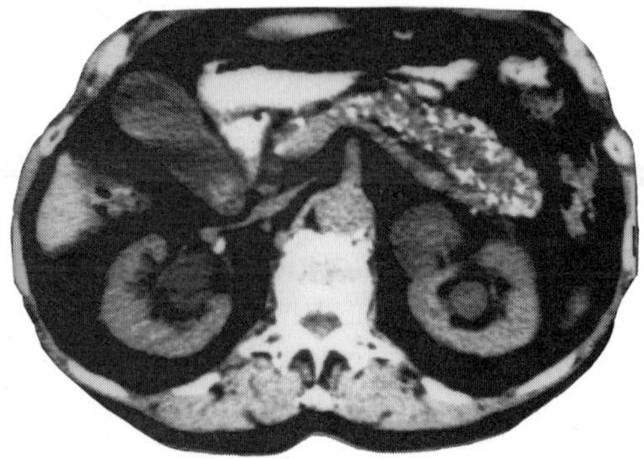

Fig. 13.7 Pancreatic calcification in chronic pancreatitis

This obese 55-year-old man had a long history of severe abdominal pain and alcohol abuse. Pancreatic calcification was not visible on a plain abdominal X-ray but extensive calcification is clearly seen on this CT scan

14 APPENDICITIS

Introduction

Appendicitis is the most common cause of abdominal sepsis in developed countries and appendicectomy is the most common emergency surgical operation. In the UK, 1.9 females per thousand have the operation each year compared with 1.5 males, and one in 6 or 7 people eventually undergo the operation. Surprisingly, the incidence of appendicitis has fallen by about 50% over the last 10 years.

Appendicitis can occur at any age but is most common below 40, especially between the ages of 8 and14. It is very rare below the age of two. Appendicitis is rare in rural parts of underdeveloped countries, but in the cities, the incidence approaches that of the West. This rapid change in susceptibility is probably related to much reduced intake of dietary fibre.

Acute appendicitis typically presents with abdominal pain. Despite lay impressions, a positive diagnosis is often difficult to make. This is partly because of the wide range of differential diagnoses. Sometimes a non-inflamed appendix is found at operation. Some of these operations will have been performed unnecessarily but a small proportion are unavoidable if acute appendicitis cannot be excluded beforehand.

Fig. 14.1 Surgical anatomy of the appendix

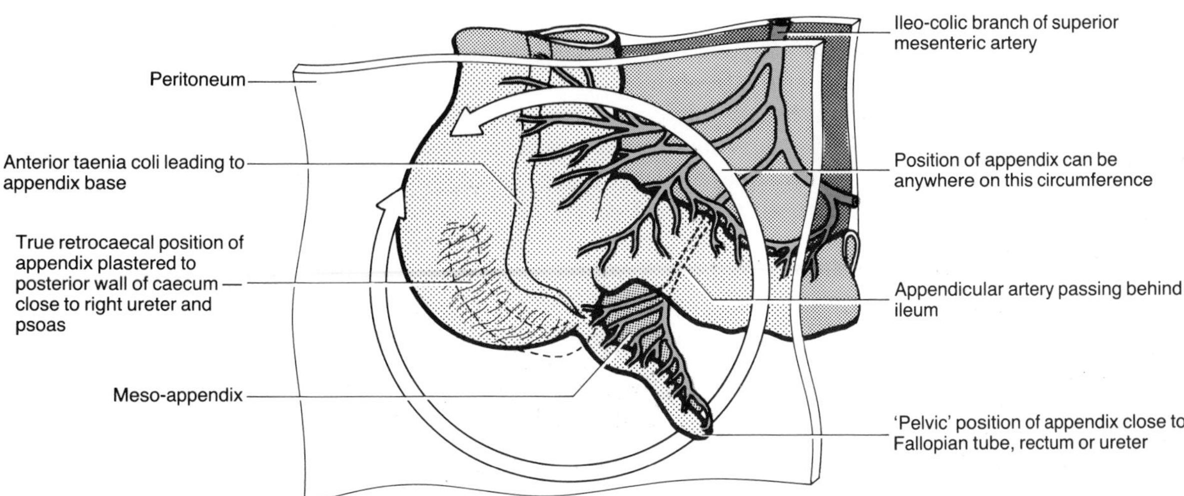

ANATOMY OF THE APPENDIX

The appendix is a blind-ending tube arising from the caecum at the meeting point of the three taeniae coli, just distal to the ileocaecal junction. The base of the appendix thus lies in the right iliac fossa, close to McBurney's point. This is two-thirds of the way along a line drawn from the umbilicus to the anterior superior iliac spine (see Figure 14.9 later). In most cases, the appendix is mobile within the peritoneal cavity, suspended by its mesentery *(meso-appendix)* with the appendiceal artery in the free edge. This is effectively an end-artery, with anastomotic connections only proximally.

The appendix has been described as lying in several 'classical' sites, but apart from the true retrocaecal appendix, the organ probably floats in a broad arc about its base (see Figure 14.1). Only inflammation will fix it in a particular place. In about 30% of appendicectomies, the appendix lies over the brim of the pelvis ('pelvic appendix'). This is adjacent to the bladder and rectum in males and to the uterus, Fallopian tubes and bladder in females. In some cases, the appendix lies retroperitoneally behind the caecum and is often plastered to it by fibrous bands. Thus, an inflamed retrocaecal appendix may irritate the right ureter and psoas muscle, and may even lie high enough to simulate gall bladder pain.

Histologically, the appendix has the same basic structure as the large intestine. Its glandular mucosa is separated from the loose vascular submucosa by the delicate muscularis mucosae. Beyond the submucosa is the main muscular component. The appendix is covered externally by the serosal layer (the visceral layer of peritoneum) which contains the large blood vessels and becomes continuous with the serosa of the mesoappendix. When the appendix lies retroperitoneally, there is no serosal covering. A prominent feature of the appendix are its collections of lymphoid tissue in the lamina propria. This lymphoid tissue, which often has germinal centres, is particularly marked in childhood but diminishes with increasing age.

The mucosa contains a large number of cells of the gastrointestinal endocrine system. These mainly secrete 5 hydroxytryptamine and were formerly known as argentaffin cells. Carcinoid tumours, which commonly occur in the appendix, arise from these cells.

PATHO-PHYSIOLOGY OF APPENDICITIS

Appendicitis is probably initiated by obstruction of the lumen by impacted faeces or a faecolith. This explanation fits with the epidemiological observation that appendicitis is associated with a poor dietary fibre intake.

In the early stages of appendicitis, first the mucosa becomes inflamed. This inflammation eventually extends through the submucosa to involve the muscular and serosal (peritoneal) layers. A fibrinopurulent exudate forms on the serosal surface and extends to any adjacent peritoneal surface, e.g. bowel or abdominal wall, representing a localised peritonitis.

By this stage the necrotic glandular mucosa sloughs off into the lumen of the appendix which becomes distended with pus. Finally, the end-arteries supplying the appendix become thrombosed and the infarcted appendix becomes gangrenous or necrotic. This usually occurs distally and the appendix begins to disintegrate. Perforation soon follows and faecally contaminated appendiceal contents spread into the peritoneal cavity. Unless the spilled contents are enveloped by omentum, resulting in a localised abscess, spreading peritonitis develops. The evolution of appendicitis is illustrated histologically in Figure 14.2.

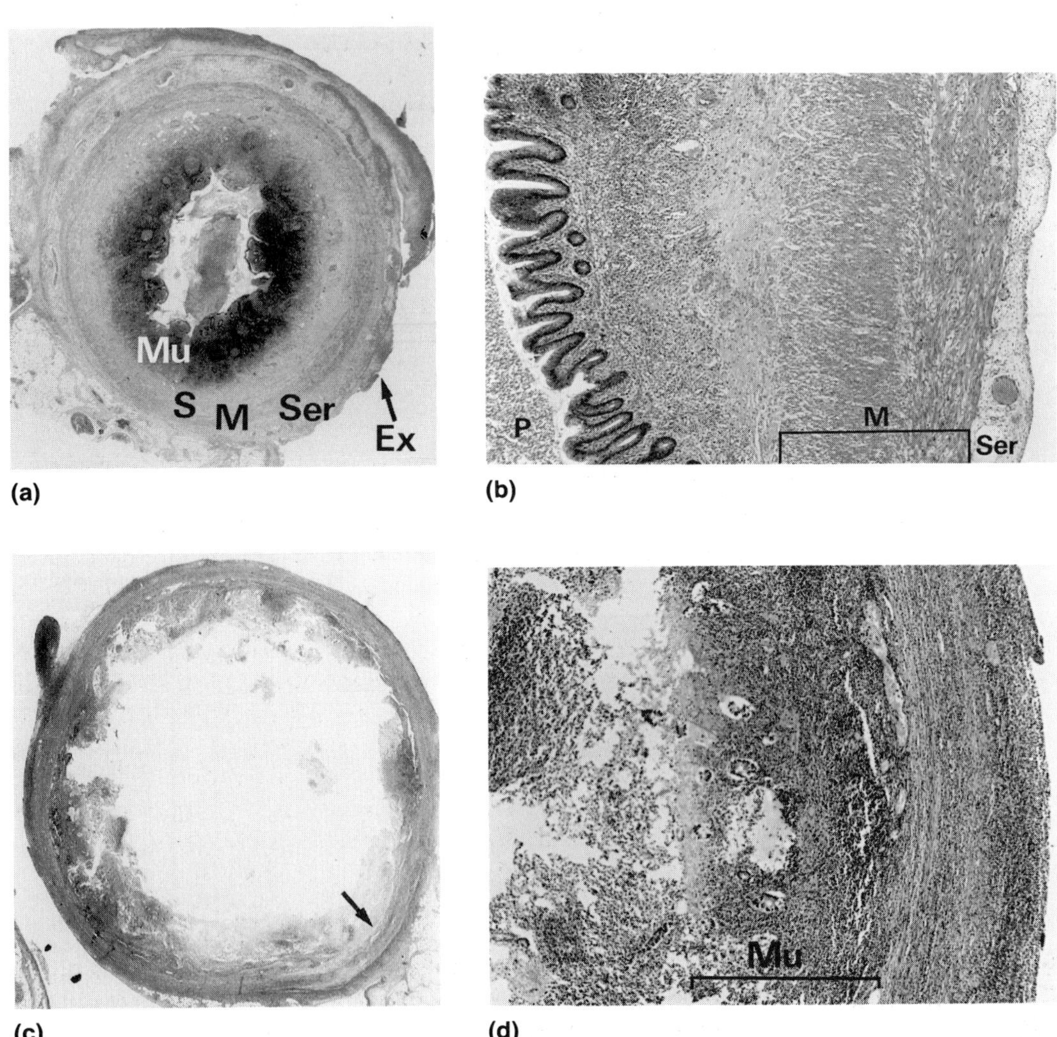

Fig. 14.2 Acute appendicitis — histopathology

(a) Acutely inflamed appendix, with the mucosa **Mu** swollen and intensely infiltrated with acute inflammatory cells. The inflammation extends through the submucosa **S**, muscularis **M** and serosal layers **Ser**, resulting in a fibrinous inflammatory exudate **Ex** on the external surface. **(b)** This is a higher magnification of the wall of specimen (a). Pus **P** can be seen in the lumen, and a moderate degree of inflammation extends into the muscular wall **M** and serosa **S**. The latter is considerably thickened by oedema and coated with a layer of fibrinous exudate. **(c)** This micrograph shows a dilated gangrenous appendix, the mucosa having completely sloughed. The appendicular wall is thin and appears about to perforate at one point (arrowed). **(d)** Higher magnification of the wall of specimen (c), showing further detail of the necrotic mucosa **Mu**

PATHOPHYSIOLOGY AND CLINICAL FEATURES

The pathophysiological evolution of appendicitis and the corresponding symptoms and signs are illustrated in Figure 14.3.

Fig. 14.3 Pathophysiology and clinical manifestations of acute appendicitis

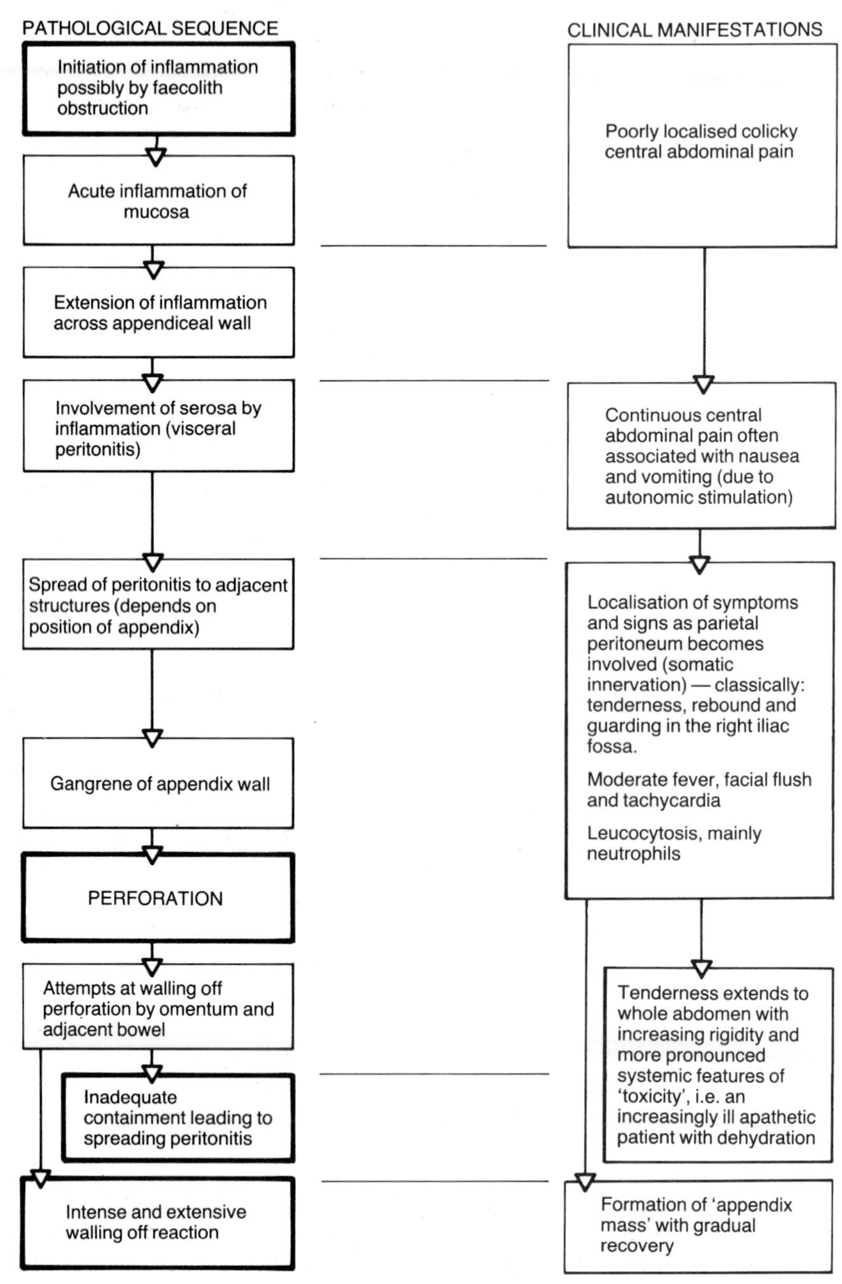

'Classic' appendicitis

Acute appendicitis classically begins with poorly localised, colicky central abdominal pain; this is probably caused by smooth muscle spasm in reaction to faecolith obstruction. Anorexia and often vomiting commonly accompany the pain at this stage. Later, the pain becomes constant as inflammation becomes established.

As inflammation progresses through the appendiceal wall to involve the parietal peritoneum (which is innervated somatically), the pain typically becomes localised to the right iliac fossa. Signs of local peritonitis, i.e. tenderness and guarding, can be elicited at this stage. This classical picture is seen in less than half of all cases, because the localising symptoms and signs vary with the anatomical relations of the inflamed appendix.

Other presentations

If the appendix lies in the pelvis near the rectum, it may cause local irritation and diarrhoea. If it lies near the bladder or ureter, inflammation may cause urinary symptoms of frequency, dysuria and (microscopic) haematuria. These may readily be mistaken for urinary tract infection. An inflamed retrocaecal appendix produces none of the usual localising symptoms or signs, but may irritate the psoas muscle causing involuntary right hip flexion and pain on extension. A high retrocaecal appendix may cause pain and tenderness below the right costal margin. An inflamed appendix near the Fallopian tube causes pelvic pain suggestive of an acute gynaecological disorder like salpingitis or torsion of an ovarian cyst.

The early phase of poorly localised pain typically lasts for a few hours until peritoneal inflammation produces localising signs. If untreated, the inflamed appendix becomes gangrenous after 12–24 hours and perforates, causing spreading peritonitis. The whole abdomen becomes rigid and tender and there is marked systemic toxicity. Perforation is particularly common in children. Sometimes, the pathological sequence is extremely rapid and the patient presents with sudden peritonitis.

In older patients, a gangrenous or perforated appendix may be contained by omentum or loops of small bowel. This results in a palpable mass containing a central abscess known as an *appendix mass*. As with any significant abscess, there is a tachycardia and swinging pyrexia. An appendix mass usually resolves spontaneously over two to six weeks. In the elderly, an appendix abscess tends to become walled-off by loops of small bowel. This may cause symptoms and signs which are not recognisable as appendicitis. These include non-specific abdominal pain and features of small bowel obstruction due to local paralytic ileus. Occasionally, appendicitis may present in a most unusual way. Examples include discharge of an appendix abscess into the Fallopian tube presenting as a purulent vaginal discharge, and inflammation of an appendix lying in an inguinal hernia presenting as an abscess in the groin.

MAKING THE DIAGNOSIS OF APPENDICITIS

Acute appendicitis is a clinical diagnosis, relying almost entirely on the history and physical examination. Investigations are only useful in excluding other differential diagnoses. If possible, the diagnosis should be made and the appendix removed before it becomes gangrenous and perforates. On the other hand, unnecessary appendicectomies must be kept to a minimum.

Diagnosis of acute appendicitis poses little difficulty if the patient exhibits the classical symptoms and signs summarised in Figure 14.4. The problem in diagnosing appendicitis occurs when the symptoms and signs are atypical. The patient may present at a very early stage, or the symptoms and signs may have some other pathological cause. At least two out of every three children admitted to hospital with suspected appendicitis do not have the condition.

Fig. 14.4 Cardinal features of acute appendicitis

Abdominal pain for less than 72 hours
Vomiting 1–3 times
Facial flush
Tenderness concentrated in the right iliac fossa
Rebound tenderness in the right iliac fossa
Anterior tenderness on rectal examination
Fever between 37.3 and 38.5° C
No evidence of urinary tract infection on urine microscopy

If the evidence for acute appendicitis is insufficient and no other diagnosis can be made, the patient should be kept under observation, admitted to hospital if necessary and re-examined periodically. Eventually, the patient settles or the diagnosis becomes clear.

Special points in the history and examination

Acute appendicitis typically runs a short course, between a few hours and about two days. If symptoms have been present for longer, appendicitis is unlikely unless an 'appendix mass' has developed. A recent or current sore throat or viral-type illness favours the diagnosis of mesenteric adenitis (inflammation of the mesenteric lymph nodes analagous to viral tonsillitis). Urinary symptoms suggest urinary tract infection but may also occur with pelvic appendicitis.

The patient with appendicitis is typically quiet, apathetic and flushed; the lively child doing jigsaw puzzles almost never has appendicitis! Oral foetor may be present but is not a reliable sign of appendicitis. Cervical lymphadenopathy tends to suggest a viral origin for the abdominal pain. Mild tachycardia and pyrexia are typical of appendicitis but a temperature much over 38° C makes the diagnosis of acute viral illness or urinary tract infection more likely.

Signs of peritoneal inflammation in the right iliac fossa are often absent in the early stages of the illness. The patient should be asked to cough, blow the abdominal wall out and draw it in; all of these cause pain if the parietal peritoneum is inflamed. In children, it may be difficult to interpret apparent tenderness, especially if the child cries and refuses to cooperate. This can usually be overcome by distracting the child's attention whilst palpating the abdomen through the bed clothes or even with the child's own hand under the examiner's hand.

Rebound tenderness can best be demonstrated by gentle percussion of the right iliac fossa. Pain on percussion is a reliable sign of local peritonitis. Anterior peritoneal tenderness on rectal examination (i.e. pelvic peritonitis) supports the diagnosis of appendicitis, provided other signs are consistent. In pelvic appendicitis, it may be the only abdominal sign. Lack of rectal tenderness does not, however, exclude appendicitis.

Differential diagnosis

The differential diagnosis of acute appendicitis theoretically includes all the causes of an acute abdomen shown in Figure 7.1. However, the main conditions of practical importance are summarised in Figure 14.5, along with the main features distinguishing them from acute appendicitis. These other conditions rarely need operation. Certain uncommon conditions such as Yersinia ileitis and inflamed Meckel's diverticulum are not included in the list since they can only be distinguished from appendicitis at laparotomy.

Fig. 14.5 Main differential diagnoses of acute appendicitis

Urinary tract infection (cystitis or pyelonephritis) — can be excluded if there are not significant numbers of white blood cells or bacteria on urine microscopy.

Mesenteric adenitis — inflammation and enlargement of abdominal lymph nodes, probably viral in origin, and often associated with an upper respiratory infection or sore throat. Symptoms and signs may be similar to those of early appendicitis but without rectal tenderness. Fever is typically higher than in appendicitis (i.e. greater than 38.5 deg C) and settles rapidly

Constipation — may cause colicky abdominal pain and iliac fossa tenderness. There is no fever and the rectum is loaded with faeces

Gynaecological disorders

— the pain of ovulation (Mittelschmerz) may cause right iliac fossa pain. It occurs at the mid-point of the menstrual cycle and there is often a history of similar pain in the past. There are no signs of infection and the pain settles quickly

— salpingitis causes lower abdominal pain, often with a vaginal discharge. Digital vaginal examination typically reveals adnexal tenderness, and moving the cervix from side to side induces pain ('cervical excitation'); these features can be elicited by rectal examination in the virginal patient

— torsion of, or haemorrhage into a right ovarian cyst may produce symptoms like appendicitis, but there is no fever. A tender mobile mass may be palpable in the right suprapubic region or on vaginal examination. This diagnosis can be confirmed with ultrasound

Perforation of another abdominal viscus — a perforated Meckel's diverticulum may present exactly like appendicitis. Necrotic small bowel from strangulation usually presents with intestinal obstruction

Acute pancreatitis — pain is predominantly central. If there is tenderness in right iliac fossa, it will also be present in the epigastrium. If in doubt, the serum amylase should be measured

Nonspecific abdominal upset — vague abdominal pain and tenderness which may be associated with vomiting and diarrhoea. Usually improves steadily during a period of observation

The equivocal diagnosis

If acute appendicitis can be diagnosed confidently on clinical grounds, no further investigations are required, unless there are secondary problems such as anaemia or dehydration. These require full blood count and electrolyte estimations. There are no diagnostic tests specific for appendicitis but certain investigations are useful where the diagnosis is in doubt.

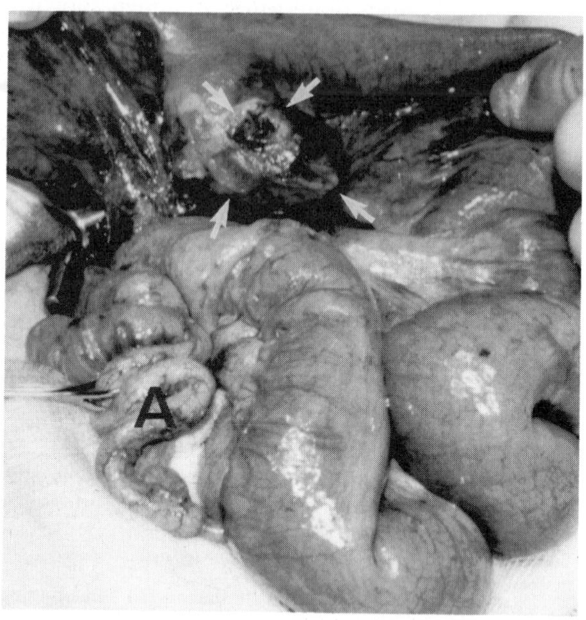

Fig. 14.6 Perforated Meckel's diverticulum

This 16-year-old male presented with symptoms and signs of acute appendicitis. At operation, the perforated Meckel's diverticulum (arrowed) was found. Note the diverticulum is short and wide and situated on the anti-mesenteric border of the ileum. Note also the normal appendix **A** in the foreground

The white blood count is usually unhelpful, as a modest rise occurs in many conditions, and if there is a great rise (to over 15 000), the clinical diagnosis of appendicitis is usually obvious. Urine microscopy must be performed if there is any suggestion of a urinary tract infection.

Abdominal X-rays are not needed unless there is confusing evidence of abdominal pathology after a period of observation. The presence of a single fluid level in the right iliac fossa suggests local adynamic obstruction due to appendicitis, but this is an uncommon finding. In adults with an equivocal diagnosis of appendicitis, the serum amylase should be measured because the early features of appendicitis and pancreatitis can be similar. There is no place for barium enema in the diagnosis of appendicitis.

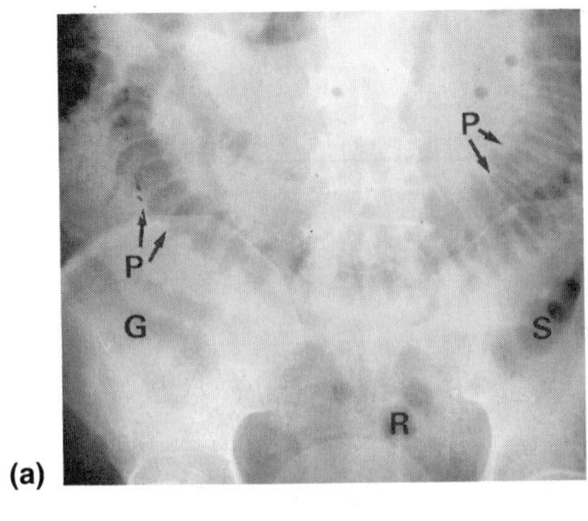

(a)

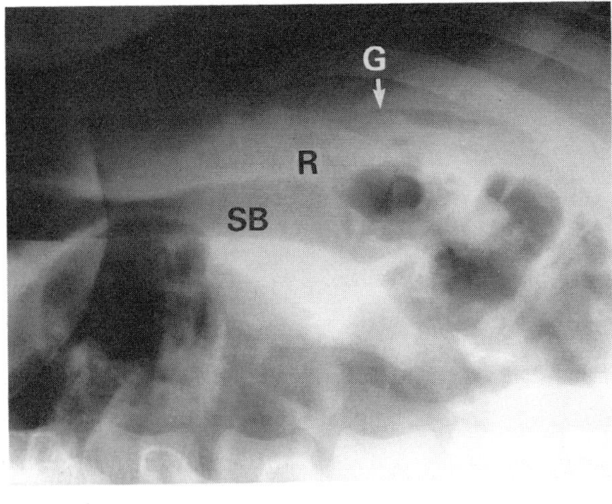

(b)

Fig. 14.7 Perforated gangrenous sub-hepatic appendix

This 12-year-old boy presented with two days' abdominal pain and vomiting. On examination, there was tenderness in the right side of the abdomen. There was also abdominal distension resonant to percussion and obstructed bowel sounds, which indicated possible small bowel obstruction. **(a)** Supine plain abdominal film showing grossly dilated small bowel filling the centre of the abdomen. The plicae semilunares **P** can be seen to completely cross the lumen, characterising dilated small bowel. There is a little gas in the rectum **R** and sigmoid colon **S**. These signs are diagnostic of small bowel obstruction. There is some free gas **G** visible in the right iliac fossa suggesting perforation. **(b)** A decubitus plain abdominal film (right-side upwards) in another similar patient shows a featureless loop of small bowel **SB**, which is adynamic due to nearby inflammation. The radio-opacity **R** is a faecolith in the appendix (*appendolith*) and the linear radiolucency **G** is free gas under a Riedel's lobe of the liver. At operation, the appendix was found to be gangrenous and perforated, but was lying in a high position close to the liver

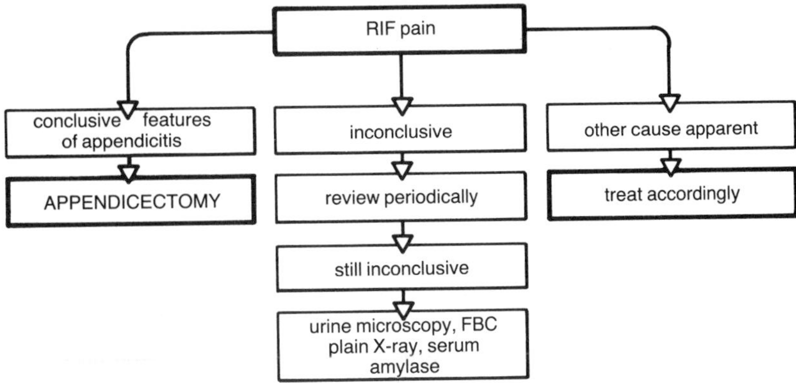

Fig. 14.8 Summary—management of suspected appendicitis

PROBLEMS IN DIAGNOSIS OF APPENDICITIS

The very young

Appendicitis is rarely seen below two years of age, but when it does occur, the 'typical' abdominal symptoms and signs are obscure or absent. An infant or toddler may display signs of sepsis without revealing the abdominal origin.

Abdominal X-rays may demonstrate dilated loops of bowel and fluid levels. Generalised peritonitis supervenes rapidly in this age group because the abdominal defence mechanisms, in particular the 'wrapping' effect of the greater omentum, are rudimentary. Laparotomy is usually indicated in an ill infant with abdominal signs.

The elderly

Appendicitis tends to develop more slowly and pursue a more prolonged course in the elderly. The appendix wall becomes fibrotic with age and the area is more readily walled-off by omentum and adherent small bowel. Many cases probably resolve spontaneously. In those who reach hospital, the history is often as long as a week. Symptoms and signs of obstruction may be present. These include vomiting, colicky abdominal pain and obstructed bowel sounds. A mass may be palpable if the patient is relaxed and not too tender but often can only be palpated under general anaesthesia. Abdominal X-rays may reveal fluid levels in the right iliac fossa.

Pregnancy

Appendicitis occurs at least as often during pregnancy as at other times but the diagnosis can be difficult. The appendix is displaced upwards by the enlarging uterus so that abdominal pain and tenderness are in a much higher position than usual. Diagnosis and management of the pregnant patient must be shared with an obstetrician. Mortality from appendicitis for both mother and fetus rises as the pregnancy progresses; this is as high as 9% for the mother and 20% for the fetus in the third trimester!

The 'grumbling' appendix

Recurrent bouts of right iliac fossa pain occur in some children and are often labelled as 'grumbling appendix'. Appendicular pathology is probably the cause in very few of these cases. Persistent chronic inflammation of the appendix probably does not occur, but recurrent bouts of appendicular colic or low-grade acute appendicitis undoubtedly do. These children may have several abortive admissions for abdominal pain and it may eventually be justifiable to remove the appendix to allay parental anxiety. A non-inflamed appendix containing a faecolith (assumed to have caused the pain) is often found. If attacks of pain persist after appendicectomy, the likelihood of organic pathology is remote.

APPENDICECTOMY

Whilst the incidence of acute appendicitis has remained steady over the past 50 years, the annual death rate has fallen dramatically. In 1934, there were 3193 deaths from appendicitis in the UK, whereas in 1982, there were 110 deaths. The improvement results from several factors including better general nutrition, earlier presentation, better preoperative preparation and better anaesthesia. Deaths that now occur are usually due to dehydration and electrolyte changes which are unrecognised or ineffectively treated before surgery. Infective complications of appendicitis have dramatically fallen since the 1970s because of the widespread use of prophylactic antibacterial agents.

Antibiotic prophylaxis

Most intra-abdominal septic complications and wound infections occur in perforated or gangrenous appendicitis. The majority of the infecting organisms are anaerobic and the infections can largely be prevented by prophylactic metronidazole. Rectal suppositories are just as effective as intravenous metronidazole but need to be given two hours before operation. Aerobic organisms are involved in a smaller number of cases and some surgeons therefore advocate additional prophylaxis with an antibiotic such as cefotaxime.

Technique of appendicectomy

The principle steps in appendicectomy are illustrated in Figure 14.9 and should be understood by any doctor called upon to assist in the operation.

A low skin crease incision *(Lanz)* rather than the higher and more oblique one centred on McBurney's point is now favoured as it gives a better cosmetic result. The superficial fascia (well marked in children) is then incised and the three musculo-aponeurotic layers of the abdominal wall are split along the line of their fibres. This produces the 'grid-iron' incision, described as such because the fibres of external oblique and internal oblique run at right angles to each other. The peritoneum is then opened and may reveal pus or mucopurulent watery fluid. The appendix is located digitally and delivered into the wound, although further exploration may be needed if it does not lie in the immediate vicinity. A retrocaecal appendix will require mobilisation of the caecum by dividing the peritoneum along its lateral side.

Once the appendix has been delivered into the wound, its blood supply in the mesoappendix is divided between clips and ligated. The appendix base is crushed with a haemostat which is then reapplied more distally. A ligature (usually catgut) is then tied around the crushed area. After this preparation, the appendix is then excised. A 'purse-string' suture is placed in the caecum near the appendix base, the appendix is inverted and the suture tied. If the appendix was perforated or gangrenous, or if pus was found, thorough peritoneal toilet is performed. A sump sucker is guided down into the pelvis with a finger to suck out any fluid, and the area is then swabbed out with gauze to remove any adherent infected material. Any pus left in the pelvis predisposes to subsequent pelvic abscess.

The peritoneum is usually closed with 2/0 chromic catgut. The internal oblique, then external oblique, are each closed with two or three sutures of 0 or 1 chromic catgut. Drainage is not usually recommended unless there is a thick-walled infected abscess cavity which will not collapse.

Postoperatively, oral fluids followed by solids are gradually increased over a few days unless vomiting or other complications occur. Intravenous fluids are rarely needed.

The 'lily-white' appendix

If the appendix is found not to be inflamed at operation (colloquially termed 'lily-white'), it should always be removed because an appendicectomy scar leads

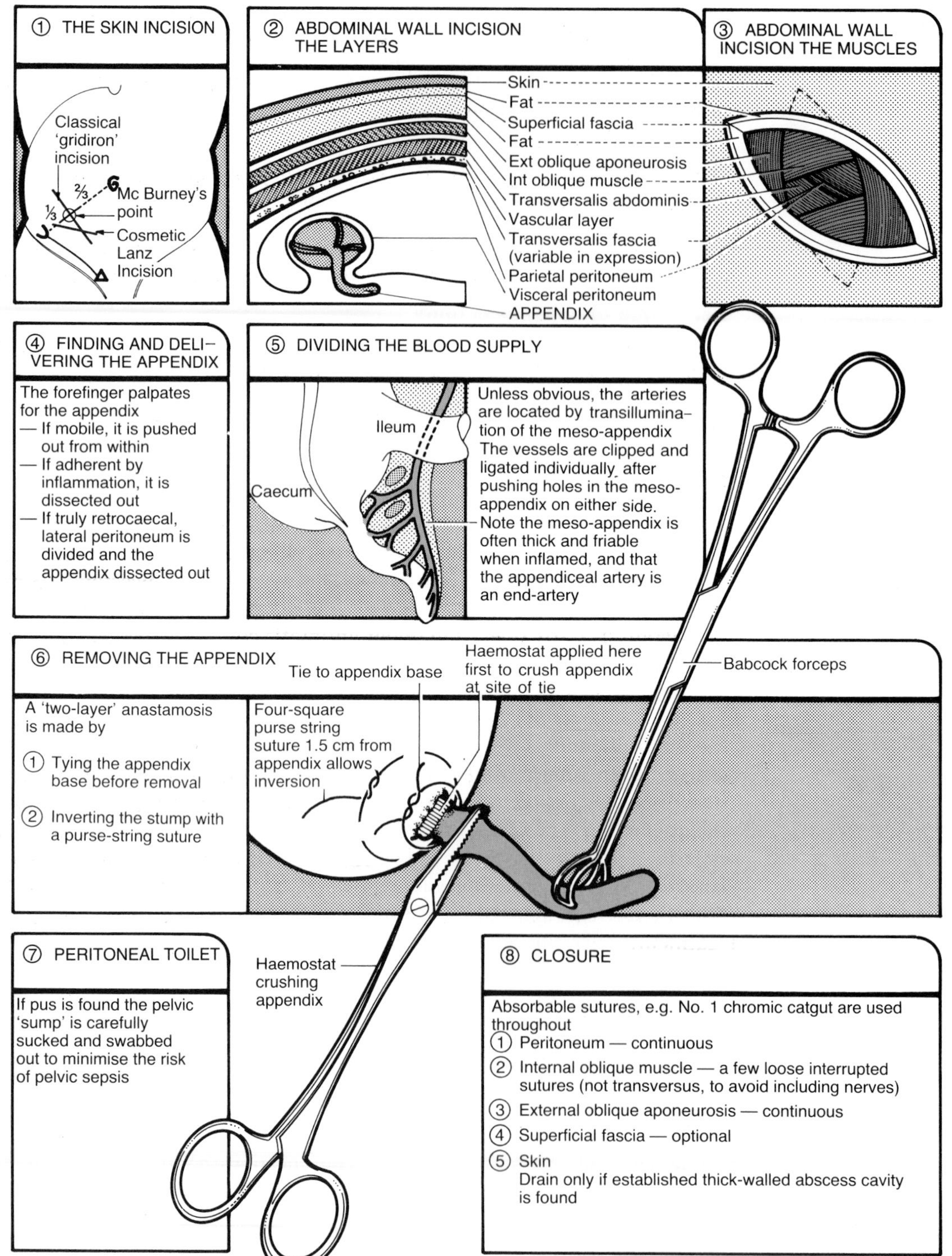

Fig. 14.9 Appendicectomy — operative technique

doctors to assume in future that the appendix has been removed. The abdomen is explored as allowed by the incision to search for a cause for the symptoms:

- Mesenteric lymph nodes in children may be grossly enlarged by mesenteric adenitis — probably viral in origin
- The terminal ileum may be thickened and reddened by Crohn's disease or by Yersinia ileitis — the appendix is removed but the bowel is left alone. If possible, an enlarged mesenteric node is removed for histological examination
- An inflamed Meckel's diverticulum may be found within 30 cm of the ileocaecal valve — if inflamed, this is removed but a wide mouthed non-inflamed diverticulum is usually left alone
- Both ovaries can usually be palpated — ovaries may be twisted, inflamed or enlarged or an inflamed Fallopian tube may be seen
- Rarely, cholecystitis, hydronephrosis or leaking aneurysm are found

The appendix mass

A vigorous response to appendicitis may result in a mass in the right iliac fossa, often with fever. Usually the patient has few systemic symptoms or signs of ill health. A conservative regime followed by interval appendicectomy six weeks later (*Ochsner-Sherren regime*) was advocated in pre-antibiotic days but is now less favoured. Early operation under antibiotic cover is now performed more frequently.

Yersinia ileitis

An uncommon cause of right iliac fossa pain and fever, clinically identical to acute appendicitis, is acute inflammation of the terminal ileum by the organism *Yersinia pseudotuberculosis*. The diagnosis can only be made at operation, when the terminal ileum is seen to be bright red and thickened by the inflammatory process. Sometimes the appearance may be difficult to distinguish from Crohn's disease. Yersinia ileitis is a self-limiting condition and requires no treatment.

15 COLORECTAL CARCINOMA AND POLYPS

Introduction

Cancer of the colon and rectum is the second most common malignancy in the Western world in both sexes. Most originate in the glandular mucosa and are therefore *adenocarcinomas*. Other forms of malignancy in the large bowel such as carcinoid tumour or lymphoma are rare. Squamous carcinoma occurs in the anal canal skin (Chapter 18) but these are rare and not usually difficult to distinguish clinically from rectal tumours.

Use of the term polyp may cause more confusion than understanding! The term should be used to describe any localised lesion protruding into the bowel lumen from the wall and should not be used to imply any specific pathology; this conforms with the use of the term elsewhere in the body, e.g. nasal polyps (usually allergic in origin), endometrial polyps (hyperplastic), polyps of *Peutz–Jehger syndrome* (hamartomatous).

POLYPS

Polyps are a common finding in the large bowel. Their great importance is in relation to malignant change. The majority of colorectal polyps are adenomas (i.e. benign neoplasms) but all have a malignant potential. Furthermore, a polyp may already have undergone malignant change, yet still be at an early and potentially curable stage. Thus for practical purposes, any colorectal polyp must be considered malignant or premalignant until proved otherwise. Hence the terminological difficulty.

A simple pathological classification of large bowel polyps is shown in Figure 15.1.

Polyps typically present with rectal bleeding, and sometimes iron deficiency anaemia due to occult blood loss. Distal lesions may occasionally produce tenesmus or they may prolapse through the anus. Many polyps cause no symptoms, at least in their early stages, and remain undiagnosed or are found incidentally on barium enema examination.

Adenomatous polyps

Adenomas have two basic morphological forms, globular *pedunculated* polyps with stalks of variable length, and broad-based (*sessile*) lesions. Histologically, three patterns of growth are recognised: tubular adenomas, villous adenomas and tubulo-villous adenomas.

Fig. 15.1 Pathological classification of colorectal polyps

Neoplasms

Adenomas — very common, all potentially malignant
Early carcinomas — common
Lymphomas — rare
Leiomyomas and leiomyosarcomas — rare
Lipomas and liposarcomas — rare
Carcinoid tumours — rare

Hyperplasias

Metaplastic mucosal polyps — common
Lymphoid aggregations — common in young children

Hamartomas

Angiomas (related to angiodysplasias) — uncommon
Juvenile polyps — uncommon, found only in children. No malignant potential

Inflammatory polyps

'Pseudopolyps' of ulcerative colitis

a. Tubular adenomas

These are small pedunculated or sessile lesions in which the adenoma cells retain a tubular form similar to normal colonic mucosa. Tubular adenomas have the least potential for malignant transformation. The exception is when multiple tubular adenomas occur throughout the large bowel in the rare familial disorder of *polyposis coli* (also known as *adenomatous polyposis*). In this condition there is a very high risk of early malignant transformation.

b. Villous adenomas

Villous adenomas are usually sessile and frond-like (papilliferous) lesions which tend to secrete mucus. This may be so copious as to be the main presenting complaint. Moreover, symptomatic hypokalaemia may develop (though rarely) because so much potassium-containing mucus is lost. The epithelial component of villous adenoma is more dysplastic than tubular adenoma and there is a greater potential for malignant change.

c. Tubulo-villous adenomas

Histologically, these lesions are intermediate between tubular and villous adenomas and include the majority of colonic polyps. Most are pedunculated, and the stalk is covered with normal colonic epithelium. The length of the stalk varies from about 0.5–10 cm and is probably due to peristalsis dragging the tumour mass distally.

The degree of epithelial dysplasia in adenomatous polyps is highly variable. In benign lesions the abnormality, by definition, is confined to the epithelium. Early malignant change, at successive stages, is represented by invasion of tumour cells through the basement membrane and then into the muscularis mucosae and submucosa. In apparently benign lesions, there may be small areas of frank malignancy, and careful histological examination is essential if

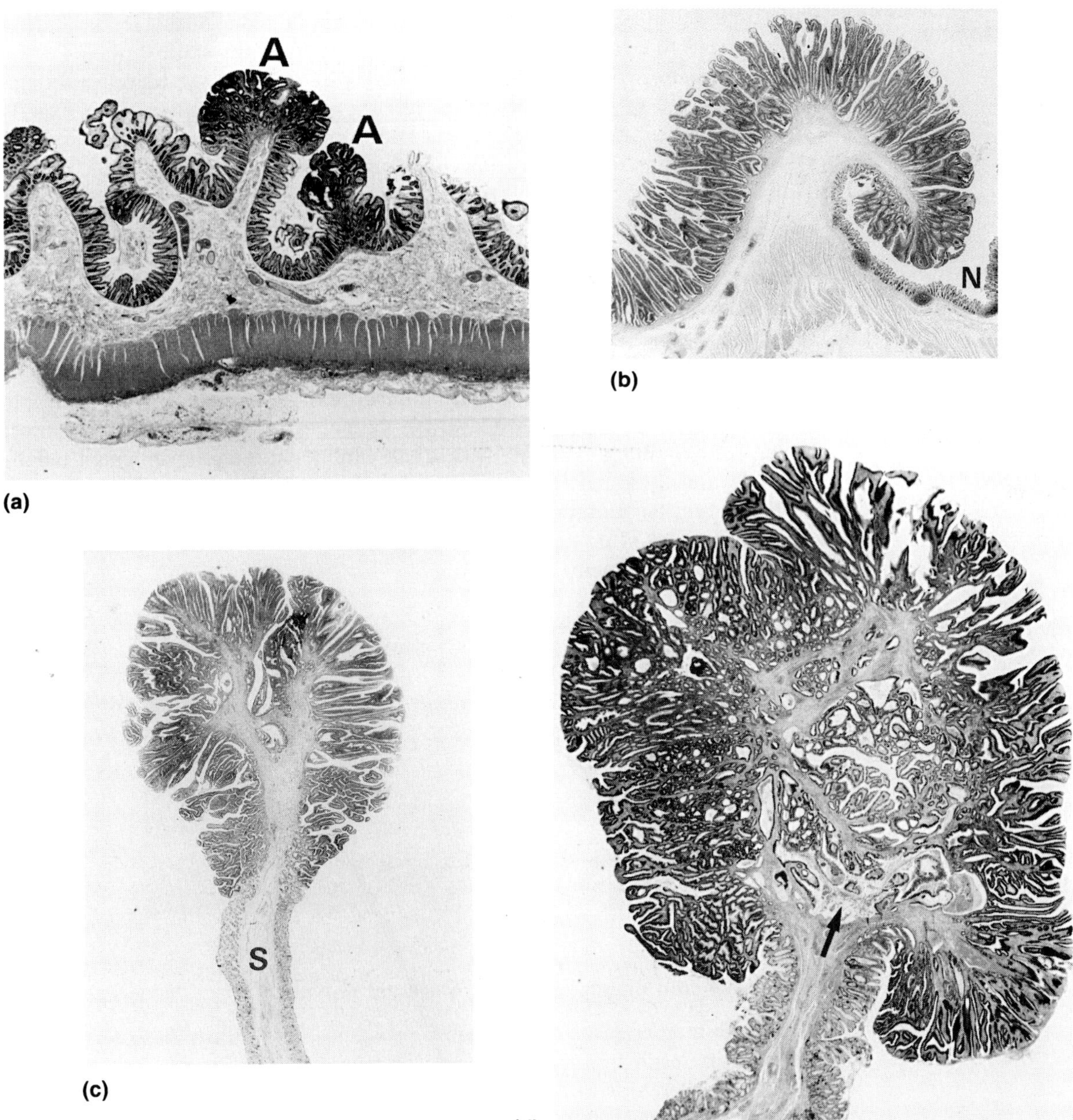

Fig. 15.2 Adenomatous colonic polyps — histopathology

Low power H & E photomicrographs showing: **(a)** Two small benign tubular adenomas **A** from the bowel of a 24-year-old man who had his entire colon removed for familial polyposis coli (see later). Note the tubular growth pattern of the tumour cells reminiscent of the surrounding normal mucosa; **(b)** Benign villous adenoma showing typical broad base and papilliferous growth pattern. Note the abrupt change to normal mucosa **N**; **(c)** Benign tubulo-villous adenoma on a long stalk **S** which is covered by normal colonic mucosa. High power examination showed that the tumour cells were confined by the basement membrane, confirming the benign nature of the lesion; **(d)** Malignant change in a tubulo-villous adenoma as evidenced by tumour invasion of the fibrous stroma of the polyp (arrowed) these are not to be overlooked. This is important in pedunculated lesions, where it is crucial to establish whether there is invasion of the stalk.

Adenomatous polyps may occur in any part of the large bowel, although three-quarters of them arise in the rectum and sigmoid colon. This exactly parallels the distribution of carcinomas, and provides strong evidence to support the view that most cancers develop from polyps. Adenomas are clinically important because they tend to cause rectal blood loss (visible or occult) and because they may undergo malignant change. If adenomatous polyps are discovered, the whole large bowel must be examined, preferably by fibre-optic colonoscopy. All polyps should be removed for histological examination ('excision biopsy') but as a general rule, the larger the lesion, the more likely it is to be malignant. Only 1% of polyps smaller than 1 cm in diameter are malignant whereas about half of those larger than 2.5 cm are malignant.

Adenomas, especially villous adenomas, tend to arise singly but multiple polyps may be present in up to 20% of patients. Multiple adenomas are most often tubulo-villous. Patients with frank carcinoma often have benign polyps as well, and these may become malignant later. This explains why the whole colon should be examined before colectomy wherever possible, and why long-term follow-up after treatment of large bowel cancer often includes colonoscopy or barium enema examination.

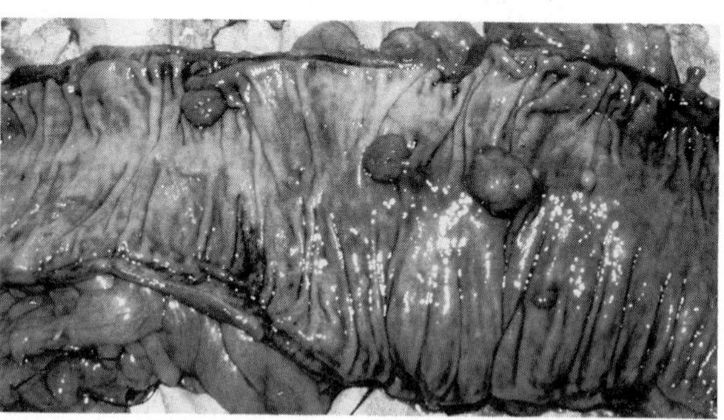

Fig. 15.3 Multiple colonic adenomatous polyps

This length of opened descending colon is from a 64-year-old man who presented with an invasive carcinoma of the rectum. Several adenomatous polyps of various sizes can be seen; the larger polyps have malignant potential

Diagnosis and management of colorectal polyps

Diagnosis may be made at sigmoidoscopy (rectoscopy); nearly half of all polyps are within reach of the 25 cm rigid instrument. Fibreoptic sigmoidoscopy enables the left side of the colon to be examined as far as the splenic flexure, the area of greatest risk, and any polyps can be removed at the same time by diathermy snare. This is becoming more popular, not least because the examination can be performed in the outpatient clinic with minimal bowel preparation.

Barium enema examination reveals most polyps of significant size, and is the examination of first choice for the transverse and right side of colon. However, it may be technically impossible to demonstrate the whole colon in sufficient detail and the caecum is particularly difficult to see well. If a barium enema demonstrates polyps or is technically unsatisfactory, colonoscopy should be performed. Polyps can be excised using a diathermy snare passed around the stalk or sessile base. Pedunculated lesions less than 2 cm in diameter can

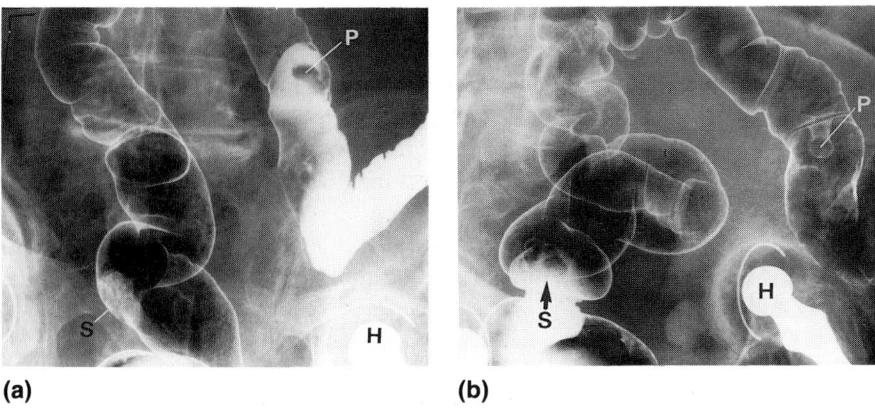

Fig. 15.4 Colonic polyps

This 65-year-old man presented with rectal bleeding. On sigmoidoscopy, a large polypoid lesion was seen in the upper rectum. The X-rays show two views of the rectum and sigmoid colon during a barium enema (note the hip prosthesis **H**). Both views show the sessile rectal lesion **S**, which was visible at sigmoidoscopy. In addition, a pedunculated polyp **P** was found in the sigmoid colon. Notice the difference in appearance of this polyp in single contrast (a) and double contrast (b). No other polyps were demonstrated in the large bowel. Sigmoidoscopic biopsies showed no malignancy, but the lesions looked suspicious and were removed by resecting the upper rectum and sigmoid colon. Histology showed the rectal lesion was an adenoma, but it had early invasive carcinoma in one area. The sigmoid polyp proved to be a benign tubulo-villous adenoma

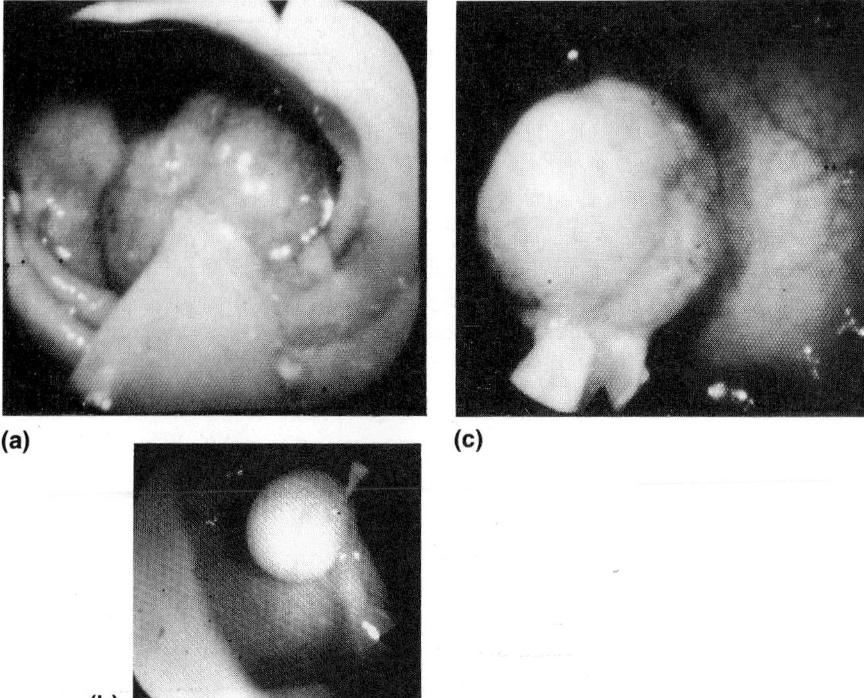

Fig. 15.5 Colonoscopic snaring of a polyp

(a) A 2-cm polyp on a long stalk in the sigmoid colon. **(b)** The snare loop has been tightened around the stalk of the polyp before applying diathermy current to remove it and coagulate the blood vessels in the stalk. **(c)** The excised polyp being withdrawn, while held in forceps, along with the colonoscope. Unfortunately, endoscopic photographs do not reproduce well in books and in practice the appearance would be more clear-cut than shown here

usually be removed with ease but larger ones or sessile lesions may require snaring in several pieces. Histology is mandatory to establish whether the lesion is malignant and whether it has been completely removed.

If a malignant polyp has been incompletely removed, then bowel resection is required. After removal of dysplastic or frankly malignant polyps, most patients are routinely endoscoped every one or two years.

ADENOCARCINOMA OF COLON AND RECTUM

Pathology and clinical presentation

Colorectal carcinomas exhibit a wide range of differentiation, which broadly correlates with their clinical behaviour and prognosis. These carcinomas are initially exophytic (i.e. growing outwards from the mucosa) and later ulcerate and progressively invade the muscular bowel wall. Eventually, the tumour involves the serosa and surrounding structures. Stromal fibrosis causes narrowing, which is responsible for the common acute presentation of large bowel obstruction.

Large bowel carcinomas metastasise mainly via lymphatics and via the blood stream. Lymphatic spread is sequential, first to mesenteric nodes and then to para-aortic nodes. Occasionally lymph node involvement may be responsible for the clinical presentation. For example, para-aortic nodes may present as a palpable mass or cause duodenal obstruction. Other enlarged nodes may compress the bile ducts in the porta hepatis causing jaundice.

Haematogenous spread is predominantly to the liver. It usually follows lymphatic spread, and therefore a patient with only early lymph node involvement has a better chance of avoiding liver metastases. However, it is important to note that hepatic involvement often occurs without lymphatic spread. The effects of liver secondaries often cause death, even after an apparently successful resection of the primary cancer. Haematogenous spread to other sites such as lung or bone is uncommon, as are systemic manifestations. By the time of diagnosis, as many as 25% of patients with colorectal cancer already have widespread metastases.

Mode of growth and clinical presentation of large bowel carcinoma depend to some extent on the site of origin of the lesion:

- Tumours of the capacious caecum rarely cause obstruction and may grow large before they produce symptoms. They usually cause occult bleeding and typically present with iron deficiency anaemia and a palpable mass in the right iliac fossa

- Lesions elsewhere in the colon or rectum ulcerate earlier, perhaps due to intraluminal pressure and stool trauma. Progressive encirclement of the bowel wall encroaches on the lumen producing an annular stenosis. The tumour usually presents with a change in bowel habit or as an emergency with large bowel obstruction, which may be partial or complete. There is usually occult blood loss. Blood may be visible in the stool, the appearance depending on how far the lesion is from the anus

- Lesions (carcinomas or polyps) in the lower two-thirds of the rectum may be perceived as a mass of faeces. This stimulates a persistent defaecation response, causing the symptom of tenesmus

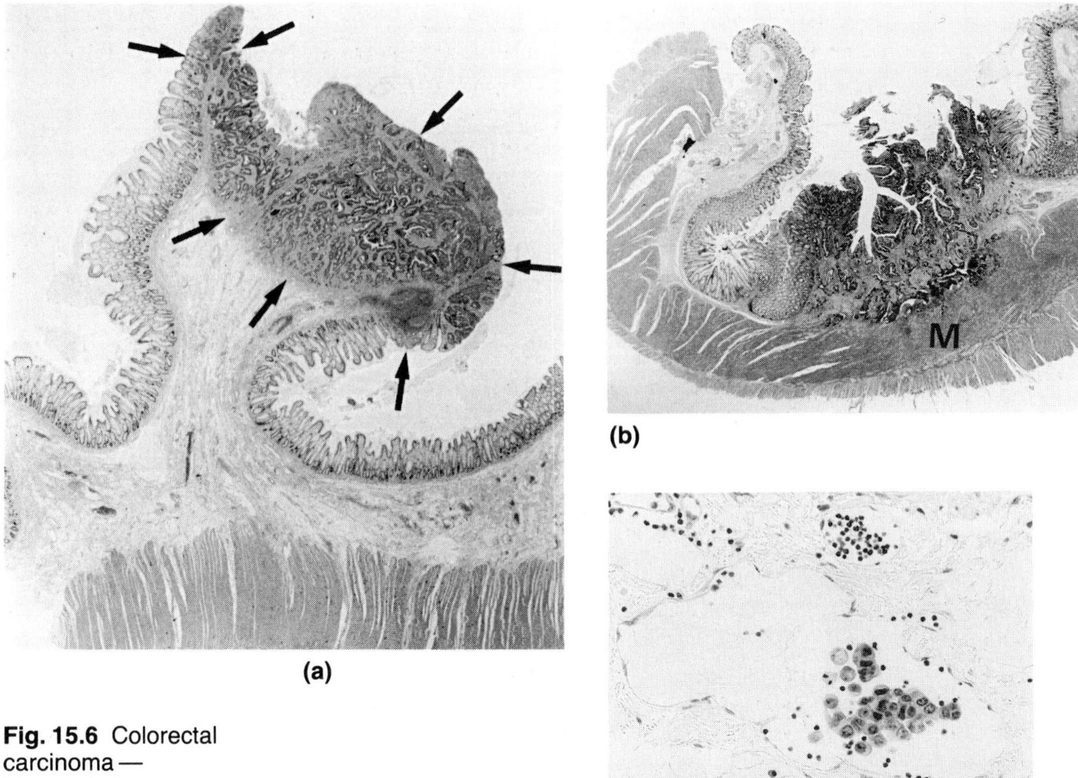

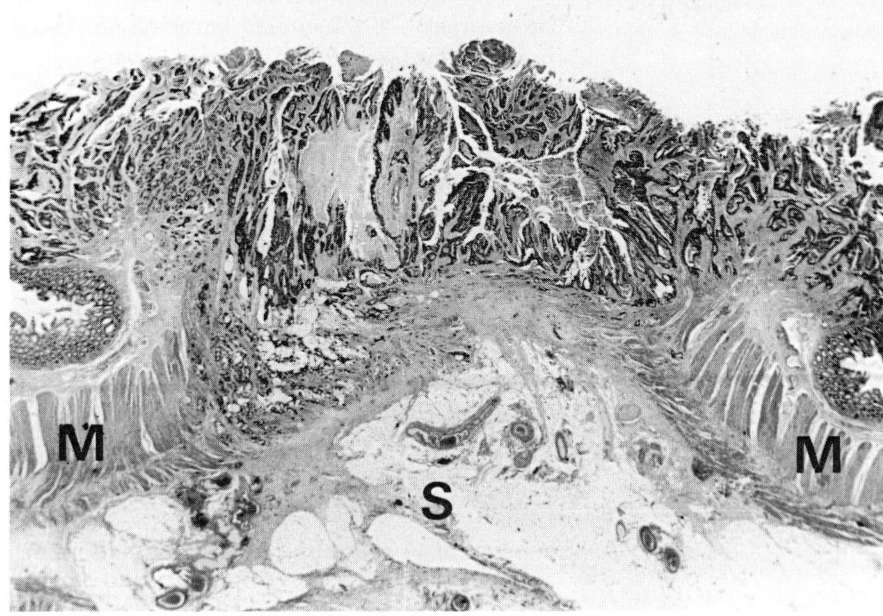

Fig. 15.6 Colorectal carcinoma — histopathology

(a) Early invasive carcinoma (outline arrowed) confined to the mucosa. **(b)** Ulcerating carcinoma extending into the underlying circular layer of smooth muscle **M**. **(c)** High power view of the connective tissue of the serosa in the same specimen as in (b) showing a clump of tumour cells in a lymphatic vessel, thus indicating that the tumour cells have actually penetrated through the full thickness of the bowel and probably to regional lymph nodes. **(d)** Deeply invasive carcinoma extending through the muscular layer of the bowel wall **M** into the serosa **S**

- A carcinoma anywhere in the colon (but rarely in the rectum) may perforate and present as an emergency with peritonitis. Occasionally a malignant fistula occurs into stomach, bladder, uterus, vagina or to the skin

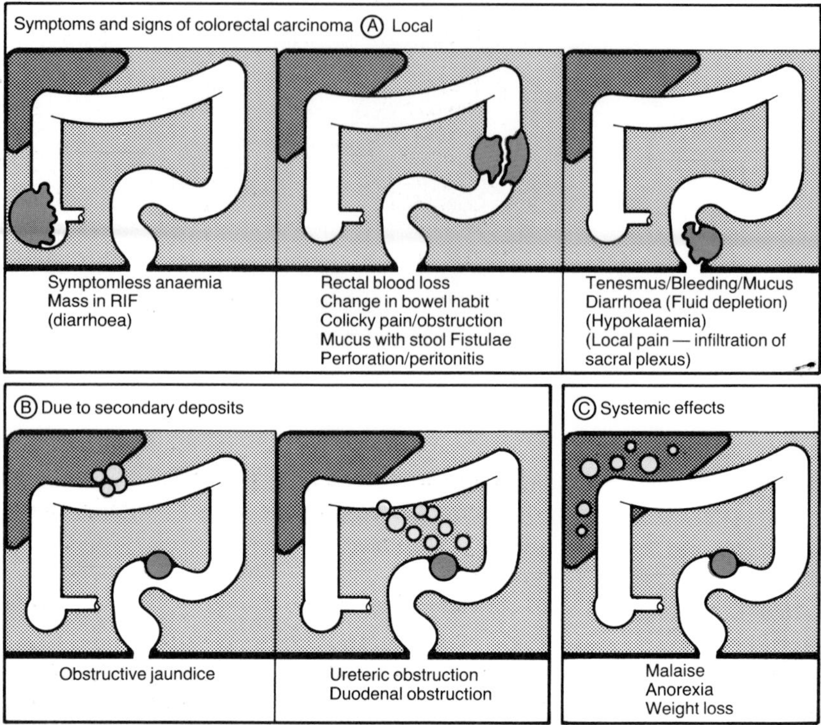

Fig. 15.7 Symptoms and signs of colorectal cancer

Epidemiology of colorectal carcinoma

Colorectal cancer is responsible for about 18 000 deaths in the UK every year. Almost one third arise in the rectum. As shown in Figure 15.8, colorectal cancer is the second most common cause of cancer death in males and the third most common in females. The disease is rare before the age of 40, except when associated with familial polyposis coli. It is common beyond the age of 60. There is little difference in incidence between the sexes.

The aetiology of most colorectal carcinomas is unknown, but a small proportion are secondary to malignant change in polyposis coli and long-standing ulcerative colitis. Colorectal cancer is a disease of developed countries, almost unknown in rural third world communities. This was first highlighted by Denis Burkitt in the early 1970s and led to the belief that our Western low fibre, high fat diet is in some way responsible. It is well established that the Western diet results in a much slower gut transit time. It may be that carcinogens in the stool thereby maintain contact with the bowel mucosa for longer.

Investigation of suspected colorectal carcinoma

General examination may show features which suggest malignant disease, e.g. obvious weight loss, anaemia, abdominal distension, supraclavicular nodes,

Fig. 15.8 Death rates from colorectal cancer compared with other malignancies (UK 1984)

MALES		FEMALES	
Ranking	Percentage of all cancer deaths	Ranking	Percentage of all cancer deaths
1. Lung	36	1. Breast	19
2. Colon & rectum	**11**	2. Lung	15
3. Prostate	8	**3. Colon & rectum**	**13**
4. Stomach	8	4. Stomach	6
5. Bladder	4	5. Ovary	6
6. Pancreas	4	6. Pancreas	4
7. Oesophagus	3	7. Cervix	3
8. Leukaemias	3	8. Oesophagus	3
9. Brain	2	9. Leukaemias	2
10. Others	20	10. Others	28
All cancers	100	**All cancers**	100

hepatomegaly or an abdominal mass. Rectal examination is mandatory as many carcinomas occur in the lowest 12 cm of the large bowel and can be reached with an examining finger. In addition, tumours in the sigmoid colon may be palpable through the rectal wall. The degree of fixation of a rectal tumour to surrounding structures can also be evaluated digitally, and this gives some indication of operative difficulty. Finally, the glove should be inspected for blood and mucus, and stool consistency.

Rigid sigmoidoscopy and proctoscopy are performed at the initial consultation; proctoscopy may show local causes for rectal bleeding. About 50% of colorectal cancers lie within reach of the rigid sigmoidoscope and can be biopsied. A barium enema should be arranged, even if a tumour has been identified at sigmoidoscopy, because synchronous tumours or potentially malignant adenomatous polyps may also be present. Fibreoptic sigmoidoscopy or colonoscopy may be necessary to obtain a histological diagnosis of more proximal lesions. Radioisotope or CT scanning of the liver is often performed to seek metastases. Finally, if there is a risk of ureteric involvement by local spread, an IVU is a useful preoperative investigation.

Many patients, especially the elderly, present as emergencies with complete large bowel obstruction. This typically takes several days to develop. Plain abdominal X-rays often show bowel dilated by gas down to the level of obstruction and empty of gas beyond it. Sigmoidoscopy may confirm the diagnosis of carcinoma; if not, an 'instant' barium enema (i.e. without bowel preparation) will usually do so, and will exclude pseudoobstruction.

Management of colorectal carcinoma

Surgical resection is the main treatment for colorectal carcinoma. Radiotherapy and chemotherapy are seldom indicated. For small tumours localised to the bowel wall, resection offers an excellent chance of complete cure. The cure rate falls markedly with invasion through the bowel wall but cures can still be achieved. Even in very extensive tumours, palliative resection is usually still worthwhile to relieve obstruction or prevent continuing blood loss.

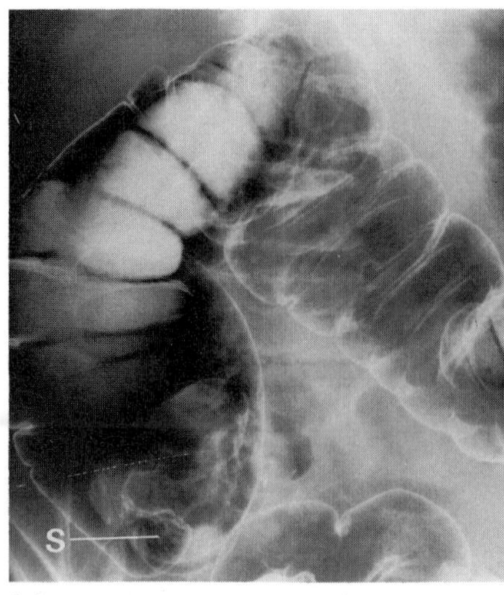

(a)

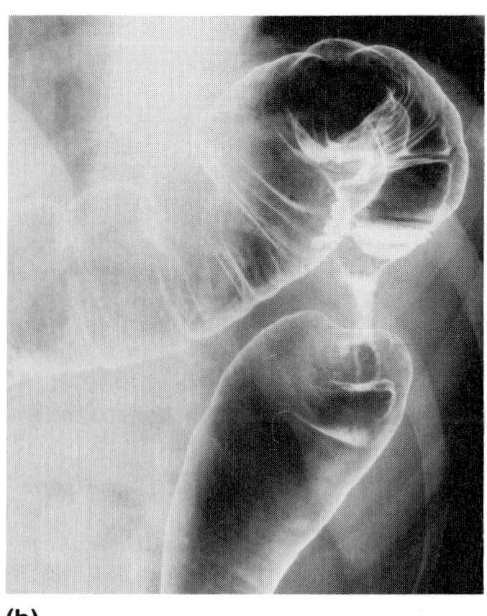

(b)

Fig. 15.9 Caecal and colonic carcinomas

Barium enema examinations. **(a)** Proliferative carcinoma arising on the medial wall of the caecum in a 73-year-old man with an iron deficiency anaemia and a mass in the right iliac fossa. Note the lesion is growing out into the lumen and is recognised by the overlapping double shadows **S**. **(b)** Typical 'apple-core' lesion just distal to the splenic flexure in a man of 39 who complained of rectal bleeding. With this degree of stenosis, it was surprising that he had no change in bowel habit. Acute obstruction would probably have soon occurred if the tumour had not been recognised and resected. The patient is unusually young for colorectal carcinoma

Staging

Staging of colorectal cancers largely depends on the findings at laparotomy and histological examination of the resected specimen. The most widely used system is based on *Dukes' classification*, which he first used for rectal carcinomas and later for colonic carcinomas. This is illustrated in Figure 15.10. Staging of colorectal carcinoma seldom influences treatment but it does give the statistical probability of cure. In fact, survival is largely determined by the presence or absence of liver metastases. Indeed, small metastases impalpable at operation can often be detected by CT scanning, and the investigation may provide additional prognostic information.

Operations for colorectal cancer

The principles of colorectal tumour resection are as follows:

- The affected segment of bowel is removed with a margin of normal bowel. A minimum of 5 cm clear each side of the tumour removes local lymphatics likely to be involved. For rectal tumours, where lymphatic drainage is virtually all in a proximal direction, a distal clearance of 1 cm is usually adequate. This allows the anal sphincter to be preserved in many patients with rectal carcinoma

- The precise lines of resection are determined by the distribution of mesenteric blood vessels. There must be a good blood supply to the cut ends of bowel to ensure healing. Many surgeons first perform proximal ligation of the venous drainage, to minimise the risk of tumour embolisation from handling during resection

- A wedge-shaped section of mesentery is resected en bloc with its lymph nodes to remove the primary field of lymphatic drainage. If there are obvious lymph node metastases, these are usually included in the resection specimen

Fig. 15.10 Staging of colorectal carcinoma based on Dukes' classification and survival rates from treated colorectal cancer

Dukes' A — Tumour confined to the bowel wall with no extension into the extrarectal or extracolic tissues and no lymph node metastases

Dukes' B — Tumour spread into the extrarectal or extracolic tissues by direct continuity but without lymph node metastases

Dukes' C — Lymph node metastases. This category is subdivided into:

C1 in which only a few nodes are involved near the primary growth, leaving proximal nodes free from metastases

C2 in which there is a continuous string of involved nodes up to the proximal limit of resection

Stage D — This is a later addition to Dukes' staging, based on clinical rather than pathological evidence. These patients are found at operation to have distant metastases or such extensive local or nodal spread that the lesion is surgically incurable whatever the pathological staging

Survival rates — all stages together
Approximately half of all patients with colorectal cancer are incurable at presentation; all of these die within 5 years. Of the other half who undergo radical surgery with the aim of cure, 50% are alive and well 5 years later. Very few patients surviving 5 years die later of recurrent disease

5-year survival rates after operation for colorectal cancer, by Dukes' stage, corrected for deaths not due to the disease

Dukes' A — 97%
Dukes' B — 80%
Dukes' C_1 — 65%
Dukes' C_2 — 35%

- In most cases, the cut ends of bowel can be rejoined at the same operation without the need for a colostomy. The method used depends on the site of the anastomosis and whether there is much disparity in diameter between the ends to be joined. Standard operations vary with the site of the tumour, and each is modified according to the operative findings. Details of technique vary from surgeon to surgeon, but an outline of standard operations is given in Figure 15.11. The technique of right hemicolectomy is illustrated in Figure 15.12

Fig. 15.11 Standard operations for rectal cancer

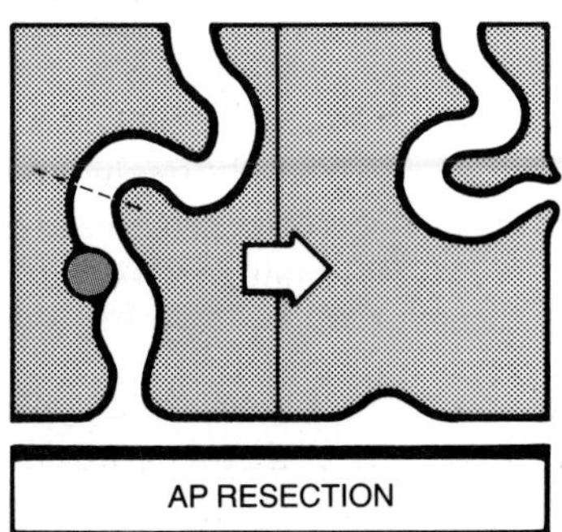

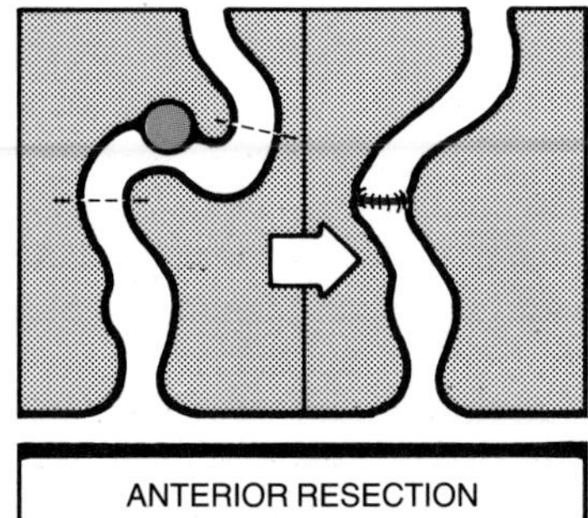

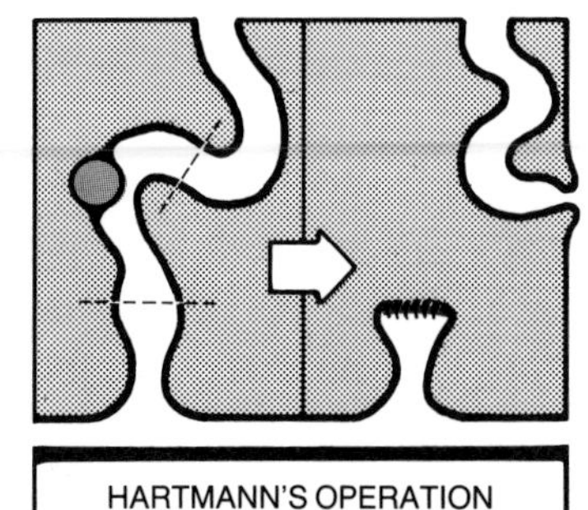

Fig. 15.12 Principles of right hemicolectomy

① Divide lateral peritoneum

② Reflect ascending colon forwards on its mesentery identifying and preserving ureter and retroperitoneal duodenum

③ Select points at which to divide bowel, retaining as much ileum as possible; ensure good blood supply to colon by transilluminating mesocolon, aiming to retain a good vessel close to line of section

④ Divide greater omentum

⑤ Ligate and divide vessels of mesentery

⑥ Anastomose cut ends of ileum and colon

⑦ Repair defect in mesentery

④
⑥ ③
②
⑤
①
⑥

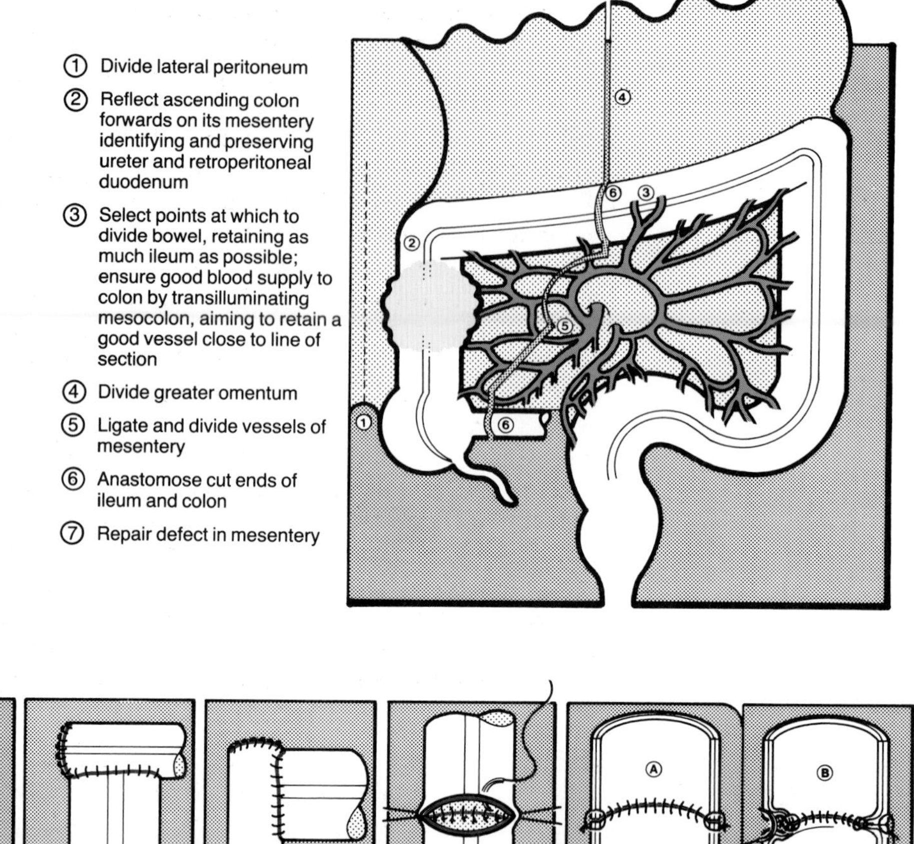

Ⓐ
Ⓑ
① End-to-end anastomosis when bowel ends of similar diameter (usual type)
② End-to-side anastomosis where proximal end is greater in diameter than distal end, e.g. bowel obstruction
③ Side-to-end anastomosis where distal end is greater in diameter than proximal end, e.g. right hemicolectomy
④ Single-layer anastomosis. Often used in rectum. Posterior sutures placed from inside bowel. Sutures include full thickness of bowel wall
⑤ Two-layer anastomosis
First-layer Ⓐ is an 'all-coats' suture.
Second-layer Ⓑ is an inverting layer including only the sero-muscular coat

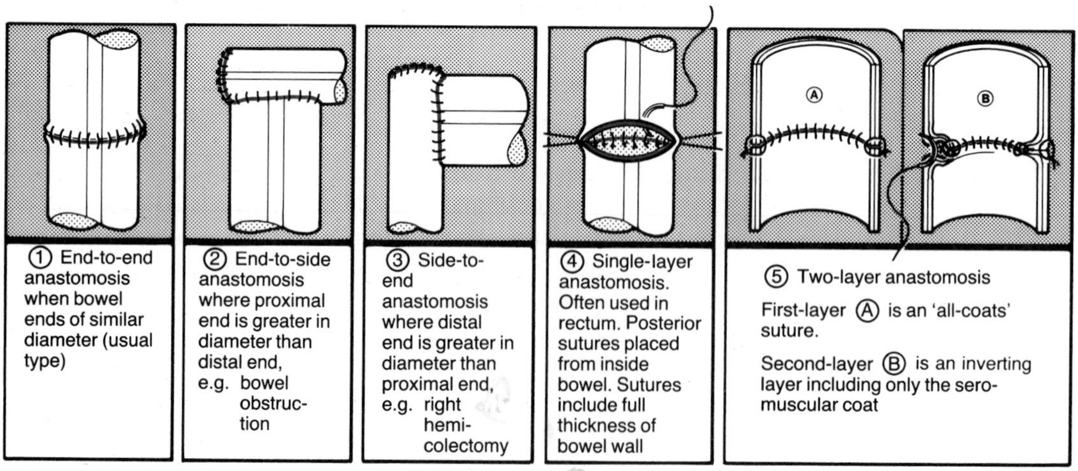

Fig. 15.13 Standard methods of large bowel anastomosis

Management of advanced disease and recurrence

The primary tumour is usually resected to relieve local effects even when distant metastases have been diagnosed. Most of these patients die within a year, and only about one in ten survives two or three years; none survives five years.

The commonest site of distant metastasis is the liver. Liver metastases can be discovered at operation (*synchronous*) or later on ultrasound or CT scanning (*metachronous*). In most cases, there are multiple liver metastases in both lobes by the time of diagnosis, but occasionally a few metastases are confined to a single anatomical lobe. In the latter group, liver resection can sometimes be performed to remove metastatic disease. This offers the only hope of cure, but is only appropriate in the tiny proportion of patients who have fewer than two metastases in one lobe of the liver and no cancer elsewhere. The metastases may be excised locally, or the affected liver lobe removed by partial hepatectomy. About 20% of these patients survive 5 years. Liver resections for metastases are rarely performed, however, because few patients fulfil the criteria for operation just described.

Patients with liver metastases seldom become jaundiced, since this only occurs when the parenchyma is almost completely destroyed or major bile ducts are compressed. This is usually a late event and treatment is rarely worthwhile unless gall stones are the cause. Colorectal tumours sometimes metastasise to bone, particularly the lumbar spine, and painful lesions may be palliated by radiotherapy.

Colorectal carcinomas are relatively unresponsive to current chemotherapeutic regimes. Occasionally 5-fluorouracil will control painful liver metastases. Colorectal carcinomas do respond to radiotherapy but its application is limited by the difficulty of directing the radiation beam at the tumour without damaging surrounding bowel. Radiotherapy is useful for palliative treatment of recurrent pelvic cancer following removal of the rectum. This is a common problem and causes intractable perineal pain. Occasionally a fungating mass grows in the anal region or buttocks and this is very distressing.

FAMILIAL POLYPOSIS COLI

Polyposis coli (adenomatous polyposis) is a rare autosomal dominant disorder characterised by multiple tubular adenomatous polyps throughout the colon and rectum. The polyps first develop in adolescence. They are usually asymptomatic but may present with rectal bleeding or change in bowel habit. The polyps are initially benign but malignant change almost invariably occurs in early adulthood, often in more than one polyp at the same time. Patients presenting with this condition should have all their close relatives screened, in adolescence if possible, by sigmoidoscopy and barium enema investigation to detect those affected by polyposis early. Once familial polyposis coli has been diagnosed, the whole colorectal mucosa should be removed. *Pan-proctocolectomy* with ileostomy is the standard treatment. An alternative to ileostomy is the creation of a *Park's pouch*. In this operation, a reservoir of ileum is fashioned in the pelvis and connected to the anus. The anal sphincter mechanism is preserved and thus the patient is usually continent and can control evacuation.

COMPLICATIONS OF LARGE BOWEL SURGERY

Infection arising from faecal contamination is the main early complication of large bowel surgery. Contamination may result from perforation prior to operation, inadvertent faecal spillage during the operation, or anastomotic leak or breakdown postoperatively. Three main types of infection occur: wound infection and dehiscence, intraperitoneal abscess and generalised peritonitis. Large bowel surgery has always been associated with a high risk of infective complications, particularly in emergency operations, but these have been dramatically reduced by preoperative mechanical bowel cleansing and prophylactic antibiotics.

Fig. 15.14 Specific complications of large bowel surgery

Early complications

Wound infections — abscess and cellulitis

Intra-abdominal abscess — at site of surgery, pelvic or subphrenic

Anastomotic leak or breakdown

Inadvertent damage to other organs e.g. ureters, bladder, duodenum or spleen

Stoma problems — sloughing or retraction

Later complications

Diarrhoea — due to short bowel

Division of pelvic parasympathetic nerves — causes impotence

Small bowel obstruction — due to pelvic peritoneal adhesions or tangling of small bowel with colostomy or ileostomy

Bowel cleansing techniques

The objective is to clear the bowel of all faecal material and to reduce the bacterial flora. This is achieved by a combination of the following procedures:

- Withdrawal of solid foods. The patient is limited to fluids or a low fibre diet for a few days preoperatively
- Purgation. This may be with stimulant laxatives (e.g. castor oil, sodium picosulphate) or osmotic laxatives (e.g. magnesium sulphate mixture, mannitol)
- Enemas and distal bowel washouts. Antiseptic agents like povidone iodine may also be used
- 'Bowel sterilisation' with non-absorbed oral antibacterial agents like neomycin. These must be given if mannitol is used, to prevent bacterial fermentation and formation of gases which may explode with diathermy

When there is complete obstruction, only distal washouts and enemas can be given. For incomplete obstruction, purgation must be used with great care to avoid precipitating acute obstruction.

Prophylactic antibiotics

A variety of faecal commensals and other organisms cause abdominal sepsis after large bowel surgery. These include E. coli and the other Enterobacteriaceae (gram negative aerobes), Bacteroides and related organisms (gram negative anaerobes), Staph. aureus (gram positive aerobes), Strep. faecalis (gram positive anaerobic 'enterococci') and the Clostridia (gram positive anaerobes). The antibiotic combination for prophylaxis is chosen to cover the main organisms, and popular regimes are shown in Figure 15.15. It is important to achieve high circulating blood levels at the time of operation, perhaps continuing for 12–24 hours afterwards. The first dose is usually given with the premedication or at anaesthetic induction.

Fig. 15.15 Prophylactic antibiotic regimens for large bowel surgery

Cephalosporin (e.g. cefazolin, cefotaxime) plus metronidazole (i.v. or p.r.)
Gentamicin plus penicillin G plus metronidazole
Ampicillin plus metronidazole
Mezlocillin alone (rarely recommended)

COLONIC ANGIO-DYSPLASIAS

Colonic angiodysplasias have only recently been recognised as a common cause of acute or chronic rectal bleeding and iron deficiency anaemia. They are tiny hamartomatous vascular lesions in the colonic wall and produce bleeding out of proportion to their size. Their origin is unknown but since they occur later in life, they are more likely to be acquired than congenital.

If bleeding is acute and is occurring rapidly, selective mesenteric arteriography may demonstrate the source of bleeding. In chronic or recurrent haemorrhage, the lesions can be visualised by colonoscopy, but are invisible on barium enema. This underlines the importance of thorough colonoscopy in patients with unexplained gastrointestinal blood loss. The lesions can often be treated by electrical coagulation via the colonoscope. If unsuccessful, the affected segment is resected. Similar lesions occur more rarely in the small bowel and bleed in the same way.

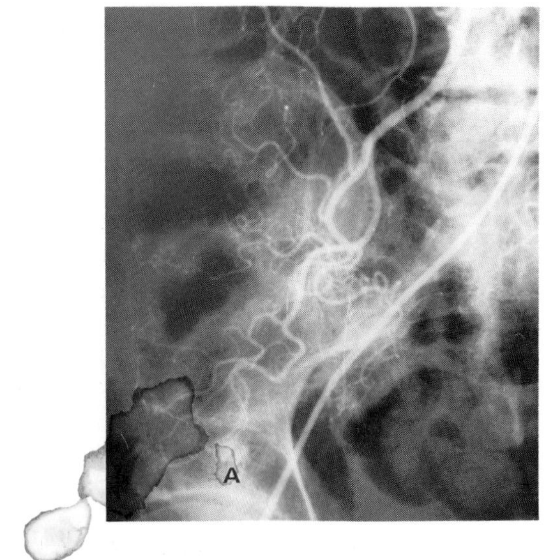

Fig. 15.16 Caecal angiodysplasia

This 63-year-old man had been admitted to hospital on 12 occasions for rectal bleeding or anaemia and received a total of 77 units of blood by transfusion. This selective arteriogram was performed on the most recent admission, and shows an abnormal mass of blood vessels **A** in the caecum typical of angiodysplasia. This part of the bowel was resected and the patient had not re-bled three years later

STOMAS

Indications and general principles

It is often necessary to divert the faecal stream onto the anterior abdominal wall via a stoma. The effluent is collected in a removable plastic bag attached by adhesive to the abdominal skin. Stomas are named according to the part of the bowel opening onto the abdominal wall, i.e. *ileostomy* or *colostomy*. The more distal the location of the original lesion, the more likely is a stoma to be required. The majority of stomas are performed in cancer surgery, although they are sometimes necessary in inflammatory bowel disease and diverticular disease. The indications for stomas and the principles of stoma design and aftercare are similar for all these conditions.

Stomas may be permanent or temporary. Wherever possible, the need for a stoma should be anticipated before operation and discussed with the patient. This is done to ensure that informed consent is obtained and to prepare the patient for what is often perceived as a 'fate worse than death'. In many health districts, specialist 'stoma nurses' are employed to assist in planning and aftercare. Preoperatively, they counsel the patient, who is encouraged to try out a dummy appliance and talk to other stoma patients. The stoma nurse will also identify and mark the most suitable and comfortable site for the stoma appliance. This takes into account the patient's occupation and leisure activities, clothing and ability for self-care.

a. Permanent stomas

This is necessary when there is no distal bowel segment remaining after resection, or for some reason the bowel cannot be rejoined. A colostomy is required after *abdomino-perineal resection* of a low rectal or anal canal tumour. An ileostomy (Figure 15.17) is required after excision of the whole colon and rectum (*pan-proctocolectomy*), unless a pelvic reservoir is constructed. The usual indications are inflammatory bowel disease or familial polyposis coli.

Permanent stomas must be carefully sited to facilitate long-term management. They are usually below the belt line. Permanent colostomies are usually fashioned in the left iliac fossa and ileostomies in the right iliac fossa.

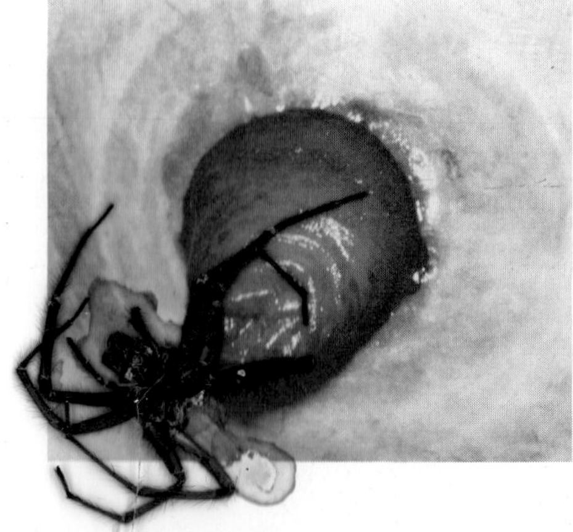

Fig. 15.17 Ileostomy
This ileostomy is in the right iliac fossa in a young man who had a pan-proctocolectomy for ulcerative colitis several years previously. Note the protruding ileostomy spout, fashioned by everting the bowel wall at the time of operation. This allows the effluent to drop directly into the appliance bag without eroding the skin. Note also the impression of the sealing ring around the stoma

b. Temporary stomas

A stoma is often required temporarily to divert the faecal stream away from a more distal part of the bowel. When the distal bowel problem has resolved, the colostomy is closed.

Firstly, a colostomy may be created as an emergency measure to relieve complete distal large bowel obstruction causing proximal dilatation. A particular application is when the ileo-caecal valve has remained competent, resulting in extreme caecal dilatation and imminent rupture. The obstructing lesion may be removed at the same operation or later as an elective procedure.

Secondly, a stoma may be used to protect a more distal anastomosis which is at particular risk of leakage or breakdown. Common examples are: a technically difficult low anastomosis (flatus and faeces may leak), an anastomosis performed after resection of an obstructing lesion (distension may compromise the blood supply), emergency resection involving unprepared bowel (solid faeces in the lumen) or elective surgery where the bowel has not been adequately cleared of faeces.

Thirdly, a temporary colostomy may be used to 'rest' a more distal segment of bowel involved in an inflammatory process such as a pericolic abscess, acute Crohn's disease or a colo-vesical or colo-vaginal fistula.

Types of stoma

The way in which a stoma is fashioned depends on its purpose. The main types of stoma are described below and illustrated in Figure 15.18. Colonic stomas are designed with the bowel mucosa lying flush with the skin. Small bowel stomas are fashioned with a 'spout' of bowel protruding about 5 cm, to ensure that the irritant small bowel contents enter the ileostomy appliance directly rather than flowing onto the skin.

Fig. 15.18 Principal types of ileostomy and colostomy

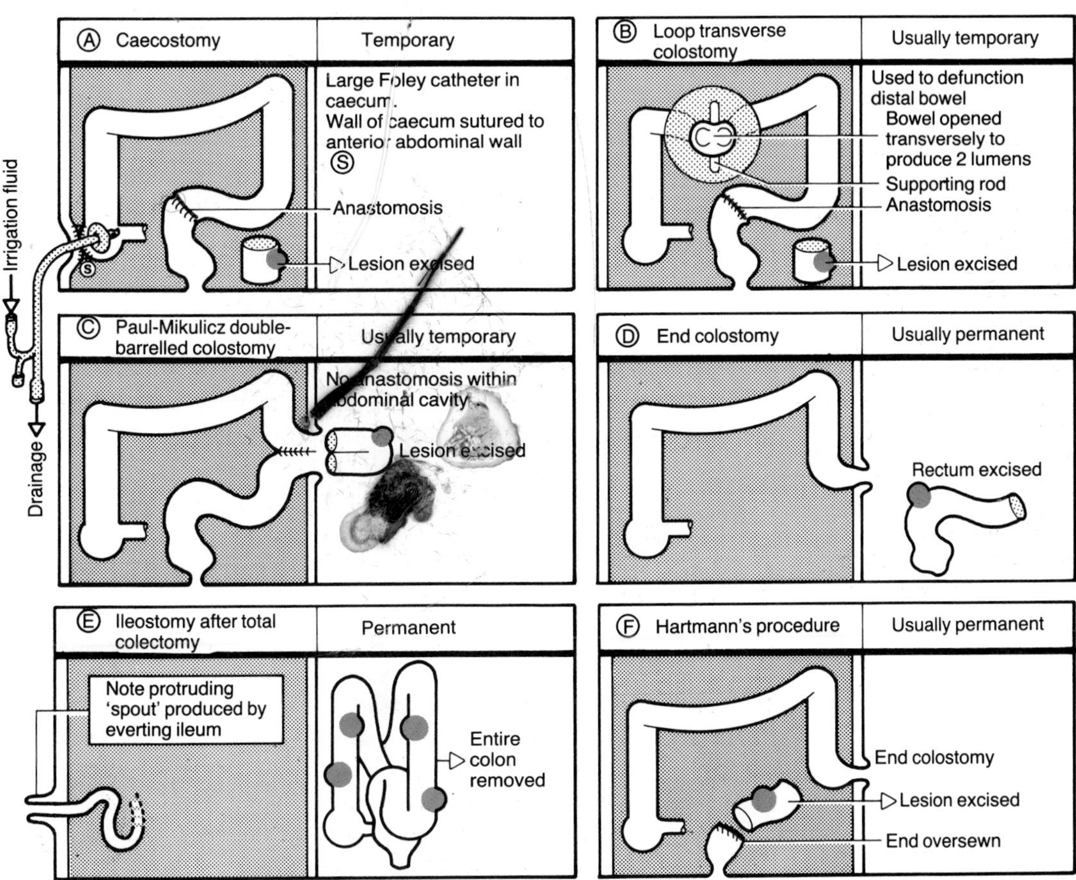

a. Caecostomy

A connection is established between the skin and the caecum and is held open with a large balloon catheter. Its sole function is to decompress the bowel of gas; it is inappropriate for diversion of the faecal stream. Caecostomy is rarely used now because it frequently becomes blocked with faeces and requires regular irrigation to maintain patency.

b. Loop stoma

This type of stoma is designed so that both the proximal and distal segments of bowel drain onto the skin surface. This deflects proximal effluent onto the skin and provides a 'blow-off' valve for the distal loop. Since the distal loop no longer has any functioning capacity, such stomas are often described as 'defunctioning' stomas. They are mainly used as a temporary measure.

A loop of bowel (usually colon) is brought through a single skin aperture and held above the skin surface by a 'bridge' of plastic or a glass rod. An incision is then made in the side of the exteriorised loop which opens both proximal and distal loops. The 'bridge' is usually removed after about a week; this allows overspill of effluent into the distal loop and re-establishes partial function. When the stoma is closed, weeks or months later, the skin and bowel are separated, the bowel incision closed or a section of bowel resected and the loop dropped back into the abdomen. The most common form of loop colostomy is the transverse colostomy, situated in the right upper quadrant.

c. Double ended stoma

This is a variant of the loop stoma and is used if complete and prolonged defunctioning is required. The 'bridge' is fashioned from a pedicle of abdominal wall skin, which remains in place until the stoma is closed.

d. Double stoma

This is the ultimate form of defunctioning stoma. The bowel ends are completely divided. Both proximal and distal ends are brought separately to the skin surface to drain into separate appliances.

e. Single end stoma

This type of stoma is most commonly used to 'resite the anus' onto the abdominal wall. It is a permanent stoma, fashioned after pan-proctocolectomy or removal of the rectum and anal sphincter (i.e. abdomino-perineal resection).

f. Hartmann's procedure

This technique is increasingly used after emergency resection of rectosigmoid lesions where primary anastomosis is inadvisable because of gross inflammation or faecal contamination. Hartmann's procedure may also be used in frail or debilitated patients. The lesion is resected, the proximal loop is made into an end colostomy and the distal remnant closed with sutures or staples. The residual rectum is thus completely defunctioned, but its secretions still pass through the anus. Several months later, when local inflammation has resolved, the bowel may be reconnected. The development of circular stapling instruments has simplified reconnection and is the main reason for the increasing use of Hartmann's operation. The colostomy is identical to the end colostomy following an abdomino-perineal resection. The colostomy is so well tolerated that some patients prefer to keep it permanently rather than undergo another major operation.

The term *double-barrelled colostomy* does not apply to any of those described above, but was applied to the stoma resulting from the old *Paul–Miculicz operation*, now rarely used. This operation enabled safe resection of colonic lesions before the days of modern surgery. At the first operation, the lesion and nearby colon was mobilised so it could be brought completely outside the abdominal wall (exteriorisation). The two limbs of the loop were sutured together for about 10 cm deep to the abdominal wall to resemble a double-barrelled shotgun. After a few days (once it has sealed to the skin), the exteriorised bowel was cut off flush with the skin leaving a double stoma. Later, the spur between the two stomas was crushed using an *enterotome* and the colostomy gradually closed spontaneously.

Fig. 15.19 Complications of ileostomy and colostomy

Early complications

Mucosal sloughing or necrosis of the terminal bowel due to ischaemia — requires reoperation and refashioning of the stoma

Obstruction of stoma due to oedema or faecal impaction — relieved by exploration with a gloved finger and sometimes glycerine suppositories or softening enemas

Persistent leakage between skin and appliance causing skin erosion and patient distress — due to inappropriate location of stoma (e.g. over skin crease). May require resiting operation

Late complications

Prolapse of bowel — requires refashioning of stoma

Parastomal hernia — due to abdominal wall weakness. Requires resiting of stoma

Retraction of a 'spout' ileostomy — requires reoperation and fashioning of a new ileostomy

16 CHRONIC INFLAMMATORY DISORDERS OF THE BOWEL

Introduction

The term *inflammatory bowel disease* is often used to describe two chronic remittent bowel disorders, *ulcerative colitis* and *Crohn's disease*. These share many pathophysiological and clinical features. Both conditions usually present with chronic diarrhoea, but recurrent bouts of abdominal pain are peculiar to Crohn's disease.

Although ulcerative colitis and Crohn's disease are relatively common in developed countries, they must be distinguished from parasitic infestations which produce chronic inflammation of the colon. Infestations, such as *amoebiasis* and *giardiasis*, are much more common in underdeveloped countries or may be contracted on overseas travel; they are described briefly at the end of the chapter. *Antibiotic-associated colitis* and *ischaemic colitis* are also included here.

Drug therapy plays an important part in management of ulcerative colitis and Crohn's disease, and so most patients are initially investigated and treated by physicians. The majority of patients can be managed as outpatients but acute exacerbations or complications may necessitate hospital admission. Surgery is usually indicated when medical management has failed or when complications such as obstruction, haemorrhage or perforation occur.

Epidemiology and aetiology of inflammatory bowel disease

Despite a wealth of studies, epidemiological, clinical and laboratory, the aetiology of the inflammatory bowel diseases remains obscure. Whilst ulcerative colitis and Crohn's disease are considered to be separate disease entities, diagnosis is not always clear-cut. Their clinical and pathological features overlap so much that in 10–15% of cases, clear distinction cannot be made. The diseases may share some aetiological factor or may even represent different facets of the same disease.

Despite problems of accurate diagnosis, epidemiological studies indicate that ulcerative colitis and Crohn's disease are relatively common in the developed communities of Western Europe, North America, Australasia and South Africa. The incidence appears to be much lower in Southern and Eastern Europe and Japan. The diseases are rare in most of Africa, Asia and South America. In the West, the incidence of Crohn's disease appears to have increased over the past 50 years, while ulcerative colitis has remained static or even declined.

Most cases of inflammatory bowel disease develop in the late teens and twenties with little difference between males and females. Social class seems to be irrelevant as does urban versus rural living. In the USA, white people are three times more susceptible to ulcerative colitis than black people and five times more susceptible to Crohn's disease.

Dietary factors, infective agents and autoimmunity have been proposed in the aetiology of inflammatory bowel diseases but none has been clearly implicated; 6–8% of patients with ulcerative colitis and 14–30% of those with Crohn's disease have first degree relatives who have the same condition. There is a high concordance of Crohn's disease in monozygous twins, though this is not so for ulcerative colitis. The conclusion is that both conditions have a polygenetic hereditary predisposition, with the more complete genotype tending to Crohn's disease and the less complete to ulcerative colitis. A genetic link between the two diseases is supported by the association of both conditions with a range of non-gastrointestinal disorders. The most common is ankylosing spondylitis, which is associated with the HLA B27 haplotype.

Infection appears to play a part in some cases of both ulcerative colitis and Crohn's disease as many cases follow an acute attack of gastroenteritis. One strain of E.coli has been implicated in causing an acute colitis very similar to ulcerative colitis, and it seems likely that other organisms, as yet unidentified, may be found responsible for these acute inflammatory disorders.

ULCERATIVE COLITIS

Ulcerative colitis is an inflammatory disorder of the mucosa and submucosa of the large bowel. It is characterised by recurrent acute exacerbations and intervening periods of quiescence or chronic low-grade activity. The severity of symptoms corresponds to the level of disease activity. Systemic features affect a small proportion of patients, and these include anaemia, inflammation of joints (arthropathy) and of the uveal tract of the eye (uveitis and iritis). The disease always involves the rectum but often extends in continuity to involve a variable length of colon. In nearly 20% of all cases (but only those with pancolitis), the distal end of the ileum is secondarily affected; this is described as *backwash ileitis*.

Pathophysiology

Initially, the colonic mucosa becomes acutely inflamed. Neutrophils accumulate in the lamina propria and within the tubular colonic glands to form small, highly characteristic *crypt abscesses*. This is followed by sloughing of the overlying mucosa to produce small superficial ulcers. If the inflammatory process persists, the ulcers coalesce into extensive areas of irregular ulceration. Residual islands of intact but oedematous mucosa project into the bowel lumen; these inflammatory lesions are called *pseudopolyps*. The inflammation is confined to the mucosa and submucosa, only extending into the muscular wall and peritoneal surface in fulminating colitis.

Acute inflammatory episodes range from several days' to several months' duration. After subsiding, they recur months or even years later. During quiescent periods, the acute inflammation resolves and the mucosa regenerates. The lamina propria however, remains swollen by a chronic inflammatory infiltrate of lymphocytes and plasma cells. The colonic glands show a marked reduction in the number of mucin-secreting goblet cells, histologically termed 'goblet cell depletion'.

After the disease has been present for some time, dysplastic changes appear in the epithelium. After prolonged or repeated episodes of inflammation, the epithelium becomes even more dysplastic, and may develop adenocarcinoma. In young patients with total colitis for ten years, the risk of developing carcinoma is about 10%. The diagnosis of cancer may have been delayed if symptoms are mistaken for a relapse of colitis. Tumours in such patients are often particularly aggressive.

In long standing colitis, the mucosa and submucosa undergo fibrosis, resulting in loss of haustration and a shortened colon. This has a characteristic radiological appearance.

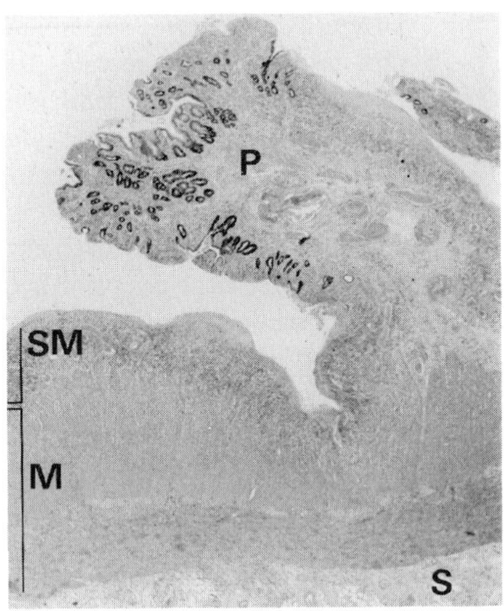

Fig. 16.1 Ulcerative colitis — histopathology

Typical pseudopolyp **P** of ulcerative colitis showing complete loss of mucosa from the surrounding area, leaving bare the underlying submucosa **SM** which is swollen and heavily infiltrated with leucocytes. Note the relatively normal muscular wall **M** and serosa **S**

Clinical features of ulcerative colitis

Acute inflammatory attacks are marked by loose blood-stained stools streaked with mucus. Diarrhoea may be severe, the patient suffering up to 20 loose stools per day, often preceded by cramping abdominal pain. In many patients, the urge to defaecate is so precipitate that incontinence ensues unless a lavatory is immediately available. Fear of incontinence keeps many patients at home and may profoundly limit social life and employment. This, rather than the frequency of defaecation, is the worst handicap in ulcerative colitis.

Any attack of ulcerative colitis may be fulminant, and the patient may become prostrated by dehydration, severe electrolyte disturbance and blood loss. Occasionally, acute inflammation spreads into the muscular bowel wall, paralysing its function and leading to progressive dilatation and eventually patchy necrosis. The patient is systemically ill with high fever, marked tachycardia and dehydration. This process, known as *toxic megacolon*, culminates in perforation and fatal peritonitis unless emergency colectomy is performed.

Fig. 16.2 Systemic manifestations of ulcerative colitis

Weight loss — frequent during exacerbations

Anaemia — typically chronic and non-specific

Elevated ESR — useful measure of disease activity

Arthropathy — sacroileitis/ankylosing spondylitis or rheumatoid-like arthritis, especially of large joints (approximately 20% of cases)

Uveitis and iritis — painful red eye or eyes (approximately 10%)

Skin lesions — erythema nodosum, i.e.tender red nodules on the shins (uncommon), pyoderma gangrenosum, i.e. purulent skin ulcers (rare)

Sclerosing cholangitis — progressive fibrosis of intrahepatic biliary system leading to cirrhosis, progressive liver failure, jaundice and eventually death (rare)

Ulcerative colitis is a systemic disorder sometimes accompanied by one or more non-gastrointestinal manifestations, summarised in Figure 16.2. During active phases of the disease, ESR is elevated and moderate anaemia is common. The anaemia is normochromic and normocytic, described as 'anaemia of chronic disease'. A similar non-specific anaemia is found in other chronic inflammatory disorders like rheumatoid disease. An arthropathy of large joints akin to ankylosing spondylitis or rheumatoid arthritis occurs in up to 20% of patients. Joint involvement does not necessarily occur when the colitis is active and may even precede its initial presentation. Tests for rheumatoid factor in serum are negative. Both ulcerative colitis and Crohn's disease can cause this *seronegative arthropathy*.

Clinical examination and investigation

The typical patient referred for investigation of suspected ulcerative colitis is a young adult who gives a history of several weeks of frequent loose stools, later streaked with blood and mucus. The attack often starts as gastroenteritis or traveller's diarrhoea, but it fails to settle. Careful questioning often elicits a history of similar attacks. There is sometimes a history of associated symptoms like arthropathy or uveitis.

General examination commonly reveals anaemia but abdominal examination is usually unremarkable. Rectal examination, followed by proctoscopy and sigmoidoscopy, is mandatory to palpate, inspect, and if necessary biopsy, the rectal mucosa. Other diseases of the rectum and anus such as carcinoma and benign solitary ulcer must be excluded. Ulcerative colitis always involves the rectum and extends proximally for a variable distance. Thus, diseased bowel is always accessible to sigmoidoscopic diagnosis. The diseased mucosa ranges in appearance from mildly hyperaemic and easily traumatised, to more severe involvement with extensive patchy ulceration. Biopsies should be taken from representative areas. Typically, blood-streaked loose faeces leak down into the lumen during examination.

At least three separate fresh stool samples should be microscoped and cultured to exclude bacterial or parasitic causes of diarrhoea, as these conditions may closely simulate ulcerative colitis.

Contrast radiology in suspected ulcerative colitis

If the clinical picture and histological findings are consistent with inflammatory bowel disease, the extent and degree of colonic involvement are assessed by barium enema examination. Radiological appearances are illustrated in Figure 16.3.

Flexible endoscopy

Colonoscopy, using flexible fibre-optic endoscopes up to 180 cm long, enables direct inspection of the entire colonic mucosa and the taking of multiple biopsies. It is a useful adjunct to radiological examination and permits excision or biopsy of polyps or other suspicious lesions (e.g. inflammatory pseudopolyps) to exclude malignancy. Furthermore, colonoscopy is used for periodic surveillance for dysplastic change in patients with long-standing total colitis, who have an increased risk of developing carcinoma.

Proctitis

In ulcerative colitis, the mucosal abnormality usually extends beyond the reach of the sigmoidoscope. Some patients with colitic symptoms however, have inflammation confined to the lower rectum. The mucosa often has a granular appearance and the condition is described as *proctitis* or *granular proctitis*. Its cause is unknown and its course self-limiting, though it tends to recur at times of stress, often at protracted intervals. Proctitis usually responds to short courses of local corticosteroid therapy. It is probably pathologically distinct from ulcerative colitis and does not precede it clinically. Barium enema is required if lesions higher up the colon such as carcinoma or Crohn's disease cannot be excluded on clinical grounds.

Fulminant ulcerative colitis

Attacks of ulcerative colitis may sometimes be fulminant, with extremely frequent watery, blood-stained stools and systemic illness. The attack may progress to perforation, even in the absence of toxic dilatation of the colon, and an urgent colectomy may be necessary in anticipation of this. Fulminant bloody diarrhoea with prostration, similar to a severe attack of ulcerative colitis, may also occur in infective colitis, e.g. salmonella, cholera or amoebiasis, and such diagnoses should be excluded by microbiological examination of the stool.

Whatever the cause, patients with acute colitis require urgent hospital admission and resuscitation including fluid, electrolyte and blood replacement. Sigmoidoscopy and biopsy are performed to establish the diagnosis. Plain abdominal radiography is performed to look for colonic dilatation as occurs in toxic megacolon. This tends to be greatest in the transverse colon and a diameter exceeding 6 cm indicates imminent perforation. In the absence of megacolon, plain radiography may demonstrate other features of acute ulcerative colitis, as shown in Figure 16.4. An urgent barium enema may be performed without bowel preparation ('instant enema') if diagnosis is in doubt and there is no evidence of toxic dilatation on plain film. Colonoscopy is rarely indicated in such fulminant cases and carries the risk of perforation.

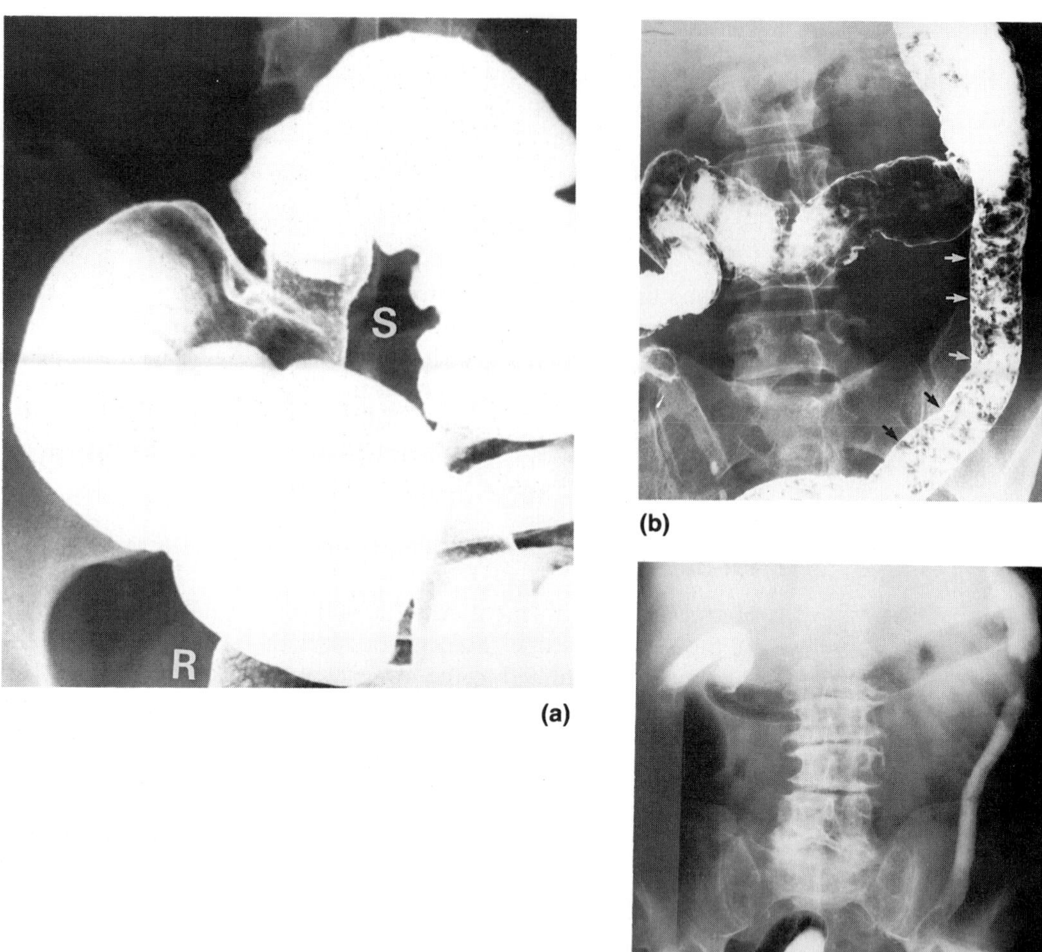

Fig. 16.3 Radiological appearances of ulcerative colitis

(a) This 35-year-old woman presented with a three month history of blood-streaked diarrhoea and the passage of mucus per rectum. Sigmoidoscopy showed marked superficial ulceration and biopsy confirmed ulcerative colitis. This barium enema showed extensive ulceration of the rectum **R** and lower sigmoid colon **S**, although this is a subtle sign. It is shown here only by fuzziness of the bowel wall caused by barium filling the mucosal ulcer craters. The rest of the colon was normal. Ulcerative colitis always affects the rectum and a variable amount of colon proximal to that, but always in continuity. **(b)** Severe and long standing ulcerative colitis in a man of 50. The whole colon is affected (pan-colitis) with loss of the normal haustral pattern. There is extensive pseudopolyp formation, particularly in the descending and sigmoid colon, manifest by multiple small filling defects. Prolonged severe ulceration stimulates mitotic activity and is probably responsible for dysplastic changes and eventual malignant change that may occur in long-standing severe ulcerative colitis. **(c)** 'End-stage' or 'burnt out' ulcerative colitis in a 70-year-old farmer. He had suffered episodic, but not incapacitating, diarrhoea for 34 years, but presented on this occasion because of urgency and incontinence. Sigmoidoscopy showed only moderate rectal ulceration. This barium enema shows a typical smooth, shortened 'lead pipe' colon, with complete loss of haustration. The apparent stricture below the splenic flexure is an underfilling artefact. He failed to respond to medical treatment and underwent pan-proctocolectomy and ileostomy

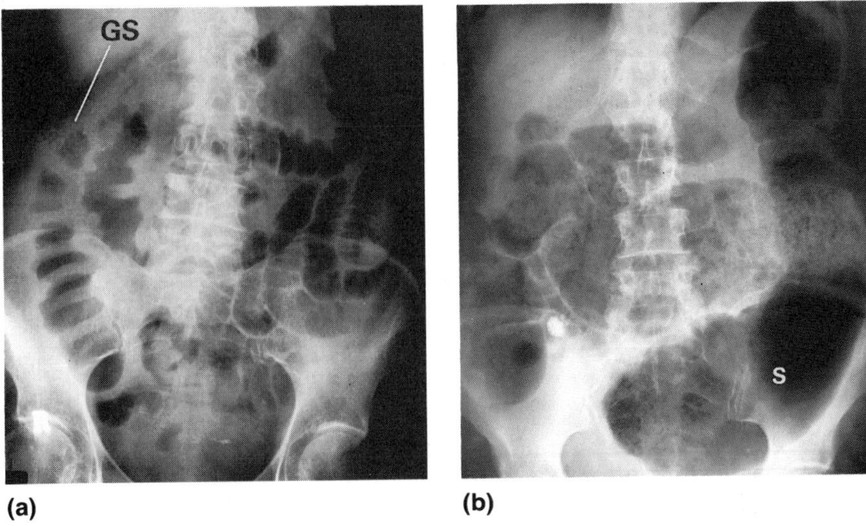

Fig. 16.4 Acute ulcerative colitis and toxic megacolon (**GS** = gallstones)

(a) This 44-year-old woman presented with fulminant ulcerative colitis. She was prostrated by frequent diarrhoea and consequent electrolyte abnormalities. This plain supine radiograph shows acute right-sided colitis. The caecum, ascending colon and proximal transverse colon are affected. In this area, there is absence of the normal 'convex outward' pattern and there are thick folds crossing the bowel lumen. This appearance is caused by oedema of the bowel wall. **(b)** This patient presented in a similar way but became toxic while in hospital undergoing intensive medical treatment. There was an increasing tachycardia and fever, and abdominal tenderness. Serial plain abdominal radiographs showed an increasing diameter of the left colon. This film shows the sigmoid colon **S** dilated to 10-cm and in imminent danger of perforation. This is known as *toxic dilatation of the colon*; it occurs most commonly in ulcerative colitis and usually affects the transverse colon

Management of ulcerative colitis

The management of ulcerative colitis not only varies from patient to patient but also from episode to episode. The choice of treatment depends on the severity of individual attacks, the amount of colon involved, the extent of chronic symptoms, and the risk of long-term complications. The treatment options for ulcerative colitis are summarised in Figure 16.5.

Fig. 16.5 Main treatment measures for ulcerative colitis

Local corticosteroid preparations (e.g. prednisolone suppositories and enemas, hydrocortisone foam) — employed in all cases of active disease

Systemic corticosteroids — suppress moderate or severe exacerbations (oral or intravenous administration according to severity of disease)

Oral (or sometimes rectal) sulphasalazine — long-term maintenance therapy to minimise relapse

Surgical removal of the colon
- emergency operation: incipient or actual perforation, serious haemorrhage, failure to improve on medical treatment
- elective operation: failure of medical treatment, risk of malignancy

a. Steroids

Mild to moderate attacks can usually be controlled with locally-active rectal steroid preparations once or twice daily. This may be in the form of prednisolone enemas or hydrocortisone foam. Steroid foam is more easily retained and just as effective as steroid enemas. Short courses of high dose oral corticosteroids are used for more severe exacerbations (e.g. prednisolone 60 mg daily for two weeks, phased out over the next month). Intravenous administration is advisable in seriously ill patients. There is no evidence that 'bowel rest' (i.e. nil-by-mouth) and total parenteral nutrition (TPN) is of any value in ulcerative colitis. Immunosuppressive drugs, especially azathioprine, are occasionally tried in patients who fail to respond to corticosteroids.

b. Sulphasalazine

Sulphasalazine, usually given orally, is a combination of a sulphonamide and aminosalicylic acid. It dissociates in the large bowel to release aminosalicylic acid, which is the therapeutic agent. The drug is widely used for long-term disease control and substantially reduces the severity and frequency of attacks. Sulphasalazine is usually well tolerated but may cause nausea and vomiting, allergic manifestations such as skin rashes or rarely, serious blood dyscrasias. Temporary infertility may be a problem in males. Rectal preparations of sulphasalazine are available but offer no therapeutic advantage.

c. Other supportive measures

Anti-diarrhoeal agents such as codeine phosphate or loperamide and bulking agents like methylcellulose may help to reduce stool frequency.

Patients with moderately severe, chronic disease frequently become anaemic and lose weight, in part because of persistent loss of protein in the stool. These problems may be helped by medical treatment, a high calorie, high protein diet, and oral iron supplements.

d. Surgery in ulcerative colitis

Surgery is required in only about 20% of patients with ulcerative colitis. Urgent colectomy may be required in fulminant cases which fail to respond to intensive medical treatment or which progress to toxic megacolon, perforation or haemorrhage. Another indication for surgery is the patient with chronic disabling symptoms. These include intractable diarrhoea with urgency, recurring anaemia, failure to maintain adequate weight and nutrition, and in children, failure to thrive and growth retardation (which are aggravated by steroid therapy). Finally, colectomy is advisable to pre-empt malignant change, especially if there is biopsy evidence of dysplasia. This applies mainly in total colitis, the risk being greatest in long-standing persistent disease, particularly when it has started in childhood.

As a general principle, surgery for ulcerative colitis requires removal of the entire large bowel and is thus, by definition, curative. *Pan-proctocolectomy* is the standard operation but the patient is left with a permanent ileostomy. Not only is this psychologically distressing, especially for a young person, but there is also a risk of permanent surgical damage to the pelvic autonomic nerves causing male impotence.

In recent years, sphincter preserving operations have been introduced by which a permanent ileostomy can be avoided and continence preserved. Their advantages may result in a wider role for surgery in the future. The favoured operations at present are versions of *Parks' pouch*. In this operation, the short rectal stump remaining after total colectomy is first stripped of mucosa. Then a reservoir is fashioned from several loops of terminal ileum. The outlet of the reservoir is brought down through the denuded rectal stump and anastomosed to the anal margin. The most refined techniques give total continence and allow bowel evacuation in the normal way.

CROHN'S DISEASE

Crohn's disease is a chronic relapsing inflammatory disorder of the gastrointestinal tract. It potentially affects any part of the tract, but usually affects the small bowel, the large bowel or both together. In contrast to ulcerative colitis, the inflammation involves the whole thickness of the bowel wall. The disease may affect one or more discrete segments of the bowel *('skip lesions')* with intervening parts of the bowel completely spared.

The terminal ileum is most commonly affected; in up to half of all cases, the disease is confined to the terminal ileum. When Dr Crohn first described the condition in 1932, he thought it only affected the terminal ileum, hence the original name 'terminal ileitis'. Later, it became clear that other segments of the bowel could also be affected. The ensuing name, *regional enteritis*, is still widely used in the USA. The large bowel is affected in at least 25% of cases, either alone or in association with disease elsewhere in the gastrointestinal tract. Crohn's disease may also affect the perianal region, whether or not the large bowel is involved. Occasionally, the disease involves the stomach or duodenum; oesophageal and oral involvement have also been reported. With each exacerbation, old or new areas may become involved. The disease tends to run a protracted but unpredictable course.

Pathophysiology and clinical consequences

The essential pathological feature of Crohn's disease is chronic inflammation in the affected segment, which extends diffusely through the entire thickness of the bowel wall. The wall becomes grossly thickened by inflammatory oedema, especially in the submucosa. The epithelium remains largely intact but is criss-crossed by deep *fissured ulcers*. These ulcers, and the intervening areas of dome-shaped mucosa and submucosa, give a typical 'cobblestone' surface appearance.

Granulomas containing multinucleate giant cells are usually scattered throughout the inflamed bowel wall as well as in local lymph nodes. Although granulomata are diagnostic of Crohn's disease, they are not always found. Longstanding inflammation leads to progressive fibrosis of the thickened bowel wall, which encroaches on the lumen, producing elongated strictures.

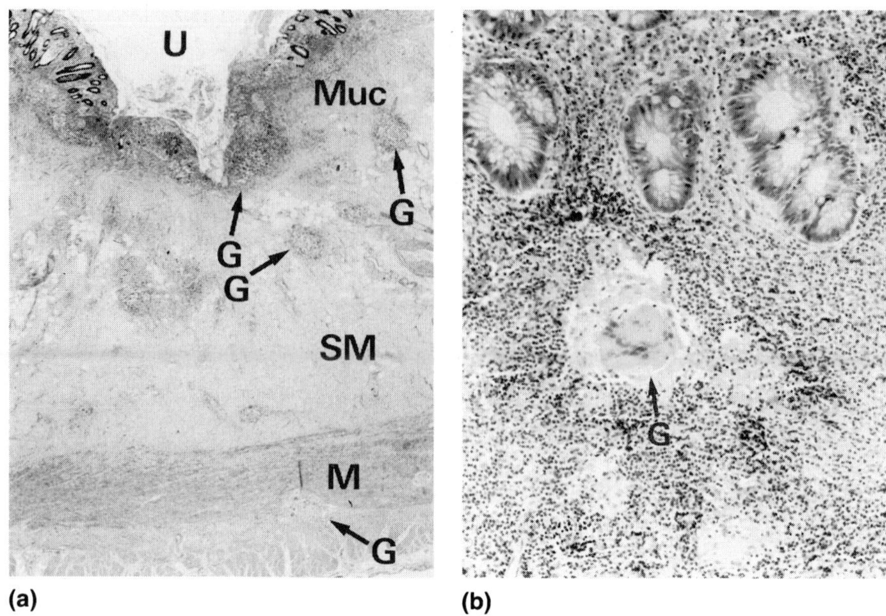

Fig. 16.6 Crohn's disease — histopathology

(a) Specimen of resected bowel from a 36-year-old woman showing a typical fissured ulcer **U** and several granulomas **G** scattered at various levels through the mucosa **Muc**, the markedly swollen submucosa **SM** and muscular wall **M**.
(b) Rectal biopsy specimen from a 27-year-old man with intermittent diarrhoea and anaemia; it shows marked mucosal inflammation and a small granuloma **G** containing multinucleate giant cells, thus enabling a diagnosis of Crohn's disease to be made

a. Effects of mucosal inflammation

Mucosal inflammation causes diarrhoea which may be streaked with mucus and blood if the colon is involved. The luminal narrowing results in partial obstruction which causes abdominal pain. This is usually grumbling and colicky, but there may be acute episodes of more severe pain and vomiting which precipitate hospital admission. Pain is a prominent feature in Crohn's disease, in contrast to ulcerative colitis, whereas bowel symptoms are less debilitating.

If the small bowel is inflamed, digestive and absorptive functions may be affected. Extensive disease results in a general malabsorption causing protein-calorie malnutrition, iron and folate deficiency, anaemia and diarrhoea. In children, Crohn's disease may cause marked growth retardation. Ileal inflammation disrupts bile salt reabsorption. Excess bile salts in the faeces cause colonic irritation (and more diarrhoea) while diminished recirculation of bile salts may result in gall stone formation. Terminal ileal involvement may also reduce vitamin B_{12} absorption, but serious deficiency usually only occurs after surgical resection.

b. Effects of transmural inflammation

Crohn's disease involves the full thickness of the bowel wall, and additional problems result if serosal inflammation extends to adjacent structures. If inflamed bowel impinges on the parietal peritoneum, pain becomes localised and more severe, and signs of local peritonitis develop. Indeed, Crohn's disease affecting the terminal ileum may simulate acute appendicitis. If the patient is operated upon, the appendix may be normal but the terminal ileum is inflamed and the bowel wall abnormally thick to palpation. Alternatively, the appendix and caecum may also be inflamed. The diagnosis of Crohn's disease can be made if other 'skip lesions' are found in the small bowel, if typical histological changes are found in excised mesenteric lymph nodes or if postoperative small bowel barium studies show characteristic lesions. Yersinia ileitis has a similar clinical presentation but the disease is acute, completely reversible and confined to the terminal ileum.

Fulminant colonic Crohn's disease occasionally results in toxic dilatation, clinically identical to ulcerative colitis, but this presentation is rare.

Serosal inflammation may cause a segment of diseased bowel to adhere to nearby abdominal structures. If these become matted together by the inflammatory process, several complications may occur. Firstly, tough, fibrotic post-inflammatory adhesions may form. These are rarely symptomatic, but constitute a formidable obstacle if operation is needed later. Secondly, the bowel may perforate causing localised abscess formation (pericolic or pelvic); free perforation is rare. Thirdly, fistulae may develop between diseased bowel and other hollow viscera causing unusual clinical phenomena. For example, a gastro-colic fistula may result in faecal vomiting, an ileorectal fistula may aggravate diarrhoea. Entero-vesical fistulae cause severe urinary tract infections and pneumaturia (passage of 'soda-water' urine), and fistulae between bowel and uterus or vagina leads to vaginal passage of faeces. Entero-cutaneous fistulae between bowel and skin occasionally develop as a complication of bowel resection for Crohn's disease.

c. *Perianal inflammation*

Perianal inflammation is common in Crohn's disease. Symptoms include recurrent perianal abscesses, characteristic blueish, boggy 'piles' and antero-lateral anal fissures. The last two are quite distinct from ordinary haemorrhoids and posterior anal fissures. Multiple fistulae commonly develop between rectum and perianal skin. These are sometimes so numerous as to cause a 'pepper pot'

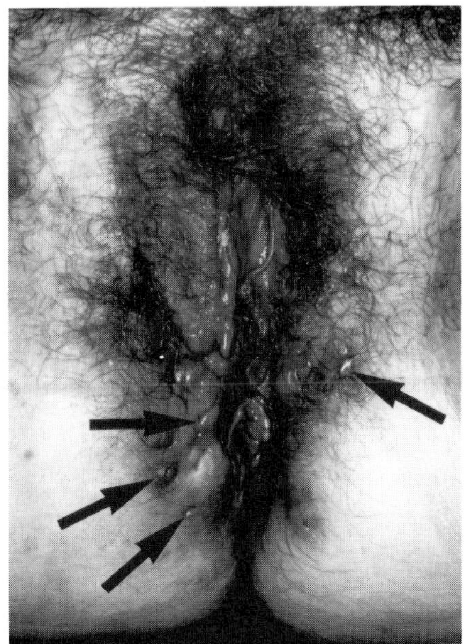

Fig. 16.7 Multiple anal fistulae in Crohn's disease

This 30-year-old woman had several 'skip lesions' of Crohn's disease in her small bowel and was troubled by recurrent perianal sepsis. This photograph shows a typical 'pepper-pot perineum', with several fistulous openings (arrowed) seen around the circumference of the anus. Anal skin tags are also visible

or 'watering can' perineum. Paradoxically, this is more often associated with small bowel disease than colorectal disease.

d. Systemic features

Like ulcerative colitis, Crohn's disease is a systemic disorder and has a similar range of non-gastrointestinal manifestations (see Figure 16.2, earlier). These are relatively uncommon and not necessarily related to disease activity in the gut. Nevertheless, exacerbations of Crohn's disease are commonly accompanied by a general feeling of ill-health which may be as distressing as the bowel symptoms. This feature is much less common in ulcerative colitis.

Clinical examination

Crohn's disease symptoms are often similar to ulcerative colitis, especially when large bowel is involved. Nevertheless, abdominal pain, weight loss and general malaise are more typical of Crohn's disease. Diarrhoea is usually less distressing and less likely to contain blood.

Physical examination may reveal generalised wasting and anaemia and sometimes other features like arthropathy. On abdominal examination, there may be areas of tenderness, an inflammatory mass or the scars of previous surgery. The perianal skin should be examined for fissures, fistulae, Crohn's 'piles' (Figure 16.8) or scarring from previous disease. Diseased rectal mucosa, with its typical firm surface nodularity may be felt on digital examination. Previous anal disease may be manifest by stenotic scarring. Sigmoidoscopy is usually normal but there may be mucosal oedema if the rectum is involved. In more severe cases, the typical 'cobblestone' appearance with fissured ulceration may be seen. Biopsies may be positive even when the mucosa is apparently normal.

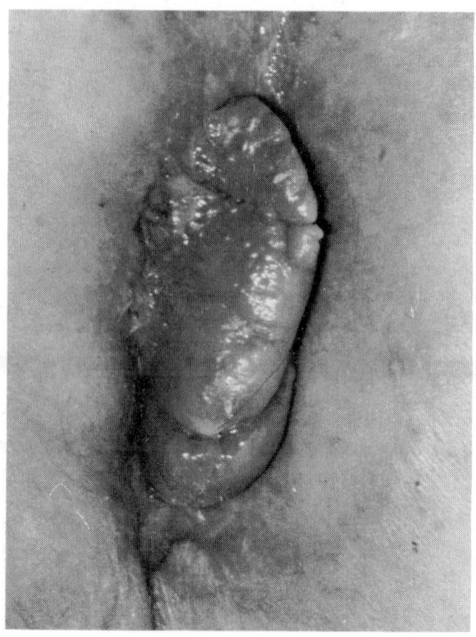

Fig. 16.8 Crohn's 'piles'

This appearance is typical of Crohn's 'piles'. They are pale and oedematous in contrast to ordinary haemorrhoids

Approach to investigation

Investigation of suspected Crohn's disease is similar to ulcerative colitis in respect of the large bowel, but follows a different pattern when there is small bowel disease.

Isotope scanning using radioactive Indium-labelled white blood cells is useful as an initial assessment of the extent of disease and indicates which parts of the bowel to examine radiologically. Abnormalities on barium enema may be difficult or impossible to distinguish from ulcerative colitis. The definitive diagnosis in these patients may depend on histological examination of a surgical specimen or a clinical course characteristic of Crohn's disease.

Barium 'follow-through' is the traditional method of examining the small bowel but is being supplanted by 'small bowel enema'; the latter, despite its name, is performed via the oral route, and involves the controlled instillation of barium into the duodenum through a nasogastric tube. Typical radiological appearances of Crohn's disease include narrowing of the lumen due to mural oedema and fibrosis, nodularity and cobblestoning of the mucosal surface, deep fissured ulceration extending into the muscular wall, spiky 'rose thorn' ulcers and possibly evidence of fistula formation. Radiological changes in small and large bowel are shown in Figure 16.9. Colonoscopy may enable a histological diagnosis to be obtained in colonic disease.

Management of Crohn's disease

Drug therapy for Crohn's disease is empirical and employs a similar range of drugs as for ulcerative colitis. Drug treatment for acute attacks is often effective but there is no maintenance therapy of proven value, although dietary modification (see below) shows some promise in this respect.

Topical steroid enemas and foams are of some benefit in acute distal colonic disease but have little value in perianal disease. In the latter case, secondary bacterial infection is probably responsible for much of the pain and purulent discharge. Treatment with oral metronidazole for one to two months often helps to alleviate symptoms.

High-dose oral corticosteroids (30–60 mg daily for several weeks) are used for acute attacks of Crohn's disease to induce remission. They are less successful than in ulcerative colitis and have no place in long-term maintenance therapy. Immunosuppressive drugs, e.g. azathioprine are occasionally used as steroid-sparing agents for intractable cases that are unsuitable for surgery. Elemental diets, supplying all nutritional requirements in a simple molecular form that can be absorbed from the proximal small bowel, are probably as effective as corticosteroids in inducing remission, but this has not yet been proved by a clinical trial. *Elemental diets* are unpalatable and expensive, and are chiefly indicated in patients with extensive small bowel disease or entero-cutaneous fistulae. Total parenteral nutrition and complete bowel rest (i.e. nil by mouth) can induce remission in acute Crohn's disease, in contrast to its lack of success in ulcerative colitis.

Dietary modification is in vogue for the long term management of Crohn's disease, in the hope of preventing acute exacerbations and avoiding the need for surgery. There is some evidence that food intolerance plays a part in provoking acute attacks. If the offending foods can be identified and avoided,

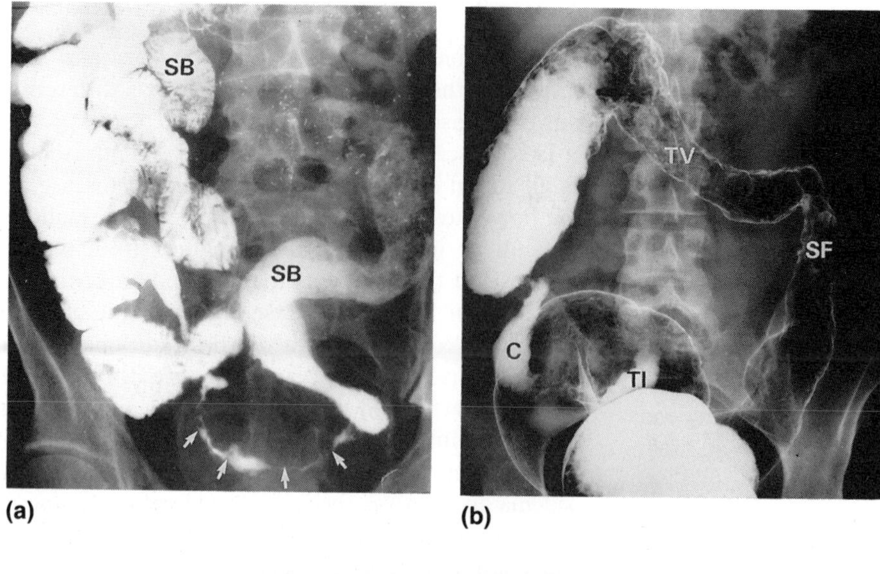

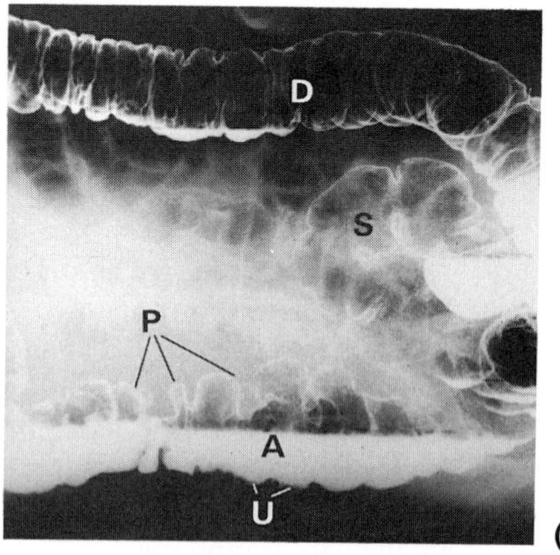

Fig. 16.9 Crohn's disease

(a) This man of 51 had recurrent attacks of colicky abdominal pain, with diarrhoea and loss of weight. This barium follow-through examination shows one of the characteristic radiological appearances of Crohn's disease. The terminal ileum is extremely narrowed by inflammation of the whole wall thickness (arrowed); this is known as the *string sign of Kantor*. This causes the symptoms and signs of partial obstruction. This film also shows dilatation of small bowel **SB** proximal to the stricture. **(b)** This man of 48 presented with eight months of diarrhoea and feeling generally unwell. The barium enema shows Crohn's disease of the terminal ileum **TI**, caecum **C**, transverse colon **TV** and splenic flexure **SF**. The descending colon and sigmoid are normal. Here, the features of Crohn's disease are discontinuous *skip lesions* with normal bowel between, a ragged luminal outline due to ulceration, and loss of haustration. **(c)** Decubitus view during barium enema (left-side up) showing Crohn's disease in the ascending colon **A** with a normal descending colon **D** and sigmoid **S** (the transverse colon is not included on the film). In the original film, in single contrast, the right-hand border of the ascending colon showed fine spiky 'rose-thorn' ulcers **U** whilst the left-hand border shows typical pseudo-diverticula **P** caused by fibrotic stricturing

there is less likelihood of an operation being necessary. An *exclusion diet* is developed by starting with an elemental diet and gradually introducing different categories of food at intervals until reactions are provoked. Such foods are excluded in the future.

Sulphasalazine does not reduce the rate of relapse but occasionally produces a response in severe colonic disease. Anti-diarrhoeal drugs and bulk-forming agents may help to control fluid stools and urgency. Supportive treatment is often required for complications such as anaemia and malnutrition.

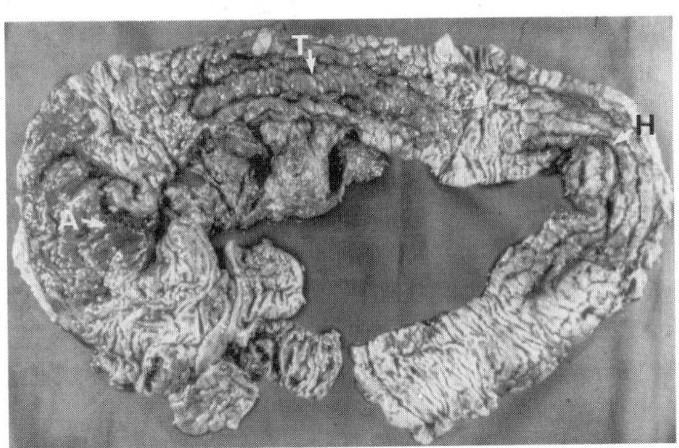

Fig. 16.10 Large bowel affected by Crohn's disease

This sub-total colectomy specimen was removed from a man of 54 with a long history of weight loss, diarrhoea and abdominal pain. There are three 'skip lesions' typical of Crohn's disease, in the ascending colon **A**, the transverse colon **T** and the hepatic flexure **H**

Surgical management of Crohn's disease

Surgery plays a larger part in Crohn's disease than ulcerative colitis but no matter how much bowel is removed, it does not influence subsequent recurrence elsewhere.

The main indications for surgery may be summarised as follows:

- Acute exacerbations unresponsive to steroids
- Acute complications e.g. abscess, perforation, major haemorrhage
- Persistent local ileal disease
- Intolerable long-term symptoms, e.g. abdominal pain, perianal disease, general ill-health
- Entero-cutaneous fistulae and symptomatic internal fistulae

The choice of operation depends on the site and extent of disease. Surgery for small bowel disease is limited to resection of the diseased segment with a small margin of normal tissue, followed by end-to-end anastomosis. If ileal Crohn's disease is a chance finding at appendicectomy, the affected segment is best left alone. For large bowel disease, the entire colon is generally removed (panproctocolectomy with ileostomy). This is because there are usually several colonic 'skip lesions' and recurrence is likely. A blind rectal stump may be left in situ if unaffected by disease in order to reduce the extent of the operation.

Recurrent disease often necessitates further surgery. Abscesses are usually treated by simple drainage with resection of the affected bowel at the same time or later. Fistulae between abdominal viscera are treated by removal of the diseased bowel. In contrast, entero-cutaneous fistulae, usually a complication of recent surgery, are a more formidable problem since they are often associated with complicating factors like intra-abdominal sepsis and septicaemia, gross fluid and electrolyte abnormalities, and a hypercatabolic state. Patients with entero-cutaneous fistulae require intensive medical care and strategic surgical intervention before definitive treatment of the fistula is possible.

Until recently, bypass operations were commonly performed, leaving inflamed segments of bowel in situ. The rationale was that diseased bowel would heal once 'rested'. The results and complications, including blind loop syndromes, were much worse than for resection and the technique has therefore been abandoned.

Fig. 16.11 Comparative features of ulcerative colitis and Crohn's disease

PATHOLOGY	ULCERATIVE COLITIS	CROHN'S DISEASE
Inflammation	Recurrent acute inflammation with intervening quiescent phases	Chronic relapsing inflammation
General distribution	Continuous involvement of affected part of colon	Skip lesions in any part of GI tract
Rectal involvement	Always	About 25%
Ileal involvement	Backwash ileitis only	Involved in 80% of cases; exclusive to ileum in 50% of cases
Depth of wall involved	Mucosa only	Transmural, including serosa
Mucosal changes	Widespread irregular superficial ulceration with or without pseudopolyps	Fissured ulceration causing 'cobblestone' appearance
Granuloma formation	Absent	Characteristic but not always present
Mesenteric adenopathy	Reactive hyperplasia only	Lymph nodes often enlarged; granulomata may be present
Fibrosis of wall	Minimal	Marked

MAIN CLINICAL FEATURES		
Diarrhoea	Severe during acute attacks, often causing incontinence	Less prominent
Rectal bleeding	Very common	Less common
Abdominal pain	Mild cramping 'pre-defaecation' pain with diarrhoeal attacks	Dominant feature — persistent or grumbling pain with severe acute attacks
Abdominal mass	Very rare	Relatively common
General debility	Unusual	Characteristic
COMPLICATIONS		
Strictures	Rare	Common and often multiple
Fistulae	Rare	Common
Anal and perianal lesions	Uncommon	Common
Massive haemorrhage	Occurs in fulminant disease	Rare
Intestinal obstruction	Rare	Incomplete obstruction Common
Perforation	Complication of toxic megacolon	Free perforation rare but perforation causing local abscess formation or internal fistula common
Toxic megacolon	May occur in fulminant attacks	Rare
Malignant change	High risk	Low risk
MANAGEMENT		
Local steroids	All active disease	Less effective
Systemic steroids	Severe exacerbations	Severe exacerbations
Sulphasalazine	Long term maintenance	Generally ineffective
Exclusion diets	No value	Promising — undergoing clinical trials
Immunosuppressives	Occasionally in intractable cases — 'steroid sparing'	In desperation — rarely effective
Surgery	Uncommon — usually in long–standing disease to prevent malignancy or in fulminant colitis	Commonly required

OTHER CHRONIC INFLAMMATIONS OF THE COLON

AMOEBIC COLITIS

Entamoeba histolytica is a protozoon parasite responsible for amoebic colitis. It is an endemic bowel commensal in many underdeveloped countries, but is also found in a few people in developed countries. Most of those infected have no symptoms but they are all carriers. Less than 5% of those infected suffer amoebic colitis. In these, the organism invades the large bowel mucosa, causing chronic relapsing symptoms similar to ulcerative colitis or Crohn's disease. Encysted parasites are shed by carriers in their faeces. Infection is readily transmitted to new individuals via contaminated hands or uncooked food.

The incidence of amoebiasis is likely to increase in the West as tourism expands into endemic areas. If sufferers are mistakenly treated with systemic steroids for inflammatory bowel disease, the result may be fatal.

Pathology

Initial penetration of bowel mucosa by the parasite causes small surface erosions. Lateral spread from the depths of the crypts produces flask-shaped mucosal ulcers. These are multiple and discrete and characteristic of amoebic colitis. Amoebae can often be seen near the edge of ulcers on standard histological preparations, but can best be demonstrated when stained magenta by the Periodic acid-Schiff method. Mucosa between the ulcers is remarkably normal. Large granulomatous colonic lesions also occur. These are known as *amoebomas*.

Occasionally, rampant invasion causes widespread mucosal sloughing and muscle wall involvement. This progresses to local perforation and a pericolic abscess, or toxic megacolon leading to massive perforation and generalised peritonitis.

In any case of amoebic colitis, amoebae passing to the liver in the portal veins may occasionally produce *hepatic abscesses*. These are usually solitary and are filled with reddish-brown necrotic material, said to resemble anchovy sauce.

Clinical features of amoebic colitis

The disease usually affects the proximal colon, causing colicky abdominal pain, erratic bowel habit with episodes of blood-stained loose stools, and right iliac fossa tenderness. If the distal colon is involved, the patient suffers chronic watery diarrhoea with blood and mucus. When the entire colon is involved, there is generalised abdominal tenderness as well as systemic features like pyrexia and progressive weight loss. A large amoeboma may be palpable and must be differentiated from carcinoma or diverticular disease.

If the patient develops an amoebic liver abscess, systemic features become more marked, with general ill-health and a swinging pyrexia with sweating attacks. There is pain in the liver area and an enlarged tender liver on palpation. The abscess may rupture spontaneously into the peritoneal cavity (causing peritonitis) or through the diaphragm into the chest. Secondary lung abscesses may then rupture into the bronchi and the patient cough up 'anchovy sauce' sputum.

Diagnosis of amoebiasis

In developed countries, amoebic colitis should always be considered in the differential diagnosis of ulcerative colitis or Crohn's colitis.

Amoebic colitis can be diagnosed on histology of biopsy specimens. Alternatively, parasites containing ingested red cells can be sought in fresh stool specimens or scrapings from bowel lesions; this is diagnostic of invasive amoebiasis. Contrast radiology does not differentiate amoebic colitis from other forms of colitis.

Liver abscesses cause serological tests for amoebiasis to become positive. The lesions are readily demonstrated by hepatic ultrasound and the diagnosis confirmed by needle aspiration.

Treatment of amoebiasis

Metronidazole is the drug treatment of choice, given orally (400 mg, three times daily) or parenterally if disease is severe. When small liver abscesses are present, the dose is doubled and may eliminate them without need for surgery. Emergency surgery is occasionally necessary in fulminating amoebic colitis or less urgently for large liver abscesses.

GIARDIASIS

Giardiasis is caused by the flagellate protozoal parasite *Giardia lamblia*. It is endemic in many underdeveloped countries as well as the USSR and other Eastern European countries. The organism thrives when sanitation is poor and water supplies contaminated. Sporadic outbreaks of Giardiasis sometimes occur in developed countries, but it is most often seen in young travellers returning from long holidays abroad. In a typical attack, explosive foul-smelling diarrhoea continues for several days or a few weeks, settling spontaneously. Less commonly, the disease may take a protracted course, with chronic diarrhoea, abdominal pain and distension. There may also be anorexia, nausea and weight loss.

Diagnosis is made on stool microscopy; at least three samples from different days should be examined to ensure that the parasite is not missed. The disease responds rapidly to oral metronidazole although other antiparasitic drugs may be preferred.

ANTIBIOTIC ASSOCIATED COLITIS

Pathophysiology and clinical features

Colonic inflammation and diarrhoeal illness may be side-effects of almost any antibiotic treatment. The conditions are probably due to selective overgrowth of micro-organisms inhabiting the gut which then produce toxins which cause mucosal damage. The clinical picture may be anything from a mild attack of diarrhoea to profuse, life-threatening, haemorrhagic colitis. Pseudomembranous colitis is a particularly virulent form (see below). Antibiotic associated colitis may develop suddenly or gradually, and occasionally becomes chronic or relapsing.

Surgical patients are most commonly affected in the postoperative period. In the past, *Staphylococcal enterocolitis* was usually blamed, but it has recently been recognised that *Clostridium difficile* is responsible for some of the cases, particularly in pseudomembranous colitis.

If a surgical patient on antibiotics develops diarrhoea which is worse or more prolonged than might be expected after an operation, antibiotic-associated colitis should be suspected. Stool specimens should be examined by microscopy and culture and a sigmoidoscopic inspection and biopsy of the rectum performed. Treatment is based on the results of these tests.

Pseudomembranous colitis

In this condition, a thick fibrinous blanket of 'pseudomembrane' forms on the colonic mucosal surface as a result of intense inflammation. This harbours the proliferating Clostridium difficile, which continues to produce its toxin. The disease was responsible for serious outbreaks of hospital diarrhoea and even death until the organism could be identified and effectively treated with the antibiotic vancomycin. Almost every antibiotic is capable of causing pseudomembranous colitis, although lincomycin and clindamycin have most often been responsible. The affected patient develops worsening and eventually prostrating diarrhoea, which may be lethal in the elderly.

Both the organism and the toxin can be identified in the patient's diarrhoea stool. At the same time, other infective agents which cause diarrhoea are sought by stool microscopy and culture. Treatment includes stopping current antibiotics and giving the patient oral metronidazole. In severe or resistant cases, oral vancomycin is given. This drug is not absorbed and acts locally to penetrate the pseudomembrane.

ISCHAEMIC COLITIS

Ischaemic colitis is a condition of the elderly which usually presents with rectal bleeding. The history is characteristic: there is a bout of cramp-like abdominal

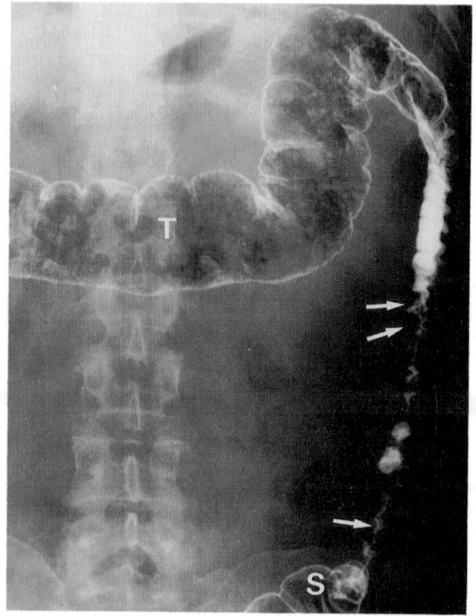

Fig. 16.12 Ischaemic colitis

This 72-year-old man presented with a bout of severe abdominal pain 48 hours before this barium enema was done. Soon after, there was a single episode of fresh rectal bleeding. The film shows typical (though extensive) changes of acute ischaemic colitis, which classically involves the first part of the descending colon. The transverse colon **T** and sigmoid colon **S** are normal. Note extremely narrowed lumen of the ischaemic segment and the characteristic thumb-printing (arrowed) caused by mucosal oedema

pain lasting a few hours, followed by an attack of rectal bleeding. Usually the bleeding is dark red, often without faeces, and occurs one to three times over about 12 hours. The episode then ceases spontaneously. The cause is transient ischaemia of a segment of large bowel, the splenic flexure being most vulnerable. Further attacks occasionally occur but most cases have no further trouble. Investigation in the acute stage by barium enema may reveal colonic oedema in the affected segment (see Figure 16.12). A rare late complication is fibrotic stricturing of the area formerly affected by ischaemia. The differential diagnosis includes acute bleeding from diverticular disease.

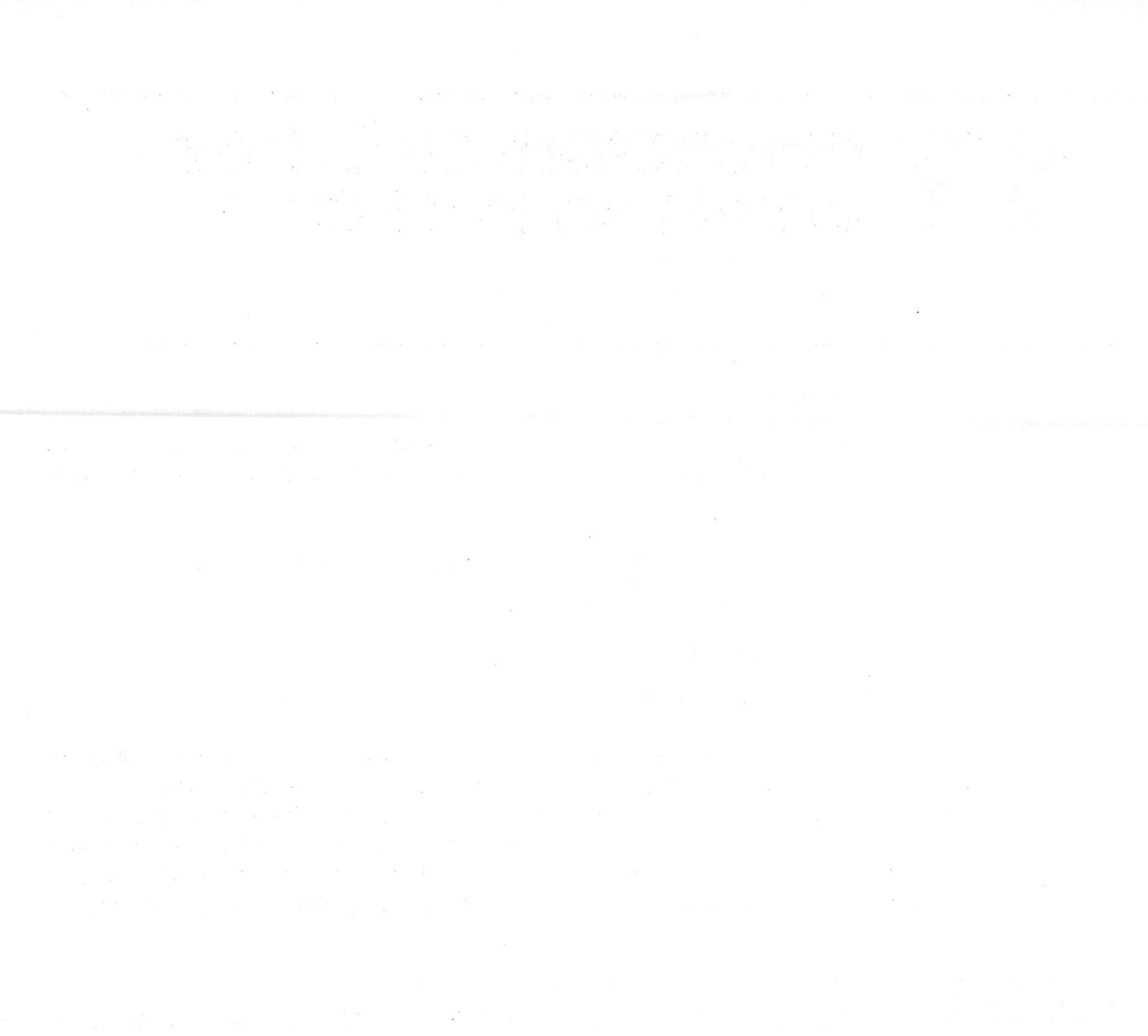

17 DISORDERS OF LARGE BOWEL DYNAMICS

Introduction

Irritable bowel syndrome, chronic constipation and *diverticular disease* all arise from disordered peristaltic function and are largely attributable to the modern refined diet.

These large bowel conditions have many symptoms in common:

- Intermittent attacks of abdominal pain
- Erratic bowel habit
- Bloating and excessive flatus

Apart from the suffering they cause, the surgical importance of these conditions is that they must be distinguished from large bowel cancer.

These conditions could be regarded as endemic in developed societies. They make considerable demands on the time of general practitioners, physicians and surgeons, yet they are largely preventable. One hundred years ago, they were unknown in the West, as they are still in undeveloped rural communities.

MODERN DIET AND DISEASE

Epidemiological observations

Not much scientific attention was paid to diet-related disease until the 1970s. Then, the ideas of Surgeon Captain T.L. Cleeve, a Royal Navy physician, and later the remarkable epidemiological observations of Denis Burkitt, a long time missionary surgeon in Africa, began to be published. Now the subject of diet is not only respectable but has made enormous contributions to the understanding and management of many common diseases. Many diseases common in Western society such as irritable bowel syndrome, diverticular disease, appendicitis and colorectal cancer are largely unknown in the underdeveloped world. This difference is almost certainly related to diet. Thus, it follows that a dietary history is important in evaluating patients with such conditions, and dietary change is an important part of their management.

Over millions of years as 'hunter-gatherers', humans subsisted on a staple diet of vegetables and fruits, grains, legumes and nuts, supplemented by small quantities of meat and fish. The human gastrointestinal and metabolic systems are thus perfectly adapted to this diet. During the brief period of the last 100 years, the average Western diet has dramatically changed, largely due to increasing affluence, fashion, convenience and food processing. The last decade has seen similar trends in the more affluent pockets of the Third World, particularly in the cities. The modern diet compared with the hunter-gatherer diet contains many more calories. These are largely in the form of refined carbohydrate and fats, especially saturated animal fats. Equally important, the modern diet contains far less unabsorbable fibre residue.

Mechanisms of disease caused by modern diet

Whilst the increase in calories and nutrients have brought many benefits, there have been just as many problems. The modern diet has had a deleterious effect on both bowel function and metabolism, particularly of lipids. This has led to a multiplicity of disorders. The ways in which modern diet induces disease are outlined in Figure 17.1. In relation to diseases of the bowel, the most important factors are faecal volume and consistency and gastrointestinal transit time. The average Western adult passes between 80 and 120 gm of firm stool each day with a transit time of about three days. Transit time is commonly as long as two weeks in the elderly. In contrast, rural dwellers in the Third

Fig. 17.1 Mechanisms by which refined diet may cause disease

1. **Slowed gastrointestinal transit time**
— increases duration of contact between stool and bowel mucosa. This increases contact of carcinogens, predisposing to colorectal cancer

2. **Increased intra-abdominal pressure due to straining at stool**
— obstructs venous return making haemorrhoids and varicose veins more likely
— predisposes to hiatus hernia, inguinal hernia and rectal prolapse

3. **Reduced bulk and more solid consistency of faeces**
— makes peristalsis less effective and constipation more likely
— increases intraluminal pressure predisposing to diverticular disease
— hard stool increases friction, causing anal fissure and haemorrhoids
— small stool bulk increases concentration of carcinogens
— may contribute to pathogenesis of appendicitis by obstruction

4. **Decreased loss of bile salts in the faeces**
— increased bile salt pool predisposes to gall stone formation
— increased bile salts in bowel which may result in formation of carcinogens

5. **Change in bacterial flora of the bowel**
— may result in formation of carcinogens
— may be implicated in appendicitis

6. **Increased refined carbohydrate intake**
— predisposes to diabetes
— contributes to excess calorie intake causing obesity

7. **Increased dietary fat intake, particularly saturated animal fats**
— predisposes to atherosclerosis
— predisposes to gall stone formation
— contributes to excess calorie intake and obesity

8. **Increased absorption of dietary fat due to reduced binding by fibre**
— increases fat absorption and blood lipid levels

9. **Obesity**
— weakens abdominal wall muscles predisposing to hiatus hernia, abdominal wall hernias and vaginal prolapse

World, with a diet similar to that of the hunter-gatherer, pass between 300 and 800 gm of much softer stool each day. The average transit time is less than a day and a half.

Increasing dietary fibre content

A substantial increase in daily dietary fibre intake is an essential part of the management of many bowel conditions and the prevention of others. Figure 17.2 lists the readily available foods with a high fibre content which can be eaten daily with little effort and no extra expense. Increasing the fibre content of the normal diet almost inevitably leads to reduced consumption of refined carbohydrates and saturated animal fats, and lower total energy intake. Patients should be advised to introduce dietary fibre gradually as a sudden increase is likely to cause abdominal discomfort and distension and increased production of flatus. Bulking agents (*ispaghula husk* preparations) can be taken in the early stages to achieve a rapid result while avoiding these unpleasant side effects.

Fig. 17.2 Foods with a high fibre content

Whole grain and bran-enriched breakfast cereals, e.g. muesli, All Bran, Weetabix (not corn flakes, puffed rice, etc)

Wholemeal bread (not white or 'brown')

Other whole wheat products, e.g. pasta, wholemeal pastry, digestive biscuits

Other whole grains, e.g. brown rice, sweet corn

Pulses of any kind, e.g. haricot beans (including canned 'baked beans'), kidney beans, chick peas, other dried beans and lentils

Potatoes (skins should be left on)

Unpeeled fruit and vegetables (actually low in fibre compared with grains and pulses)

IRRITABLE BOWEL SYNDROME

Irritable bowel syndrome has only recently been accepted as a pathological entity although the symptom complex has been described in the past under other names such as 'spastic colon'. The condition is very common, particularly in young to middle-aged women.

Clinical features

The typical patient complains of episodic 'cramping' abdominal pain occurring at any time of day and lasting from about 15 minutes to several hours. The pain is unrelated to meals or other provoking factors. It may occur anywhere in the abdomen but tends to occur peripherally, i.e. in either iliac fossa or the epigastrium, and usually recurs in the same general area in any one patient.

Symptoms occur daily for weeks at a time, and then resolve for weeks or months, only to return later. The patient may admit that symptoms are worse at times of stress and are absent during weekends and holidays. The pain may provoke an urge to open the bowels and evacuation may bring some relief from the pain. An erratic bowel habit is a characteristic feature of irritable bowel syndrome. Passage of loose stools alternates with constipation with small hard stools that look like rabbit pellets. Patients may also complain of abdominal distension and excess flatus.

Pathophysiology and aetiology

The pathophysiology of irritable bowel syndrome is poorly understood but a low fibre diet seems to play a part. Colonic motility studies in these patients show abnormal rises in intraluminal pressure and disordered peristalsis, resulting in segmenting, non-propulsive contractions. The small volume of faeces (because of little residual fibre) thus becomes excessively dehydrated and fragmented. Food intolerance (wrongly called food allergy) may play a part but there is little evidence for this as yet. Psychological factors are probably important; patients tend to be tense and introspective. Perhaps the condition represents an imbalance in gut hormonal and autonomic control systems, both centrally and locally mediated.

Management of irritable bowel syndrome

There is no specific test for irritable bowel syndrome. Diagnosis is made on the basis of a typical history after excluding other disorders and often after a trial of treatment. In the young patient, where carcinoma is unlikely, abdominal and rectal examination (including sigmoidoscopy) is all that is required. These will be normal, except perhaps for mild tenderness in the area of pain. In a patient over the age of 50, the diagnosis is unlikely. Before the diagnosis of irritable bowel syndrome can be made, carcinoma and diverticular disease must be excluded by sigmoidoscopy and barium enema or colonoscopy.

Treatment involves reassurance, adjusting the diet to include adequate fibre, and prescribing bulking agents and antispasmodic drugs such as mebeverine. Codeine phosphate is useful as an analgesic for occasional use. This treatment will produce rapid relief of symptoms and confirms the diagnosis. For selected patients, relaxation therapy may be useful.

CONSTIPATION

Clinical features

Whether they regard it as a problem or not, many patients suffer from chronic constipation. Constipation is difficult to define but the essence is an inability to evacuate the bowels with sufficient frequency, ease, completeness or satisfaction. Perception of the norm varies greatly: some patients insist that daily evacuation is essential whilst others tolerate a bowel movement only once a week.

From a medical viewpoint, evacuation less than twice a week is probably abnormal. In the uncomplaining elderly, defaecation may occur much less frequently, causing vague discomfort and anorexia, and predisposing to urinary retention, incontinence and urinary tract infection. Severe constipation may lead to faecal impaction and complete bowel obstruction. Faecal fluid may intermittently escape past the impacted faecal mass and cause soiling, overflow incontinence or apparent ('spurious') diarrhoea.

Abdominal pain may be the presenting symptom of constipation. The pain may be sufficiently severe to result in emergency hospital admission with suspected appendicitis (usually children) or intestinal obstruction (usually the elderly). As many as 25% of patients in these age groups admitted with abdominal pain are diagnosed as suffering from constipation. There is no fever, tachycardia or vomiting, and signs of peritoneal inflammation are absent. There may however be mild abdominal tenderness. The faeces-loaded left side of the colon often forms a palpable column which may indent and have a putty-like consistency. Rectal examination usually reveals a mass of faeces, although in the elderly the faeces may be impacted higher up. Thus, an empty rectum does not exclude constipation.

Pathophysiology of chronic constipation

For surgeons, chronic constipation is mainly a problem of children and the elderly. Patients present both as emergencies and in the out-patient clinic. For general practitioners and gastroenterologists, constipation is more a problem of young women. In most cases, the cause is a combination of low fibre diet, poor fluid intake, obesity, inactivity and persistent failure to respond promptly to the urge to defaecate. Long term use of *purgative drugs* renders the bowel temporarily or even permanently atonic. Some drugs, particularly *codeine* and *opiates*, slow large bowel motility, whilst other drugs such as *aluminium hydroxide mixtures* and *iron preparations* solidify the stool. Constipation is a characteristic feature of *hypothyroidism* and is also seen in *hypo-* and *hypercalcaemia*.

Management of constipation

Diagnosis in children can usually be made on history and clinical examination; successful treatment confirms the diagnosis. If chronic severe constipation persists despite treatment, the diagnosis of *ultra-short segment Hirschsprung's disease* (see Chapter 31) should be considered. In the elderly, carcinoma or the complications of diverticular disease should be excluded by sigmoidoscopy and barium enema once the constipation has been treated.

In severe constipation, immediate treatment involves the following local measures, in order of desperation!

- Lubricant glycerine suppositories
- Stimulant suppositories (e.g. bisacodyl)
- Small phosphate enemas (disposable or 'mini' enemas)
- Stool softening arachis oil enemas
- Large volume soap and water enemas ('high, hot and a helluva lot')
- Manual disimpaction (may require general anaesthetic)

Oral laxatives of any kind are contraindicated if there is any suggestion of bowel obstruction.

Management of chronic constipation involves treating the acute problem as above or with oral laxatives (see Figure 17.3), followed by long term prophylactic measures. Patients should be encouraged to increase dietary fibre and fluid intake and to heed the urge to defaecate. Bulking agents may be appropriate in the medium term.

Fig. 17.3 Oral laxative agents

1. Stimulant/irritant laxatives, e.g. danthron, bisacodyl, senna derivatives
2. Faecal softeners and lubricants, e.g. dioctyl, liquid paraffin
3. Osmotic laxatives, e.g. lactulose, mixtures of magnesium hydroxide or magnesium sulphate
4. Proprietary preparations, e.g. Milpar, Ex-lax
5. Strong laxatives for single dose use — for bowel preparation or very stubborn constipation, e.g. sodium picosulphate (stimulant), mannitol solution (osmotic)

Note: bulking agents do not have a laxative effect in the short term

SIGMOID VOLVULUS

Pathophysiology

Patients with long standing chronic constipation tend to develop a capacious, elongated and relatively atonic colon, especially in the sigmoid region. This is sometimes described as *acquired* or *idiopathic megacolon*.

Occasionally, the huge sigmoid loop, heavy with faeces and distended with gas, becomes twisted on its mesenteric pedicle to produce a closed loop obstruction. If this sigmoid volvulus is not corrected, venous infarction ensues, followed by perforation and catastrophic faecal peritonitis. This full picture is uncommon but when it occurs, there is often a history of several episodes of transient obstruction which could represent incomplete volvulus. Some episodes of abdominal pain diagnosed as constipation may in fact be sigmoid volvulus, resolving spontaneously as constipation is treated. Volvulus of the caecum, small bowel or stomach, however, is unrelated to constipation.

Fig. 17.4 Mechanism of sigmoid volvulus

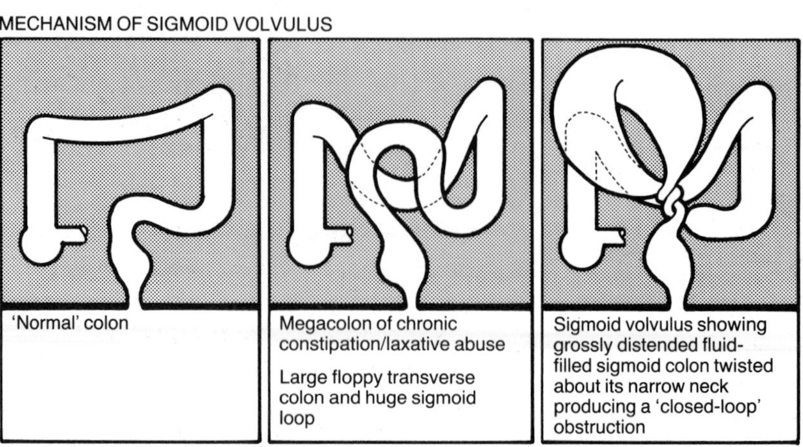

Clinical features of sigmoid volvulus

Sigmoid volvulus is rarely seen except in the elderly, the mentally handicapped and long-stay patients in mental institutions. The patient is 'off-colour' with abdominal distension and a variable degree of abdominal pain. There is also absolute constipation (of both faeces and flatus) for at least 24 hours. On digital examination, the rectum is commonly empty but capacious. The abdomen is visibly distended and tympanitic but barely tender. This is true even if the colon has reached the stage of venous infarction. Once perforation occurs, the full picture of faecal peritonitis will be apparent.

Management of sigmoid volvulus

Plain abdominal X-ray usually shows a single grossly dilated sigmoid loop, often reaching the xiphisternum (see Figure 17.5). An erect film may reveal a characteristic 'inverted U' of bowel gas in the upper abdomen, with fluid levels at the same height in the two bowel limbs in the lower abdomen; an abdominal lateral decubitus X-ray may reveal two parallel fluid levels running the full length of the abdomen.

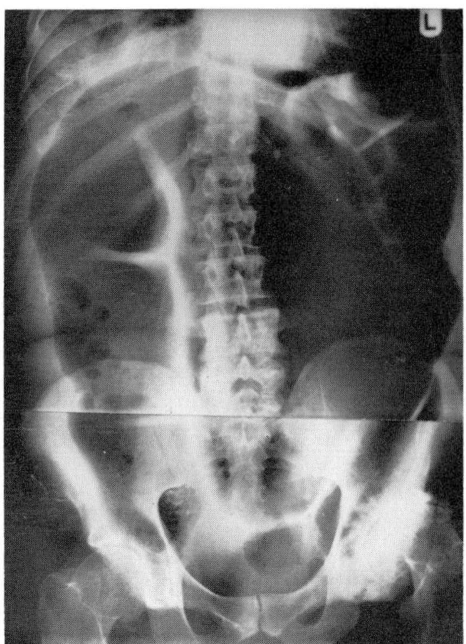

Fig. 17.5 Sigmoid volvulus

This patient was a man of 65 who had lived in a mental hospital for many years; he was not taking any regular medication. He had several previous attacks of abdominal pain which were undiagnosed. On this occasion, he was admitted to hospital without abdominal pain but with huge abdominal distension and absolute constipation. He was so distended that two separate films (joined together here) had to be taken to include the whole abdomen! These supine radiographs show an enormous gas filled loop of bowel ascending from the pelvis (an important diagnostic feature) up to the lower thorax. This loop overlies the liver and the descending and ascending colon. The major differential diagnosis is colonic pseudo-obstruction (adynamic obstruction), which occurs in elderly patients on psychotropic or anti-Parkinsonian drugs

If volvulus is diagnosed, a sigmoidoscope is passed as far as possible into the rectum and a *flatus tube* inserted through it. The end of the flatus tube is then gently manipulated through the twisted bowel into the obstructed loop. If this is successful, there is a gush of liquid faeces and flatus, relieving the obstruction. The flatus tube can be left in-situ for 24 hours to maintain decompression, discourage retwisting and allow recovery of the bowel wall vascular supply. Despite this, volvulus may recur later.

If plain X-ray and sigmoidoscopy does not confirm volvulus but large bowel obstruction is still suspected, a *limited barium enema* is performed, without bowel preparation. This differentiates volvulus from other causes of obstruction such as carcinoma and diverticular disease. Pressure from the barium enema may cause the bowel to untwist, releasing a torrent of faeces and flatus.

If a volvulus cannot be released, operation is performed urgently. In most cases, the gut is still viable but sigmoid colectomy is often required to prevent recurrence. The usual procedure is to bring the two divided ends of bowel out onto the abdominal wall to form a *double-barrel colostomy*, rather than risk a primary anastomosis in dilated and unprepared colon. For recurrent volvulus, *sigmoid colectomy* or suturing the bowel to the abdominal wall to prevent twisting may be performed electively.

DIVERTICULAR DISEASE

Diverticular disease is a common condition caused by chronic lack of dietary fibre. It occurs in at least one third of the population over the age of 60. Females are affected more often than males. (In semantic terms, the singular is *diverticulum* and the plural *diverticula*, not *diverticulae*; the adjectival form is *diverticular*.)

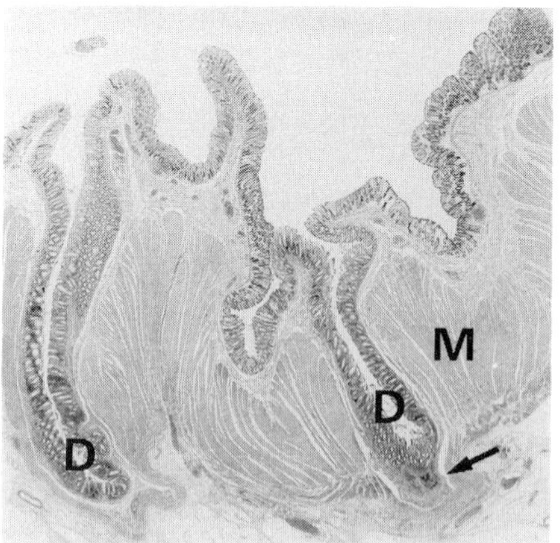

Fig. 17.6 Diverticular disease — histopathology

Low power photomicrograph (H & E) showing a portion of sigmoid colon with two diverticula **D**. The one on the right has a small abscess (arrowed) at its base. Note the marked thickening of the smooth muscle **M**, a characteristic feature of diverticular disease

Pathophysiology of diverticular disease

Chronic constipation causes hypertrophy of the muscle of the colonic wall. The functional sphincter at the rectosigmoid junction probably fails to relax to decompress the proximal bowel. Increased intraluminal pressure results in pockets of mucosa herniating through weak points in the bowel wall. These potential defects are where mucosal blood vessels penetrate the wall from outside, between the longitudinal muscle bands (taeniae coli). The sigmoid colon is most affected by diverticular disease, the condition extending for a variable distance proximally. Isolated diverticula sometimes occur alone in the caecum but these may be a congenital abnormality.

The presence of diverticula is probably unimportant; this asymptomatic condition was formerly described as 'diverticulosis'. Individual diverticula may, however, become inflamed, probably as a result of obstruction of the narrow outlet. This results in the formation of a small *diverticular abscess* which effectively lies outside the bowel wall. The microscopic anatomy is demonstrated in Figure 17.6.

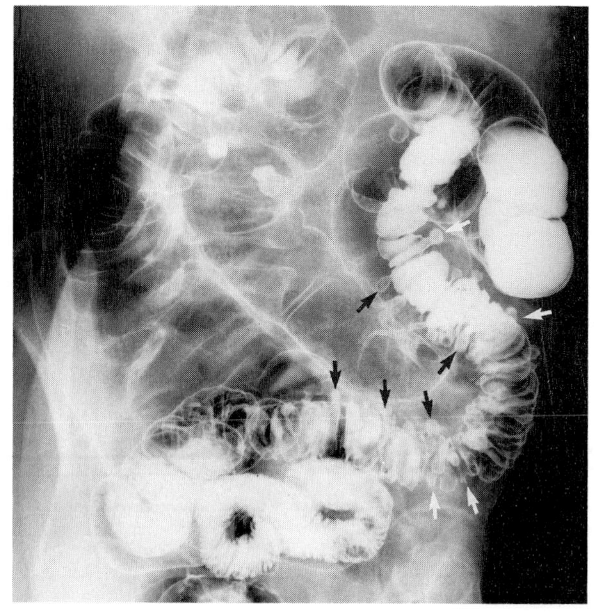

Fig. 17.7 Diverticular disease

Barium enema showing the typical appearance of multiple diverticula (arrowed) in the sigmoid and descending colon in a 77-year-old woman. A few diverticula are also present in the transverse colon

Complications of diverticular disease

Diverticular inflammation may lead to a variety of complications:

- Spreading pericolic inflammation
- Pericolic abscess
- Intraperitoneal perforation
- Fistula formation into other abdominal or pelvic structures
- Acute rectal haemorrhage
- Fibrous bowel strictures
- Bowel to bowel adhesions

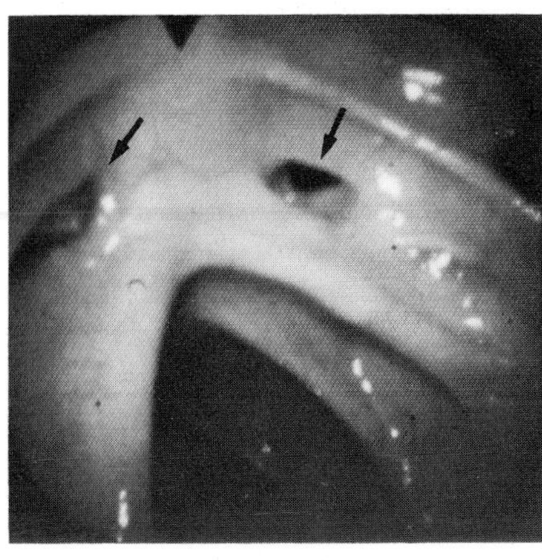

(a)

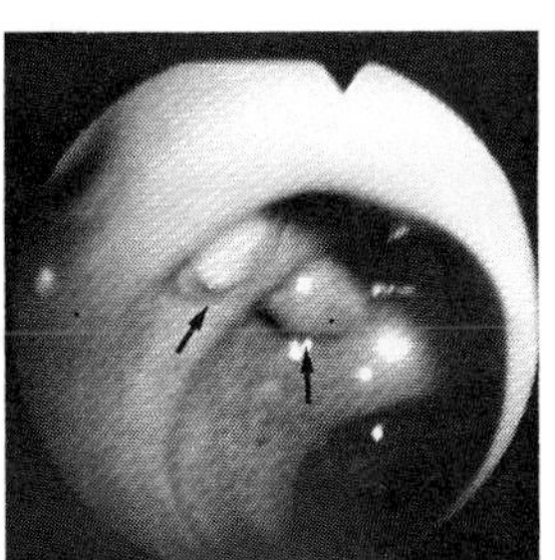

(b)

Fig. 17.8 Colonoscopic view of diverticula

(a) Diverticular orifices (arrowed) are easily seen with the wide-angle lens of a colonoscope.
(b) Faecoliths (arrowed) are often seen protruding into the bowel lumen through diverticular orifices

Clinical presentations of diverticular disease and their management

The pathological consequences of diverticular inflammation are described together as *diverticulitis* and are summarised in Figure 17.9. The majority of patients with diverticula are asymptomatic, and diverticula are a common incidental finding when the colon is investigated by barium enema or colonoscopy. The typical appearances are shown in Figures 17.7 and 17.8.

Fig. 17.9 Clinical presentations of diverticular disease

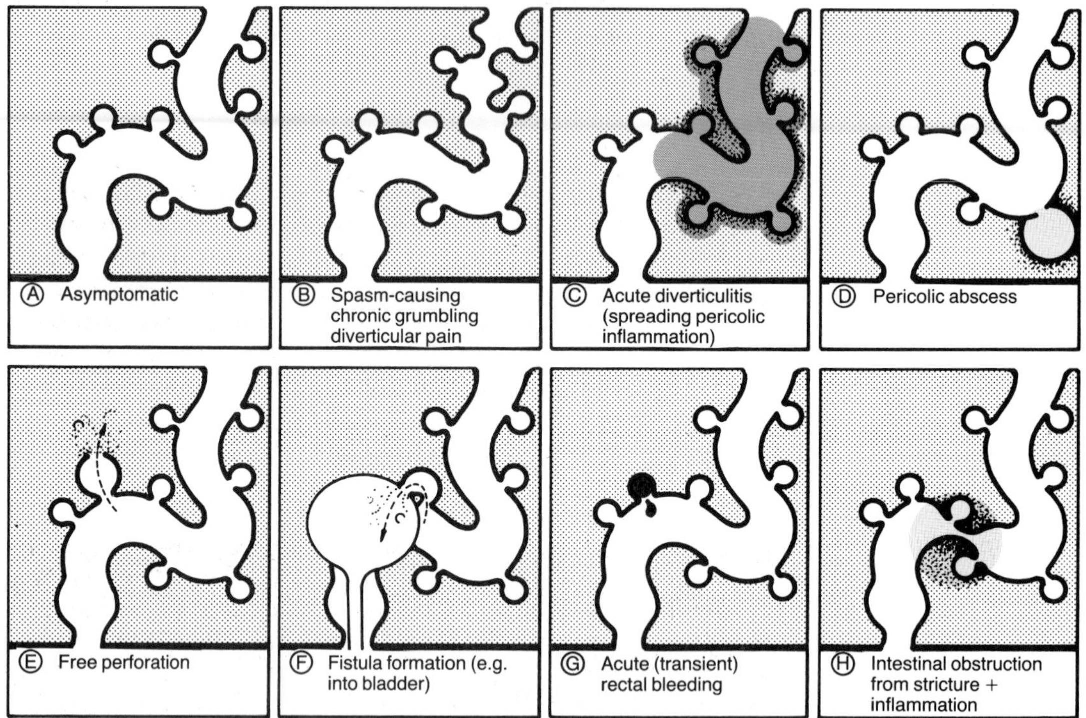

a. Chronic grumbling diverticular pain

This is probably the most common manifestation of diverticular disease, and is usually managed in general practice. Peridiverticular inflammation is chronic and low-grade. Local irritation causes bowel wall spasm causing chronic pain and erratic bowel habit. There is chronic constipation with small pellet-like faeces, punctuated by episodes of diarrhoea. On examination, there is little to find, except perhaps mild left iliac fossa tenderness and faecal loading. Barium enema is often performed to confirm the diagnosis and exclude malignancy.

In most patients, symptoms can be relieved by a high fibre diet and bulking agents. In the recent past, however, before the importance of dietary fibre was realised, many patients with severe chronic symptoms were subjected to colectomy, with all its attendant complications.

b. Acute 'diverticulitis' (i.e. spreading pericolic inflammation)

This represents local extension of the inflammation described in the last paragraph. The local inflammation is extensive however, and involves the pericolic tissues and parietal peritoneum. Typically, the patient complains of continuous left iliac fossa pain and is systemically ill with a pyrexia and tachycardia. Abdominal findings range from mild left iliac fossa tenderness to obvious local peritonitis.

Antibiotic treatment is directed against the usual faecal organisms. In severe cases, a combination of intravenous antibiotics such as gentamicin, benzyl penicillin and metronidazole is used, and the bowel 'rested' by stopping oral intake and giving intravenous fluids. Less severe cases can be managed at home with oral antibiotics, e.g. metronidazole and amoxycillin or a cephalosporin.

c. *Pericolic abscess*

Pericolic abscess represents a further extension of the pathological process just described. The clinical presentation is similar at first but fails to resolve with antibiotics. The patient suffers persistent pain and tenderness, a swinging pyrexia, and incomplete obstruction due to spasm of the bowel wall muscle. Sometimes a pericolic abscess presents as septicaemia or 'pyrexia of unknown origin'. The pericolic abscess may spontaneously drain into the bowel, producing an attack of purulent diarrhoea; the condition then resolves. Diagnosis of a pericolic abscess can often be made by ultrasound. A barium enema may show leakage of contrast into the abscess cavity (see Figure 17.10).

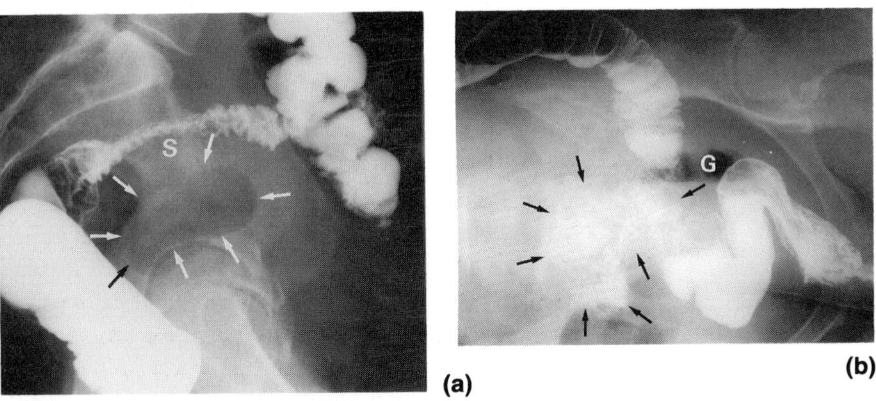

Fig. 17.10 Pericolic abscess due to perforated diverticular disease

Barium enema films from a 49-year-old woman who presented with abdominal pain and tenderness, a mass in the left iliac fossa and a swinging pyrexia. She was treated with antibiotics but the pyrexia failed to settle. **(a)** Right lateral view of recto-sigmoid region showing marked narrowing of the distal sigmoid **S** due to spasm and inflammatory oedema. The radiolucent area antero-inferiorly (outline arrowed) represents a bubble of gas in a large pelvic abscess. **(b)** Lateral decubitus film (left-side upwards) of the same patient taken later during the same examination. This shows barium which has leaked into the abscess cavity (outline arrowed). Note also a fluid level with a gas bubble **G** above it, within the abscess. At laparotomy, a large pericolic and pelvic abscess was found to be walled off. This was drained, the sigmoid colon excised and the end of the descending colon brought out as a terminal colostomy in the left iliac fossa. The rectal stump was oversewn. Three months later, the bowel was reconnected.

Antibiotic therapy, as for acute diverticulitis, is the first line of treatment. Ideally, this contains the abscess, allowing it to drain spontaneously into the bowel. If antibiotic treatment fails, operation is required. This is a major procedure involving diversion of the faecal stream via a colostomy, and exploration and drainage of the abscess. In addition, the affected segment of bowel must be removed. This is best done at the first operation if the inflammation is not too extensive and the surgeon is sufficiently experienced. If not, resection is performed electively several months later when inflammation has subsided. The colostomy is closed at the same time or later.

d. *Diverticular perforation*

A small, asymptomatic diverticular abscess may rupture spontaneously, i.e. perforate, resulting in the escape of bowel contents into the peritoneal cavity. The patient presents with an acute abdomen but the severity of clinical signs depends on the size of the perforation. This may be anything from a pinhole size, allowing only bowel gas and a little fluid to escape, to a hole up to a centimetre in diameter causing widespread faecal peritonitis and septicaemia. With small perforations, the symptoms and signs may be little more than those of acute diverticulitis; diagnosis is made by the presence of free gas under the diaphragm on an erect chest X-ray.

Treatment involves immediate parenteral antibiotics to prevent septicaemia, followed by laparotomy to perform peritoneal toilet, diversion of the faecal stream and resection of the diseased bowel, as previously described.

e. *Fistula formation into other abdominal or pelvic structures*

Fistula formation occurs when an inflamed diverticulum lies in close proximity to another hollow viscus. An inflammatory adhesion develops between them, and the diverticulum then ruptures into the other viscus, leaving a persistent channel between the two. A fistula between the large bowel and a loop of small bowel causes diarrhoea. A vesico-colic fistula causes pneumaturia and severe urinary tract infection. A fistula into the female reproductive

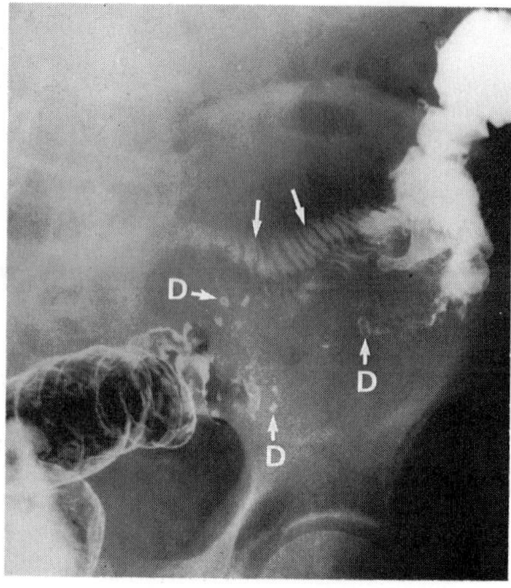

Fig. 17.11 Diverticular fistula into the distal ileum

Barium enema of a 61-year-old man with a recently erratic bowel habit, who presented with pain and tenderness in the left iliac fossa. The X-ray shows the sigmoid colon, although part of it is poorly filled with barium which is only seen in the diverticula **D**. There is a loop of small bowel which contains contrast (arrowed) which indicates the presence of a colo-ileal fistula caused by peri-diverticulitis

system causes a purulent vaginal discharge. Diverticular disease is the most common cause of these kinds of fistulae but they may also be caused by Crohn's disease or sometimes colorectal cancers.

Surprisingly, fistulae rarely show up on barium enema examination. Diagnosis is made on the history, at operation or at cystoscopic examination in the case of bladder fistulae. Surgical treatment involves excision of the affected segment of bowel.

f. Acute rectal haemorrhage

Diverticular disease may present with an episode of acute rectal bleeding, probably from erosion of a bowel wall artery by a small diverticular abscess. Blood loss is variable but the bleeding almost always stops spontaneously. Typically, the patient complains of having passed a mass of fairly fresh blood instead of the expected stool and is admitted to hospital urgently. The main differential diagnosis is ischaemic colitis but other causes of rectal bleeding such as carcinoma and haemorrhoids must be considered.

Management is rarely surgical. After any necessary resuscitation, the patient is kept under observation for several days, by which time it is safe to perform a barium enema.

g. Intestinal obstruction

Diverticular disease occasionally presents with complete large bowel obstruction due to a combination of acute inflammatory thickening, muscle hypertrophy and spasm. Incomplete obstruction, presenting as severe consti-

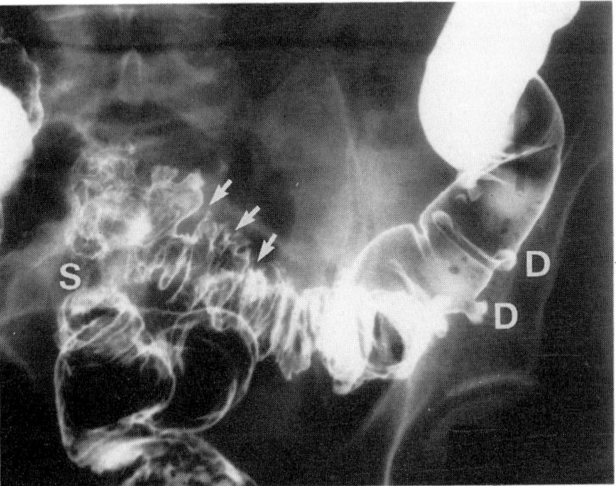

Fig. 17.12 Diverticular stricture in the sigmoid colon

This 64-year-old man suffered several attacks of diverticulitis which settled with antibiotics. This frontal view of a barium enema shows diverticula **D** in the upper sigmoid colon and circular muscle hypertrophy in the distal sigmoid colon (arrowed) typical of diverticular disease. There is a stricture **S** near the colorectal junction. This stricture does not show the typical 'shouldering' of a carcinoma, although this could not be excluded on barium enema. Colonoscopy confirmed that it was benign. This patient later had a severe attack of diverticulitis which required surgery and a Hartmann's operation was performed

pation, is much more common. Chronic diverticular inflammation sometimes causes isolated fibrous strictures, particularly in the sigmoid colon, which cause intermittent bouts of constipation. When seen on a barium enema (see Figure 17.12), such strictures must be distinguished from malignancy or Crohn's disease. This usually requires colonoscopy.

When acute diverticular inflammation involves the pericolic tissues, small bowel may become entangled in the process. Thus, adynamic small bowel obstruction may be the presenting feature.

18 ANAL AND PERIANAL DISORDERS

Introduction

Anal and perianal disorders make up about 20% of all outpatient surgical referrals. Although trivial in pathological terms, these conditions are extremely distressing and embarrassing. Patients often put up with symptoms for a long time before seeking medical advice. The common anal symptoms are summarised in Figure 18.1 and their interpretation is discussed in Chapter 6.

Fig. 18.1 Common anal symptoms

Anal bleeding
Anal pain and discomfort
Perianal itching and irritation
'Something coming down'
Perianal discharge

Disorders of the anus and perianal area are illustrated in Figure 18.2. Haemorrhoids and other common benign anal conditions must be distinguished from carcinoma of the rectum and the rare carcinoma of the anus, particularly in older patients. Most anal and perianal conditions can be treated on an outpatient basis, although abscesses and haemorrhoids that have become strangulated or thrombosed may present as surgical emergencies.

Anatomy of the anal canal

The anal canal is approximately 4 cm long, surrounded by the anal sphincter mechanism. The upper half of the anal canal is lined by a continuation of the rectal glandular mucosa. This gives way abruptly to stratified squamous epithelium (modified skin) at the *dentate (pectinate) line*. The mucosa of the upper part of the anal canal is thrown into 6–10 longitudinal folds, the *columns of Morgagni*, each containing a terminal branch of the superior rectal artery and vein. The folds are most prominent in the left lateral, right posterior and right anterior quadrants where the veins form prominent venous plexuses. The lymphatics of the upper part of the anal canal drain to the pelvic and abdominal lymph node chain, whereas the lower part of the anal canal drains to the inguinal lymph nodes. The glandular mucosa is relatively insensitive, in contrast to the highly sensitive lower anal canal skin.

The anal sphincter mechanism has three constituents, the *internal sphincter, external sphincter* and *puborectalis*. The internal sphincter represents a downward but thickened continuation of the rectal wall musculature. The encircling

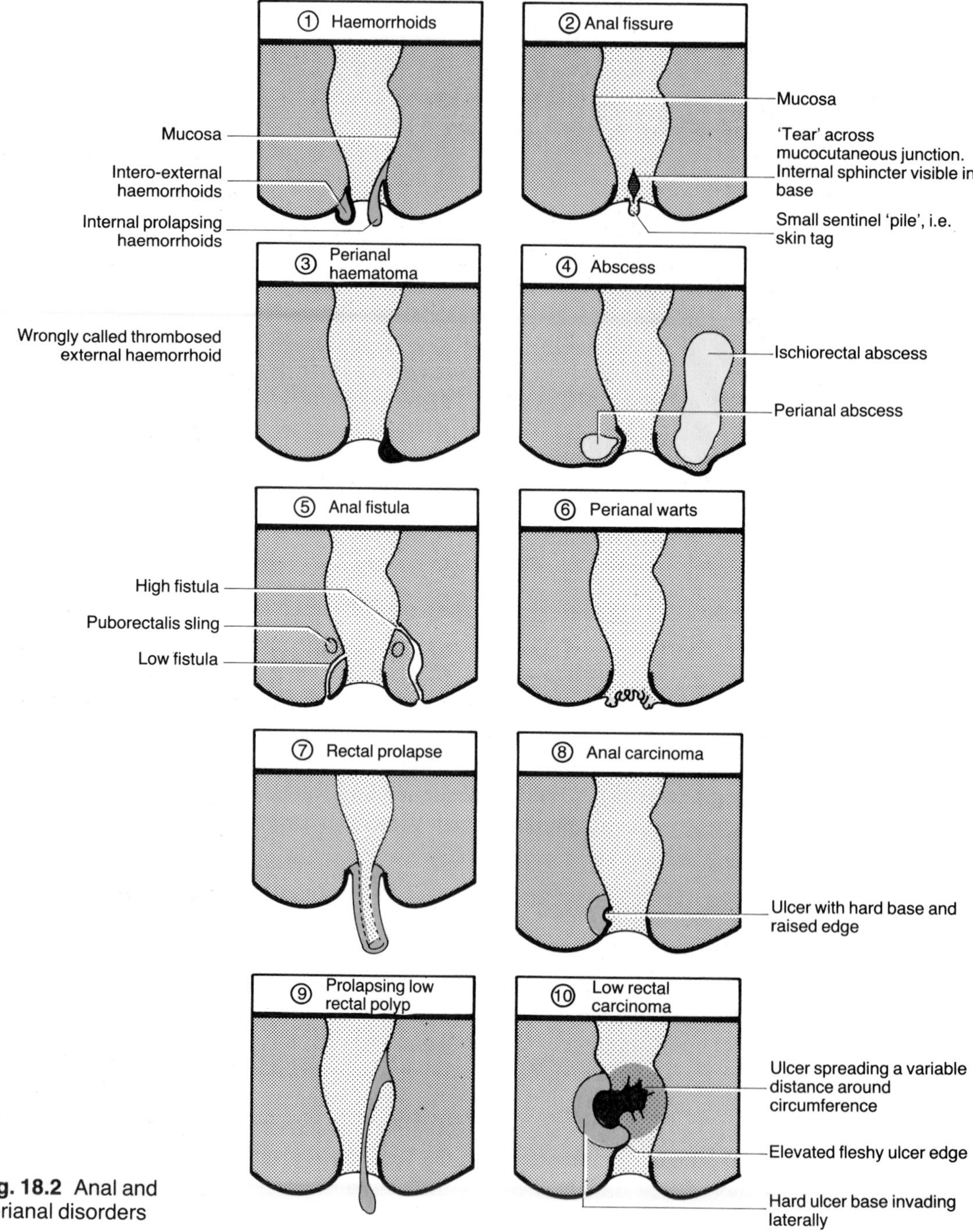

Fig. 18.2 Anal and perianal disorders

external sphincter and the puborectalis sling (which is part of levator ani) arise from the pelvic floor. The mechanism of continence is complex but the most important factor is the angle maintained by the action of puborectalis.

Fig. 18.3 Anatomy of the anal canal

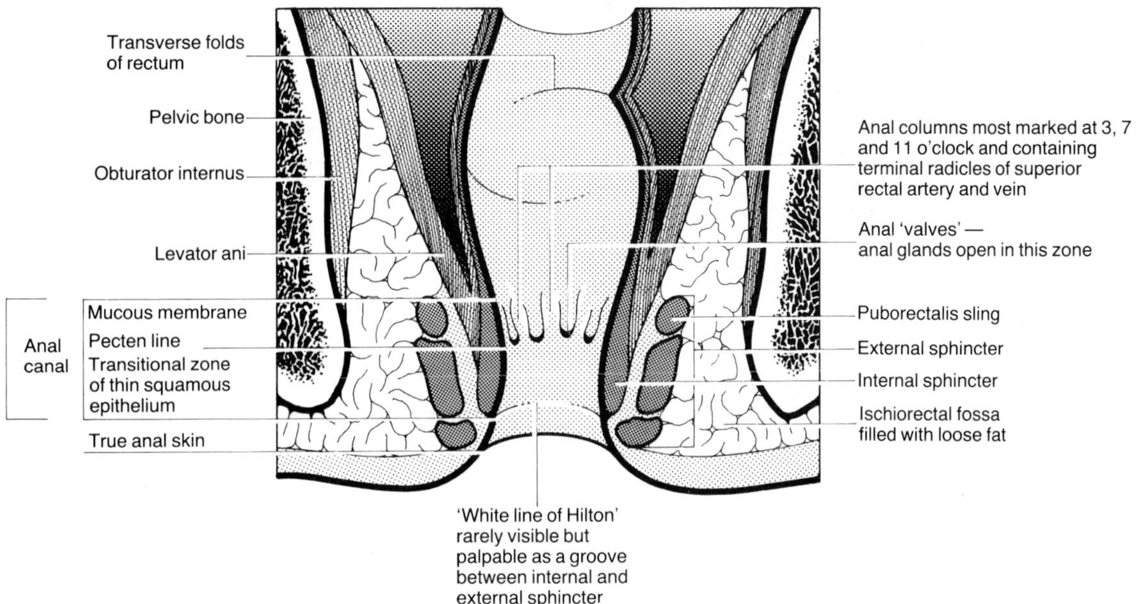

The pink rectal mucosa becomes a darker reddish-blue colour in the anal canal where it overlies the submucosal venous plexus. The anal columns are not readily visible on proctoscopy but the transition between glandular mucosa and anal skin is clearly visible.

HAEMORRHOIDS

Haemorrhoids (piles) are extremely common, affecting nearly half of the population at some stage in their lives. Men tend to suffer more often and for longer periods, whereas women are particularly susceptible in late pregnancy and the puerperium. Lack of fibre in the modern 'civilised' diet is probably the most important aetiological factor; haemorrhoids are almost unknown in undeveloped countries.

Pathogenesis

Haemorrhoids represent excessive enlargement of the venous plexuses at the lower ends of the anal mucosal columns. Haemorrhoids are usually located in the three, seven and eleven o'clock positions when viewed with the patient in the lithotomy position. These correspond to the anatomical positions of the three most prominent anal columns.

Haemorrhoids are caused by straining to pass small hard stools. Increased intra-abdominal pressure inhibits venous return and the venous plexuses become engorged. The bulging mucosa is then dragged distally by the hard stool. Furthermore, persistent straining at stool causes the pelvic floor to sag downwards, extruding the anal mucosa and causing a minor degree of prolapse. Venous engorgement and mucosal prolapse are probably the main mechanisms in pregnancy-related haemorrhoids. Oestrogens mediate venous dilatation, and the fetus obstructs pelvic venous return.

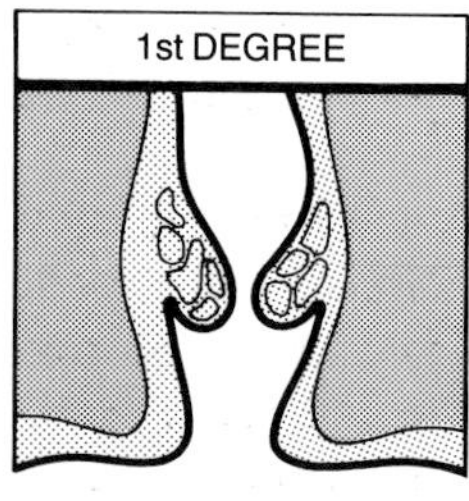

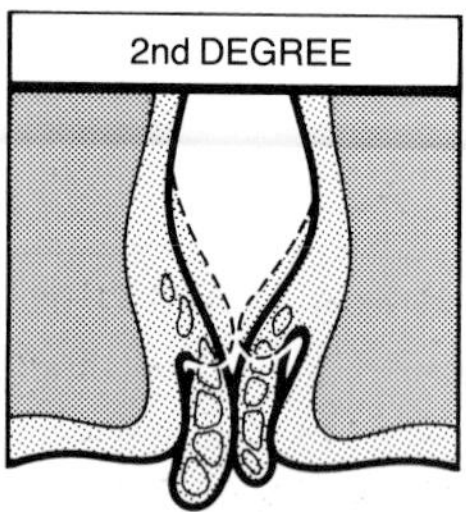

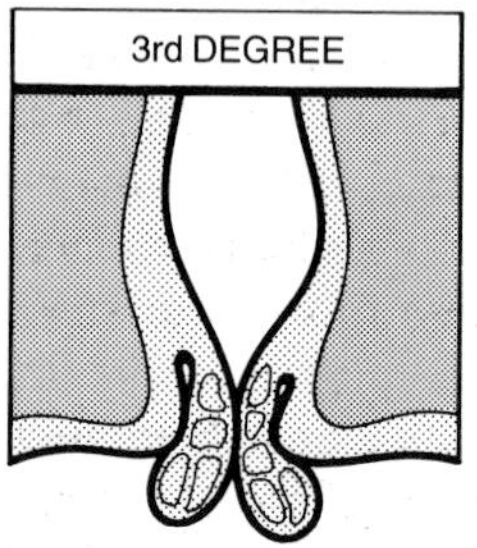

Fig. 18.4 Classification of haemorrhoids

Haemorrhoids are classified into first, second and third degrees according to the extent to which they prolapse through the anal canal. *First degree piles* never prolapse, *second degree piles* prolapse during defaecation but then return spontaneously into the anal canal, whilst *third degree piles* remain outside the anal margin unless replaced digitally (Figure 18.4). Most haemorrhoids can be described as 'internal' because they are covered by glandular mucosa. Large neglected haemorrhoids may extend beneath the stratified squamous epithelium so that their lower part becomes covered by skin. These are correctly described as 'intero-external' haemorrhoids, or more commonly 'external piles'.

Any haemorrhoids may bleed from stool trauma during defaecation. Large haemorrhoids may thrombose if they prolapse and their venous return is obstructed by sphincter tone. Such piles then become solid and cannot be effectively replaced within the anal canal. In extreme cases, the haemorrhoid undergoes venous infarction and ulceration. The local pain and irritation caused by haemorrhoids results in increased anal sphincter tone and spasm, thus aggravating the problem of defaecation and prolapse. Some surgeons argue that chronic inflammation results in fibrosis within the perianal tissues, restricting anal dilatation during defaecation. Long standing haemorrhoids appear to atrophy, probably by thrombosis and fibrosis, leaving small *skin tags* at the anal margin.

Clinical presentation of haemorrhoids

Haemorrhoids often produce symptoms intermittently. Attacks last from a few days to a few weeks, often with complete freedom from trouble between times. Episodes of constipation are often a precipitating factor.

The symptoms of haemorrhoids are:

- Perianal irritation and itching (pruritus ani)
- Aching discomfort and pain exacerbated by defaecation
- Haemorrhoidal prolapse
- Rectal bleeding

Most patients reaching the surgeon have already tried various anaesthetic and sedative creams and suppositories, self-administered or prescribed by the general practitioner. Reasons for referral are persistent symptoms and the need to exclude malignancy as a cause of bleeding.

Mucus secreted by the glandular epithelium and low-grade secondary infection by faecal bacteria or candida cause both the skin maceration and perianal irritation. Scratching and application of creams keep the area wet and exacerbate the problems.

External piles or skin tags may be visible in the anal area. Digital examination is essential to exclude carcinoma and provides a useful measure of anal tone. Haemorrhoids, however, are not palpable since they empty with pressure from the examining finger. *Proctoscopy* is necessary to demonstrate internal piles, which are seen bulging into the lumen as the proctoscope is withdrawn.

Sigmoidoscopy is essential if there is a history of bleeding or any symptoms suspicious of malignancy; occasionally a rectal polyp on a long pedicle will be diagnosed in this way.

Thrombosed or strangulated haemorrhoids present with acute pain and most patients are admitted to hospital as an emergency. The diagnosis is usually obvious on inspection as an oedematous, congested purplish mass is seen at the anal margin. Tight spasm of the anal sphincter makes digital rectal examination extremely painful. Strangulated haemorrhoids are even more painful than thrombosed haemorrhoids, and the strangulated mass may be necrotic or even ulcerated.

Conservative management and prevention of haemorrhoids

A high fibre diet is the most important means of preventing and treating haemorrhoids. A change in diet may be supplemented initially with a bulking agent. In addition, the patient should be strongly encouraged to spend minimal time in defaecating and to avoid straining. Some patients regularly spend a long time on the lavatory reading. This ritual easily leads to unnecessary straining at the end of defaecation, when mild haemorrhoid or mucosal prolapse is interpreted as incomplete evacuation of faeces. Prolonged straining occasionally leads to the formation of a '*solitary ulcer*' in the posterior wall of the proximal anal canal, which may be clinically indistinguishable from a malignant ulcer.

In many patients with symptomatic haemorrhoids, these simple measures are enough to relieve the symptoms.

Pruritus ani can be helped greatly if the perineum is washed and dried after defaecation and kept dry by applying simple talcum powder. If haemorrhoids prolapse at defaecation but do not return spontaneously to the anal canal (third degree haemorrhoids), symptoms can be relieved if the prolapsed haemorrhoids are replaced digitally after defaecation. Many creams, suppositories and other topical preparations are available with or without prescription, and are very widely used. Many contain local anaesthetic agents and steroids. They are useful to help a patient recover from an episode of haemorrhoidal symptoms but do nothing to treat the underlying condition. Overuse causes maceration of the perianal skin and predisposes to secondary infection.

Surgical treatments for haemorrhoids

a. Injection

First degree haemorrhoids (which do not regress with dietary change and avoidance of straining), and most second degree haemorrhoids are best treated by injection. An irritant solution is injected submucosally around the pedicles of the three major haemorrhoids. This provokes a fibrotic reaction, effectively obliterating the haemorrhoidal veins and causing atrophy of the haemorrhoids.

The procedure can be performed on an outpatient basis and does not require any anaesthetic. The haemorrhoids are first assessed by external inspection, both with the patient at rest and 'straining down'. A proctoscope is then inserted to its full length so that the distal end of the proctoscope lies beyond the external sphincter and projects into the lower rectum. The instrument is then slowly withdrawn and the haemorrhoids are seen to bulge into the lumen. The proctoscope is reinserted as before and 3–5 ml of 5% phenol-in-oil is injected just beneath the mucosa. Usually three injections are given, near the site at which each haemorrhoidal vein leaves the haemorrhoidal plexuses, i.e. at positions three, seven and eleven o'clock, as viewed with the patient in the lithotomy position. A specially designed aspirating syringe and a shouldered needle are used to avoid injecting directly into a vein or injecting too deeply. Injection is painless provided the needle is placed correctly into the neck of the haemorrhoid; direct injection into the haemorrhoid itself is extremely painful. Injection may be repeated on two to three occasions at intervals of four to six weeks.

Fig. 18.5 Technique of injecting

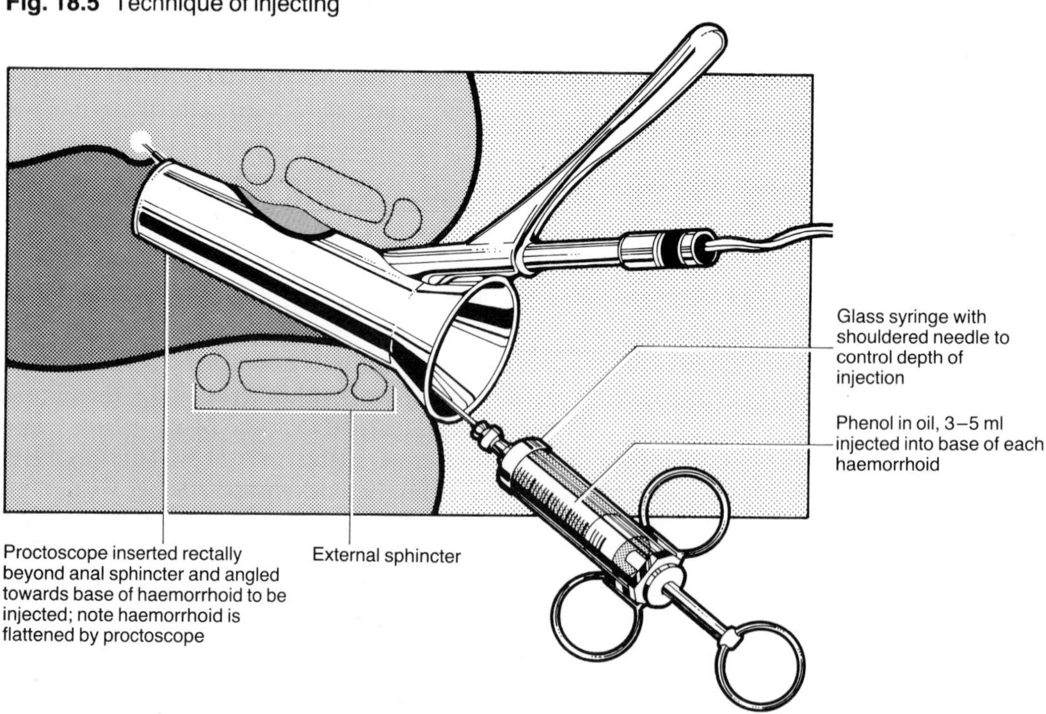

b. Banding

An alternative to injection is the application of *Barron's bands* to obliterate the haemorrhoidal vessels (see Figure 18.6). Contrary to popular belief, the bands are not placed around the stalk of prolapsing haemorrhoids; this would be unbearably painful because of the somatic innervation of anal skin. Instead, a cone of mucosa just above the haemorrhoidal neck is picked up in special forceps and drawn into the banding instrument. The bands are then released around the base of the cone, constricting the haemorrhoidal vessels. The result is that the haemorrhoid slowly shrinks.

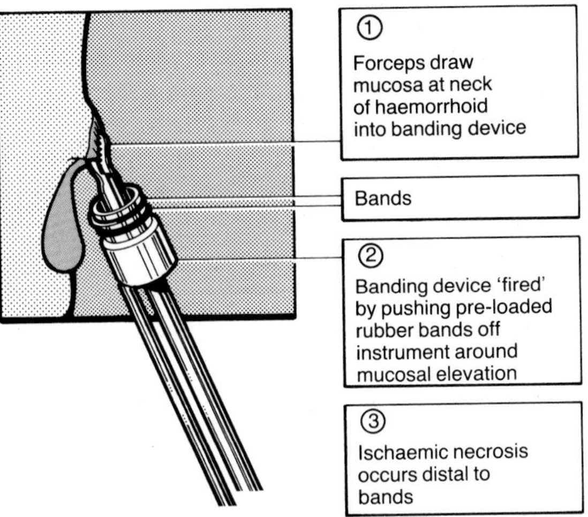

Fig. 18.6 Barron's banding technique for haemorrhoids

c. Lord's stretch

This technique, which has become popular in recent years, involves manual dilatation of the anal sphincter under general anaesthetic. The procedure reduces anal sphincter tone by controlled tearing of the encircling sphincter muscle, and is believed to break down fibrotic bands which might prevent normal anal dilatation during defaecation. If performed in an uncontrolled manner, anal stretch may cause permanent incontinence, especially in the elderly.

d. Haemorrhoidectomy

Haemorrhoidal excision is indicated for third degree haemorrhoids and for lesser degrees when other treatments have failed. The operation most commonly performed is the one described by Milligan and Morgan, as shown in Figure 18.7, in which the haemorrhoidal masses are excised, together with overlying mucosa and some skin. This leaves skin and mucosal defects which heal by secondary intention and wound contraction. A skin bridge must be preserved between each wound to prevent the serious late complication of anal stenosis.

Before operation, stool softeners such as bulking agents and gentle laxatives, should be given to avoid postoperative constipation. The painful early postoperative period can be greatly eased by caudal analgesia, given at operation.

The treatment of choice for thrombosed or strangulated piles is urgent haemorrhoidectomy. Prophylactic antibiotics should be given because of the greater risk of infection in necrotic tissue. Thrombosed or strangulated piles are sometimes treated conservatively with ice packs and analgesics. Alternatively, pain can be relieved by anal dilatation under anaesthetic, but this leaves an even larger prolapsed haemorrhoidal mass which shrinks slowly over two or three weeks. Hospital stay and recovery period are both shorter with urgent haemorrhoidectomy than with either conservative approach.

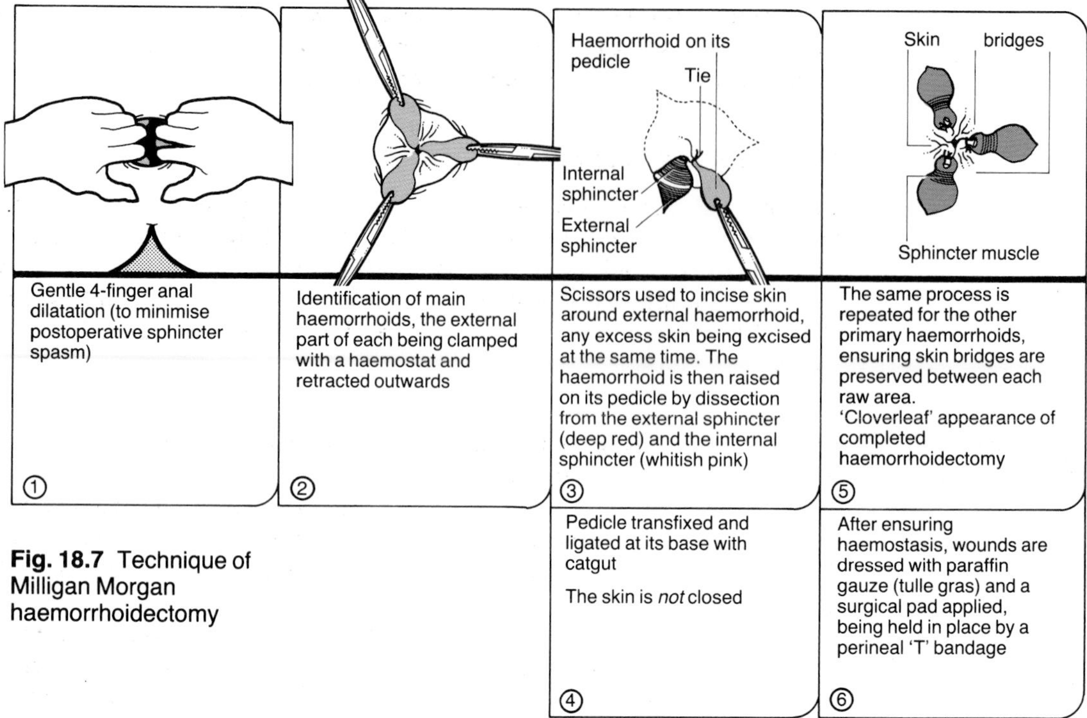

Fig. 18.7 Technique of Milligan Morgan haemorrhoidectomy

ANAL FISSURE

An anal fissure is a longitudinal tear in the mucosa and skin of the anal canal caused by passage of a large, constipated stool. The tear is nearly always in the midline of the posterior anal margin. The fissure causes sphincter spasm and acute pain during defaecation, which persists for up to an hour. The result is a fear of defaecation which aggravates the constipation. Sometimes, there is a small amount of fresh bleeding at defaecation. This history is diagnostic of an anal fissure. The fissure is concealed by the anal spasm but a small skin tag (*sentinel pile*) may be seen at the superficial end of the fissure. Rectal examination is extremely painful and rarely possible.

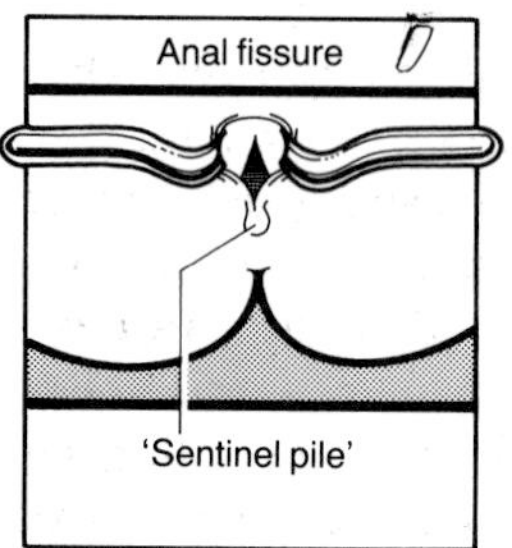

Fig. 18.8 Anal fissure

Chronic anal fissure **F** with a 'sentinel pile' **P**. These fissures are typically posteriorly located, as in this patient

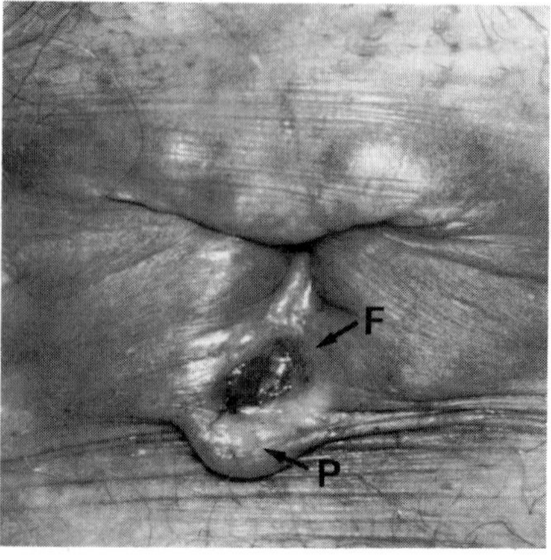

Patients sometimes manage to tolerate the pain of an acute fissure by using local anaesthetic creams, and then present with a chronic anal fissure. Anal sphincter spasm, however, prevents the fissure from healing.

Management of anal fissure

Anal fissure may be managed conservatively; the patient uses local anaesthetic gel and inserts a plastic anal dilator twice daily. Immediate relief can, however, be obtained by surgery. This involves either an *anal stretch* or a *lateral submucous (internal) sphincterotomy*, a minor operation. The fissure heals rapidly after either procedure. Dietary advice should be given to help prevent recurrence.

PERIANAL HAEMATOMA

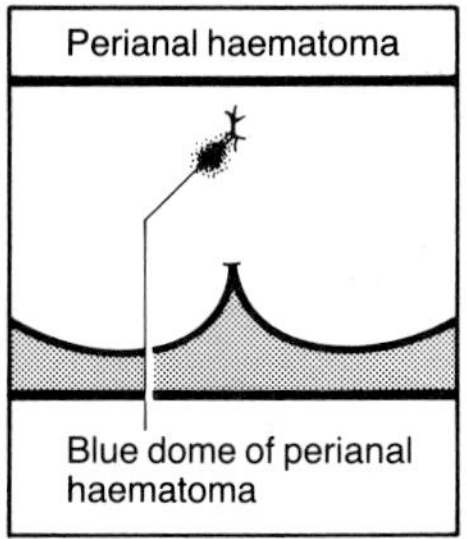

Fig. 18.9

Perianal haematoma is another acutely painful condition with a history similar to that of anal fissure. It is caused by rupture of a blood vessel beneath the anal skin, either spontaneously or after straining at stool. On examination, a small blue-black hemispherical bulge is seen in the skin near the anal margin. The condition is often described as a *thrombosed external pile* but it is in fact unrelated to haemorrhoids.

Most perianal haematomas subside over a few days and patients need only oral analgesia. Topical anaesthetic creams are not absorbed by the skin and are useless. If pain is intolerable, the haematoma may be incised and drained under anaesthesia.

ABSCESSES IN THE PERIANAL REGION

Abscesses in the anal area are extremely common surgical emergencies. They present with severe and constant perianal pain, tenderness and swelling.

Perianal abscesses begin as acute purulent infections of the anal glands. These lie between the internal and external anal sphincters, and drain into tiny pits at the bases of the anal columns along the dentate line. The ducts through which they drain are very narrow, and duct obstruction by faeces may initiate the infection. If an abscess remains confined between the two anal sphincter layers, a small *intersphincteric abscess* results, and the only symptom may be anal pain. There is often a localised area of tenderness on rectal examination.

Fig. 18.10

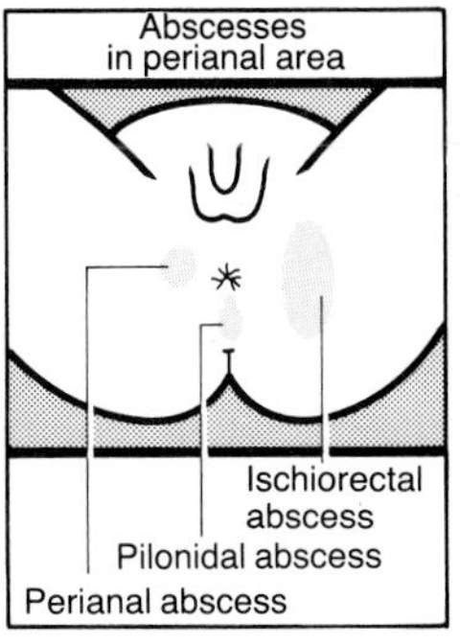

Infection of the anal glands tends to spread laterally through the external sphincter into the tissue beneath the perianal skin, forming a *perianal abscess*. At this point, there is little barrier to the spread of infection into the loose fibro-fatty tissue of the ischiorectal fossa, and a neglected or inadequately treated perianal abscess may develop into a much larger *ischiorectal abscess*. Further spread may involve the pararectal tissues above the pelvic floor resulting in a *pararectal abscess*.

If a perianal abscess is seen early, oral antibiotic treatment may abort the infection. Over the last two decades, the widespread use of antibiotics in this way by general practitioners has greatly reduced the number and severity of cases reaching the surgeon. Established abscesses require incision and drainage, which is performed under general anaesthesia through the perianal skin. Large ischiorectal abscesses require packing to keep the neck of the cavity open whilst granulation tissue gradually fills the space from its depths. Incising a perianal abscess carries a risk of creating an *anal fistula* (see below) if the abscess already communicates with the anal canal. These connections are not usually detectable at the time of surgery but a wound discharge persisting for several weeks suggests the presence of a fistula.

Pilonidal abscesses occur in the skin of the natal cleft. If near the anal margin, they may simulate a genuine perianal abscess. Treatment is by incision and drainage, but further procedures are usually required to treat the associated pilonidal sinus (see Chapter 28).

ANAL FISTULA

Anal fistulae usually develop as a complication of perianal, ischiorectal or pararectal abscesses. The fistula tracks from the lower rectum or upper anal canal through the abscess site to the perianal skin at the point of previous drainage. The communication between abscess cavity and bowel is established by spontaneous drainage into the bowel either before surgical drainage or after incomplete surgical drainage. Thus any abscess in the anal region should be drained early and thoroughly.

The patient typically complains of an intermittent discharge in the perianal region. On examination, a small papilla of granulation tissue is seen on the skin within 2–3 cm of the anal margin (see Figure 18.11). This clinical picture is diagnostic of an anal fistula; unfortunately, this apparently trivial skin lesion may be dismissed as a pustule or an incompletely healed perianal abscess.

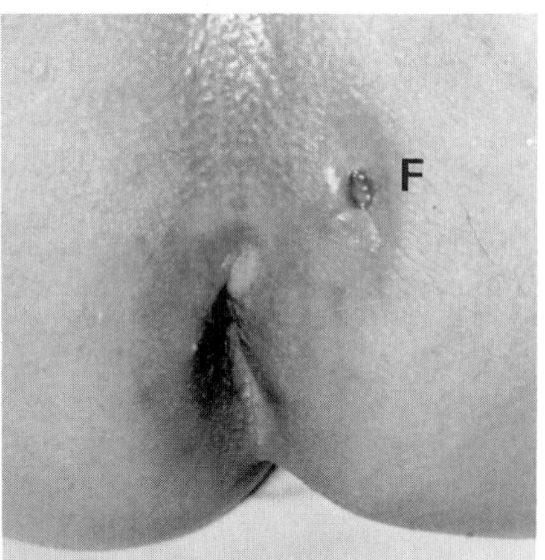

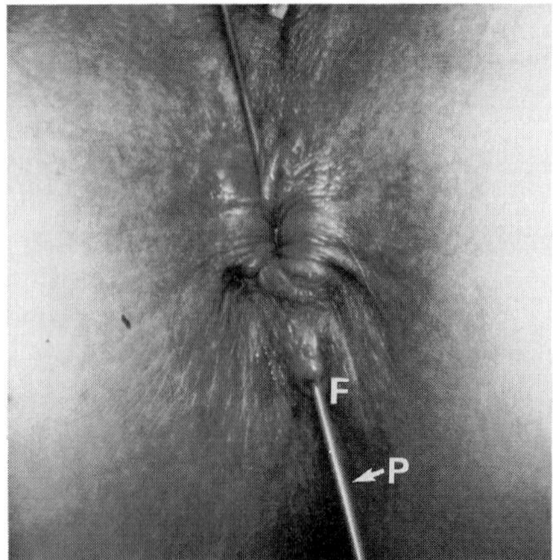

Fig. 18.11 Anal fistula
(a) The external opening of a typical anal fistula **F**. Note that it is in the scar left by drainage of a perianal abscess three months previously. **(b)** A different patient at operation. A probe **P** has been passed from the skin surface through a low anal fistula **F** to emerge low in the anal canal. Treatment consisted simply of cutting down onto the probe, thus laying open the fistula along its length. The wound was then left to heal by secondary intention

Most anal fistulae are simple and relatively superficial, the internal orifice beginning below puborectalis; these are known as low anal fistulae. Assessment requires examination under anaesthetic. A malleable probe is gently manipulated through the fistula to demonstrate the internal orifice. If this is not found, blue dye can be injected into the external orifice and may be seen to emerge in the anal canal. If the fistula is situated entirely below the puborectalis muscle (which is palpable at operation), it is laid open by cutting down onto the probe with a scalpel, transsecting the anal margin and the whole length of the fistula. The wound heals spontaneously by secondary intention. There is no loss of faecal continence, but flatus may be less well controlled.

If the fistula lies above puborectalis, surgical treatment is difficult and highly specialised because of the need to preserve the functional integrity of puborectalis.

Anal fistulae may sometimes occur as a manifestation of *Crohn's disease*. Such fistulae tend to be multiple and in the most extreme cases form a 'pepper pot' perineum (see Figure 16.7).

ANAL WARTS

Warts in the perianal region have the same pathology and viral aetiology as warts elsewhere but are transmitted by sexual activity. Referral to a genitomedical unit may be appropriate if other sexually transmitted diseases are suspected.

In small numbers, anal warts can be treated by topical applications of *podophyllin*. When large numbers are present, surgical excision under general anaesthetic is the only practical option. This involves meticulous excision of each individual wart by electrocautery. The normal skin between the warts is carefully preserved to avoid delayed healing and the disastrous complication of anal stenosis.

Fig. 18.12 Anal warts

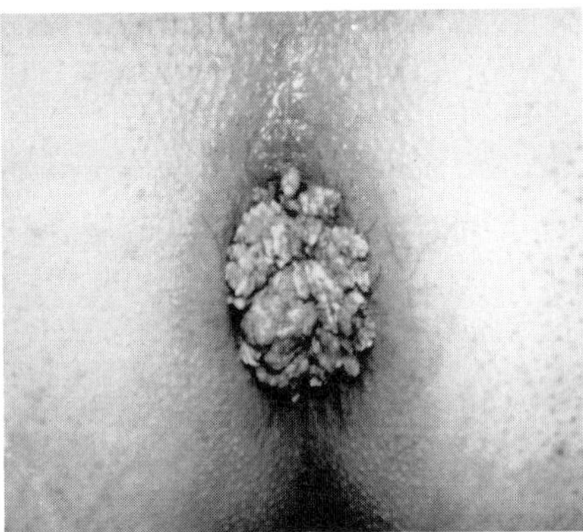

RECTAL PROLAPSE

Rectal prolapse is mainly seen in young children and the elderly. In children, it is usually a relatively minor and self-correcting problem. In the elderly, it is a chronic problem with no easy surgical solution. In pathophysiological terms, a rectal prolapse is a hernia of the rectum through the pelvic floor. In effect, the mucosa and muscle wall intussuscept through the anal canal. In the early stages, the prolapse occurs only with defaecation and retracts spontaneously. At a later stage, the rectum may prolapse when the patient merely stands up. The patient thus becomes socially isolated.

In childhood, rectal prolapse usually occurs around the age of two years. It tends to occur during toilet training and causes parental anxiety. Parents should be reassured that the prolapse will return spontaneously after defaecation, although gentle manipulation may be required. These children should be given a high fibre diet and taught not to strain during defaecation. More sophisticated treatment is rarely required.

In the elderly, rectal prolapse is either remarkably well tolerated, or else concealed. The patient becomes accustomed to reducing the prolapse manually after defaecation and rarely complains about it. A high fibre diet makes little difference to the problem since the anatomical defect will never recover spontaneously. If the prolapse occurs on standing or if incontinence develops, the patient will require surgical treatment.

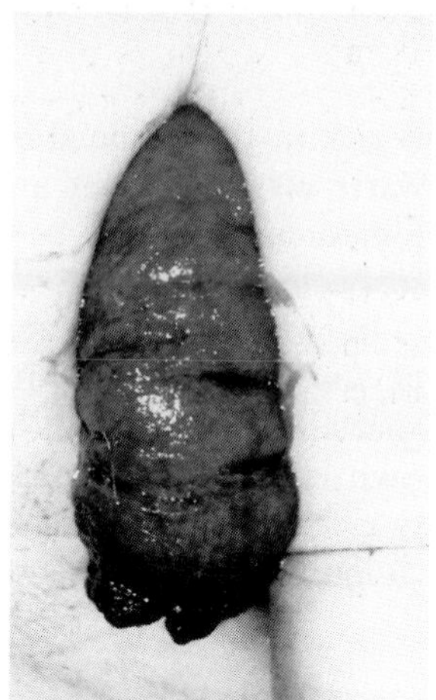

Fig. 18.13 Rectal prolapse

This complete rectal prolapse was in an 80-year-old woman. It emerged spontaneously whenever she stood, causing considerable discomfort and inconvenience, to say the least!

Management of rectal prolapse

The usual surgical procedure for rectal prolapse is an abdominal operation to secure the rectum within the abdominal cavity or pelvis. The most common operations are the *Wells operation* and the *Ripstein rectopexy*. In the former, a sheet of synthetic Ivalon sponge is wrapped around the rectum and sutured to the sacral concavity. The material provokes an intense fibrotic response which holds the rectum in place. The risk of infection associated with the Ivalon sponge operation is largely avoided by the Ripstein rectopexy. This operation involves hitching the rectum up to the sacral promontory with a polyester fabric sling. This operation may help to improve faecal continence, but a sphincter repair operation may be necessary later if incontinence remains a problem.

For the elderly or the infirm, where abdominal operation is contraindicated, a subcutaneous circum-anal silicone rubber ring may be inserted. This is a minor operation but is apt to fail because the ring is too tight (causing constipation) or too loose (allowing recurrent prolapse).

CARCINOMA OF THE ANUS

Carcinoma of the anus is an ulcerating *squamous cell carcinoma* arising from the stratified squamous epithelium of the lower half of the anal canal. It is uncommon and forms less than 5% of all ano-rectal malignancies. It is mainly a disease of the elderly. Since the symptoms (fresh rectal bleeding, anal pain, discomfort and discharge) are similar to those of haemorrhoids and other common benign anal conditions, the patient may ignore the symptoms and the doctor may miss the diagnosis. Metastasis of anal carcinoma is to the inguinal lymph nodes, reflecting the drainage of the anal canal skin. Occasionally, malignant melanomas and other rare tumours arise in the perianal area.

On palpation, squamous carcinoma feels hard and woody due to invasion of perianal tissues. This is in contrast to the other perianal conditions described above. Diagnosis is confirmed by proctoscopic biopsy.

The standard surgical treatment is *abdomino-perineal resection* of rectum and anus with a permanent end colostomy in the left iliac fossa. Inguinal lymph node metastases usually respond well to radiotherapy. More distant metastasis is rare. In elderly and infirm patients, palliative radiotherapy to the primary lesion may be all that is appropriate.

LOW RECTAL POLYPS AND CANCER

Rectal adenomas and other polyps may sometimes develop a long pedicle and be dragged down into the anal canal. If they appear at the anal verge, they may be mistaken for haemorrhoids. This emphasises the importance of proper investigation by proctoscopy and sigmoidoscopy in patients with persistent haemorrhoid-like symptoms. Treatment is by excision with a diathermy snare, the specimen being sent for histological examination.

Adenocarcinomas arising low in the rectum may sometimes present with perianal bleeding and discharge. Again, these symptoms should be properly investigated rather than dismissed as haemorrhoids.

19 DISORDERS OF THE GROIN AND MALE GENITALIA

Introduction

Groin lumps and swellings account for about 10% of surgical outpatient referrals.

In both sexes, the commonest lumps in the groin are *hernias*, either inguinal or femoral. Both are caused by abdominal contents protruding through defects in the abdominal wall. In the male, the testis descends into the scrotum via the inguinal canal, and this area remains potentially weak throughout life; inguinal hernias are therefore more common in males. If large, an *inguinal hernia* may present as a scrotal lump rather than a groin lump. In the female, the uterine round ligament pursues a similar course to the spermatic cord in the male; this explains the occasional occurrence of inguinal hernias in females. The femoral canal, below the inguinal ligament, is another potential weakness in the abdominal wall and may give rise to a *femoral hernia*.

Enlarged lymph nodes due to infection or malignancy also cause groin lumps or swellings. Less common are vascular abnormalities such as a *saphena varix* or a *femoral artery aneurysm*. Very rarely nowadays, a *psoas abscess* may track beneath the inguinal ligament to present in the groin.

The embryology and anatomy of the groin, testis and perineum provide a good starting point for understanding many surgical problems in this area and are explained in Figures 19.1 to 19.4.

Testicular tumours of germ cell origin are uncommon, but are important because curative treatment is now available for most of them. The embryology of testicular descent determines the lymphatic drainage of the testis, which is different from that of the scrotal skin.

When pain in the groin or scrotum is the main presenting symptom, the usual cause is a newly developed inguinal hernia, a strangulated inguinal or femoral hernia, an acute infection of the scrotal contents or testicular torsion. All but the first of these are acute surgical emergencies.

Disorders of the penis are uncommon in adults, but the most important is carcinoma. In children, penile disorders are either developmental or minor inflammatory conditions; these are discussed in Chapter 31. Disorders of the female genitalia are usually seen by gynaecologists.

The important disorders of the groin and genitalia are summarised in Figure 19.5, together with their anatomical and clinical significance.

Fig. 19.1 Structure of the inguinal and femoral canals

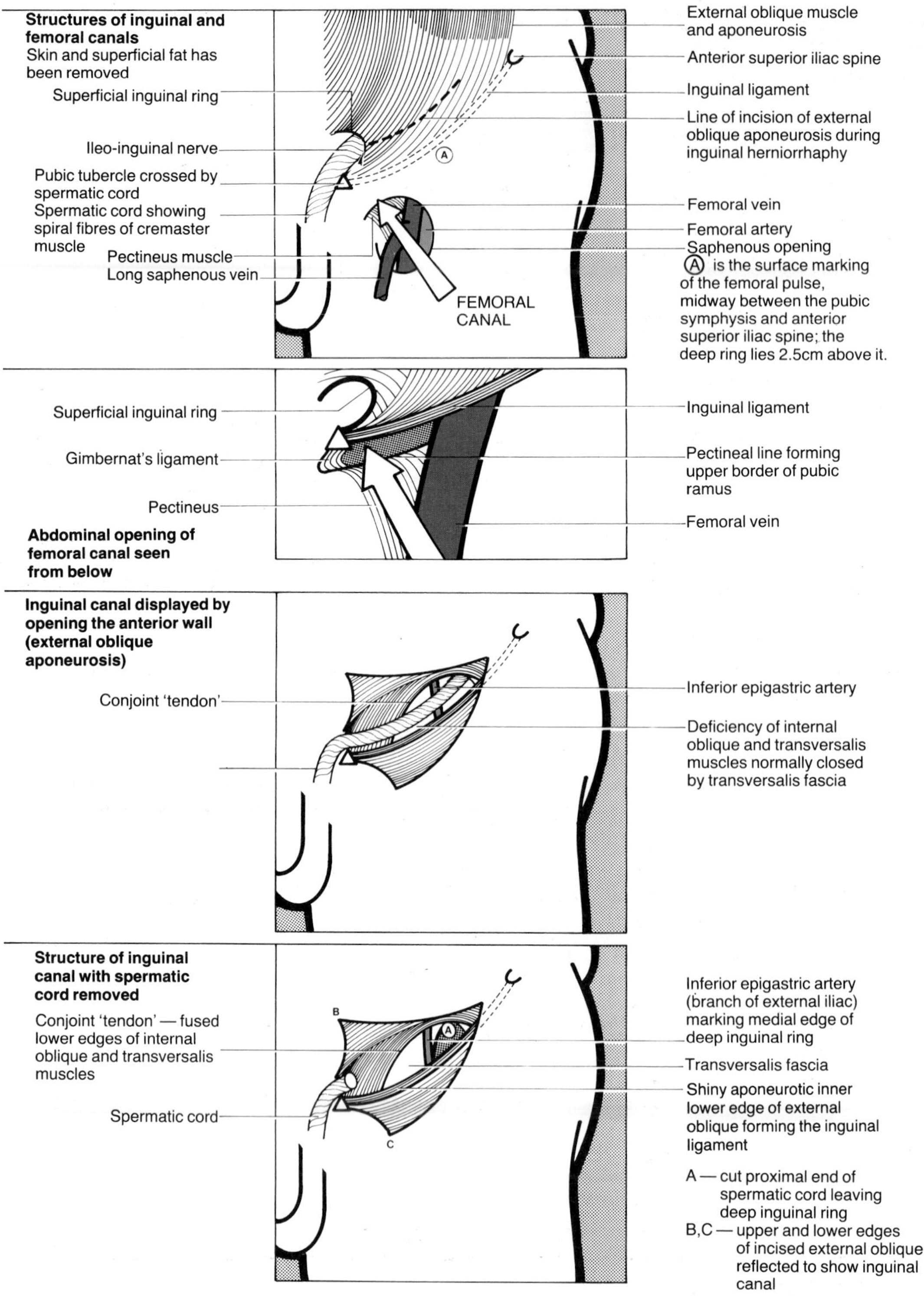

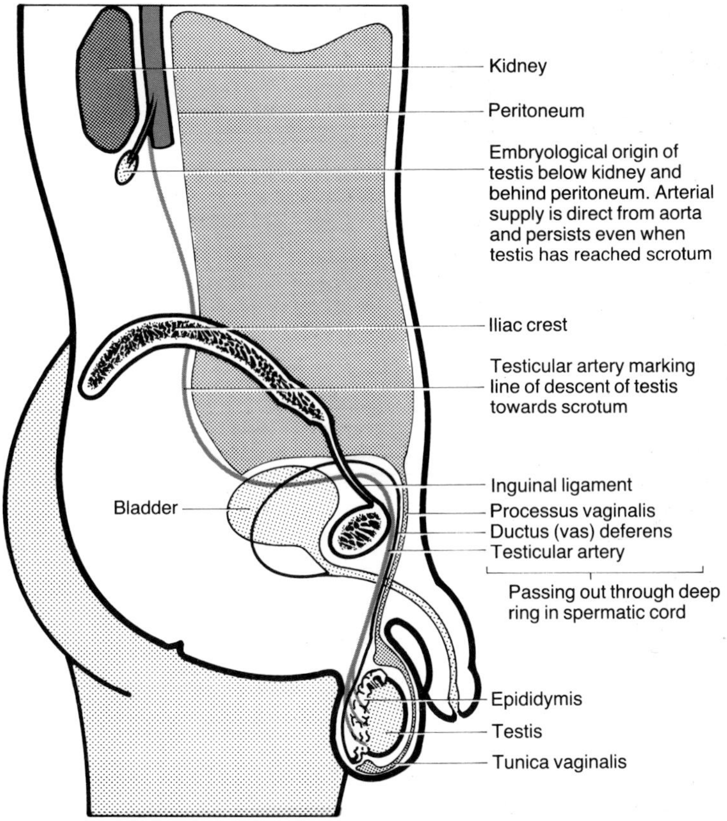

Kidney
Peritoneum
Embryological origin of testis below kidney and behind peritoneum. Arterial supply is direct from aorta and persists even when testis has reached scrotum
Iliac crest
Testicular artery marking line of descent of testis towards scrotum
Bladder
Inguinal ligament
Processus vaginalis
Ductus (vas) deferens
Testicular artery
Passing out through deep ring in spermatic cord
Epididymis
Testis
Tunica vaginalis

Fig. 19.2 Embryological descent of the testis

Fig. 19.3 The sapheno-femoral venous junction

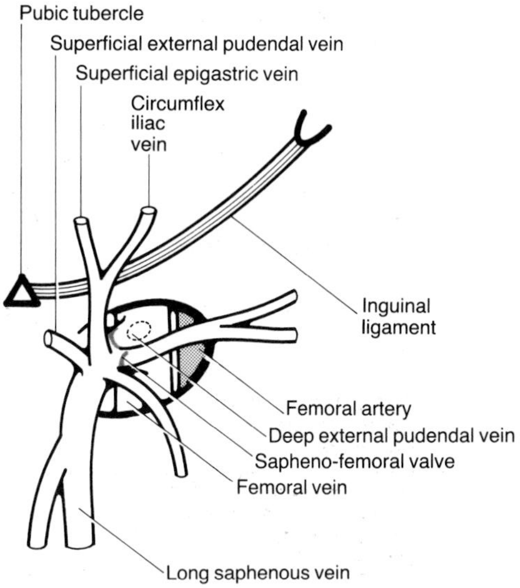

Pubic tubercle
Superficial external pudendal vein
Superficial epigastric vein
Circumflex iliac vein
Inguinal ligament
Femoral artery
Deep external pudendal vein
Sapheno-femoral valve
Femoral vein
Long saphenous vein

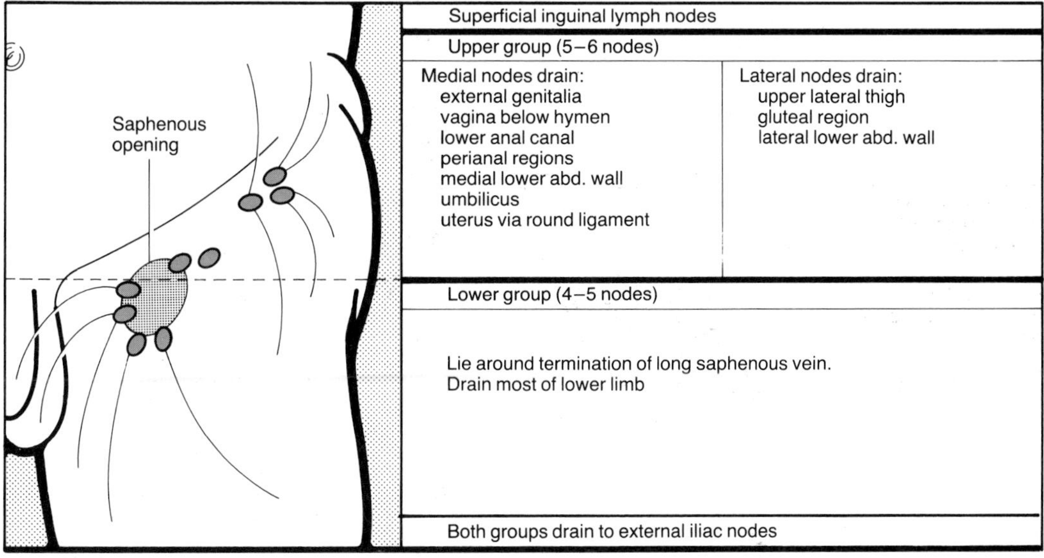

Superficial inguinal lymph nodes	
Upper group (5–6 nodes)	
Medial nodes drain: external genitalia vagina below hymen lower anal canal perianal regions medial lower abd. wall umbilicus uterus via round ligament	Lateral nodes drain: upper lateral thigh gluteal region lateral lower abd. wall
Lower group (4–5 nodes)	
Lie around termination of long saphenous vein. Drain most of lower limb	
Both groups drain to external iliac nodes	

Fig. 19.4 Lymph nodes of the groin

Fig. 19.5 Summary — disorders of the groin and scrotum and their clinical features

DISORDER	ANATOMICAL/ DEVELOPMENTAL BASIS	CLINICAL FEATURES
1. Groin lumps and swellings		
a. Inguinal hernias		
— Direct	Simple bulging of abdominal contents due to inadequate support given by weak posterior wall of inguinal canal	Discomfort; lump disappears on lying down; risk of incarceration if large; low risk of strangulation
— Indirect	Passage of abdominal contents, often including bowel, through inguinal canal towards scrotum or labium majus	Potential for incarceration and strangulation; much more common in men
b. Femoral hernia	Passage of abdominal contents often including bowel into femoral canal	Likely to become incarcerated or strangulated
c. Inguinal lymph-adenopathy	Inguinal nodes drain lower limb, abdominal wall below umbilicus, anal canal, scrotal skin, penis (but not testes, which drain to para-aortic and para-iliac nodes)	Enlarged nodes indicate infection, lymphoma or secondaries in drainage area
d. Saphena varix	Dilatation of long saphenous vein superficial to deep fascia before it enters the femoral vein	Can be mistaken for femoral hernia but empties on pressure and disappears on lying down, unlike femoral hernia
e. Femoral artery aneurysm	Dilatation of common femoral artery just below inguinal ligament	Classical clinical sign is expansile pulsation; could be mistaken for femoral hernia
f. Psoas abscess	Tuberculous abscess of lumbar vertebra tracking down inside sheath of psoas muscle	Presents as swelling or 'cold abscess' below inguinal ligament. Rare nowadays but may be confused with lymph nodes
2. Testicular disorders		
a. Incompletely descended testis	Failure of complete descent from retroperitoneal site into scrotum; testis may be arrested at any point of descent or in an ectopic site	Mainly a problem of infancy and childhood requiring orchidopexy; possible cause of lump in groin; predisposition to malignancy; fertility may be impaired
b. Torsion of testis	Rotation of testis in scrotum; twists in the spermatic cord result in venous obstruction which may culminate in infarction; recurrent incomplete torsion may occur	Complete torsion causes severe acute scrotal pain (and sometimes abdominal pain); partial torsion may cause episodic pain

Fig. 19.5 continued

DISORDER	ANATOMICAL/ DEVELOPMENTAL BASIS	CLINICAL FEATURES
c. Inflammation of epididymis or testis	'Epididymo–orchitis' is a term often used incorrectly for acute epididymitis. Usually caused by common urinary tract pathogens.	Acute epididymitis is painful; must be distinguished from testicular torsion
	Acute orchitis is often viral (mumps)	Testicular pain and swelling
	Chronic orchitis may be caused by tuberculosis or syphilitic gumma	Usually presents as painless testicular enlargement
d. Testicular tumours	Derived from germ cells of testis; metastasise via lymphatics to para-iliac and para-aortic nodes or via blood stream, commonly to lung	Presents as painless swelling of testis usually with small secondary hydrocoele
3. Disorders of other scrotal contents		
a. Hydrocoele	Abnormal collection of fluid in space around testis; in children may still be in communication with peritoneal cavity (communicating hydrocoele)	Presents as a painless scrotal swelling which transilluminates; testis may be difficult to palpate within it until fluid is drained
b. Haematocoele	Collection of blood around testis; usually late result of trauma or surgery	Presents as hydrocoele but does not transilluminate
c. Varicocoele	Dilatation of pampiniform venous plexus of spermatic cord	Presents as a scrotal swelling separate from testis and epididymis; feels like a 'bag of worms'. Disappears on lying down, thus patient must be examined standing
d. Epididymal cyst and spermatocoele	Cyst derived from epididymal tissue	Epididymal cyst presents as a scrotal swelling which transilluminates; separate from the testis, often multiloculated. Spermatocoele is unilocular, in cord or epididymis, and may be transilluminable
e. Torsion of hydatid of Morgagni	Torsion of epididymal appendage	May present late as a small hydrocoele; in the acute phase, presents as scrotal pain and oedema and may simulate testicular torsion

DIAGNOSIS OF PROBLEMS IN THE GROIN AND SCROTUM

A lump in the groin or scrotum is the most common presenting symptom. This may or may not be painful. The groin and scrotum must both be examined when either is swollen to discover the anatomical origin of the swelling. The patient must also be examined while standing, to avoid missing an inguinal hernia which reduces spontaneously or a varicocoele which empties when the patient is supine.

LUMP IN THE GROIN

Lumps in the groin are examined in the same way as lumps elsewhere but there are certain special points to note as follows:

The relationship of the groin lump to the inguinal ligament

The position of the lump in relation to the inguinal ligament should first be identified. The ligament is not visible but stretches between two palpable bony prominences: the anterior superior iliac spine laterally and the pubic tubercle medially (see Figure 19.1 earlier). Usually, the iliac spine is easily found but the pubic tubercle can be difficult to locate, especially in obese patients. The pubic tubercle can be found by palpating out from the midline along the upper border of the pubic symphysis (care is needed as the spermatic cord can be tender) or by invagination of the scrotum with the index finger from below upwards, passing deep to the cord as it crosses the tubercle (see Figure 19.7).

The pubic tubercle is higher than might be imagined from the skin contour. Similarly, the inguinal ligament does not correspond to the crease between lower abdomen and thigh. Rather, the inguinal ligament is a centimetre or more above the crease. As shown in Figure 19.6, inguinal hernias always originate above

Fig. 19.6 Significance of the relationship of groin lumps to the inguinal ligament

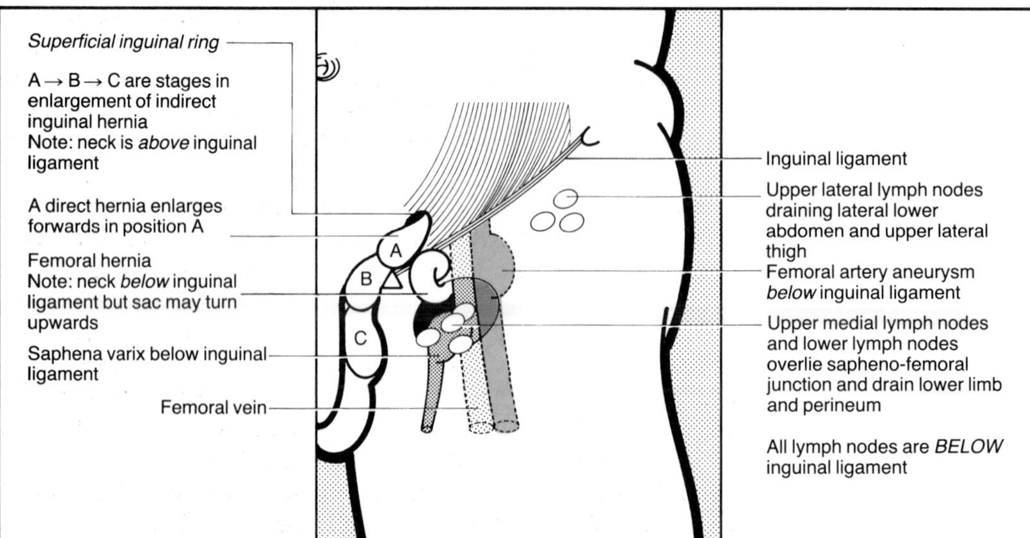

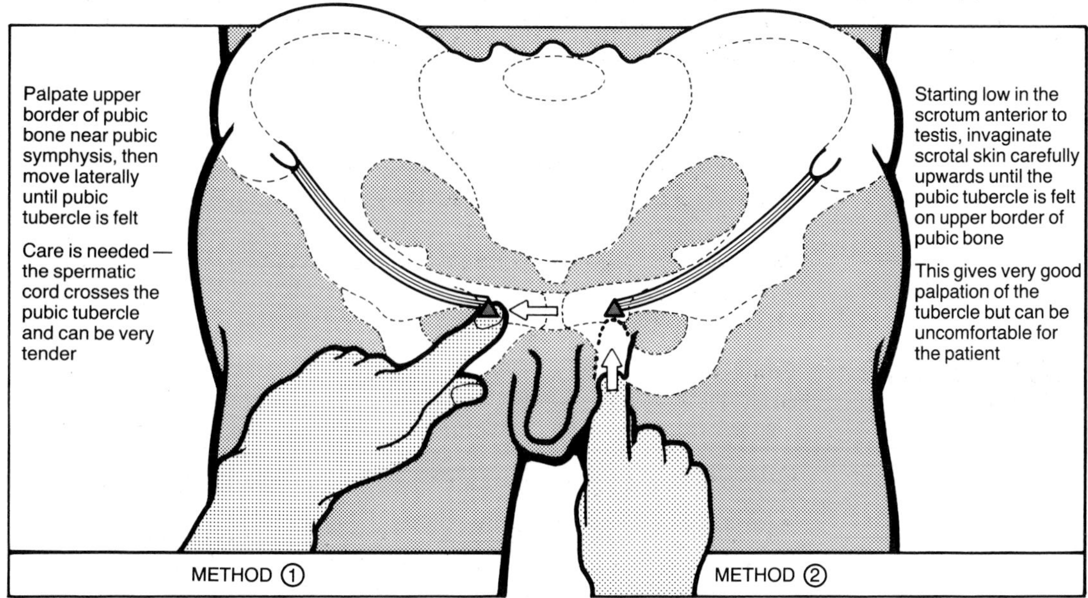

Fig. 19.7 Digital palpation of the pubic tubercle

the inguinal ligament, whereas femoral hernias, saphena varices and femoral artery aneurysms always arise below it. Enlarged inguinal lymph nodes are usually below the inguinal ligament. Psoas abscesses originate well above the inguinal ligament but track down within the psoas sheath to present below the inguinal ligament.

The consistency and reducibility of the lump

The consistency and reducibility of a groin lump can be useful diagnostic features. Hernias are usually soft but the most reliable diagnostic sign is whether the lump reduces spontaneously when the patient lies flat or with gentle manipulation. Most inguinal hernias are at least partially reducible, although long-standing hernias gradually become irreducible because of adhesions within the sac. These are said to be *incarcerated*. Another characteristic of an inguinal hernia is a palpable expansile impulse when the patient coughs. If bowel is present (and the hernia is not strangulated) auscultation will reveal bowel sounds. In contrast, femoral hernias are usually irreducible and have no cough impulse since the femoral canal is so narrow. Bowel sounds are not heard unless the hernial orifice is so large as to admit a large and reducible mass of bowel. This is rare, however.

Distinguishing between direct and indirect inguinal hernias may be clinically difficult and is of little operative importance. Despite this, it is a useful exercise in eliciting clinical signs and is frequently asked in student examinations! By definition, an *indirect inguinal hernia* is one in which the hernial sac leaves the abdomen via the deep (internal) inguinal ring to enter the inguinal canal. Thus, if the hernia can be completely reduced, finger pressure over the deep ring (2 cm above the femoral pulse) will prevent it reappearing on coughing. In contrast, a *direct inguinal hernia* leaves the abdomen through a weakness in the posterior wall of the inguinal canal, i.e. medial to the deep ring, and so cannot be controlled by digital pressure over the deep ring.

Enlarged inguinal nodes vary in consistency, number and size depending on the pathological cause; they are not reducible. A saphena varix is very soft and completely disappears on palpation, refilling when pressure is released. Femoral artery aneurysms, however, are firm and pulsatile. These vascular conditions must be diagnosed correctly as injudicious operation could be catastrophic!

SCROTAL LUMPS AND SWELLINGS

A lump or swelling in the scrotum may be:

- A solid mass arising from one of the components of the scrotal contents or spermatic cord. These anatomical structures include testis, epididymis, epididymal appendage, ductus (vas) deferens and pampiniform venous plexus
- A collection of fluid in the tunica or processus vaginalis (hydrocoele)
- An inguinal hernia extending along the embryological path of testicular descent

Origin of a scrotal lump

The first clinical objective is to determine whether the swelling arises in the groin, in the spermatic cord itself, or in the scrotum. This is achieved by palpating the spermatic cord at the neck of the scrotum. In the case of a hernia, the spermatic cord is much thicker than normal and the hernia can be shown to communicate with the abdominal cavity. Spermatic cord swellings (varicocoele or cyst) are usually easy to recognise. If the lump is scrotal, the spermatic cord is normal in diameter.

Testicular and epididymal lumps

When the abnormality is scrotal, an attempt is made to palpate the testis and epididymis separately, and find their relationship to the lump. If the testis is enlarged or there is a lump within it, this must be regarded as a primary tumour until proven otherwise by excision biopsy. Testicular swellings due to lymphoma, leukaemia or granulomatous infections (e.g. tuberculosis or syphilitic gumma) tend to be softer, but this is an unreliable sign. Any testicular pathology may cause a little fluid to accumulate in the tunica vaginalis resulting in a small *secondary hydrocoele*. This rarely interferes with testicular palpation.

Lumps in the epididymis (cysts, chronic bacterial epididymitis or rarely, tuberculous granulomata) are discrete from, but attached to an otherwise normal testis. Tiny focal lumps in the epididymis are rarely clinically important. Infective lesions cause diffuse thickening of the epididymis, whereas epididymal cysts are almost always located at its upper pole. Epididymal cysts are filled with clear fluid and therefore transilluminate. Transillumination is demonstrated by shining a strong beam of light (torch or fibreoptic cable) through the scrotum in a partly darkened room. If the lesion is fluid-filled, it will glow (except in the case of blood). About 10% of cysts in the epididymis, and most of those in the cord, are filled with an opalescent fluid containing spermatozoa. These spermatocoeles are usually recognisable by the brilliance of their transillumination.

Other scrotal lumps and swellings

Slow accumulation of fluid within the tunica vaginalis produces a *primary hydrocoele* surrounding the testis. These are common in the elderly. They are often ignored by the patient until they become very large (300 ml or more) because they cause no pain. The testis is not palpable separately from the swelling but occasionally, the hydrocoele is lax enough to allow the testis to be palpated through it; more often the hydrocoele is too tense for this. Diagnosis is confirmed if the swelling transilluminates. In young boys, the tunica vaginalis may sometimes remain in continuity with the peritoneal cavity via a *patent processus vaginalis*. This is so narrow that herniation does not occur but it allows peritoneal fluid to accumulate by gravity during the day. This causes a scrotal swelling which disappears overnight, and is known as a *communicating hydrocoele*.

Fig. 19.8 Causes of a lump or swelling in the scrotum

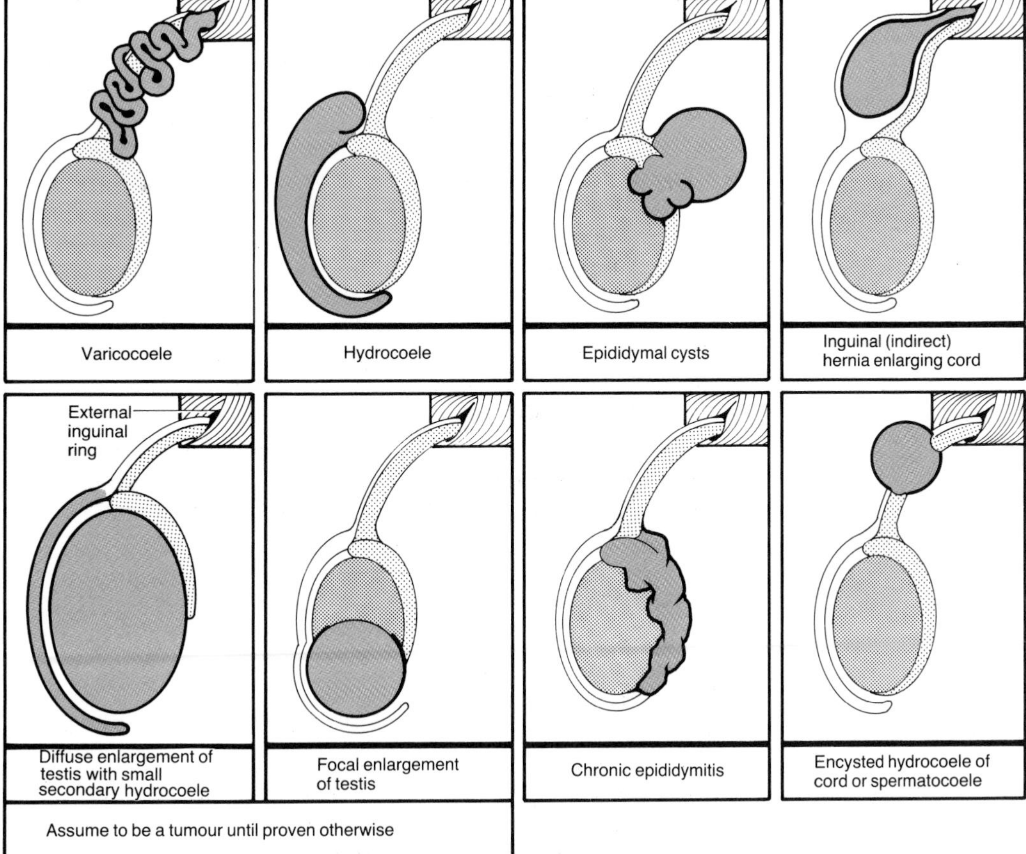

Abnormalities of the spermatic cord are usually varicocoeles or cysts. Varicocoeles are common, often asymptomatic, and represent dilatation of the venous network making up the pampiniform plexus. They feel like a 'bag of worms' on palpation and disappear in the supine position. Cysts of the cord are usually small, spherical and transilluminable. They represent either an encysted hydrocoele arising from a remnant of the processus vaginalis, or a spermatocoele.

GROIN AND SCROTAL PAIN

Acute pain

Several common conditions may present with acute pain in the groin or scrotum. These are listed in Figure 19.9 with their typical signs and symptoms. A strangulated hernia will be readily diagnosed by finding an irreducible hernia which is tender and often red. Strangulated hernias, particularly femoral hernias, sometimes present with abdominal pain or signs of obstruction but without localised pain. This emphasises the importance of examining the hernial orifices in every patient with an acute abdomen.

Testicular torsion must always be excluded if there is acute scrotal pain since the testis can be saved if operation is performed promptly; an exploratory operation is mandatory if torsion of the testis cannot be confidently excluded. Torsion occurs mainly in adolescents and occasionally in young adults. The main differential diagnosis at all ages is acute bacterial epididymitis. Torsion of an epididymal appendage (hydatid of Morgagni) produces symptoms similar to testicular torsion but less severe; surgical exploration is still required to exclude the latter.

Fig. 19.9 Common causes of acute pain in the groin and scrotum

Strangulated inguinal or femoral hernia — painful, irreducible, tender groin lump. Sometimes presents as intestinal obstruction or abdominal pain

Torsion of the testis — sudden onset of unilateral scrotal pain with or without poorly-localised abdominal pain. In early cases, the testis is high in the scrotum, exquisitely tender and the cord is thickened. Later these signs are often obscured by oedema. The opposite testis often lies horizontally (bell-clapper testis)

Torsion of the epididymal appendage (hydatid of Morgagni) — sudden onset of unilateral scrotal pain; the testis hangs normally. There is tenderness only at its upper pole and minimal overlying oedema

Acute epididymitis — moderate or severe scrotal pain and tenderness with marked redness and oedema. Often preceded by symptoms of urinary tract infection. Urine usually contains white cells and organisms

Haematocoele following trauma or scrotal surgery (e.g. vasectomy) — history may be diagnostic although torsion is sometimes precipitated by trauma

Chronic pain

When chronic pain in the groin or scrotum occurs without any other clues in the history and no swelling, it is often difficult to diagnose and treat.

Groin pain may be caused by inflamed inguinal lymph nodes secondary to infection in their field of drainage. Strained muscle attachments to the bony pelvis sometimes cause groin pain; this particularly affects the hip adductor attachments near the pubic tubercle. Groin pain may also be referred from a diseased hip joint. An early inguinal hernia sometimes causes groin pain before the hernia becomes clinically detectable.

Chronic scrotal pain is most often due to inflammation. It can often be traced back to a vasectomy, although the cause is often obscure and the treatment ineffective. Patients present weeks or months after the operation, complaining of localised tenderness at the operation site or a general ache in one side of the scrotum. If there is a small tender lump due to a stitch granuloma, this is easily cured by excision.

Pain is also a feature of chronic bacterial epididymitis, which usually follows an acute episode.

Recurrent, incomplete testicular torsion may cause transient episodes of severe pain in the inguino-scrotal region or poorly-defined lower abdominal pain. In such cases, the anatomical relationship of the testis to the tunica vaginalis is often abnormal so the testes lie horizontally rather than vertically when the patient is standing. Such 'bell-clapper' testes are susceptible to torsion.

THE MISSING OR ECTOPIC TESTIS

Scrotal examination may reveal one or both testes to be absent. The problem is very common in children but is sometimes discovered by chance in adults. The testis is very rarely missing but lies somewhere along the normal path of testicular descent, usually in the inguinal canal or occasionally within the abdomen. Such incompletely descended testes (often called undescended testes) are usually small and atrophic and are predisposed to malignant change; indeed an inguinal mass may sometimes be a testicular tumour. Previous orchidectomy, sometimes performed during surgery of recurrent inguinal hernias, should be excluded.

Occasionally, an adult testis may become displaced towards the inguinal canal following trauma or surgery. The testis is normal in size but fixed in position by adhesions. If there were other major injuries, the scrotal injury may have been overlooked.

Trauma, including operations for hernia or incompletely descended testis, may damage the blood supply and cause testicular atrophy. The resulting testis is abnormally small and soft. When both testes are small, the cause is usually hypoplasia, androgen insufficiency or oestrogen therapy for prostatic carcinoma.

DISORDERS OF THE GROIN

INGUINAL HERNIA

Inguinal hernia is one of the most common complaints in general surgical outpatients' departments. In a typical district general hospital, inguinal hernias account for about 7% of outpatient consultations and about 12% of operating theatre time.

As shown in Figure 19.10, inguinal hernias occur twice as often as femoral hernias in females. In males, inguinal hernias are much more common (97.5% inguinal versus 2.5% femoral) because of the potential abdominal wall weakness caused by testicular descent. Femoral hernias occur twice as often in females as in males.

Fig. 19.10 Relative incidence of inguinal and femoral hernias

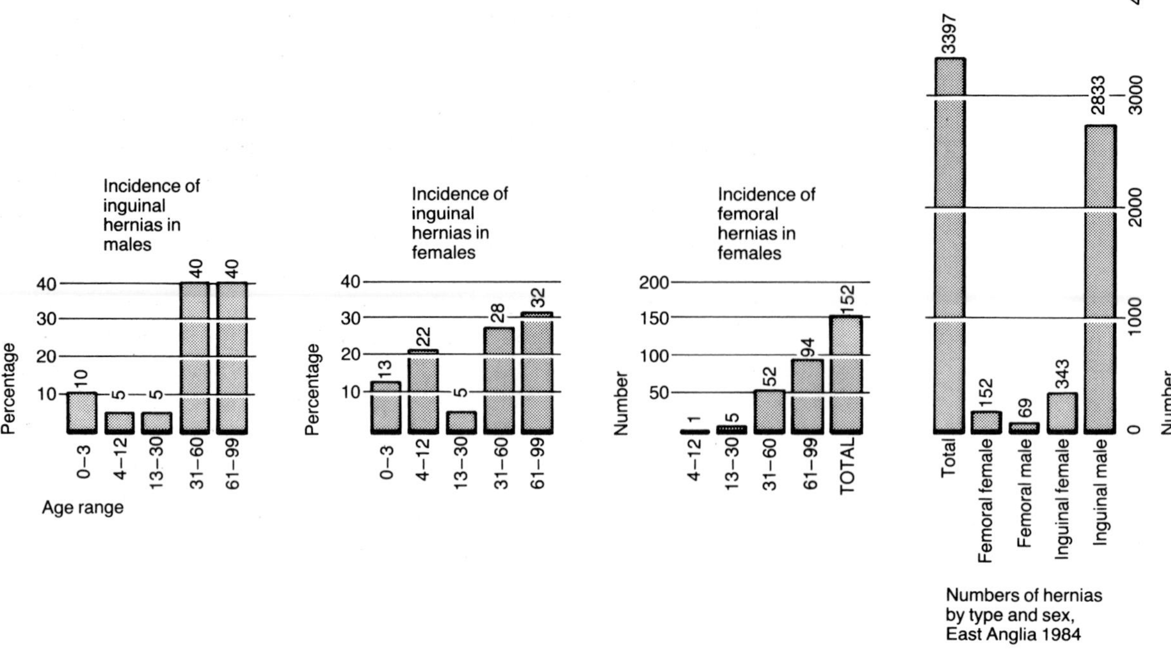

Inguinal hernias occur at any age. In childhood, they are always of developmental origin. In males, hernias are most common under the age of five and from middle age onwards. A smaller peak occurs in the late teens and early twenties. Hernias in these young men are probably a result of congenital predisposition, exacerbated by work or sport. Inguinal hernias should be repaired early to reduce the risk of strangulation and the need for emergency operation.

Anatomical considerations

Further detail of the surgical anatomy of the inguinal and femoral canals is shown in Figure 19.11. In this diagram, the external oblique aponeurosis (or fascia), which forms the anterior wall of the inguinal canal, appears opened as it would after the first stage of a hernia repair operation.

Fig. 19.11 Relations of the deep inguinal ring

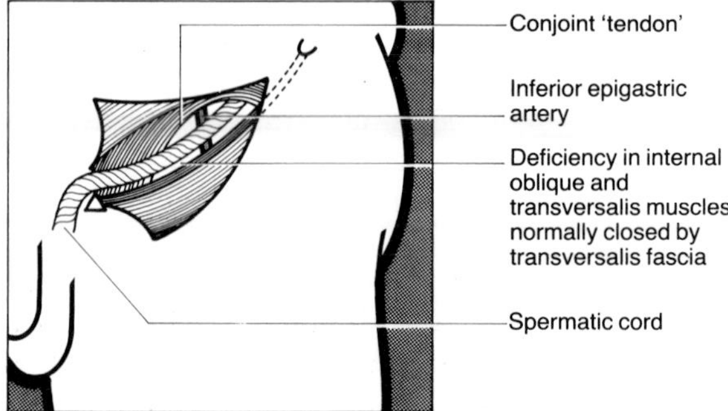

The external oblique aponeurosis has been split obliquely from the external ring along the line of its fibres for about 5 cm laterally and the cut edges reflected upwards and downwards to expose the inguinal canal. Note that the internal oblique and transversus abdominis muscles are deficient above the medial half of the inguinal ligament. Their inferior borders fuse in this area to form the conjoint tendon. This 'tendon', which is usually just the fused lower edge of the muscles, forms a shallow arch stretching from the lateral half of the inguinal ligament to the pubic crest. The D-shaped defect in the muscular abdominal wall leaves the transversalis fascia as the only restraint to herniation of the abdominal contents. It is normally particularly strong in this area.

The spermatic cord passes through the transversalis fascia in the most lateral part of the muscular defect. The inferior epigastric artery passes upwards immediately medial to it. Thus, the deep (internal) ring is bounded by inguinal ligament below, conjoint tendon above and laterally, and the inferior epigastric artery medially. The posterior wall of the inguinal canal consists of transversalis fascia and the medial insertion of the conjoint tendon.

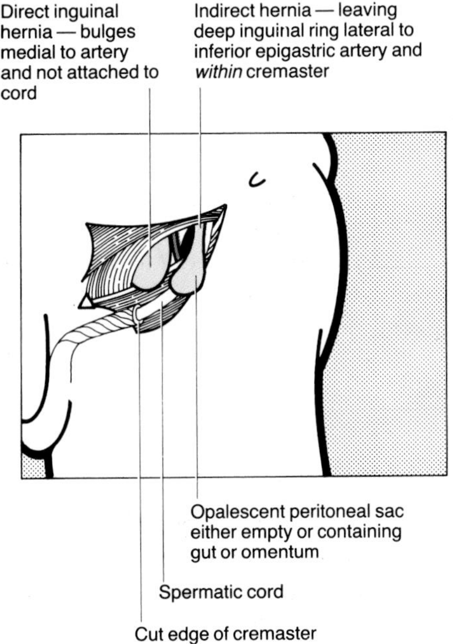

Fig. 19.12 Direct and indirect inguinal hernias

Mechanisms of inguinal hernia formation

Inguinal herniation may be direct or indirect. A direct hernia protrudes directly through the transversalis fascia and enters the inguinal canal through its posterior wall. An indirect hernia leaves the abdomen via the deep inguinal ring to follow an oblique course along the inguinal canal through the abdominal wall (see Figure 19.12). In either case, the herniated abdominal contents are contained within a sac of peritoneum. The hernia may merely consist of peritoneum and its associated extraperitoneal fat, but the sac usually contains omentum or small bowel. Less commonly, the sac contains large bowel or appendix, or rarely bladder. Occasionally, the sac contents are diseased, e.g. large bowel carcinoma, appendicitis or peritoneal secondaries, and this may be the reason for the emergency operation at which the condition is discovered.

Clinically distinguishing between direct and indirect hernias is often difficult, and is unimportant except in clinical examinations. Sometimes an indirect and a direct hernia occur together on the same side.

In an indirect hernia, the peritoneal sac may represent a patent or reopened processus vaginalis. It may extend as far as the tunica vaginalis surrounding the testis. It is easy to accept that indirect hernias have a congenital origin in children or in young muscular men, but this is less convincing in flabby older men.

Direct hernias tend to bulge forwards and rarely enter the scrotum. They are usually found in older patients with deficient muscles and weak transversalis fascia. The neck of the direct sac tends to be broad, in contrast to the narrow neck of an indirect hernia, confined by the borders of the deep ring. Indirect inguinal hernias are therefore more liable to strangulate.

Sometimes a retroperitoneal structure 'slides' down the posterior abdominal wall and herniates directly or indirectly into the inguinal canal, dragging its overlying peritoneum with it. Thus, *sliding hernias* lie behind and outside the peritoneal sac (see Figure 19.13). Diagnosis can only be made at operation.

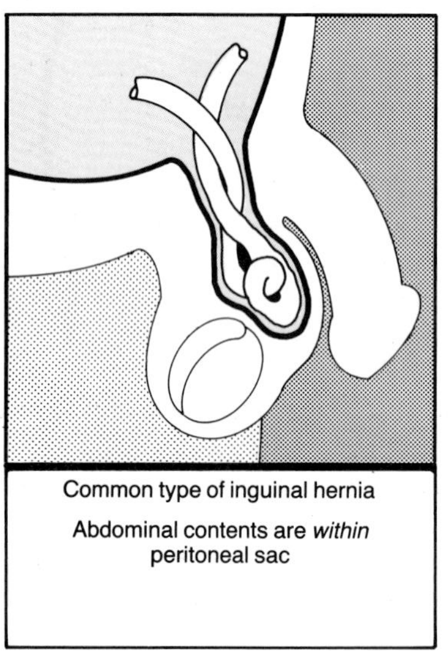

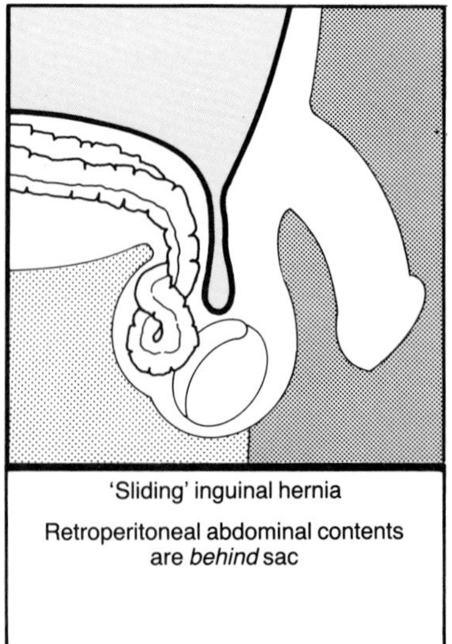

Fig. 19.13 Common and sliding inguinal hernias

Rarely, herniation occurs through a fascial defect at the lateral border of rectus abdominis. The hernial sac comes to lie interstitially between the layers of internal and external oblique. This is known as a *Spigelian hernia*. It has some of the clinical characteristics of an inguinal hernia but the bulge lies above and medial to the position of an inguinal hernia, and may be difficult to palpate because it is covered by one or more layers of the abdominal wall (see Figure 19.14).

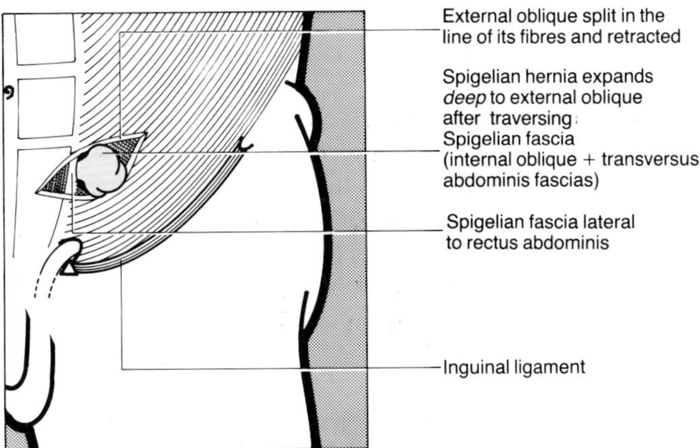

Fig. 19.14 Spigelian hernia

Natural history of inguinal hernia

Inguinal hernias usually develop slowly, although aggravated by any condition which raises intra-abdominal pressure, e.g. obesity, constipation, straining at micturition or chronic coughing. In adults, a single episode of increased intra-abdominal pressure, e.g. heavy lifting, may 'rupture' the abdominal wall, resulting in the sudden appearance of a direct hernia. In infants, a bout of severe coughing may precipitate an acute indirect hernia.

Initially, the peritoneal sac and its contents are completely reducible into the abdominal cavity. This usually occurs spontaneously when the patient lies down, but larger hernias may need manipulating by the patient if they are to be reduced. The longer a hernia remains and the larger it becomes, the more difficult it is to reduce. This increases the likelihood of fibrous adhesions developing within the sac which prevent complete reduction. An irreducible hernia which is not strangulated is described as *incarcerated*.

Hernial strangulation

Strangulation occurs if the hernial contents become constricted by the neck of the sac or by twisting. Obstruction of venous return then leads to swelling and later to arterial obstruction. If strangulation is not relieved by manual or operative reduction, infarction follows. The strangulated inguinal hernia first becomes irreducible and then tender. Symptoms and signs of bowel obstruction then develop over the next few hours.

Management of inguinal hernias

Inguinal hernias in adults should ideally be repaired by *herniorrhaphy*. Elective repair, performed soon after diagnosis, reduces the risk of strangulation and minimises stretching of the abdominal wall musculature. This probably lowers the rate of recurrence. If age or infirmity makes an operation hazardous, a *truss* may be the treatment of choice.

With time, an enlarging hernia may become irreducible. Provided that there are no problems with it, urgent operation is not essential. Some patients give a history of episodes in which the hernia becomes temporarily irreducible. These episodes may be accompanied by local pain and tenderness or even symptoms of bowel obstruction (vomiting, colicky abdominal pain, distension and absolute constipation). This is an indication for urgent operation. More severe and prolonged symptoms usually precipitate emergency admission to hospital, in which case strangulation must be assumed to have occurred, and operation should be performed urgently.

Very large 'wheelbarrow' hernias are invariably of long standing and are found in elderly men. They only present if size has become a handicap, if bowel has strangulated within the hernia or if the anatomical distortion interferes with micturition. Bowel adhesions may make operation difficult and postoperative wound infections are common. Despite this, surgery for strangulation cannot be avoided. If the hernia is not strangulated, a bag truss (see below) may be the most appropriate treatment.

Inguinal hernia repair

The herniorrhaphy techniques shown in Figure 19.15 are the most commonly used, although most surgeons have their own variations. Non-absorbable suture materials must be used for the abdominal wall repair to prevent recurrence. The operation is usually performed under general anaesthesia, although epidural or spinal anaesthesia may be used in patients with poor cardiovascular or respiratory function. In the severely compromised patient for whom a truss is unsuitable, inguinal herniorrhaphy can be performed (often with difficulty) under local anaesthesia; indeed some surgeons recommend repair under local anaesthesia for most inguinal hernias.

Complications of herniorrhaphy are unusual but scrotal haematoma or wound infection occasionally occur soon after operation. Late complications include chronic groin pain due to inadvertent trapping of the ilio-inguinal nerve in the repair and testicular atrophy caused by inadvertent damage to the testicular artery.

In infants, the patent processus vaginalis is merely ligated and excised (*herniotomy*); formal repair of the abdominal wall defect is usually unnecessary. If the defect is enormous, a single stitch to narrow the medial side of the deep ring should be used.

Recurrent inguinal hernia

Even when a recognised operative technique is competently performed, hernias recur in about 3% of cases. The rate is greatly increased when inadequate attention has been given to operative principles. Apart from technical failure, recurrence is probably due to inherently poor musculature, chronic cough, urinary obstruction, constipation or resumption of heavy work too soon after repair.

During the first postoperative week, patients should avoid activities likely to strain the repair, such as heavy lifting or driving a car. Over the next few weeks, they should gradually return to normal activity. Return to work depends on the physical nature of the job, but usually varies from two to six weeks.

Fig. 19.15 Inguinal hernia repair

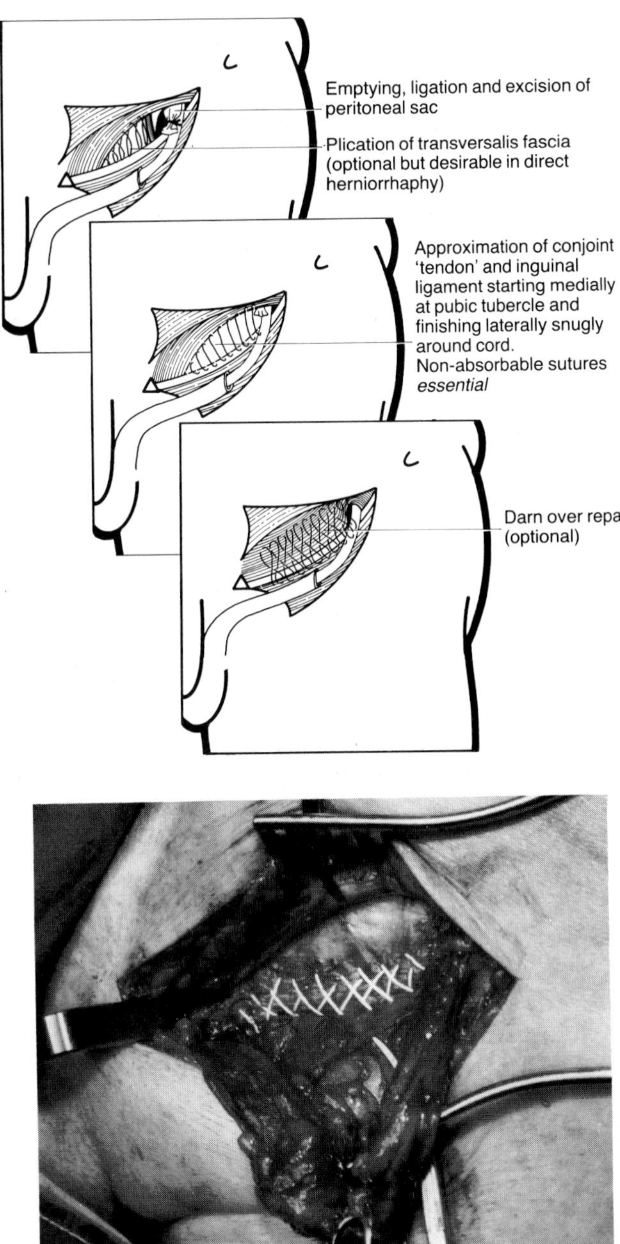

Trusses

A truss may be used to control certain types of hernia when surgery is either inappropriate or unacceptable to the patient. A pressure truss can be safely used if the hernia is easily reducible and can be kept reduced and free of symptoms. Pressure trusses made of padded webbing have superceded various spring contraptions. For very large hernias which cannot be reduced, a 'bag truss' can be used to support the hernia.

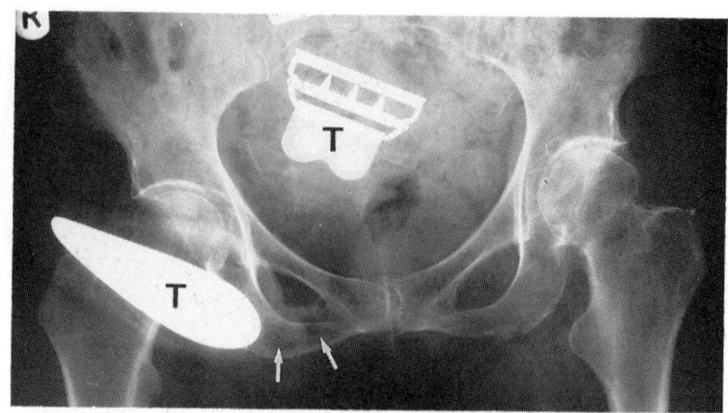

Fig. 19.16 Truss with unreduced inguinal hernia

X-ray of the pelvis in an 82-year-old woman following a fall causing a fractured neck of the left femur. She happened to be wearing a truss **T** for a long-standing, large right inguinal hernia. This was not kept reduced by the truss as indicated by the presence of bowel gas (arrowed) in the inguinal area

FEMORAL HERNIA

Femoral hernias are formed by protrusion of peritoneum into the potential space of the femoral canal. The sac may contain abdominal viscera (usually small bowel) or omentum. In males, inguinal hernia is 40 times more common than femoral hernia, but in females, inguinal hernia is only twice as common. Increased intra-abdominal pressure and other factors related to pregnancy may be important in females since the incidence of femoral hernia is higher in parous than nulliparous women. In both sexes, femoral hernia is assumed to be acquired; no evidence of a congenital sac has ever been found. Thus, femoral hernias, unlike inguinal hernias, are rare in children.

Clinical features

A femoral hernia is usually small, appearing as a grape-sized lump immediately below the inguinal ligament and just lateral to its medial attachment to the pubic tubercle. The anatomy of the femoral canal is shown in Figure 19.2, earlier. If a femoral hernia becomes large, it tends to be deflected upwards and may seem to arise above the inguinal ligament. This explains the importance of careful examination to determine the origin of the hernial neck.

Since the femoral canal is narrow, a cough impulse can rarely be detected, and the hernia is usually irreducible. Thus, small femoral hernias may be difficult to distinguish from other lumps arising in the femoral canal such as a lipoma or enlarged Cloquet's lymph node. However, a hernia is deeply fixed whereas the others tend to be more mobile.

Strangulated femoral hernia

In contrast to strangulated inguinal hernia, there are usually no localising symptoms and signs in strangulated femoral hernia, and the classic presenting features are those of distal small bowel obstruction. The diagnosis of strangulated femoral hernia is easily missed unless the femoral region is carefully examined for a lump, which is usually small and often unimpressive.

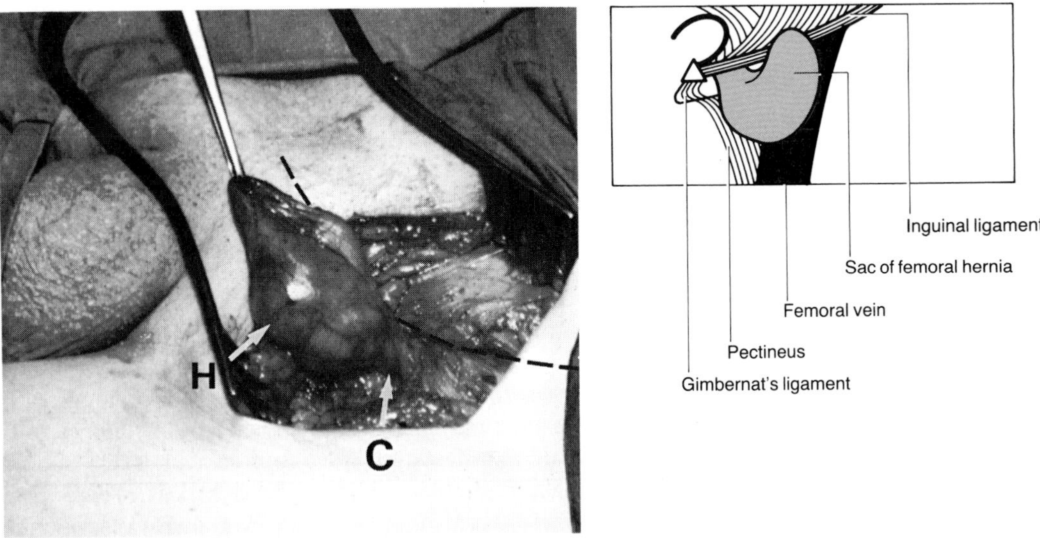

Fig. 19.17 Femoral hernia

An average sized femoral hernia **H** at operation. The patient's genitalia are to the right. The line of the inguinal ligament is marked with an interrupted line and the opening of the femoral canal is seen at **C**

In nearly 30% of strangulated femoral hernias, only part of the bowel circumference is trapped in the hernial sac. Although the bowel lumen remains patent and the patient continues to pass flatus, peristalsis is sufficiently disrupted for other signs of obstruction to occur. This is known as *Richter's hernia*.

Management of femoral hernia

The abdominal orifice of the femoral canal is small and indistensible. Consequently, abdominal contents finding their way into the canal strangulate much more readily than they do in inguinal hernias. Thus, all femoral hernias, even if asymptomatic, must be repaired without delay. Use of a truss is dangerous.

Elective repair is performed by emptying and excising the peritoneal sac. The femoral canal is then closed with non-absorbable sutures. The canal can be exposed by several different methods. The most common are the femoral or low approach, the *Lotheissen* or high approach via the inguinal canal, and the *McEvedy* or transrectus, extraperitoneal approach.

ENLARGED INGUINAL LYMPH NODES

The lymph nodes of the inguinal region are clustered into the three anatomical groups shown in Figure 19.4. These drain the lower abdominal wall, perineum (including vulva and vagina), anal canal, penis and scrotal skin and the whole lower limb. The testes, derived from the retroperitoneal area, drain to the upper para-aortic nodes within the abdomen rather than the inguinal nodes.

Inguinal lymph nodes may become secondarily enlarged as a result of local disease in their field of drainage. Examples include infections of the foot, skin diseases, venereal infection or tumours. Inguinal lymph node enlargement may also be part of a generalised lymphadenopathy in lymphoma or a systemic infection such as glandular fever. Multiple small hard ('shotty') nodes are commonly found, especially in men, and are accepted as normal. These nodes probably result from minor infections of the lower limb, and are easily palpable in males because they have less subcutaneous fat.

Clinical features

Enlarged inguinal lymph nodes present with pain or a lump in the groin but are often discovered incidentally. Enlarged lymph nodes are recognised by their anatomical position and by excluding hernias or vascular abnormalities. Enlarged nodes are usually mobile but when infiltrated by tumour, become fixed to the surrounding tissues. If enlarged and fixed inguinal lymph nodes are found, the history may need to be reviewed for clues as to the origin. A history of systemic manifestations of lymphoma or AIDS should be sought. These include malaise, periodic fevers and weight loss. There may be a history of a 'mole' or 'wart' having been removed, even many years before. If this was a malignant melanoma or squamous carcinoma, it could now have metastasised. Other symptoms of tumour that could metastasise to inguinal lymph nodes should be sought. For example, anal pain or bleeding might indicate an anal carcinoma.

The examination should include palpating lymph nodes in the neck and axillae, and palpating the liver and spleen. The skin of the whole drainage field should be examined closely, paying particular attention to the perineum and the feet, including between the toes and beneath the toenails. The examination may reveal infection, squamous cell carcinoma or malignant melanoma. Rectal examination is mandatory to exclude anal carcinoma. A blood test for HIV may be indicated.

If enlarged lymph nodes cannot be explained by simple local factors, a node should be surgically removed for histological examination. If only a single node is enlarged, histology often shows non-specific reactive changes. The patient usually recovers fully and a diagnosis is never made.

SAPHENA VARIX

A saphena varix is a dilatation of the long saphenous vein in the groin, just proximal to its junction with the femoral vein. The varix is thought to be caused

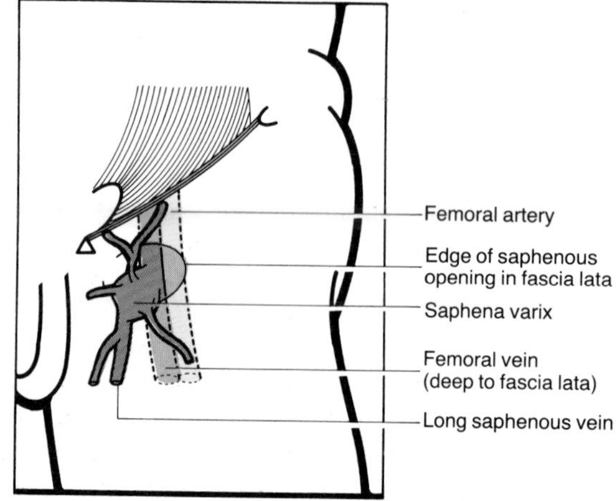

Fig. 19.18 Saphena varix

by valve incompetence at this point; there are usually varicose veins elsewhere in the long saphenous system.

The varix can reach the size of a golf ball or even larger. On examination, the swelling is soft and diffuse. The diagnostic feature is that it empties with minimal pressure and refills on release. A cough impulse is invariably present.

Treatment is a high saphenous ligation, as for saphenofemoral incompetence associated with varicose veins (see Chapter 26).

FEMORAL ARTERY ANEURYSM

Femoral aneurysms are uncommon as a cause of a lump in the groin. They may occur as part of generalised aneurysmal disease of the abdominal aorta, iliac and lower limb arterial system but more often occur in isolation.

Diagnosis is made on clinical examination: the lump lies below the midpoint of the inguinal ligament and has a characteristic expansile pulsation. The management of aneurysms is discussed in Chapter 26.

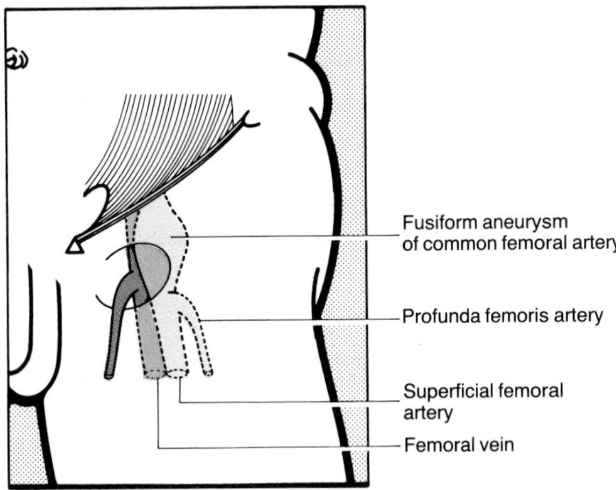

Fig. 19.19 Femoral aneurysm

DISORDERS OF THE SCROTUM AND TESTIS

TESTICULAR TUMOURS

Testicular tumours are the most common tumours in males between the ages of 20 and 40. In males of all ages, they comprise about 1% of all malignancies. About one new case occurs in 20 000 males per annum.

Most testicular tumours are derived from germ cells: *seminomas* are derived from spermatocytes and *teratomas* are derived from multipotent germ cells. Maldescended testes are at least thirty times more likely to become malignant than normally descended testes.

The testes may also be involved in other forms of malignancy: lymphoma, chronic lymphocytic leukaemia or, in children, acute lymphoblastic leukaemia. These rarely present as lumps in the testis but the surgeon may be asked to perform a testicular biopsy as part of the monitoring process. Rarely, tumours may arise from cells of the testicular stroma, e.g. Leydig cells. These tumours present as excess hormone secretion rather than testicular lumps.

Pathology of testicular tumours

Seminomas

Seminomas make up more than half of malignant testicular tumours. Their peak incidence is between the ages of 30 and 45 years. The cut surface of seminomas is typically pale, creamy-white and homogeneous. Histologically, the tumour cells are uniform and tightly packed.

Teratomas

Teratomas are slightly less common than seminomas and their peak incidence is a decade earlier. Since they are derived from multipotent cells, teratomas may contain tissue from all three germ cell layers, ectoderm, mesoderm and endoderm. Teratomas exhibit a wide range of differentiation. Well-differentiated tumours contain a collection of tissues resembling mature adult tissues, in particular, squamous epithelium (ectodermal), cartilage and smooth muscle (mesodermal) and respiratory epithelium (endodermal). Consequently, the cut surface of teratomas often appears variegated, with cystic areas and areas of necrosis and haemorrhage; this is easily distinguished from seminoma with the naked eye.

In poorly differentiated teratomas, no organoid elements are apparent, and for this reason they are sometimes described as *embryonal carcinomas*. A variant contains tissues with malignant syncitio- and cytotrophoblastic features. These are known as *trophoblastic teratomas* or *choriocarcinoma*. Some poorly differentiated teratomas contain areas of seminoma, but one or the other tumour types usually predominates. These mixed tumours behave as teratomas and should be treated as such.

Figure 19.20 shows the current classification of primary malignant testicular tumours used in the UK. Other classifications are used in other countries. All classifications are frequently updated as new information emerges.

Fig. 19.20 Classification of malignant testicular tumours (Testicular Tumour Panel and Registry of the Pathological Society of Great Britain and Ireland

Seminoma

Differentiated teratoma (TD)

Malignant teratoma intermediate (MTI)

Malignant teratoma undifferentiated (MTU) — also known as embryonal tumour (USA)

Sub-variant: Malignant teratoma trophoblastic (MTT) — also known as choriocarcinoma

Teratoma with seminoma (MTU + S)

Clinical features of testicular tumours

Malignant testicular tumours usually present as a painless, progressively enlarging testicular lump. If the capsule becomes involved, a *secondary hydrocoele* may develop but this is usually small and does not hinder palpation of the lump.

Both tumour types spread via lymphatics to para-aortic nodes at the level of L1/2. Spread is then proximally along the lymphatic chain and thoracic duct to the supraclavicular nodes and systemic circulation. Lung secondaries are particularly common in teratomas. Poorly differentiated testicular tumours metastasise early and may present as enlarged cervical lymph nodes or with chest symptoms. The primary testicular lesion may be very small or even impalpable.

Testicular tumours, particularly the poorly differentiated teratomas, secrete *alpha-fetoprotein (AFP)* and *human chorionic gonadotrophin (HCG)*. The levels correlate closely with tumour bulk. Thus, serial measurements of AFP and HCG are valuable in monitoring disease progress and the success of therapy.

Diagnosis and staging

A testicular lump must be assumed to be tumour until proven otherwise. The history is rarely helpful but may include an episode of trauma which merely drew attention to the lump. On examination, the testis is either diffusely enlarged or contains a discrete lump which is firm and non-tender. A small hydrocoele may be present. General examination may reveal evidence of metastases. Enlarged para-aortic nodes can rarely be palpated unless they are

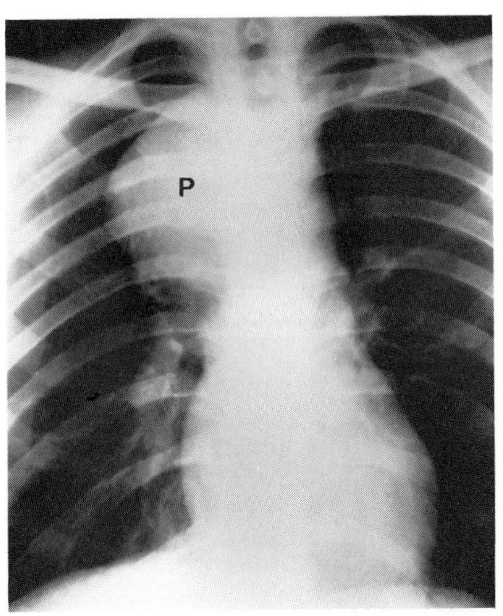

(a)

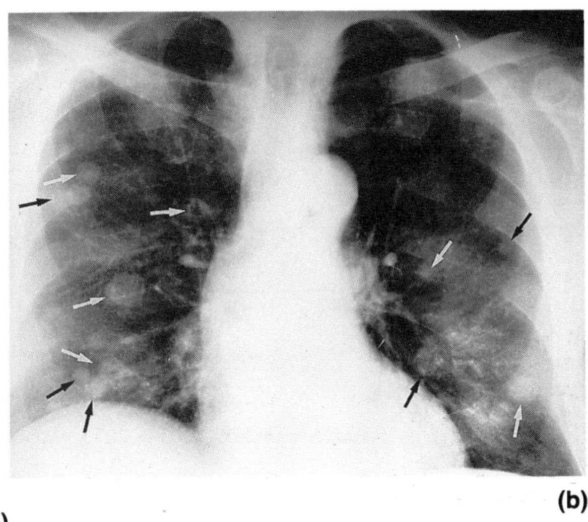
(b)

Fig. 19.21 Metastatic testicular tumours

(a) This 24-year-old man presented with a small testicular lump. An orchidectomy was performed and the cut surface of the tumour was cystic and haemorrhagic. Histology confirmed the expected diagnosis of testicular teratoma. This chest X-ray shows a large mediastinal mass which represents a grossly enlarged paratracheal lymph node **P**. Para-aortic node involvement occurs in teratoma but not seminoma. This patient's disease was defined as stage III because there were no pulmonary metastases. **(b)** Multiple bilateral pulmonary metastases (arrowed) in a 27-year-old man with a testicular swelling. The cut surface of the orchidectomy specimen was homogeneous and histology confirmed seminoma. Pulmonary metastases occur in both teratoma and seminoma, and in either case indicate stage IV disease

huge, but malignant cervical nodes will be palpable. Inguinal nodes are not involved unless the tumour has spread to the scrotal skin. This is rare except when biopsy or orchidectomy has been performed through a scrotal incision, which is considered bad surgical practice.

Initial investigations are chest X-ray (to look for para-aortic node involvement and lung secondaries) and plasma radioimmunoassay for tumour markers. The levels of AFP and HCG rise in proportion to tumour mass.

If there is a reasonable suspicion of tumour, the next step is direct examination of the testis. This is done surgically via an inguinal approach to avoid involvement of the scrotal skin. The spermatic cord is temporarily clamped to prevent venous spread of tumour cells, and the testis is then brought out for visual examination and palpation. If the testis is obviously malignant, orchidectomy is then performed and a length of cord excised. If there is any doubt, the testis is incised in the saggital plane ('bivalving') so that the cut surfaces can be examined. A seminoma has a pale, homogeneous, fleshy appearance, whereas a teratoma is typically heterogeneous with cystic, necrotic and haemorrhagic areas. If the appearance is that of tumour, the testis and a length of cord is excised. If doubt still remains, a biopsy is taken and examined immediately by frozen section.

Once a tissue diagnosis has been made, the degree of spread must be assessed to establish the stage of the tumour. CT scanning is the best way to establish the sites and the involvement of abdominal and thoracic lymph nodes, as well as the presence of pulmonary secondaries. CT scanning has virtually superceded lymphangiography, which is invasive and unreliable. A method of staging testicular tumours is shown in Figure 19.22.

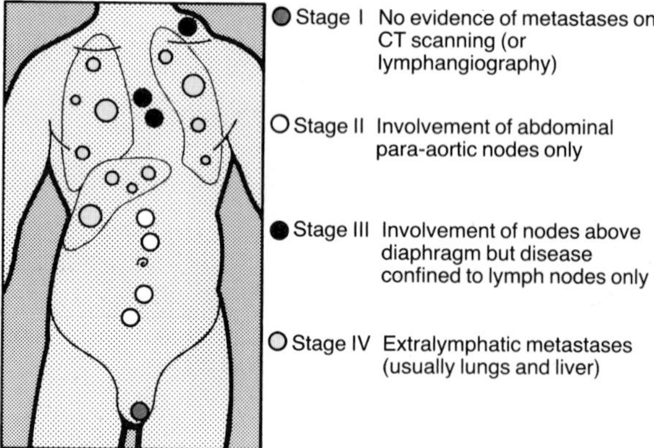

Fig. 19.22 Stages of spread of testicular tumours

Prognosis of testicular tumours

The management of testicular tumours has been revolutionised in the past 20 years by the development of new chemotherapeutic regimens, and the use of CT scanning and sensitive tumour markers to stage and monitor disease progress. For stage I and stage II disease, total cure is now a realistic prospect in 90% of cases. For more advanced disease, cure is less likely but 5-year survival rates approaching 70% are now being achieved.

Treatment of testicular tumours

Orchidectomy, the only appropriate treatment for the primary tumour, is usually performed as part of the diagnostic process. The other testis is usually unaffected and can be preserved.

Metastatic disease is highly responsive to chemotherapy, which is now recommended in all cases with metastases. Radiotherapy was widely used for advanced disease, but recent studies have shown that its use should be restricted to low-dose irradiation of bulky deposits of seminoma before they are surgically removed. Seminomas are much more radiosensitive than teratomas. Extensive, large-field irradiation should be abandoned because of the risks of severe or even fatal bone marrow suppression. Occasionally, surgical debulking of residual tumour after chemotherapy is also indicated.

Success of these treatments can be monitored by sequential CT scans and plasma assay for tumour markers. Recurrent disease is treated by further radiotherapy, chemotherapy or surgery.

Treatment of malignant testicular tumours may result in sterility. If appropriate, semen should be collected and stored before treatment so that artificial insemination may be performed later.

Fig. 19.23 Summary: treatment of testicular tumours

1. Removal of the affected testis — usually performed as part of the diagnostic process
2. Chemotherapy — for all cases of metastatic disease in both seminoma and teratoma
3. Radiotherapy — local irradiation of bulky metastases in seminoma
4. Debulking surgery for lymph nodes treated by chemotherapy — sometimes necessary

INFLAMMATION OF THE EPIDIDYMIS AND TESTIS

Bacterial infections

The most common inflammatory disorder of the scrotal contents is bacterial epididymitis. This usually spreads from a urinary tract infection involving the bladder via the vas deferens. Coliforms, pyogenic staphylococci and faecal streptococci are the organisms most often responsible. Epididymitis is often incorrectly referred to as orchitis or epididymo-orchitis. The testis is rarely infected, although the surrounding inflammation may cause testicular tenderness. Epididymitis is painful and usually begins acutely. It may be clinically indistinguishable from testicular torsion and present as a surgical emergency.

On examination of a patient with acute epididymitis, the affected side of the scrotum and its contents are swollen, oedematous and tender, and the scrotal skin is red and warm. It may be difficult to palpate the testis and epididymis separately once the infection has become established.

Treatment is with broad spectrum antibiotics for at least a month. The infecting organism may be identified by urine cultures.

Persistent or chronic epididymitis may cause the patient to present with chronic scrotal tenderness. This usually follows an initial acute episode. Chronic epididymitis may also result from inadequate antibiotic therapy of an acute episode.

Tuberculosis

Tuberculosis may involve the epididymis through blood stream spread from a pulmonary focus. Occasionally, a tuberculous urinary tract infection may spread to the epididymis. The whole length of the epididymis is typically thickened, non-tender and 'cold'. In contrast to bacterial epididymitis, the epididymis is readily distinguished from the testis on palpation. If untreated, the testis may also become involved. The epididymal swelling may be the presenting complaint.

Diagnosis requires analysis of serial early morning urine specimens (EMUs) for Mycobacteria. If tuberculosis is diagnosed, a search must be made for pulmonary and urinary tract disease (see Chapter 24).

Syphilis

Tertiary gummatous syphilis may involve the testis, producing diffuse, non-tender enlargement; this is now extremely rare. There is usually a history of primary and secondary lesions. Sometimes a gumma is found unexpectedly during investigation of a suspected testicular tumour.

Granulomatous orchitis

Granulomatous orchitis is a common, non-infective inflammatory disorder of the testis. It mainly occurs after trauma or surgery involving the spermatic cord, e.g. vasectomy. Clinically, the testis becomes diffusely firm and enlarged and may be indistinguishable from tumour.

On sectioning, the testis has a pale homogeneous appearance. Histological examination shows a diffuse chronic inflammatory cell infiltrate with numerous granulomata containing giant cells. The seminiferous tubules are atrophic or completely destroyed. The cause of this condition is unknown but it may be a response to extrusion of spermatozoa into the testicular interstitium.

HYDROCOELE

Primary hydrocoele

A hydrocoele is an excessive collection of fluid in the tunica vaginalis, the serous space surrounding the testis. Like the peritoneal cavity, the tunica vaginalis normally contains a small amount of serous fluid which is produced and reabsorbed at the same rate.

Simple hydrocoeles may develop in adulthood, particularly in the elderly, by the slow accumulation of serous fluid. Presumably, they are caused by impaired reabsorption. Such hydrocoeles may reach a huge size, containing several hundred millilitres of fluid. The lesion is otherwise asymptomatic. On examination, the swelling is soft and non-tender and the testis cannot be palpated. The presence of fluid is demonstrated by transillumination.

Provided there is no suspicion of tumour, the hydrocoele can be tapped, i.e. aspirated with a needle and syringe. The fluid obtained is clear and straw-

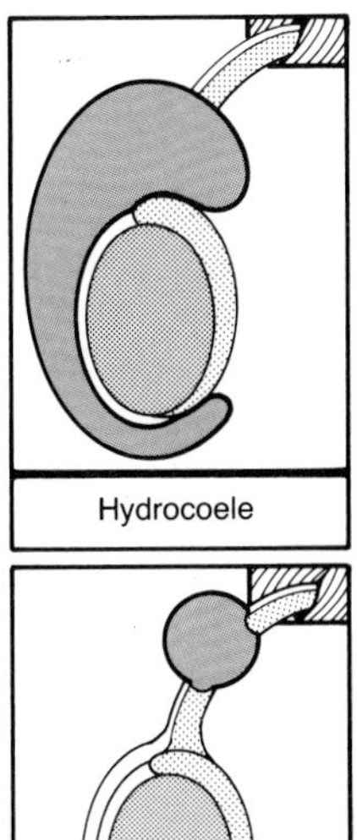

Fig. 19.24

coloured. After aspiration, a normal testis should be palpable. Clear fluid and a normal testis confirm the diagnosis.

After aspiration, fluid reaccumulates over the following months and the hydrocoele will therefore need periodic aspiration or operation. For younger patients, operation is usually preferred, whereas the elderly or unfit can have aspirations repeated when the hydrocoele becomes uncomfortably large. After aspiration, 6% aqueous phenol (10–20 ml) can be injected and this often inhibits reaccumulation. Several treatments may be necessary.

Rarely, a hydrocoele develops in a remnant of the processus vaginalis somewhere in the course of the spermatic cord. This hydrocoele also transilluminates, and is known as an *encysted hydrocoele of the cord*.

Secondary hydrocoele

Hydrocoeles may develop secondarily to tumour or inflammation of the testis. In most cases, the hydrocoele is small and the testis can be palpated to reveal the primary abnormality. If tumour is a possibility, aspiration must not be performed. Otherwise, tumour cells may spread to the scrotal skin and its lymphatic field.

Fournier's scrotal gangrene

Occasionally, elderly men develop an acute unilateral infection in the tunica vaginalis, which rapidly spreads outwards to cause spreading gangrene of the scrotal skin (see Figure 19.25). There is often an associated septicaemia. Most patients have a pre-existing primary hydrocoele which becomes infected, probably via the bloodstream. Infection is with a mixture of anaerobic strep-

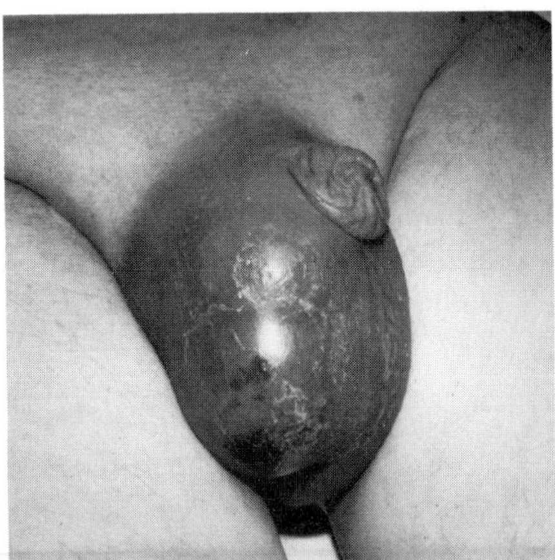

Fig. 19.25 Fournier's scrotal gangrene

This 81-year-old man presented with scrotal pain and a rapidly rising temperature. The right side of the scrotum was red and oedematous on admission to hospital; within two hours, the black necrotic areas seen at the lower pole appeared and rapidly extended. He was treated with intravenous antibiotics and wide surgical opening of the scrotum to remove all necrotic tissue. The patient had a pre-existing hydrocoele

tococci and other faecal organisms. Treatment includes intravenous antibiotics and urgent surgical excision of the necrotic tissue, with the wound being left open to heal by secondary intention.

EPIDIDYMAL CYST AND SPERMATOCOELE

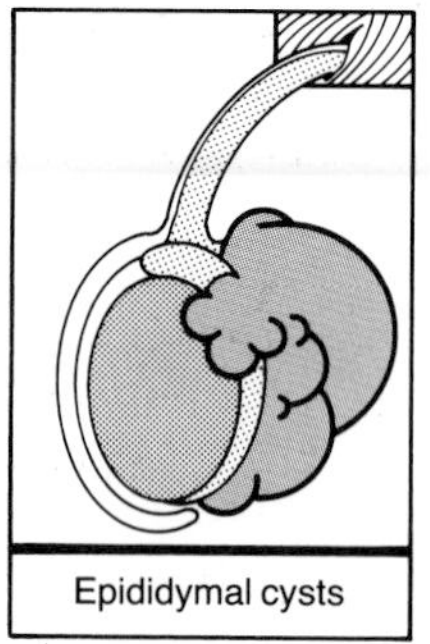

Fig. 19.26 Epididymal cysts

Multiple cysts may develop in the upper pole of the epididymis and present as a painless scrotal swelling. One cyst is usually larger than the others. Epididymal cysts affect a slightly younger age group than do hydrocoeles. The testis can usually be palpated separately from the cysts, which lie posteriorly near the upper pole of the testis. Epididymal cysts transilluminate.

Less common is the spermatocoele, a single cyst containing spermatozoa. Spermatocoeles usually occur in the head of the epididymis. Here they are clinically similar to epididymal cysts but transilluminate very brightly. Spermatocoeles occasionally occur in the spermatic cord.

These lesions are usually treated by excision although this may result in obstruction to the passage of sperm. If a patient with an abnormality on the other side wishes to remain fertile, excision may be contraindicated.

VARICOCOELE

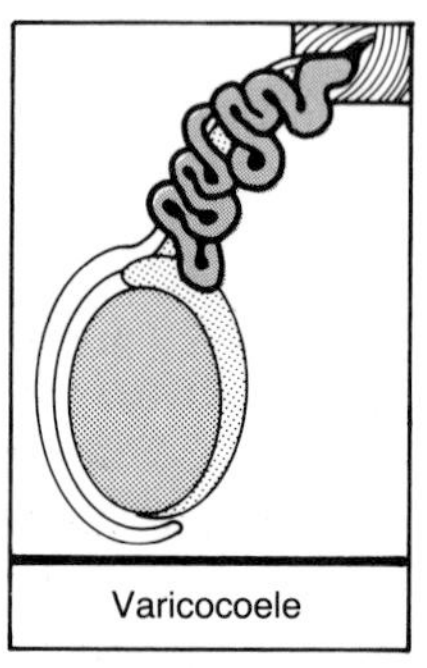

Fig. 19.27 Varicocoele

Varicocoele represents gross dilatation and tortuosity of the veins of the pampiniform plexus of the spermatic cord. The cause is unknown, but since the condition is much more common on the left, it may result in some way from the different venous drainage on the two sides. On the left, the testicular vein drains into the high pressure renal vein, whereas the right testicular vein drains directly into the inferior vena cava.

Varicocoele is common, affecting as many as 8% of young adult males. It is usually asymptomatic but is often discovered during investigation for infertility. Varicocoele results in a raised scrotal temperature which may inhibit normal sperm function. In the supine position, the distended veins collapse and are impalpable. Varicocoele can only be diagnosed if the patient is examined while standing, at which time the varicocoele feels like 'a bag of worms'.

Rarely, a varicocele may be caused by obstruction of the left renal vein by an invading renal adenocarcinoma. If the history of varicocoele is short, then investigation for renal adenocarcinoma may be appropriate.

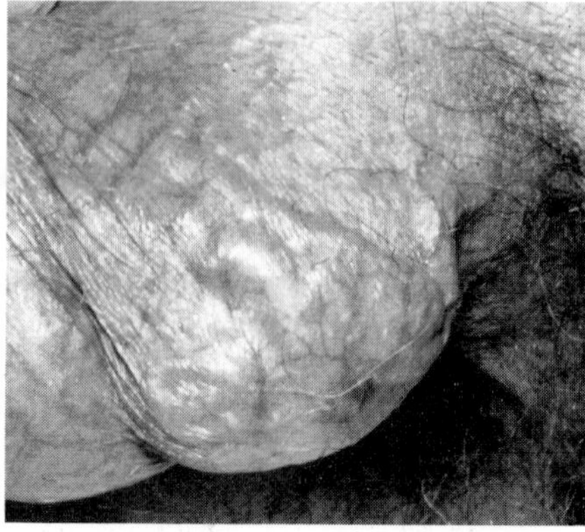

Surgical treatment is only necessary if a varicocoele causes pain or the patient is infertile. The testicular vein is ligated at the deep inguinal ring proximal to its many tributaries.

MALDESCENT OF THE TESTIS

The testis may fail to descend normally from the posterior abdominal wall into the scrotum, where it should lie at birth in the full-term infant. If the testis is not in the scrotum, it usually lies at some point along its normal path of descent, most commonly in the inguinal canal. Alternatively, it may be found in an ectopic position, most commonly in the superficial inguinal pouch just above the external inguinal ring.

Maldescended testes are often structurally abnormal, and this may be responsible for the failure of descent. The maldescended testis is known to be at increased risk of malignancy. This may also be due to developmental abnormalities. Despite surgical correction at an early age, the risk of malignancy is believed to persist.

In developed countries, the condition is usually identified during early childhood and corrected (see Chapter 31).

A few cases of absent testis are missed, however, and present in adulthood with:

- An 'absent' testis
- A groin lump which is the testis, or a testicular tumour
- Groin pain due to acute or recurrent torsion

TORSION OF THE TESTIS OR EPIDIDYMAL APPENDAGE

Testicular torsion

The testis is normally suspended in the scrotum in a near vertical position, anchored by the spermatic cord and by attachments to the posterior wall of the scrotum. This prevents rotation of the testis. Minor anatomical variations producing a narrow-based pedicle or a horizontal ('bell-clapper') lie, may allow the testis to become twisted about its axis within the tunica vaginalis. When this occurs, the veins in the pampiniform plexus are compressed causing venous congestion. After a few hours, venous infarction will occur unless the torsion is corrected. Trauma during sport may sometimes initiate the process of torsion.

Torsion of the testis is a surgical emergency requiring prompt diagnosis and urgent surgical treatment if the testis is to be saved.

Testicular torsion presents with a sudden onset of severe testicular pain and poorly localised central abdominal pain and sometimes vomiting. The abdominal pain occurs because the testis retains its embryological nerve supply within the abdomen. In the early stages of torsion, the affected testis is tender, slightly swollen and drawn up into the neck of the scrotum where the cord may be palpably thickened. With these features, the diagnosis is seldom in doubt. At a later stage, the overlying scrotal skin tends to become red and oedematous, making accurate palpation difficult. At this point, torsion may be difficult to distinguish clinically from acute epididymitis.

Torsion of the epididymal appendage (hydatid of Morgagni)

At the upper pole of the testis is a small embryological remnant known as the hydatid of Morgagni. This may similarly undergo torsion and produce symptoms akin to those of testicular torsion. The symptoms are quite out of proportion to the size of the infarcted tissue. Infarction of the hydatid is of no consequence, except that it must be distinguished from testicular torsion. This may only be possible at operation.

Fig. 19.28 Torsion of the testis and hydatid of Morgagni

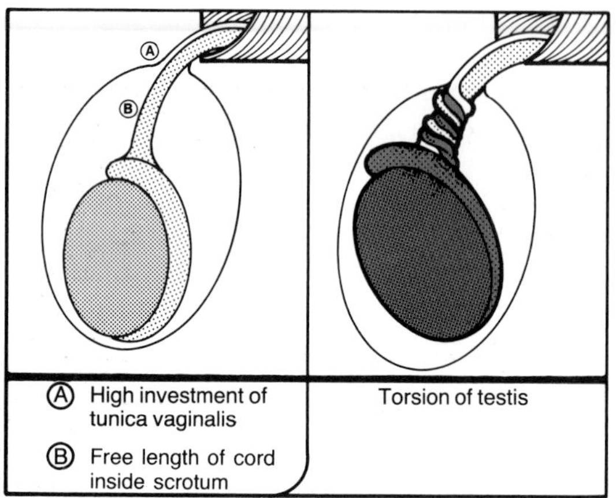

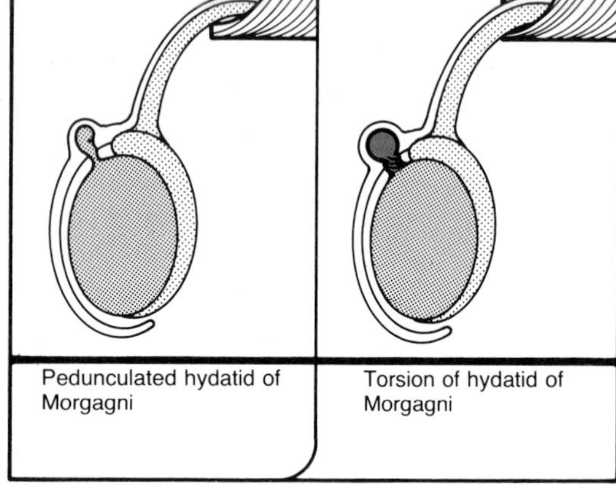

Management of suspected testicular torsion

If testicular torsion is seen at an early stage, it is sometimes possible to untwist the testis without operation. The testis is gently rotated in one direction or, if pain increases, in the opposite direction. Successful reduction relieves the emergency, but the testis should later be surgically secured to prevent recurrence.

If the testis cannot be untwisted, operation is imperative as soon as possible. There are few surgical emergencies where time is of such crucial importance. A scrotal incision is made and the testis is examined and untwisted. If the testis is black and fails to recover its colour, it is necrotic and should be removed. If some colour is restored, the testis is best left, although it may later atrophy. The untwisted testis is then sutured to the tunica vaginalis or placed into a dartos pouch to prevent recurrence. Both testes should be secured since predisposition to torsion is usually bilateral.

TRAUMA TO THE TESTIS

The testes may be injured during contact sports or fights. The tunica albuginea may remain intact or split. The testis is extremely painful in either case. If the tunica remains intact, a testicular haematoma results; if it splits, the testicular parenchyma bursts and bleeds into the tunica vaginalis cavity, resulting in a haematocoele.

If pain is severe and persistent, the scrotum can be explored surgically. Pain from a testicular haematoma can be relieved by incision of the tunica albuginea. Evacuating a haematocoele, however, may be impossible because blood tends to infiltrate the tissues.

MALE STERILIS-ATION

Male sterilisation by vasectomy is a simple, effective method of birth control. It can be performed under local anaesthesia at little cost and requires no special equipment. The essential prerequisite is that the couple involved should have already completed their family, since reversal is technically difficult and unreliable. The technique of vasectomy is illustrated in Figure 19.29.

Fig. 19.29 Technique of vasectomy

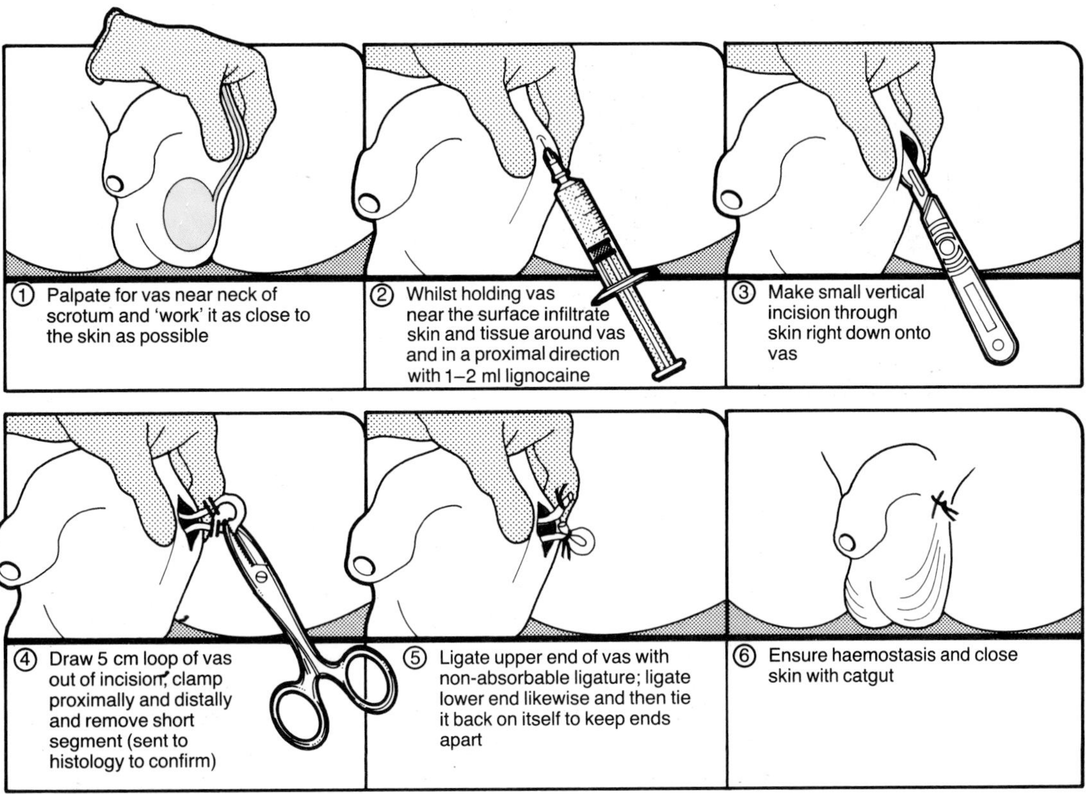

Technique of vasectomy Note: Each side is dealt with separately

Most techniques involve removal of a section of the vas (ductus) deferens and ligation or cauterisation of the cut ends. For medico-legal reasons, the nature of the excised portion is often confirmed histologically. Spermatozoa remain in the proximal duct system for several months after vasectomy. Thus, the operation cannot be considered a success until at least two successive sperm counts about a month apart are negative. Despite correct operative technique and negative sperm counts, however, there is a late failure rate of about one case in every 500. Failure is due to spontaneous reconnection of the vas, and is proved by a positive sperm count; note the problems of determining paternity in the case of unexpected pregnancy!

DISORDERS OF THE PENIS

Introduction

Problems with the foreskin (prepuce) are common and form the majority of surgical disorders of the penis. They include *balanoposthitis* (inflammation of the glans and foreskin), *phimosis* (stricture of the preputial meatus), *paraphimosis* (acute constriction of the glans by a tight retracted foreskin) and *balanitis xerotica obliterans* (idiopathic sclerosis of the foreskin).

Carcinoma of the penis, obviously important, and *Peyronie's disease* (idiopathic fibrosis of the corpora cavernosa) are both rare. Congenital abnormalities of the penis are usually recognised and treated in childhood.

CARCINOMA OF THE PENIS

Carcinoma of the penis is rare in developed countries and almost unknown in circumcised males. Poor hygiene and the accumulation of smegma are known aetiological factors but there is growing evidence of a viral aetiology linked to that of carcinoma of the uterine cervix in females (genital wart virus).

Histologically, the tumours are squamous cell carcinomas, usually well differentiated, which arise from the inner surface of the foreskin or glans penis in the region of the coronal sulcus. The tumour invades locally and tends to invade the distal urethra. Metastatic spread is to the inguinal lymph nodes. *Erythroplasia of Queyrat* is the term given to severe dysplasia and carcinoma-in-situ of the glans and may represent a precursor of frank invasive carcinoma.

Fig. 19.30 Stages in the spread of carcinoma of the penis

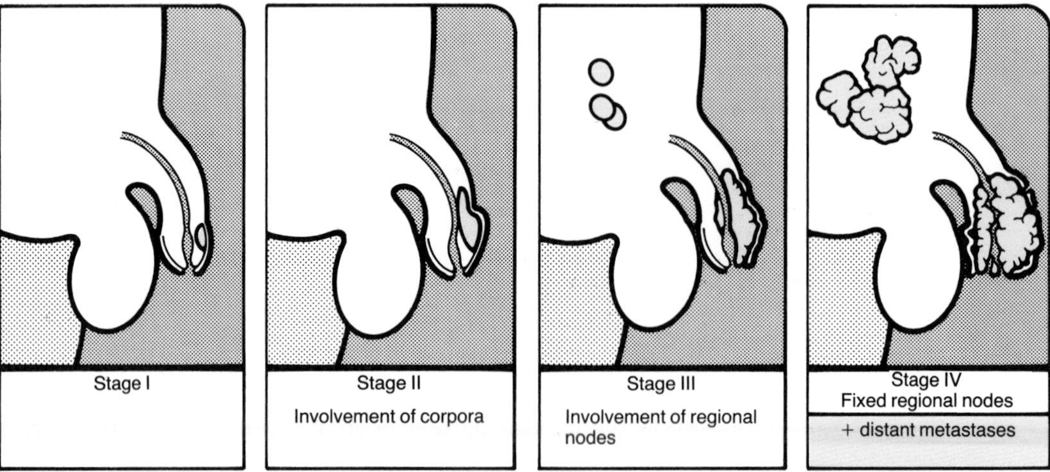

Most cases of carcinoma of the penis are found in the elderly. The disease is usually well advanced before an irregular lump, bleeding or discharge is noticed. In uncircumcised males, the lesion may be hidden by the foreskin. Figure 19.30 illustrates staging of the disease.

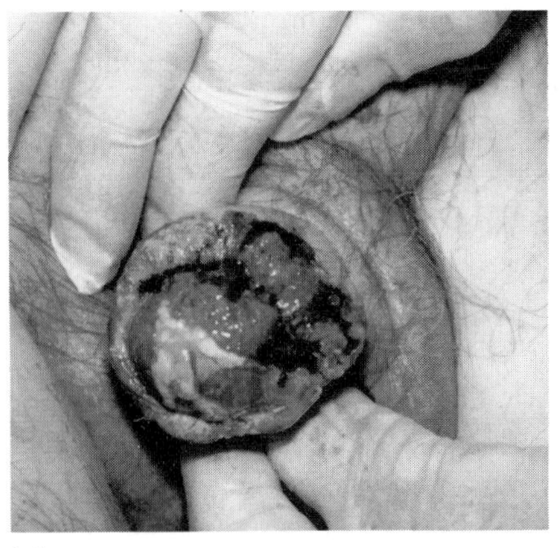

(a)

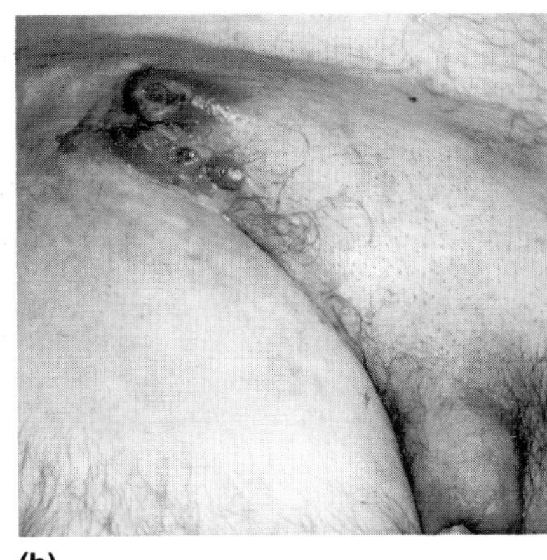

(b)

Fig. 19.31 Carcinoma of the penis

(a) An obvious carcinoma of the penis, revealed when the foreskin is retracted. Unfortunately, this patient already had extensive spread to the inguinal lymph nodes as shown in photograph **(b)**

Surgical excision usually requires at least partial amputation of the penis, and block dissection of the inguinal lymph nodes if they are involved. Radiotherapy can be used in stage I disease if the urethra is not involved and for palliation in stage IV disease.

FORESKIN PROBLEMS IN ADULTS

Phimosis

The most common foreskin problem in adults is a tight foreskin which will not retract fully and causes pain on intercourse. This is called phimosis and is usually caused by fibrosis of the foreskin. This fibrosis is probably due to chronic or recurrent low-grade Candida infection. This is aggravated by attempts at retraction which cause minor tears of the inner epithelial lining. Phimosis may be accompanied by stenosis of the urethral meatus, also due to recurrent inflammation and fibrosis.

Balanoposthitis (balanitis)

The correct term balanoposthitis refers to overt inflammation of the glans penis and foreskin (Greek: balanos = gland, posthe = foreskin); the short form balanitis, however, has passed into common usage. The condition occurs most commonly in children. Inflammation is most often caused by candida or faecal bacteria, but this problem rarely reaches the surgeon.

Balanitis xerotica obliterans is a fibrotic condition of the foreskin of unknown aetiology which produces a thickened, stenosed, often depigmented foreskin which is often adherent to the glans. It occurs in later life and is relieved by circumcision.

Paraphimosis

If a phimotic foreskin is forcibly retracted, the tight meatal band may lodge in the coronal sulcus making reduction impossible. This is known as paraphimosis. Progressive oedema of the glans penis and foreskin then exacerbates the difficulty of reduction. It may occur at any age, but is particularly common in elderly infirm men in whom the foreskin is not correctly pulled forward after retraction for catheterisation or washing the glans (female nurses and junior doctors are the main culprits!). Paraphimosis also occurs in children and adolescents experimenting with foreskin retraction.

In most cases, the foreskin can be reduced by manual compression of the glans and foreskin. A local anaesthetic jelly is applied for lubrication and pain relief. Sometimes, it may be necessary to incise the tight ring under local or general anaesthesia to effect reduction. Circumcision is performed at a later date when the oedema and inflammation have resolved.

Circumcision

Circumcision is indicated for phimosis, paraphimosis, recurrent balanitis and balanitis xerotica obliterans. The surgical technique is shown in Figure 19.32. During operation, the urethral meatus should be checked for stenosis. If present, a *meatotomy* may be required. Haemorrhage is an occasional early postoperative problem and usually requires surgical re-exploration. At one time, oestrogens were given orally to prevent erections in the postoperative period, as erections were believed to contribute to postoperative haemorrhage. Post-operative bleeding, however, can best be prevented by meticulous haemostasis at operation.

Fig. 19.32 Technique of circumcision

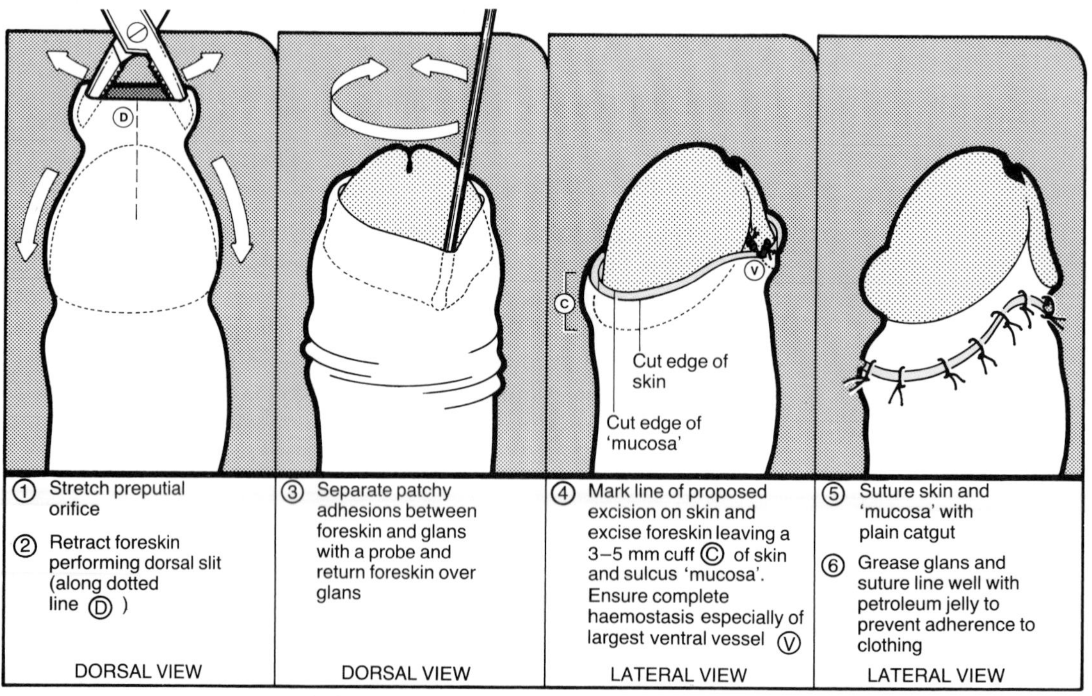

PEYRONIE'S DISEASE

This disease of unknown aetiology occurs in young adults. Slowly progressive asymmetrical fibrotic plaques develop in the fascia surrounding the corpora cavernosa of the penis. The corpus cavernosum urethrae (corpus spongiosum) including the glans is spared. The plaques may become calcified and visible on X-ray. The condition causes the penis to bend towards the affected side on erection making intercourse difficult and painful. There may be spontaneous partial resolution with time.

In severe cases, the plaques are surgically excised, allowing symmetrical erection. Various medical treatments, including steroid injections, have been tried but their efficacy is uncertain.

20 SYMPTOMS, SIGNS AND INVESTIGATION OF URINARY TRACT DISORDERS

Introduction

Urinary tract disorders are common and comprise a significant part of the workload of family practitioners, general physicians, paediatricians and surgeons. In recent years, the specialty of urology has become well established, especially in larger centres. Despite this, the general surgeon still deals with many routine urological problems, especially in smaller hospitals, where they make up about 25% of the surgical workload.

Disorders of the prostate account for at least half the workload in urological surgery. The main conditions are benign prostatic hypertrophy and prostatic carcinoma, both a major cause of morbidity in ageing males. The remaining surgical disorders of the kidney and urinary tract can be divided into five broad groups: tumours, stone disease (urolithiasis), infections, congenital abnormalities and finally, local and systemic disorders which secondarily involve the urinary tract.

This chapter deals with the symptoms, signs, approach to investigation and diagnosis of urinary tract disease. The various disease entities are then discussed in the following five chapters.

SYMPTOMS OF URINARY TRACT DISEASE

Introduction

The common symptoms of urinary tract disease fall into six categories:

- Abdominal pain
- Passage of blood in the urine (haematuria)
- Pain associated with micturition (dysuria)
- Disorders of micturition such as frequency or hesitancy
- Retention of urine
- Urinary incontinence
- Passage of bowel gas in the urine (pneumaturia)

Outflow of urine from the kidney may sometimes become impeded by obstruction of the urinary tract, and this may interfere with renal function. If there is chronic obstruction to bladder outflow or bilateral upper tract obstruction, the patient may develop renal failure without any localising symptoms.

Benign prostatic hypertrophy is the most common prostatic disorder, and usually presents with symptoms of bladder outflow obstruction (i.e. disorders of micturition or urinary retention or both) and sometimes with haematuria. Prostatic obstruction predisposes to bladder infections or stones, and the patient may present with these. Carcinoma of the prostate is less common. It may present with bladder outflow obstruction similar to benign prostatic hypertrophy or it may be discovered because of symptoms from metastases, such as bone pain. Infection of the prostate (prostatitis) is uncommon and usually presents with chronic perineal pain.

The important urinary tract tumours, stone diseases and infections are briefly outlined in Figure 20.1. Any of these disorders may present with haematuria. Some of the conditions cause urinary obstruction and abdominal pain. The severity and character of the pain is determined by the site and degree of obstruction and, perhaps most important, the rapidity of onset. Disorders which cause urinary stasis also predispose to urinary tract infection.

Many different congenital abnormalities may involve the kidneys, ureters, bladder, urethra and genitalia, either alone or in combination. Most of the serious abnormalities are recognised at birth or in early childhood. The exceptions are polycystic disease and medullary sponge kidney, which usually present in adulthood. Less serious congenital abnormalities such as duplex systems often predispose to urinary tract infections because of abnormal flow dynamics. These abnormalities may be discovered at any age during the investigation of recurrent urinary tract infections. Congenital disorders which present mainly in adulthood are discussed in Chapter 25 and those presenting mainly in childhood in Chapter 31.

The urinary tract sometimes becomes secondarily involved in local inflammatory conditions such as Crohn's disease or diverticular disease. Fistulae may form, resulting in the passage of flatus or faeces in the urine or both (pneumaturia and faecuria). Retroperitoneal fibrosis, diverticulitis, tumours of the prostate, cervix or colon, and sometimes aortic aneurysms, may secondarily involve the ureters and cause upper urinary tract obstruction.

ABDOMINAL PAIN

Most urinary tract diseases cause symptoms obviously referrable to the urinary tract. When urinary symptoms are associated with abdominal pain, the cause is usually found to arise in the urinary tract. Urinary tract disorders may, however, cause abdominal pain without urinary symptoms; the diagnosis is then not so obvious and other characteristic clinical features must be sought.

Pain arising from the kidneys and upper tract

Renal inflammation or stretching of the renal capsule causes pain in the renal angle, the posterior space between the lowest rib and the iliac crest. This area may also be tender to palpation or percussion.

If there is obstruction to urinary outflow, there may also be a slight fullness of the normal loin concavity, visible on careful inspection. Renal stones,

Fig. 20.1 Pathophysiology and clinical features of urinary tract tumours, stones and infections

DISEASE	PATHOPHYSIOLOGY	CLINICAL FEATURES
i) Tumours		
Renal adenocarcinoma (also known as renal carcinoma)	Occurs in adults. Derived from renal tubular cells	Presents with haematuria, a mass or constitutional signs such as pyrexia or polycythaemia
Nephroblastoma (Chapter 31)	Developmental origin; usually diagnosed before age 5	Presents as an abdominal mass with or without pain and haematuria
Transitional cell carcinoma	May arise in transitional epithelium anywhere from pelvicalyceal system to urethra, but most common in bladder	Usually presents with haematuria. Predisposes to urinary tract infections. May cause ureteric obstruction
Squamous cell carcinoma (very uncommon)	Arises in metaplastic squamous epithelium. Secondary to chronic stone irritation, especially in bladder. Also arises de novo in squamous epithelium of distal urethra (very rare)	As for transitional cell carcinoma
Adenocarcinoma of bladder (very rare)	Arises from columnar epithelium of urachal remnant	As for transitional cell carcinoma
ii) Stone disease		
Stones may develop in pelvicalyceal system or bladder. Pelvicalyceal stones can pass into the ureter	Stones in situ may cause irritation of urinary tract epithelium	Present as pain or haematuria or recurrent infection
	Renal stones may cause chronic pelviureteric or ureteric obstruction either directly or by fibrotic strictures	Present as chronic pain (due to back pressure), or recurrent infection
	Renal stones may cause total ureteric obstruction as they pass down the tract	Present as acute colicky pain often with renal tenderness
iii) Infections		
a) 'Common' infections due to bowel organisms	Develop either via blood stream or lower urinary tract (ascending infection) Any urinary tract abnormality or stasis predisposes to infection	Typically presents with dysuria and frequency with or without haematuria
b) Tuberculosis (uncommon)	Kidney involvement via bloodstream from pulmonary or other primary disease. May spread via urine to ureters and bladder	May present as haematuria or persistent sterile pyuria, or an incidental finding in pulmonary tuberculosis
c) Schistosomiasis (very common in some underdeveloped countries)	Induces chronic inflammation and fibrosis in bladder wall leading to gross bladder distortion and stones	Presents with haematuria and various symptoms of infection and bladder fibrosis
d) Urethritis	Caused by gonococcus or chlamydia ('non-specific urethritis'). Sexually transmitted	Presents with urethral discharge and dysuria

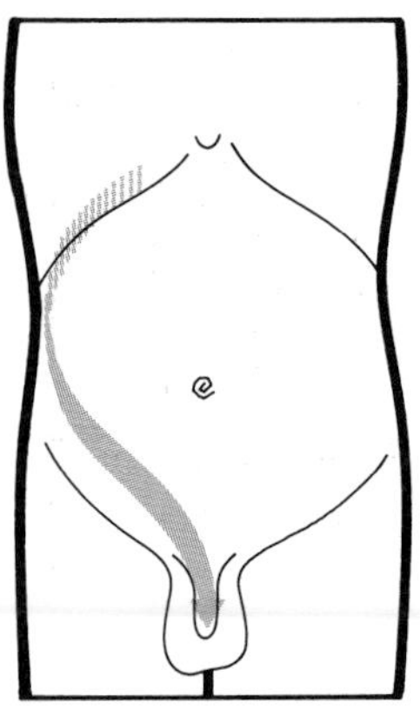

Fig. 20.2 Renal pain and its referral

tumours or polycystic disease may cause dull and persistent loin pain even without obstruction.

In acute infections such as pyelonephritis or bladder infection, the pain is more severe and is usually associated with systemic features and urinary tract symptoms.

Acute obstruction and distension of the pelvicalyceal system produces excruciating loin pain which often radiates to the hypochondrium or groin. If the ureter is obstructed, the pain is colicky (due to ureteric peristalsis) and often radiates down to the iliac fossa and groin. When obstruction is low in the ureter, the pain may radiate to the genitalia. This pain is known as *renal* or *ureteric colic*.

Pain arising from the bladder

Pain originating in the bladder (e.g. in cystitis) is felt in the suprapubic area. Pain may be referred to the penis or vulva if the bladder trigone is involved. In adults, clear-cut urinary symptoms such as dysuria and frequency are usually also present, but children often complain only of pain, making the diagnosis less obvious. Dysuria is usually the predominant symptom of urethral disorders, but pain arising in the male urethra (e.g. in venereal infections) is usually referred to the tip of the penis. Finally, the pain of prostatic inflammation (prostatitis), is usually felt deep in the perineum. The prostate is tender on rectal examination.

Pain simulating urinary tract disease

Pain from other abdominal pathology may sometimes mimic pain arising from the urinary tract. Biliary tract pain may be referred to the right thoraco-lumbar region, while posterior duodenal ulcers and pancreatic disease may cause pain in the central lumbar region. An expanding or leaking abdominal aortic aneurysm may sometimes mimic the pain of urinary tract disease, particularly if a ureter is compressed. Diseases of the thoraco-lumbar spine such as metastatic cancer, tuberculosis, spondylosis and disc lesions, may also simulate upper urinary tract disorders. In women, pain arising from the ovaries or genital tract (e.g. pelvic inflammatory disease) may be confused with bladder pain.

HAEMATURIA

Patients may notice blood or even clots in the urine (*frank haematuria*) but more often, blood is discovered on 'dipstick' testing or microscopy of a midstream urine specimen (*microscopic haematuria*). Haematuria is often episodic rather than persistent, whatever the cause.

Causes of haematuria

Tumours are the most common cause of frank and microscopic haematuria and must be suspected, even if another possible cause is found. Haematuria from tumours is typically painless. Irritation from infection or stones may also cause bleeding, but this is usually accompanied by pain or dysuria. If the urethra is obstructed by prostatic enlargement, straining at micturition may cause bleeding from dilated veins at the bladder neck.

Fig. 20.3 Causes of haematuria

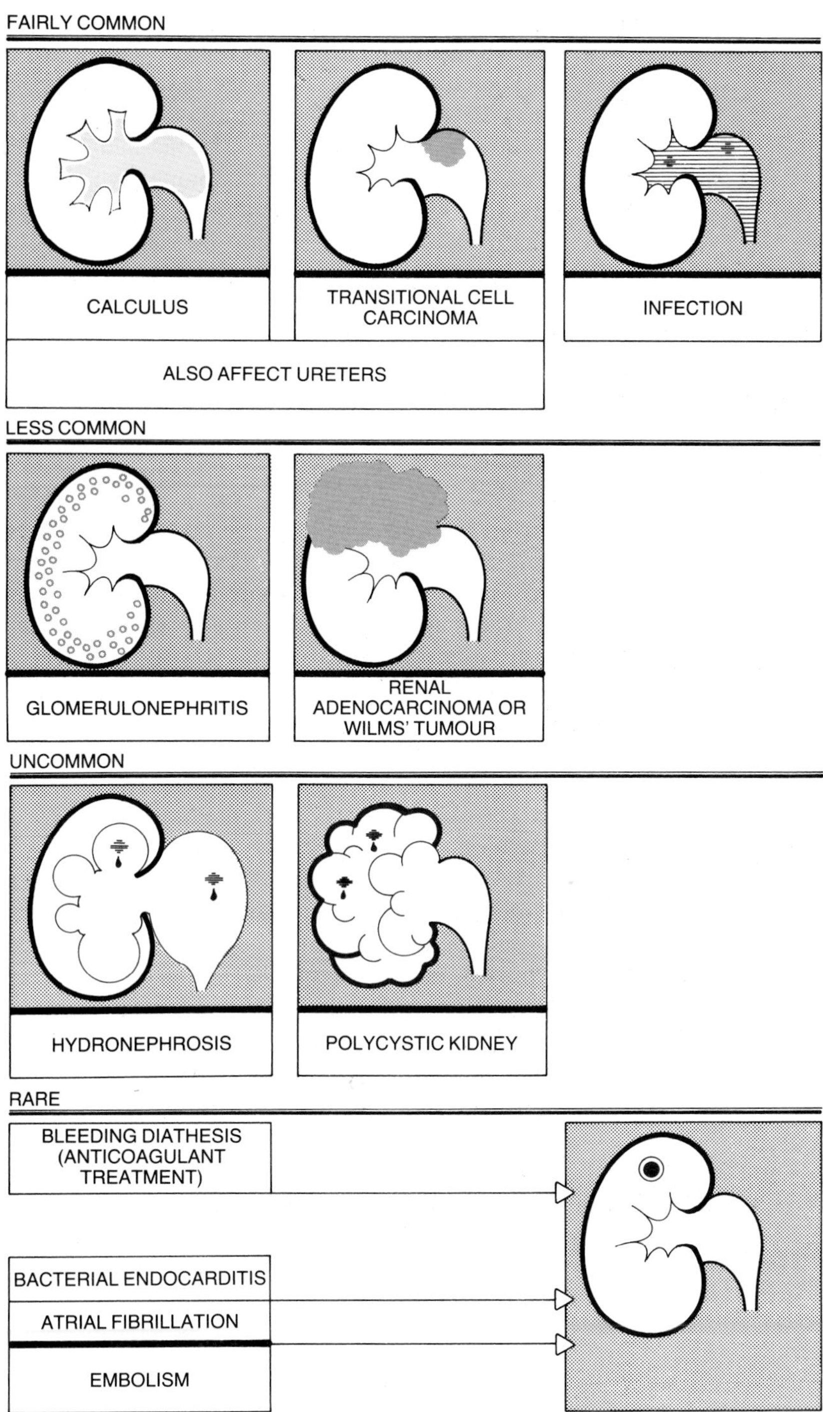

Trauma to a normal kidney may cause frank haematuria if considerable force has been applied, but microscopic haematuria is common after minor trauma in contact sports and rarely indicates a significant injury. Enlarged kidneys from any cause are more susceptible to trauma. In hydronephrosis or polycystic kidneys, minor blunt trauma may cause gross haematuria.

Sometimes, urine becomes red with haemoglobin rather than blood. This may be induced by vigorous exercise in young people such as prolonged marching in soldiers (*march haemoglobinuria*). These patients are believed to have defective red cell membranes which makes them more vulnerable to trauma. Exercise haemoglobinuria is self-limiting and requires no treatment.

Haematuria also occurs in renal parenchymal inflammations such as glomerulonephritis or arteritis. Renal haematuria may also be caused by microemboli settling in the kidneys, as in atrial fibrillation or infective endocarditis. Any urinary tract disorder with a potential for haematuria is more likely to be revealed when a patient is on anticoagulant therapy or develops a bleeding diathesis.

Diagnostic features of haematuria

Gross bleeding results in the passage of clots, whose shape may indicate their origin. Clots that form in the ureter are long and stringy, while clots formed within the bladder are more globular.

The stage of micturition at which blood appears is sometimes diagnostically useful. Blood from the kidneys, ureters or bladder wall will completely mix with the urine, and be present throughout the urinary stream. Urethral bleeding may leak out independently of micturition, or be seen only at the beginning of the urinary stream. Blood arising from the bladder neck or posterior urethra may sometimes present as terminal haematuria.

Dipstick testing is often the first step in the diagnosis of occult haematuria. Because this test is highly sensitive, a positive result should be confirmed by urine microscopy, which can also check for infection. Microscopic haematuria may represent a significant lesion anywhere in the urinary tract and must always be taken seriously. Often, however, a cause is never found for isolated episodes of microscopic haematuria.

DYSURIA

Dysuria describes pain or discomfort on micturition, often accompanied by difficulty in voiding. The pain is often described as 'burning' or 'scalding' and likened to 'passage of broken glass'. Any irritation of the urethra may cause dysuria. The most common cause is urinary tract infection, but urethral instrumentation, or the presence of a catheter, also commonly cause dysuria.

DISORDERS OF MICTURITION

The normal bladder has a capacity of about 350 ml. When this is reached, the detrusor muscle undergoes reflex contraction, initiating the desire to void. Micturition is normally initiated by conscious sphincter relaxation; involuntary detrusor contraction then empties the bladder completely.

Frequency of micturition

This is defined as the frequent passage of small quantities of urine, but with a normal daily urine volume. If severe, frequency may sometimes result in incontinence.

There are four main causes of frequent micturition:

- *Bladder irritation* — infection is the most common cause of urinary frequency and is usually accompanied by dysuria. The patient feels an almost constant need to pass urine regardless of the amount of urine in the bladder
- *Incomplete emptying of the bladder* — this is most commonly caused by bladder outlet obstruction as in prostatic hypertrophy, but it may also be caused by neurological disorders such as multiple sclerosis or spinal trauma. Voiding is incomplete so the bladder soon reaches full capacity again. The increased volume of residual urine in the bladder after micturition predisposes to infection
- *Detrusor instability (the unstable bladder)* — in this condition, the voiding reflex is activated before the bladder is properly filled. Small volumes of urine are thus passed more frequently
- *Small or indistensible bladder* — this is a rare cause of frequency and may be due to surgical resection or inflammatory fibrosis such as tuberculosis or idiopathic interstitial fibrosis

Frequency must be distinguished from *polyuria*, in which the amount of urine produced is excessive, and micturition therefore occurs more often. In polyuria, therefore, normal volumes are passed at more frequent intervals. Polyuria is usually accompanied by polydipsia (excessive drinking). Excess urine production is not a surgical problem; it most commonly results from diabetes mellitus, less commonly from renal failure and occasionally from diabetes insipidus.

Nocturia

Nocturia describes the need to pass urine with abnormal frequency at night. The patient may wake with the urge to void hourly, if not more frequently. Nocturia usually accompanies frequency or polyuria unless the symptoms are psychogenic in origin. Patients with cardiac failure may experience nocturia as peripheral oedema is returned to the general circulation in the supine position and renal perfusion is thereby increased.

Urgency

Urgency is the sudden desire to void, which if ignored, may result in incontinence. Urgency results from irritation of the bladder neck as in cystitis, or from the abnormal entry of urine into the proximal urethra as in prostatic enlargement. Other urinary symptoms are usually present.

Hesitancy

Difficulty in initiating micturition, known as hesitancy, usually occurs in males. In extreme cases, the patient may have to stand for several minutes before urinary flow begins. The usual cause is prostatic obstruction, which prevents entry of sufficient urine into the proximal urethra to initiate sphincter relaxation.

Poor urinary stream

Urinary stream is often reduced when there is urethral obstruction. The most common cause is prostatic enlargement, which may limit the urine flow to a dribble despite straining. Occasionally, a poor stream may be caused by a urethral stricture, in which case other urinary symptoms are minimal or absent.

Post-micturition dribbling

This symptom occurs when urine flow does not cease completely at the end of micturition. Dribbling may simply involve the leakage of a few drops of urine or be so severe as to amount to incontinence. Post-micturition dribbling results from abnormal sphincter function, and is especially common when voiding is incomplete. This symptom occurs most commonly in prostatic obstruction along with other urinary symptoms. When occurring in isolation, the symptom may denote weakness of the pelvic floor, especially in women.

'Prostatism'

This term is often applied to the symptoms of hesitancy, poor stream, frequency, urgency, nocturia and post-micturition dribbling. Any of these symptoms may occur in prostatic obstruction, but the term should be avoided because it implies a diagnosis, and may prejudice proper evaluation of symptoms.

RETENTION OF URINE

Urinary retention means the inability to void when the bladder is full. It occurs when the sphincter is unable to relax or when there is proximal urethral obstruction. Both factors may occur together.

Acute retention

In its simplest form, acute urinary retention can occur in normal individuals, usually males, particularly postoperatively. At this time, fluid overload, drugs, pain, the supine posture, anxiety or embarrassment are responsible. Similar factors may precipitate an episode of acute retention in individuals with asymptomatic prostatic enlargement. Occasionally acute retention is caused by an obstructing blood clot (clot retention) or stone.

Chronic retention

Chronic retention may occur with abnormalities of structure or function of the bladder muscle or sphincter mechanism. Less commonly, it is caused by persistent urethral obstruction. In chronic retention, voiding of urine is often incomplete. The problem progresses until the residual volume approaches maximum bladder capacity. Voiding then usually occurs by 'overflow' and the bladder tends to become abnormally distended. When obstruction is prolonged and severe, the bladder muscle hypertrophies, bladder diverticula may develop, and back pressure on the kidneys may cause uraemia and renal failure. At any stage, complete cessation of flow, i.e. *acute-on-chronic retention*, may be precipitated by overfilling, urinary tract infection, or severe constipation. The most common cause of chronic retention is prostatic enlargement.

PNEUMATURIA

Pneumaturia is the passage of gas mixed with urine. It is caused by perforation of gut into the urinary tract, or vice versa, resulting in fistula formation. The commonest causes are diverticular disease and Crohn's disease, although it sometimes occurs in carcinoma of colon or bladder. Gross urinary tract infection is inevitable. The patient typically complains of symptoms of urinary infection (dysuria and frequency) and may also describe bubbles or even faeces in the urine.

Fig. 20.4 Causes of vesico-colic fistulae

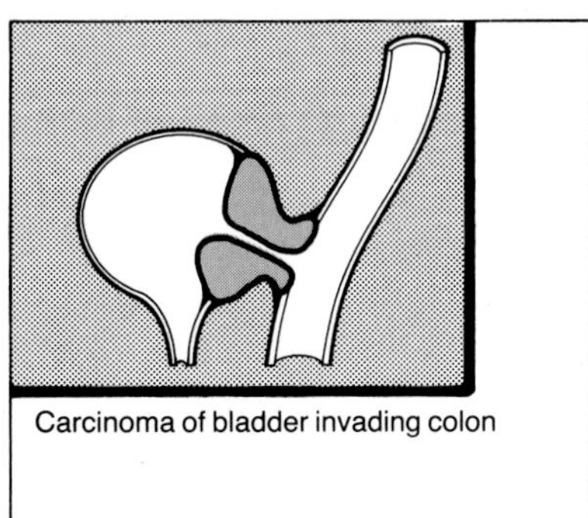

Carcinoma of bladder invading colon

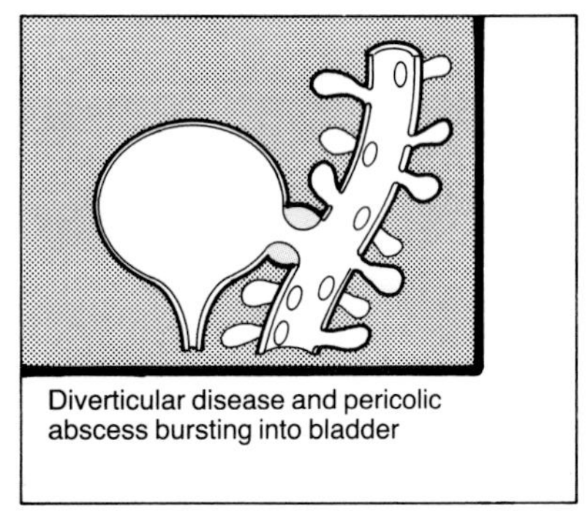

Diverticular disease and pericolic abscess bursting into bladder

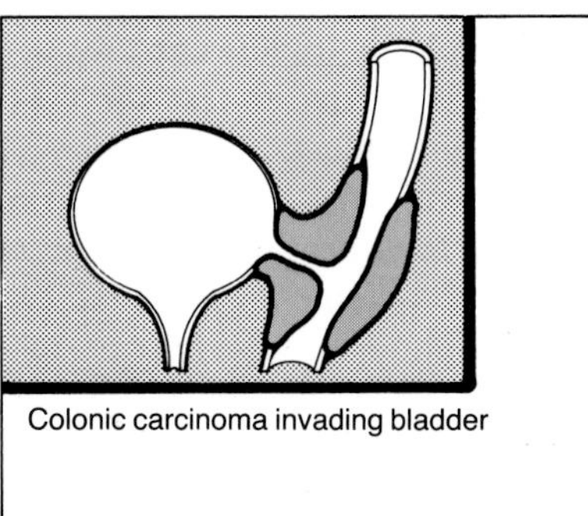

Colonic carcinoma invading bladder

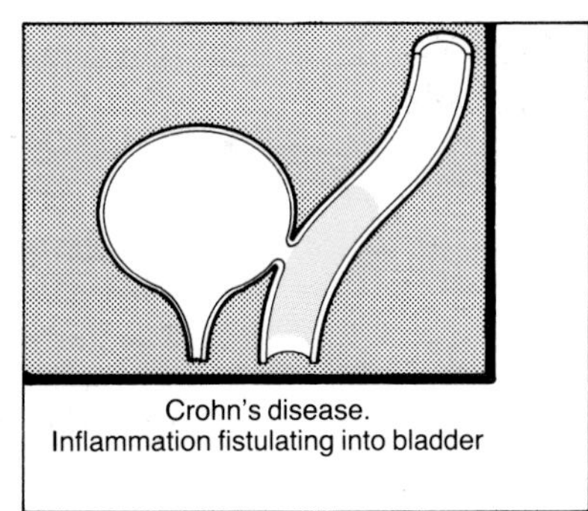

Crohn's disease.
Inflammation fistulating into bladder

URINARY INCONTINENCE

Involuntary passage of urine is a distressing and socially debilitating symptom. It may occur in a variety of disorders with a structural or functional abnormality of the bladder or sphincter mechanism. The normal bladder has a capacity of approximately 350 ml. During filling the detrusor muscle relaxes so that the intravesical pressure does not rise until bladder capacity is approached. Once the bladder is filled, voiding occurs by detrusor contraction and sphincter relaxation. Both are mediated via a spinal reflex at the level of S3,4. Superimposed on this system is an inhibitory mechanism under cortical (conscious) control, which delays voiding if it is socially inappropriate. Conscious control, including nocturnal control, develops during early childhood. Nocturnal incontinence is known as *enuresis*.

The pathophysiology of incontinence can be divided into three categories based on disorders of structure and function. Some disease processes may produce incontinence by more than one mechanism.

1. Loss of cortical control

Loss of inhibitory control over reflex voiding may occur in disease of the cortex, such as senile atrophy (dementia), or in disease of the spinal cord above the sacral reflex level, such as multiple sclerosis. Traumatic paraplegia is a common cause of complete loss of cortical control. The resulting incontinence may be described as the *supra-sacral neurogenic bladder*. The bladder fills to normal capacity and then empties spontaneously, and more or less completely, leaving little residual urine.

2. Disorders of sacral reflex control of detrusor and sphincter function

If the sacral reflex arc is damaged on its afferent or efferent sides, reflex contraction of the detrusor and relaxation of the sphincter are lost. This may occur in low spinal trauma or nearby disease, such as myelomeningocoele, diabetic neuropathy or invasive pelvic tumours. The bladder consequently becomes grossly distended and urine passively overflows causing constant dribbling incontinence. This can be alleviated considerably by regular manual emptying of the bladder, achieved by applying abdominal pressure. This form of incontinence may be described as a *sacral neurogenic bladder*. The large residual volume of urine strongly predisposes to infection.

In some patients, typically middle aged women, the reflex control of detrusor activity becomes hypersensitive so that the voiding reflex is initiated when the bladder volume is well below full capacity. The cause is unknown. This hypersensitivity results in small volumes of urine being passed frequently, and often so precipitously as to produce *urge incontinence*. The condition is known as *irritable bladder syndrome* or *detrusor instability*, a minor but distressing form of incontinence.

Bladder infection produces excessive sensory irritation and activation of the voiding reflex. In young children and the elderly, this may be responsible for incontinence without the usual symptoms of infection.

Persistent bladder outflow obstruction, from prostatic enlargement for example, causes progressive stretching of the bladder and in some way damages the voiding reflex. The result is a hugely distended, flaccid (hypotonic) bladder. Dribbling overflow incontinence may persist even when the obstruction has been removed.

3. Structural abnormalities of the bladder or sphincter

Many disorders may directly interfere with normal detrusor or sphincter function. In some cases, an additional contributory factor is damage to the afferent or efferent components of the neurogenic reflex mechanism.

The most common condition in this category is *stress incontinence*, in which the sphincter is weak. Any sudden increase of pressure on the bladder (while coughing, sneezing or laughing, for example) causes small quantities of urine to leak out. Stress incontinence is usually seen in parous women and results from pelvic floor damage during childbirth. There is often a degree of uterine prolapse and cystocoele.

Prostatectomy (transurethral or abdominal) may damage the sphincter, as may locally invasive tumours or pelvic fractures which involve the proximal urethra. Tuberculosis, radiotherapy and *idiopathic bladder fibrosis (interstitial cystitis)* may cause severe bladder contraction and frequency to the point of incontinence.

Incontinence is a feature of several rare congenital abnormalities such as epispadias or ectopic ureter opening into the vagina. These should be excluded in a child who fails to develop continence.

Fig. 20.5 Summary: causes of incontinence

Loss of cortical control
a. cortical disease
b. spinal cord disease, i.e. suprasacral neurogenic bladder

Abnormalities of the sacral reflex mechanism
a. sacral neurogenic bladder
b. detrusor instability
c. infection producing bladder hyperactivity
d. hypotonic bladder

Detrusor or sphincter abnormalities
a. stress incontinence
b. post-prostatectomy
c. tumour invasion
d. urethral trauma
e. contracted bladder
f. rare congenital abnormalities

HAEMOSPERMIA

Haemospermia describes the presence of blood in semen. A cause is rarely found and is assumed to be minor trauma to the genital tract. Inflammation of the prostate (prostatitis) sometimes causes haemospermia, accompanied by perineal pain.

APPROACH TO DIAGNOSIS OF URINARY SYMPTOMS

SPECIAL POINTS IN THE HISTORY

A detailed history of the urinary tract symptoms should be taken, together with a general history to elucidate any systemic causes or contributing factors, e.g. diabetes or multiple sclerosis.

In patients with haematuria, the occupational history may be important. Exposure to aniline dyes and other industrial chemicals that were once widely used in the rubber and cable industries, greatly increased the risk of transitional cell carcinoma of the urinary tract.

Haematuria can also be caused by infestation with Schistosoma, which is endemic in parts of the Middle East and Africa. A history of residence or travel in affected regions should therefore be sought. Similarly, tuberculosis is common in underdeveloped countries and can easily be overlooked in immigrants.

PHYSICAL EXAMINATION

General examination

A full general examination should pay special attention to a sallow complexion and signs of weight loss which may indicate uraemia, particularly if accompanied by a uriniferous smell and scratch marks. Blood pressure must be measured in every case as hypertension may be a feature of pyelonephritis, renal artery stenosis, polycystic kidneys or glomerulonephritis.

Abdominal examination

Abdominal inspection may reveal asymmetry due to a huge renal mass; this may be a nephroblastoma in a child or polycystic kidneys in an adult. In chronic retention, a large, lop-sided bladder may be visible. The loins should be carefully in spected from behind: a subtle fullness may indicate a renal mass or upper tract obstruction.

A bimanual technique is used when examining the abdomen for urinary tract disease. One hand palpates the subcostal region anteriorly while the other hand is placed in the renal angle to push the kidney forward onto the palpating hand. The kidneys are impalpable unless they are enlarged or displaced, except in a very thin patient. A renal mass will usually move with respiration and, because it is retroperitoneal with gut anteriorly, should also have an overlying area of resonance to percussion. The main causes of an enlarged kidney are hydronephrosis, polycystic disease, renal cell carcinoma and, in children, nephroblastoma (Wilms' tumour). Loin tenderness is uncommon in non-acute renal disorders except in chronic perinephric abscess. Tenderness is usually found in acute conditions, such as pyelonephritis or acute obstruction. Renal tenderness can be distinguished from vertebral tenderness by gently tapping the spinous processes. This will cause pain if the tenderness is vertebral.

The lower abdomen is palpated for the bladder. A distended bladder is felt as a soft mass arising from the pelvis, sometimes asymmetrically. It is dull to percussion and pressure on it may induce an urge to void. A suprapubic mass in the male usually indicates urinary retention, but occasionally it is a colonic carcinoma, a huge bladder tumour or stone. In the female, ovarian masses, pregnancy or uterine fibroids are more common causes of a suprapubic mass than urinary retention.

Auscultation of the abdomen may occasionally reveal a bruit in the upper abdomen radiating to the renal angles. This is characteristic of renal artery stenosis.

Rectal examination

Rectal examination should be performed in both sexes. To exclude gynaecological masses, a vaginal examination should also be done in females. In the male, the prostate is palpated per rectum for size, shape and consistency. The normal prostate is about 3 cm in diameter and weighs 10–15 gm. When moderately enlarged, it is approximately the size of a golf ball and weighs about 30–40 gm; when greatly enlarged, the prostate may weigh as much as 800 gm. When the prostate gland is this large, its upper edge may well be out of reach

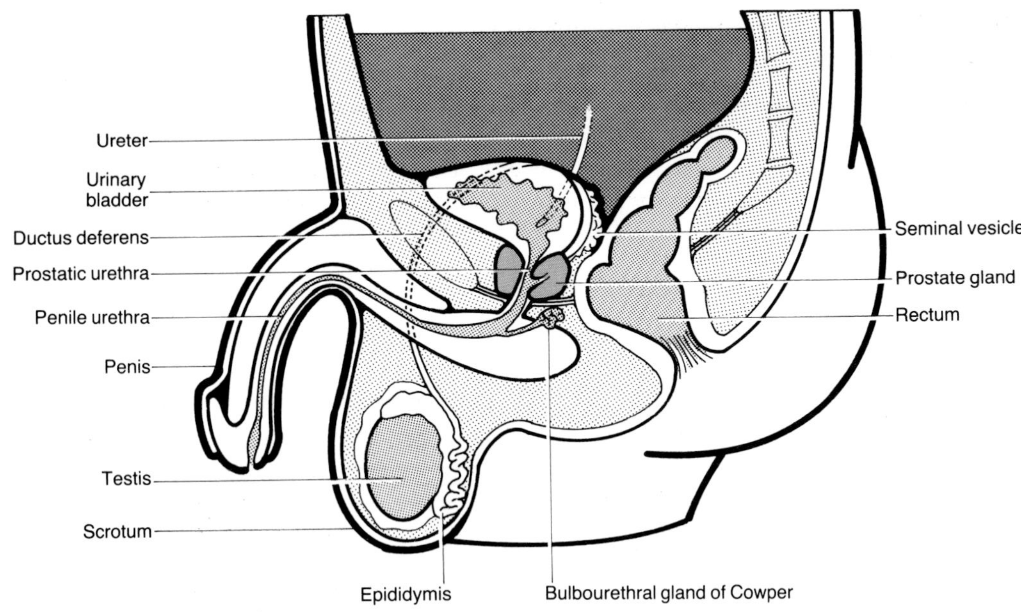

Fig. 20.6 Relationship of prostate to rectum and peritoneal cavity

of the examining finger. Note that most prostatectomy operations leave a capsular remnant so that the prostate appears unaltered on palpation.

The severity of prostatic obstructive symptoms depends on the extent of encroachment upon the urethra and not the prostatic diameter. In some cases, an enlarged median lobe lying posteriorly above the bladder outlet may act as a flap valve, intermittently obstructing urine outflow.

On palpation, the normal prostate has a smooth surface and a firm consistency, and is divided into two lateral lobes by a midline groove. In prostatic hyperplasia, enlargement is usually symmetrical, and the midline groove is maintained. Consistency remains normal. In contrast, a prostate infiltrated with carcinoma is irregular and asymmetrical. There are often hard nodules, and the median groove may be lost. In advanced cases, the tumour may be felt invading laterally into the pelvis or forward around the rectum. Digital examination is only reliable in distinguishing benign from malignant prostatic enlargement in gross cases. If carcinoma is suspected, *transrectal needle biopsy* is usually performed at the time of rectal examination. Prostatic tenderness is uncommon and may indicate prostatitis.

INVESTIGATION OF SUSPECTED URINARY TRACT DISEASE

In common conditions like prostatic hyperplasia or urinary tract infection, the diagnosis is evident from the history and examination. Investigation is limited to confirming and refining the diagnosis before treatment is initiated. Symptoms such as haematuria, however, suggest several diagnostic possibilities and require further investigation. Urothelial tumours frequently enter the differential diagnosis and must be excluded.

Fig. 20.7 Palpation characteristics of the prostate

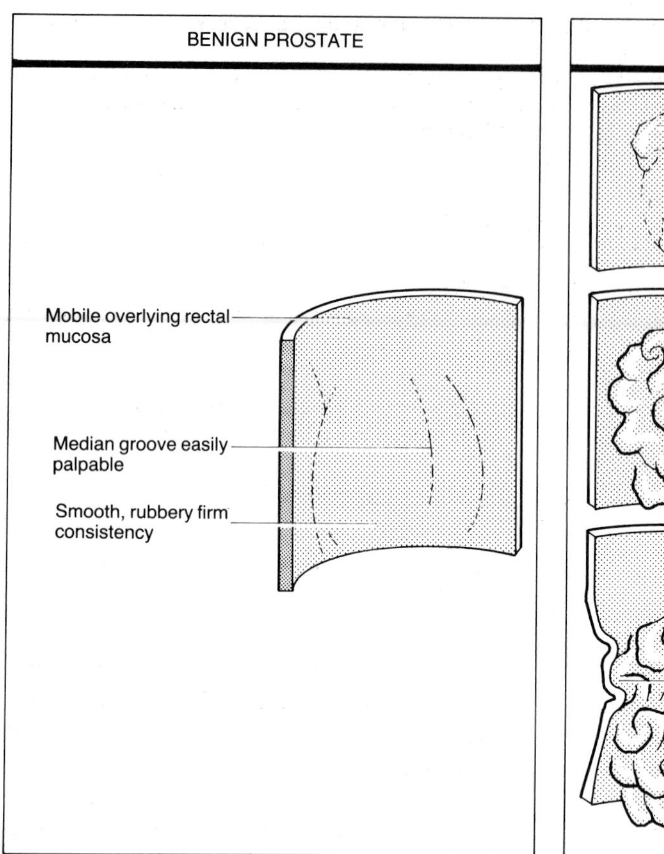

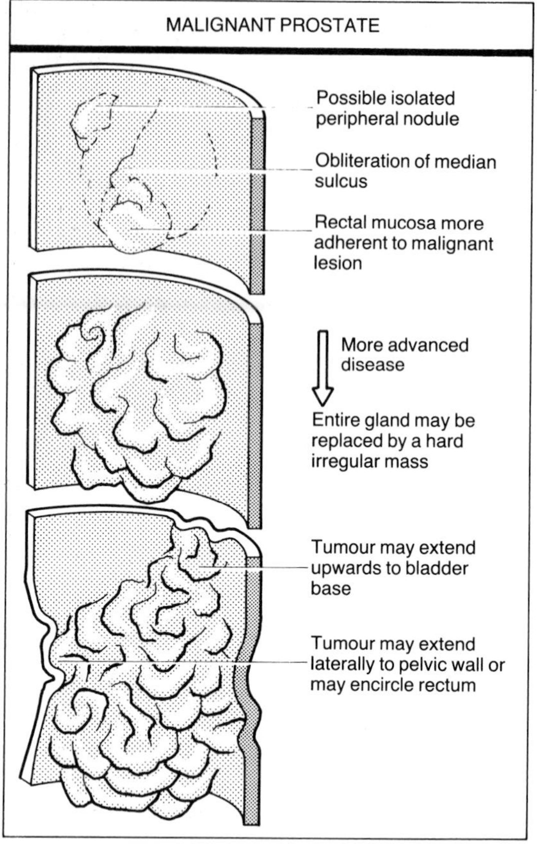

A simple approach to investigation of urinary tract disease is to consider the following questions:

- Are any blood tests likely to be helpful in diagnosis?
- What urine tests are indicated?
- Where is the lesion?

Are any blood tests likely to be helpful in diagnosis?

The blood tests which can be useful in diagnosing urinary tract disease are summarised in Figure 20.8.

What urine tests are indicated?

Any urinary symptoms should prompt collection of a clean midstream urine specimen (MSU) for microscopy and bacteriology. Microscopy will show the presence or absence of significant numbers of red blood cells (microscopic haematuria), white cells (pyuria) and bacteria (bacteriuria).

Bateriuria of more than 5×10^5 per cubic millimetre is considered to indicate significant infection. The urine is cultured to identify the organisms, and the organisms tested for antibiotic sensitivity. *Sterile pyuria* is characteristic

Fig. 20.8 Blood tests useful in diagnosing urinary tract disease

Full blood count
— hypochromic microcytic anaemia: chronic iron deficiency anaemia due to haematuria
— normochromic normocytic anaemia: chronic renal failure (lack of erythropoietin), chronic inflammatory disorders, e.g. tuberculosis
— polycythaemia : renal adenocarcinoma
— leucocytosis : infection

ESR
— raised in chronic and acute infections
— raised in renal adenocarcinoma

Urea, electrolytes and creatinine
— impaired renal function in bilateral obstructive uropathy or chronic renal failure in hypertension, diabetes, etc

Acid phosphatase
— raised in metastatic carcinoma of prostate, but rarely raised if carcinoma is confined to the gland (despite former belief, rectal examination does not affect acid phosphatase level)

Alkaline phosphatase (bone isoenzyme)
— raised in multiple bony metastases from any type of tumour

Calcium, phosphate, uric acid and parathyroid hormone levels
— useful investigations in stone disease

of urinary tract tuberculosis. If present, three early morning urine specimens should be examined for acid-fast bacilli and cultured. *Bacteriuria without significant pyuria* usually indicates contamination of the urine specimen. *Casts* found on microscopy suggest a nephritic process.

Urine cytology is a useful screening test for urothelial tumours in people at high risk, particularly those who have been exposed to industrial carcinogens. Some centres use cytology for long term followup of patients with treated bladder cancer.

Fig. 20.9 Typical MSU reports

(a) Haematuria **(b)** and **(c)** overleaf

Date of onset 2/52
Antibiotics Current / Intended } nil
Clinical Details
Intermittent haematuria. No pain
Signed

PATIENT STATUS
Please tick box
NHS (circled)
PP
OSV
CAT 2
Consultant/G.P.

Surname
Hospital No.
Forenames
Date of Birth 2 Oct 1940
Ward/Address

USE BALLPEN FIRMLY

MICROSCOPY			T. Vaginalis	
Pus Cells	0 /hpf	Gr. Pos. Cocci	Gr. Pos. Rods	
Red Cells	> 25 /hpf	Gr. Neg. Rods	Gr. Neg. Cocci	
Epithelial Cells		Yeasts	Vincents	
Casts	1. no growth			
Crystals	2.			
	3.			
Glucose	G%			
Protein trace	mg%			

1	2	3	4	5	6	7	8	9	10	11	12	13	14	15	16	17	18
AMP/AMOX	CEPHALEXIN	SULPHONAMIDE	NITROFURANTOIN	NALIDIXIC ACID	COTRIM/TRIMETH	TETRACYCLINE	ERYTHROMYCIN	PENICILLIN	FLUCLOX	FUCIDIN	NEOMYCIN	METRONIDAZOLE	GENTAMICIN	CEFOTAXIME			

S — Sensitive R — Resistant M — Intermediate

Phoned:

Specimen Request	Date taken	Received	Lab. No.	Reported
MSU Micro, C & S				

BACT.

Fig. 20.9 (cont.)

Date of onset 4 days
Antibiotics Current / Intended } nil
Clinical Details: burning dysuria, frequency
Signed

PATIENT STATUS — Please tick box: (NHS) | PP | OSV | CAT 2
Consultant/G.P.

Surname | Hospital No. | Forenames | Date of Birth 18. 6. 28 | Ward/Address

USE BALLPEN FIRMLY

MICROSCOPY			T. Vaginalis	1 AMP/AMOX	2 CEPHALEXIN	3 SULPHONAMIDE	4 NITROFURANTOIN	5 NALIDIXIC ACID	6 COTRIM/TRIMETH	7 TETRACYCLINE	8 ERYTHROMYCIN	9 PENICILLIN	10 FLUCLOX	11 FUCIDIN	12 NEOMYCIN	13 METRONIDAZOLE	14 GENTAMICIN	15 CEFOTAXIME	16	17	18
Pus Cells >50 /hpf	Gr. Pos. Cocci		Gr. Pos. Rods																		
Red Cells >100 /hpf	Gr. Neg. Rods		Gr. Neg. Cocci																		
Epithelial Cells ±	Yeasts		Vincents																		
Casts —	1. >10⁵ orgs/ml Enterococci			S		R	S		R												
Crystals —	2.																				
Bacteria ++	3.																				

Glucose — G% | S — Sensitive R — Resistant M — Intermediate
Protein ++ mg% | Phoned:
Specimen Request: MSU C & S | Date taken | Received | Lab. No. | Reported | BACT.

(b) MSU indicative of urinary tract infection

Date of onset 3/12
Antibiotics Current / Intended } none
Clinical Details: Pain (L) loin, Evening fevers, Frequency
Signed

PATIENT STATUS — Please tick box: (NHS) | PP | OSV | CAT 2
Consultant/G.P.

Surname | Hospital No. | Forenames | Date of Birth 12/4/50 | Ward/Address

USE BALLPEN FIRMLY

MICROSCOPY			T. Vaginalis	1 AMP/AMOX	2 CEPHALEXIN	3 SULPHONAMIDE	4 NITROFURANTOIN	5 NALIDIXIC ACID	6 COTRIM/TRIMETH	7 TETRACYCLINE	8 ERYTHROMYCIN	9 PENICILLIN	10 FLUCLOX	11 FUCIDIN	12 NEOMYCIN	13 METRONIDAZOLE	14 GENTAMICIN	15 CEFOTAXIME	16	17	18
Pus Cells >25 /hpf	Gr. Pos. Cocci		Gr. Pos. Rods																		
Red Cells 0 /hpf	Gr. Neg. Rods		Gr. Neg. Cocci																		
Epithelial Cells 0	Yeasts		Vincents																		
Casts	1. no growth																				
Crystals	2.																				
	3.																				

Glucose G% | S — Sensitive R — Resistant M — Intermediate
Protein trace mg% | Phoned:
Specimen Request | Date taken | Received | Lab. No. | Reported | BACT.

(c) MSU showing 'sterile pyuria' (possible tuberculosis)

WHERE IS THE LESION?

1. Suspected upper tract lesions

Ultrasound

Renal ultrasound is a valuable non-invasive technique for investigating a suspected renal mass. Ultrasound is particularly useful in differentiating solid from cystic lesions, and for demonstrating dilatation of the renal pelvis. If bladder pathology is suspected, the bladder can easily be examined at the same time. The bladder is particularly well seen if it is distended with urine; patients should be advised to take copious fluids before the investigation is performed.

Intravenous urography

Intravenous urography (IVU) is the traditional radiographic technique for demonstrating the urinary tract, although it provides poor assessment of function. Renal function is best investigated by radionuclide scanning. An IVU involves intravenous injection of an aqueous solution of iodinated benzoic acid which is rapidly filtered by the glomeruli and excreted. This radiopaque solution opacifies the urinary system, demonstrating the renal parenchyma, the renal pelvis and the ureteric anatomy. The cortical concentration of contrast (*nephrogram*) gives an indication of the shape, thickness and bilateral symmetry of the renal cortex.

Cysts and tumours of the kidneys are usually revealed by the distortion of normal anatomy they cause, although they are often indistinguishable from each other by this investigation. Tumours opacify with contrast to a variable extent and sometimes show a characteristic 'vascular blush'.

If the collecting system (renal pelvis, calyces and ureter) is dilated, this is usually easily seen, and the level of an obstruction can often be demonstrated. When obstruction is almost complete, films may have to be taken at long intervals since back pressure delays cortical excretion.

Congenital abnormalities of the pelvicalyceal system, such as duplex systems, are often found incidentally. Transitional cell tumours may show as filling defects in collecting systems or bladder. If an abnormality is seen in the kidney or renal pelvis, *tomography* can be performed during the same examination to reveal more structural detail. If renal excretion is poor, as in chronic renal failure or gross obstruction, IVU examination may be improved by using a high dose infusion of contrast. However, this is a dangerous technique in diabetic nephropathy as it may precipitate acute renal failure.

Arteriography

If a renal mass is demonstrated by IVU and found to be solid on ultrasound, arteriography may be performed to outline the vasculature of the lesion. Characteristic vascular patterns are often found in renal adenocarcinoma. *CT scanning*, however, is more reliable for investigating renal masses and is gradually superceding arteriography for this purpose.

Special contrast investigations

When obstruction or urothelial tumour of the upper tract is suspected, the collecting system may be outlined by one of two methods. Contrast media may be instilled, either by cystoscopic cannulation of the ureter (*retrograde ureterography*) or *percutaneous puncture* of the renal pelvis.

Radionuclide scanning

Radionuclide scanning techniques can be used to assess differential renal function. They are particularly useful in monitoring kidney function after relief of obstruction (see p. 38).

2. Suspected lower tract lesions

Radiography and ultrasound

Plain abdominal X-rays and IVU have little use in investigating lower urinary tract disorders, with the exception of bladder stone and chronic retention. In patients with bladder outlet obstruction, the volume of residual urine after voiding has traditionally been estimated from an IVU. However, ultrasound is now safer, more accurate and cheaper. The volume of this residual urine is an important factor in deciding whether operation is necessary.

Cystourethroscopy

When a bladder tumour or urethral pathology is suspected, cystourethroscopy (cystoscopy) is the investigation of choice. It allows direct visual examination, biopsy and immediate treatment if appropriate. Cystoscopy is usually performed under general or regional anaesthesia which also permits deep bimanual palpation.

Other investigations

If clinical examination suggests local spread of a bladder or prostatic tumour, *CT scanning* may be used to assess the extent of invasion. In carcinoma of the prostate, *radionuclide scanning* is valuable for diagnosing bony metastases. For suspected urethral obstruction, *contrast urethrography* can be used to localise the site of obstruction or stricture. If a colo-vesical fistula is suspected, *barium enema* may demonstrate the colonic lesion responsible (but rarely the fistula itself!).

When investigating incontinence, *cystometrography* can be used to assess the relationship between bladder pressure and volume. This is particularly useful in distinguishing between urge and stress incontinence in women.

Fig. 20.10 Summary : investigations for localising urinary tract pathology

INVESTIGATION	INDICATIONS	FINDINGS
Plain erect abdominal X-ray ('KUB' film)	Suspected stone disease, ureteric colic	Renal calcification; stones in kidney, ureter and bladder
	(incidental finding)	Abnormal renal size, shape and position
Ultrasound scanning	Renal masses	Differentiates solid from cystic renal lesions
	Suspected upper tract obstruction	Shows dilatation of renal pelvis or ureters
	Symptoms of bladder outflow obstruction	Estimates bladder volume
Intravenous urography (with or without tomography)	Chronic renal disease and chronic urinary obstruction	Shape and thickness of renal cortex (nephrogram)
	Haematuria	Non–functioning part of cortex and distorted anatomy if tumour present
	General investigation of urinary symptoms	Morphology of upper tract and bladder
Renal arteriography	Renal mass suspicious of tumour	Abnormal renal vasculature typical of renal tumour
CT scanning	Palpable loin mass, differentiation of a pelvic mass from a prostatic or bladder tumour	Size, nature and extent of invasion of lesions
Special contrast examinations of upper tract, e.g. retrograde or percutaneous ureterography	Obstruction of upper urinary tract	Site and perhaps nature of obstruction
Micturating cystography	Recurrent urinary tract infections or failure to thrive in children	Severity of vesico–ureteric reflux
Radionuclide renal scans	Investigation of low urine output, or differential renal function (e.g. renal artery stenosis)	Renal morphology, excretory function (total and differential), presence and sites of obstruction
Radionuclide bone scans	Bone pain in prostatic carcinoma	Bony metastases

(continued over)

Fig. 20.10 (cont.)

Cystourethroscopy (with or without biopsy or resection)	Haematuria	Urothelial tumours of urethra or bladder
	Investigation of bladder neck obstruction and treatment e.g. transurethral resection of bladder neck or prostate	
	Diagnosis and treatment of bladder stones	
Cystometrography	Investigation of incontinence	Nature of incontinence
	Sometimes used in assessment of bladder outflow obstruction	

21 DISORDERS OF THE PROSTATE

Benign prostatic hypertrophy and carcinoma of the prostate are the most common prostatic disorders. Infection of the prostate, or prostatitis, is a poorly defined and a less common condition.

Anatomical considerations

The normal prostate gland is small, about 3 cm in both length and diameter. Its weight is about 10 gm. The gland is situated immediately below the bladder neck, so that the first 3 cm of the urethra pass through the gland. Thus, the walls of the proximal urethra are composed of glandular tissue and this part is known as the *prostatic urethra*. The urethra then penetrates the muscles of the pelvic floor, which incorporate the sphincter mechanism. Prostatic hypertrophy and carcinoma may, therefore, cause urethral obstruction, and carcinoma may invade and disrupt the sphincter mechanism.

The posterior aspect of the gland is palpable rectally (as seen earlier in Figure 20.7) where a *median groove* can readily be identified. This groove is described as dividing the gland into two lateral lobes. The median groove tends to be obliterated in prostatic carcinoma but is usually exaggerated in benign hypertrophy.

When the prostatic urethra is examined cystoscopically, an important landmark is the *veru montanum* (urethral crest), an elongated mound on the posterior wall. At its midpoint is a small depression, the prostatic utricle (the embryological representative of the uterus), into which the two ejaculatory ducts open. The posterior part of the gland above the ejaculatory ducts is known as the *median lobe*. If this becomes hypertrophied it tends to form a pedunculated mass (often described as the 'middle lobe') in the floor of the bladder; this may act as a flap-valve obstructing the bladder outlet.

As seen in Figure 21.1, the bulk of the normal prostate consists of up to 50 *glandular lobules*. These converge into about 20 separate ducts which open into the prostatic urethra lateral to the veru montanum. In addition to this glandular tissue proper, there is a zone of small *paraurethral glands* immediately adjacent to the urethra. It is these glands and their supporting tissue which tend to enlarge greatly from middle age onwards causing benign prostatic hypertrophy; the prostatic glandular tissue proper then becomes compressed beneath the fibrous outer capsule. In contrast, carcinoma of the prostate arises in the prostatic glandular tissue proper at the periphery, usually spreading into adjacent structures rather than obstructing the centrally located urethra.

The prostate gland is invested by a fascial sheath with a rich *venous plexus* between it and the gland capsule. This venous plexus may be the source of

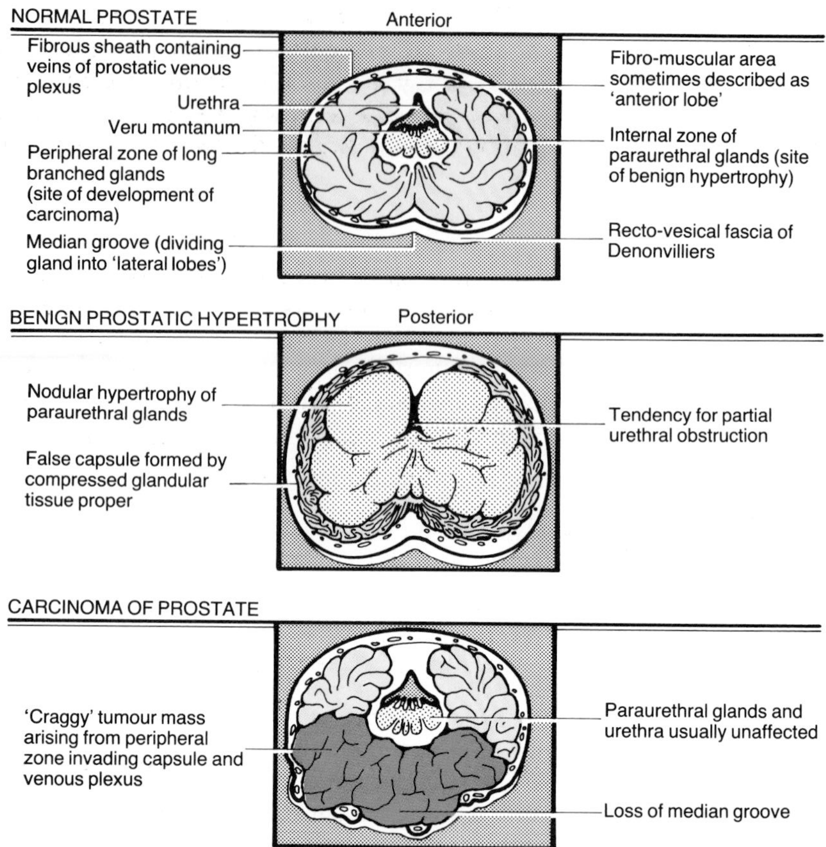

Fig. 21.1 Horizontal sections through normal, hypertrophic and malignant prostate glands

considerable haemorrhage during and after prostatic surgery. Direct connections between this plexus and the extradural venous plexus of the vertebrae provide an easy route for haematogenous dissemination of prostatic carcinoma. Posteriorly, the prostatic capsule is fused with the dense *fascia of Denonvillier*, which tends to act as a barrier to direct spread of carcinoma from the prostate to the rectum or vice versa.

BENIGN PROSTATIC HYPERTROPHY

Benign prostatic hypertrophy is a common finding in elderly men. The majority have no symptoms, or mild symptoms considered to be part of the normal ageing process. In about 20% of men over 60, however, hypertrophy produces such severe symptoms that surgical treatment has to be considered.

Pathophysiology

In pathological terms, the paraurethral glands undergo *nodular hyperplasia*. This causes progressive symmetrical enlargement of the gland up to many times its normal size. In gross cases, the hypertrophied gland may weigh as much as 800 grams. The prostatic glandular tissue proper is compressed to form a false capsule at the periphery. Occasionally, the process is predominantly fibrotic, resulting in a small dense gland.

The severity of symptoms in benign prostatic hypertrophy is not directly proportional to the size of the gland but to the degree of encroachment on the prostatic urethra and the resulting obstruction of urinary outflow.

In some cases, hypertrophy of the bladder neck muscle alone causes the same symptom complex, but the two can only be distinguished at cystoscopy.

Clinical features

The symptoms of bladder outlet obstruction are summarised in Figure 21.2. They usually develop gradually until they come to interfere with daytime activity and sleep. At any time, *acute retention of urine* may occur. This is commonly precipitated by bladder overfilling after excess fluid intake, classically beer, but is also a hazard of many general surgical operations on older men. In some patients, the severity of prostatic symptoms fluctuates from month to month, making it difficult to decide whether an operation is necessary.

Fig. 21.2 Symptoms of bladder outlet obstruction

Hesitancy
Poor stream
Frequency
Urgency
Nocturia
Post-micturition dribbling

Complications of bladder outlet obstruction

Bladder outflow obstruction progressively interferes with the patient's ability to empty his bladder. The volume of *residual urine* increases gradually over weeks and months (i.e. chronic retention), and the intravesical pressure rises. The threshold for the voiding reflex is therefore reached more quickly, and calls to void increase in frequency. The stagnant residual urine is prone to infection, and this may exacerbate the symptoms. In some cases, the bladder becomes vastly distended and atonic, leading to *overflow incontinence*. In other cases, the detrusor muscle undergoes hypertrophy in an attempt to overcome the outflow obstruction. The normally smooth bladder lining then becomes trabeculated. With a further rise in pressure, the depressions between the muscle bands deepen and eventually form *bladder diverticula*. Stasis in the diverticula predisposes to stone formation.

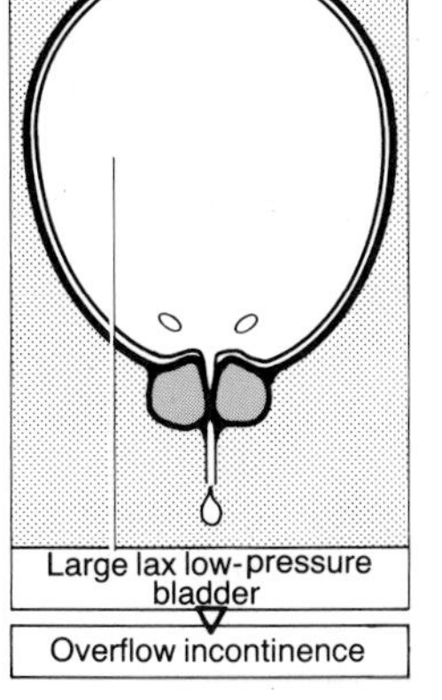

Fig. 21.3 Atonic bladder due to outlet obstruction

A small proportion of patients with bladder outlet obstruction experience only minimal local symptoms. Meanwhile however, rising intravesical pressure is transmitted back into the ureters and kidneys causing hydronephrosis, and later, progressive renal parenchymal damage. These patients tend to present with severe systemic illness. Their renal failure may be accompanied by anaemia, dehydration, acidosis and infection. Bladder outflow obstruction is easily overlooked unless the bladder is examined for distension.

Principles of management of benign prostatic hypertrophy

The principles of management of bladder outlet obstruction, believed to be due to benign prostatic hypertrophy, are outlined in Figure 21.5.

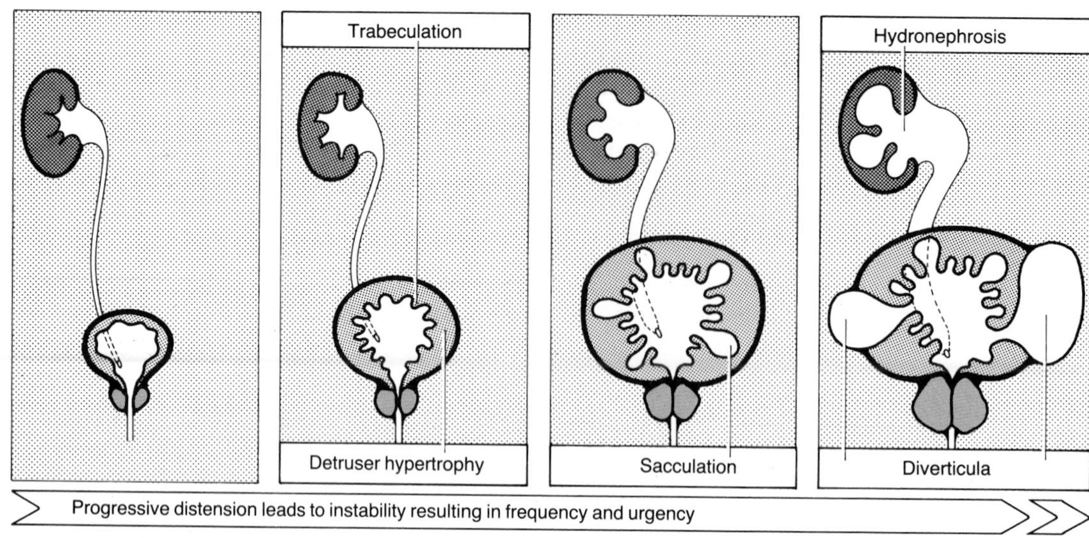

Fig. 21.4 Back pressure effects of bladder neck obstruction

Fig. 21.5 Management of chronic bladder outflow obstruction

1. Assess the symptoms and the need for operation from the history
2. Estimate the severity of bladder outlet obstruction by ultrasound, possibly by intravenous urography and sometimes by cystometrography
3. Investigate the disturbance of upper tract function by renal function tests, ultrasound and perhaps IVU
4. Exclude urinary tract infection by urine microscopy and culture
5. Exclude prostatic carcinoma clinically and if necessary by needle biopsy
6. Treat renal failure and other systemic problems
7. Consider whether catheter drainage of the bladder is desirable

If operation appears necessary:

8. Diagnose the cause and extent of obstruction by cystoscopy
9. Resect benign prostatic hypertrophy or bladder neck hypertrophy transurethrally, or obtain biopsy material by the same method if carcinoma seems likely
10. Consider other operative measures such as open prostatectomy or excision of diverticula where appropriate

1. Diagnosis

A detailed history is first taken to assess the nature of the symptoms and how much they interfere with the patient's life. This, in addition to the patient's general condition, will be the principal factor determining the need for operation. The abdomen is examined for bladder size and the prostate palpated rectally. These, however, will only reveal gross abnormalities.

The next step is to investigate the effects of outlet obstruction on the bladder, by estimating the volume of residual urine. Traditionally, IVU has been used for this but ultrasound is more reliable, quicker, less invasive and cheaper. Occasionally, when urinary symptoms are severe but residual volume is insignificant, the alternative diagnosis of irritable bladder syndrome should be investigated. Urine flow and bladder pressure should be measured during voiding by *cystometrography*.

Renal function is assessed by estimating plasma urea, creatinine and electrolytes. If these are abnormal, further metabolic investigations may be necessary. Upper tract distension can be demonstrated reliably by ultrasound.

Urinary infection alone may be responsible for the symptoms, or may have precipitated an episode of urinary retention. A midstream specimen of urine should therefore be examined by microscopy and culture. It is important that infection be eradicated if surgery is intended because of the risk of septicaemia.

Carcinoma of the prostate should be suspected if the prostate feels nodular. Transrectal needle biopsy should be performed because a diagnosis of carcinoma will alter management. Serum prostatic acid phosphatase is often measured in these patients, but is only elevated if there are bony metastases.

2. *Relief of chronic retention and obstructive effects on the kidney*

If there is a large volume of residual urine (750 ml or more), the patient is usually catheterised to effect bladder drainage. This allows bladder tone to recover over the course of a few days. Drainage also allows any reversible component of renal failure to correct itself. Fluid and electrolyte balance is monitored and restored by infusion of intravenous fluids if necessary. A severely ill patient may need blood transfusion, intravenous antibiotics and other preparatory measures before surgery can be contemplated.

3. *Cystoscopy*

Despite all the above investigations, the nature of bladder outlet obstruction can only be accurately assessed by direct cystoscopic examination. This is true even when open prostatectomy is intended. At the same time, the bladder is examined for trabeculation, diverticula, tumours and stones. In most cases, transurethral resection (TUR) of obstruction is immediately performed under the same anaesthetic. Histological examination of resected prostate may reveal unsuspected carcinoma (see prostatic carcinoma, later).

4. *Transurethral resection of prostate (TURP)*

Transurethral prostatectomy reduces postoperative morbidity compared with open abdominal operation and requires a shorter hospital stay.

Bladder outlet obstruction is most commonly caused by benign prostatic hypertrophy. The aim of surgery is to remove the bulk of the gland and leave the compressed normal peripheral tissue. This protects the subcapsular venous plexus which might otherwise bleed catastrophically. 'Chips' or 'divots' of tissue are excised with the resectoscope using a *cutting diathermy wire loop*. The operation is performed with continuous *glycine* irrigation; saline or water would be absorbed and induce systemic fluid and electrolyte disturbances. As shown in Figure 21.6, the gland is progressively chipped away, taking great care to preserve the sphincter mechanism immediately distal to the veru montanum. Prostatic chippings are sent for histology and unsuspected carcinoma is sometimes diagnosed.

When obstruction is caused by bladder neck hypertrophy, the muscle is divided by making a longitudinal incision at the bladder neck using a cutting point on the resectoscope. The prostate is not resected.

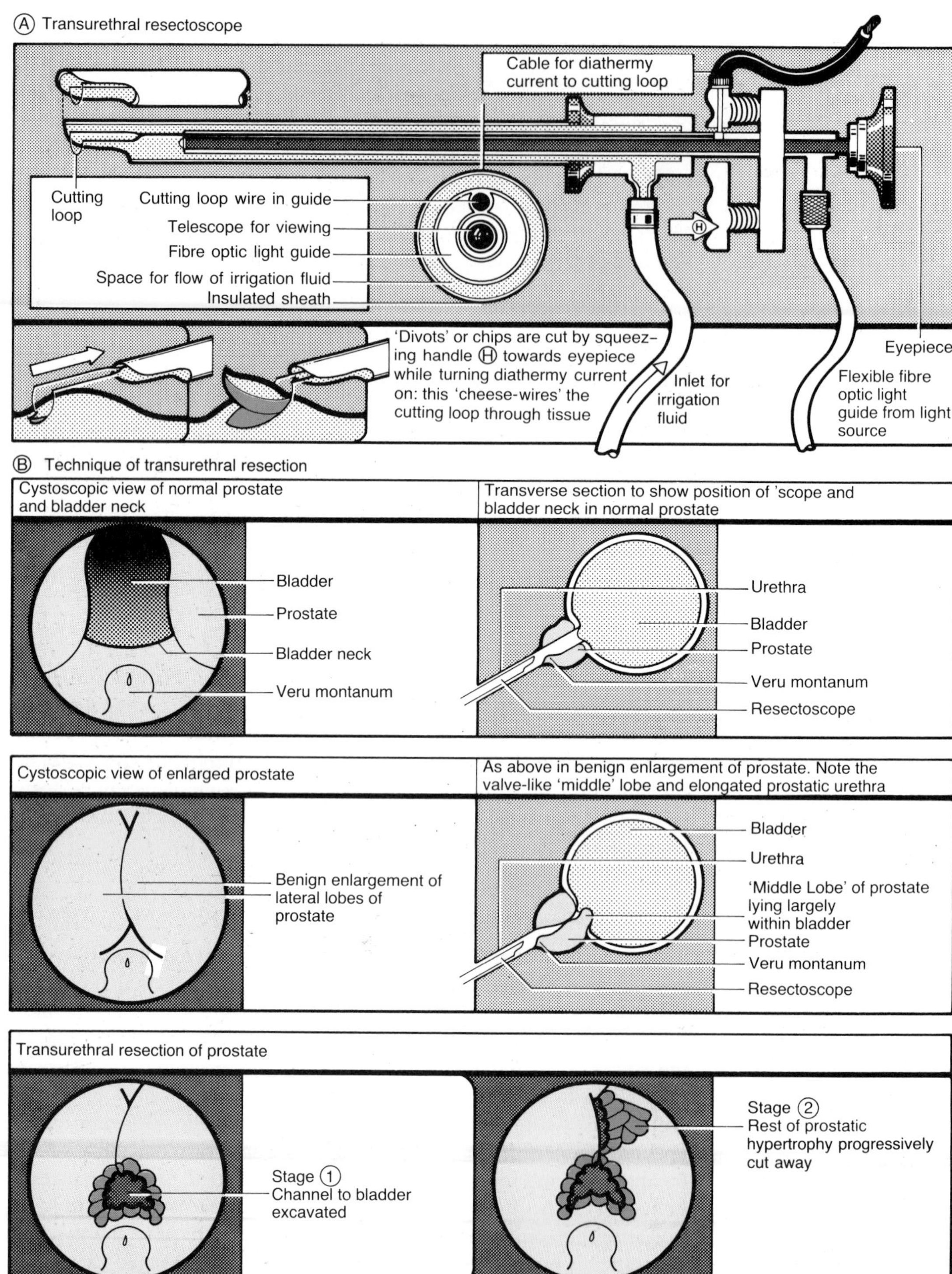

Fig. 21.6 Transurethral prostatectomy

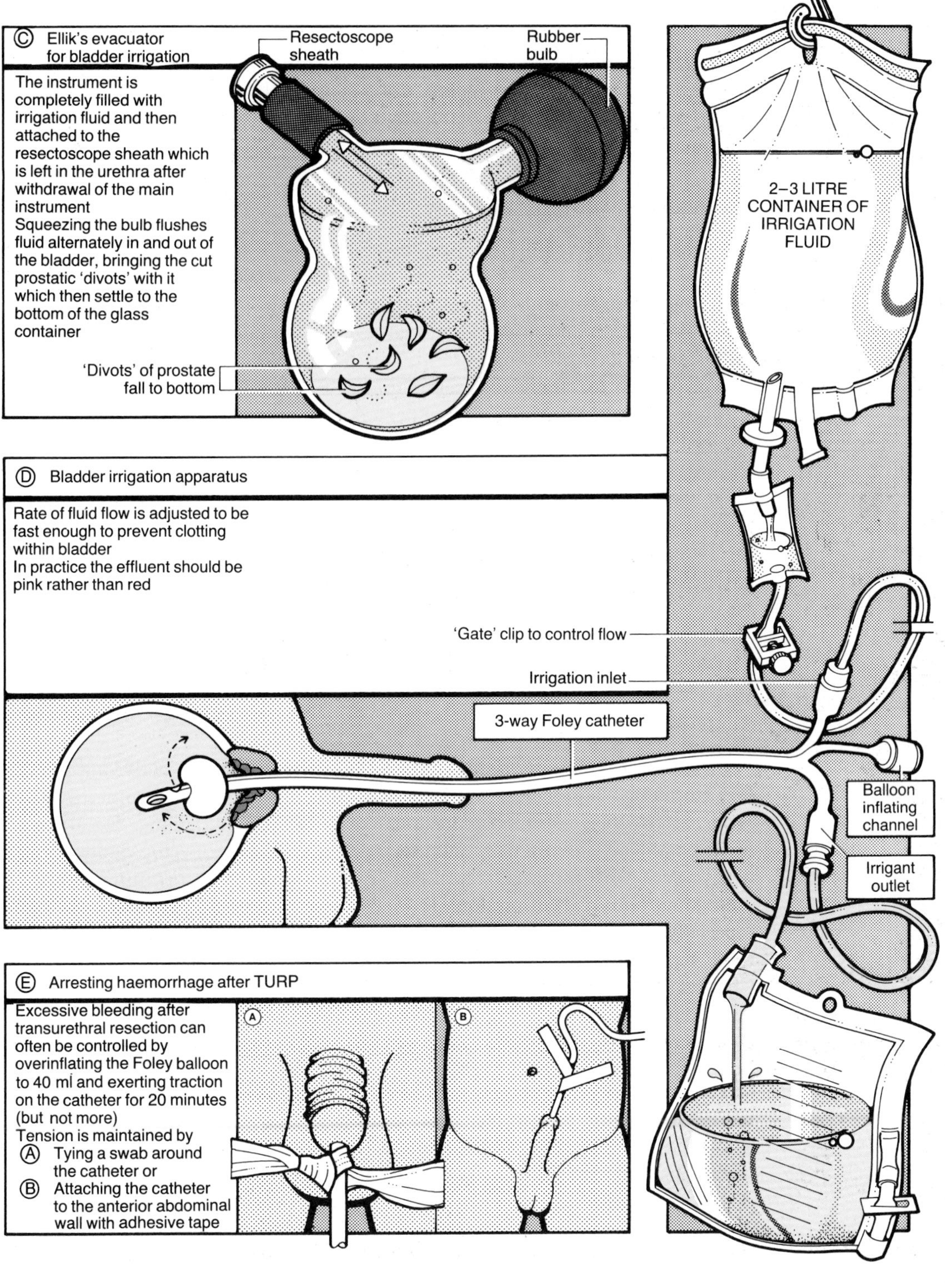
Ⓒ Ellik's evacuator for bladder irrigation
Resectoscope sheath
Rubber bulb
The instrument is completely filled with irrigation fluid and then attached to the resectoscope sheath which is left in the urethra after withdrawal of the main instrument
Squeezing the bulb flushes fluid alternately in and out of the bladder, bringing the cut prostatic 'divots' with it which then settle to the bottom of the glass container
'Divots' of prostate fall to bottom
2–3 LITRE CONTAINER OF IRRIGATION FLUID
Ⓓ Bladder irrigation apparatus
Rate of fluid flow is adjusted to be fast enough to prevent clotting within bladder
In practice the effluent should be pink rather than red
'Gate' clip to control flow
Irrigation inlet
3-way Foley catheter
Balloon inflating channel
Irrigant outlet
Ⓔ Arresting haemorrhage after TURP
Excessive bleeding after transurethral resection can often be controlled by overinflating the Foley balloon to 40 ml and exerting traction on the catheter for 20 minutes (but not more)
Tension is maintained by
Ⓐ Tying a swab around the catheter or
Ⓑ Attaching the catheter to the anterior abdominal wall with adhesive tape
Ⓐ
Ⓑ

5. Retropubic prostatectomy

Retropubic prostatectomy is used when the gland is so large that transurethral resection is not practical. The abdominal retropubic approach is also widely used by general surgeons untrained in the technique of cystoscopic resection. Occasionally, an open operation is necessary to deal with bladder diverticula or huge stones when they accompany prostatic hypertrophy.

Complications of prostatectomy

Prostatectomy invariably disrupts the mechanism at the bladder neck which prevents semen entering the bladder during ejaculation. Thus, patients usually fail to ejaculate through the penis after prostatectomy *(retrograde ejaculation)*, although erection and orgasm are unaffected. Maintaining fertility is not usually important in this older age group, but if necessary, urine can be filtered to recover sperm for artificial insemination.

Moderate haematuria can be expected after transurethral prostatectomy in the first postoperative weeks. Occasionally, this is severe enough to cause *clot retention*.

Recovery of complete urinary continence is sometimes delayed following prostatectomy but only occasionally is there permanent damage to the sphincter mechanism.

Operation greatly improves the quality of life in most patients. Even in patients over 80, postoperative morbidity and mortality is acceptably low. Nevertheless, a small proportion of severely debilitated, immobile or demented patients are better managed by long-term catheterisation.

Acute urinary retention and its management

Acute urinary retention usually appears suddenly in patients with long standing symptoms of bladder outlet obstruction. It can complicate chronic retention. Acute retention is commonly precipitated by bladder overfilling, faecal loading or urinary tract infection. Sometimes, acute retention develops unexpectedly in a patient with minimal symptoms. Acute retention is a common cause for emergency surgical admission. It is also a common postoperative problem, especially in males, and it may occur at any age, even in the absence of bladder neck hypertrophy or prostatic enlargement. Management is described in Chapter 33.

a. Diagnosis of acute retention

Acute retention must be distinguished from anuria but the diagnosis is usually not difficult. The patient is acutely distressed and in pain with an easily palpable bladder. A history of symptoms suggestive of chronic retention or bladder outlet obstruction should be sought, together with details of previous episodes or prostatic surgery.

b. Catheterisation

Retention is usually treated by *urethral catheterisation*. This is usually a simple procedure and can be performed in a clean clinical area. Strict aseptic precautions must be taken to avoid introducing infection. Certain factors should discourage an attempt at simple urethral catheterisation. These include previous prostatectomy or known urethral stricture, a history of difficult catheterisation or a non-retractile foreskin. For these patients, an experienced opinion should be sought to decide whether *suprapubic catheterisation* or urethral catheterisation under general anaesthesia with a metal introducer or other instruments should be attempted. If a surgeon with urological training is available, cystourethroscopy and appropriate surgical treatment may be performed immediately.

c. Evaluating the underlying cause and any precipitating factors

After relieving the acute retention, the catheter is usually left in situ for a day or two until the patient has been fully assessed. The initial decision is whether to attempt a *trial without catheter*, i.e. test whether the patient can void urine satisfactorily when the catheter is removed, or whether to proceed directly with an operation. Any urinary tract infection must be vigorously treated before a trial without catheter or an operation.

The indications for cystourethroscopy, and prostatectomy or bladder neck resection are:

- A huge volume of retained urine diagnostic of chronic retention
- Raised levels of plasma urea and creatinine which improve after catheterisation — this indicates chronic obstructive uropathy
- Previous episodes of acute retention
- Bladder outflow obstruction caused by carcinoma of prostate
- Failure of 'trial without catheter'

d. 'Trial without catheter'

The catheter should be removed early in the morning so that if the trial is unsuccessful, the catheter can be replaced before bedtime. Success is judged by the passage of reasonable volumes of urine with each voiding, i.e. more than about 100 ml. The patient must be regularly examined to ensure that the bladder is not becoming distended by retained urine. If it is, this indicates chronic retention with overflow. Unsuccessful trial without catheter is an indication for cystourethroscopy and probable surgical treatment on the next available operating list.

Indwelling catheters and their management

The majority of patients with permanent catheters are elderly men with bladder outflow obstruction, where surgery is contraindicated or has failed.

Indications for permanent catheterisation include:

- Unfitness for prostatectomy

- The elderly, severely debilitated, demented or immobile patient with incontinence
- Incontinence due to external sphincter damage by previous prostatectomy or invasive carcinoma
- 'Sacral neurogenic bladder', e.g. in multiple sclerosis

The major problems of long-term catheterisation are recurrent catheter blockage and infection. Catheters readily become blocked by epithelial debris or by gradual accretion of calculus. They must be changed regularly every 6–10 weeks. In most cases, this can be done at home by the general practitioner or community nurse, if sterile packs are available from a hospital. Infection, once established, is difficult to eradicate in the presence of a catheter. In elderly patients, low grade infection is present almost constantly and causes little discomfort; antibiotics should only be prescribed if local symptoms become troublesome or systemic signs of infection develop.

In paraplegic patients, however, ureteric reflux predisposes to recurrent upper urinary tract infections. These infections lead to progressive renal failure and death at an early age. For these patients, special care is taken to avoid introducing infection. Urine specimens should be examined regularly, microscoped and cultured, and if infection does develop it must be treated promptly.

CARCINOMA OF THE PROSTATE

Carcinoma of the prostate is common after the age of 70 years. Fortunately, the tumour grows slowly and remains asymptomatic in most cases and the diagnosis may only be made incidentally or at autopsy. Even when symptomatic, the disease tends to pursue a prolonged course, and most patients die of other diseases.

Carcinoma arises peripherally in the prostatic glandular tissue proper rather than the paraurethral tissues. Transurethral resection or open prostatectomy for benign prostatic hypertrophy leaves a compressed remnant or pseudocapsule of glandular tissue. The potential for carcinomatous change in this must not be overlooked.

Pathology and clinical features

Prostatic tumours are adenocarcinomas with a variable degree of differentiation. This is reflected in their behaviour and the aggressiveness of their local and metastatic spread. Most of these tumours are well differentiated and remain confined within the capsule. They slowly invade adjacent prostatic tissue and sometimes involve the bladder neck or sphincter mechanism. In many cases, the prostate is already enlarged by benign hypertrophy. Early on, the patient is either asymptomatic or has symptoms of bladder outlet dysfunction identical to those of benign hypertrophy. In the latter case, diagnosis is usually made incidentally after histological examination of TURP specimens.

Rectal palpation of a malignant prostate typically reveals an irregular surface with hard nodules. In many cases, however, the gland appears normal or is smoothly enlarged as in benign hypertrophy.

Tumour spread outside the prostatic capsule substantially worsens the prognosis. By this stage significant symptoms have developed. Local spread may involve surrounding pelvic tissues, in particular the rectum (causing change in bowel habit), or the bladder and ureters (causing urinary obstruction or incontinence). At this stage, the tumour is obvious on rectal palpation. It may be invading laterally into the pelvic walls or encircling the rectum. In very advanced cases, the pelvis may be frozen solid with tumour. Occasionally, pelvic spread presents with a major deep venous thrombosis affecting the lower limb.

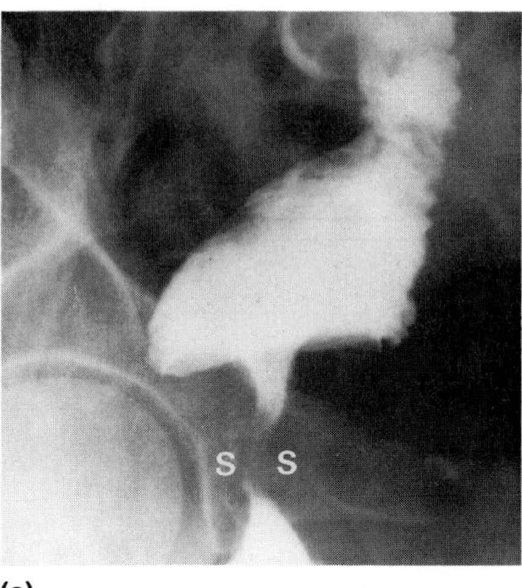

(a)

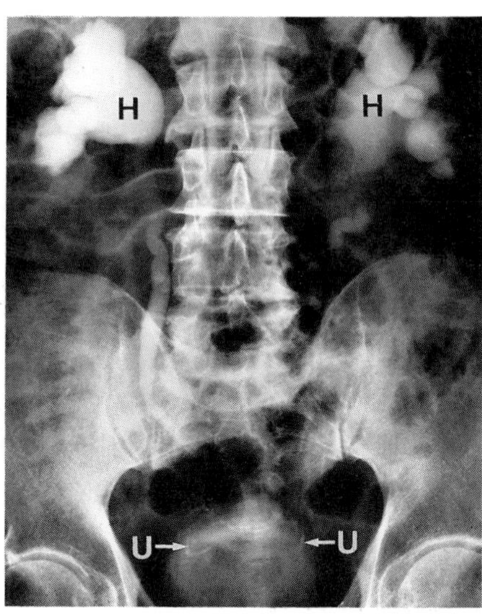

(b)

Fig. 21.7 Local effects of advanced prostatic carcinoma

(a) Barium enema from a 76-year-old man with known prostatic carcinoma who developed a change in bowel habit. The tumour has compressed and invaded the rectal wall circumferentially causing a marked stricture **S**.
(b) Intravenous urogram from another elderly man with advanced prostatic carcinoma. He presented with renal failure due to retroperitoneal spread of tumour which had caused bilateral distal ureteric obstruction. Note the gross bilateral hydronephrosis **H**; on the original film, the distal ureters can be seen to narrow at **U**

Distant spread of prostatic carcinoma mainly occurs via the bloodstream. Tumour cells have ready access to the venous plexus immediately beneath the prostatic capsule. Metastases have a proclivity for bone, especially the pelvis and spinal column. This may be so because of their direct venous anastomoses with the prostatic plexus. Bone metastases cause skeletal pain and may be responsible for pathological fractures, e.g. vertebral crush fractures or fractured neck of femur. Bony lesions are typically sclerotic (i.e. dense, appearing white on X-rays) rather than osteolytic (as in most other bony secondaries) and have a characteristic radiological appearance as shown in Figure 21.9.

Fig. 21.8 Summary: modes of presentation of carcinoma of prostate

Asymptomatic — incidental finding of nodular prostate on rectal examination
Symptoms of bladder outflow obstruction — tumour found histologically after transurethral prostatectomy for benign hypertrophy or suspected clinically by finding nodular prostate on rectal examination
Symptoms of spread to surrounding pelvic tissues, e.g. change in bowel habit, loss of continence
Symptoms of bony metastases, e.g. bone pain, pathological fractures

Approach to investigation of suspected prostatic carcinoma

Prostatic bladder outlet obstruction may be caused by benign hypertrophy or less commonly, carcinoma. It may be impossible to distinguish between the two clinically, unless the prostate feels malignant or there are obvious bony metastases. Carcinoma is therefore often unsuspected. Diagnosis depends on histology; needle biopsy is performed if the prostate is nodular or craggy, otherwise, the obstruction is treated by transurethral resection of the prostate and the chippings are examined histologically. A small proportion of patients, particularly the elderly, will thus be discovered to have carcinoma. Open prostatectomy on a patient with unsuspected prostatic carcinoma can be difficult. The gland is usually hard and fibrous, without the clear plane of cleavage found in benign hypertrophy.

If rectal examination of the prostate leads to suspicion of tumour, transrectal needle biopsy (e.g. Trucut) of nodular or hard areas is performed. Serum prostatic (tartrate labile) acid phosphatase is often measured, but this is only elevated if disease is locally extensive or if metastases are present; a normal result does not exclude a diagnosis of carcinoma.

Plain X-rays are indicated if skeletal pain is a symptom. Prostatic bony metastases are characteristically sclerotic, giving a patchy cotton-wool appearance as shown in Figure 21.9. Some lesions, however, are radiolucent. A radioisotope bone scan may be performed when plain X-rays are negative or equivocal.

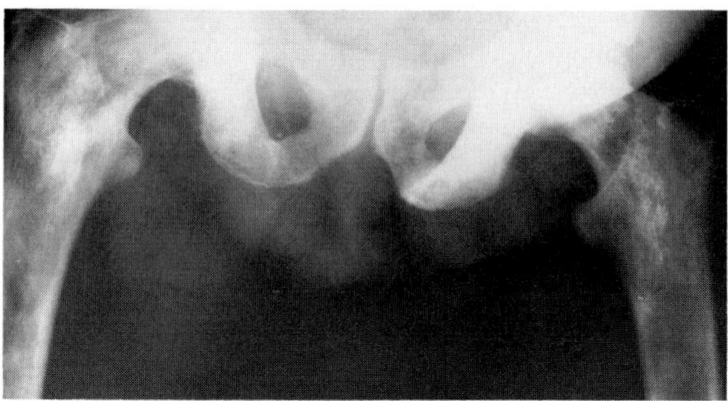

Fig. 21.9 Bony metastases from prostatic carcinoma

This 82-year-old man had disseminated prostatic cancer. Note the typically mixed osteosclerotic and osteolytic lesions in the upper femurs and ischial arch, giving a 'moth-eaten' appearance. The same appearance is often found in the ribs

Management of prostatic carcinoma

There is no effective cure for carcinoma of the prostate, although if the disease is confined to the gland, total prostatectomy would theoretically eliminate it. However, the risks and side effects of this operation are unacceptably high, and include massive haemorrhage and permanent incontinence. Since the effects of local disease can readily be controlled by other means, total prostatectomy is no longer performed.

The goals of treatment in carcinoma of the prostate are to control symptoms and inhibit disease progression. It must be remembered that prostatic carcinoma grows slowly in the majority of patients and that the disadvantages of some treatments outweigh the benefits. For this reason, early tumours are treated by local resection (transurethrally) and more advanced cases, both local or systemic, by hormonal manipulation.

The rate of growth of prostatic carcinoma is controlled by circulating testosterone. Reducing testosterone or opposing it chemically provides effective palliation in most cases for both local and metastatic disease.

Hormonal manipulation

There are four options, each of which amounts to castration, i.e. prevents secretion of testosterone from the testes:

- Removal of both testes by *subcapsular orchidectomy*. This is a quick and simple scrotal operation. The testicular capsules are left in-situ and fill with blood clot, which preserves the scrotal contour. There are minimal side effects and no serious long-term sequelae
- Administration of an oral oestrogen dose sufficient to suppress testosterone production. *Stilboestrol*, in a dose of 3 mg daily, is now the usual regimen. This dose, though considerably lower than previously used, is equally effective treatment, but can still cause thrombo-embolic complications and fluid retention. Vascular complications may be arterial (e.g. stroke or myocardial infarction) or venous (e.g. deep venous thrombosis and pulmonary embolism). Fluid retention may precipitate cardiac failure. Other common side effects are nausea and vomiting, loss of libido and gynaecomastia. The serious risks of oestrogen therapy must be weighed against the harmful effects of the tumour itself, and compared with alternative treatments with fewer disadvantages
- Monthly injections of depot LHRH (luteinising hormone releasing hormone). This newly developed treatment releases endogenous luteinising hormone from the anterior pituitary. Testicular synthesis of testosterone is initially enhanced but rapidly exhausted, thus lowering circulating testosterone levels. The treatment is expensive but may be preferred to orchidectomy
- Anti-androgen drugs, such as cyproterone acetate, antagonise the action of testosterone at cellular level. This treatment may prove to be more effective because it blocks testosterone from both testes and adrenals

Symptoms of urinary outflow obstruction are often relieved by hormonal therapy but TURP may become necessary. There is a risk of permanent incontinence, however, if carcinoma has invaded the sphincter mechanism.

Fig. 21.10 Summary: management of prostatic carcinoma

Histological diagnosis by rectal biopsy or incidentally after TURP for symptoms of bladder outlet obstruction

No active treatment for asymptomatic disease

Hormonal manipulation
— bilateral orchidectomy or
— administration of oestrogens (stilboestrol) or
— administration of LHRH
— administration of anti-androgen drugs, e.g. cyproterone acetate

Transurethral resection for persistent bladder outlet obstruction

Radiotherapy to control local symptoms or painful bony metastases

Radiotherapy to the gland and surrounding structures may control symptoms caused by pelvic spread when hormonal manipulation has been unsuccessful. The side effects (including radiation proctitis or small bowel damage) may be serious. Radiotherapy is an effective treatment for painful localised bony metastases.

PROSTATITIS

This uncommon disorder represents inflammation of the prostate gland, usually caused by coliform bacteria. Instrumentation or infection of the urinary tract may be predisposing factors. Prostatitis may present acutely or in a chronic form.

Acute prostatitis

Acute prostatitis is characterised by perineal pain and fever. Glandular swelling may also cause bladder outflow obstruction and urinary frequency. The prostate is tender to rectal examination and prostatic massage may cause exudation of pus from the urethra. The latter is a valuable diagnostic feature. Treatment is with oral antibiotics, such as amoxycillin or co-trimoxazole, which are usually continued for two to three weeks.

Chronic prostatitis

Chronic prostatitis presents with chronic, low-grade perineal and suprapubic pain. Symptoms and signs are often vague and ill-defined and the diagnosis is sometimes made on inadequate grounds, without considering a possible psychosexual cause for the presenting symptoms. Treatment is with appropriate antibiotics according to culture and sensitivity of urethral pus. Antibiotics should be continued for several weeks. Response may be poor, especially if the diagnostic criteria were weak. Infective prostatitis may be the first presentation of diabetes mellitus, so the blood sugar should always be checked.

22 TUMOURS OF THE KIDNEY AND URINARY TRACT

Introduction

Two types of tumour arise from the renal parenchyma. *Adenocarcinomas* are confined to adults, and are also known as renal cell carcinomas and by the old names of hypernephroma and Grawitz tumour. *Nephroblastomas* (Wilms' tumour) are developmental in origin and present in infancy or early childhood.

Tumours of the transitional cell epithelium lining the urinary tract (urothelium) are common. They arise anywhere in the tract, including the pelvicalyceal system of the kidney, the ureters, the bladder and occasionally the urethra. These *transitional cell carcinomas*, which occur exclusively in adults, are most common in the bladder. Squamous cell carcinomas sometimes occur in the urinary tract, and probably arise from metaplastic squamous epithelium caused by chronic irritation from stones or schistosomiasis. Squamous cell carcinomas occasionally arise in the squamous epithelium at the urethral meatus. Very rarely, an adenocarcinoma may develop in the bladder from glandular epithelial remnants of the embryological urachus.

RENAL ADENOCARCINOMA

Pathology

Renal adenocarcinoma is twice as common in males as in females; it rarely develops before puberty, but may occur at any age thereafter. The incidence rises after the age of 40.

Renal adenocarcinoma originates in the renal tubules. Characteristically, the tumour cells are large and polygonal with clear cytoplasm due to accumulation of glycogen and lipid. For this reason, these tumours are sometimes known as clear cell carcinoma. In other variants, the cells are granular and stain more intensely.

Renal adenocarcinomas probably vary in their degree of malignancy. Small isolated tumours are often found incidentally on IVU examination or at autopsy. Tumours less than 2 cm in diameter are regarded by some pathologists as benign, since evidence of local invasion or distant metastases is rarely found in these small tumours. Bilateral tumours are present in about 5% of cases. Larger tumours invade surrounding tissues and may spread to para-aortic lymph nodes. A characteristic feature of renal adenocarcinoma is invasion of the larger tributaries of the renal vein and growth as a long cord along the lumen into the inferior vena cava (Figure 22.1). From here, tumour emboli reach the lungs, typically giving rise to large round discrete 'cannonball' secondaries. Occasionally, isolated metastases occur in the brain, bone and elsewhere.

Fig. 22.1 Venous spread of renal adenocarcinoma

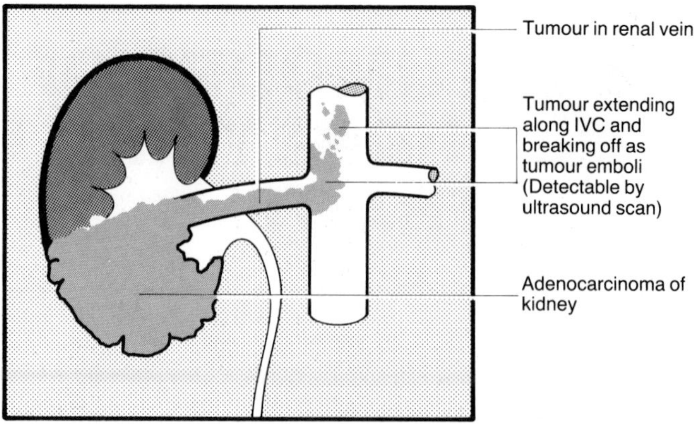

Clinical features

Haematuria, frank or microscopic, is the most common presenting feature of renal adenocarcinoma and occurs in at least 60% of cases. Chronic haematuria may result in iron deficiency anaemia. Less commonly, loin pain or a renal mass leads to the diagnosis.

Renal adenocarcinoma can also present in a variety of unusual ways. Some tumours secrete excess erythropoietin which causes polycythaemia. Hypertension may result from excess renin production. Similarly, ectopic production of parathormone may cause hypercalcaemia. Renal adenocarcinoma may cause pyrexia and should be considered in patients with a pyrexia of unknown origin. In most cases, the ESR is elevated. As with other malignancies, metastases may be the presenting feature, for example, cannonball secondaries on a chest X-ray.

Fig. 22.2 Presenting features of renal adenocarcinoma

Frank haematuria
Microscopic haematuria
Iron deficiency anaemia
Loin pain
Renal mass
Elevated ESR
Hypertension
'Pyrexia of unknown origin'
Polycythaemia
Hypercalcaemia
Secondary lesions (e.g. 'cannon-ball' lesions on chest X-ray, pathological fractures)

Approach to investigation

When a renal adenocarcinoma is suspected, intravenous urography is usually the first investigation. The plain abdominal control film may show an abnormal renal outline: tumour is suggested by a mass in the renal cortex, often with distortion or separation of the calyces.

When a mass suspicious of renal adenocarcinoma has been found on an IVU, the next step is to determine whether the mass is solid or cystic. Ultrasound

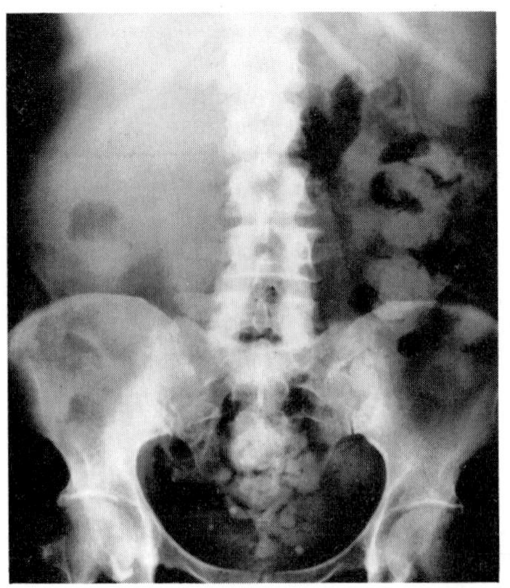

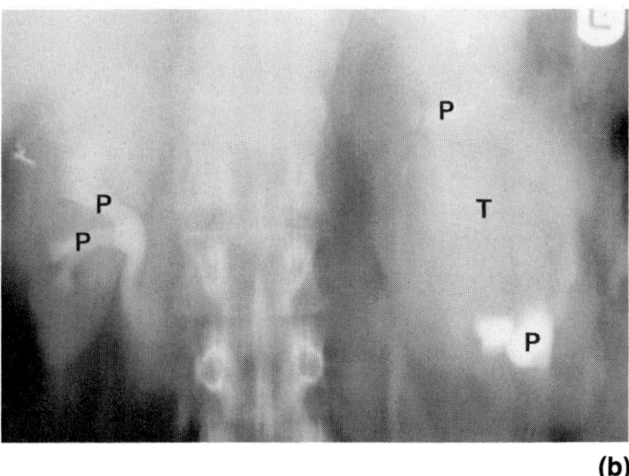

Fig. 22.3 Renal adenocarcinoma

(a) This 50-year-old man presented with painless haematuria. The plain abdominal film shows a large soft-tissue mass in the right loin which obscures the psoas shadow. **(b)** Tomogram taken during intravenous urography of a 58-year-old woman presenting with haematuria. The shape of the pelvicalyceal system **P** on the right is normal, but on the left it is grossly distorted by a tumour **T** in the middle of the kidney

is simple and reliable for this purpose. If the mass is cystic, it is most likely a simple benign cyst. If solid, it must be assumed to be a tumour. If there is tumour invasion of the large veins, this can often be demonstrated preoperatively using ultrasound. CT scanning is similarly valuable in assessing invasion of the perinephric tissues and metastasis to regional lymph nodes.

Before the advent of ultrasound and CT scanning, arteriography was widely used to demonstrate tumour circulation. This confirmed the diagnosis and gave some indication of tumour size and spread. Arteriography is still sometimes used to demonstrate the arterial anatomy, particularly when the other kidney is missing or bilateral renal tumours are suspected and a partial nephrectomy may have to be performed to preserve some renal function. Inferior vena cavography is sometimes useful if venous extension of tumour is suspected on ultrasound.

A chest X-ray is usually taken, and will show most pulmonary metastases. No other screening investigations are worthwhile.

Management of renal adenocarcinoma

In most patients, the kidney involved by tumour is *excised* (*nephrectomy*). The incision and the extent of resection is chosen according to the extent of tumour spread into surrounding structures, for example, the renal capsule, the perinephric fat or the para-aortic lymph nodes. When the tumour has breached the capsule or involves regional lymph nodes, local radiotherapy is usually given postoperatively.

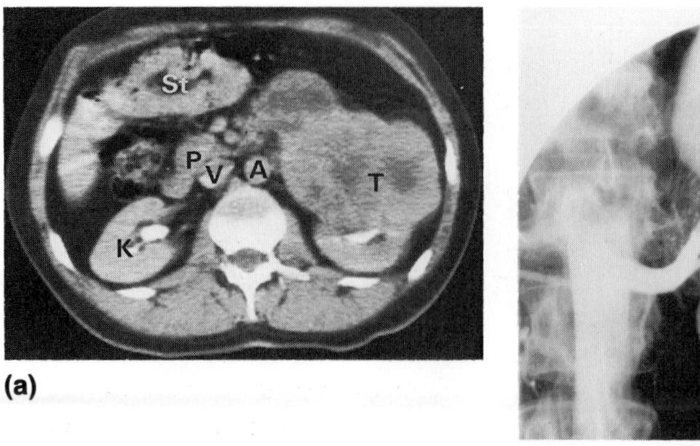

Fig. 22.4 Renal adenocarcinoma

(a) CT scan showing huge left renal tumour **T** in a 62-year-old man with left loin pain and a palpable mass; note the variable density of the tumour due to areas of necrosis and haemorrhage. Note also the normal right kidney **K**, aorta **A**, pancreas **P**, inferior vena cava **V** and stomach **St**. **(b)** Left renal arteriogram from a 68-year-old woman in whom a renal mass was demonstrated on intravenous urography. The arteriogram outlines the normal renal vasculature and shows a large crescentic mass of abnormal vessels in the upper pole (outline arrowed) typical of renal adenocarcinoma. Only part of the tumour vasculature is demonstrated, the rest having been destroyed by necrosis within the tumour

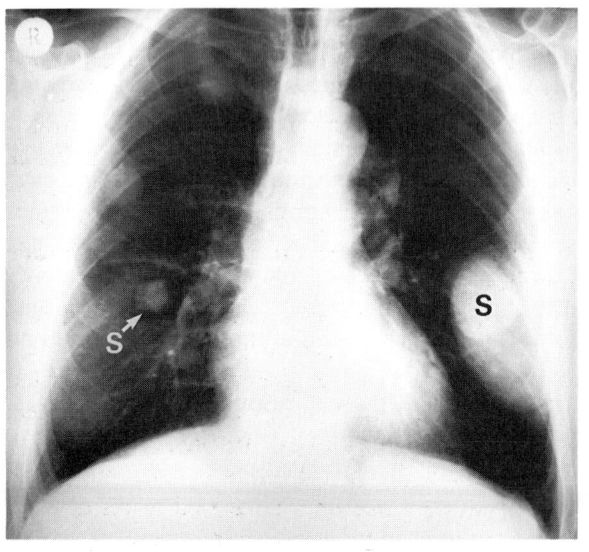

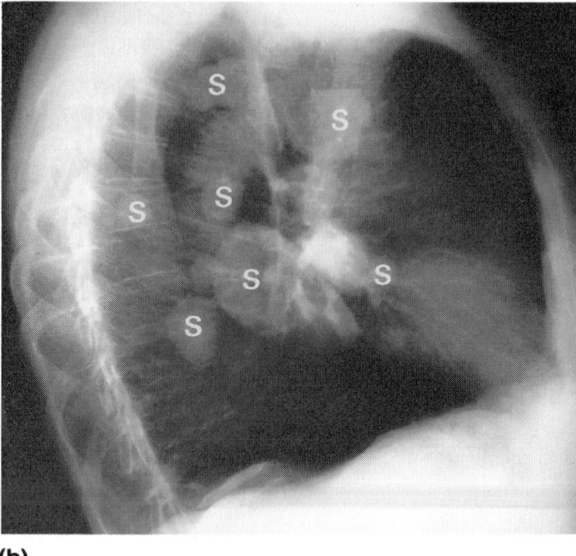

Fig. 22.5 Pulmonary metastases from renal adenocarcinoma

(a) P–A and **(b)** lateral chest X-rays from the same patient as in Figure 22.4(b), showing multiple 'cannon-ball' secondary lesions **S** of various sizes. These are typical of renal adenocarcinoma

Isolated pulmonary or cerebral metastases are sometimes amenable to surgical excision, which often results in cure. For multiple metastases, chemotherapy may be used for palliation.

TRANSITIONAL CELL CARCINOMA

Epidemiology and aetiology

Tumours of the urothelium are common. Histologically, they are transitional cell carcinomas. Most arise primarily in the bladder, but they also occur in the pelvicalyceal system and ureters and rarely in the urethra. Urothelial tumours are uncommon below the age of 50 and their incidence increases with age. Men are affected three times more often than women. Transitional cell carcinoma occurs about as often as gastric cancer in men, and are about one quarter as common as lung cancer. Transitional cell carcinoma is at least four times as common as renal adenocarcinoma.

Urothelial cancers are strongly associated with exposure to carcinogens, which were widely used in the rubber, cable, dye and printing industries. Exposure to these carcinogens causes a 20–60 times increased risk of developing urothelial cancer. The tumours develop as long as 25 years after exposure and so a detailed occupational history should be taken in suspected cases. These carcinogens are excreted in the urine, and the prolonged exposure of the bladder to urine compared with the rest of the tract probably explains why urothelial tumours most often arise in the bladder. Cigarette smoking is associated with a four-fold increase in incidence of urothelial tumour and is probably caused by urinary excretion of inhaled carcinogens.

Pathology

Histologically, well-differentiated tumours resemble normal transitional epithelium. Less differentiated tumours become increasingly unlike their tissue of origin so that the most anaplastic tumours can only be classified as urothelial because they are known to have arisen in the urinary tract. The degree of differentiation tends to be reflected in the tumour morphology as seen at cystoscopy. Well differentiated tumours form papillary frond-like lesions, whereas more aggressive tumours form plaque-like lesions which invade underlying muscle and surrounding tissues.

Most aetiological factors predispose the whole urothelium to malignant transformation. Consequently, urothelial tumours are often multifocal and there may already be multiple tumours at the time of presentation. An affected individual is at high risk of developing further tumours, despite complete eradication of the earlier tumour. When the primary tumour is in the pelvicalyceal system or ureter, there is a high risk of tumour developing later anywhere in the urothelium distal to the primary. This is said to result from 'seeding' of tumour cells shed from the proximal lesion, but is more likely due in some way to the multicentric nature of the disease.

Clinical features

Transitional cell carcinoma usually presents with painless haematuria. An upper tract lesion may cause ureteric colic (clot colic) and long stringy clots in the urine. If bleeding is gross, clots may cause ureteric obstruction. Rapid bleeding from a bladder tumour may cause clot retention, i.e. acute retention of urine due to clot obstruction. Tumours arising near a ureteric orifice in the bladder commonly cause unilateral ureteric obstruction resulting in hydronephrosis. Rarely, bilateral obstruction causes uraemia. Bladder tumours also predispose to infection. Therefore, recurrent unexplained urinary tract infections require investigation to exclude tumour. Tumour invasion near the bladder neck may cause incontinence but haematuria or infection usually precede these symptoms.

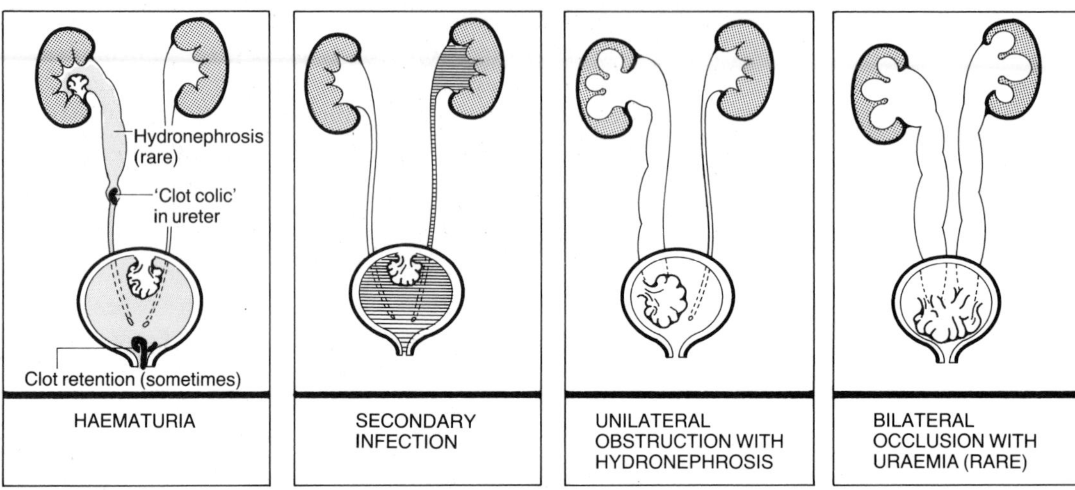

Fig. 22.6 Presenting features of urothelial tumours

Investigation of suspected transitional cell carcinoma

Confirmed haematuria in the absence of infection must be investigated. Intravenous urography outlines the upper tracts; a filling defect in the collecting system or ureter is suspicious of a urothelial tumour. A renal adenocarcinoma causing haematuria will usually be demonstrated by an IVU.

IVU is followed by cystoscopy, the only reliable method for examining the lining of the bladder and urethra. Cystoscopy may reveal blood emanating from one of the urethral orifices if there is an upper tract tumour. When bladder tumours are found at cystoscopy, diagnosis and initial therapy go hand in hand. Where possible, lesions are completely excised down to muscle using a *resectoscope*. The resected tissue is then sent for histological examination. This defines the degree of differentiation and the depth of tumour invasion into the bladder wall. Transitional cell lesions must be treated as malignant even if they look histologically benign.

Staging of transitional cell tumours

Staging of bladder tumours is achieved by a combination of palpation under anaesthetic and histology. For small and superficial lesions, histology will show the extent of bladder wall invasion and whether the tumour has been completely

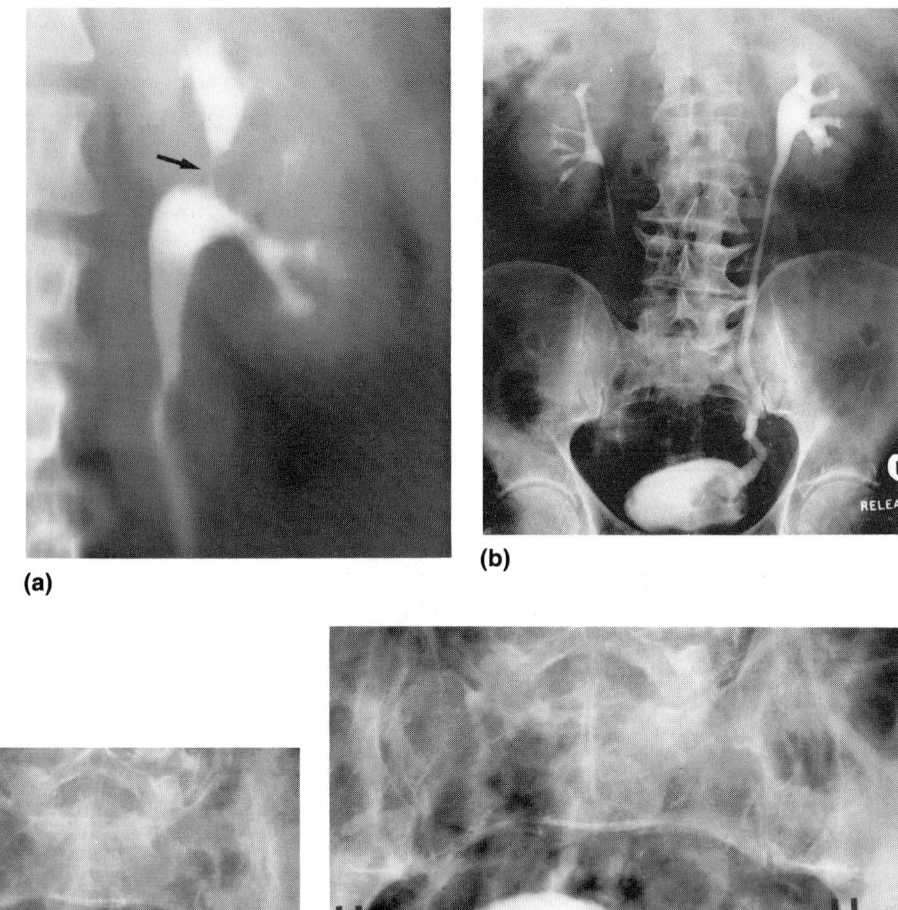

(a) (b)

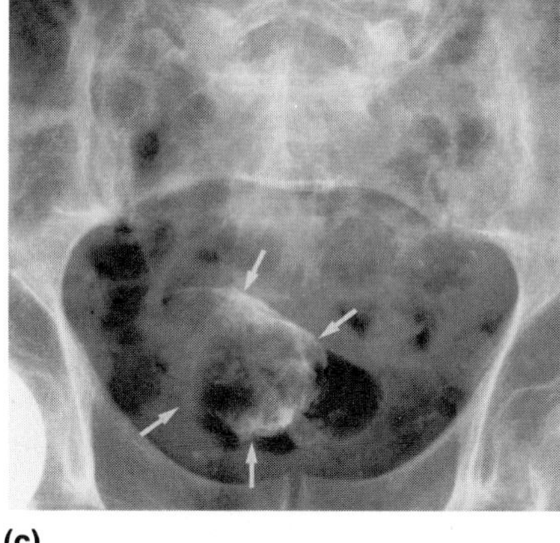

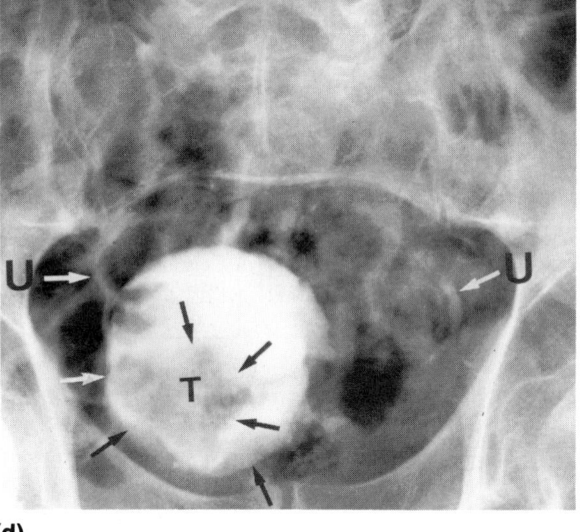

(c) (d)

Fig. 22.7 Urothelial tumours at different sites

(a) This woman of 64 presented with persistent microscopic haematuria; left renal tomogram during intravenous urography showing a stricture in the upper pelvicalyceal infundibulum (arrowed) caused by a urothelial tumour. **(b)** Intravenous urogram of a 67-year-old man complaining of loin pain and haematuria; on the left there is hydronephrosis and ureteric obstruction caused by a bladder tumour at the vesico-ureteric orifice. **(c)** Plain X-ray of the pelvis in an 84-year-old man with recurrent urinary tract infections; note the calcified lesion in the bladder (arrowed), typical of calcification on a large bladder tumour. In a woman, this appearance would more likely be due to a calcified uterine fibroid. **(d)** Intravenous urogram of the same patient showing a large filling defect due to the tumour **T** in the bladder (outline arrowed). Note also the position of the ureters **U** containing contrast

removed. For larger or deeper lesions, bimanual palpation of the bladder between a finger in the rectum and a hand on the anterior abdominal wall should be performed, before and after resection of the tumour. This gives an idea of the extent of bladder wall penetration and spread into the pelvis. Spread outside the bladder wall may be confirmed by CT scanning, which will demonstrate the extent and direction of spread.

The clinical system used in staging bladder tumours is illustrated in Figure 22.8 (the **'T'** system). In addition, some pathologists grade transitional cell tumours of the urinary tract in two ways: the **'P'** system classifies the extent of invasion on gross anatomical and histological grounds and the **'G'** system grades the lesion according to the degree of differentiation (G_1 = well differentiated, G_2 = moderately differentiated and G_3 = poorly differentiated or undifferentiated). Thus, a pathologist may report a transitional cell tumour as P_1G_1 or P_1G_3 or P_2G_3, and so on. Up to clinical stage T_2, the pathological system is more accurate than the clinical system.

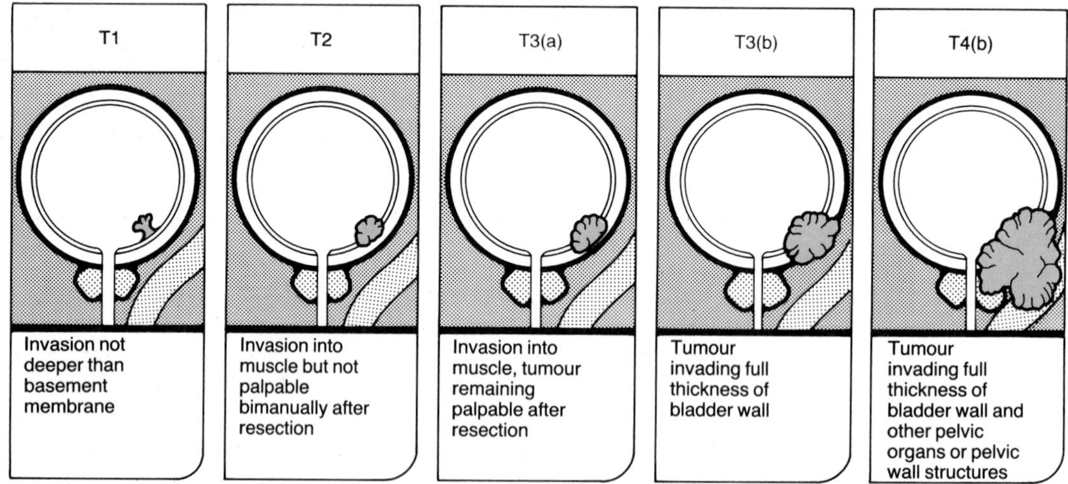

Fig. 22.8 System for staging bladder tumours. Note: stage T3(b) indicates tumour invasion of prostate gland

Management of transitional cell carcinomas

Bladder tumours

Transitional cell tumours of the bladder display a range of morphological types from small discrete, often multiple, frond-like lesions through to extensive papilliferous or flat tumours. The first type is usually still at an 'in situ' or very early invasive stage, and the tumours used to be known as papillomas before their malignant potential was fully realised. Initial management of bladder tumours is usually aimed at complete removal of tumour by *cystoscopic resection*, even with large lesions. Further management depends on the stage of tumour spread.

As shown in Figure 22.9, bladder tumours classified as T_1 can usually be completely resected. If the lesions are too numerous or widespread for resection, *topical chemotherapy* may be more effective. Cytotoxic drugs such as adriamycin are instilled in to the bladder. An alternative treatment is to cause

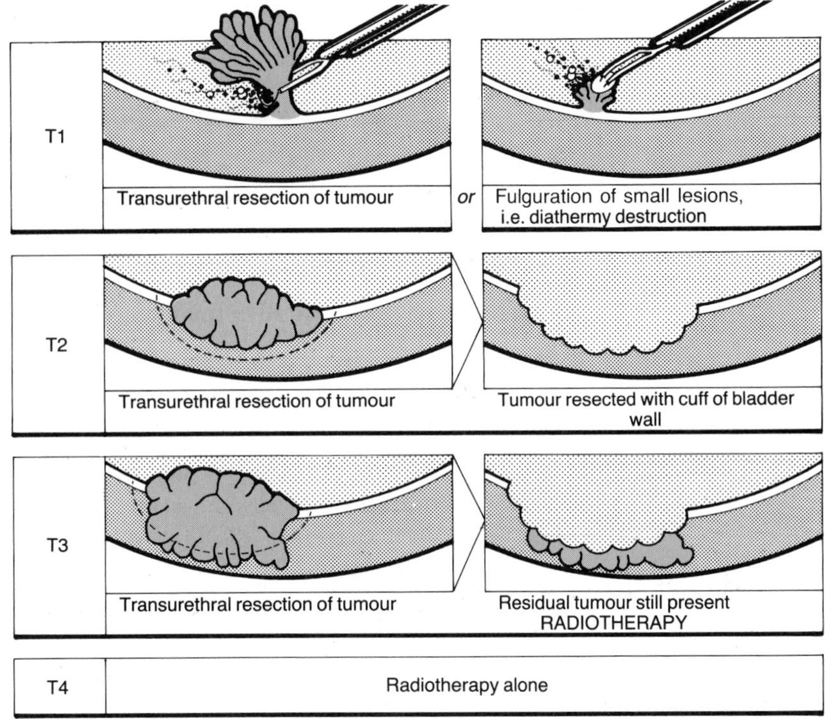

Fig. 22.9 Cystoscopic management of bladder tumours

pressure necrosis of the tumours; this is performed by inflating a *Helmstein balloon* in the bladder for several hours under regional anaesthesia.

Lesions defined as stage T_2 by histology have, by definition, been completely removed cystoscopically and no further treatment is required.

T_3 tumours have invaded too deeply for complete resection, given the risk of bladder perforation. Residual tumour (palpable after resection as a thickening in the bladder wall) is treated by radiotherapy.

T_4 tumours are usually incurable; even total cystectomy rarely eliminates the whole lesion. Radiotherapy offers palliation and is valuable in controlling pain and haematuria.

Transitional cell tumours of the upper tract

Transitional cell carcinomas of the pelvicalyceal system and ureter are uncommon. Treatment requires excision of the whole upper tract on the affected side. This includes the kidney, ureter and a cuff of bladder wall surrounding the distal ureter, to prevent recurrence of tumour.

Urethral tumours

Bladder tumours occasionally involve the urethra by direct spread. Very rarely a primary lesion may occur in the urethra; a urethral stricture may be a predisposing factor. Management is by cystoscopic excision. The surrounding penile vasculature allows early spread via the blood stream and thus the prognosis is poor.

Unusual tumours of the urinary tract

The rare squamous cell carcinomas of the urinary tract are diagnosed and treated along similar lines to transitional cell carcinomas. The exception is a distal urethral lesion which is managed in the same way as penile carcinoma (see Chapter 19). The extremely rare adenocarcinomas of the bladder can often be excised, since they arise solely in the urachal remnant.

Follow up and control of recurrent disease

Patients who have had curative treatment for urothelial tumours (i.e. bladder stages T_1 to T_3 and all upper tract lesions), must be followed up for life. The goal is to detect recurrence of the original tumour (the staging system is not completely reliable) or to diagnose new primary lesions at an early stage. The factors which induced the initial lesion make the remaining urothelium liable to undergo malignant change. It is not always easy to distinguish between small recurrences and new primaries; all of them tend to be called 'recurrences'.

Follow up involves regular 'check' cystoscopies. Initially, these are performed at 3-month intervals, and the interval gradually extended to once a year if no further tumour is discovered. After several years free of tumour, cystoscopy may be replaced by annual urine cytology. This method may also be used for screening individuals with a high occupational risk.

Recurrent lesions are managed in the same way as the first lesion, i.e. according to the stage of bladder wall invasion. The exception is when the initial management involved radiotherapy. For these patients, cure is improbable and palliative surgery (ranging from diathermy to total cystectomy) may be necessary to treat intractable problems such as severe haemorrhage.

23 STONE DISEASE OF THE URINARY TRACT

Introduction

Stone disease, second only to prostatic disease, accounts for a major part of the urological workload. Stones occur in all parts of the urinary tract, including the pelvicalyceal system of the kidney, the ureters and the bladder. Stones most commonly cause symptoms by obstruction or by predisposing to urinary tract infections.

The pattern of stone disease has changed remarkably over the last century. Bladder stones were once extremely common, particularly in children, and were one of the few conditions successfully treated by surgery before the advent of anaesthesia and antisepsis. 'Cutting for stone', or *lithotomy* (lithos = stone), was often performed by itinerant surgeons. They used a perineal approach to the bladder, placing the patient in the manner still described as the *lithotomy position*. A bladder sound (i.e. a curved bougie) was placed in the bladder to find the location of the stone. Meanwhile, fascinated onlookers held down the wretched patient for the surgeon's theatrical ministrations. The operation was often completed in seconds!

Nowadays, upper tract calculi are much more common than bladder calculi and the incidence is rising. The stones range from the uncommon *staghorn calculi* which fill the pelvicalyceal system, to small stones which may enter and obstruct the ureter. Acute ureteric obstruction causes severe pain and presents as the surgical emergency *ureteric colic*. Most stone disease is, however, asymptomatic or else presents non-urgently to the outpatient clinic.

In developed countries stone disease is now rare in childhood. As shown in Figure 23.1, stone disease has a peak incidence in early adulthood, and declines slowly thereafter. Males are affected two and a half times as often as females.

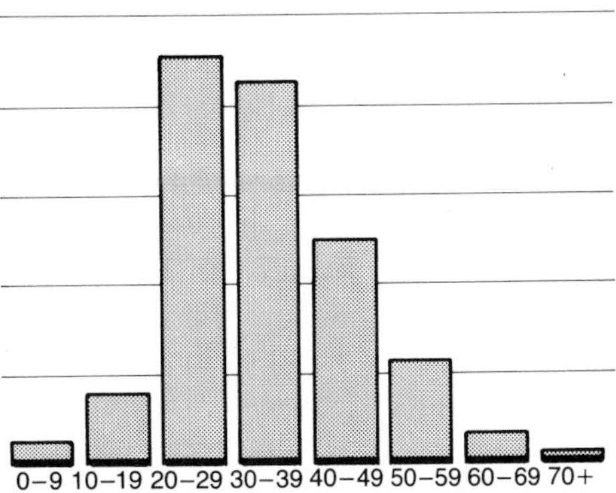

Fig. 23.1 Relative incidence of stone disease by age in developed countries

Right and left upper tracts are equally affected. There is a high incidence of recurrent stones.

PATHO-PHYSIOLOGY OF STONE DISEASE

Chemical composition

Urinary calculi consist of crystalline compounds with a small proportion of matrix similar to ground substance. One constituent often predominates but sometimes there is a mixture of constituents. In other cases, the central nucleus of the stone and the surrounding bulk of the stone may each be composed of different constituents. Thus, it is often difficult to reconcile the chemical classifications used in different analytical studies. Figure 23.2 provides a simple chemical classification showing the relative frequency of the different types of stone, as well as their important clinical characteristics and aetiology. Calcium is present in at least 70% of stones, either as oxalate or phosphate compounds, or both.

Mechanisms of stone formation

In a minority of patients with stones, there is a definable underlying disorder causing excessive urinary excretion of the major constituent of the stone. Examples include *hyperparathyroidism*, *hyperoxaluria*, *gout*, *cysteinuria* and *xanthinuria*. In a further minority of cases, there is a specific predisposing factor such as chronic infection. Urea-splitting bacteria, e.g. Proteus, predispose to magnesium-ammonium-phosphate stones.

In the majority of cases (in which the stones contain calcium), no specific cause is evident. Some of these patients excrete excessive calcium (*idiopathic hypercalciuria*) without being hypercalcaemic. In such people, there is possibly increased absorption of calcium from the gut and increased excretion in the urine. Experimental evidence suggests that some of the remaining patients are deficient in a factor which normally prevents stone formation.

In other patients there may be obvious or occult *urinary stasis* in the upper tract (e.g. hydronephrosis or horseshoe kidney) or in the lower tract (e.g. prostatic hypertrophy or neurogenic bladder). Stasis becomes a particularly important predisposing factor when associated with recurrent or chronic infection. Finally, *diseased tissue* such as necrotic papillae (occurring in diabetes or analgesic nephropathy) may calcify. If sloughed off into the renal pelvis, this calcified tissue can act as a nidus for calculus formation. Similarly, *foreign bodies* in the bladder act as foci for calcification. These may be inserted by the patient, e.g. ball point pens or hair clips, or be accidentally left behind after instrumentation or surgery (e.g. sutures, catheter fragments). *Schistosome ova* are responsible for bladder stones in some undeveloped countries.

Idiopathic stone disease is probably not caused by a single factor but by *interaction of several factors*. The following examples illustrate some of these factors. Bladder stones composed of urate were once common in boys in England and are still common in some parts of Africa, Turkey and India. They are believed to be due to the combined effects of protein, vitamin A and trace element deficiency, dehydration and gastroenteritis. All these factors lead to a small volume of concentrated acid urine, which encourages uric acid to precipitate. Another factor is *prolonged immobilisation*, e.g with multiple frac-

Fig. 23.2 Chemical composition, clinical features and aetiology of urinary tract stones

CHEMICAL COMPOSITION	%	CLINICAL FEATURES	AETIOLOGY
Calcium oxalate	40	3 types of stone are described : — small smooth 'hempseed' stones — small irregular 'mulberry' stones — small spiculate 'jack' stones	Most cases are idiopathic; predisposing factors include urinary stasis, infection and foreign bodies. Some are due to metabolic disorders: —hyperparathyroidism causing hypercalcaemia rather than hypercalciuria —hyperoxaluria (rare inherited disorder)
Mixed calcium oxalate and phosphate stones	15	as above	Some are due to disorders associated with hypercalcaemia, e.g. sarcoidosis, multiple metastases, multiple myeloma, milk–alkali syndrome, overtreatment with vitamin D
Calcium and phosphate (hydroxyapatite)	15	as above	Some patients excrete abnormally large amounts of calcium (idiopathic hypercalciuria, but without hypercalcaemia)
Magnesium ammonium phosphate	15	Typical of large 'staghorn' calculi of pelvicalyceal system & some bladder stones	Caused by chronic infection by organisms capable of producing urease. This enzyme splits urea, forming ammonia if the urine is alkaline
Uric acid	8	Stones tend to absorb yellow and brown pigments. Pure stones are radiolucent	Occur in primary gout, and hyperuricaemia following chemotherapy for leukaemias and myeloproliferative disorders. Childhood urate bladder stones occur in some underdeveloped countries when urine pH is low
Cystine or xanthine	2	Excess urinary excretion of cystine or xanthine. Pure stones are radiolucent	Autosomal recessive inherited disorders

tures or paraplegia, which causes generalised skeletal decalcification and increased calcium excretion. If there is also poor fluid throughput and incomplete bladder emptying, stone formation is likely.

The clinical problem of urinary stones should not be confused with calcification of the renal parenchyma which is a feature of tuberculosis and medullary sponge kidney. These and similar diseases can usually be diagnosed by their characteristic X-ray appearance.

Fig. 23.3 Predisposing factors in stone formation

Idiopathic (most common)

Stasis of urine, e.g congenital abnormalities, chronic obstruction

Chronic urinary infection (urea-splitting organisms, e.g. Proteus, cause alkaline urine and the development of magnesium-ammonium-phosphate stones, typically the 'staghorn' calculi of the renal pelvis).

Excess urinary excretion of stone-forming substances, e.g. idiopathic hypercalciuria (calcium stones), hyperparathyroidism (calcium stones), hyperoxaluria (oxalate stones), gout (uric acid stones), cysteinuria (cysteine stones), xanthinuria (xanthine stones)

Foreign bodies, e.g. fragments of catheter tubing, self-inserted artefacts, parasites (schistosome ova)

Diseased tissue, e.g. renal papillary necrosis

Multifactorial, e.g. prolonged immobility, children in the third world

CLINICAL FEATURES OF STONE DISEASE

Urinary tract stones produce their deleterious effects in three main ways:

- By obstructing urinary flow
- By predisposing to infection
- By causing local tissue damage

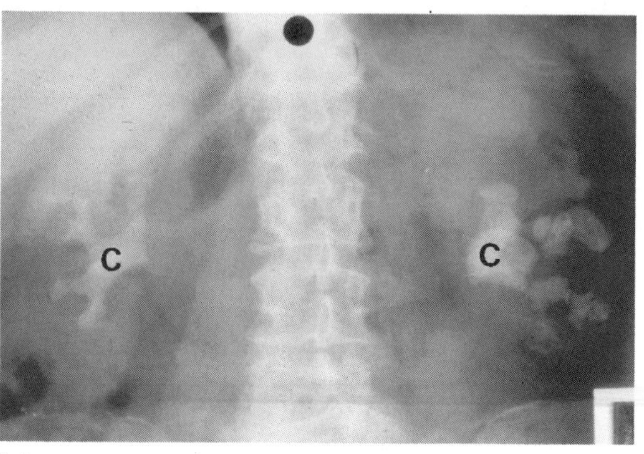

(a)

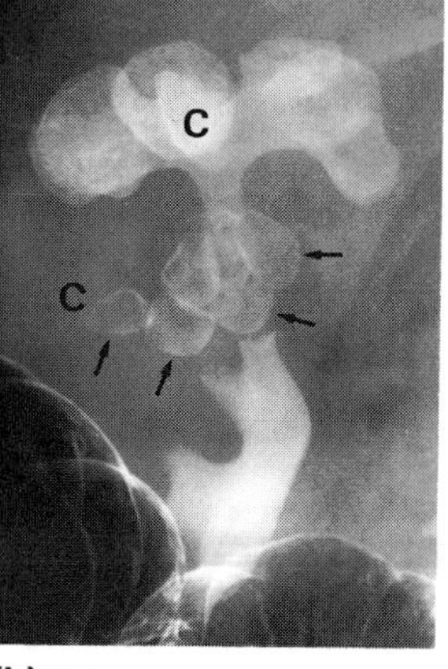

(b)

Fig. 23.4 Staghorn calculi

Plain abdominal X-rays showing
(a) Asymptomatic bilateral 'staghorn' calculi **C** found incidentally in a 61-year-old woman.
(b) Huge 'staghorn' calculus **C** in upper and middle parts of the right kidney; an incidental finding in a 69-year-old woman during barium enema; note also the multiple radio-opaque facetted gallstones (arrowed), also asymptomatic!

The nature of the problem depends on the size, morphology and site of the stone. Many stones cause no problems at all but represent a potential problem. Other stones produce marked pathological effects which may present acutely, chronically or not at all.

Pelvicalyceal obstruction

Obstruction of a calyx or calyces causes local urinary obstruction (*hydrocalyx*), typically causing chronic or recurrent loin pain. Similar pain may also be caused by chronic, incomplete obstruction of the pelviureteric junction (PUJ) or ureter. The result is *hydronephrosis*. More severe obstruction may cause progressive renal parenchymal damage and diminished renal function; if both kidneys are affected, the patient may develop renal failure.

Passage of stones into the ureter

If small renal stones pass into the ureter, there are several possible outcomes:

- Stones may pass to the bladder and exit via the urethra causing minor symptoms. The patient may pass 'gravel', for example, and experience dysuria and sometimes haematuria
- Stones may pass to the bladder and there act as a nidus for a large bladder stone. Bladder stones occasionally cause outlet obstruction and urinary retention
- A stone may impact in the ureter, causing chronic partial obstruction and eventually hydroureter. This typically presents as loin pain but, suprisingly, may be asymptomatic

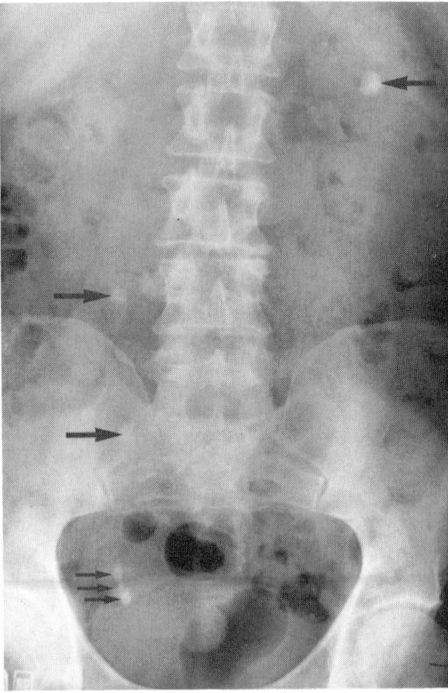

(a)

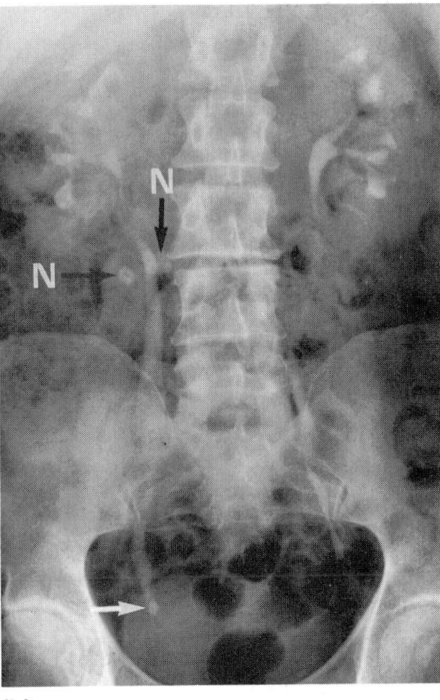

(b)

Fig. 23.5 Recurrent urinary tract stones

This man aged 40 had a two-year history of passing small stones and 'gravel' in the urine. **(a)** Plain abdominal X-ray showing what appear to be several stones (arrowed) in the right ureter and a further stone (arrowed) in the upper pole of the left kidney. **(b)** IVU of the same patient showing partial obstruction at the lower end of the right ureter (arrowed); note that two of the radiopaque objects on the right side lie outside the area of contrast and thus probably represent calcified mesenteric lymph nodes **N**; metabolic studies showed that this patient has idiopathic hypercalciuria

- A stone may impact in the ureter, causing sudden complete obstruction. The patient experiences extremely severe, unilateral colicky pain (*ureteric colic*) often with loin tenderness

Predisposition to infection

Urinary tract stones predispose to infection by causing urinary stasis, by preventing proper 'flushing' of the tract, and by providing a niche for bacterial multiplication. Pelvicalyceal or ureteric stones may cause acute pyelitis or pyelonephritis and occasionally perinephric abscess. Bladder stones predispose to cystitis and ascending infections.

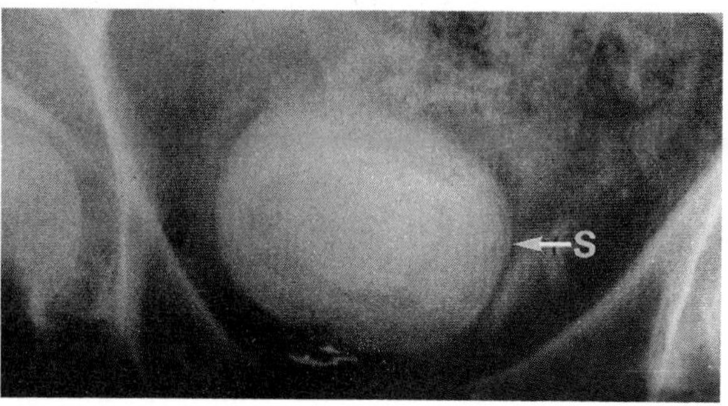

Fig. 23.6 Bladder stone

Massive bladder stone **S** in an 85-year-old man with benign prostatic hypertrophy and recurrent urinary tract infections; such stones are rare nowadays

Local irritation

Stones may also present because of their irritant effects on local tissues. Simple inflammation may cause bleeding and thus present as *haematuria*. Chronic inflammation may lead to fibrosis; if this occurs at a narrow part of the tract, typically the PUJ or ureter, a *stricture* may form. Prolonged irritation of the bladder mucosa by stone may cause *squamous metaplasia* and eventually *squamous carcinoma*.

Fig. 23.7 Summary: presentations of stones in the urinary tract

Incidental finding on X-ray
Loin pain
Ureteric colic
Passage of small stones in the urine
Cystitis
Pyelonephritis
Haematuria
Impaired renal function

When investigating a patient with urinary tract stones, the objectives are:

- To confirm a stone is present
- To locate the stone or stones
- To evaluate any deleterious effects of the stone(s) on renal function and urinary tract morphology
- To identify any structural disorders of the urinary tract acting as local predisposing factors
- To identify any metabolic predisposing factors

Methods of investigation

In general, the above objectives will be met by performing the following investigations. For convenience, they are conducted concurrently:

- Urine microscopy, culture and sensitivity
- Tests of renal function, i.e. plasma urea, electrolyte and creatinine estimation
- Plain abdominal X-ray ('KUB') — 90% of stones are radiopaque
- IVU — shows the effects of stone obstruction (see Figure 23.8)
- Renal ultrasound — to demonstrate hydronephrosis (rarely stones themselves)
- Special contrast techniques — occasionally required e.g. percutaneous (antegrade) pyelography
- Biochemical analysis of any recovered stones
- Tests for metabolic disorders (for recurrent stones), i.e. serum calcium, phosphate, uric acid and alkaline phosphatase; 24-hour urinary excretion of calcium, uric acid and cysteine

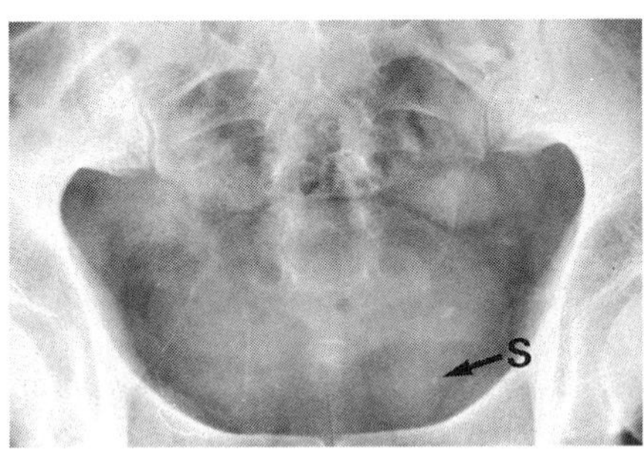

(a)

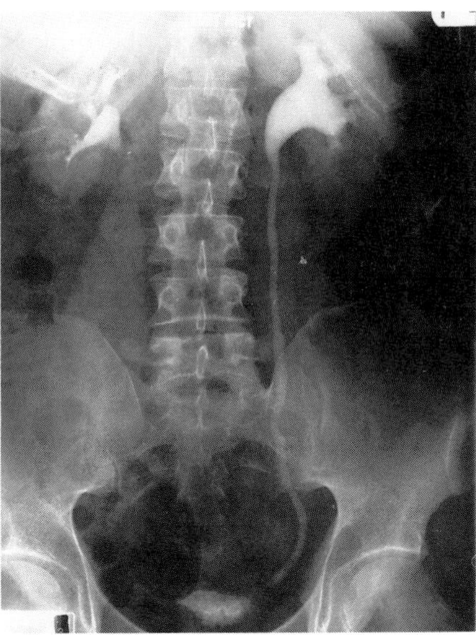
(b)

Fig. 23.8 Emergency IVU in ureteric colic

This 37-year-old man presented with left ureteric colic. **(a)** 'Control' film showing small radiopacity **S**, probably a stone, in the area of the left vesico-ureteric junction. **(b)** IVU showing dilated left pelvicalyceal system and contrast-filled ureter down to the area of the stone. This confirms an obstruction at the vesico-ureteric junction

Indications for stone removal

The finding of a urinary tract stone is not an automatic indication for its removal. The indications for stone removal are summarised in Figure 23.9. Small stones in the pelvicalyceal system often remain unchanged and asymptomatic for many years and can safely be observed by annual radiography. Stones of 0.5 cm or less in diameter often pass right through the tract, although in doing so, they may produce severe but short-lived symptoms like ureteric colic, dysuria or haematuria.

Fig. 23.9 Indications for removal of urinary tract stones

Obstruction of urinary flow
Infection
Persistent or recurrent pain
Stones likely to cause future obstruction or infection
Small 'metabolic' stones likely to grow rapidly in size

Methods of stone removal

Stones can be removed by cystoscopic methods, open surgery or a variety of recently introduced percutaneous and less invasive techniques. The choice of technique depends on the size, nature and site of the stone, the availability of expertise and special equipment, and whether there is a need to correct congenital or acquired structural abnormalities.

a. Cystoscopic techniques

Cystoscopic methods are suitable for most bladder stones and for impacted stones in the lower third of the ureter (see Figure 23.10). Bladder stones can be broken into small framents (*litholapaxy*) using a *lithotrite*, a modification of the cystoscope, incorporating stone-crushing jaws. The fragments are then washed out by irrigation.

A *Dormia basket* is used to remove low ureteric stones which are less than 0.5 cm in diameter. This involves passing a special catheter into the ureter under cystoscopic vision; the catheter used has a mechanism for capturing the stone (see Figure 23.10). This method does not always succeed, so the patient must be prepared for open surgery to follow immediately, should the attempt fail. Recently, a new instrument called a *ureteroscope* has been developed for passing into the ureter. The ureteric orifice is first dilated cystoscopically and then the slender rigid ureteroscope is passed. It can be used to help capture difficult stones with a Dormia basket or used to apply destructive ultrasonic or electro-hydraulic probes.

b. Open surgical methods

Open surgery was often required for removing stones in the pelvicalyceal system (*pyelolithotomy*), ureter (*ureterolithotomy*), and for certain bladder stones (*cysto-lithotomy*). Many of these applications have been superceded by endoscopic and percutaneous techniques, described below.

Ureterolithotomy is used when Dormia basket extraction is not indicated or has been unsuccessful. Surgery is indicated if there is also an anatomical abnormality which predisposes to stone formation. Examples are bladder diverticula, pelviureteric junction obstruction or ureteric stricture.

c. Percutaneous techniques

Direct access to the renal pelvis can be obtained percutaneously under radiological or ultrasound control. This allows creation of a track from the loin into

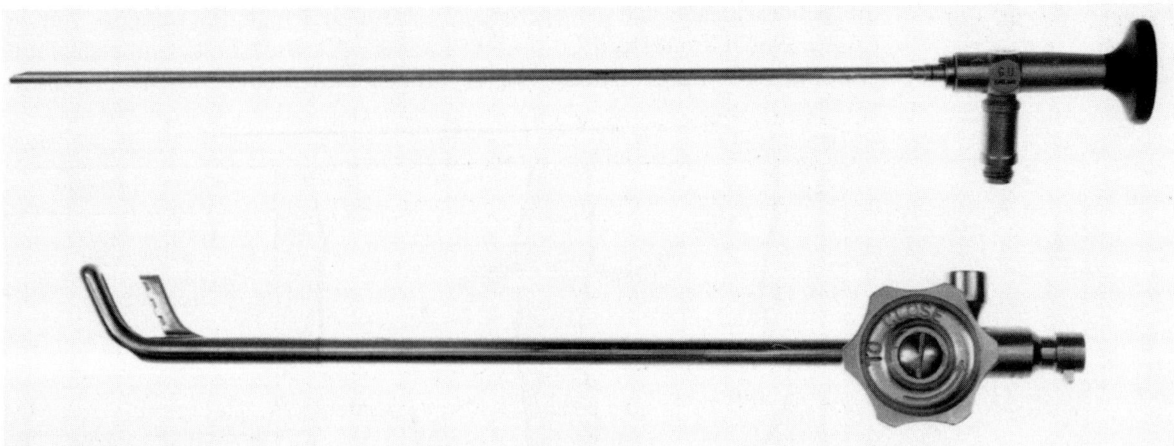

(ai)

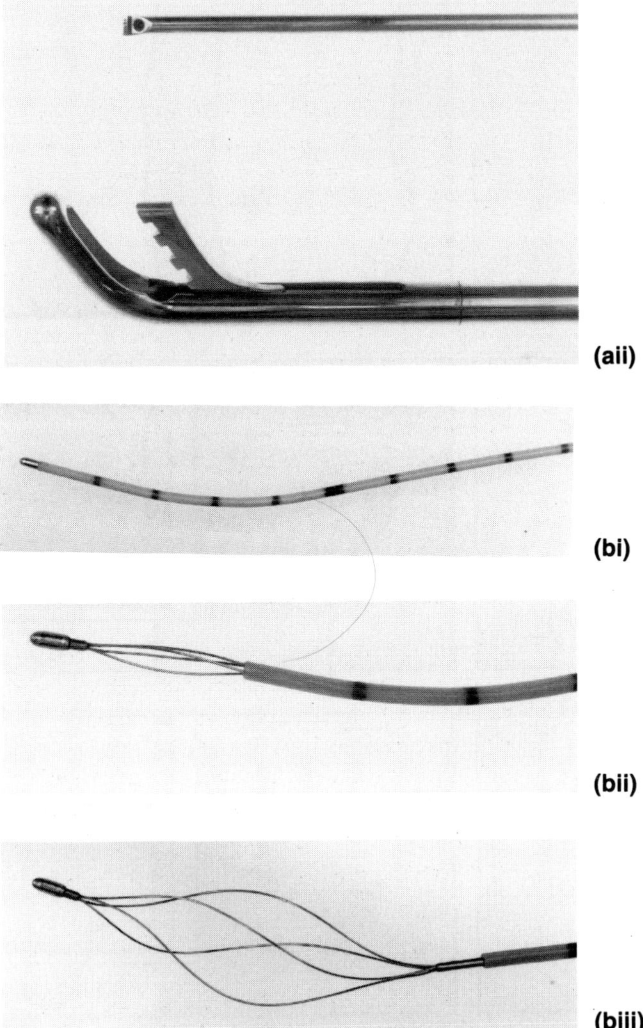

(aii)

(bi)

(bii)

(biii)

Fig. 23.10 Instruments for urinary stone removal

(a) Lithotrite. The telescope fits through the centre of the lithotrite, allowing direct vision as stones are crushed between the jaws. Note: the jaws are closed before passing the instrument into the bladder via the urethra. **(b)** Dormia basket. The upper photograph shows the instrument fully closed, in which state it is passed through the cystoscope and into the ureter. Note the centimetre markings on the sheath. The basket is advanced beyond the stone and then opened by pushing the centre wire from the proximal end. The middle photograph shows the instrument partially open and the lower photograph shows it fully open. When open, the whole instrument is gradually withdrawn until the stone lodges within the wire basket. The centre wire is then drawn back until the stone is firmly held within the basket and the whole instrument withdrawn complete with stone

the pelvicalyceal system (*nephrostomy*), through which instruments can be passed. Small stones can be retrieved using a Dormia basket or a steerable grasping tool. Larger stones can be broken into fragments with electrohy-

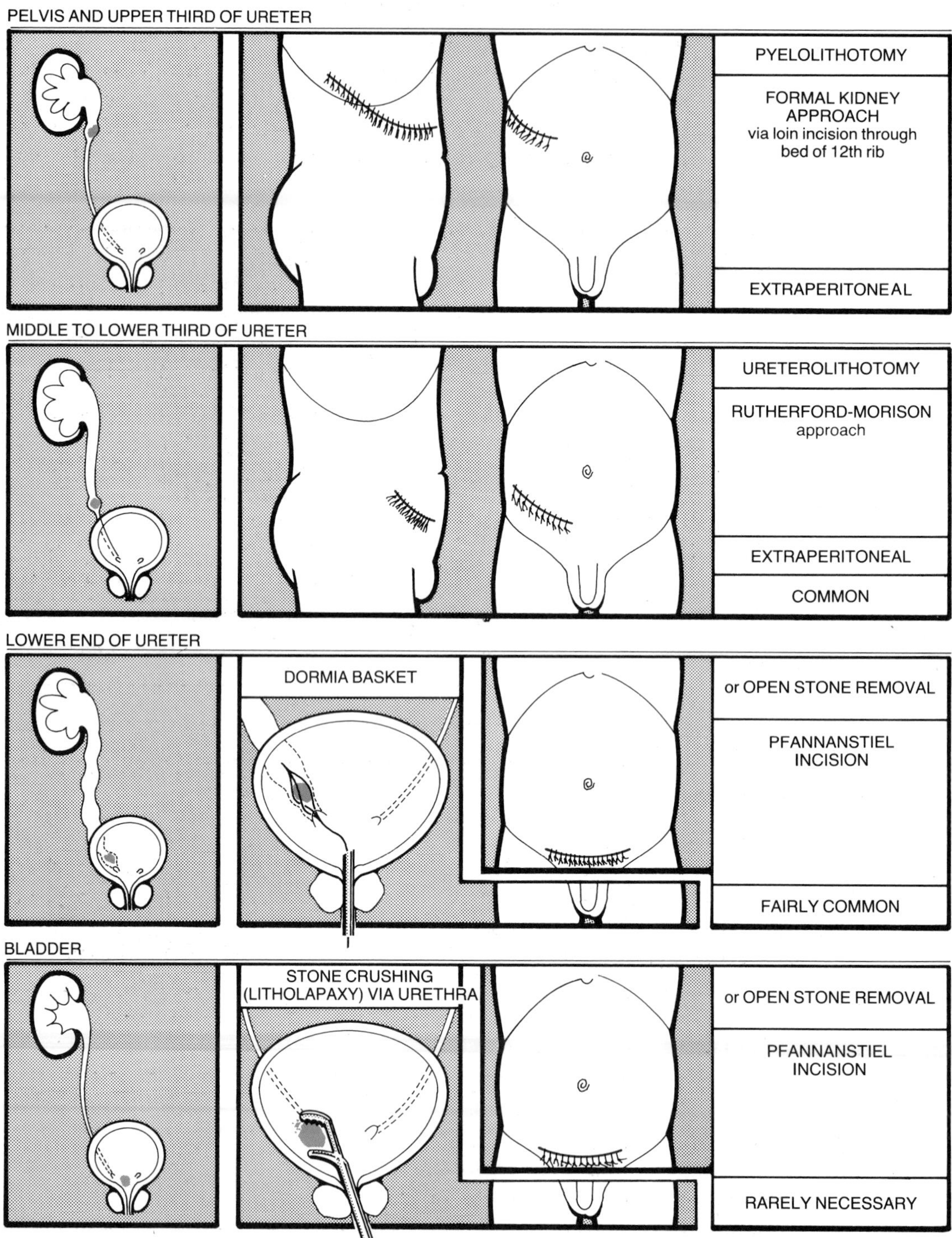

Fig. 23.11 Conventional surgical approaches for removal of urinary tract stones

draulic probes, after which the fragments can be lifted out with special instruments. Afterwards, the nephrostomy track closes spontaneously.

d. Non-invasive stone removal technique

Recently, a non-invasive method of stone destruction has been devised using external application of a shock wave. This is known as *lithotripsy*. The patient's trunk is immersed in a bath of water, and a series of shock waves (500–2000 shocks) are then focussed radiologically. The method requires general anaesthesia and extremely expensive equipment, and its availability is limited.

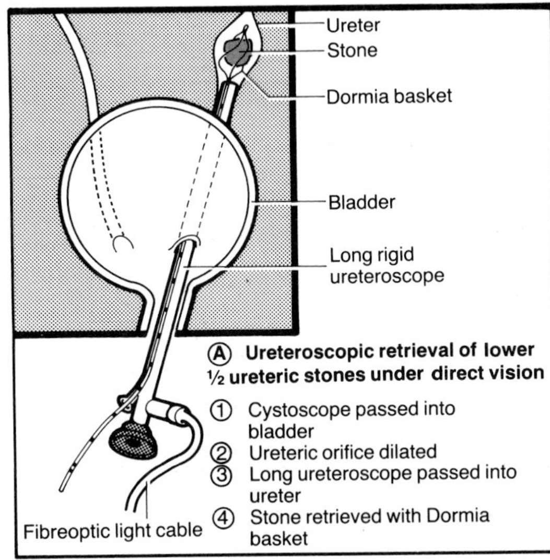

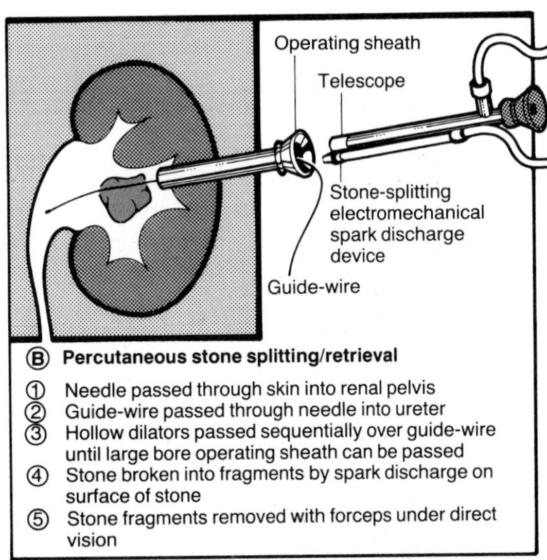

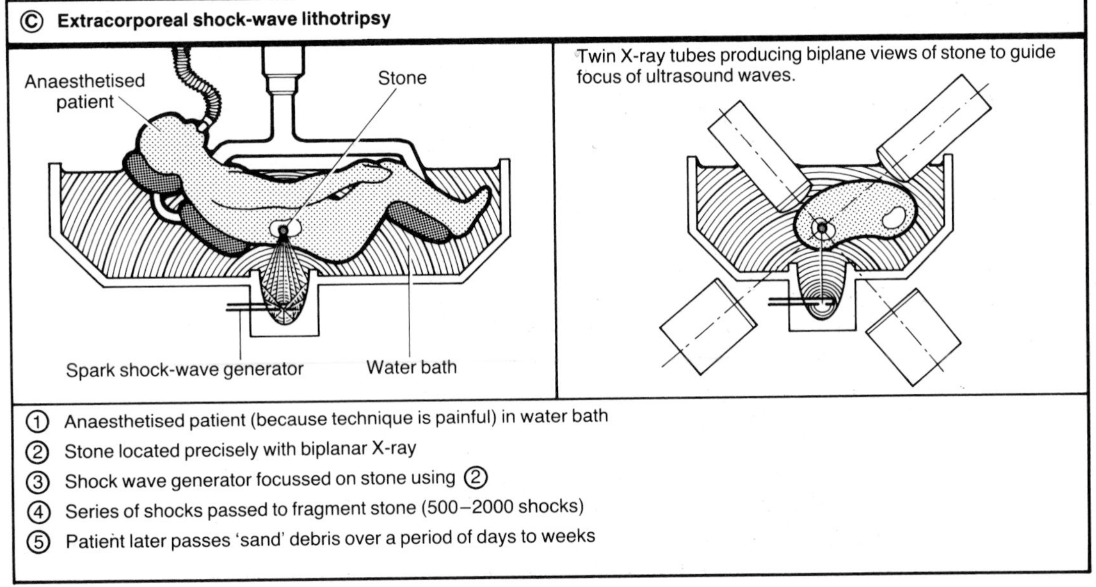

Fig. 23.12 Modern methods of urinary tract stone removal

Management of acute ureteric colic

Ureteric colic occurs when a stone causes sudden obstruction of the ureter. It typically presents with a sudden onset of severe unilateral colicky pain radiating from the loin to the groin or tip of the penis. The pain is due to waves of ureteric peristalsis and episodes may last from several minutes to half an hour. At the peak of the pain, the patient writhes in agony. Indeed, the pain of ureteric colic can be so severe and incapacitating that flying officers known to have stones are grounded until the stones are removed. Most patients are seen urgently by their general practitioner or brought straight to the accident and emergency department. Intramuscular opiate analgesia is given as soon as possible to settle the pain. The patient may be pain free when first seen by the surgical staff, but the pain history is usually diagnostic. Occasionally, ureteric colic is not as severe but is more persistent. Then, it may simulate other acute abdominal conditions.

Investigation of ureteric colic

Ureteric colic almost always causes *microscopic haematuria*, and the first investigation is 'dipstick' testing of the urine for blood. A positive result reinforces the diagnosis. An IVU should then be performed urgently to confirm or refute the diagnosis (see Figure 23.8 earlier).

The characteristic radiological features of acute ureteric obstruction are:

- *Delay* at all phases of the passage of contrast through the kidney and collecting system on the affected side; the more severe the obstruction, the longer the delay. If there appears to be no excretion, further X-rays are taken every few hours for about 24 hours; contrast will usually eventually pass into the system, demonstrating the site of obstruction
- *Dilatation* of the collecting system above the point of obstruction

Treatment of ureteric colic

Most patients with ureteric colic require strong analgesics initially. These are usually opiates given by injection or non-steroidal anti-inflammatory drugs by suppository. Many patients settle on a single dose but two or three doses may be required. In most cases, the stone gradually passes down the ureter and into the bladder. Each stage of movement is accompanied by an attack of colic. All specimens of urine should be filtered so that any stones passed can be seen and preserved for analysis. If there is complete obstruction of the ureter, or there is infection above an obstructing stone, urgent surgery may have to be performed. In other cases, where pain persists, plain abdominal X-rays will usually record any change in position of the stone. If the stone is very large, it may have to be surgically removed. If the stone appears to be small enough to pass spontaneously, yet fails to progress, the patient can safely be allowed home if the criteria for urgent surgery mentioned above are not fulfilled. The IVU can be repeated after a week or two and a decision taken about the need for operation at that time.

Management of metabolic abnormalities

Hyperparathyroidism is the only stone-forming metabolic abnormality which can be corrected by surgical treatment. Other metabolic causes of urolithiasis may be amenable to dietary modification or drug therapy. For example, dietary calcium should be reduced in idiopathic hypercalciuria; tea, coffee, chocolate, strawberries and rhubarb should be avoided in hyperoxaluria.

The drug *allopurinol* may be given for hyperuricaemia (gout) and is routinely given during chemotherapy for leukaemia. Allopurinol inhibits xanthine oxidase, an enzyme involved in synthesis of uric acid.

Long-term follow up of patients with urinary tract stones

For many patients, a urinary tract stone is a single phenomenon with no apparent predisposing cause. Long-term follow up for these patients is not usually required. Patients with stones that do not need removing, or with recurrent stones, require long-term follow up with regular plain abdominal X-rays. Any patients with stone disease should probably be advised to increase fluid intake, although the value of this is disputed.

Patients with metabolic or anatomical abnormalities which predispose to stone formation also need long-term follow up.

24 URINARY TRACT INFECTIONS

Introduction

Urinary tract infections are a common problem in surgery. They may be responsible for abdominal pain or urinary tract symptoms which present for diagnosis. More often, urinary tract infection is a secondary problem. It may occur postoperatively, particularly if a urinary catheter has been used, or it may complicate surgical disorders of the urinary tract such as tumours or stones. Infections are usually caused by common bacteria of faecal origin.

Urinary tract infections may also be caused by special organisms, in particular *Mycobacterium tuberculosis*. Urinary tract infection with the tubercle bacillus, in it early stages, may produce the same symptoms and signs as ordinary bacterial infection. Tuberculosis is easily overlooked unless specifically sought.

On a world-wide basis, other organisms are more important causes of urinary tract infection, most notably the nematode *Schistosoma*. This causes severe bladder disease in underdeveloped countries.

Infections of the urethra are usually transmitted by sexual intercourse. Gonococcus and Chlamydia are the organisms most commonly involved. A late result of gonorrhoea in males is fibrous urethral stricture.

The most common cause of urethral stricture is trauma. This may follow prolonged catheterisation, instrumentation of the urethra or pelvic fractures with urethral involvement.

COMMON BACTERIAL INFECTIONS OF THE LOWER URINARY TRACT

Pathophysiology

The common infections of the urinary tract, i.e. those caused by faecal organisms, involve either the bladder or the upper tract (kidney, pelvicalyceal system and ureter) or both together.

The bladder is infected most often, with females being particularly susceptible; probably half of all females are affected at one time or another. Infection rate rises with pregnancy, multiparity and especially increasing age. In females, the infecting organisms probably enter via the urethra which is only 3 cm long. Organisms easily spread from the perineal skin, particularly during sexual intercourse.

Normally, the bladder is flushed clean by the frequent passage of newly produced urine, preventing the multiplication of bacteria in the urinary tract. Stasis of urine for any reason, such as incomplete bladder emptying, dehydration or immobility, interferes with this mechanism and predisposes to infection. Urethral instrumentation greatly predisposes to infection in either sex.

Faecal bacteria may also reach the urinary tract from the bloodstream. This may explain why infections develop without an obvious urethral source in immobilised or constipated elderly patients.

Clinical features

Typical symptoms of bladder infection are *dysuria*, *frequency*, *urgency* and a sensation of *incomplete bladder emptying*. The term 'cystitis' is often used by patients to mean symptoms from this list; however, infection is not always the cause of symptoms and, to prevent confusion, the term is probably best avoided. Even when infection is present, the symptoms may be trivial or absent, and this may make diagnosis difficult. Abdominal pain may be the only symptom; consequently, patients with abdominal pain should have their urine tested routinely.

In the elderly or the very young, there are often no localising symptoms, and the patient is just non-specifically unwell. In any ill patient in these age groups, the urine must be examined. A sudden onset of enuresis or urinary incontinence should also suggest bladder infection in children and the elderly.

Fig. 24.1 Presentations of bladder infection

Dysuria with frequency and urgency of micturition (very common)

Lower abdominal pain (common — usually children or young adults)

Unexpected development of incontinence (common in the elderly)

Development of enuresis in a previously 'dry' child

Non-specific ill-health in previously well infants or the elderly (including PUO and septicaemia)

Bacteriological diagnosis

Urinary tract infection is confirmed by examining a 'mid-stream' specimen of urine (MSU). The specimen is centrifuged and the unstained sediment is then examined microscopically for white blood cells ('pus cells') and bacteria. The specimen is also cultured to identify the causative organism and determine antibiotic sensitivity. Bacterial contamination of urine specimens is common; a 'significant' infection is therefore defined as one in which pus cells are abundant and there are more than 100 000 organisms per ml of urine. Coliform organisms are almost always responsible, the usual culprits being *E. coli*, *Proteus spp.*, *Strep. faecalis* and *Pseudomonas* (particularly in debilitated and catheterised patients).

Significant numbers of pus cells in the urine without bacterial growth most commonly results from patients taking antibiotics. If this is not the case, a stone or tuberculosis must be suspected and investigated. Infection often causes frank or occult haematuria; this only warrants further investigation if it persists after the infection is treated.

Some female patients experience typical symptoms of urinary infection, but no evidence of bacterial infection is found despite multiple laboratory exam-

Fig. 24.2 Typical MSU report of urinary tract infection

Date of onset 4 days
Antibiotics Current } nil
Intended
Clinical Details
burning dysuria
frequency

Signed

PATIENT STATUS
Please tick box
NHS (circled)
PP
OSV
CAT 2
Consultant/G.P.

Surname | Hospital No.
Forenames | Date of Birth 18. 6. 28
Ward/ Address

USE BALLPEN FIRMLY

MICROSCOPY

Pus Cells > 50 /hpf	Gr. Pos. Cocci		Gr. Pos. Rods		T. Vaginalis
Red Cells > 100 /hpf	Gr. Neg. Rods		Gr. Neg. Cocci		
Epithelial Cells ±	Yeasts		Vincents		
Casts —	1. > 10⁵ orgs/ml Enterococci				
Crystals —	2.				
Bacteria ++	3.				
Glucose — G%					
Protein ++ mg%					

	1 AMP/AMOX	2 CEPHALEXIN	3 SULPHONAMIDE	4 NITROFURANTOIN	5 NALIDIXIC ACID	6 COTRIM/TRIMETH	7 TETRACYCLINE	8 ERYTHROMYCIN	9 PENICILLIN	10 FLUCLOX	11 FUCIDIN	12 NEOMYCIN	13 METRONIDAZOLE	14 GENTAMICIN	15 CEFOTAXIME	16	17	18
1.	S		R	S		R												
2.																		
3.																		

S — Sensitive R — Resistant
M — Intermediate

Phoned:

Specimen Request MSU C & S | Date taken | Received | Lab. No. | Reported | BACT.

inations of urine. Non-specific urethral inflammation from the trauma of intercourse may be responsible; this is probably the cause of 'honeymoon cystitis'.

Management of bladder infections

Antibiotic therapy is the principal treatment for bladder infection, initially chosen on a 'best guess' basis. Ideally, an MSU specimen should be collected for microscopy, culture and sensitivities ('M, C & S') before therapy is commenced. If the initial antibiotic choice is inappropriate or unsuccessful, then the results of urine culture may suggest a more suitable alternative. An MSU should be repeated about six weeks after treatment, even if the infection appears to clear quickly. If there is doubt whether the infection has been eliminated, the MSU should be repeated several days after completion of the course of antibiotics.

Patients who have had urinary tract infections should be encouraged to increase their fluid intake. Indeed, this is often effective in dealing with early or mild symptoms and will probably cause many infections to resolve without drugs. Potassium citrate mixture may be given to diminish urinary acidity and relieve dysuria.

In pregnancy, where there is a great risk of infection ascending into the upper tracts, the urine should be tested routinely; any evidence of significant bacterial growth requires antibiotic treatment, whether or not the patient is symptomatic.

Recurrent bladder infections

Patients who suffer recurrent infections tend to fall into three groups as follows. Those in the first two groups can usually be managed without surgery.

a. The elderly, debilitated and infirm

These patients often have a multiplicity of simple predisposing factors such as constipation, incontinence, an indwelling catheter, poor fluid intake and diminished resistance. Correction of these and good nursing care (e.g. regular changes of indwelling catheter and bladder irrigation) may break the pattern.

b. Young and middle-aged women

Many of these patients can be helped by simple hygiene measures. These include 'wiping from front to back' after micturition or defecation, frequent and complete emptying of the bladder, increasing urine flow by greater fluid intake, and emptying the bladder soon after intercourse.

c. Patients with unexpected urinary tract infections

This group includes children or young men with a single episode of urinary infection, any patients in the first two groups who fail to respond to simple measures, and anyone with recurrent urinary infections. These patients require investigation (e.g. IVU) and are often found to have a structural abnormality or pathological condition which encourages bacterial proliferation. Bladder stone or prostatic hypertrophy are commonly responsible. These predisposing conditions can often be corrected surgically. In many patients, however, no predisposing factor can be found.

As with isolated episodes of infection, recurrent infections are treated with antibiotics, but bacteriological investigation assumes a greater importance. In some patients, long-term, low dose antibiotic or antiseptic therapy is necessary to prevent recurrence.

The 'urethral syndrome'

This syndrome is only found in women and is characterised by episodic or persistent dysuria, frequency or urgency. Urinary symptoms occur without demonstrable infection or local anatomical abnormality such as uterine prolapse. The cause is not known, and the condition may be indistinguishable from recurrent urethral trauma due to sexual intercourse. Urethral dilatation under general anaesthetic may be successful in relieving symptoms. Dysuria may also be a symptom associated with *atrophic vaginitis* in peri- and postmenopausal women; this may be relieved by topical application of oestrogens to the vagina and introitus.

Some patients, particularly women and girls, experience persistent or recurrent low-grade symptoms, notably frequency and urgency. No cause is found, although some cases can be attributed to habit, psychogenic or psychosexual factors.

UPPER URINARY TRACT INFECTIONS

Pathophysiology

Infections of the pelvicalyceal system (*acute pyelitis*) and renal parenchyma (*acute pyelonephritis*) arise either by upward extension of a lower tract infection or via the blood stream (haematogenous). *Ascending infections* occur most commonly when an abnormality causes ureteric reflux or stasis. Such conditions include ureteric obstruction, abnormal peristalsis (as in megaureter) and congenital incompetence of the cysto-ureteric antireflux mechanism. During pregnancy, the ureter becomes unusually dilated because of hormonal influences, and this may contribute to the increased incidence of urinary infections during this time.

Haematogenous infection is often responsible when there is urinary stasis in the upper tract. Common causes are stones in the renal pelvis or obstruction of the pelviureteric junction (PUJ). In such cases, lower tract infection is a secondary phenomenon.

What initiates a renal infection is often unclear but pre-existing renal damage is a strong predisposing factor.

Pathological examination of an acutely infected kidney shows extensive neutrophilic infiltration of the renal parenchyma, often with small abscesses. Usually only one kidney is involved and the causative organisms are coliforms, as in other urinary tract infections.

Clinical features

The classic clinical features of acute pyelonephritis are unilateral loin pain and tenderness. The patient is generally unwell with systemic features of infection, i.e. pyrexia and tachycardia. The urine is usually cloudy, and microscopy and culture confirm the presence of pus cells and bacteria. There may also be typical symptoms of bladder infection. Often, the symptoms and signs are less specific, and the patient presents with unilateral abdominal pain or discomfort. This may be mistaken for early acute appendicitis unless the urine is examined. Pyelonephritis may present without localising signs, especially in infants and the elderly, but patients are more unwell than in bladder infection and may even be septicaemic.

Fig. 24.3 Presenting features of acute pyelonephritis

- Unilateral loin pain and tenderness
- Less specific abdominal pain and discomfort
- Dysuria and cloudy, strong-smelling urine
- Haematuria
- Pyrexia and tachycardia
- Septicaemia (especially young children and the elderly)

Management of upper urinary tract infections

Diagnosis is made on the basis of clinical symptoms, signs and urine examination. Blood is also taken for culture when there are systemic signs of infection.

Treatment is with antibiotics, initially on a 'best-guess' basis. Dosage and route of administration depend on the severity of the illness; severe cases are given intravenous antibiotics.

Once the acute illness has been successfully treated, further investigation, usually intravenous urography, may be indicated in the search for predisposing factors. In children, investigation should include a micturating cystogram or radionuclide excretion scintigram to identify ureteric reflux (see Chapter 31).

Complications of acute pyelonephritis

Pyonephrosis

Severe infections may be complicated by obstruction of the pelvi-ureteric outlet, resulting in the accumulation of pus in the renal pelvis (pyonephrosis). If untreated, this will destroy the renal parenchyma. Treatment involves surgical or percutaneous drainage followed by *pyeloplasty*.

Perinephric abscess

Sometimes, particularly when a large 'staghorn' calculus is present, the accumulating pus may discharge through the renal capsule into the surrounding fat, resulting in a perinephric abscess. This presents as a slowly expanding mass in the loin, often with only low-grade local and systemic symptoms. Urine investigation will reveal pyuria, whilst ultrasound and radiology will show a non-functioning renal mass containing fluid-filled areas. A renal calculus may also be seen. A perinephric abscess sometimes develops by haematogenous infection of a traumatic perinephric haematoma. The treatment of perinephric abscess is drainage, often followed later by nephrectomy.

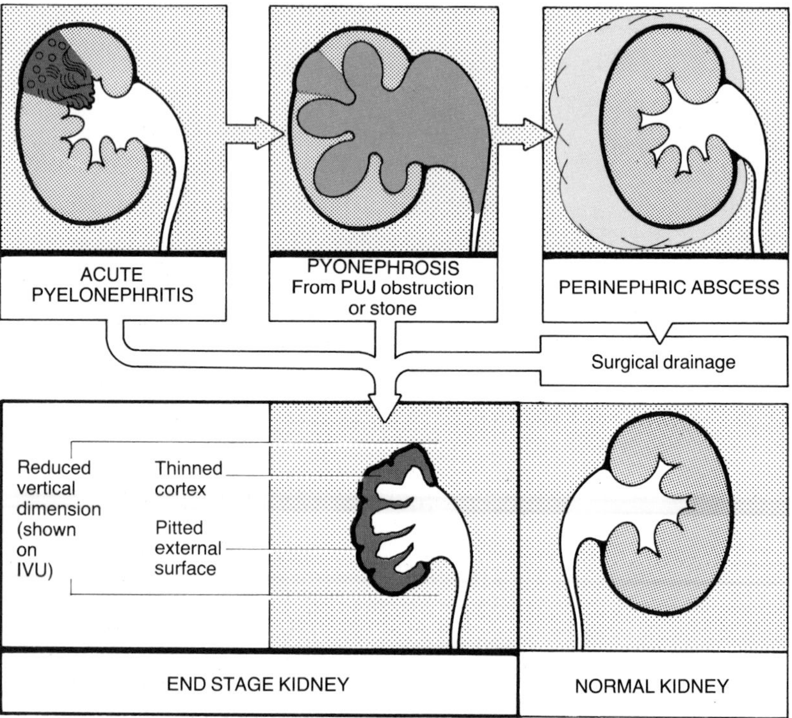

Fig. 24.4 Consequences of untreated renal infection

GENITO-URINARY TUBERCULOSIS

Pathophysiology

About 4% of patients with tuberculosis have involvement of the genito-urinary system. In developed countries, incidence is highest in debilitated elderly patients, often with a history of treated tuberculosis. The other vulnerable group is immigrants from Third World countries.

Mycobacteria reach the kidney or epididymis via the bloodstream, causing typical centrally-caseating granulomatous lesions which may later calcify. From the kidney, direct spread may occur to the ureter (causing a fibrous stricture) or to the bladder. Tuberculosis of the bladder usually begins around a ureteric opening and spreads more widely to cause patchy ulceration of the bladder wall, and later fibrotic contraction. Young adults are most commonly affected.

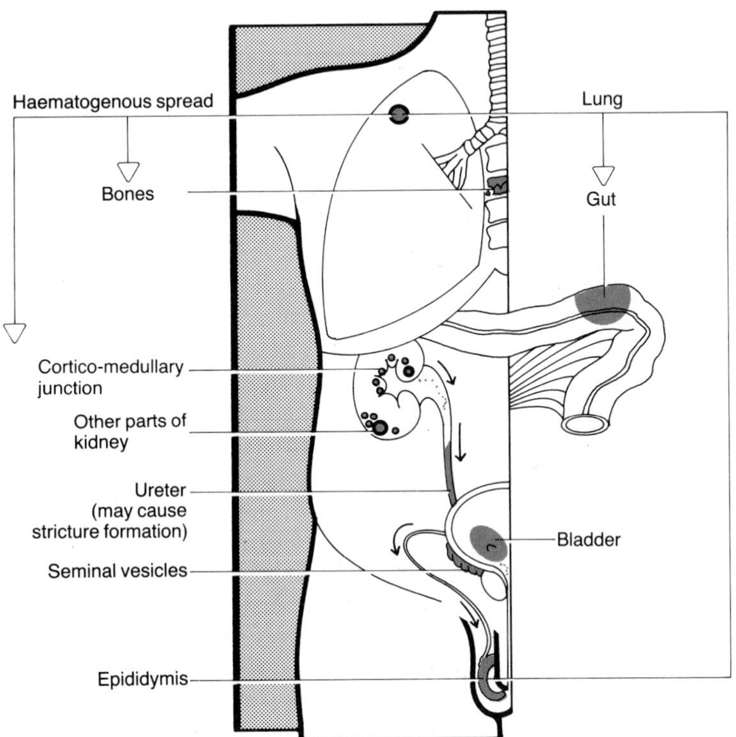

Fig. 24.5 Spread of tuberculosis to the genito-urinary tract

Clinical features and investigation

Urinary tract tuberculosis is often asymptomatic, and diagnosed during investigation of 'sterile pyuria'. If there are symptoms, the usual ones are painless urinary frequency, nocturia and sometimes haematuria. There may also be systemic features such as weight loss and night sweats, and respiratory symptoms if the lungs are affected.

When urinary tuberculosis is suspected, at least three early morning urine (EMU) specimens must be stained and cultured for tubercle bacilli (AFB). All of the first urine passed in the morning is collected and then centrifuged to concentrate the small number of organisms. A negative result does not, however, exclude urinary tuberculosis. Blood is tested for anaemia, lymphocytosis and elevation of ESR, and biochemical indicators of renal function. A chest X-ray is taken to search for pulmonary disease. Renal calcification may be seen on plain abdominal X-ray (such as the control film of an IVU), while urography may show renal abnormalities or ureteric strictures.

Management

Chemotherapy, as for pulmonary tuberculosis, is the mainstay of treatment. Surgery may be required later to treat ureteric strictures or a contracted bladder, or to excise damaged kidney tissue (partial or total nephrectomy).

SCHISTOSOMIASIS

Pathology

Schistosomiasis (bilharzia) is the most important parasitic disease of the urinary tract. It causes chronic inflammatory lesions in the bladder which lead to severe fibrotic damage. Schistosomiasis also predisposes to stone formation and squamous carcinoma.

Three Schistosome species, *S. haematobium, S. mansoni and S. japonicum*, have a wide tropical distribution and are important human pathogens. The most destructive bladder disease, however, is caused by *S. haematobium*. This species is endemic to tropical and North Africa (particularly the Nile valley), and is also found in some Middle Eastern and Southern European countries. Increasing worldwide travel makes it likely that the disease will be seen more in travellers from Western countries.

The Schistosome has a sophisticated life-cycle which is dependent on poor sanitation. Humans (the main definitive host) are infected by working or bathing in contaminated water. The free-swimming adult forms (*cercaria*) penetrate the skin, usually of the feet, and pass through the venous circulation and lungs to the systemic arterial circulation, which disseminates them throughout the body. In the hepatic portal veins, male and female worms copulate. The females, crammed with fertilised ova, then find their way via the mesenteric veins to the venous plexuses of the pelvic viscera, notably the bladder, where the ova are released. Aided by lytic enzymes, the ova then pass through the bladder wall into the urine and thence to the external environment.

On reaching water, the ova release immature ciliated forms (*miracidia*) which enter the intermediate host, a species of freshwater snail. The miracidia mature in the snail's liver before they are released as a new generation of adult cercarial worms. At this point, they are ready to enter human hosts, thus completing the life cycle.

Clinical presentations of schistosomiasis

Initial skin penetration may cause mild local inflammation. Subsequently, the phase of haematogenous spread may cause general malaise, low-grade pyrexia and eosinophilia. About two months later, ova invading the bladder mucosa cause local inflammation, manifest as frequency and haematuria at the end of micturition. The early symptoms may be trivial, and in low-grade infestations, may pass unnoticed.

The main damage caused by schistosomiasis in the bladder is due to an intense chronic inflammatory reaction to dead ova which have not passed out in the urine, and are sequestered in the bladder mucosa. Small granulomatous 'pseudotubercles' develop around each ovum, and these later becoming fibrotic and calcified. Heavy or recurrent infestations result in a variety of destructive lesions including *ulcers, papillomata, cysts, giant granulomata* and *severe bladder contracture*. All predispose to secondary bacterial infection and formation of bladder stones. Squamous metaplasia is common and strongly predisposes to *squamous carcinoma*.

Fig. 24.6 Clinical features of schistosomiasis

Skin rash
Low-grade systemic illness with eosinophilia
Urinary frequency and terminal haematuria
Chronic inflammation of the bladder
Bladder fibrosis and contracture
Bladder stones
Squamous carcinoma of the bladder

Management of schistosomiasis

Bladder or ureteric calcification is almost diagnostic of schistosomiasis. Diagnosis is confirmed either by microscopic examination of urine for ova (these are best found in the last few ml of a mid-morning specimen of urine) or more reliably by cystoscopic biopsy of bladder lesions.

Treatment involves long courses of chemotherapy to eradicate the parasites. Unfortunately, many of the cheap, established drugs are potentially toxic *antimony compounds*. Treatment is monitored by regular urine microscopy for ova. Surgery is often necessary later to correct or palliate residual deformities of the lower urinary tract.

About 5% of the world's population is affected by various forms of Schistosomiasis and prevention must be the cornerstone of disease control. Improved sanitation and clean water supplies are essential. Ironically, the rapid expansion of water conservation and irrigation schemes tends to spread the disease to previously unaffected populations. Overall, the prospects remain grim.

URETHRAL INFECTIONS AND STRICTURES

Urethral infections

The only clinically significant infections of the urethra are sexually transmitted diseases. The most common are *gonorrhoea* and '*non-specific urethritis*', the latter caused by chlamydial infection. The acute condition usually presents with a urethral discharge and dysuria. The surgical importance of urethritis, particularly gonoccoccal, is that it may lead, months or years later, to a fibrous stricture in the posterior urethra. Fortunately, the condition is becoming uncommon as primary antibiotic therapy is more readily available and effective.

Urethral stricture

Urethral strictures are now most commonly caused by inflammation resulting from prolonged catheterisation. These strictures involve the distal urethra or meatus. Strictures may also be a complication of traumatic instrumentation, in which case the membranous urethra is most vulnerable. A few strictures result from urethral tearing or rupture following displaced pelvic fractures. These usually require open surgical repair.

The characteristic symptom of urethral stricture is a progressive diminution in urinary stream. This may be accompanied by symptoms of bladder outlet obstruction, i.e. frequency and urgency, if there is any associated chronic retention. Diagnosis is made by direct inspection using a cystourothroscope.

Strictures may be short, elongated or multiple. Treatment is either by stretching or tearing the scar tissue with dilators passed along the urethra or, more satisfactorily, by cutting the stricture longitudinally with a urethrotome under direct urethroscopic vision. More difficult strictures may require open surgical treatment. Recurrence after treatment is not only frequent, but almost to be expected; skilled urological follow up is therefore desirable.

Urethral strictures may cause life-long disablility and most can be avoided by extreme care of the urethra during catheterisation and urethral instrumentation. 'Routine' catheterisation appears to be an irresistable temptation to all but urologists! As a general rule, the urethra should not be catheterised or interfered with unless absolutely essential. A catheter or other urological instrument should be 'hammered into place with a feather'.

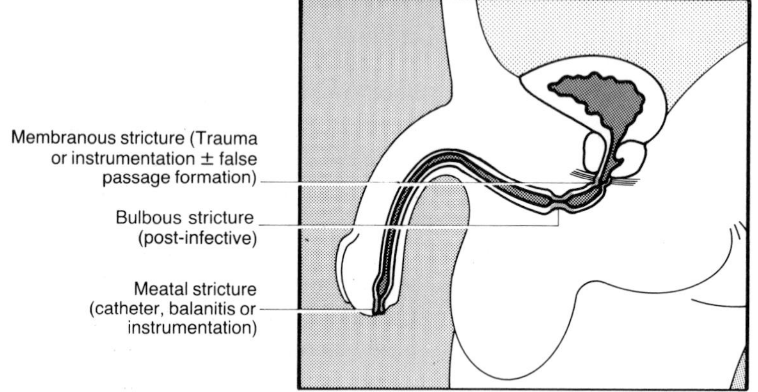

Fig. 24.7 Common sites of urethral strictures

25 CONGENITAL DISORDERS AND DISEASES SECONDARILY INVOLVING THE URINARY TRACT

Introduction

Most serious congenital disorders of the kidneys and urinary tract present at birth or in early childhood; these are described in Chapter 31. The exception is polycystic kidney which usually presents in adulthood. There are also a number of lesser abnormalities of the upper tract, e.g. duplex systems or medullary sponge kidney, which interfere with normal flow dynamics and predispose to infection. These are usually discovered during investigation of recurrent infections. Finally, asymptomatic abnormalities like unilateral renal agenesis, renal cysts or horseshoe kidney, may be discovered incidentally during investigations or surgery.

A systematic summary of the important congenital disorders is presented in Figure 25.1, highlighting those conditions which present in adulthood.

POLYCYSTIC KIDNEYS

The adult polycystic kidney syndrome is an autosomal dominant disorder characterised by multiple, bilateral cysts of the renal parenchyma. The cysts slowly expand, compressing and damaging the kidney. Thus adult polycystic kidney may present with *hypertension* or progressive *chronic renal failure*. The enlarged cystic kidneys may cause loin pain or may be discovered incidentally on abdominal examination. These kidneys are particularly vulnerable to even minor trauma and *haematuria* is a common presentation.

Many patients eventually require renal transplantation. Some patients also have multiple cysts in the liver and sometimes in the pancreas. They present with massive abdominal swelling due to gross liver enlargement.

MEDULLARY SPONGE KIDNEY

This rare disorder is caused by cyst-like dilatation (*ectasia*) of the collecting ducts of the renal medulla and may affect one or both kidneys. The cysts tend to become calcified, giving a characteristic radiographic appearance of streaky linear calcification in the renal papillae. Because of intrarenal stasis of urine, medullary sponge kidney predisposes to recurrent infection and stone formation. Patients rarely present before adulthood.

DUPLEX SYSTEMS

The urinary collecting system may be duplicated to a greater or lesser extent. The duplication always affects the renal end of the system and extends distally.

Fig. 25.1 Congenital abnormalities of the urinary system (conditions presenting in adulthood are highlighted)

NATURE OF ABNORMALITY	PRESENTATION
a. Kidney	
Bilateral agenesis (Potter's syndrome)	Oligohydramnios in pregnancy, stillborn infant with characteristic appearance of face and ears
Unilateral agenesis, aplasia or *hypoplasia*	Usually an incidental finding at any age. Often some abnormality on other side
Multicystic kidney: usually unilateral dysplasia of kidney with multiple cysts	Usually presents in the neonate as abdominal mass. Fatal if bilateral
Infantile polycystic disease: bilateral inherited disorder in which multiple small cysts replace renal parenchyma. Liver and pancreatic cysts often present also	Usually presents as gross abdominal distension in the neonate due to huge non–functioning kidneys. Invariably fatal
Medullary sponge kidney: cystic dilatation of collecting ducts of one or more medullary pyramids in one or both kidneys	May be found incidentally or during investigations for urinary infection. Cysts tend to become calcified and have characteristic X–ray appearance
Adult polycystic kidney: autosomal dominant disorder with multiple cysts throughout the renal parenchyma	Usually presents after age 30 with chronic renal failure, hypertension, haematuria or recurrent urinary tract infections
Solitary cysts: usually develop at one pole	Often incidental finding. May present with loin swelling or pain
Horseshoe kidney: fusion of lower poles of kidneys preventing normal developmental ascent	Often found incidentally but may cause hydronephrosis due to pelvi-ureteric obstruction
Ectopic kidneys and *abnormalities of rotation* due to failure of developmental ascent	Found incidentally or due to complications such as pelvi–ureteric obstruction
b. Pelvicalyceal system and ureters	
Pelvic hydronephrosis: dilatation of pelvicalyceal system due to congenital stenosis at pelviureteric junction	Usually presents in childhood or adolescence with loin pain or mass
Megaureter: abnormality of peristalsis of lower ureter resulting in gross proximal dilatation	Presents in young children with recurrent urinary tract infections
Ureterocoele: cystic dilatation of intravesical part of ureter due to stenosis of ureteric orifice	Incidental finding or causes infection or symptoms of obtruction

Fig. 25.1 (cont.)

NATURE OF ABNORMALITY	PRESENTATION
Vesicoureteric reflux: unilateral or bilateral abnormality of ureteric insertion into bladder	Presents in children as recurrent pyelonephritis which can cause severe damage to developing kidney
Duplex systems: partial or complete duplication of a ureter	Often incidental finding or cause of recurrent infection
Ectopic ureter: ureter does not open into the bladder but into some other part of the genital tract e.g.vagina	In females presents as dribbling incontinence and in males as recurrent urinary tract infections
c. Bladder and urethra	
Bladder hypoplasia: associated with some hypospadias in boys and ectopic ureters in girls	Bladder distends once ureters or hypospadias is corrected
Urachal abnormalities i.e. cyst, sinus, patent urachus: due to persistence of urachal remnants	Patent urachus usually presents in childhood with urine dribbing from umbilicus. Cysts and sinuses may present in adulthood. Adenocarcinoma sometimes develops in the urachal remnant
Bladder diverticulum: forms by herniation of mucosa through defect in muscular wall. Usually due to bladder outlet obstruction in adults. In children, it results from congenital urethral valves	Usually presents as recurrent urinary tract infection
Bladder exstrophy: incomplete closure of lower abdominal wall in midline	Gross abnormality of genito–urinary system obvious at birth
Urethral valves: usually occur in posterior urethra causing varying degrees of obstruction. More distal valves cause less obstruction	Severe cases present in the neonate with gross obstructive effects, renal failure and infection. Milder cases present later with recurrent infection
Epispadias: urethral meatus located in abnormal position somewhere on dorsum of penis. Often associated with major abnormality of penis	Obvious at birth
Hypospadias: urethra opens in abnormal position on ventral aspect of penis due to defective urethral fold. Distal urethra hypoplastic and shortened	Major cases obvious at birth. Minor abnormal cases have downward deviation of urinary stream. Sometimes a degree of chordee (downward bend of the penis)

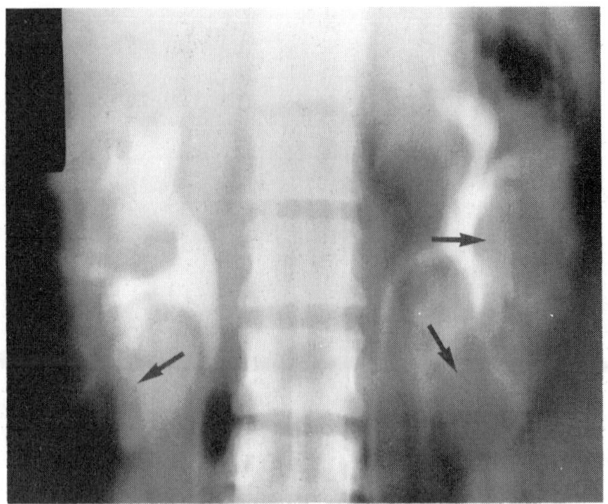

Fig. 25.2 Polycystic kidneys

IVU tomogram from a 52-year-old woman with hypertension and microscopic haematuria; both kidneys exhibit multiple lucent areas in the nephrogram representing cysts (arrowed) and the pelvicalyceal systems are slightly compressed

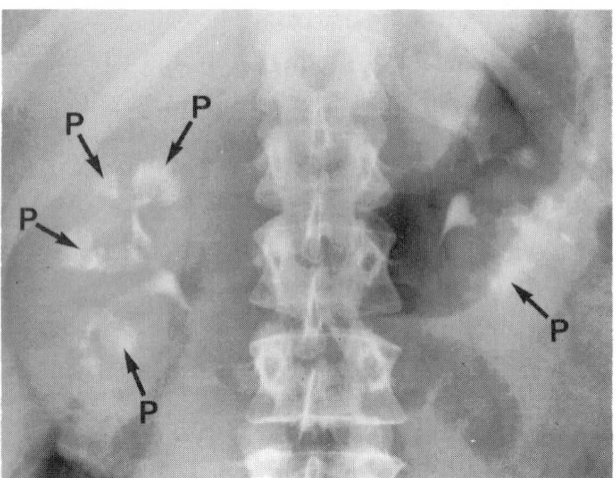

Fig. 25.3 Medullary sponge kidney

Bilateral medullary sponge kidney on an IVU from a 55-year-old woman with recurrent urinary tract infections; the renal papillae **P** have a typical 'flared' appearance and retain contrast because of the dilated collecting ducts. No radiopacity was visible on the control film although it can be seen in a considerable proportion of cases due to calcification in the ectatic ducts of the papillae

Complete duplex ureter is relatively common and may result in renal damage (see Figure 25.4). The ureter draining the upper pole of the kidney joins the bladder below the orifice of the lower pole ureter; this ureter has a defective anti-reflux mechanism at its junction with the bladder, thus predisposing to infection and renal parenchymal damage, stone formation and stenosis. Lesser degrees of duplication are usually discovered by chance on IVU.

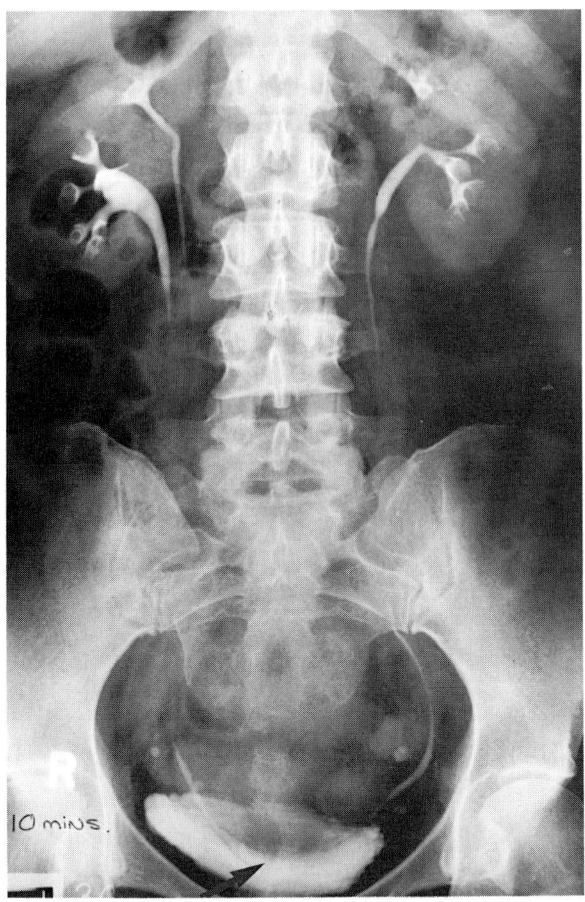

(a)

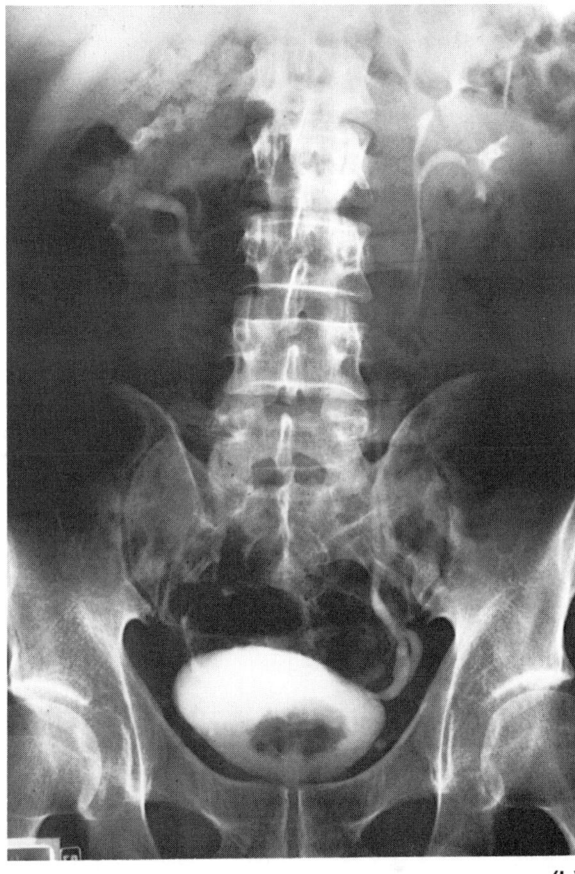

(b)

Fig. 25.4 Duplex systems

(a) Duplication of the ureters on the right side; only one ureter can be seen passing as far as the bladder, the vesico-ureteric junction being associated with a small, elongated ureterocoele (arrowed). **(b)** Complete left duplex system with both ureters visible all the way down to the bladder. **(c)** Partial duplication on the left side, the upper moiety of which exhibits the medullary sponge abnormality; this 25-year-old man presented with multiple ureteric stones and the other abnormalities were incidental findings

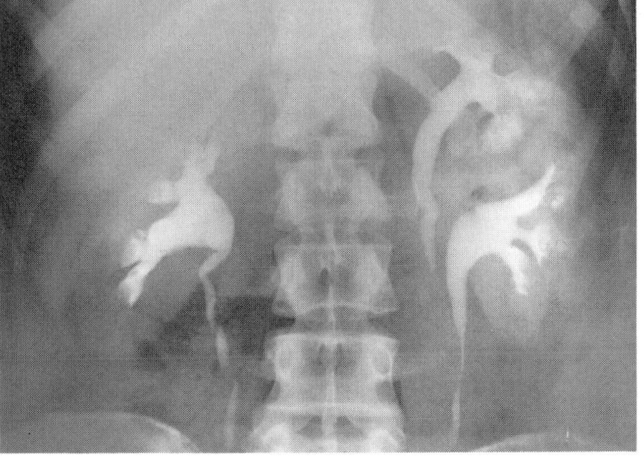

(c)

Fig. 25.4 (cont.)
Duplex systems

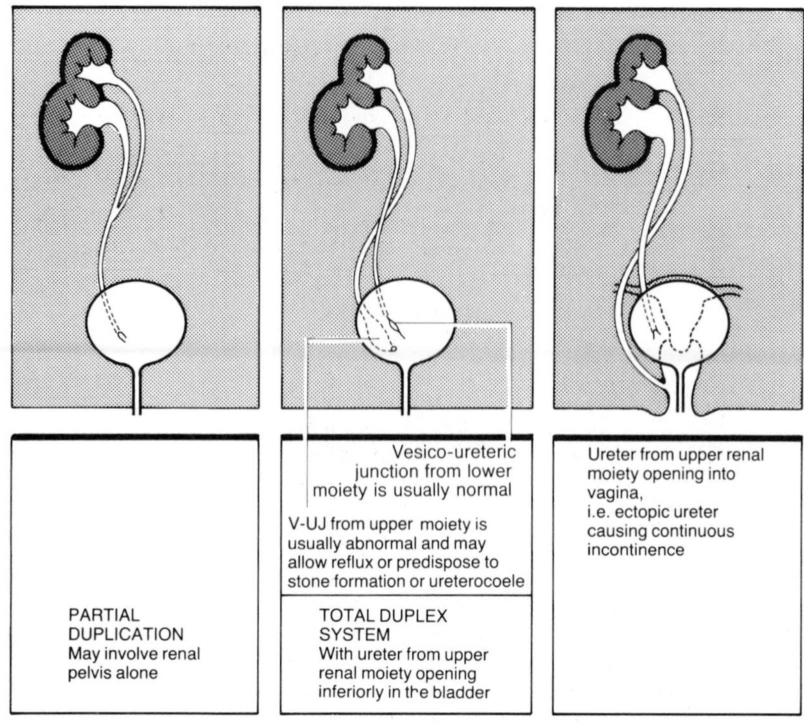

SOLITARY RENAL CYSTS

Isolated cysts of the renal parenchyma are a common developmental abnormality, rarely symptomatic, being found incidentally during renal ultrasound or IVU investigation. Their importance lies in distinguishing them from solid tumours; this is easily done with ultrasound. Occasionally such cysts cause pain or swelling. Treatment is by percutaneous aspiration under ultrasound control.

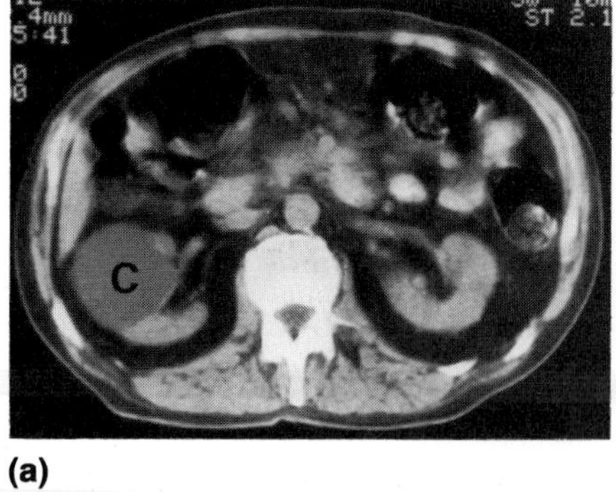

(a)

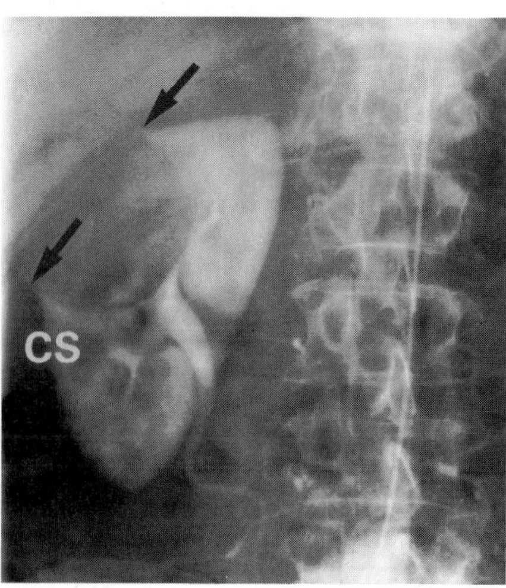

(b)

Fig. 25.5 Solitary renal cyst

(a) CT scan showing right renal cyst **C**. This was a chance finding in a woman of 45 being investigated for pancreatic pain. No treatment was necessary.
(b) Another solitary renal cyst found by chance, this time on an aortogram. In this film, contrast has been injected into the aorta ('flush aortogram') rather than selectively; the typical 'claw sign' **CS** (arrowed) of a simple cyst is shown

HORSESHOE KIDNEY

This abnormality is caused by fusion of the two developing kidneys at their lower poles. Normal embryological ascent is prevented by the inferior mesenteric artery, so that the isthmus of the kidney comes to lie across the aorta at the level of the 3rd or 4th lumbar vertebra. The condition is usually a chance finding on IVU investigation or at abdominal aortic surgery, when it may cause serious operative difficulties. Horseshoe kidney is sometimes associated with PUJ obstruction, which may lead to the diagnosis. Occasionally, a horseshoe kidney causes problems during pregnancy.

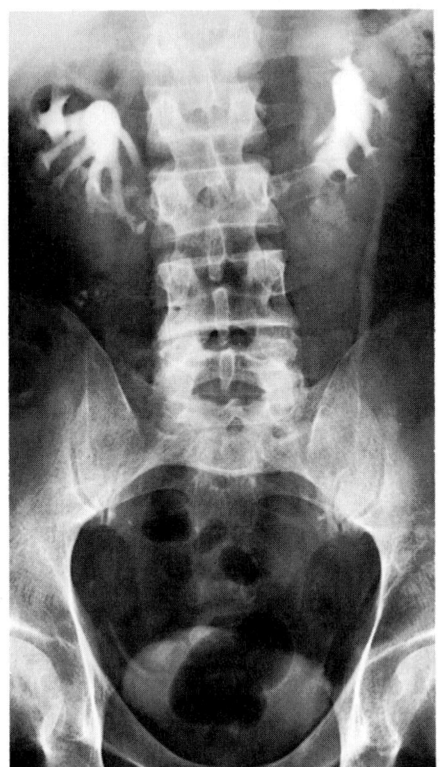

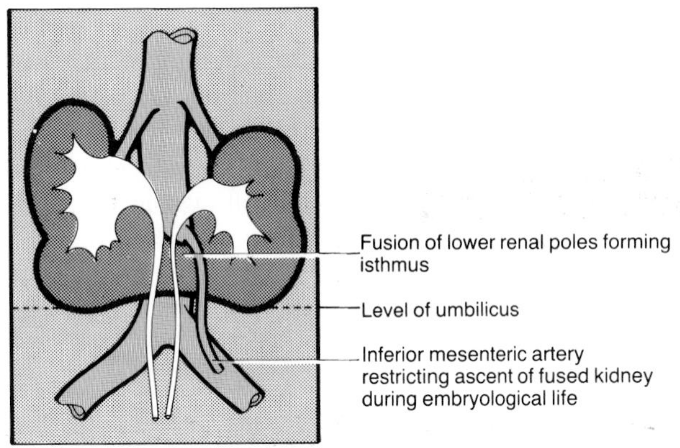

Fig. 25.6 Horseshoe kidney

Horseshoe kidney shown on IVU from a 51-year-old woman with recurrent urinary tract stones; the pelvicalyceal systems are oriented obliquely, converging inferiorly, because of the isthmus being stretched over the vertebral column. Each pelvis and ureter is more medially placed than normal and the whole renal mass lies much lower than normal kidneys; the isthmus of a horseshoe kidney can rarely be demonstrated by IVU or ultrasound

RENAL ECTOPIA AND OTHER RENAL ABNORMALITIES

A variety of other renal abnormalities (including ectopic kidneys, rotational abnormalities, unilateral agenesis, aplasia or hyperplasia) may be found unexpectedly on investigation or at surgery. These abnormalities may confuse diagnosis and sometimes result in surgical mishap, e.g. excision of a pelvic kidney mistaken for an ovarian tumour. Note that transplanted kidneys are usually sited in the iliac fossa!

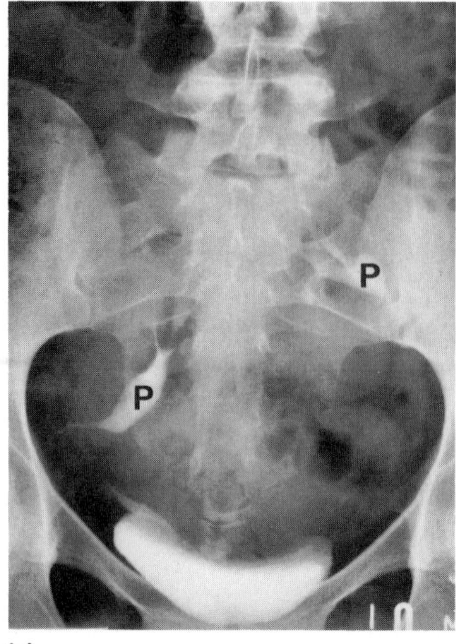

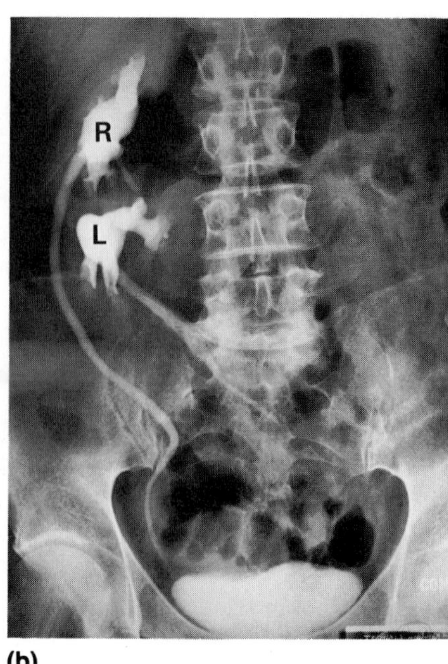

(a) (b)

Fig. 25.7 Ectopic kidneys

(a) A 48-year-old woman with recurrent urinary tract infections; IVU shows abnormal pelvicalyceal systems **P** of bilateral pelvic kidneys. **(b)** Another middle-aged woman with recurrent urinary tract infections; the left kidney **L** is ectopically located on the opposite side and is fused to the right kidney **R** ('crossed renal ectopia')

URACHAL ABNORMALITIES

During development, the urogenital sinus communicates with the allantois via the urachus. Occasionally, this tract persists as a fistula between bladder and umbilicus. Sometimes the fistula does not open until adulthood. Similarly, a remnant may form a blind urachal sinus opening at the umbilicus or result in a urachal cyst in the midline of the lower abdomen. These structural abnormalities may then become infected. Very rarely, an adenocarcinoma develops in a urachal remnant in the bladder vault or in other urachal remnants.

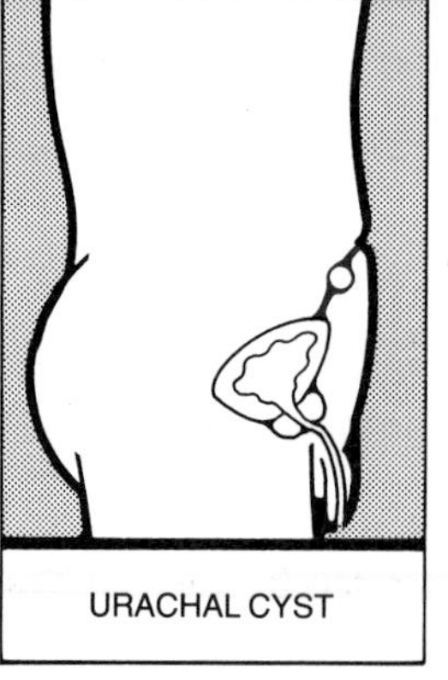

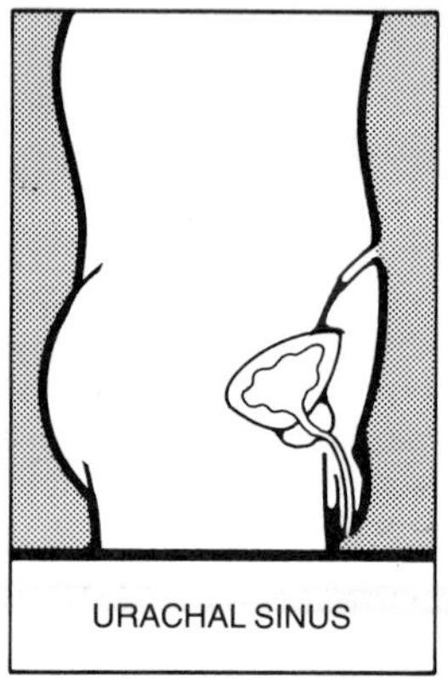

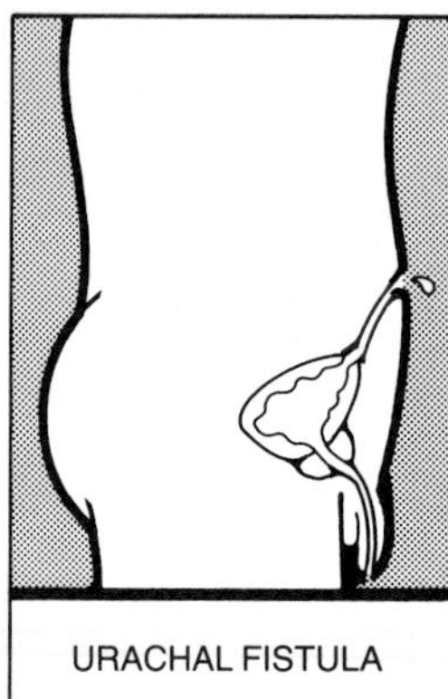

Fig. 25.8 Urachal abnormalities

DISEASES SECONDARILY INVOLVING THE URINARY TRACT

Introduction

A variety of abdominal disorders such as tumours, inflammatory bowel disease, aneurysms and retroperitoneal fibrosis may secondarily involve the urinary tract. These conditions affect the urinary tract by obstructing one or both ureters or occasionally by causing a fistula between bowel and urinary tract. Obstruction of one ureter alone may be asymptomatic, although it may cause loin pain or predispose to infection; bilateral involvement usually presents with renal failure, either acute or chronic.

Of tumours outside the urinary tract, advanced *carcinoma of the uterine cervix* most commonly produces bilateral obstruction because of the close anatomical relationship of the ureters to the cervix. This closeness makes the ureters vulnerable even at straightforward hysterectomy. Carcinomas of the ascending colon or rectosigmoid colon suprisingly rarely obstruct the right or left ureter respectively. Most ureteric damage in relation to large bowel cancer results from surgical operations to remove them.

Inflammatory disease which involves the bowel serosa may extend to involve nearby structures such as the ureters and bladder, and this may lead to fistula formation. This is important in *Crohn's disease* and *diverticular disease*. A fistula between bowel and urinary tract presents as severe urinary infection, often with pneumaturia or faecuria.

An expanding abdominal mass may compress one or both ureters and cause symptoms from partial obstruction; sometimes *aorto-iliac aneurysms* are responsible. A much more common cause of ureteric compression is *pregnancy*, which tends to cause bilateral megaureter both hormonally and by pressure effects. The main clinical significance of bilateral megaureter is that it predisposes to upper tract infection. Thus, significant bacteriuria in pregnancy, symptomatic or not, should be treated with antibiotics.

RETRO-PERITONEAL FIBROSIS

This rare and obscure condition is characterised by progressive, intense fibrosis of the connective tissue behind the peritoneal cavity. The cause is unknown (i.e. idiopathic) in the majority of cases, but some drugs such as *methysergide* may induce the condition; it may sometimes be associated with an inflammatory aortic aneurysm. Retroperitoneal fibrosis often causes hypertension by its effect on the kidneys.

Retroperitoneal fibrosis compresses both ureters, causing bilateral hydronephrosis and eventually renal failure. Sometimes it is associated with inferior vena caval obstruction. Diagnosis is usually made on IVU, which shows bilateral hydronephrosis (see Figure 25.9). The fibrotic process also draws the ureters closer together in the midline. The ESR is characteristically elevated.

Treatment usually requires dissection of the ureters from the retroperitoneal tissue (*ureterolysis*). The ureters are then resited within the peritoneal cavity to try to prevent recurrent obstruction. A biopsy of the retroperitoneal tissue should be taken to exclude tumour and confirm the diagnosis. If obstruction recurs, steroid therapy may suppress the condition.

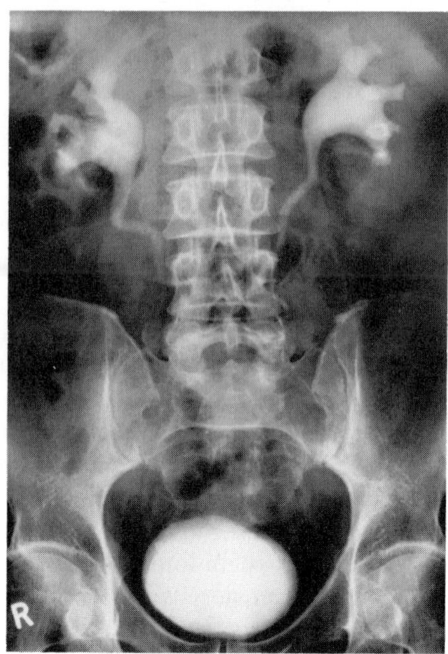

Fig. 25.9 Retroperitoneal fibrosis

This man aged 62 presented with back pain. The IVU shows bilateral hydronephrosis due to ureteric compression; note how the ureters are tapered and characteristically drawn medially by the fibrotic process

26 VASCULAR DISORDERS

Introduction

The term 'vascular disease' is usually taken to mean disease of the arterial system, but it does include diseases of veins. The active management of arterial disease has really only developed since the 1950s. Since arterial surgery involves special techniques uncommon to general surgery, a new sub-specialty of *vascular surgery* has evolved since then. Despite this, the principles of diagnosis and management should be understood by all clinicians. The first reason is that complications of arterial disease are seen across the field of medicine. The second reason is that *varicose veins* make up the largest group of vascular problems, and most cases are managed by general surgeons.

Chronic lower limb ulcers are usually managed by general practitioners but the more difficult cases are referred to dermatologists or surgeons. Many of these ulcers represent a late complication of past deep venous thrombosis. The majority of the remainder are caused by arterial insufficiency or diabetes, and a few by ulcerating tumours. In developed countries, infection rarely plays a primary role. In intractable cases, persistent ulceration may be due to a combination of factors.

The bulk of arterial surgery is concerned with *lower limb ischaemia*, which is caused mainly by atherosclerotic obstruction. In a minority of cases the primary disorder is arterial thrombosis or embolism. The symptoms and signs of arterial insufficiency in the lower limb depend on the degree of ischaemia.

There are three main clinical presentations of lower limb ischaemia:

- *Intermittent claudication* — relatively mild ischaemia produces muscular pain only on exercise which is relieved by rest
- *Rest pain* — severe ischaemia presents with pain in the affected foot which becomes intolerable over a few days or weeks
- *Critical ischaemia* — severe ischaemia may progress to dry or wet gangrene of one or more toes or foot ulceration. At this stage, the viability of the whole limb is threatened. Critical ischaemia may develop very rapidly if thrombosis or embolism occurs, with the leg suddenly becoming cold, numb and painful. Emergency surgery is required if the limb is to be saved

Most arterial and venous disorders of the lower limbs can be easily recognised, but in the acutely painful limb, differentiating between arterial insufficiency and venous thrombosis may be difficult. Furthermore, non-vascular disorders, such as cauda equina compression, may be misdiagnosed as being of vascular origin. Whatever the cause of the acutely painful limb, assessing the arterial element is an essential preliminary.

Aneurysms of the abdominal aorta, ileo-femoral and popliteal arteries are an important complication of atherosclerosis. All aneurysms may rupture or leak, or thrombose causing distal ischaemia. Although some aneurysms present in these ways, the majority present as a painless pulsatile mass. The way an aneurysm is managed depends on its site and its potential for serious complications.

Occasionally, similar arterial problems arise in the upper limb. Arterial problems in other parts of the body that may require surgical intervention are *carotid artery disease and renal artery stenosis.*

VASCULAR DISORDERS OF THE LOWER LIMB – GENERAL CONSIDERATIONS

PATHO-PHYSIOLOGY

Vascular disorders of the lower limb are caused mainly by atherosclerosis, thromboembolism, complications of diabetes mellitus, and thrombotic and varicose disorders of the venous system. In some patients, especially the elderly, a variety of causes may interact. For vascular disorders in particular, accurate diagnosis depends largely on clinical evaluation rather than special investigations. Symptoms and signs are best interpreted by understanding the underlying pathophysiological processes. These are outlined in Figure 26.1.

SYMPTOMS AND SIGNS IN THE LOWER LIMB

The principal symptoms and signs of lower limb vascular disease are pain, changes in skin texture, changes in skin colour and temperature, ulceration and swelling. The diagnostic importance of these is outlined in the following section.

Pain

Pain in the lower limb is most commonly due to trauma or musculo-skeletal disorders. Surgical patients with lower limb pain have either minor pain and discomfort associated with varicose veins, or have more severe pain caused by ischaemia and obliterative arterial disease.

Intermittent claudication

Ischaemia most commonly presents as muscular pain which develops during exercise and increases in severity. Symptoms usually predominate in one limb and the patient commonly limps with the pain, which accounts for the descriptive term 'intermittent claudication' (Latin: claudicare = to limp). The patient is forced to stop walking, whereupon the pain subsides, usually within a minute or two. If exercise is then resumed, the pain recurs at about the same walking distance.

The pain of intermittent claudication is almost always in the calf, whatever the level of the causative arterial obstruction. The pain may extend into

Fig. 26.1 Pathophysiology and clinical consequences of vascular diseases affecting the lower limb

BASIC DISEASE	PATHOPHYSIOLOGICAL PROCESS	CLINICAL MANIFESTATIONS
1. **Atherosclerosis and its complications**		
a. Obliterative disease — luminal narrowing by atherosclerotic plaques, with chronic exacerbation or sudden occlusion by superimposed thrombus. Affects aorta and large distributing vessels.	i. Arterial supply adequate at rest but inadequate to supply metabolic demands of muscles, especially calf muscles, during exercise. Foot and popliteal pulses usually not palpable. Femoral pulses present in the majority of cases	Pain in leg muscles on walking, quickly relieved by rest, i.e. 'intermittent claudication'. Onset usually insidious
	ii. Arterial supply inadequate even at rest resulting in ischaemia of all tissues. Blood supply just sufficient to sustain viability of the limb, although extreme peripheries may undergo patchy necrosis. Skin particularly vulnerable, becoming atrophic with reactive dilatation of peripheral microvasculature. Pressure or trauma (accidental or surgical) may easily cause ulceration, severely impaired healing and risk of spreading infection	Pain, typically in the foot, at rest — worse at night or on elevation of limb and relieved by hanging the leg down. Symptoms develop over days or weeks. Skin of peripheries red to purple and dusky. Skin also shiny and taut due to dependent oedema (since patients tend to sleep with feet hanging down). Skin of foot becomes pale on elevation and red on dependency (Buerger's test). May be patches of dry gangrene or ulceration at extremity of toes
	iii. Acute severe ischaemia due to thrombotic obstruction of diseased vessel. Leads to necrosis within 6–8 hours	Sudden onset of pallor, paralysis, paraesthesia and numbness of foot or leg, with variable level of pain. Skin slowly becomes blue and blistered as necrosis supervenes. Symptoms and signs are identical to acute embolic occlusion
b. Aneurysmal dilatation — mainly affects aorta and ileo–femoral arteries and less commonly the popliteal artery	i. Progressive aneurysmal dilatation which may eventually be self-limiting if hypertension controlled	Asymptomatic — discovered by chance on plain abdominal X-ray or as a pulsatile mass in abdomen, groin or popliteal fossa
	ii. Sudden rupture of aneurysm (usually into peritoneal cavity)	Acute, usually fatal, cardiovascular collapse
	iii. Leakage of aneurysm (usually into retroperitoneal tissues)	Ill–defined back or abdominal pain often simulating uteric obstruction or other abdominal emergencies. Often accompanied by transient collapse. Sometimes, a recent history of similar episodes. Pulsatile abdominal mass usually palpable

Fig. 26.1 (cont.)

BASIC DISEASE	PATHOPHYSIOLOGICAL PROCESS	CLINICAL MANIFESTATIONS
	iv. Dissection along tunica media (almost always begins in thoracic aorta) obstructing major branches, i.e. mesenteric, renal and iliac arteries	Characterically presents with shock and severe chest pain radiating to the back. Renal artery involvement results in anuria. Usually fatal and rarely reaches the surgeon
	v. Sudden occlusion of aneurysmal vessel due to thrombosis (aneurysmal popliteal artery)	Symptoms and signs of acute severe ischaemia of the leg. Mass in the popliteal fossa (usually not pulsatile by this stage)
c. Emboli arising from atherosclerotic lesions (obliterative or ulcerating) or from within aneurysms	Emboli of atheroma or mural platelet thrombi (usually small) passing to extreme peripheries. Showers of emboli may occur at recurrent intervals	Sudden onset of severe, highly localised pain in digits. Development of small reddish-blue areas of skin necrosis which do not blanch on pressure
2. **Cardiac disease**		
a. Thrombo-embolism secondary to myocardial infarction, ventricular aneurysm, atrial fibrillation, mitral valve disease (especially rheumatic)	Emboli (usually large masses of mural thrombus) become detached and impact at bifurcations of distributing system. These cause acute, critical ischaemia distally (usually below the knee)	Sudden onset of symptoms and signs of acute severe ischaemia. If occlusion is by a hugh *saddle embolus* across the aortic bifurcation, then both limbs are affected. Often atrial fibrillation or a recent history of myocardial infarction
b. Poor cardiac output, e.g. acute myocardial infarction, cardiac failure	Results in inadequate perfusion of all peripheral tissues and exacerbates any pre-existing arterial insufficiency. Claudication may be converted to critical ischaemia	Rapid development of severe ischaemic signs in legs, usually bilateral. Patient is usually elderly, with severe (often terminal) cardiovascular disease
3. **Diabetes mellitus**		
Diabetic neuropathy. Diabetes is also associated with accelerated atherosclerosis, and predisposition to infection	Pre-existing diabetic sensory neuropathy predisposes to traumatic injury and ulceration. Effects are exacerbated by abnormal glucose metabolism leading to necrosis of deep tissues usually complicated by pyogenic infection Arterial supply may already be compromised by atherosclerosis	Typical presentation is a deep, painless, infected ulcer with a characteristic 'punched out' appearance; these are described as *perforating ulcers*. Surrounding tissues are usually well perfused (pink and warm). Peripheral pulses are often palpable but there is generalised sensory impairment. Ulcer is often recent, over a bony prominence and preceded by minor trauma. Infection may spread deeply and rapidly causing extensive limb-threatening necrosis and septicaemia

Fig. 26.1 (cont.)

BASIC DISEASE	PATHOPHYSIOLOGICAL PROCESS	CLINICAL MANIFESTATIONS
4. **Venous disorders**		
a. Deep venous thrombosis predisposed by pregnancy, oral contraceptive pill, major surgery, trauma, obesity, abdominal or pelvic malignancy, immobility	Spontaneous thrombosis in the deep venous system of the calf; tends to extend proximally into the ilio-femoral veins. Obstructs venous return both in the short and long term. Organisation and recanalisation may relieve the obstruction but cause valvular incompetence of the deep venous system, causing chronic venous hypertension. This obstructs capillary flow causing back-pressure ischaemia. Leakage of plasma proteins results in interstitial fibrin deposition which inhibits metabolite exchange. Leakage of blood results in subcutaneous deposition of haemosiderin. Combined effects may produce atrophy of skin and subcutaneous fat, subcutaneous fibrosis, poor healing capacity and predisposition to ulceration	Classical presentation is acute pain and swelling of calf and ankle with exquisite tendernes in calf muscle. Dorsiflexion of the ankle causes pain the calf (*Homan's sign*). The leg is usually warm and of normal colour but pulses may be impalpable due to oedema. If ilio-femoral veins are involved as well, the thigh is also swollen. Note: many small deep venous thromboses are completely asymptomatic. A late complication is post-thrombotic (or *post-phlebitic*) *limb* with chronic brawny oedema of the leg. The ankle is narrow due to subcutaneous fat atrophy (*lipo-dermatosclerosis*) and skin is atrophic, scaly and pigmented (*varicose eczema*). Skin above the medial malleolus most vulnerable and may become chronically ulcerated after minor trauma
b. Superficial venous thrombosis, i.e. *phlebitis*. Usually occurs in dilated varicose veins; more common in pregnancy. Occasionally presents as *thrombophlebitis migrans* in patients with underlying malignancy elsewhere	Spontaneous thrombosis in tortuous dilated superficial veins; excites an inflammatory response in the vessel wall and surrounding tissues	Rapid onset of acute, highly localised pain and tenderness, associated with varicose veins in the long saphenous system. Overlying skin is red and oedematous; underlying veins are hard and nodular
c. Varicose veins — incompetent function of valves between deep and superficial venous systems, including the sapheno-femoral valve. The basic abnormality may be in the vessel wall	Blood is forced through the incompetent valves from the deep venous system to the superficial system causing slowly progressive tortuous dilatation of superficial veins. Venous stagnation may cause chronic skin changes and sometimes ulceration. Dilated vessels are vulnerable to trauma and may bleed profusely	Slowly progressive development of prominent, purple, dilated, tortuous superficial veins. The patient often complains of aching pains, especially after long period of standing. Patients may be upset by the cosmetic appearance or, if there is a family history, fear at progression or ulceration. Pain relieved by elevation. Women more often affected than men; varicosities normally first appear during pregnancy

the thigh or even buttock if walking is continued, and this indicates obstruction of arteries above the inguinal ligament. Absent foot pulses, or foot pulses which become impalpable after exercise, may be the only clinical signs.

Provided a thorough history is taken, there is only one condition which might reasonably be mistaken for arterial claudication. This is *cauda equina claudication*, which is caused by compression of the cauda equina within the spinal canal by either central disc protrusion or spinal stenosis. Pain in the lower limb is also brought on by exercise, but there are important differences: the claudication distance is variable, the pain takes thirty minutes or so to subside and there is usually a history of low back pain. On examination, there is usually some evidence of a lower motor neurone lesion such as diminished or absent lower limb tendon reflexes.

Rest pain

With more severe arterial obstruction, ischaemic pain may occur when the patient rests in bed. This rest pain occurs usually in the skin of the foot and is burning in character. It is probably caused by a number of factors working together. These include the loss of gravity assistance to arterial supply in the horizontal position, the physiological reduction in cardiac output at rest, and the reactive dilatation of skin vessels to warmth. Consequently, the pain is relieved by hanging the leg over the side of the bed or even walking around. In acute critical ischaemia, when blood flow in the periphery is virtually absent, there may be no pain in the most severely affected area, presumably due to peripheral nerve ischaemia. There may, however, be severe pain more proximally where the tissue is less ischaemic.

The pain of deep venous thrombosis is usually less severe than that of severe ischaemia. Physical examination will usually distinguish between the two conditions. In deep vein thrombosis, the limb is warm, pulses are detectable and there is no colour change (except in very severe cases). Swelling is often a feature of deep venous thrombosis but is not found in acute arterial ischaemia.

Changes in skin texture

Changes in skin *texture*, *colour*, *pigmentation* or *temperature* (and the distribution of these changes) help to distinguish between the different types of lower limb vascular disorders. In the chronic disorders, the epidermis may be thin and atrophic because of deficient oxygenation and nutrition; this explains the use of the term *trophic changes*.

In arterial insufficiency, whatever the level of obstruction, the effects are most evident at the extreme periphery, i.e. the foot and toes. In contrast, the skin changes caused by chronic venous insufficiency are most severe around the medial side of the ankle above the malleolus, and are almost never seen on the foot. Furthermore, in venous disease, the cutaneous fat around the ankle may become thinned by atrophy and hardened by fibrosis (lipo-dermatosclerosis or, less accurately, *fat necrosis*). The leg above the ankle is oedematous. In extreme cases, there may be marked constriction at the ankle giving rise to a *beer-bottle leg*.

Changes in skin colour and temperature

Colour change may suggest the underlying disease process, particularly if temperature change is also considered. Many people, particularly the elderly, suffer from cold feet in cold weather. If both feet are pale when cold and have normal pulses, this is normal arteriolar constriction for temperature conservation.

The acutely cold foot

The main pathological reason for a foot becoming acutely cold and white is a sudden complete arterial occlusion. This event is usually unilateral unless the abdominal aorta or both iliac arteries become obstructed. There are ischaemic changes in the foot extending a variable amount up the leg.

The cardinal clinical features of acute critical ischaemia are:

- Pain — variable in intensity, usually at the junction of perfused and ischaemic tissue
- Paraesthesia or anaesthesia of the periphery (i.e altered or absent skin sensation)
- Paralysis of calf muscles. The patient is unable to flex or extend the toes or ankle. This only occurs if ischaemia is extreme
- Pallor of the extremity. The ischaemic area is initially white, but later becomes blue when necrosis occurs
- Pulselessness of the extremity. Foot pulses are absent and popliteal and femoral pulses may be lost, according to the level of occlusion

(As an aide memoir, the features of acute limb ischaemia are known as the five P's: **P**ain, **P**araesthesia, **P**aralysis, **P**allor and **P**ulselessness. Not all of these are present all of the time).

If the foot becomes dusky purple and fails to blanch on pressure, surgically irretrievable necrosis has occurred. These changes always involve the foot but may extend proximally (though rarely above the knee). The upper limit of the necrotic area is usually well demarcated from the proximal viable tissue. Blistering of the skin begins 24–48 hours after infarction.

Colour change is unusual in deep venous thrombosis but massive pelvic vein thrombosis may cause colour changes mistaken for arterial occlusion. Massive thrombosis is now unusual and occurs mainly in high-risk patients. Massive thrombosis was once much more common, especially during late pregnancy or the early puerperium. The condition was known as *white leg of pregnancy* or *phlegmasia alba dolens*. The whole of the lower limb is affected, with pain, pallor and massive swelling of the leg and thigh. In contrast to arterial occlusion, the limb is warm and pulses are detectable despite the oedema. A rare but more serious variant is *blue leg* or *phlegmasia caerulia dolens* which represents incipient venous infarction.

The chronically cold foot

In chronic arterial insufficiency (severe claudication or rest pain), the onset of a dusky skin colour in the toes or foot suggests incipient tissue necrosis (*pre-gangrene*). If finger pressure is applied to ischaemic skin, the rate of colour return gives some indication of skin perfusion.

Necrosis following chronic ischaemia tends to be patchy and localised due to the protective effect of a developed collateral circulation. Once necrosis occurs, blood flow ceases and skin becomes mottled blue over the next few hours. Now, finger pressure does not produce blanching and pigmentation is fixed. Such necrosis is usually confined to a toe or a limited part of the forefoot. The necrotic area slowly becomes hard, black and mummified (*dry*

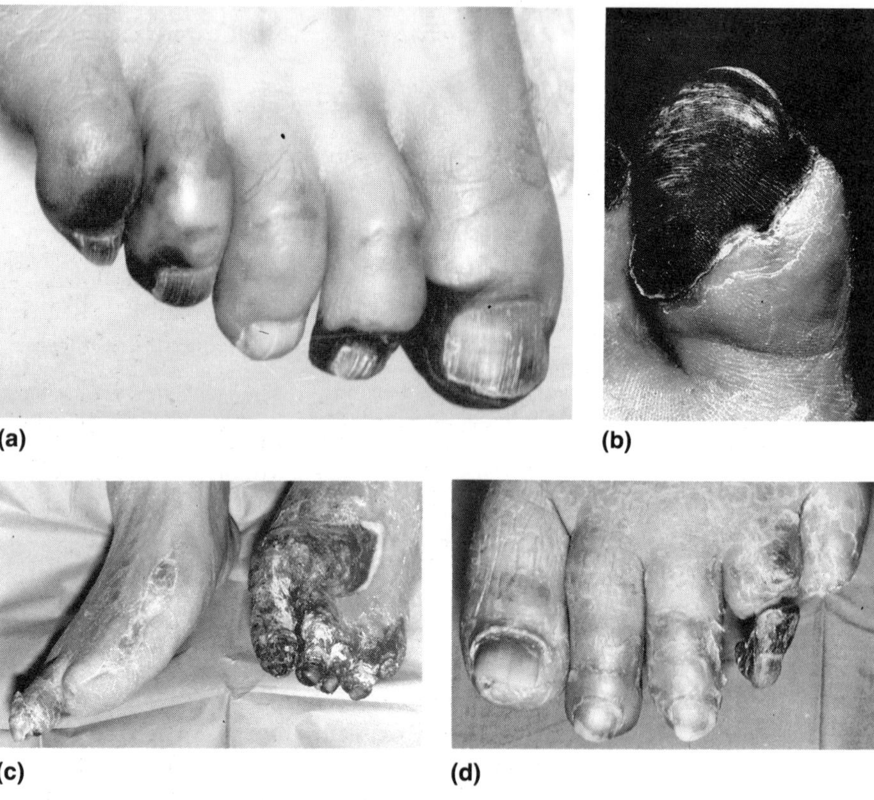

(a) (b) (c) (d)

Fig. 26.2 Necrosis resulting from severe ischaemia

(a) Early necrosis of tips of toes resulting from acute occlusion of the right common iliac artery three days before this photograph. The patient had pre-existing widespread obliterative atherosclerosis of the lower limb. **(b)** The same patient as in (a), showing a clear line of demarcartion of the necrotic toe tip. This photograph was taken two months after an emergency aorto-popliteal bypass graft. **(c)** This elderly diabetic woman had long standing severe peripheral arterial disease. There is established necrosis ('dry gangrene') with mummification in the left forefoot. The right foot had been similar, but the onset of infection ('wet gangrene') persuaded the reluctant patient to undergo arterial reconstructive surgery. A right femoro-popliteal bypass graft was performed and the necrotic tissue amputated three months before this photograph was taken. **(d)** Auto-amputation of necrotic toe tips in a patient with peripheral ischaemia resulting from polycythaemia rubra vera. Note the tip of the fifth toe has been shed and the fourth is retained only by the bony phalanx

gangrene) and eventually separates spontaneously from the viable tissue (see Figure 26.2). Skin slowly heals the defect. If the necrotic area becomes infected, the tissue becomes boggy and ulcerated and the infection and gangrene spread proximally (*wet gangrene*). Wet gangrene requires urgent surgical treatment.

Redness of the skin indicates that oxygenated blood is present in the capillaries. This usually implies there is no venous congestion or obstruction. With arterial ischaemia, there is reactive dilatation of the microvasculature to hypoxia. This is a physiological attempt to extract the maximum oxygen from whatever blood is reaching the area. Thus severely ischaemic skin may be red but paradoxically cool.

Buerger's test for severe ischaemia involves high elevation of the leg for a minute or two. Because the peripheral arterial pressure is inadequate to overcome the effects of gravity, the leg then becomes white. When the leg is hung down, it gradually becomes bluish-red and turgid as blood flow returns.

Fig. 26.3

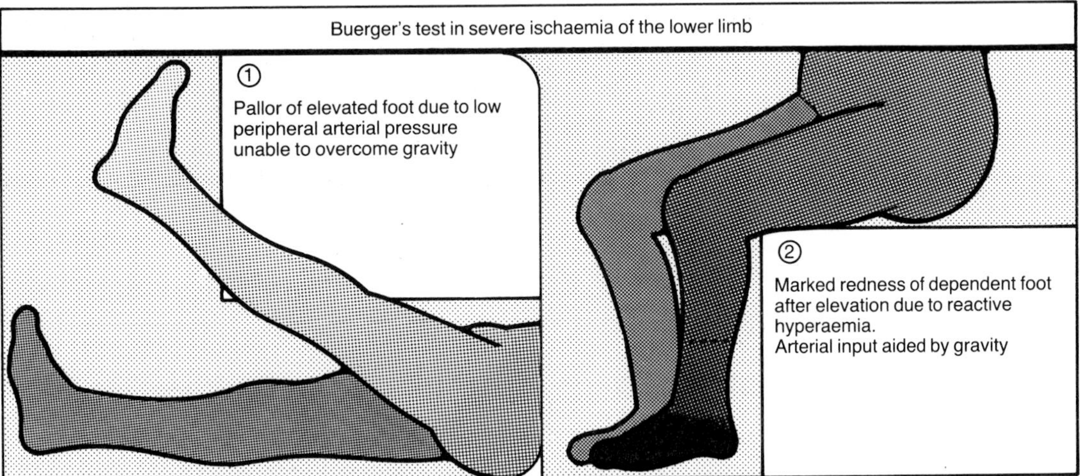

The warm foot

Inflammatory dilatation of the microcirculation also causes skin redness, but the skin is warm and slightly swollen because of enhanced blood flow. An example is low-grade bacterial *cellulitis* which may be seen in diabetes, mild arterial in sufficiency, venous disease or arise unexpectedly. Note that if infection develops in a severely ischaemic limb, the usual signs of inflammation may not develop and the extent of infection may be underestimated. If the blood supply is later restored surgically, signs of inflammation then develop.

Abnormal pigmentation

In a post-thrombotic limb, the valves of the deep veins have been destroyed by organisation and recanalisation after deep venous thrombosis. This prevents the leg muscles acting as a venous return pump and causes chronic venous insufficiency. The erect posture then causes venous stagnation, increased venous pressure in the leg and chronic leg swelling. Red cells extravasate into the tissues

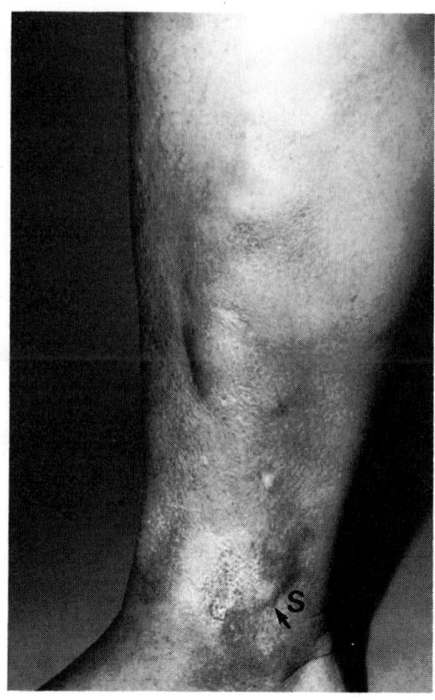

Fig. 26.4 Skin changes of chronic venous insufficiency

This 53-year-old woman suffered a deep vein thrombosis during her second pregnancy many years before. The leg is pigmented around the ankle and this tissue is woody to palpation (lipodermatosclerosis). The scar of a healed varicose ulcer **S** is seen above the medial malleolus

and haemosiderin deposits cause brown skin pigmentation. This condition, accompanied by dry, scaly, atrophic skin, is described as *varicose eczema* (see Figure 26.4).

Ulceration

Chronic ulceration of the lower limb is a common problem particularly in the elderly. The causes are summarised in Figure 26.5.

Fig. 26.5 Causes of chronic leg ulcers

Previous deep venous thrombosis
Varicose veins
Chronic arterial insufficiency
Diabetic neuropathy
Traumatic flap lacerations over shin
Pressure sores
Sensory neuropathies
Tropical and other infections
Malignant tumours

Effective treatment depends on clinical evaluation of the following factors, discussed in detail below:

• History of the origin and evolution of the ulcer

• The site of the ulcer

- The characteristics of the ulcer
- The nature of the surrounding tissues
- Relevant regional findings
- The patients general condition

History of the ulcer

Details of the initial skin lesion and the circumstances in which it occurred may provide diagnostic clues. *Minor trauma* may be the initiating incident but failure to heal can usually be attributed to abnormal skin nutrition. The causes include chronic venous insufficiency, arterial ischaemia and diabetic neuropathy. The ulcer often begins insidiously with minor breakdown in a patch of atrophic skin. In venous insufficiency, the skin often 'weeps' plasma.

In the elderly or in patients on long term steroid therapy, minor trauma to the tibia may produce a V-shaped *flap laceration*. This invariably fails to heal because of poor blood supply both to the flap and the underlying tissue. Suturing a flap laceration increases tension and compounds local ischaemia; the result is even greater tissue loss and ulceration. The most effective management is early excision of the flap and immediate split skin grafting.

In tropical countries, traumatic injuries and burns readily become infected. If they are not medically treated, these injuries develop into large chronic tropical ulcers. The infecting organisms are a mixture of spirochaetes and fusiform bacteria.

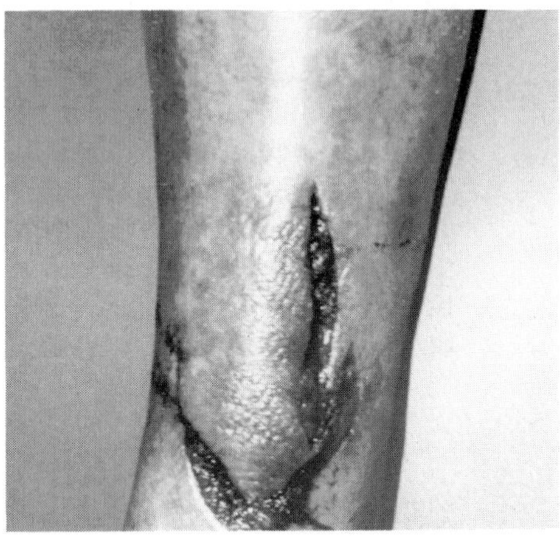

Fig. 26.6 Flap laceration

This wound was caused by a fall in which the patient's shin was scraped on a stone step. It is tempting to suture such a wound but if this is done, the flap will invariably undergo necrosis. Most of these types of wounds require split skin grafting

The duration of the ulcer, its healing, and subseqent recurrence or other changes give further clues to the diagnosis. Ischaemic ulcers present early because pain soon becomes intolerable and the ulcer refuses to heal. In contrast, post-thrombotic and varicose ulcers are rarely painful and usually fluctuate between healing and breakdown. Rarely, squamous carcinoma develops in a longstanding ulcer and is recognised by proliferative change at the ulcer margin. These are known as *Marjolin's ulcers* and were first described following burns which failed to heal. Primary skin malignancies on the leg may ulcerate, but these usually begin as a skin lump.

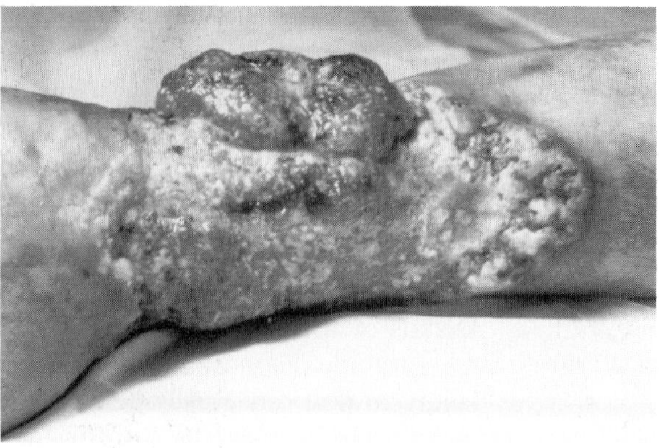

Fig. 26.7 Squamous carcinoma developing in a chronic venous ulcer

If a patient with a leg ulcer has claudication or rest pain, this suggests an ischaemic cause. Diabetic ulcers tend to be painless because of a sensory neuropathy (which may be the main predisposing cause). Previous deep venous thrombosis makes venous insufficiency the likely cause.

Site of the ulcer

The site of the ulcer on the lower limb may reveal its cause. Post-thrombotic and varicose ulcers typically arise just above the medial malleolus (the 'gaiter' area) and may extend circumferentially around the leg. They rarely occur in other sites. Diabetic (neuropathic) ulcers always occur on the foot, either as perforating ulcers on the sole beneath the metatarsal heads or at other bony prominences; these include the toes, the ball of the great toe and the malleoli.

Ulcers due to arterial insufficiency may occur anywhere below the mid calf, including the usual sites of venous or diabetic ulcers. *Pressure ulcers* occur mainly in debilitated, elderly or unconscious patients, especially at the back of the heel (see Figure 33.9, later). Even minutes in one position on a hard casualty trolley or operating theatre table may initiate skin necrosis. Pressure ulcers usually begin as a well-circumscribed patch of skin discolouration, which becomes necrotic and later ulcerates. The heels of vulnerable patients should be regularly inspected to avoid this complication.

Characteristics of the ulcer

Most ulcers are shallow, involving only the skin and subcutaneous fat. Diabetic ulcers, however, tend to penetrate deeply into the foot, where there is underlying necrotic and infected tissue. The base of any ulcer usually contains slough and fibrin but granulation tissue may be visible beneath. The slough should not be removed unless arterial insufficiency can be excluded, as this could aggravate ischaemia. If there is proliferating tissue in the ulcer, this should be biopsied.

The edge of most chronic lower limb ulcers slopes towards the base with no specific diagnostic features, although epithelial proliferation inwards from the edge suggests healing. Diabetic ulcers have a characteristic 'punched-out' edge with abrupt transition from normal skin to the necrotic crater. Malignant ulcers may have a raised margin.

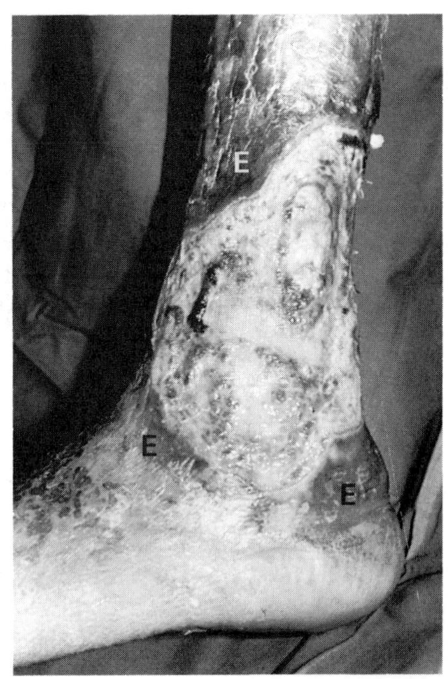

Fig. 26.8 Varicose ulcer

This shows the lateral part of an enormous ulcer which virtually encircles the ankle; note the surrounding varicose eczema **E**. The patient, an elderly woman, had suffered a deep venous thrombosis in her 20s soon after her first child was born. This ulcer was painless but discharged coplous inflammatory exudate and was chronically infected with *Pseudomonas*

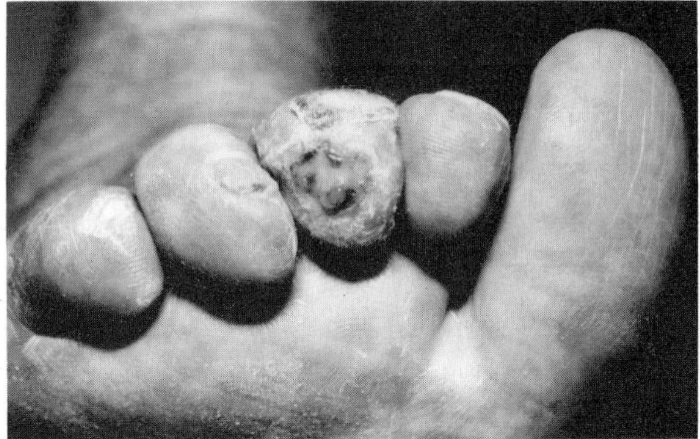

Fig. 26.9 Ischaemic ulcer

Punched-out ulcer on the tip of the third toe in a patient with severe rest pain. The foot was pale and cool. No pulses were palpable below the femoral and the ankle systolic pressure, measured by Doppler ultrasound, was 30 mmHg

Nature of the surrounding tissues

The characteristics of the surrounding tissues indicate the background on which the ulcer has formed. These characteristics include colour, texture and perfusion (shown by temperature, blanching response, venous filling and Buerger's test) as well as swelling and pigmentation.

Regional features

Regional examination should search for diagnostic clues, e.g. inguinal lymphadenopathy (infection or malignancy), varicose veins or superficial venous thrombosis.

The patient's general state of health

General history and examination may give diagnostic clues but are easily overlooked. Cardiac failure or arrhythmias may contribute to both arterial and venous insufficiency. Maturity onset diabetes may have recently developed, so the urine and blood sugar should always be tested. A diagnosis of diabetes may not mean that diabetic neuropathy is the cause of the ulceration; diabetics often have accelerated atherosclerosis and therefore arterial ulcers. Neuropathic complications and secondary infection are also common.

Swelling of the lower limb

Swelling of the lower limb may be bilateral or unilateral. The causes are summarised in Figure 26.10. Systemic causes, and conditions listed under 'sluggish venous return' cause bilateral swelling. The other causes tend to produce swelling of only one limb. Most causes of unilateral swelling are chronic and painless, except for acute deep venous thrombosis and cellulitis.

Fig. 26.10 Causes of swelling of the lower limb

a. Local causes

Sluggish venous return, e.g. immobility, pregnancy, prolonged sitting in a chair, inefficient calf muscle pump (paralysis due to polio or paraplegia)
Acute obstruction of venous return, e.g. deep venous thrombosis
Destruction of valves in deep venous system following previous deep venous thrombosis
Congenital lymphatic aplasia or hypoplasia, e.g. Milroy's disease
Cellulitis (usually streptococcal)
Lymphatic obstruction by filariasis (in tropical Africa)

b. Regional causes

Venous obstruction by pelvic mass, e.g. advanced pregnancy, ovarian cyst, pelvic malignancy
Lymphatic obstruction by malignant involvement of inguinal or more proximal nodes or after block dissection or radiotherapy
Inferior vena caval obstruction

c. Systemic causes

Congestive or right-sided cardiac failure
Hypoalbuminaemia e.g. malnutrition, nephrotic syndrome
Fluid overload

ARTERIAL DISORDERS OF THE LOWER LIMB — SPECIFIC CLINICAL ENTITIES AND THEIR MANAGEMENT

CHRONIC LOWER LIMB ISCHAEMIA

Chronic lower limb ischaemia presents as either intermittent claudication or severe ischaemia. The latter causes rest pain, ulceration or gangrene.

Intermittent claudication

Intermittent claudication is the classical symptom of chronic lower limb ischaemia with cramping pain in the lower limb muscles on walking which is quickly relieved by rest. The calf is almost always involved, but in more proximal arterial disease, the pain ascends into the thigh or even buttock if walking continues. On resting, the pain resolves within a minute or two, after which the patient can walk a similar distance before the pain recurs. The *claudication distance* may range from 50 to several hundred metres; once established, it remains remarkably constant.

The first symptoms appear unexpectedly and are often attributed to musculoskeletal causes. When symptoms persist for several weeks or more, the patient seeks medical advice. Most patients are male, aged from 50–70 years and are in otherwise good health. There may be a history of myocardial infarction or angina. Nearly all are, or have been, cigarette smokers. Claudication may be precipitated by polycythaemia, or by beta adrenergic blocking drugs, which are often prescribed in such patients to control hypertension.

Local examination is usually unremarkable, apart from absent peripheral pulses on the affected side. The dorsalis pedis, posterior tibial and popliteal pulses are almost invariably absent, and the femoral pulse is absent in about 25% of patients. Systematic examination should seek other signs of atherosclerosis, as summarised in Figure 26.11. These may have an important bearing on management and prognosis.

Fig. 26.11 General examination of the arteriopath

Observe whether the patient can lie flat during examination (? orthopnoea)

Inspect skin and mucous membranes for signs of polycythaemia, anaemia or cyanosis

Examine for signs of cardiac failure — jugular venous pressure and lung bases

Auscultate for cardiac murmurs

Auscultate for arterial bruits in carotids, subclavians (in supraclavicular fossa), renals (in epigastrium or posteriorly in loins), mesenterics (in epigastrium) and femorals

Measure blood pressure in both arms

Palpate the abdomen for aortic aneurysm

Inspect skin of legs for ischaemic changes and signs of arterial embolism

The natural history of intermittent claudication

About one third of patients experience spontaneous remission of all or most of their symptoms over a year or two without any treatment. A further third remain stable in the long term, with tolerable symptoms. The remaining third are either severely disabled by restriction of walking ability or else progress to more severe ischaemic symptoms like rest pain. Indeed, about 10% of the total would progress to necrosis and amputation if untreated. It is well established that stopping cigarette smoking greatly improves the outcome.

Epidemiological studies show that patients with intermittent claudication have only half the life expectancy of unaffected people of the same age. Most die of other manifestations of atherosclerosis such as ischaemic heart disease and stroke.

When reconstructive arterial surgery became more widespread in the 1960s, most patients with moderate or severe claudication were considered to need surgical treatment. Since then, better understanding of the natural remission rate of intermittent claudication, and its benign nature as regards limb loss, has led to a great reduction in the proportion of patients offered surgery.

Critical ischaemia and rest pain

Critical ischaemia is defined as arterial insufficiency severe enough to threaten the viability of the foot or leg. It may develop suddenly and acutely from embolic or thrombotic occlusion of major distributing vessels, in which case it demands surgical treatment within hours. More commonly, critical ischaemia develops insidiously over days or weeks. The cause is progression of atherosclerotic narrowing, so that arterial blood flow can barely maintain adequate tissue oxygenation and nutrition.

The first manifestations of critical ischaemia develop in the skin of the foot; these include:

- Rest pain
- Failure of trivial injuries to heal
- Extreme vulnerability of ischaemic feet to pressure sores
- Patchy skin necrosis
- Development of ischaemic ulcers

Critical ischaemia may develop after a period of deteriorating intermittent claudication. More commonly, there is no history of claudication. In general, patients are older and less physically active than typical claudicants. If left untreated, a small proportion of patients will improve slightly (probably as more collateral vessels open up) but the majority progress to extensive necrosis. Once deeper tissues of the foot become necrotic, local defences are overwhelmed. The result is spreading infection (wet gangrene) and ultimately, death from septicaemia. This sequence of events is rarely permitted to run its full course since rest pain usually becomes so severe that vascular reconstruction or amputation becomes essential. Extremely elderly debilitated patients may be managed with opiate analgesia as for the terminally ill, since any form of surgery would be likely to be fatal.

Approach to investigation and management of chronic lower limb ischaemia

The treatment options for chronic lower limb ischaemia range from advice about smoking, through drug therapy and minor surgical procedures to extensive reconstructive operations. These are summarised in Figure 26.12. The approach to treatment is usually decided after initial clinical assessment; further investigation is then decided according to treatment options.

Fig. 26.12 Treatment options for chronic lower limb ischaemia

Mild to moderate claudication
No active treatment except advice to stop smoking or lose weight

Disabling claudication

Balloon angioplasty

Reconstructive arterial surgery

Critical ischaemia

Intravenous drug therapies, such as prostacycline, vasodilators (naftidrofuryl oxalate)

Lumbar sympathectomy (surgical or by phenol injection)

Balloon angioplasty

Reconstructive arterial surgery

Amputation (below, through or above knee)

Terminal pain relief

a. Mild to moderate claudication

Most patients with mild or moderate claudication do not require reconstructive surgery. The symptoms often improve spontaneously, especially if the patient stops smoking and loses excess weight. Simple advice to walk more slowly will often greatly extend the claudication distance. Care of the feet and appropriate footwear should be strongly emphasised.

Numerous oral 'vasodilator' drugs are prescribed for claudication but none has withstood critical evaluation and they are not recommended.

Investigation of this group of patients is usually unnecessary apart from a full blood count to exclude *polycythaemia* and *thrombocythaemia*. In polycythaemia rubra vera, soft thrombi can develop in the lower limb and cause arterial insufficiency. Systemic manifestations of atherosclerosis, such as hypertension, angina or arrhythmias, should be investigated and treated if appropriate.

b. Disabling claudication

The main indications for further investigation of claudication are symptoms severe enough to warrant surgical intervention. Worrying symptoms are marked exercise restriction in younger patients or markedly worsening symptoms, especially if they are associated with proximal arterial obstruction (as shown by absent femoral pulses). Treatment is by balloon angioplasty or reconstructive surgery.

The simplest investigation is walking the patient along a corridor to test claudication distance. Resting ankle systolic blood pressure can be measured using a *Doppler ultrasound blood flow detector*. Ankle pressure in patients with claudication usually ranges from 50–120 mmHg, whereas normal pressure is slightly above systolic pressure measured at the brachial artery. More sophisticated evaluation uses a motorised treadmill and measurements of ankle pressures before and after exercise (see Figure 26.13). The drop in ankle pressure after exercise gives an indication of the severity of arterial disease. In some hospitals, all claudicants are investigated in this way as a baseline evaluation. This allows objective assessment of further disease and the response to conservative or operative treatment.

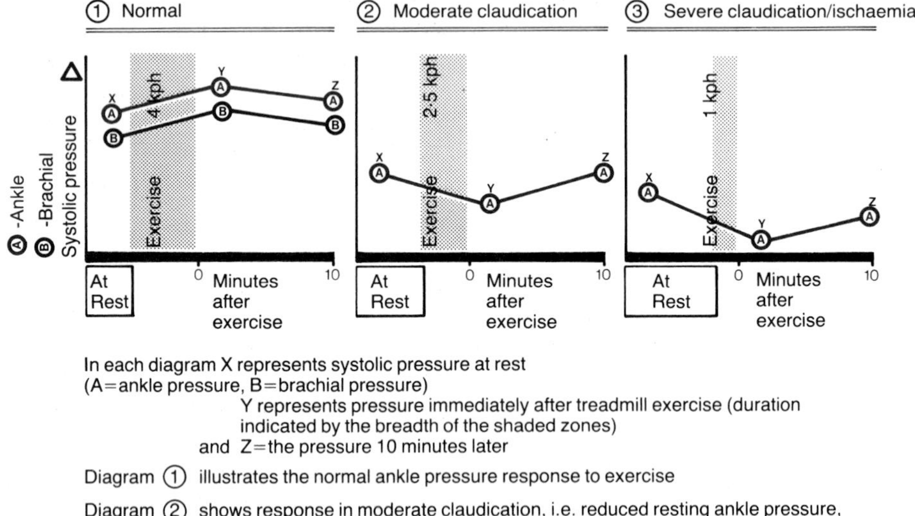

Fig. 26.13 Ankle pressure response to exercise in intermittent claudication

In each diagram X represents systolic pressure at rest (A=ankle pressure, B=brachial pressure)
Y represents pressure immediately after treadmill exercise (duration indicated by the breadth of the shaded zones)
and Z=the pressure 10 minutes later

Diagram ① illustrates the normal ankle pressure response to exercise

Diagram ② shows response in moderate claudication, i.e. reduced resting ankle pressure, reduced exercise tolerance, ankle pressure fall and recovery within 10 minutes

Diagram ③ shows the response in severe claudication or severe ischaemia

c. Critical ischaemia

In patients with critical ischaemia, Doppler measurement of resting ankle pressures is useful; these patients can rarely walk enough to test exercise tolerance. Resting ankle systolic pressure in these patients is rarely above 60 mmHg; a pressure below 40 mmHg indicates impending gangrene.

Arteriography

Arteriography is often wrongly used for assessment of chronic arterial insufficiency. It does not measure the rate of blood flow to the tissues, nor the dynamic circulatory responses to exercise. Arteriography does provide a two-dimensional map of the arterial system, and demonstrates the site and severity of vessel stenoses and occlusions. Arteriography should therefore be reserved for those patients in whom reconstructive surgery or balloon angioplasty is intended.

A recent development in angiography is electronic processing of the radiological image which 'subtracts' the bony image and enhances the arteriographic profile. Much smaller doses of contrast are required, which can be given intravenously rather than intra-arterially, thus simplifying the procedure. This technique, known as *digital subtraction angiography* (DSA), lacks the resolution of conventional arteriography but has several advantages. Because it is relatively non-invasive and therefore safer than conventional arteriography, it can be used repeatedly for disease follow up. It can also be used for screening of doubtful cases where conventional arteriography could not be justified.

Intravenous drug therapies

There are no drugs which can reverse atherosclerosis, but there has been extensive research into drugs to improve peripheral perfusion or tissue viability in the short term. The goal is to allow time for the natural development of a collateral circulation. A *guanethidine block*, given by intravenous injection into a limb excluded from the circulation by a tourniquet, sometimes gives temporary relief of rest pain. *Papaverine* has a similar but even more transient effect; it is sometimes used to treat acute arterial spasm. *Naftidrofuryl oxalate* and the prostaglandin, *prostacycline*, have shown encouraging results but their side effects, and the need for intravenous injection, have limited their usefulness. The race is now on to find an effective oral drug!

Sympathectomy

Blood flow in the skin (but not muscle) is controlled by the sympathetic nervous system. Thus, even if the major arterial supply is inadequate, rest pain in the skin may sometimes be relieved by *sympathetic blockade*. This can be performed by *surgical excision* of part of the lumbar sympathetic chain via an extraperitoneal approach or, less invasively, by *translumbar injection of 6% aqueous phenol*. This is done under local anaesthesia and usually with radiographic control.

Unfortunately, only about 15% of patients obtain sufficient relief of symptoms to avoid a reconstructive operation or amputation. Regrettably, there is no way of selecting in advance those who will benefit. Sympathectomy is often helpful in healing ulcers where ischaemia is present with some other factor such as chronic venous insufficiency, but it is of no proven value in intermittent claudication.

Balloon angioplasty

In the 1950s, Dotter experimented with techniques for dilatating local arterial stenoses with graded metal bougies. For technical reasons, the methods were not widely adopted. More recently, *Gruntzig* developed a balloon dilatation technique in which a polythene balloon, incorporated in the end of a catheter, is introduced percutaneously into the femoral artery. The balloon is placed across the stenosis using a guide wire under arteriographic control. The balloon is finally inflated to a high pressure, crushing the atheroma into the arterial wall and relieving the obstruction. The technique is effective for isolated short stenoses, particularly in the iliac vessels, and avoids the need for major surgery in many patients. Unfortunately, the method is less useful for distal vessels. A similar technique is increasingly used for localised coronary artery stenosis instead of coronary artery bypass surgery.

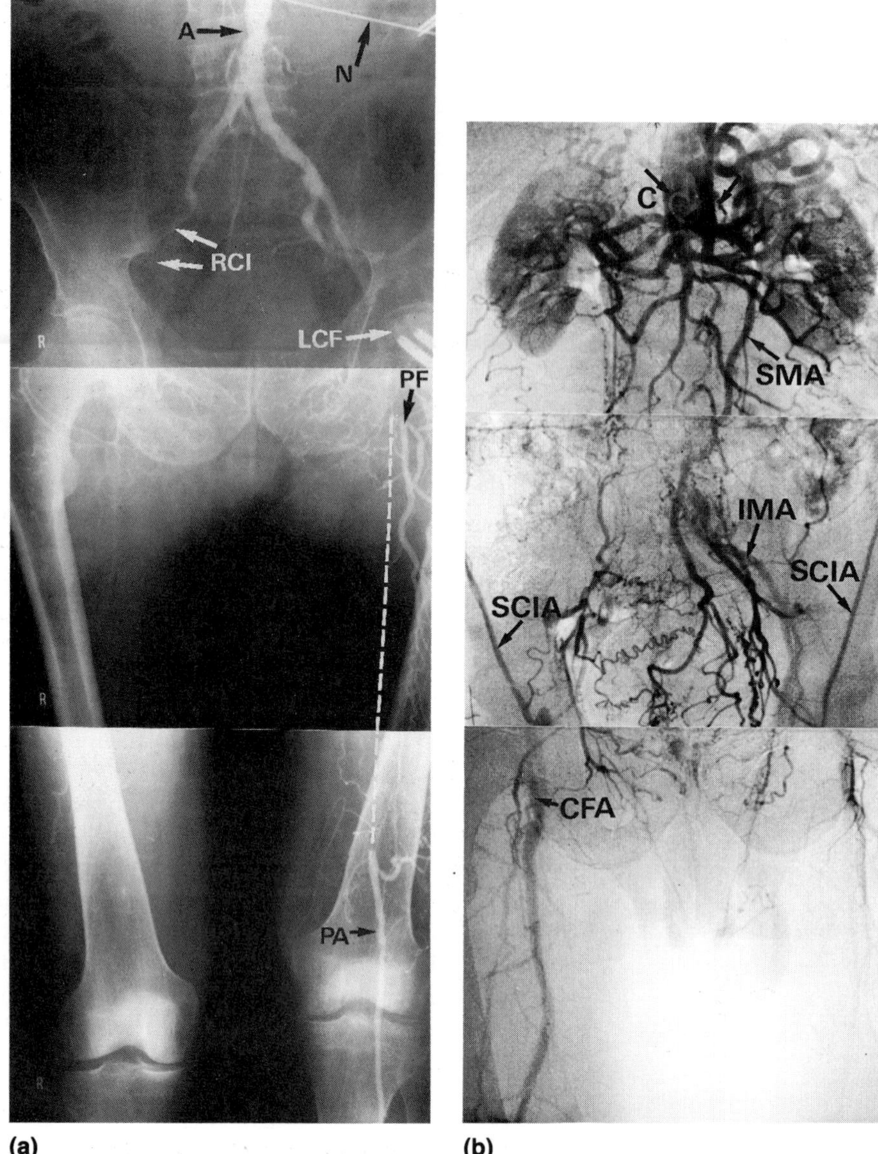

Fig. 26.14 Typical patterns of arterial disease

(a) This 71-year-old man presented with ischaemic rest pain in his right foot and severe bilateral intermittent claudication. Neither femoral pulse was palpable and so this aortogram was performed by the translumbar route with the patient prone. The needle **N** punctured the aorta directly from the left paraspinal area. There is atherosclerotic irregularity in the lower aorta **A** and complete occlusion of the right common iliac **RCI** and left common femoral **LCF** arteries. Note the two screws visible in the left femoral head to fix a previous fractured neck of femur. On the right, there is very little collateral filling of distal vessels. On the left, the profunda femoris **PF** reconstitutes well by collaterals and, although the left superficial femoral artery is occluded (its course indicated by a broken line), the proximal popliteal artery **PA** also reconstitutes well via collaterals. **(b)** This arteriogram is a composite of several

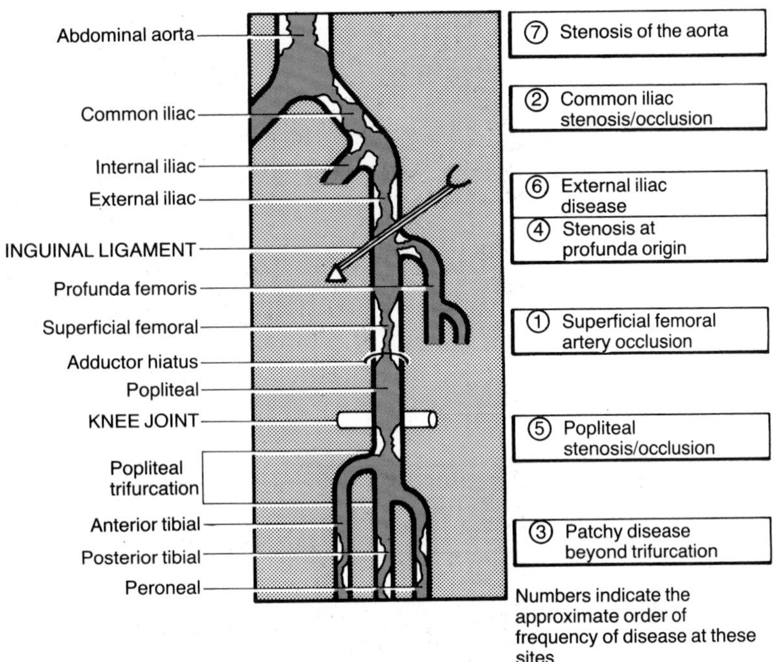

Fig. 26.14 (cont.)
subtraction films from a 63-year-old man who presented with severe bilateral intermittent claudication. His feet were well perfused at rest but his femoral pulses were not palpable. To inject contrast, a pigtail catheter **C** was placed in the aorta via the brachial artery. A complete occlusion of the aorta is demonstrated (arrowed) just below the renal arteries. The lower half of the body is thus completely supplied by collateral vessels from the superior mesenteric artery **SMA**, the inferior mesenteric artery **IMA** and lumbar arteries. Note the common femoral artery **CFA** is reconstituted by collaterals, mainly the superficial circumflex iliac arteries **SCIA**

Arterial reconstructive surgery

Arterial reconstructive surgery began in the 1950s with the open removal of atheromatous plaques and organised surface thrombus from the aorta and iliac arteries. This technique, known as *thrombo-endarterectomy*, is technically difficult and time-consuming. It has largely been replaced by *bypass grafting*, although endarterectomy remains the standard operation for carotid artery stenosis (see later).

Arterial bypass grafting was first developed during the Korean war to treat arterial trauma, using homografts from human cadavers. The initial results were excellent but within a few years, the grafts suffered from aneurysmal dilatation and rupture. This led to the use of synthetic graft materials, which are now available in a wide variety of shapes, sizes and cloths. *Knitted polyester* (Dacron) is the most popular and is the standard graft material for treating aorto-iliac obstruction.

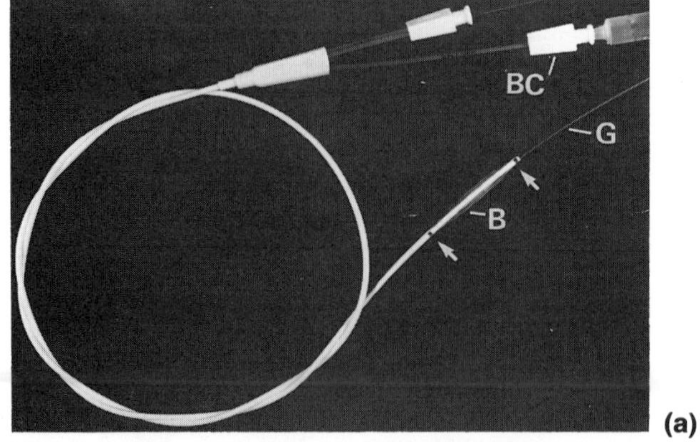

(a)

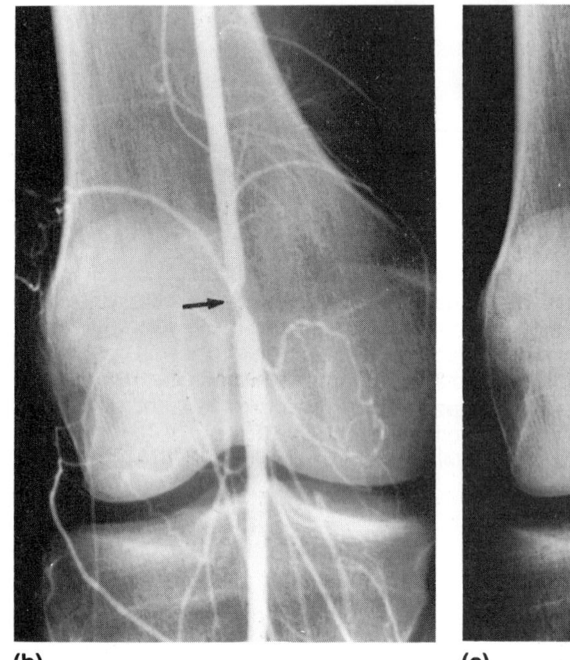

(b)

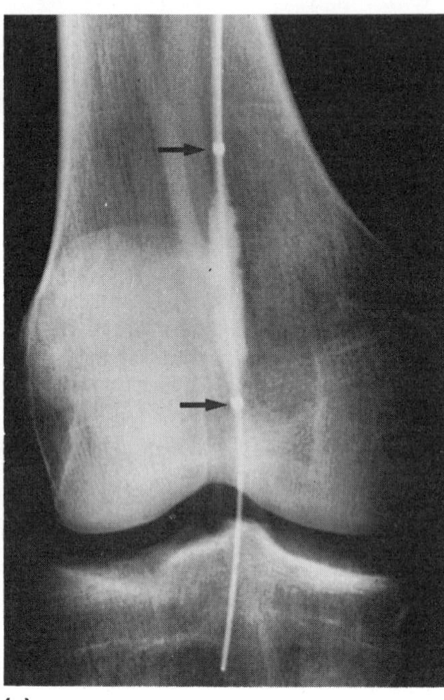

(c)

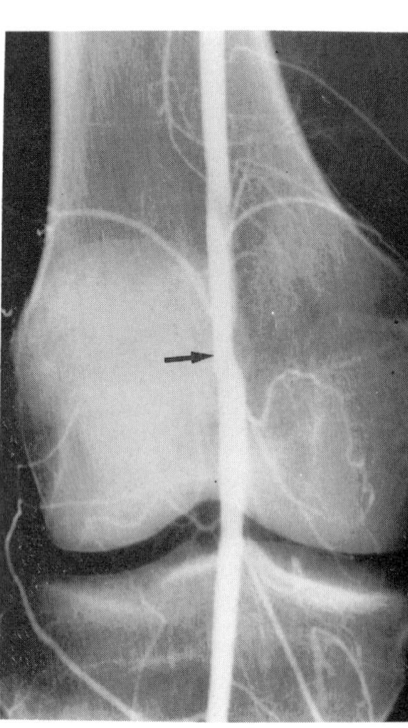

(d)

Fig. 26.15 Percutaneous transluminal angioplasty

(a) Balloon angioplasty equipment. This catheter is used for balloon dilatation of arterial stenoses. First, an artery some distance from the stenosis (usually the femoral) is punctured with a needle. A flexible guide-wire **G** is passed through the needle, along the artery and manipulated across the stenosis. The catheter is then threaded over the guide-wire until the distal balloon **B** (made of non-stretch polythene) lies within the stenosis. The balloon is then inflated to high pressure using a special syringe attached to the balloon channel **BC**. Note the radiopaque markers (arrowed) at each end of the balloon to allow it to be sited radiographically (these are also visible in Figure 26.16(b)). **(b)–(d)** Arteriograms from a 49-year-old woman presenting with ischaemic rest pain in her first toe and intermittent claudication in the calf. **(b)** Highly localised stenosis of popliteal artery (arrowed). **(c)** Gruntzig balloon catheter inflated within the stenosis; radiopaque markers at each end of balloon (arrowed) **(d)** Angiographic appearance after balloon catheter removed, showing marked improvement in stenosis (arrowed)

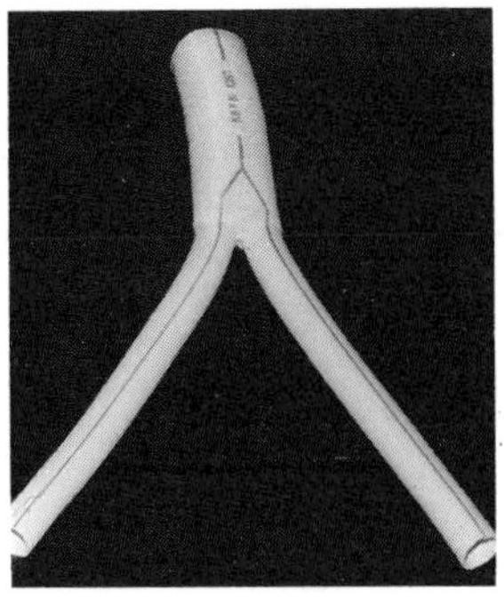

Fig. 26.16 Trouser graft for aorto-bifemoral disease

A Dacron bifurcation graft or prosthesis is used to bypass the aorto-iliac segment when it is occluded or stenosed, or to replace it when it is aneurysmal. Note the guide-line down each limb which is to ensure they are not twisted during anastomosis

Aorto-iliac disease

The most common operation for aorto-iliac obstruction is the insertion of a *trouser graft* between the infrarenal aorta and the common femoral arteries just below the inguinal ligament. Each 'trouser leg' is sewn to a femoral artery, and the diseased vessels are left in situ posteriorly (see Figure 26.17).

Femoro-popliteal disease

The other common obstruction of lower limb vessels is of the superficial femoral artery. This is relieved by connecting the patient's long saphenous vein between the common femoral artery and the popliteal artery; this is known as *autogenous femoropopliteal bypass grafting*. The usual technique is first to dissect out the long saphenous vein from groin to knee and ligate its tributaries. The vein graft is then inserted in reverse so the valves do not obstruct flow. If there is no vein suitable for grafting, synthetic materials can be used, but these have a lower long term survival. A vein graft is therefore always the first choice.

Recently, a method of vein grafting has been developed for more distal bypasses which leaves the long saphenous vein in situ. The natural taper of the vein thus remains from proximal to distal. In this technique, the valves are destroyed with a wire device known as a *valvulotome*. This method allows bypasses down to the tibial or even dorsalis pedis arteries, thus treating distal disease that was previously inoperable.

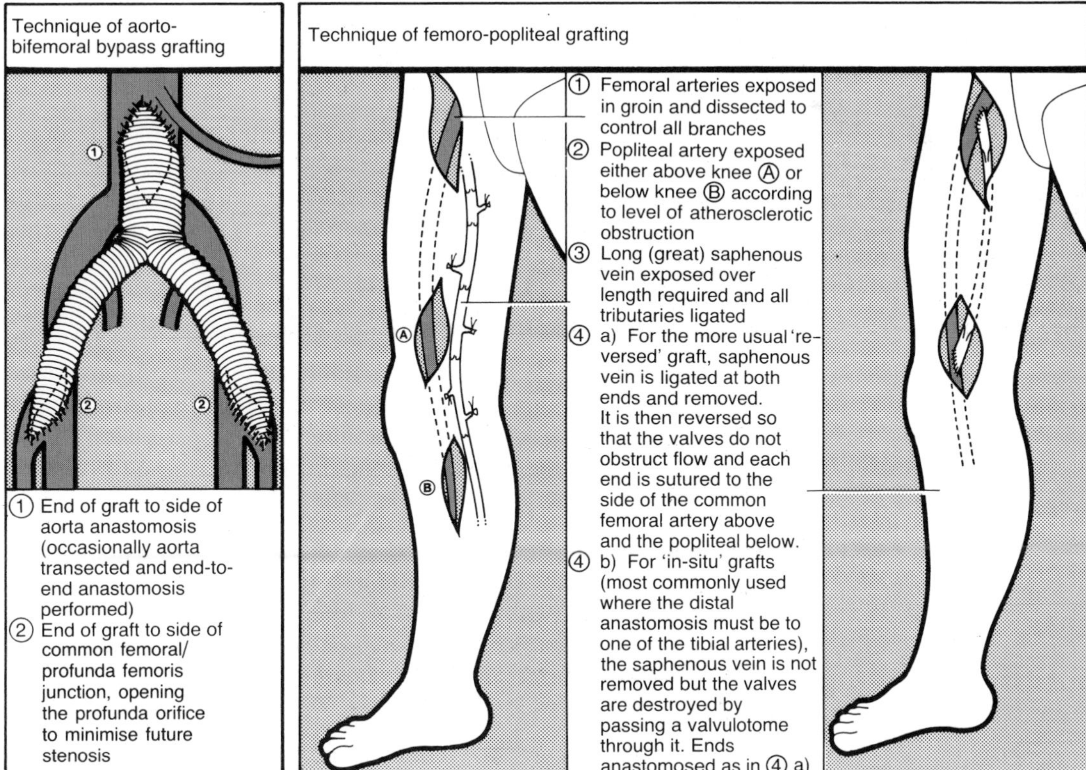

Fig. 26.17 Arterial bypass grafting

Fig. 26.18 Summary — complications of arterial surgery

Complications of generalised arteriopathy — myocardial ischaemia, cerebrovascular accidents, renal failure and intestinal ischaemia

Haemorrhage — arterial or venous

Thrombosis of the reconstructed vessels leading to profound distal ischaemia (usually a technical fault)

Embolism into renal vessels or limb vessels (particularly aneurysm surgery)

Graft infection

False aneurysm formation

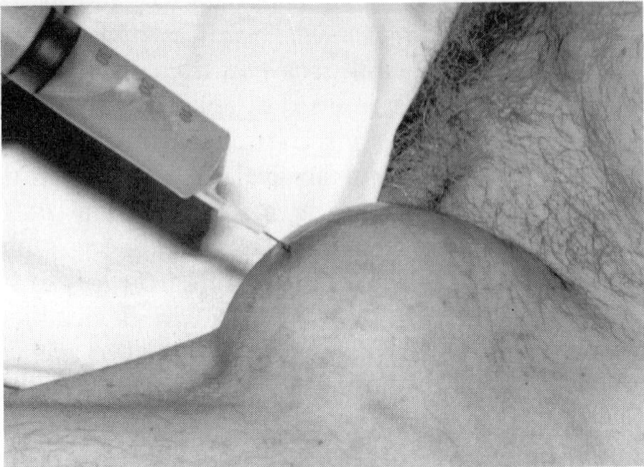

Lymphocoele in groin following graft to femoral artery. Any operation in the region of the inguinal lymph nodes can interfere with lymphatic drainage and cause an accumulation of lymph known as a lymphocoele. In this case, the lymphocoele was aspirated periodically and finally stopped refilling about six months after the original operation

Amputation

Reconstructive surgery may not be technically possible in some patients, especially those with diffuse distal arterial disease. For these patients, there may be no alternative to amputation. Reconstructive surgery is futile if there is substantial tissue necrosis and a functionally useless foot, or if there is deep spreading infection.

Two principles guide the level of amputation:

- The amputation must be made through healthy tissue. If not, there is a high risk of wound breakdown and chronic ulceration, requiring further amputation at a higher level. When amputation is for peripheral ischaemia, it is almost always necessary to amputate at mid-tibial level or above to ensure healing
- The choice of amputation level must take into account the fitting of a prosthetic limb. For this purpose, the mid-tibia (*below knee*) and lower femoral levels (*above knee*) are preferred. If the knee joint can be saved, the functional success of a prosthesis is much better. With improved prostheses, there is a renewal of interest in *through knee* amputation

The traditional 'guillotine' amputation of the battlefield simply sliced off the limb, leaving the wound to heal by secondary intention. This reduced the risk

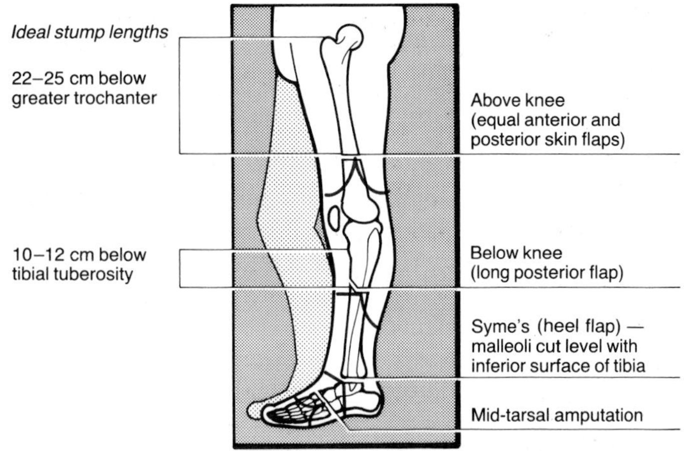

Fig. 26.19 (a) Sites of election for lower limb amputations

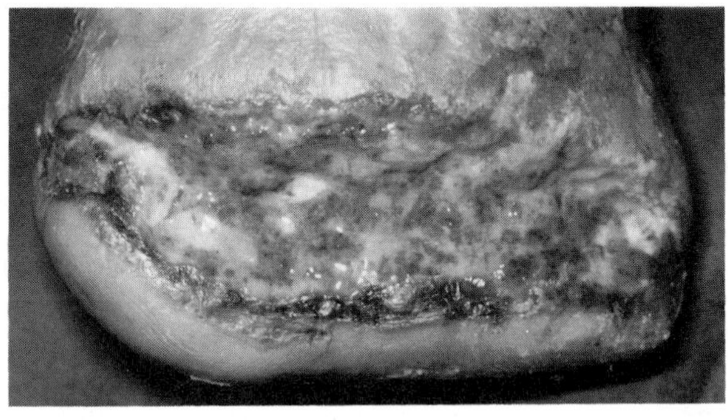

(b) Ischaemic breakdown of an amputation stump three weeks after operation. There was insufficient arterial supply to allow this to heal and an above-knee amputation had then to be performed

of fatal gas gangrene or tetanus but left a poor result for fitting an artificial limb prosthesis.

There have been considerable developments in amputation techniques in recent years. For below knee amputations, a *long posterior flap* of muscle and skin is now wrapped forward over the amputated bone and sutured in place. This results in more reliable healing and a suitably shaped and cushioned stump.

For above knee amputations, a *myoplastic flap* technique is used in which the bony amputation level is just proximal to the musculo-cutaneous amputation level. This allows the muscles to be sutured over the exposed bone end, after which the short anterior and posterior skin flaps are closed over the muscle.

ACUTE LOWER LIMB ISCHAEMIA

Pathophysiology

The lower limb may become acutely ischaemic as a result of embolism or *thrombosis*.

If a large embolus impacts in a major distributing artery, the distal blood supply is abruptly cut off. An alternative collateral network has not developed because the distal arteries are not atherosclerotic and the ischaemia is therefore all the more severe. Most large emboli originate in the heart, caused by atrial fibrillation or mitral stenosis (left atrial thrombus), or myocardial infarction (mural thrombus).

Sudden acute ischaemia may also develop if an essential distributing artery, already narrowed by atherosclerosis, becomes completely obstructed by thrombosis of its lumen. Another cause is thrombosis of a popliteal aneurysm. Occasionally, widespread thrombosis occurs in normal arteries causing acute ischaemia. This was well recognised as a complication of the *high oestrogen contraceptive pill* when it was in common use. Similar widespread thrombosis is sometimes seen as a complication of *polycythaemia rubra vera*, *thrombocythaemia* or *leukaemia*.

Emboli usually impact where the arterial lumen narrows abruptly. Impaction is especially common at branching points, in particular the aortic bifurcation (*saddle embolus*), the common femoral bifurcation and the popliteal trifurcation. Acute thrombotic occlusion causes the most catastrophic results when it occurs in the popliteal artery (which has few useful collaterals), the external iliac/common femoral arterial trunk (the axial blood supply of the lower limb) or the profunda femoris (if the superficial femoral artery is already occluded).

Clinical features of acute lower limb ischaemia

The clinical presentation of acute lower limb ishaemia is sudden onset of a cold, white foot, extending a variable distance up the leg. Nerve ischaemia causes loss of sensation and paralysis but pain may be severe at the margin of the ischaemic area. Complete numbness indicates total cessation of blood flow (the five P's — see earlier).

It is crucial that the diagnosis of complete arterial occlusion is recognised quickly because the resulting ischaemia is usually so profound that infarction occurs within hours unless urgent treatment is undertaken. Unfortunately, because pain is often not a dominant feature, the urgency of the situation may not be appreciated by the patient, nursing staff or inexperienced doctors. The onset of infarction is marked by a mottled dusky blue discolouration of the affected area. Later, the skin becomes completely blue, with blistering after about 24 hours. Infarction is irreversible.

Principles of management of the acutely ischaemic limb

Embolic ischaemia can usually be treated by the relatively simple operation of *embolectomy*. Thrombosis of diseased vessels, however, requires emergency reconstructive surgery. Distinction between these two conditions should be made before operation but this may not be possible in practice.

History and clinical examination may provide clues to the diagnosis. Evidence of mitral stenosis, an arrhythmia or recent myocardial infarction suggests embolism, whereas a history of claudication or a blood disorder points to thrombosis. Examination of the affected limb does not help to distinguish embolism from thrombosis, but the other limb provides evidence of the general condition of the peripheral arteries. For example, if the other limb is well perfused with good peripheral pulses and normal ankle systolic pressure, then

Fig. 26.20 Clinical features of acute severe lower limb ischaemia

Symptoms and signs suggesting a predisposing cause for acute ischaemia (embolism or thrombosis)

Recent chest pain or other evidence of myocardial infarction

History of rheumatic heart disease

History or finding of atrial fibrillation

Previous arterial embolism

History of intermittent claudication or other symptoms of peripheral arterial disease

Polycythaemia rubra vera (prone to intravascular thrombosis)

Aortic aneurysm (possible source of embolism)

Symptoms suggesting acute lower limb ischaemia

Sudden onset of continuous pain, usually in one periphery

Sudden and persistent coldness, usually in one periphery

Suddden numbness or paraesthesia, usually in one periphery

Signs of acute lower limb ischaemia

Unexpected coldness of the peripheral part of one (or less commonly) both legs

Pallor or blueness of the periphery; in extreme cases, the fixed pigmentation of necrosis or skin blistering

Poor peripheral capillary return after pressure blanching

Strongly positive Buerger's test (pallor on elevation, slow return of redness on dependency)

Absent lower limb pulses (particularly if known to have been present before)

Undetectable ankle pulses by Doppler or very low ankle systolic pressure

embolus is more likely. If a *saddle embolus* has become lodged at the aortic bifurcation, then both limbs are involved, although one side is usually more affected than the other. The popliteal fossa must always be examined to exclude a thrombosed popliteal aneurysm.

Blood should be examined to exclude predisposing blood disorders and several units should be cross matched. As soon as possible, the patient should be *anticoagulated* with intravenous heparin to prevent propagation of thrombus proximal and distal to the occlusion. If the diagnosis is embolism, then anti-coagulation will usually be continued later with oral warfarin.

Arteriography should be performed before surgery to indicate the site and nature of the obstruction and to plan the appropriate operation. Unfortunately, expediency is often the excuse for omitting preoperative arteriography but its omission places the patient at greater risk.

Surgical management of acute lower limb ischaemia

Embolectomy is usually performed under local anaesthetic. A groin incision provides access to the arterial system. The femoral artery bifurcation is exposed, all the vessels are temporarily clamped and an incision (*arteriotomy*) is made

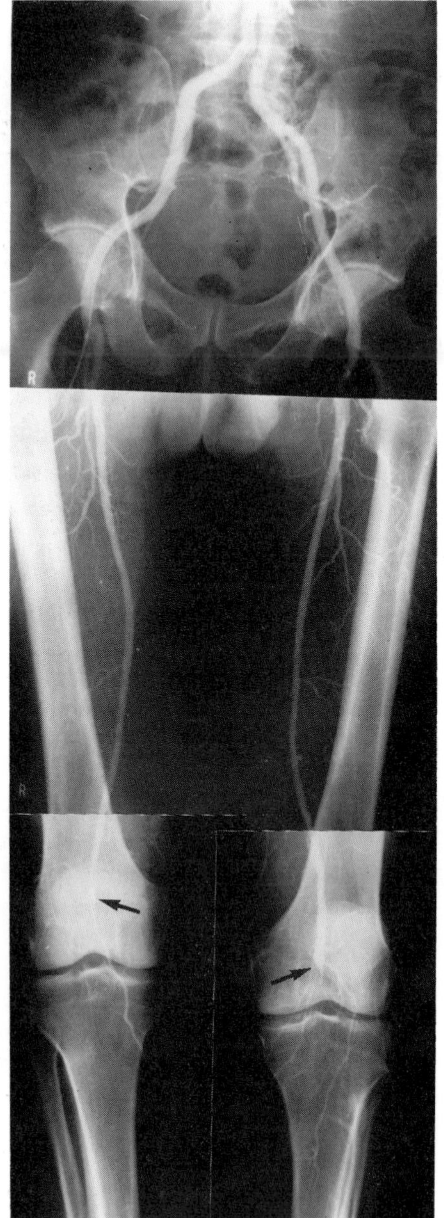

Fig. 26.21 Embolic occlusion of popliteal arteries

This 60-year-old woman presented as an emergency with critical ischaemia of both legs; she was known to have rheumatic mitral stenosis and atrial fibrillation. This aortogram was obtained by passing an arterial catheter via the right femoral artery until its tip lay above the aortic bifurcation. The iliac and femoral arteries are seen to be virtually normal but there is an abrupt occlusion (arrowed) in each popliteal artery, typical of embolism. The emboli were successfully retrieved by bilateral femoral embolectomy, immediately restoring the peripheral arterial circulation

in the common femoral artery. This in itself may reveal the obstructing clot. A *Fogarty balloon catheter* is then passed into each main vessel in turn. When the catheter has been passed as far as it will go, the balloon is inflated and the catheter drawn back to sweep out any obstructing clot. The operation is successful if clot is retrieved and blood flows back (*'back bleeding'*) from each vessel as it is unclamped. If embolectomy fails, arterial reconstruction is begun immediately.

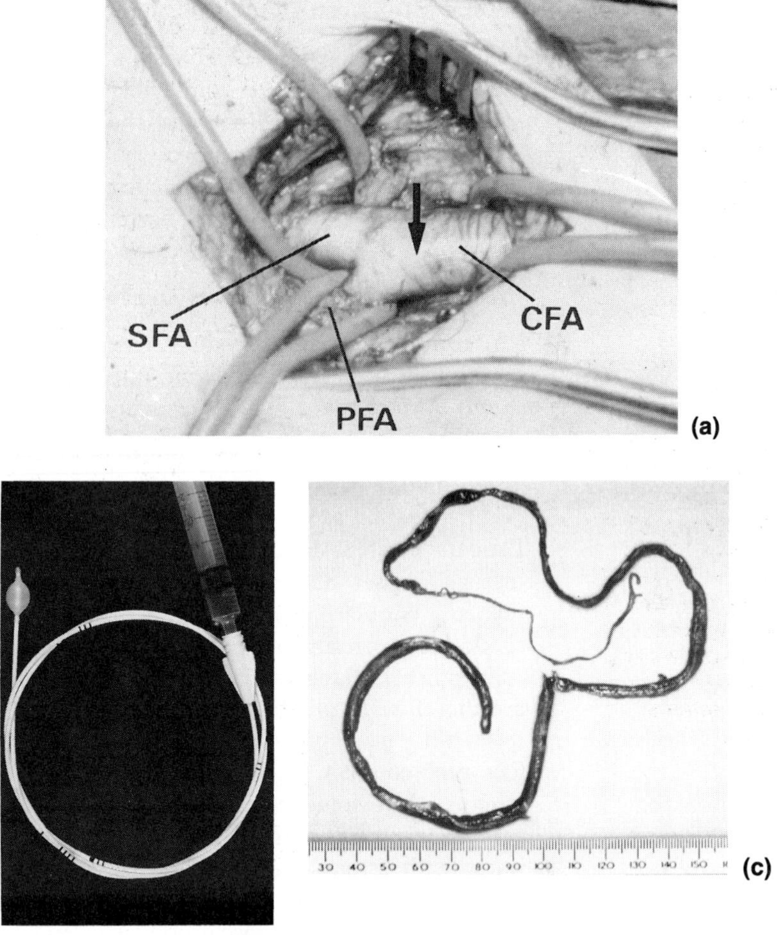

Fig. 26.22 Femoral artery embolectomy

(a) Surgical exposure of the femoral artery bifurcation, performed under local infiltration anaesthesia. The common femoral artery **CFA**, the profunda femoris **PFA** and the superficial femoral artery **SFA** are dissected cleanly and rubber slings placed around each artery. A transverse arteriotomy is made just proximal to the bifurcation (position arrowed); a Fogarty balloon catheter, shown in **(b)** is passed distally, the balloon gently inflated and the catheter withdrawn to extract embolic and thrombotic material. This is performed in stages until the catheter can be passed to ankle level and back-bleeding occurs. The procedure may have to be performed in a proximal direction as well. **(c)** An unusually long thrombus retrieved in this way

Most patients needing arterial reconstruction for acute ischaemia require a *femoropopliteal* or *femorotibial bypass* (see back to Figure 26.17).

For debilitated elderly patients who are surgically unfit, and who present with acute thrombotic ischaemia, it is worth considering treatment with *fibrinolytic agents*. Systemic treatment with streptokinase is dangerous and not recommended, but direct instillation into the clot is often successful. This is performed via an arterial catheter manoeuvred into place under radiological control from the other femoral artery. Dissolving the clot by this method usually takes 12–72 hours. Therefore, the technique is appropriate only if the degree of ischaemia will allow the limb to survive while treatment takes place.

THE DIABETIC FOOT

Pathophysiology

Diabetics are particularly prone to serious ulceration and infection of the feet. The primary disorder is believed to be within the microcirculation (*microangiopathy*).

Several factors contribute to diabetic foot problems:

- The microangiopathy is responsible for a peripheral neuropathy which affects motor, sensory and autonomic nerves. The affected motor nerves supply the small muscles of the foot and the consequent unmodified traction of calf muscles produces distortion of the morphology and weight bearing characteristics of the foot. Sensory neuropathy decreases awareness of injury from footwear and foreign bodies within shoes, and damaged autonomic nerves disrupt vascular control and cause loss of sweating
- Arterioles become narrowed and restrict capillary perfusion
- Arteriovenous communications open beneath the skin, diverting nutrient flow away from it. Damaged tissue thus heals poorly and is vulnerable to infection, even if the injury or pressure damage is only minor
- Impaired tissue energy metabolism and the glucose-rich tissue environment both favour bacterial growth

Patients most at risk of foot complications are elderly, poorly controlled, maturity onset diabetics and younger patients with long-standing type I diabetes. Similarly, patients with diabetic microangiopathic complications in the kidney or retina appear to have an increased risk of foot problems.

In general, diabetics have a marked predisposition to atherosclerosis. They are therefore at greater risk of arterial insufficiency. Atherosclerotic disease follows the usual pattern but tends to develop at a younger age. Most diabetic foot problems can be identified as being primarily neuropathic or a therosclerotic, but some patients have elements of both. This makes diagnosis and management more difficult. Typically, the *neuropathic foot* is red and warm with strong pulses, whereas the *atherosclerotic foot* is pale, cold and pulseless.

Management of atherosclerotic ischaemia is the same in diabetics as in non-diabetics. For mixed disease, the arterial insufficiency should usually be treated if there is to be any hope of healing.

Fig. 26.23 The problem of the diabetic foot

'Diabetic gangrene is not heaven-sent but earth-born' Joslin 1934

Four out of five patients with diabetic foot problems are type II diabetics

Foot problems are responsible for 47% of days spent in hospital by diabetics

Foot problems are responsible for 12% of all hospital admissions in internal medicine

In diabetics with new foot ulcers, 90% have peripheral neuropathy compared with 20% in a control group, whereas only 14% have peripheral arterial disease compared with 10% in controls (Miami 1983–4)

Patients with diabetic foot problems are incapacitated for an average of 16 weeks

Care and prevention of diabetic foot problems requires specialist surveillance and management by a dedicated team; foot ulceration in diabetics represents a failure of medical management

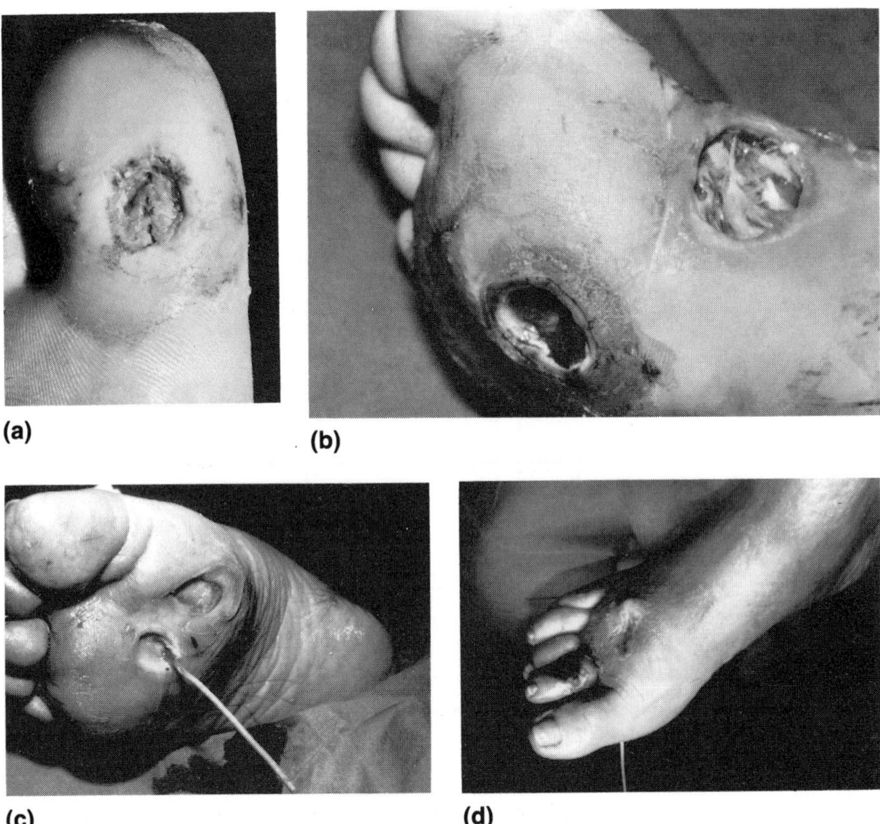

Fig. 26.24 Foot complications of diabetes
(a) Penetrating ulcer of the great toe in a young farmer with diabetic neuropathy. The ulcer was painless and contained necrotic slough. It healed after excision of the necrotic material and provision of special footwear to prevent undue pressure on the toe. **(b)** Chronic penetrating ulcers in a 60-year-old woman with maturity-onset diabetes. She had no evidence of major vessel disease but had signs of neuropathy. The deep ulcer beneath the head of the first metatarsal is characteristically surrounded with a thick keratin margin, and the ulcer on the medial side of the foot has an exposed tendon in its base. **(c)** and **(d)** Two penetrating ulcers in the sole of the foot. In (c), an ulcer is being probed and in (d), the probe can be seen to pass right through the foot to lift the skin of the dorsum. This demonstrates the extent of destruction of tissue by infection

Clinical presentations of diabetic foot complications

Foot complications of diabetes present in four main ways:

- *Painless, deeply penetrating ulcers*. These usually develop beneath the first metatarsal head or between the toes. The infecting organism is usually Staphylococcus aureus. The necrosis spreads up the web space and along the tendon sheaths. Spreading infection appears to be the predominant factor in tissue destruction
- *Painless necrosis of individual toes*. These first turn blue then later become black and mummified, and may eventually be shed spontaneously. Toe necrosis also occurs in non-diabetics with arterial insufficiency, but the diabetic necrotic toe is much more likely to become infected. If the infection is untreated, the whole limb is threatened.
- *Extensive spreading skin necrosis* associated with superficial or deep infection. This develops very rapidly and spreads proximally, threatening both limb and life
- *Chronic ulceration* of pressure points and sites of minor injury; skin perfusion is otherwise adequate

Management of the diabetic foot

a. Control of infection

As a general rule, control of infection is the first priority in the management of diabetic foot problems. Minor foot lesions in the diabetic should always be taken seriously and treated early with *oral antibiotics* and *frequent topical antiseptic cleansing*. Useful antiseptics include EUSOL, hydrogen peroxide and gentian violet.

If there is any sign of spreading infection or systemic involvement (i.e. fever, tachycardia or loss of diabetic control), the patient should be admitted to

Fig. 26.25

OPERATIONS FOR DIABETIC FEET

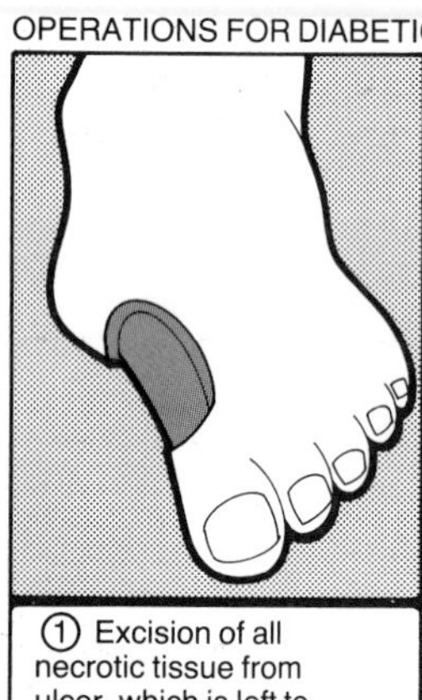

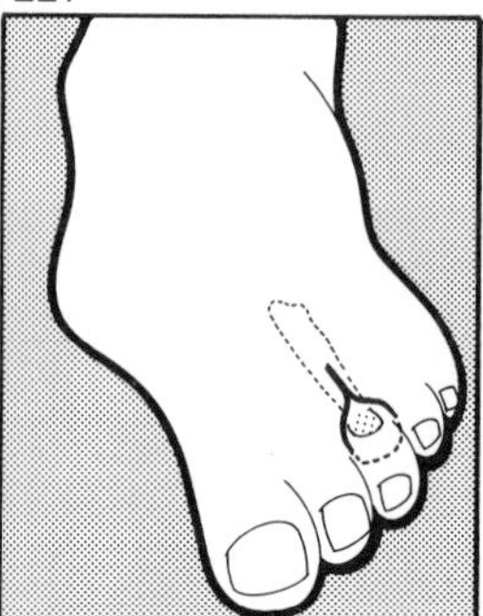

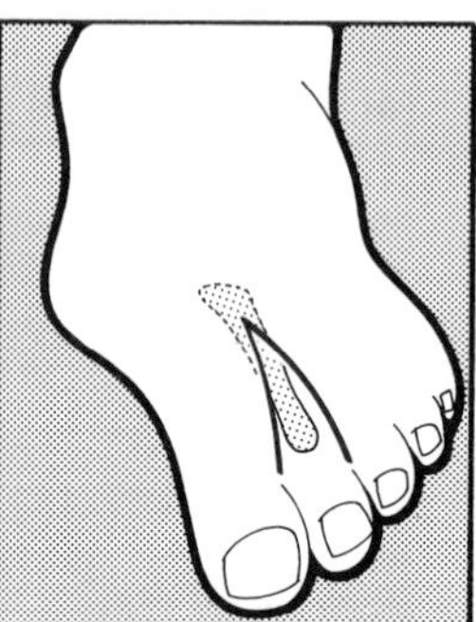

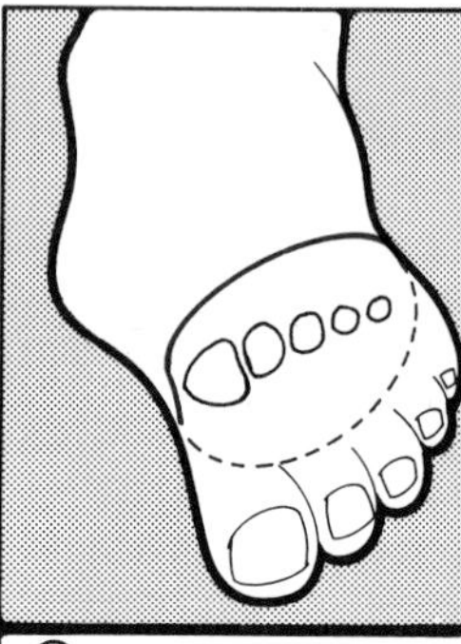

Note: The principle is to remove all necrotic tissue to eliminate infection and allow healing by secondary intention. Contrast amputations for ischaemia where level of amputation is determined by blood supply; this is not a problem in diabetic feet uncomplicated by atherosclerosis

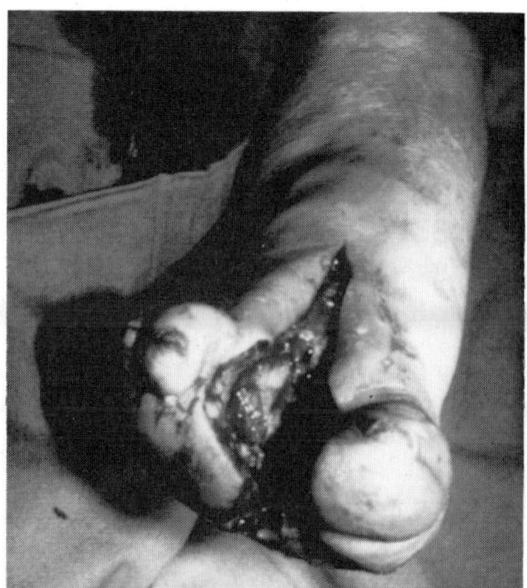

(a)

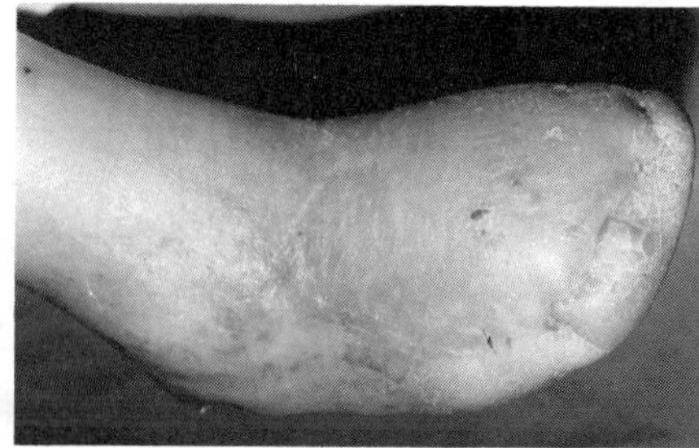

(b)

Fig. 26.25 Operations on the diabetic foot

(a) This is the same patient shown in 26.24(c) and (d). The second and third metatarsals have been excised, together with all the necrotic tissue. The wound was left open to heal by secondary intention, eventually giving a remarkably good functional result.

(b) Amputation of all toes in a patient with several necrotic diabetic toes. There was no evidence of large vessel disease

hospital for more intensive treatment. This includes parenteral antibiotics, excision of any necrotic tissue and attention to blood glucose control.

b. Removal of necrotic tissue

Surgery may involve anything from simple *desloughing* of an ulcer to major amputation. If performed correctly, these surgical procedures result in complete healing.

c. Prevention

All clinicians dealing with diabetics should place the highest priority on prevention. Detailed advice on self care should be given, and adequate chiropody services should be provided. Careful attention should be given to footwear, which may need to be specially made by a surgical fitter.

ANEURYSMS

Introduction

Aneurysms of the abdominal aorta, iliac, femoral and popliteal arteries are a complication of atherosclerosis. They are relatively uncommon, and are found mainly in patients over 70 years of age. At least a quarter of these patients have more than one aneurysm. In many patients with aneurysmal disease, all the major arteries tend to be of large diameter, but the aneurysm is a localised area of pathological excessive dilatation.

Atherosclerotic aneurysms are usually fusiform in shape, slowly expanding in diameter. As the aneurysm becomes larger, expansion accelerates with increasing risk of rupture. The majority of abdominal aortic aneurysms involve

Fig. 26.26

Patterns of aneurysm formation

Most patients with atherosclerotic aneurysms have only one but there is a tendency for most arteries to be somewhat dilated.

In at least 25% of cases there are other aneurysms either in continuity (common iliac, internal iliac) or not (femoral, 10%; popliteal, 20%)

It is rare for abdominal aortic aneurysms to extend above the renal arteries. Such cases represent a more demanding surgical procedure to replace

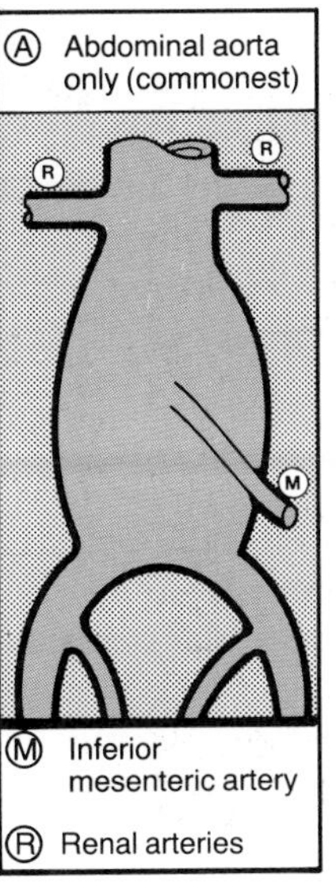

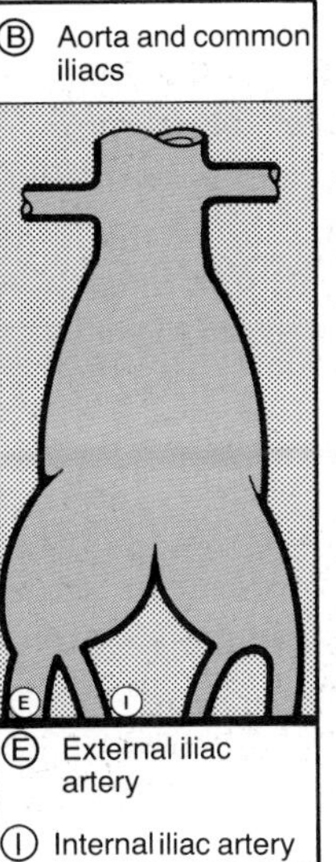

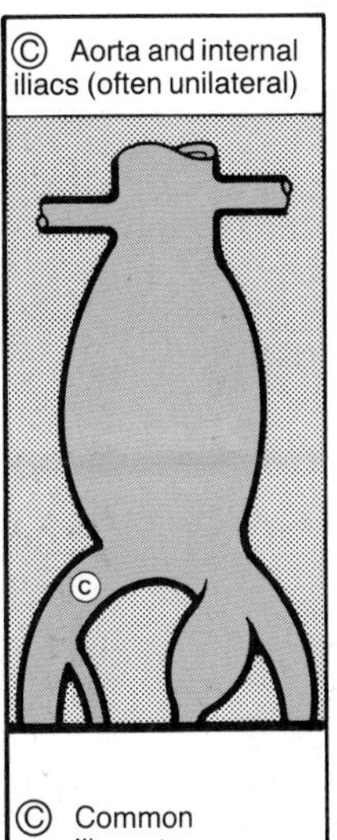

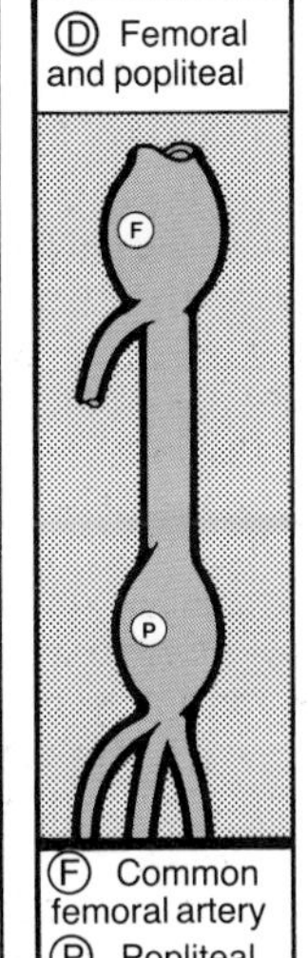

only the infrarenal aorta; some extend distally to involve one or both of the common iliac arteries and sometimes internal iliac arteries.

Clinical presentation of aneurysms

Aorto-iliac aneurysms are often found incidentally, either as a pulsatile mass on abdominal examination or on plain abdominal X-ray (see Figure 26.27). Occasionally the patient notices the pulsation. Despite this, nearly half of those reaching the surgeon develop symptoms from leakage into the retroperitoneal tissue.

Pain is the most common symptom of a leaking aneurysm. The clinical picture ranges between an 'acute abdomen' and abdomino-lumbar pain of up to a week's duration. The diagnosis is usually suggested by the finding of a pulsatile abdominal mass. The patient often exhibits transient or more severe cardiovascular collapse, which should alert the clinician to this possible diagnosis.

Intraperitoneal rupture is rapidly fatal and is probably often an unrecognised cause of sudden death in the elderly.

Femoral and popliteal aneurysms are uncommon and usually present as a pulsatile mass. Femoral aneurysms occasionally rupture and popliteal aneurysms are liable to undergo thrombosis, in which case the patient presents with an acutely ischaemic leg.

Principles of management of aneurysms

a. Indications for operation

A leaking abdominal aortic aneurysm is a surgical emergency. Less than half the patients reach hospital alive, and only about half of these survive. The majority of patients die of shock before reaching the operating theatre or else of acute renal failure after operation.

On the other hand, the mortality after elective operation for aneurysm is less than 6%. Thus, the decision to operate electively depends on the likelihood of leakage or rupture. If there are any symptoms at all which can be attributed to the aneurysm, imminent rupture must be assumed and urgent operation performed. For asymptomatic aneurysms, the risk of rupture increases disproportionately as the aneurysm dilates. Most vascular surgeons would consider operation for abdominal aortic aneurysms of 4 cm or more in diameter; 6 cm is generally considered to be critical since 75% of such aneurysms can be expected to rupture in the succeeding year.

b. Investigation

If an aneurysm is obviously leaking, there is barely time to cross match blood, let alone perform specific investigations! For non-acute cases, ultrasound or CT scanning are extremely useful for establishing the size of the aneurysm(s). Ultrasound is also used for periodic monitoring of asymptomatic aneurysms considered too small to warrant operation. Neither ultrasound nor CT scanning is completely reliable for showing the relationship of the aneurysm to the

Fig. 26.27 Abdominal aortic aneurysm

This very obese 64-year-old man complained of continuous aching back pain for two weeks.
(a) Plain abdominal X-ray showing a huge abdominal aneurysm (outline arrowed); note calcification **C** along its left hand aspect.
(b) Abdominal ultrasound scan of the same patient. This shows the aneurysm to be 11.5 cm in maximum A–P diameter, as measured between the markers **M**, **M**. **(c)** and **(d)** Normal aorta **A** shown on abdominal ultrasound scan in transverse and longitudinal section. The inferior vena cava **V** is also shown on the transverse scan (note that it is larger than the aorta), as is a lumbar vertebra **LV**

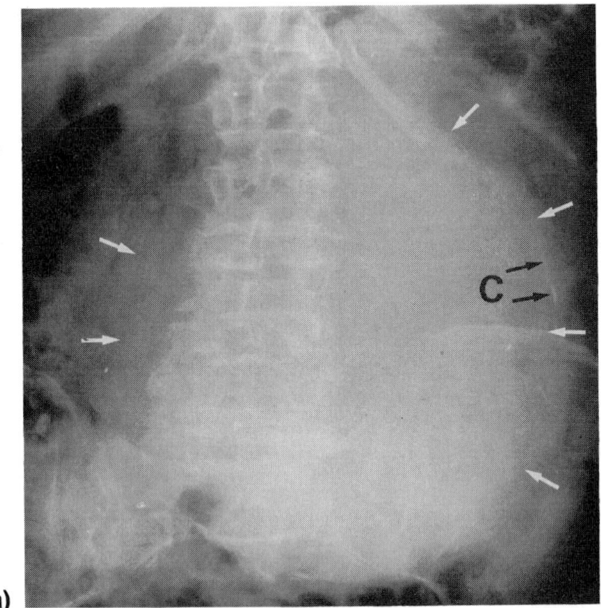

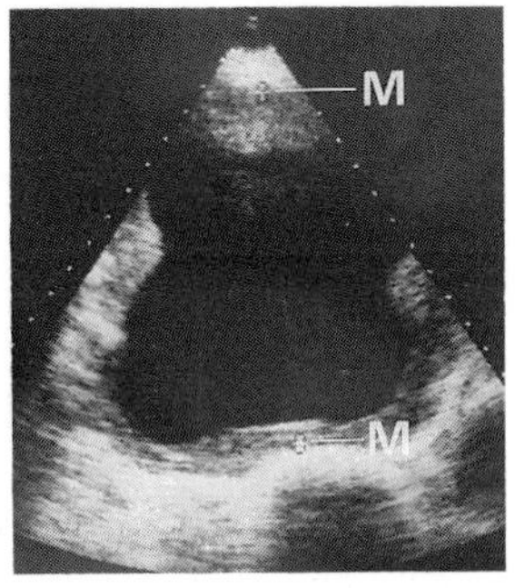

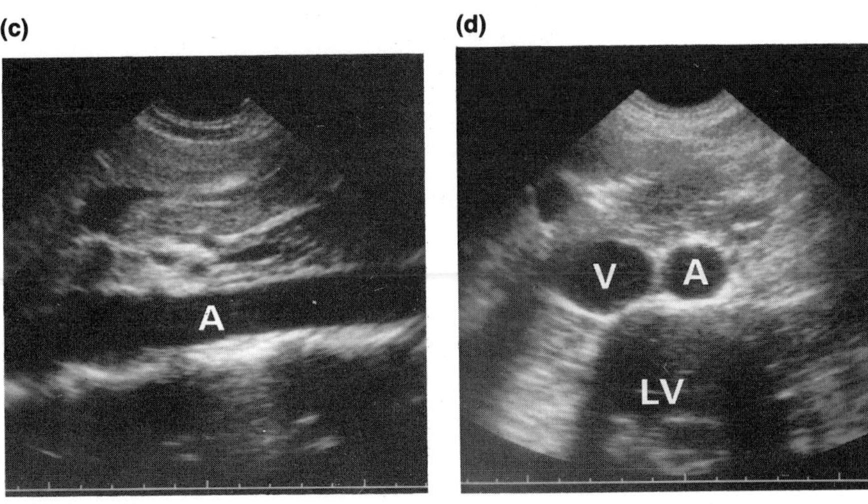

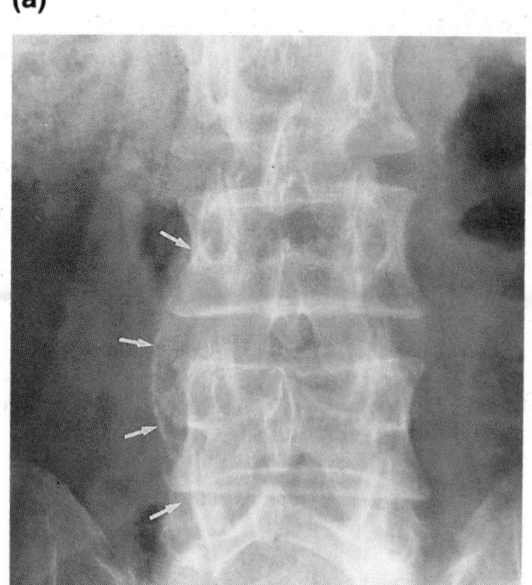

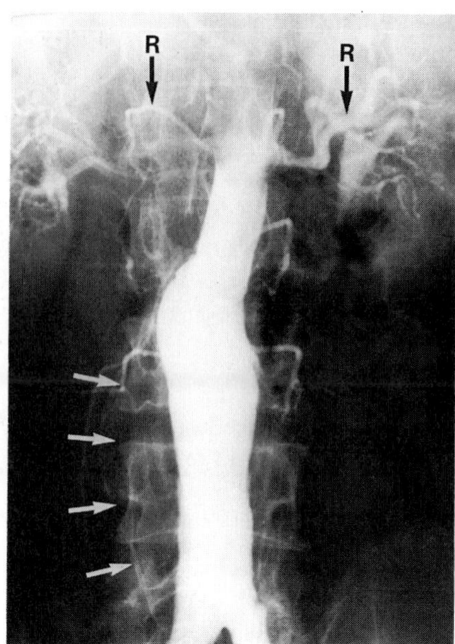

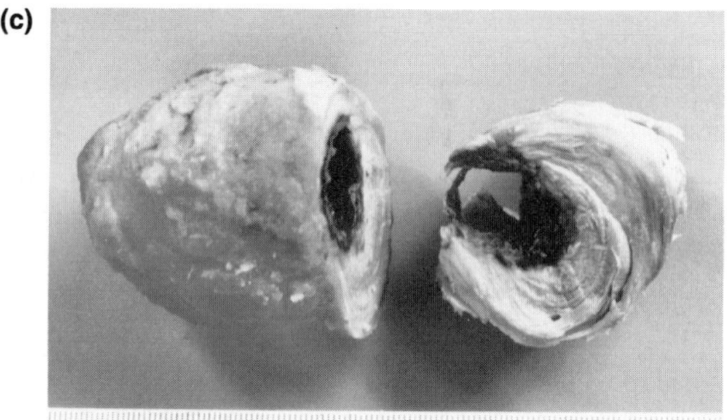

Fig. 26.28 Abdominal aortic aneurysm

A 70-year-old asymptomatic man in whom a pulsatile abdominal mass was an incidental finding.
(a) Plain A–P abdominal X-ray showing a mildly radiopaque mass in the midline with a line of calcification down its right hand margin (arrowed).
(b) Arteriogram from the same patient showing fusiform dilatation of the aorta beginning 2.5 cm below the origins of the renal arteries **R**. Note the calcification (arrowed) in the outer wall corresponding to that in (a); the space between this and the lumen of the aneurysm consists of old lamellated thrombus.
(c) This cast of thrombus was removed from within the aortic aneurysm at operation; note the false lumen and concentric lamellae of thrombus progressively laid down as the aneurysm expanded over many months

renal arteries, and arteriography may be necessary for this. The 5% of cases where the aneurysm extends above the renal arteries require a thoraco-abdominal operative approach, and the operation carries a greater risk.

Arteriography is also necessary in aneurysm patients with evidence of lower limb ischaemia.

Principles of aneurysmal surgery

The aneurysmal segment is surgically corrected by means of a graft, the technique varying according to the site. Tube or bifurcation grafts of synthetic material (usually Dacron) are used for aorto-iliac and femoral aneurysms, while autogenous saphenous vein is preferred for popliteal aneurysms.

For abdominal aneurysms, the standard approach is a long midline abdominal incision. The aorta is usually reached via the peritoneal cavity or sometimes via a retroperitoneal approach. The patient is then anticoagulated with intravenous heparin to prevent distal thrombosis and the iliac arteries and the

Fig. 26.29

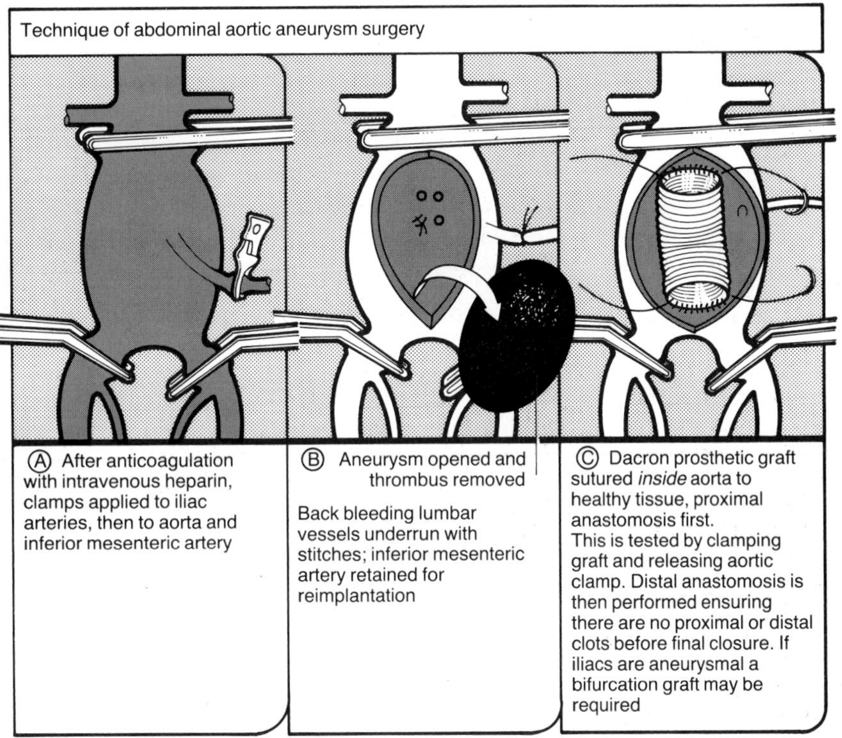

infrarenal aorta are clamped. The aneurysm is incised longitudinally and any clot within it removed. Bleeding lumbar arteries opening into the posterior aortic wall are oversewn.

The graft is then placed within the aneurysmal sac; the sac is left in situ and later closed around the graft, separating it from the gut, giving it greater strength and reducing the risk of haemorrhage from the graft anastomoses. The graft is sutured proximally just above the upper limit of the aneurysm to (relatively) normal aortic wall. Placement of the distal end likewise depends on the extent of the aneurysm and may be located in the aorta near the bifurcation, when a straight tube graft can be used, or more distally to iliac or femoral vessels, when a bifurcation graft ('trouser graft') is necessary.

Complications of arterial surgery (for summary, see Fig. 26.18)

Arterial surgery is subject to all the complications of major surgery but in addition the patients invariably have generalised arteriopathy which makes them vulnerable to serious or fatal complications during the perioperative period. Common complications include myocardial infarction, cardiac failure, acute arrhythmias, cerebrovascular accidents, renal failure and intestinal ischaemia. Therefore, patients for elective arterial surgery must undergo meticulous preoperative assessment and preparation. Any pre-existing medical conditions like cardiac failure or hypertension should be stabilised under expert advice.

Prolonged general anaesthesia and heavy operative blood loss place extra stress on a compromised cardiovascular system. Thus patients require intensive monitoring both during and after operation. This usually means central venous and peripheral arterial catheterisation for accurate pressure measurements. For patients with severe myocardial disease, a Swann-Ganz catheter is usually placed to monitor the pulmonary artery wedge pressure (equivalent to left atrial pressure) as well as cardiac output.

The local complications of arterial surgery include haemorrhage, embolism, thrombosis, graft infection and false aneurysm formation. Patients should be closely monitored in the early postoperative period, usually in an intensive care unit, so that complications can be recognised and treated early.

a. Haemorrhage

During surgical access to the affected arteries, nearby veins are vulnerable to tearing even when great care is taken in dissection. For example, the iliac veins cross deep to the iliac arteries and are often adherent to them. Venous tears are often inaccessible and thus difficult to identify and repair; they usually result in massive blood loss.

Making an arterial anastomosis is demanding under the best conditions, but is made even more difficult by friable vessels and calcified atherosclerotic plaques. In the high pressure arterial system any defect is quickly revealed, and blood sprays everywhere! Fortunately the vascular system can be remarkably forgiving, and small leaks are quickly plugged by platelets. If blood loss is massive (5–25 units), platelets and coagulation factors are consumed and haemostasis is progressively impaired (*consumption coagulopathy*). Standard blood transfusions are unfortunately of little help since stored blood is deficient in functioning platelets. In this deteriorating situation, infusion of *platelet concentrates* and *fresh frozen plasma* or preferably transfusion of *fresh blood* provide the only answers.

Patients are routinely heparinised before arteries are clamped to prevent distal thrombosis. This does not cause much of a haemostatic problem later, and if necessary the effect can be reversed by injection of *protamine*.

Postoperative haemorrhage is uncommon provided adequate haemostasis is achieved before the operation is finished and the wound closed. When bleeding does occur, it usually results from a pin-hole leak at the anastomosis. Haemorrhage is manifest by generalised signs of hypovolaemia, persistent bleeding into the drainage tubes, progressive abdominal distension or, in the lower limb, by swelling beneath the wound. Postoperative haemorrhage will often stop spontaneously following transfusion of blood and clotting factors, but if blood loss continues or there is major haemorrhage, further operation is required.

b. Embolism

In aneurysm surgery, embolism is usually caused by dislodgement of fresh or organised thrombus from the aneurysmal sac. It is largely preventable if the outflow vessels are clamped before the aneurysm is manipulated. Large emboli that lodge in femoral vessels can be retrieved with a Fogarty balloon catheter, but the more common distal emboli may cause infarction of digits or even the whole foot ('trash foot'). Infarction due to distal emboli is irreversible and usually necessitates amputation later. Dissection around a thrombus-containing aorta near the renal arteries may dislodge thrombus and cause renal artery occlusion. If bilateral, the result is acute renal failure, which is usually fatal.

c. Thrombosis

Thrombosis of the reconstructed vessels is a major problem in arterial surgery. It leads to profound distal ischaemia and results in loss of the limb unless urgently corrected. Thrombosis usually occurs if blood flow through the reconstructed vessels is sluggish.

Slow flow leading to thrombosis may arise for a variety of technical reasons:

- Unrecognised stenosis proximal or distal to the reconstruction causing poor inflow or runoff
- Poor anastomotic technique with partial luminal obstruction
- Dissection of the layers of the distal vessel wall resulting in a flap of tunica intima and media which acts as a 'flap valve' occluding the lumen
- Twisting or kinking of a graft

Thrombosis usually occurs in the first few hours after operation and becomes manifest by deterioration in the colour, temperature and pulses of the affected limb from the satisfactory state initially achieved at operation.

d. Graft infection

Infection of a synthetic graft is uncommon but can be a devastating complication. The infecting organisms are usually from the patient's own gut. Infection is minimised by meticulous asepsis, perioperative antibiotics and drainage of the wound to prevent haematoma collection. Antibiotics are normally given intravenously at anaesthetic induction and over the first 24 hours postoperatively. A cephalosporin (e.g. cefotaxime or ceftizoxime), or a combination of gentamicin and flucloxacillin, are suitable.

Graft infection should be suspected if there is recurrent pyrexia and malaise or a persistently discharging wound sinus; occasionally, the wound breaks down exposing the infected graft. Major graft infection has a bleak prognosis even when treated, with septicaemia or anastomotic failure and catastrophic bleeding as the eventual outcome. Treatment is to remove the infected graft and restore the distal circulation with an *extra-anatomic graft* (e.g. axillo-bifemoral), which bypasses the infected area.

e. False aneurysm formation

A false aneurysm is the result of a slow anastomotic leak which is confined by surrounding tissues. A slowly expanding blood-filled cavity results, which eventually ruptures or undergoes thrombosis. A false aneurysm usually presents as a palpable pulsatile mass. Occasionally a false aneurysm at the upper anastomosis with the abdominal aorta leaks into the overlying duodenum. This produces an *aorto-duodenal fistula* and presents with haematemesis. Aorto-duodenal fistulae may also result from graft infection. False aneurysms were formerly much more common because of the gradual breakdown of silk suture materials but suture durability has greatly improved with the introduction of polyester and polypropylene sutures.

Long-term follow up

All patients with atherosclerotic disease are liable to further progression of the disease and subsequent ischaemic events. Thus, most arterial surgery patients are followed up for life to monitor new disease and graft deterioration, and to enable timely intervention.

VENOUS DISORDERS OF THE LOWER LIMB

VENOUS THROMBOSIS AND THE POST-THROMBOTIC LIMB

Introduction

Deep venous thrombosis (DVT) in the lower limb most commonly results as a complication of major operations, multiple fractures, myocardial infarction and other severe illness. In the past, DVTs were commonplace after child-birth but early mobilisation has considerably reduced the incidence. About one third of DVTs present with no apparent cause and these are usually managed by physicians. Risk factors, and the clinical presentation and management of acute DVT and pulmonary embolism are discussed in Chapter 33.

Deep venous thrombosis in the lower limb is an acute local problem with the added risk of potentially fatal pulmonary embolism, but may also lead to major long-term complications in the lower limb. By and large, the severity of post-thrombotic problems in the lower limb reflects the extent of the initial DVT. The affected extremity is known as a *post-thrombotic limb* or, less accurately, a *post-phlebitic limb*.

A high proportion of patients with risk factors for deep venous thrombosis but without clinical evidence of thrombosis can be shown, with the use of sensitive radio-isotopic techniques, to have small asymptomatic thrombi in the calf veins. Such 'silent' thromboses may explain the occurrence of typical post-thrombotic changes in patients where there is no history of an acute thrombotic episode.

Anatomy of the lower limb venous system

Blood is drained from the lower limb via two separate systems. The *deep venous system* drains the deep tissues of the foot and muscles of the lower leg and thigh. These deep veins lie within the mass of lower limb muscles, and include the large *soleal venous sinuses*. Contraction of muscles during walking and other exercise provides an essential mechanism for pumping blood back towards the heart against the effects of gravity. Reverse flow is prevented by numerous valves throughout the system.

The skin and tissues superficial to the deep fascial layer of the lower limb drain mainly into the *superficial venous system* which comprises two major vessels, the *long (great) saphenous vein* and the *short (small) saphenous vein*. The long saphenous vein receives tributaries from the antero-medial aspect of the limb (and lower anterior abdominal wall), and penetrates the deep fascia in the groin to drain into the femoral vein. The short saphenous vein, which drains the posterior of the leg, passes through the deep fascia of the popliteal fossa to flow into the popliteal vein, part of the deep venous system. The superficial system has no muscular pump to aid venous return, but valves normally guard against retrograde flow, particularly at the sapheno-femoral junction and in the popliteal fossa. A number of *perforating veins* drain blood from the superficial system into the deep system; valves normally ensure one-way flow. Most of the perforators are on the medial part of the leg above the ankle but there is a fairly constant 'Hunterian perforator' in the medial mid thigh.

Pathophysiology of post-thrombotic problems

Provided fatal pulmonary embolism has not occurred, deep venous thromboses gradually undergo organisation and recanalisation. In the process, valves in the deep veins can be damaged and become incompetent, thus leading to *chronic venous insufficiency*. The syndrome usually takes years to develop; the prolonged interval makes it easy to forget this reason for trying to prevent deep venous thrombosis in hospital patients! In patients where the proximal veins have been completely occluded by thrombus, recanalisation may not occur at all or else is incomplete. This leaves venous outflow obstruction and the consequences are more marked and appear sooner.

In the normal adult limb, venous pressure at the ankle while standing is about 125 cm of water. This falls markedly during walking due to the action of the calf pump. In contrast, in the post-thrombotic limb, where deep venous valves are incompetent or, worse still, veins are occluded, ankle venous pressure remains high during calf muscle activity; this probably predisposes to incompetence of valves in the perforator veins. Blood is forced into the superficial system (perhaps causing varicose veins) but more importantly, disrupts the normal vascular dynamics of the skin and subcutaneous tissues. This may result in impairment of skin vitality and healing ability.

The following factors probably contribute to a greater or lesser extent to the clinical outcome:

- Venous stagnation restricting arterial replenishment of capillary blood
- Arteriovenous fistulae beneath the affected skin shunt blood away from the dermal capillaries
- Venous hypertension causes dilatation of the local venules and capillary network, allowing plasma proteins to leak into the interstitial spaces. Fibrin polymerises forming *pericapillary cuffs* which interfere with metabolic exchange between blood and tissues. There is also an unexplained reduction in fibrinolytic activity in both blood and tissues

The gross post-thrombotic limb is recognised by the following signs in the leg:

- Chronic swelling with brawny oedema
- Varicose veins with incompetent perforating veins
- Inflammation and haemosiderin pigmentation above the medial malleolus, known as *varicose eczema*. This may be complicated by low-grade cellulitis
- Active or healed venous ulceration above the medial malleolus
- *Lipo-dermatosclerosis* around the ankle (replacement of soft subcutaneous fat with firm collagen). This causes the 'beer-bottle leg' with oedema above and a narrow atrophic ankle below

The post-thrombotic syndrome should also be suspected when a patient presents with lesser degrees of skin change. The majority, however, will prove to have only superficial venous insufficiency or occasionally, isolated incompetence of the perforating veins.

Investigation of venous insufficiency

When a patient presents with ankle ulceration, a chronically swollen limb or typical skin change of venous insufficiency around the ankle, a post-thrombotic limb may be suspected. The diagnostic pathway is as follows:

1. Is the condition venous in origin ? — this is suggested by a history of DVT or a finding of varicose veins or beer-bottle leg. If not venous, investigate other cause of ulceration and swelling.
2. Is there deep venous insufficiency, superficial venous insufficiency (see Figure 26.32 later), or a combination of both?
3. How much of a contribution is made by superficial venous insufficiency or perforator incompetence (these factors, unlike deep venous incompetence, are likely to respond to surgery)?

When there are small areas of skin change or ulceration which correlate with the degree of superficial venous incompetence, these can be treated surgically as uncomplicated varicose veins. If there are marked skin changes, *venography* should be performed to demonstrate the anatomy of the deep venous system and the competence of valves in the deep veins and perforating veins. *Doppler ultrasound* can also be used to listen for retrograde (outward) flow through incompetent valves in the perforator veins when the calf is squeezed.

Ambulatory venous pressure can be measured at the ankle during repeated calf muscle contraction, using direct cannulation. As described earlier, high venous pressure during calf exercise is a feature of the post-thrombotic limb, however, it may also be caused by excessive pressure in the superficial venous system due to incompetence of the valve at the spaheno-femoral junction or other thigh perforators. If ambulatory venous pressure is high, the measurement is repeated with an above-knee tourniquet in place. Any lowering of the ambulatory venous pressure is then attributable to superficial venous incompetence, which can be treated by surgery. Deep venous incompetence is not generally amenable to surgery, and treatment is necessarily conservative.

Management of post-thrombotic problems

The main post-thrombotic problems requiring active treatment are chronic ulcers and cellulitis. Ulcers may develop spontaneously but are more commonly initiated by minor trauma which fails to heal, often complicated by secondary infection.

Venous ulcers

The majority of venous ulcers can be healed by simple non-operative methods, provided treatment is applied effectively and assiduously. Even if operative treatment is required, conservative measures should be used to prepare the limb. These include reducing swelling by bandaging, removing necrotic tissue from the ulcer base and controlling cellulitis. Support and gentle compression of the skin and superficial tissues is the mainstay of treatment. This may be provided by elastic bandages or correctly sized graded-compression stockings. In either case, the aim is for pressure to be greatest at the ankle (about 20 mm Hg), and reducing progressively up the limb. Great care must be taken to ensure that pressure does not cause ischaemia or abrasions over tendons or bony prominences. The main contraindication to the use of compression is severe chronic ischaemia, where pressure could further reduce arterial input.

Spreading cellulitis should be treated with systemic antibiotics. Infection confined to the ulcer is treated by simple excision of dead tissue and frequent applications of mild antiseptics such as EUSOL (Edinburgh University Solution of Lime) or hypochlorite. When the ulcer base is clean, saline alone should be used for cleaning and dressing because antiseptics may then retard granulation tissue and epithelialisation. Local applications of antibiotics have little place in the management of ulcers.

Surgical treatment may be indicated, particularly if there is superficial venous incompetence. Varicose veins should be ligated or removed. More controversial is surgical disruption or ligation of incompetent perforating veins. Intractable or large ulcers may require skin grafting once the ulcer base is clean.

If ulcers and lipo-dermatosclerosis fail to respond to treatment, and particularly if they are painful, a course of *fibrinolytic enhancement therapy* using *stanozolol* may be tried. This anabolic steroid has minimal androgenic effects and trials have shown encouraging results in difficult cases.

Long term care and prevention

The uncomplicated post-thrombotic limb is debilitating enough to the patient, who is often elderly, without the added complication of chronic venous ulceration.

As soon as the condition is recognised, the patient should be encouraged to apply compression support and to take great care to avoid even minor trauma to the limb, especially to the area above the medial malleolus.

For minor venous insufficiency, well fitting two way stretch full-length elastic stockings or tights provide adequate support but care should be taken that there is no proximal constricting band to impair venous return. In more severe venous insufficiency, graded-compression stockings are extremely valuable and may reverse the tissue damage or at least arrest its progress. In addition, they provide protection from minor trauma. Ideally they should be worn at all times except in bed. The importance of correctly fitted stockings should be emphasised; ideally, they should be supplied by an experienced surgical fitter.

In many patients, effective elastic support will be required for life. Even so, subsequent episodes of cellulitis or ulceration are likely to occur.

Axillary vein thrombosis (upper limb equivalent of DVT)

Axillary vein thrombosis is an uncommon condition usually managed by physicians, but may sometimes reach the surgeon. It usually presents with a sudden onset of swelling and aching pain in the whole arm. On examination, the hand, forearm and arm are swollen with a bluish tinge. Sensation is preserved. In most patients, no cause is found, but the condition can occur as a manifestation of visceral malignancy (*thrombophlebitis migrans*), or a blood disorder with raised viscosity, such as polycythaemia rubra vera. It is likely that some cases result from external compression of the subclavian vein between the first rib and clavicle. The usual treatment is anticoagulation to prevent propagation of thrombus and to encourage spontaneous clot lysis. Predisposing disorders should be sought. A few patients benefit from surgical excision of the first rib.

VARICOSE VEINS

Introduction

Varicose veins are dilated, tortuous and prominent superficial veins in the lower limb. Varicose veins are very common, being present in about 20% of people aged 20 and increasing to 80% at 60 years. Nevertheless, only about 12% of those affected have symptoms or develop complications. Varicose veins are one of the most common reasons for surgical referral in developed countries, particularly when improved medical services are able to cope with the volume of more serious disease and expectations for treatment are higher. The condition appears to be a disorder of modern civilisation though the reasons why are far from clear.

Pathophysiology

Abnormal communication between the deep and superficial venous systems appears to be the essential factor in the development of varicose veins. In most patients the process probably begins with failure of the valve at the saphenofemoral junction. When this happens, an uninterrupted column of blood from the heart progressively dilates the veins down the leg (see Figure 26.31). Varicose veins usually develop slowly over 10–20 years, so that in most cases, surgical treatment is not urgent. The long saphenous system is involved in about 90% of cases and the short saphenous system in 10%.

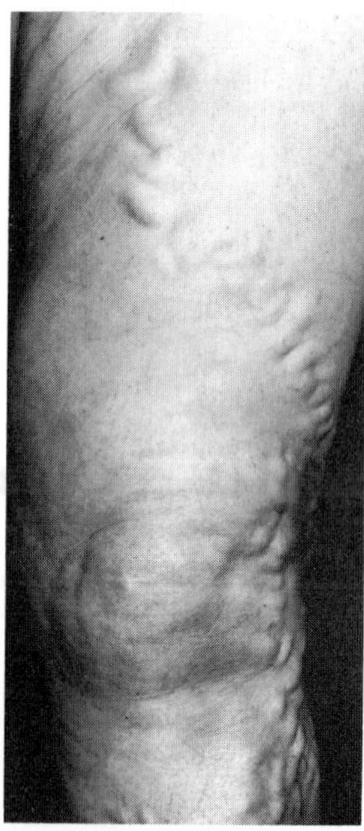

Fig. 26.30 Varicose veins

One of the typical patterns of varicosities found in long saphenous varicose veins. The dilated tortuous vein snaking down the thigh into the leg is a tributary which enters the long saphenous vein near its junction with the femoral vein

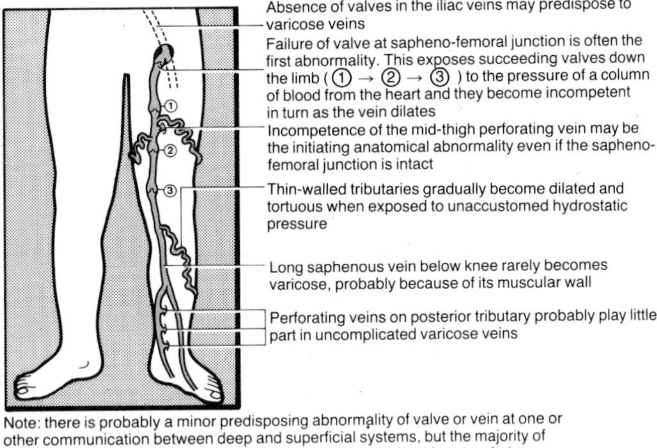

Note: there is probably a minor predisposing abnormality of valve or vein at one or other communication between deep and superficial systems, but the majority of varicose veins appear in response to the hormonal and other changes during pregnancy

Fig. 26.31 Pathophysiology of varicose veins

Women are affected about six times more often than men, with the majority of varicose veins developing during or soon after the second or third pregnancy. An important factor is probably the high level of progesterone which causes changes in the structure of collagen (which may not later recover), as well as smooth muscle relaxation. Pressure on the pelvic veins by the enlarging uterus may contribute by restricting venous return.

In some patients, hereditary factors appear to play a part, especially in men, particularly those who develop varicose veins in their teens. Predisposing

Fig. 26.32

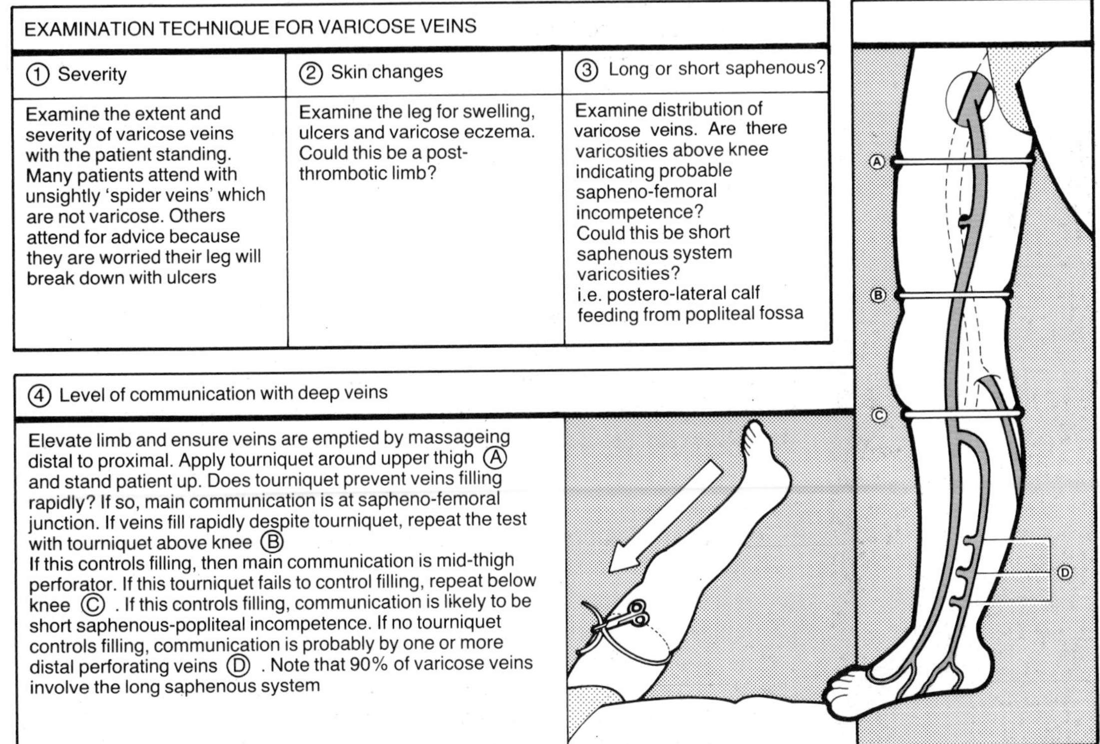

anatomical factors may include congenital lack of valves in the iliac veins or abnormal vein wall elasticity. Deep venous thrombosis plays little part in causing simple varicose veins. Rarely, multiple congenital arteriovenous fistulae cause gross varicose veins. In these patients, there is gigantism of the lower limb and often venous ulceration.

The technique of examining varicose veins is shown in Figure 26.32.

Symptoms and signs of varicose veins

The most common complaints related to varicose veins are:

- Aching legs, usually after standing all day
- Poor cosmetic appearance, especially in summer when the legs are exposed
- Fear of future leg ulcers
- Fear of varicosities progressing
- Worry about varicosities bleeding, particularly if traumatised
- Varicose eczema or ulcers
- Ankle oedema
- Recurrent superficial thrombophlebitis

Management

Many patients who consult a surgeon because of unsightly vascular markings on their legs do not have varicose veins. Instead, these are often 'spider veins' or dilated superficial venules, for which treatment is generally unsatisfactory. Covering cosmetics or perhaps laser coagulation therapy may give some benefit. Many other patients have long standing varicose veins with no complications, and merely seek reassurance that they will not ulcerate in the future. Surgical treatment is not usually necessary for these patients, but advice can be given to elevate the legs when sitting and to wear supporting elastic stockings when standing for long periods.

a. Indications for surgical treatment of varicose veins

Surgical treatment for varicose veins is to a large extent cosmetic, and operation can be planned at leisure. The main medical indications for treating varicose veins are *aching legs* after standing (particularly with unilateral ankle oedema), *haemorrhage* from a varicose vein, *superficial thrombophlebitis* and *varicose skin changes* due to superficial venous insufficiency. All of these can be treated with support bandages or stockings, but surgery is often preferable.

Injection sclerotherapy is often used for treating small cosmetically unattractive varicose veins below the knee but is unsuitable for major varicosities, particularly in the thigh.

The techniques of injection sclerotherapy and surgery for varicose veins are shown in Figure 26.33 (p. 530–531).

b. Perioperative management of the patient having varicose vein surgery

Varicose veins must be *marked out* on the legs before operation. This should be done by the surgeon who will actually do the operation. An indelible marker must be used so that marks are not washed off by the patient or by skin preparation in the operating theatre. The patient must stand, often for some minutes, to allow the veins to fill, and marking should be performed in this position. Most surgeons mark all the prominent veins that are visible or palpable. Extra marks are often added for areas needing special surgical attention like suspected perforating veins.

Any patient with a history of venous thrombosis, whether deep or superficial, should be prescribed low-dose subcutaneous heparin. Patients with other risk factors for deep venous thrombosis should have the same prophylactic treatment. The first dose of heparin should be given an hour before operation.

Immediately after operation, non-adherent dressings are applied to all the incisions, and the whole leg is bandaged firmly with crepe or other similar bandage. The next day, additional support is usually applied to the leg using elastic bandages or graded compression stockings, over the postoperative bandage. The patient should then be mobilised and encouraged to walk about. On return home, patients should keep as active as possible, walking at least a mile outside the house every day. When sitting, the legs should be elevated, and the patient should get up and walk around about every half hour. All these measures are designed to discourage venous stagnation and venous thrombosis.

UPPER LIMB ISCHAEMIA

Introduction

Ischaemia of the upper limb is rare. This is because atherosclerosis is very uncommon in the arteries supplying the upper limb. Furthermore, there is a rich collateral blood supply via the scapular anastomoses which can bypass occlusive disease of the subclavian artery. Upper limb ischaemia also occurs when the subclavian artery is compressed at the thoracic outlet, or when emboli obstruct the brachial or more distal arteries. Occasionally, vasospastic disorders like severe Raynaud's disease cause ischaemia of the fingers.

THORACIC OUTLET COMPRESSION

The subclavian artery passes through the narrow space between the first rib and the clavicle. Occasionally, this gap becomes narrowed by a healed fracture or some unknown means, so that the artery becomes compressed. This is exacerbated when the arm is held above the head. The subclavian artery also may become compressed by the upward pressure of a cervical rib, causing upper limb 'claudication' in people who habitually work with their arms above their heads. In long standing cases of subclavian compression, the artery beyond the stenosis often becomes dilated into an aneurysm (*post-stenotic dilatation*) which may collect thrombus. This may later embolise the brachial artery causing acute ischaemia.

Fig. 26.33

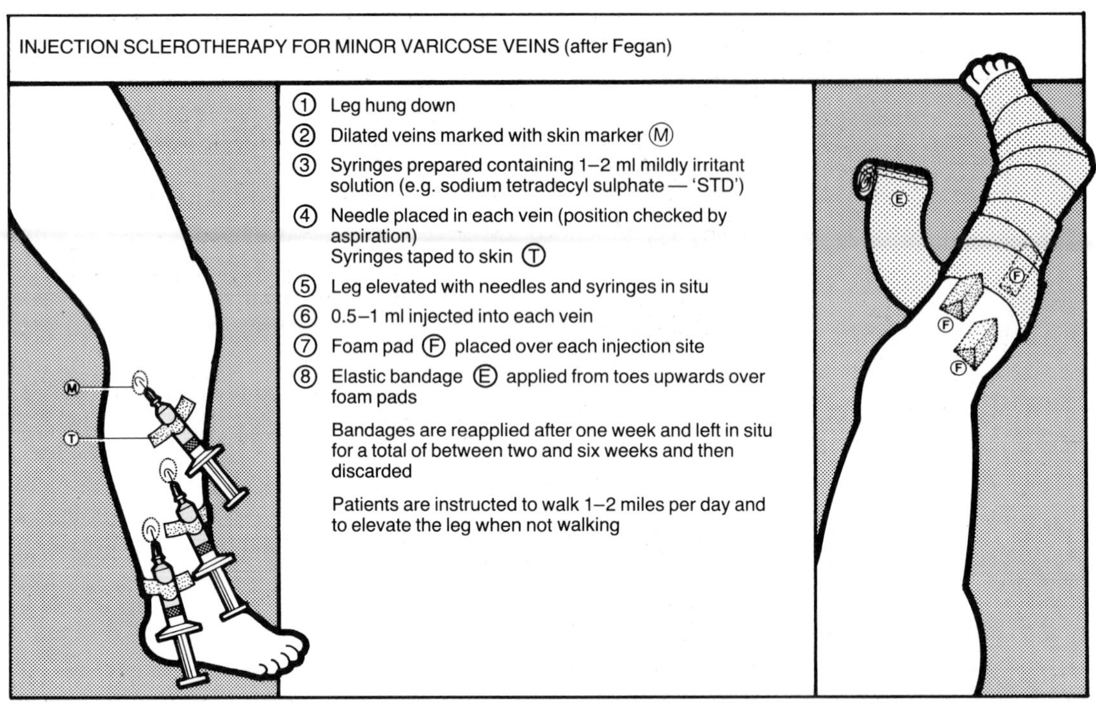
INJECTION SCLEROTHERAPY FOR MINOR VARICOSE VEINS (after Fegan)
① Leg hung down
② Dilated veins marked with skin marker Ⓜ
③ Syringes prepared containing 1–2 ml mildly irritant solution (e.g. sodium tetradecyl sulphate — 'STD')
④ Needle placed in each vein (position checked by aspiration)
Syringes taped to skin Ⓣ
⑤ Leg elevated with needles and syringes in situ
⑥ 0.5–1 ml injected into each vein
⑦ Foam pad Ⓕ placed over each injection site
⑧ Elastic bandage Ⓔ applied from toes upwards over foam pads
Bandages are reapplied after one week and left in situ for a total of between two and six weeks and then discarded
Patients are instructed to walk 1–2 miles per day and to elevate the leg when not walking
M
T
E
F

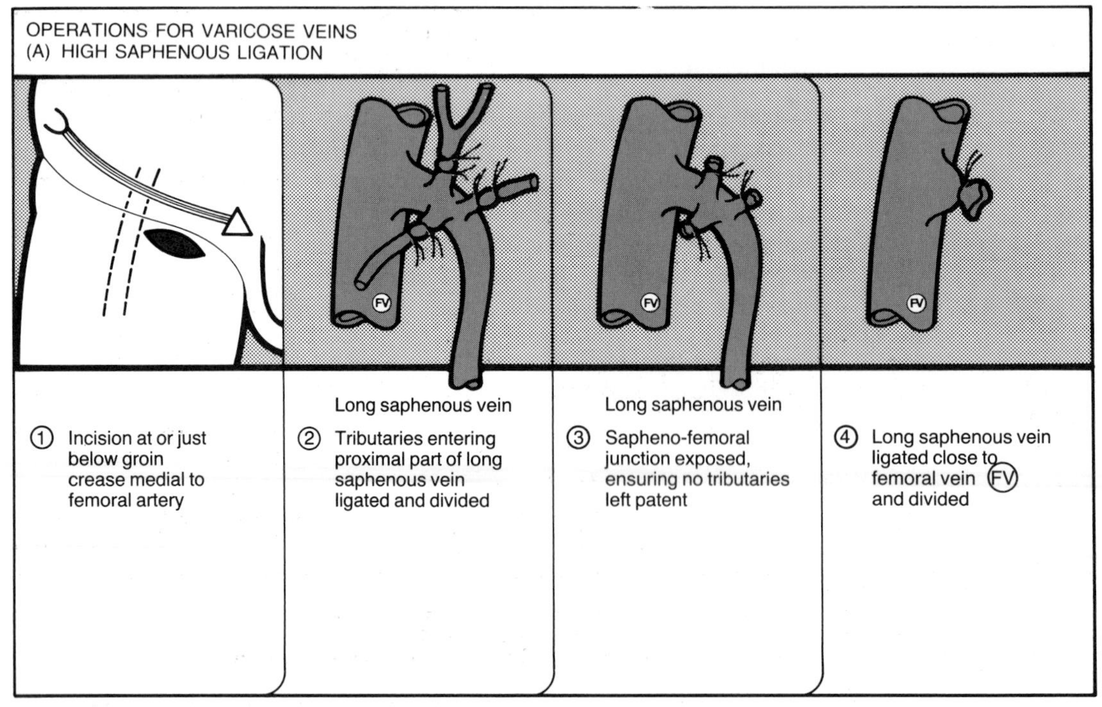
OPERATIONS FOR VARICOSE VEINS
(A) HIGH SAPHENOUS LIGATION
FV
Long saphenous vein
Long saphenous vein
① Incision at or just below groin crease medial to femoral artery
② Tributaries entering proximal part of long saphenous vein ligated and divided
③ Sapheno-femoral junction exposed, ensuring no tributaries left patent
④ Long saphenous vein ligated close to femoral vein FV and divided

Fig. 26.33 (cont.)

(B) STRIP OF LONG SAPHENOUS VEIN

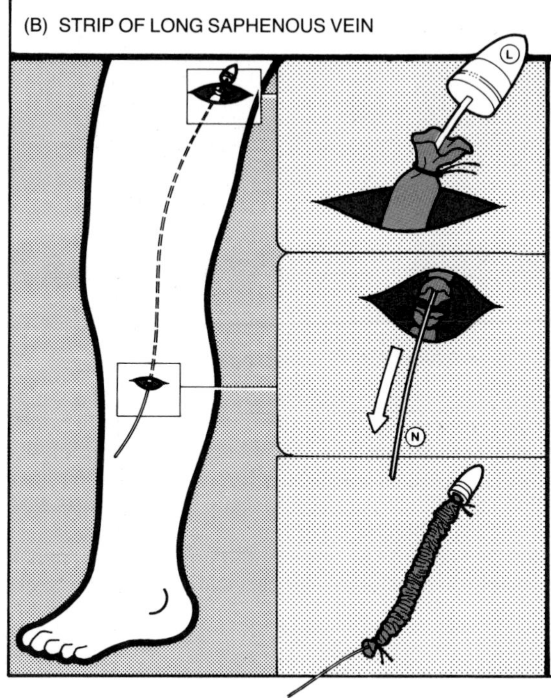

This once-routine operation is much less commonly performed nowadays and, if it is, stripping is nearly always performed only between groin and knee, the distal part (almost never itself varicose) being left in situ

The stripper is a long flexible wire with a bullet-shaped knob on the 'business' end

The entry vein (proximal or distal, according to choice) is prepared as shown and the narrow end of the stripper Ⓝ passed down or up within the long saphenous vein until it can be brought out to the surface

The vein is ligated to the wire at the bullet end Ⓛ and the narrow end is pulled smoothly and firmly, tearing off tributaries and any perforators on the way, emerging with the complete vein bunched up on the stripper

The wounds are closed and the limb firmly bandaged to prevent subcutaneous bleeding

(C) AVULSION OF VARICOSITIES

(Usually performed in addition to high saphenous ligation and strip, if the latter is performed)

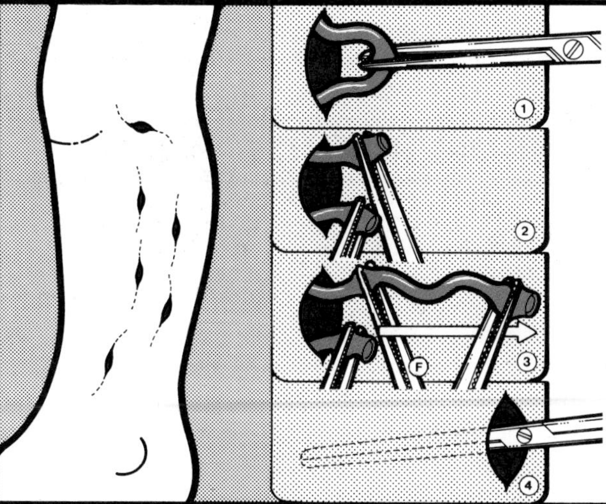

Before operation, all varicosities are marked by the surgeon with the patient standing, using an indelible spirit based fibre-tip pen.
Very small incisions are made over the marks and as much vein as possible is pulled out ('nick and pick') as follows:

Vein grasped with fine artery forceps

Second forceps applied and vein divided

One end is drawn out of wound gently and further traction applied by means of another forceps Ⓕ.
The vein will eventually break and bleeding is controlled by finger pressure and tucking a swab into the wound. The process is repeated for the other end of vein

Forceps can be passed subcutaneously to retrieve nearby varices thus reducing the number of incisions required.
Each wound is closed neatly with 'steristrips' or a fine suture and non-adherent gauze applied to each one.
The limb is bandaged firmly from toes proximally using crepe

POSTOPERATIVE MANAGEMENT
Bandages remain in place for 1–2 weeks, often with an additional elastic bandage or graded compression stocking. The limb should be elevated wherever possible when sitting.

Daily exercise by walking 1–2 miles or cycling is encouraged. Patients can usually leave hospital the day after operation

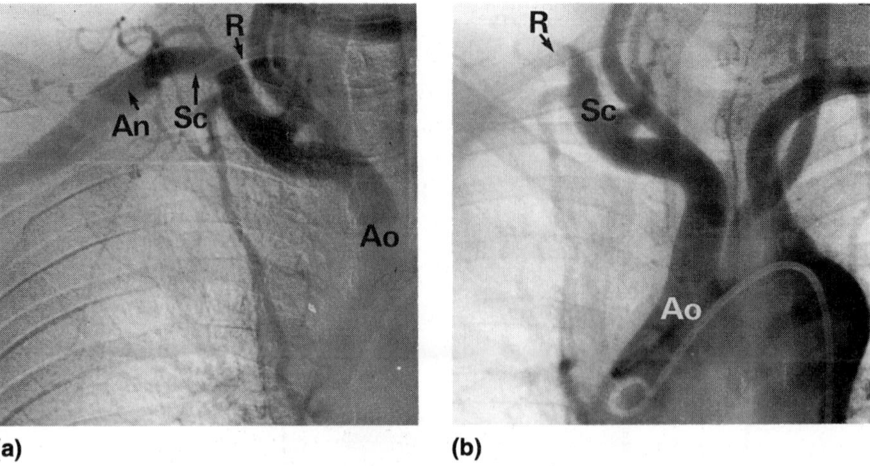

Fig. 26.34 Cervical rib causing subclavian artery compression

Subtraction arteriograms from a 65-year-old butcher who complained of a sudden onset of extreme pallor, coldness, weakness and paraesthesia in his right hand and forearm when handling meat in the cold room. **(a)** With the shoulder adducted, there is normal blood flow through the subclavian artery **Sc**. Note the presence of a cervical rib **R** and dilatation of the subclavian artery just distal to it. This was a post-stenotic aneurysm **An** containing thrombus, which gave rise to distal emboli.
(b) With the shoulder abducted and externally rotated ('the army saluting position'), subclavian blood flow is completely obstructed by the cervical rib; note the 'pigtail' catheter in the aorta **A**

Diagnosis is made by the finding of lower blood pressure in the affected arm which varies with arm posture. This is confirmed by arteriography (see Figure 26.34).

Treatment is by excision of a cervical rib if present, or else excision of the first rib. A subclavian aneurysm should be resected and replaced with a graft.

EXTRA-CRANIAL ARTERIAL INSUFFICIENCY

Introduction

Extracranial arterial disease is common and is probably responsible for about a third of all strokes. The common carotid bifurcation is the area most affected by atherosclerosis, although obstructive disease may affect the distal internal carotid in the carotid siphon. The vertebral arteries are next most commonly affected. Less commonly, the orifices of the great vessels become obstructed where they leave the aortic arch.

CAROTID ARTERY STENOSIS

Pathophysiology

Carotid artery atheroma often results in stenosis, with cerebral blood flow becoming critically impaired when luminal narrowing exceeds 75% or so. Rough atherosclerotic plaques may also be the source of platelet emboli. Small emboli

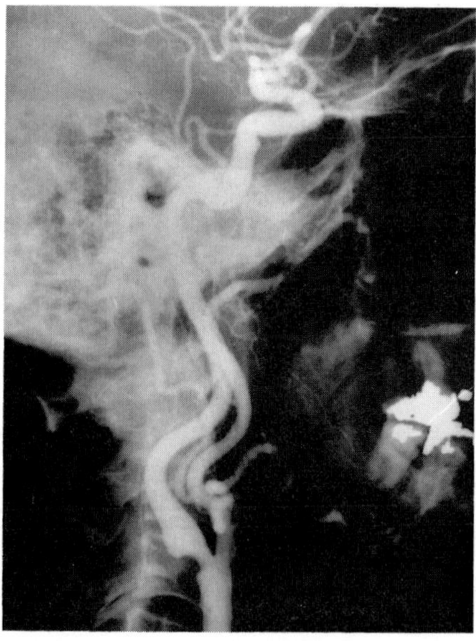

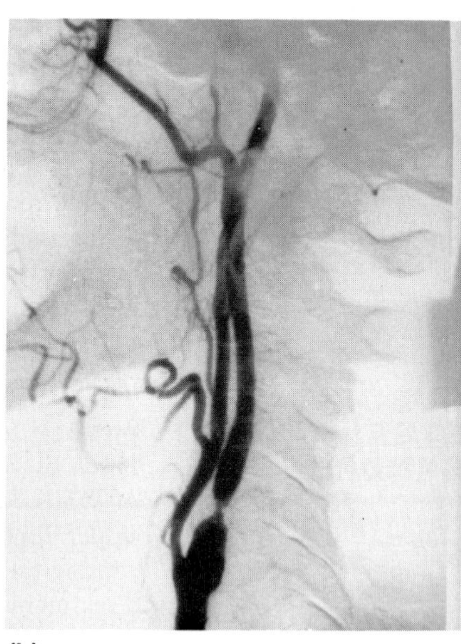

(a) (b)

Fig. 26.35 Carotid artery disease

(a) This 71-year-old man suffered two transient episodes of left hemiparesis in one week ('TIAs'). Carotid angiography shows a localised 50% stenosis of the internal carotid artery just distal to the common carotid bifurcation; this degree of stenosis would not explain the symptoms. Note the typical post-stenotic dilatation immediately beyond the stenosis. The rest of the cerebral arterial system appears normal. At operation, an ulcerated atheromatous plaque was found, which was undoubtedly the source of emboli which caused the transient ischaemic attacks. Endarterectomy was performed and the patient has been entirely well since. **(b)** Subtraction film from a carotid angiogram in a different patient. This shows a 90% stenosis in the internal carotid artery which is haemo-dynamically significant, causing cerebral ischaemia on its own account

may cause *transient ischaemic attacks* (including transient blindness, *amaurosis fugax*), whereas large emboli cause major strokes.

Investigation of suspected extracranial vascular disease

A minority of patients suffering transient ischaemic attacks or stroke are found have a *bruit* on auscultation of the carotid arteries. However, such a finding does not indicate the degree of narrowing. Indeed, a significant stenosis may be silent, as of course is complete occlusion.

Patients with strokes, asymptomatic carotid bruits and transient ischaemic attacks should initially, if possible, be investigated by non-invasive means. The preferred method is duplex scanning, an ultrasound technique which allows simultaneous imaging of the carotid arteries and measurement of blood flow velocity. If this is abnormal, carotid and vertebral angiography may be necessary (see Figure 26.35); these invasive techniques, however, carry a risk of stroke, and are therefore justifiable only if operative intervention is likely to be appropriate.

Treatment of extracranial arterial disease

The position of surgery in management of extracranial vascular disease is not yet universally established. In the UK, a conservative approach is usually adopted, whereas in many other countries, surgery is more freely offered. In the UK, most patients with transient ischaemic attacks seem to do at least as well with medical treatment as surgery (the usual medical treatment is with antiplatelet drugs, e.g. aspirin 70–150 mg daily), but a definitive answer to this problem is awaited. Patients with proven significant stenosis may be offered surgery, but many believe the long term results of surgery are disappointing even in this group. They prefer to manage their patients with medical treatment.

The usual operation for carotid artery stenosis is *endarterectomy*. The carotid bifurcation is opened longitudinally after clamping the carotid arteries. A *Javed shunt* is used to maintain cerebral perfusion; this involves placement of a tube in the common carotid below the stenosis which is inserted into the internal carotid above the stenosis, bypassing the operation site. The stenotic plaque is then removed and the carotid sutured directly or with a patch in the wall to maintain the diameter. Carotid surgery carries an appreciable rate of cerebral complications such as stroke, which many detractors maintain to be equivalent to the rate of complication without surgery.

SUBCLAVIAN STEAL SYNDROME

This unusual syndrome is caused by obstruction of the subclavian artery proximal to the origin of the vertebral artery. In consequence the subclavian is fed by retrograde flow from the vertebral artery via the carotids and circle of Willis. This situation remains tenable until there is excessive demand in the upper limb when blood is diverted ('stolen') from the cerebral circulation causing transcient cerebral ischaemia. Figure 26.36 illustrates a classic example. Treatment is to bypass the obstruction with a graft.

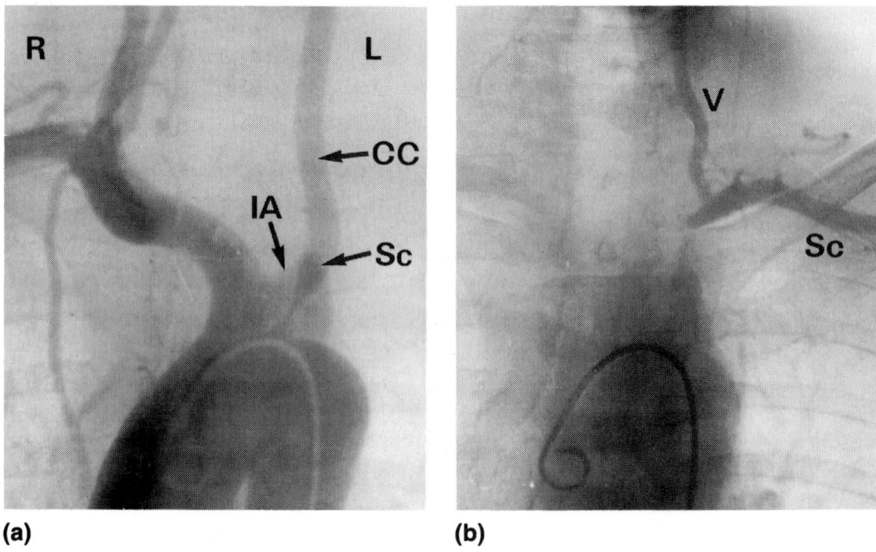

Fig. 26.36 Subclavian steal syndrome

Subtraction angiograms from a 55-year-old house painter who complained of dizziness when painting walls and ceilings. **(a)** Aortic arch (with 'pigtail' arteriogram catheter visible) showing normal right innominate artery with its subclavian and common carotid branches. On the left, the arterial anatomy is anomalous, with the common carotid **CC** arising from an innominate artery **IA** rather than direct from the aorta. The left subclavian artery **Sc** appears to be occluded beyond a short stump. **(b)** Exposure taken 4 seconds later; the aortic arch and its branches are now clear but contrast has appeared in the left vertebral artery **V** through downward flow via the circle of Willis. This has continued to fill the left subclavian artery **Sc** retrogradely. Thus there is complete obstruction of a segment of the left subclavian artery proximal to the origin of the vertebral artery. The vertebral artery thus supplies the left upper limb at the expense of the cerebral circulation, resulting in episodes of transient cerebral ischaemia at times of high vascular demand from the left upper limb

MESENTERIC ISCHAEMIA

Introduction

Blood supply to portions of the bowel may be compromised in four main ways:

- *Strangulation* — this is a mechanical problem presenting as a form of bowel obstruction. It is described in detail in Chapter 8. It may be the result of a *hernia* (see Chapter 19), *volvulus* (see Chapter 17) or *fibrous bands* resulting from previous surgery (see Chapter 33)
- *Acute thrombotic or embolic obstruction* — in pathological terms this is analagous to acute thrombosis or embolism of the lower limb, as described earlier in the chapter. The condition presents as an 'acute abdomen' and is described in Chapter 8
- *Transient critical ischaemia* — this presents as inflammation of the bowel characterised by abdominal pain and rectal bleeding. The condition is known as *ischaemic colitis* and is discussed at the end of Chapter 16
- *Chronic mesenteric artery insufficiency* — this condition, which presents as abdominal pain following eating, is analagous to intermittent claudication due to arterial insufficiency in the lower limb and is described in the next section

CHRONIC MESENTERIC ISCHAEMIA

The rare condition of chronic mesenteric ischaemia or 'gut claudication' occurs when the visceral blood supply is restricted to a point where it is adequate at rest but inadequate during active digestion. This occurs when there is gross atherosclerotic narrowing of the three main mesenteric vessels (coeliac, superior mesenteric and inferior mesenteric arteries). These patients present with severe epigastric pain on eating which causes 'fear of food'. There is always gross weight loss and sometimes an epigastric bruit.

Diagnosis is by arteriography, and a lateral projection allows the origins of the three main vessels to be seen. Treatment is by surgical reconstruction of the origins of one or more of the mesenteric arteries.

RENAL ISCHAEMIA

RENAL ARTERY STENOSIS

Pathophysiology

This uncommon condition arises in two main ways: in children and young adults, the cause is *fibromuscular hyperplasia*. In older patients, *atherosclerosis* is the usual cause. Renal artery stenosis may present with hypertension (ischaemia of one or both kidneys causes poor perfusion, thus activating the renin-angiotensin system), or functional renal impairment. It is sometimes discovered incidentally on urography as a non-functioning or poorly-functioning kidney.

Fibromuscular hyperplasia responds well to balloon dilatation, which often results in the blood pressure returning to normal. Atherosclerosis may be amenable to balloon dilatation, but the effect on hypertension is unpredictable; renal function, however, may be improved, particularly if the renal artery stenosis is bilateral.

It is important that renal artery stenosis be recognised in patients needing aortic reconstructive surgery, whether this is for occlusive or aneurysmal disease. This is because hypotension during the operation may initiate thrombotic occlusion of narrowed renal arteries. This causes post-operative renal failure. Renal artery stenosis should be treated before operation by balloon dilatation or by reconstruction combined with the aortic operation.

27 DISORDERS OF THE BREAST

Introduction

Patients with breast problems constitute 15–20% of new referrals to surgical outpatient clinics. Virtually every woman with a breast lump, breast pain or discharge from the nipple fears that she has cancer. The anxiety that results is made up of three components: the unknown course of the disease, the fear of dying, and the threat of mutilation. Previously, this often prevented women from seeking early medical advice, but in recent years public awareness about self-examination and screening, and the possible advantages of early treatment, have encouraged earlier presentation.

Many patients have friends or relatives with breast cancer and their understanding of the disease will understandably be coloured by experience. The possible effects of mastectomy on sexual attractiveness and femininity are often uppermost in a woman's mind, so psychological care should accompany every stage in the management of breast disorders.

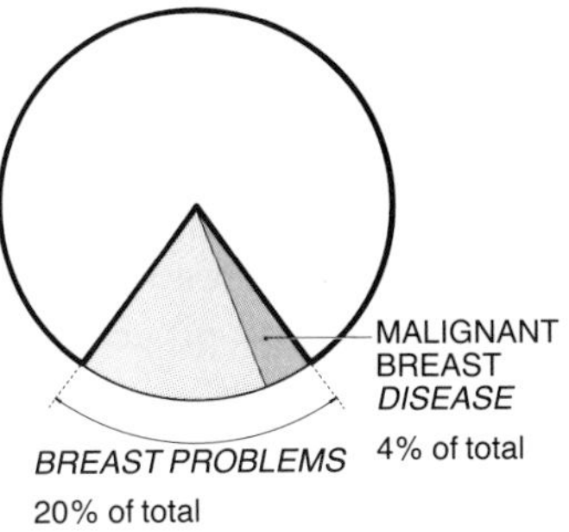

Fig. 27.1 Breast disease as a proportion of surgical out-patient referrals

Despite their fears, less than a quarter of patients presenting with breast problems to surgical outpatients departments in the UK have cancer. However, in Western societies one women in 14 will develop the disease and one in 20 will die from it. Early recognition of cancer offers the best hope of cure, so priority should be given to prompt diagnosis. This will either allay fears or allow treatment to be started as early as possible.

EPIDEMIOLOGY OF BREAST DISEASE

Breast cancer

Breast cancer is predominantly a disease of Western civilisation. It is the most common carcinoma in women and the most common cause of death in women between the ages of 35 and 55. In the UK each year, over 24 000 new cases

Fig. 27.2 Types of breast disease of surgical importance

Malignant neoplasms — *adenocarcinoma* is by far the most common. Rarely, a *sarcoma* or *metastasis* from elsewhere occurs in the breast

Benign tumour-like lesions — this category comprises the common condition known as *fibroadenoma* and the less common conditions of *intraduct papilloma* and *lipoma*

Disordered physiological responses of breast tissue — *fibroadenosis* (also known as benign mammary dysplasia, fibrocystic disease and chronic mastitis) encompasses a variety of proliferative and other changes of the breast tissues. All probably have a n underlying hormonal aetiology. *Male gynaecomastia* is a similar hormone-associated disorder

Infections — *cellulitis* and *breast abscess* are the main types of infection and usually occur during lactation

Non-infective inflammatory conditions — inflammation resulting from rupture of an ectatic duct (*mammary duct ectasia*), or the late result of trauma (*fat necrosis*)

are diagnosed and over 13 000 women die of the condition. Breast cancer is not, however, a new disease; it was recognised by the ancient Egyptians and mastectomy was certainly performed in Roman times.

Breast cancer is extremely rare before the age of 25. It reaches a high incidence in the decade from 40 to 50 and continues to increase in frequency into old age. Breast cancer in the male accounts for up to 1% of new cases. Genetic factors may be important, as women with affected grandmothers, mothers or sisters have an increased susceptibility. Worldwide differences in incidence (the exceptionally low level in Japan, for example) are more likely due to environmental than racial differences.

Childless women, or those having their first pregnancy over the age of 30, have double the breast cancer risk of women who have their first child before the age of 25. Nuns appear to be at extremely high risk. Protective factors include a short time between menarche and first pregnancy, and ovarian ablation below the age of 35. Breast feeding is said to be associated with a lower incidence of breast cancer. The epidemiology suggests that oestrogens, when unopposed by progestogens, play an important role in pathogenesis. Present evidence suggests that the oral contraceptive pill plays no part in causing breast cancer.

The only environmental factor known to promote the development of breast cancer is ionizing radiation. Women exposed to large numbers of chest X-rays for monitoring tuberculosis (which occurred in the days before modern chemotherapy) have a moderately increased risk of breast cancer, and the women of Hiroshima and Nagasaki have a high risk of developing breast cancer even now.

Non-malignant breast disease

Fibroadenosis and *fibroadenoma* account for most of the non-malignant breast disease which reaches the surgeon. Both occur almost exclusively in the reproductive years and are probably both controlled by hormonal factors. Fibroadenoma is more common in young women, while fibroadenosis usually occurs in women between 30 and 45.

Breast infections most commonly occur during pregnancy and lactation. Most are successfully treated early with antibiotics and do not reach the surgeon. If resolution is slow or incomplete, or if an acute abscess develops, surgical intervention is required.

Fat necrosis is rare and occurs in older age groups. The lump often appears long after the traumatic episode has been forgotten.

SYMPTOMS AND SIGNS OF BREAST DISEASE

The patient not only has symptoms but is often the first to notice the physical signs. The symptoms and signs are outlined in Figure 27.3 along with their diagnostic importance.

Special points in history taking

The duration of symptoms should be established, bearing in mind that a lump may have been present much longer than the woman is aware or will admit. Periodicity of pain or lumpiness in relation to the menstrual cycle suggests a hormone-related condition rather than malignant disease.

A history of previous breast problems such as cysts, abscess or trauma may provide a clue to the current diagnosis. Parity, age at first pregnancy, and history of breast feeding might alter the statistical likelihood of a lesion being malignant.

Drug history should be recorded, including present or past use of hormone preparations. These include the contraceptive pill and hormone replacement therapy (HRT) for menopausal symptoms. A causal link between the use of hormones and the development of breast cancer is unproven but cannot be discounted.

History taking especially provides the opportunity for establishing rapport with the patient, who usually fears cancer and its implications. A sympathetic approach and clear explanations lay the foundation for a trusting and co-operative relationship should malignancy be diagnosed.

Examination of the breasts

The basic examination technique is shown in Figure 27.4 and can be simplified for patient self-examination. Most women should be taught to examine their own breasts.

Breast examination involves six distinct manoeuvres:

- Observation with the patient sitting up
- Observation with the patient raising and lowering her arms
- Examination of the nipples
- Palpation of each breast quadrant
- Palpation of the axillae
- General examination for signs of distant metastases

Fig. 27.3 Symptoms and signs of breast disease

SYMPTOM OR SIGN	CLINICAL SIGNIFICANCE
1. PAIN	
—varying with menstrual cycle	Suggests physiological cause such as premenstrual tension or fibroadenosis
—independent of menstrual cycle	Not helpful in diagnosis but may occur in carcinoma, fibroadenosis or infection
2. LUMP IN THE BREAST	
—hard lump	The surface characteristics provide the most useful diagnostic information: a discrete lump with a smooth surface is most likely to be a fibroadenoma if it is solid, or a fibroadenotic cyst if it is fluctuant. An ill–defined margin and any suggestion of tethering to superficial or deep structures strongly suggests carcinoma but is sometimes due to non–infective inflammation.
—firm lump	This suggests fibroadenosis, especially if the outline is difficult to distinguish from normal breast tissue or if the breast is generally lumpy
—soft lump	Usually a lipoma or occasionally a lax cyst
3. SKIN CHANGES IN THE BREAST	
—skin dimpling	Sometimes a subtle sign but highly suggestive of carcinoma
—visible lump	Cysts, carcinoma or giant fibroadenoma
—peau d'orange (texture of orange peel)	Over a lump, this is pathognomonic of carcinoma. It is due to tumour invasion of dermal lymphatics causing dermal oedema
—redness	Usually infection especially if skin is hot. Sometimes a feature of mammary duct ectasia
—ulceration	Neglected carcinoma in the elderly (often slow growing)
4. NIPPLE DISORDERS	
—recent inversion	Suggests a fibrosing underlying lesion such as carcinoma or mammary duct ectasia
—'eczema' (rash involving nipple or areola, or both)	If unilateral, this is the classic sign of Paget's disease of the nipple, a presentation of breast cancer
—nipple discharge:	
milky	—pregnancy or hyperprolactinaemia
clear	—physiological
green	—perimenopausal, duct ectasia , fibroadenotic cyst
blood–stained	—carcinoma or intraduct papilloma

Fig. 27.4 Technique of breast examination

Inspection: the breasts should be inspected for asymmetry, skin tethering and dimpling, and changes in colour. This should be performed with the patient sitting comfortably, pressing hands on hips **(a)**, lifting arms in the air **(b)**, and pressing hands on top of the head **(c)**. *Palpation*: the patient should sit on an examination couch as shown in **(d)**, with the backrest at about 45° and rolled slightly to the contralateral side. The arm on the side to be examined should be elevated and the head rested on the pillow. The effect of these manoeuvres is to spread the breast over a greater area of the chest wall. The left hand is used to retract the breast, whilst the flat of the right hand is used to palpate the breast circumferentially by quadrants **(e), (f)**. (continued overleaf)

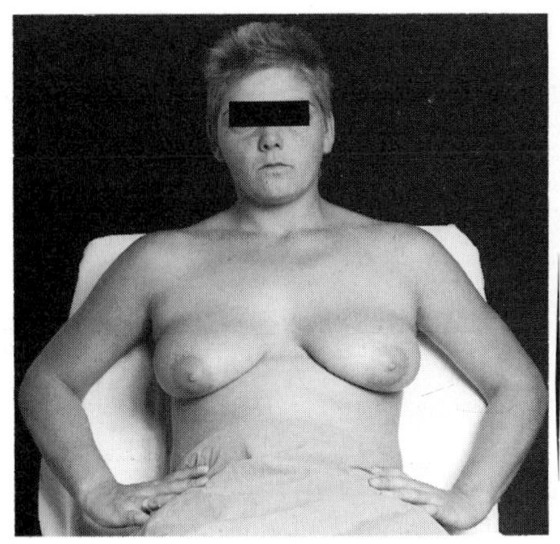

(a)

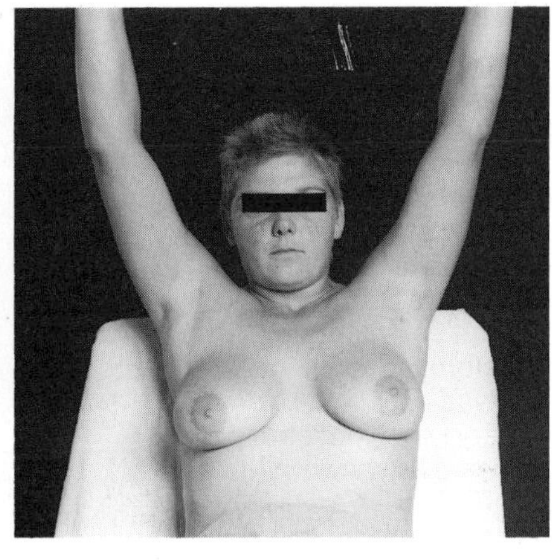

(b)

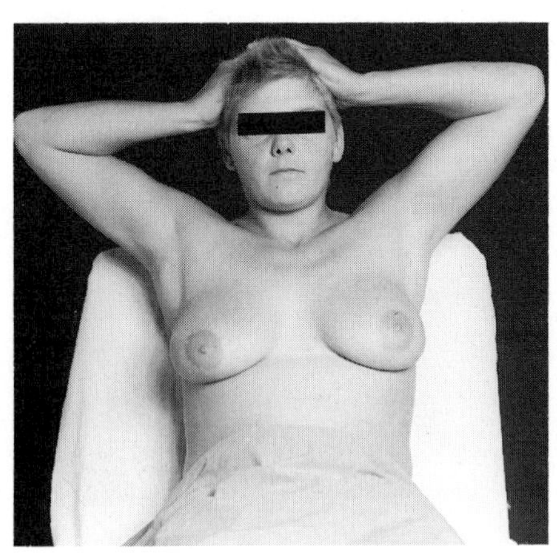

(c)

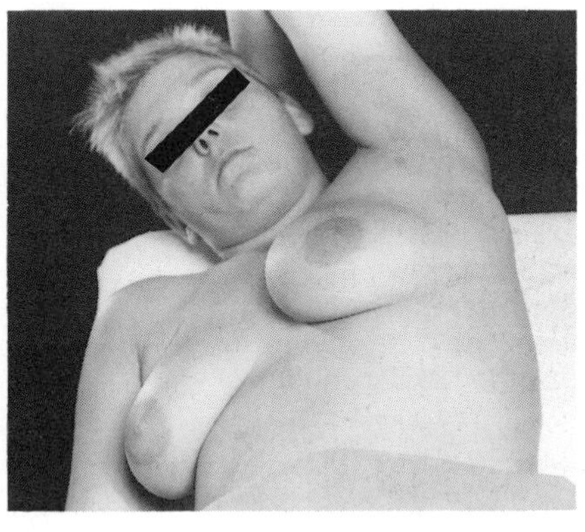

(d)

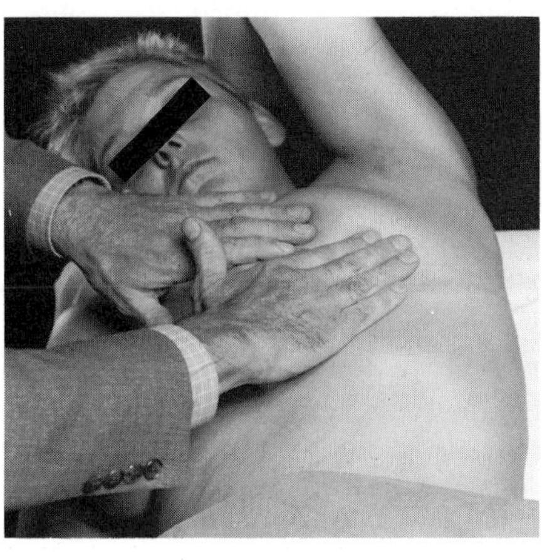

(e)

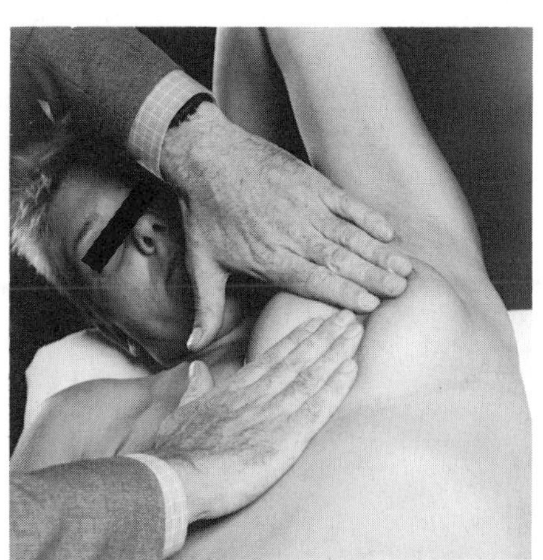

(f)

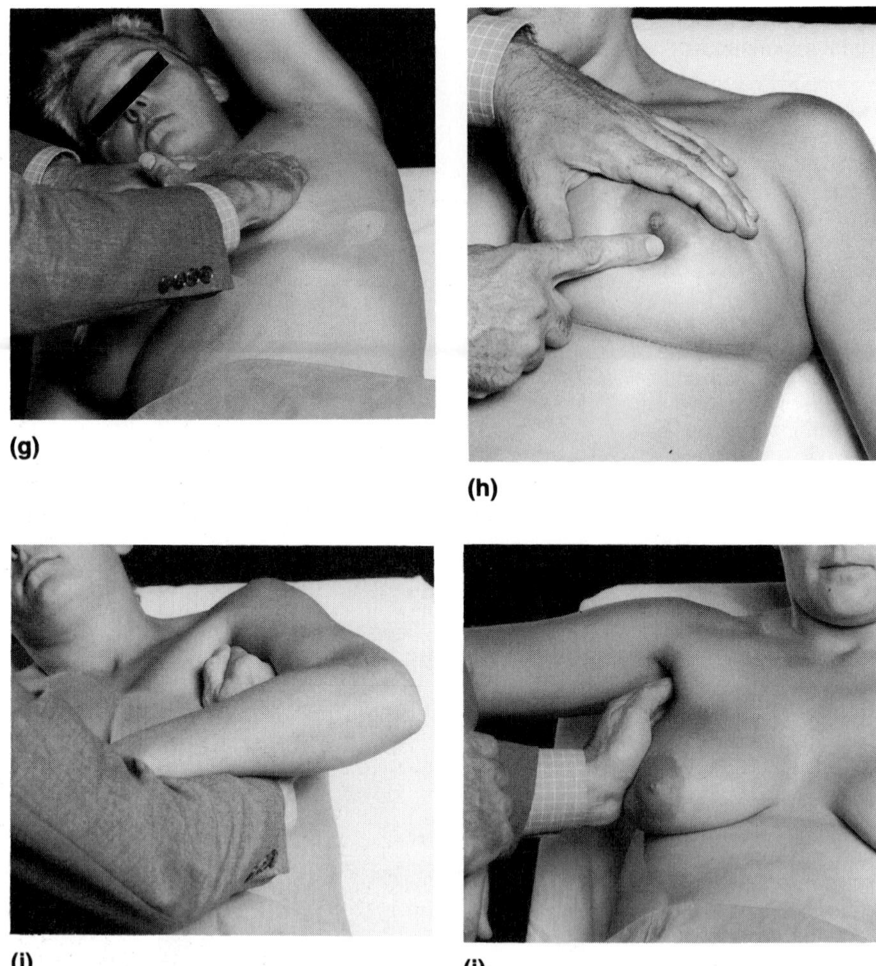

Fig. 27.4 (cont.)

The central part of the breast and the axillary tail **(g)** must also be palpated. If there is a history of nipple discharge, the areola is pressed in different areas **(h)** to identify the duct from which it emanates and therefore the segment involved. Finally, the axillary lymph nodes are palpated as shown in **(i)** and **(j)**. The left axilla is palpated with the right hand and the right axilla is palpated with the left hand. It is important to relax the axillary muscles by supporting the weight of the patient's arm as shown. The fingers of the examining hand are firmly held in a curve, pressed high into the apex of the axilla against the chest wall and drawn downwards. The hand will then 'ride over' any enlarged axillary nodes

(g) **(h)** **(i)** **(j)**

The technique of palpating the breast may need to be modified according to the type of breast being examined. Palpation with the flat of one hand is usual, but it may be more appropriate to examine large pendulous breasts between two hands. The normal breast has a wide range of textures, ranging from soft, through nodular, to hard. This underlines the difficulties of clinical evaluation of a lump or lumpiness. Suspicious physical signs should be compared with the breast on the opposite side because physiological and other hormonally induced changes tend to be symmetrical. If a lump is found, the overlying skin must be examined for mobility and tethering. Fixation of the lump to the chest wall can be assessed by having the patient tense pectoralis major. She does this by pressing her hand onto her hip.

A history of nipple discharge can often be confirmed by applying pressure over the appropriate quadrant of the breast near the areola. The position of the duct on the summit of the nipple from where the discharge emerges can then be noted. Discharges that are not obviously blood-stained should be tested for blood using urinalysis dipsticks.

Fig. 27.5 Characteristic signs of breast cancer

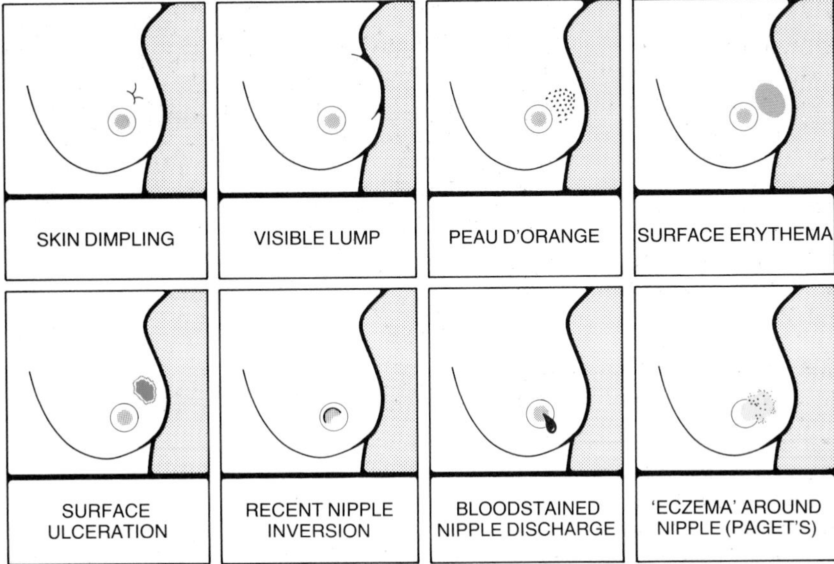

Fig. 27.6 Carcinoma of the breast

(a) and **(b)** Characteristic skin dimpling (arrowed) over breast carcinomas. This may be a subtle sign and only be visible in tangential light.
(c) Nipple retraction and widespread 'peau d'orange' resulting from a large central breast carcinoma. Peau d'orange is caused by a combination of cutaneous infiltration by tumour and skin oedema

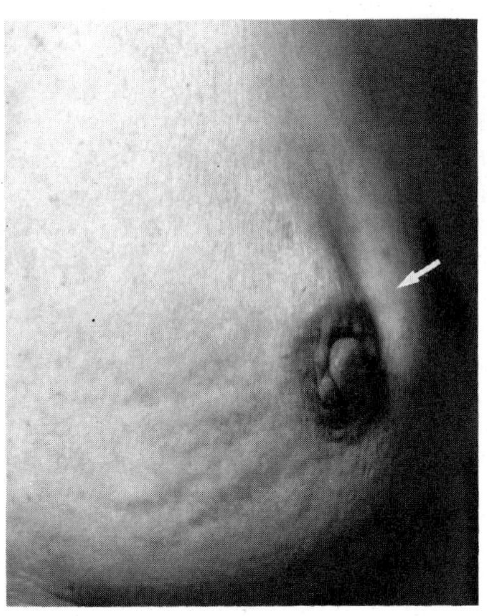

(a)

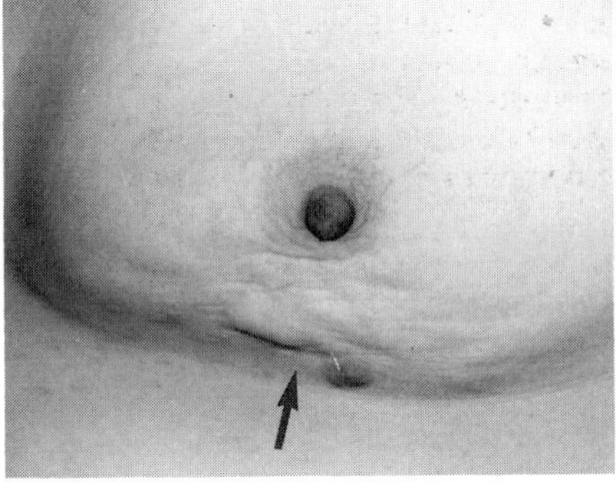

(b)

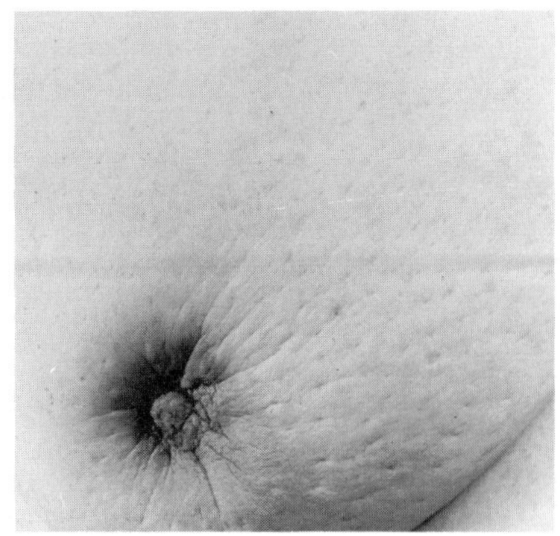

(c)

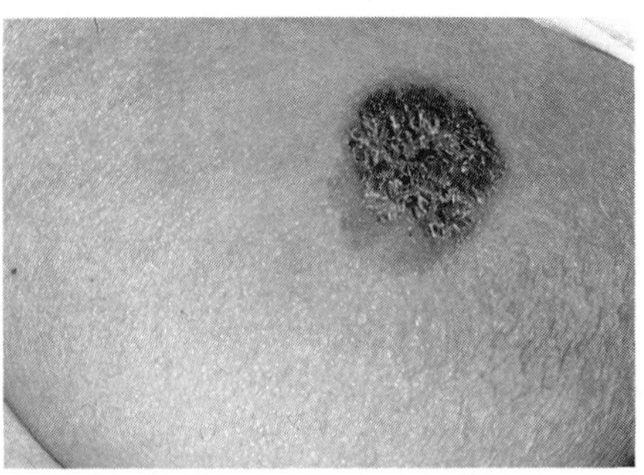

Fig. 27.7 Paget's disease of the nipple

The experienced clinician can probably detect 85% of carcinomas bigger than one cm in diameter. Nonetheless, a third of the carcinomas in asymptomatic women attending for screening will be missed. Fortunately, carcinomas are rare in women without symptoms. Similarly, even among experts, there is at least a 25% error in detecting axillary node involvement by palpation. Because of the high rate of false negative examinations, clinical suspicion alone is enough to justify further investigations.

Investigation of breast disorders

The range of investigation, short of surgical excision and histological examination, is limited. *Mammography* gives up to 95% diagnostic accuracy in the presence of a palpable lump but accuracy falls when mammography is used as a screening procedure. Mammography is unreliable in women under 40 years. The radiological features of carcinoma include a characteristic fine calcification and puckering of breast tissue. These may be quite subtle signs, however, and the definitive interpretation should be left to an experienced radiologist.

In the case of an apparently solid but discrete lump, *ultrasound* can readily distinguish between a solid mass and a cyst. If a cyst is suspected, aspiration should be attempted; any fluid obtained should be sent for cytological examination. A simple cyst will contain yellow or green fluid and the lump will disappear. If the fluid is blood-stained, or if the lump does not disappear or reappears a few days later, then a carcinoma should be suspected and the lump must be excised (see Figure 27.20 later).

If the lump is solid, a sample can be taken for histology using a special biopsy needle (e.g. Trucut). Alternatively, cells may be aspirated using a fine-needle and sent for cytological examination. These methods are finding increasing favour because of the advantages of accurate preoperative diagnosis. A negative result does not, however, exclude carcinoma.

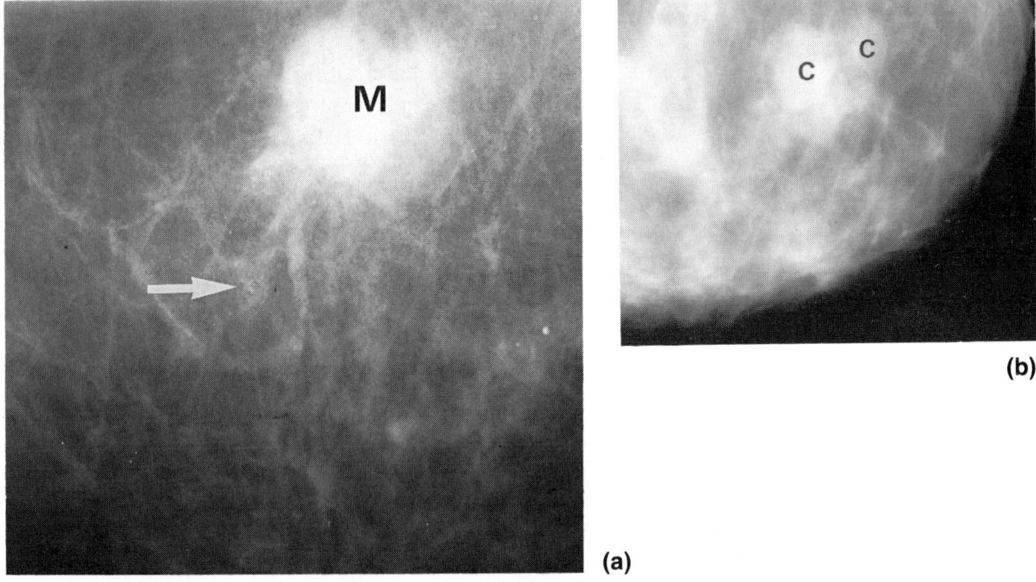

Fig. 27.8 Mammograms contrasting breast cancer and fibroadenosis

(a) An infiltrating radiopaque mass **M** is suggestive of malignancy but the nearby fine calcification (arrowed) clinches the diagnosis. Malignant micro-calcification is a subtle sign requiring careful examination of the films with magnification; it does not reproduce well in photographs. Coarser calcification is found in benign breast diseases. **(b)** This mammogram shows a fibroadenotic mass incorporating two well-circumscribed cysts **C**

IMPORTANT SURGICAL DISORDERS OF THE BREAST

CARCINOMA OF THE BREAST

Pathology

Virtually all cancers of the breast are adenocarcinomas; the exceptions are the occasional sarcoma and metastasis from elsewhere. Adenocarcinomas originate either in the epithelium of the mammary ducts or in the glands of the breast lobules. The vast majority are of ductal origin. Most breast cancers show clear evidence of invasiveness at the time of presentation. They are known as *infiltrating ductal* or *infiltrating lobular carcinomas*. In patients with breast carcinoma, other areas of the breast often contain dysplastic cells still confined within the epithelial basement membrane of duct or lobule; this 'in-situ' stage probably precedes the development of infiltrating carcinoma. A histological diagnosis of non-infiltrating intraduct or intralobular carcinoma must be interpreted with caution because this may mean that an invasive carcinoma has been inadequately sampled.

The distinction between lobular and ductal carcinoma is not merely of academic interest. Lobular carcinomas tend to arise multicentrically, so that bilateral tumours occur in a significant proportion of cases. Further, lobular carcinomas are more likely to bear oestrogen receptors and are thus more amenable to anti-oestrogen therapy.

The majority of invasive carcinomas excite a strong fibrous reaction in the stromal connective tissue, producing a hard *scirrhous* lesion. Much less commonly, there is little fibrotic response and the tumour is soft and brain-like (*encephaloid*) in texture. These tumours tend to occur in younger, particularly pregnant women. A small minority of carcinomas excite a strong lymphocytic inflammatory response; recent evidence suggests that this indicates a much better prognosis. These are now described as *medullary* carcinomas, although this term was formerly used synonymously with encephaloid carcinomas.

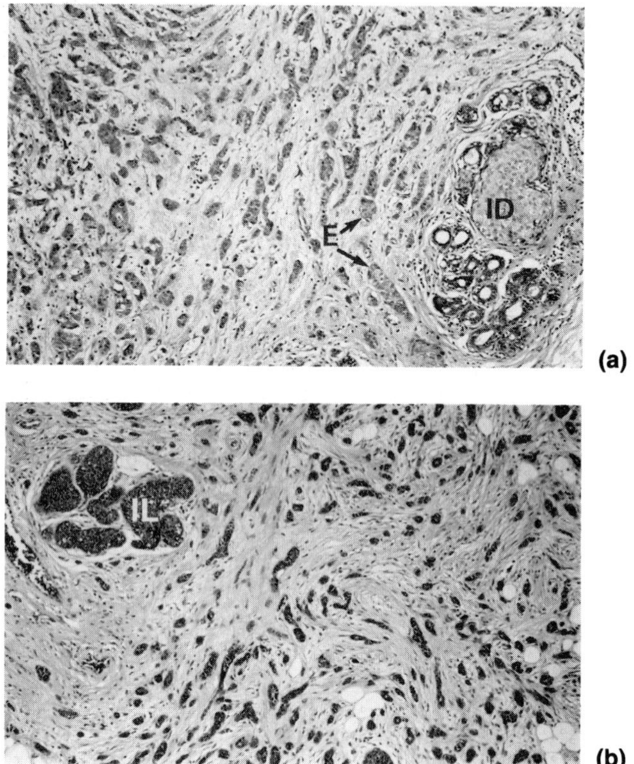

Fig 27.9
Breast adenocarcinoma — histopathology

(a) An example of infiltrating ductal carcinoma. Note the small clumps of atypical epithelial cells **E** surrounded by dense reactive connective tissue. Near the right-hand edge there is an area of intraduct (in-situ) carcinoma **ID**, the tumour cells being still surrounded by a basement membrane.
(b) This illustrates the much less common lobular form of breast carcinoma. The field is mainly occupied by infiltrating tumour with a small intralobular (in-situ) area **IL** near the left-hand edge

Some patients with breast carcinoma (usually of ductal origin) present with reddening and thickening of the skin of the nipple and sometimes areola, often followed by fissuring and ulceration. In this condition, known as *Paget's disease of the nipple*, the epidermis of the nipple and areola becomes infiltrated by huge neoplastic cells from the underlying carcinoma. These cells are believed to reach the surface by intra-epithelial spread along the mammary ducts.

Natural history of breast carcinoma

Before there is any clinical evidence of its presence, the breast tumour has usually reached at least 1 cm in diameter. Malignant cells may, however, have

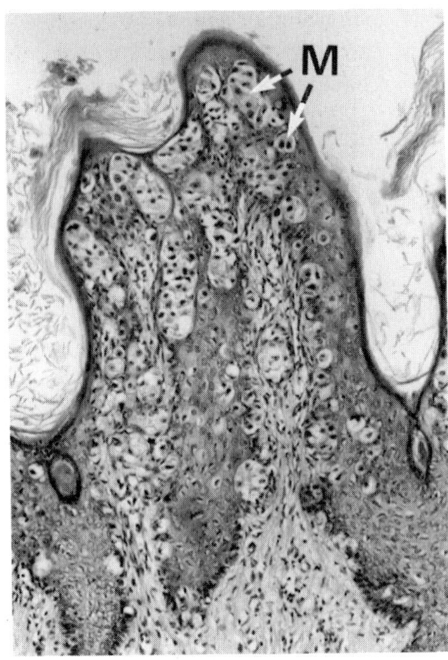

Fig. 27.10 Pagetʼs disease of the nipple — histopathology

The epidermis in and around the nipple is infiltrated by clumps of large malignant cells **M** from an underlying intraduct carcinoma

been proliferating for several years and an in-situ form may have been present for even longer. Invading locally, the tumour usually evokes an intense fibrous response in adjacent breast tissue, which is largely responsible for the mass becoming palpable.

At some stage, tumour cells enter the lymphatics and spread to the regional lymph nodes of the axillary and internal mammary groups. The nodes closest to the lesion are involved first, followed successively by other nodes in the chain. Micrometastases are present in the nodes long before they are palpable. Later, tumour cells may breach the lymph node capsules to invade the surrounding tissues. In this way, the nodes become fixed and matted together. Systemic

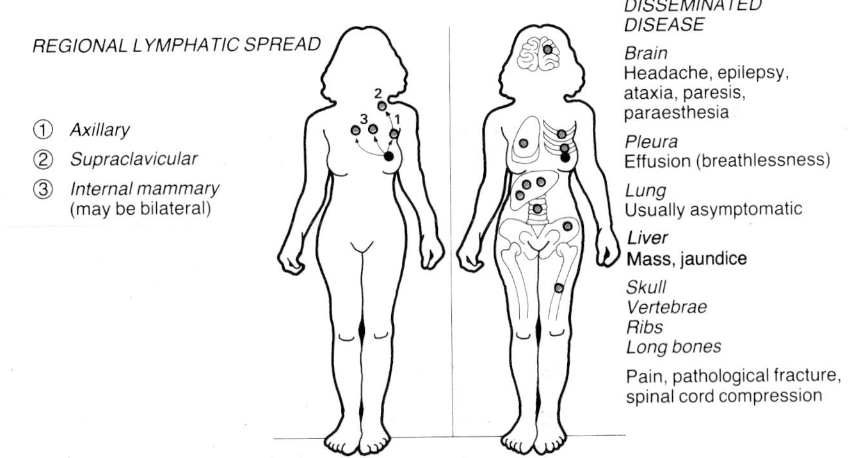

Fig. 27.11 Common sites of spread of breast carcinoma

spread may also occur very early so that even a small localised lesion may have already metastasised widely. Nevertheless, systemic spread is more likely to have occurred once regional lymph nodes are involved.

There is great variation in the behaviour of breast cancer between individuals. The disease progresses more slowly with advancing age. Indeed, 10% of untreated patients survive ten years or more. In a minority of patients, usually the young, the disease follows a much more aggressive course. Histological grade is also a useful prognostic indicator: the poorer the differentiation, the more likely is recurrence or early death. In some tumours, the cells possess oestrogen receptors which can be demonstrated by immunological techniques. These tumours are partly dependent on oestrogen for their growth. This characteristic makes possible palliative treatment by hormonal manipulation. Contrary to popular belief, pregnancy probably does not accelerate tumour growth when other factors, such as youth, are taken into account.

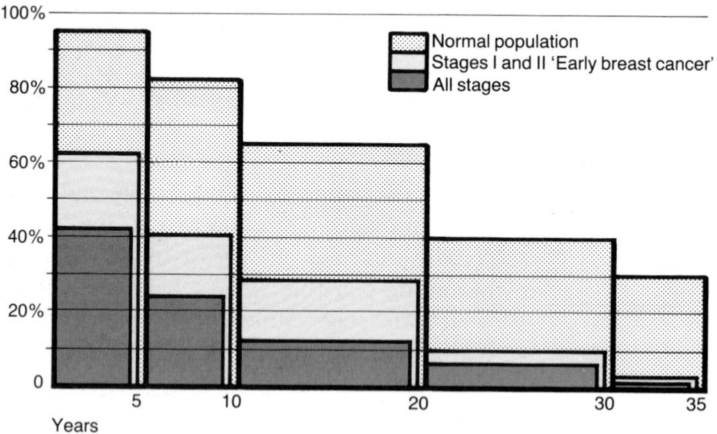

Fig. 27.12 Life expectancy after diagnosis of breast cancer

Life expectancy

Life expectancy for women with breast cancer (irrespective of the type of treatment) is shown in Figure 27.12, compared with unaffected women of equivalent ages. Two important facts emerge: women often survive many years after treatment for breast cancer, but very few are completely cured of the disease. That is, most affected women will eventually die of breast cancer unless they should die of some other disease in the meantime. Patients with a disease-free interval of five years after treatment clearly cannot be described as 'cured', as might be the case with other malignancies.

Staging of breast cancer

The purpose of staging is to define the extent of tumour spread so that prognosis can be estimated and the most appropriate treatment planned. There are several systems of staging in common use; the simplest is based on clinical

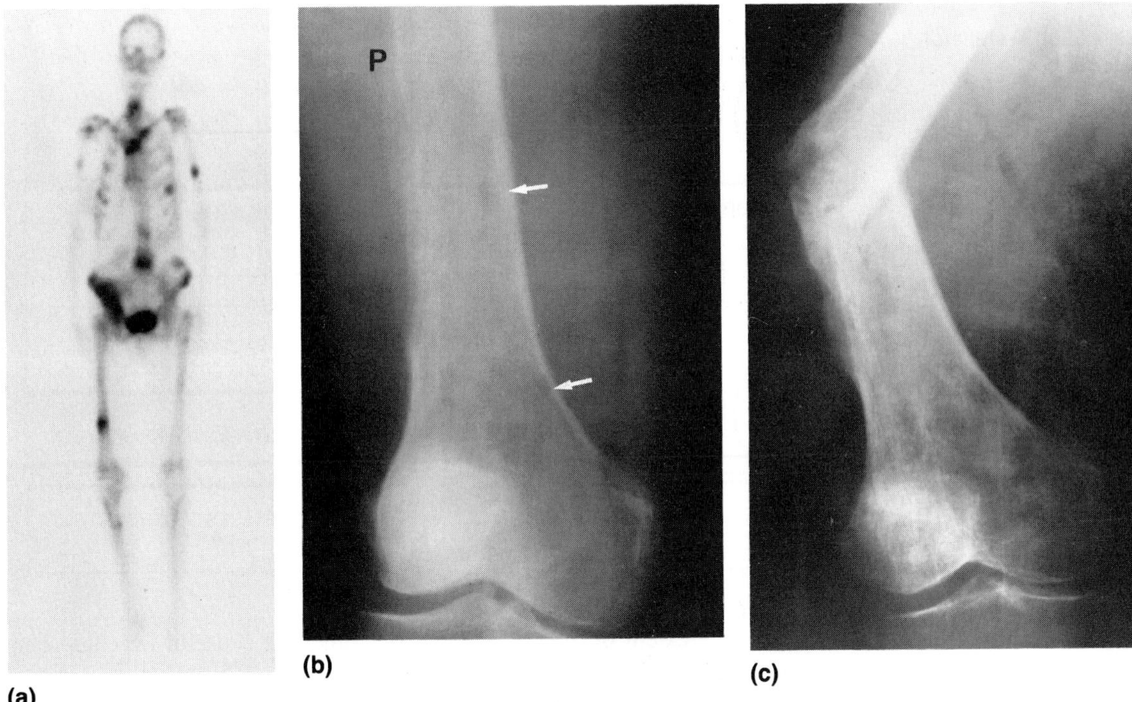

(a) (b) (c)

Fig. 27.13 Skeletal metastases from carcinoma of the breast

(a) Anterior view of radioisotope bone scan of a 48-year-old woman complaining of pain in the neck and right hip. She had had a mastectomy for carcinoma eight years previously. The scan shows large metastatic deposits in the lower cervical and lumbar spine, right pelvis, right femur and left humerus as well as several smaller deposits in the ribs and elsewhere in the skeleton. **(b)** X-ray of the lower femur in a 79-year-old woman presenting with a fungating breast carcinoma and pain in the left knee. The X-ray shows radiolucencies (arrowed) indicating bony metastasis in the distal femur and elevation of the periosteum **P** medially. Radiotherapy was arranged to alleviate the symptoms. **(c)** Some weeks later, despite treatment, the patient returned with this pathological fracture of the femur

evidence of local and systemic spread. The more sophisticated use various additional methods such as grading of tumour histology, lymph node biopsy, chest X-ray or bone scans. Unfortunately, staging is still a crude tool since microscopic spread cannot reliably be detected by these methods.

The *Manchester system* of staging (Figure 27.14) is based purely on clinical findings. Although simple, it is necessarily imprecise. The internationally accepted *TNM system* (see Figure 27.15) uses clinical and investigation results to grade local *T*umour size and extent, regional spread to lymph *N*odes, and the presence or absence of *M*etastases. This precision allows more accurate

Fig. 27.14 Manchester staging system for breast cancer

Stage	
I	Breast only
II	Nodes thought to be involved but not fixed
III	Locally advanced disease in breast or nodes
IV	Distant metastases

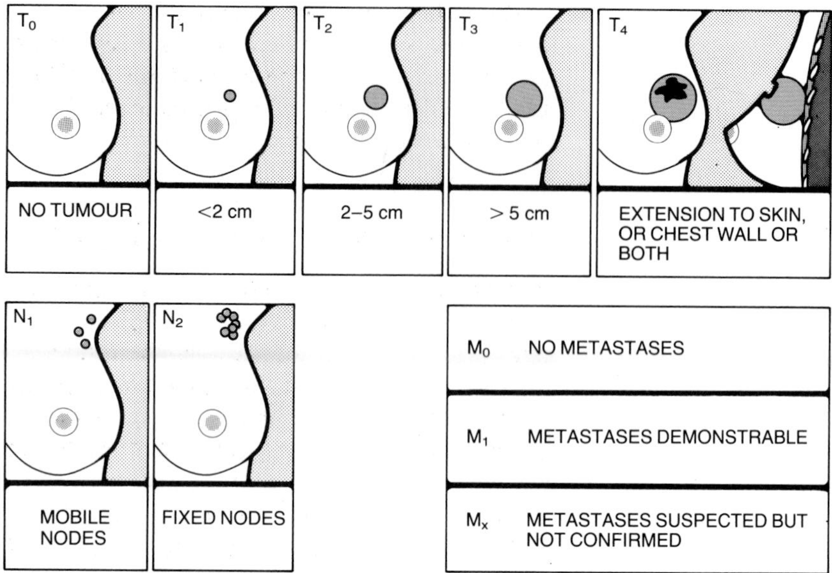

Fig. 27.15 TNM classification system for breast cancer

recording of the extent of disease at any given time and is useful for comparing responses to different treatments.

Principles of management of breast cancer

Despite extensive research into methods of treatment, the prognosis for patients with treated disease has not significantly changed over the past 30 years. No single treatment is clearly superior and this explains why specific details of management vary from one centre to another. There are, however, four universal principles of management, which are summarised in Figure 27.16.

There is a reasonable prospect of long-term survival, if not cure, in *early breast cancer* i.e. true stage I or II disease. In *advanced breast cancer*, i.e. stages III and IV, palliation is the only realistic objective, to improve the quality of life and only secondarily to extend life.

Fig. 27.16 Principles of management of breast cancer

Establish the diagnosis
Control disease in the affected breast
Prevent and treat local and regional disease
Control advanced and disseminated disease

Establishing the diagnosis

If there is clinical suspicion that a breast lump is malignant, the first priority is to obtain tissue for microscopic examination. This may be achieved by *aspiration cytology* or *needle biopsy*. More commonly, a discrete lump is completely excised with a margin of apparently normal breast tissue. The specimen is then sent for histology. This procedure, called *excision biopsy*, is also the first step in controlling local disease.

If the clinician is more doubtful about the diagnosis and does not feel surgery is justified, soft tissue radiography (*mammography*) may resolve the issue (see Figure 27.8). Other non-invasive methods of investigation include thermography and ultrasound, but the value of either has yet to be demonstrated in breast cancer diagnosis.

Control of disease in the affected breast

Removal of a discrete tumour mass along with a margin of apparently normal tissue (*lumpectomy*) might be thought to effect a cure. Bitter experience, however, has shown that 40% of these tumours recur later within the same breast. Furthermore, distant metastatic spread may have already occurred. Local recurrence occurs either because malignant cells had already penetrated beyond the margin of excision or because the remaining breast tissue is more susceptible to malignant change. The latter is particularly true for lobular carcinomas. Therefore, rational treatment must aim to eliminate tumour cells anywhere else in the affected breast. This can be achieved by surgical removal of the whole breast or by radiotherapy.

The conventional approach is to remove the entire breast (*mastectomy*) once the diagnosis is confirmed. Some surgeons prefer to prepare patients for possible mastectomy at the same operation as excision biopsy. The biopsy specimen is examined histologically in frozen sections while the patient remains on the operating table; if cancer is unequivocally demonstrated, the surgeon then proceeds to mastectomy. Unfortunately, frozen sections are not always easy to interpret. Thus, definitive diagnosis and treatment sometimes have to await histological examination of paraffin sections.

There has been a recent trend towards breast conservation in the management of breast cancer. Wide local excision of the tumour mass is performed and the remaining breast tissue is irradiated. The efficacy of this approach in preventing local recurrence is similar to that of mastectomy. Apart from its cosmetic and psychological advantages, wide local excision allows the option of later mastectomy if there is a local recurrence. Breast irradiation, following local excision, forms part of *radical radiotherapy*, designed to prevent local and regional recurrence.

Occasionally a patient presents with extensive local disease or widespread metastases. Surgery in these circumstances may be inappropriate and palliative measures such as radiotherapy may be used alone.

Prevention and treatment of local and regional disease

Even with a small primary tumour, microscopic disease may have already spread to local skin, chest wall or regional lymph nodes. Larger primary lesions may show local or regional secondary deposits at the time of initial presentation.

The management options are:

- *An expectant policy* may be adopted. This involves treating local and regional spread by surgery or radiotherapy only when it becomes clinically apparent

- *Axillary node biopsy* may be performed at the initial operation and the nodes subjected to radiotherapy only if they are histologically involved
- *Radical radiotherapy* may be given to all patients with breast cancer. This involves radiotherapy to the chest wall, as well as lymph nodes in the axillary, and perhaps supraclavicular and internal mammary groups. This may be applied after conservative surgery regardless of the apparent degree of spread
- *Surgery* may be used to excise axillary lymph nodes, whether clinically involved or not. The possible operations include *radical mastectomy* or less mutilating variants such as the *Patey modified radical mastectomy*. Since these operations take no account of spread to mediastinal and supraclavicular nodes, they are often combined with radiotherapy

Control of advanced and disseminated disease

The unexpectedly low cure rate for 'early' breast cancer is probably due to occult metastatic spread. On this basis, scientific trials of chemotherapy are being conducted for early breast cancer. Single or multiple cytotoxic drugs are used in addition to the usual surgical and radiotherapeutic techniques. Results are so far disappointing but if newer regimens are more effective, this *adjuvant chemotherapy* may become a routine part of future treatment.

All the treatments so far described attempt to achieve a complete cure. In reality, about 70% of patients presenting with early breast cancer will eventually succumb to the disease, though this may be as long as 35 years later. The control of advanced and disseminated disease at any stage can only be palliative.

Locally, tumour may spread within the breast, into the overlying skin or into the chest wall. It may even spread to the pleura causing an effusion. Systemic spread commonly causes osteolytic bone lesions which are painful and may result in pathological fracture. Secondary deposits are common in the liver but less common in the lungs and brain. These metastases tend to become troublesome only at a terminal stage of the disease. Some of these metastatic sites respond to local treatment, while others may respond to systemic therapy. These palliative treatments enable many patients to enjoy a good quality of life for several years, which is especially important to women with children.

a. Local palliation

The mainstay of local palliation is radiotherapy, provided the area has not already been irradiated. Advanced skin, breast, chest wall and lymph node disease or tumour recurrences usually respond well, as do isolated bone metastases. Pleural effusions can be aspirated or the pleural cavity obliterated by pleurectomy or instillation of tetracycline or various cytotoxic agents. Discrete lesions, for example in skin, can sometimes be removed surgically.

b. Hormonal manipulation

Systemic palliative treatment is largely confined to *hormonal manipulation*. This is designed to counteract any oestrogen-dependent characteristics of the tumour.

Hormonal treatment of breast cancer is essentially empirical:

- *Tamoxifen*, an oestrogen receptor blocker taken orally, is being widely used with good short-term results. There is also evidence of increased patient survival when the drug is used in post-menopausal women. The drug has the side-effect of causing menopausal symptoms in most women
- Surgical *oophorectomy* gives a good but temporary response in about a third of patients with intractable bone pain
- *Corticosteroids* may be used to suppress adrenal sex hormone production
- *Adrenalectomy* and *hypophysectomy* are now seldom performed because of low response rate and unpleasant side effects. Occasionally, the drug amino-glutethimide is used to perform a 'medical' adrenalectomy

c. Systemic chemotherapy

Chemotherapy, using combinations of drugs, is sometimes employed for palliation of extensive metastatic disease. Recent improvements in chemotherapeutic drugs make this option worthwhile for certain patients, for example, young women or those with hepatic involvement.

Long-term follow up

Women who have had one breast cancer have a 15% risk of developing a second tumour in the other breast at some time during their life. The risk is higher if the original lesion was a lobular carcinoma. The breast tissue in these women may have an increased susceptibility to cancer, or breast cancer may arise at the same time in multiple foci. Thus, women with breast cancer should be regularly followed up. The unaffected breast should be examined clinically, and possibly by mammography, for many years after initial treatment. Indeed, there is a trend in the USA to perform prophylactic contralateral mastectomy with cosmetic implant at the outset.

Prostheses and preoperative preparation

The cosmetic effects of mastectomy are of great psychological importance to woman and their families. Careful attention to this can alleviate distress and improve acceptance of disfigurement. Preoperative counselling by medical or specially trained nursing staff should prepare the patient for treatment.

After mastectomy, it is important that life-like prostheses are provided. Wherever possible, this should start with temporary prostheses in the immediate postoperative period. These may even be inserted before the patient leaves the operating theatre. Sometimes, reconstructive surgery using muscle flaps and

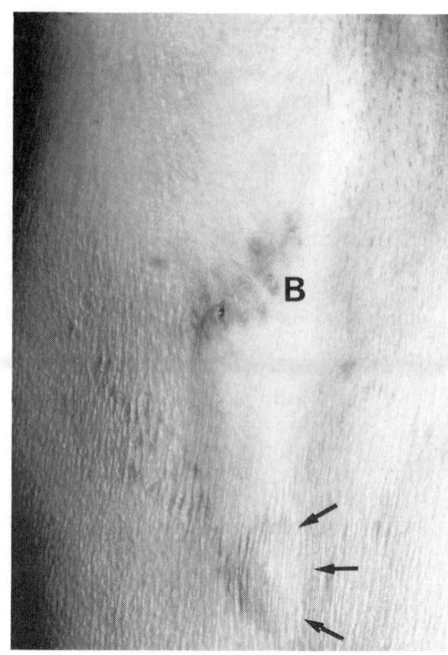

Fig. 27.17 Skin secondaries following simple mastectomy and radiotherapy

This patient presented with painless, slightly elevated nodules in the skin below the axilla three years after treatment for lobular carcinoma of the breast. In this photograph, the arm is elevated and one skin secondary can just be made out (arrowed); the site of excision biopsy of another is seen at **B**

silicone implants may be appropriate later. Self-help societies, like the Mastectomy Association, can play a valuable part in helping the patient to return to normal life.

Breast cancer in males

1% of all breast cancers occur in males. Presentation and management are similar to that in females. Chest wall and lymph node involvement may occur earlier because there is so little breast tissue, and prognosis may be worse than for females.

Fig. 27.18 Summary — major treatment options in breast cancer

Excision biopsy alone (not recommended)

Needle biopsy or aspiration cytology plus radiotherapy

Wide local excision (lumpectomy) plus radiotherapy

Simple mastectomy with or without node biopsy

Modified (Patey) radical mastectomy

Standard (Halsted) radical mastectomy

Supra-radical (Urban) mastectomy

Note: The list ranges between what is now generally regarded as inadequate treatment and excessive treatment. Treatments near the centre of the list are the most commonly used. Radiotherapy can be added to any type of mastectomy. Adjuvant chemotherapy or anti-oestrogen therapy can be combined with any of the list.

BENIGN BREAST DISORDERS

FIBRO-ADENOSIS

Pathology

Fibroadenosis is a disorder of the breast in women of reproductive age, its peak incidence occurring between the ages of 35 and 45. It probably results from disordered physiological responses to circulating hormones. In brief, the

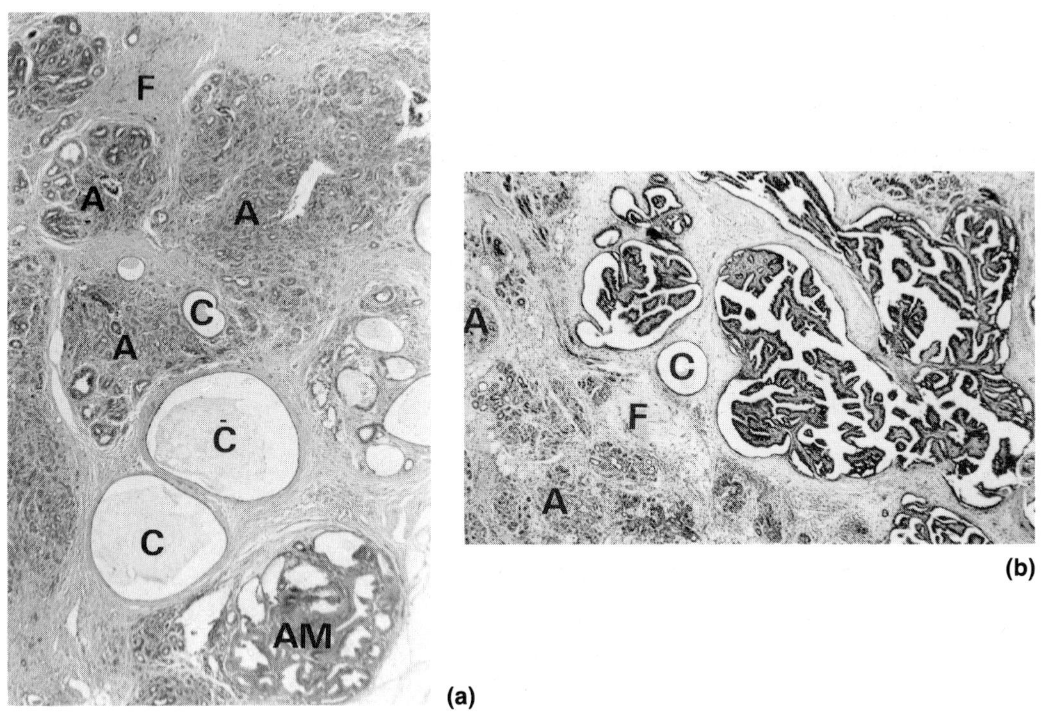

Fig. 27.19 Fibroadenosis—histopathology

These micrographs illustrate several of the common histological forms of fibroadenosis, many of which can be found in a single lesion. These are responsible for the various names applied to the condition. *Cysts* **C** of various sizes (from microscopic to several centimetres) are common. They are most often lined by simple flattened ductular epithelium. In some cysts, the lining proliferates to resemble that of apocrine sweat glands, a condition known as *apocrine metaplasia* **AM**. Sometimes the cystically dilated ducts are filled with papillary ingrowths from the duct wall, producing a condition known as *florid duct papillomatosis*. This is seen in (b). Similar but solitary lesions constitute the duct papillomas which may be found in larger mammary ducts and lactiferous sinuses. Hyperplastic proliferation of lobular acini is responsible for areas where *adenosis* **A** predominates. Variation in the density of the fibrous tissue **F** surrounding the epithelial components contributes to the general heterogeneity of the lesions. In addition, the fibrous tissue may proliferate within the lobules of hyperplastic epithelium, splitting the acini apart; this appearance is known as *sclerosing adenosis*. In older patients, the fibrous component which replaces the normal mammary fat may be the dominant feature; the epithelial component is represented by the occasional dilated (ectatic) mammary duct. This condition is known as *mammary fibrosis*

changes result from distortion and overgrowth of one or more of the various components of the breast, namely the *ducts*, the *lobules* and the supporting *fibrous tissue*. The fibrous tissue element becomes exaggerated, i.e. *fibrosis*, and the epithelial components undergo hyperplasia, i.e. *adenosis*; hence the name fibroadenosis.

Although this book uses the general term of fibroadenosis, many other descriptive terms have also been applied, including cystic mastopathia, mastitis, fibrocystic disease of the breast and cystic mammary dysplasia. Most of these terms are confusing, and some erroneously suggest that the condition is more than a simple proliferative disorder of breast tissue.

There is no evidence that fibroadenosis is a precursor of carcinoma. Fibroadenosis is common, however, and carcinoma will sometimes develop in a woman with fibroadenosis.

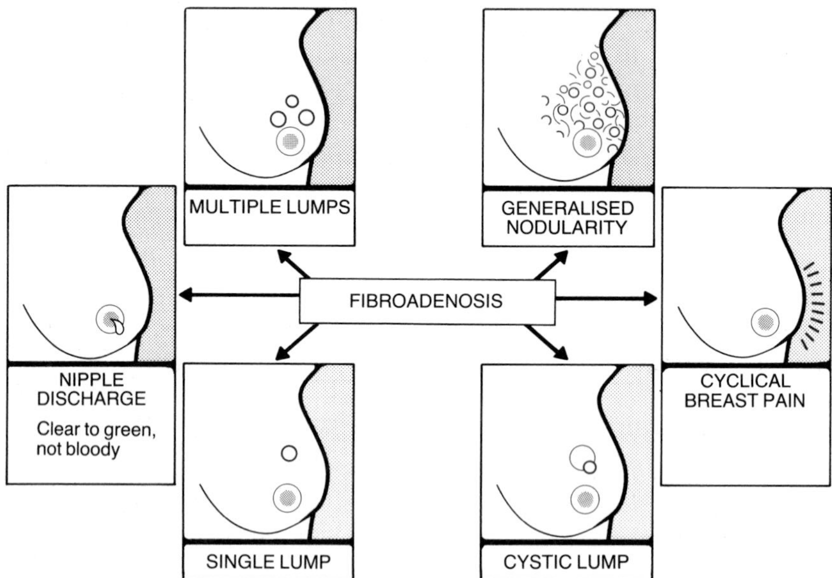

Fig. 27.20 Clinical presentation of fibroadenosis

Clinical presentation and management

Fibroadenosis usually presents as a single lump or multiple lumps in the breast, which are painful and tender premenstrually. Often pain is the presenting complaint rather than a lump. Lumpiness and tenderness are a cyclical feature of the normal breast; thus, diffuse fibroadenosis may just represent an extreme variation of the normal. Isolated lesions, however, may be difficult to distinguish clinically from carcinoma.

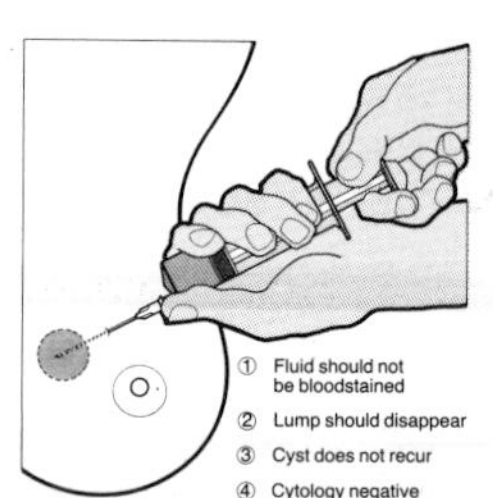

Fig. 27.21 Cyst aspiration and criteria for exclusion of cancer associated with a cyst

Breast cysts are a common form of fibroadenosis. The cysts are usually single, occasionally multiple, and they are most common in perimenopausal women. They sometimes develop with startling rapidity. On palpation, they can usually be recognised by their smooth rounded outline and characteristic tense fluctuation, similar to the texture of a 'ping-pong' ball. The diagnosis can be made by simple aspiration. Carcinoma can be excluded if the criteria shown in Figure 27.21 are satisfied. The diagnosis of fibroadenosis thus depends on excluding cancer. This is done clinically, by mammography or by excision biopsy.

Once cancer has been excluded and the patient reassured, further treatment is often unnecessary. Isolated fibroadenotic lesions may have been surgically excised (and thus treated) in the process. When pain is severe and localised to a particular area, excision of the area is justified, but if pain is more diffuse, drugs such as *danazol* and *bromocriptine* may be prescribed. Danazol inhibits pituitary gonadotrophin secretion but may have serious androgenic and other side effects which often limit its usefulness. Bromocriptine inhibits pituitary prolactin release, and has fewer side effects.

FIBRO-ADENOMA

Pathology

Fibroadenoma commonly presents in younger women as a solitary breast lump. It is considered to be a benign neoplasm, but may well represent a nodular form of fibroadenosis. The lesions are composed of epithelial and fibrous components: the epithelium forms glandular structures lined by mammary ductal cells and the connective tissue forms a loose cellular stroma. The lesions are well circumscribed by a condensed connective tissue capsule. As with fibroadenosis, there appears to be no association with breast cancer.

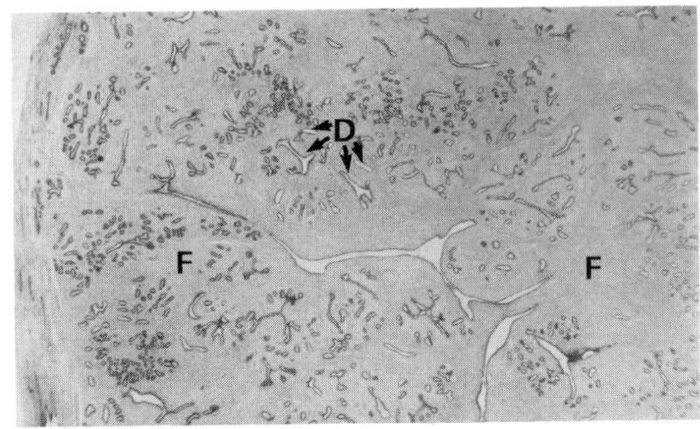

Fig. 27.22 Fibro-adenoma — histopathology

The characteristic histological features of fibroadenoma are proliferation of mammary ducts **D** and gross hyperplasia of the intervening fibrous stroma **F**

Clinical presentation and management of fibroadenoma

Unlike fibroadenosis, fibroadenomas are usually found in younger women, below the age of 30. They usually present as discrete, non-tender, highly mobile lumps. They may be found incidentally or during self examination. Small lesions are sometimes described as *breast mice* since they slip away from beneath the palpating hand. Giant fibroadenomas tend to occur in older women. Like fibroadenosis, the main clinical importance of fibroadenoma is distinguishing it from breast cancer. Excision biopsy confirms the diagnosis and provides treatment.

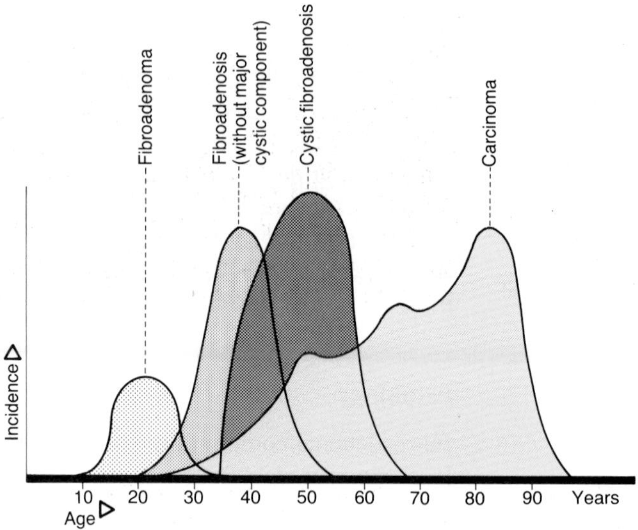

Fig. 27.23 Age incidence of common breast disorders

DUCT PAPILLOMA

Duct papillomas are localised areas of epithelial proliferation within large mammary or lactiferous ducts. They are therefore benign hyperplastic lesions rather than neoplasms.

Duct papillomas present with nipple bleeding or a blood stained discharge. The differential diagnosis thus includes intraduct carcinoma and infiltrating carcinoma. The breast is carefully palpated for lumps and a mammogram is usually performed to search for frank carcinoma. *Ductography* (see Figure 27.25) may confirm the presence of a duct papilloma. Duct papillomas are usually treated by surgical excision of the affected segment of breast (*microdochectomy*). The affected segment is identified during operation by passing a probe into the duct from where blood can be expressed.

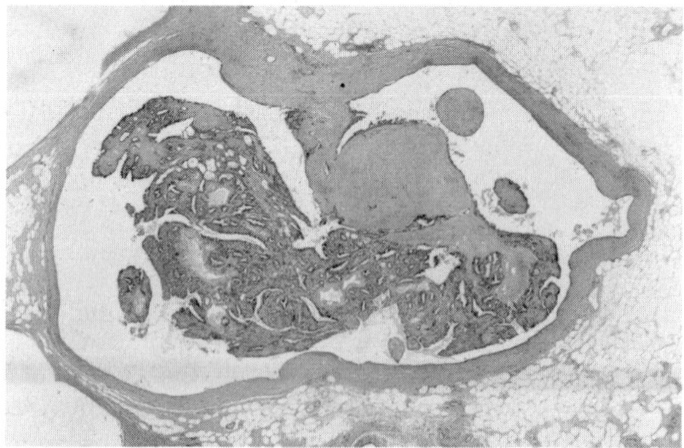

Fig. 27.24 Duct papilloma—histopathology

This micrograph shows a duct papilloma which, in pathological terms, merely represents an isolated form of florid duct papillomatosis (see Fig. 27.19b) occurring in a larger duct. The ectatic (dilated) duct is filled with a friable papillary mass which bleeds readily, causing a blood-stained discharge from the nipple

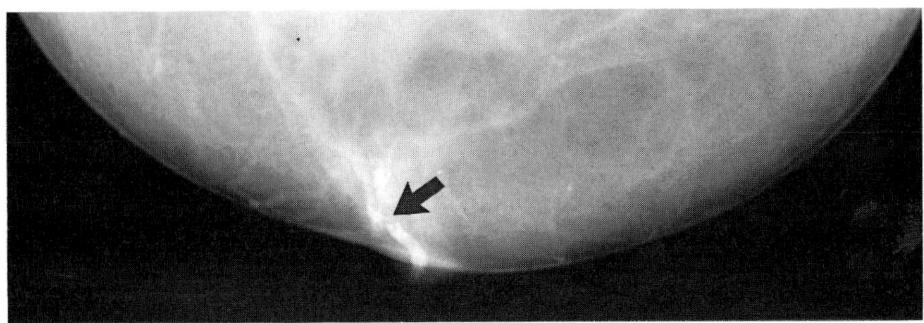

Fig. 27.25 Contrast mammogram outlining duct papilloma

This patient presented with bleeding from the nipple but no breast lump was palpable. The affected duct was injected with contrast material which outlines the duct system revealing a small defect (arrowed) which represents a duct papilloma

TRAUMATIC FAT NECROSIS

Trauma to the breast, sometimes trivial or even unnoticed, may cause necrosis of mammary adipose tissue. Initially, there is an acute inflammatory response, but if necrotic fat remains, the inflammatory picture becomes more chronic. Plasma cells appear in large numbers and macrophages take up lipid material. A fibrotic response at the margins of the damaged area produces a hard, often irregular breast lump, which may cause skin dimpling if it is close to the surface. Thus the clinical picture may be indistinguishable from carcinoma. Traumatic fat necrosis is uncommon and the diagnosis can only be made by excision biopsy.

INFECTIONS OF THE BREAST

Infections of the breast lobules present either as a diffuse cellulitis or as an abscess. The latter is often the result of inadequately treated cellulitis. Less commonly, infections arise in the sebaceous (Montgomery's) glands of the areola, where they resemble common skin boils. Deep infections occur most commonly during late pregnancy and lactation. The organism is almost invariably Staphylococcus aureus. It gains access to the breast either through cracked nipple skin or the blood stream. Stagnation of breast secretions may be a predisposing factor.

Diagnosis is usually obvious, with local and systemic signs of acute inflammation. The patient is generally unwell with a tachycardia and marked fever. The affected segment of the breast is painful and tender, red and warm. If the infection is inadequately treated, a considerable amount of breast tissue is destroyed and a large amount of pus forms. The lesion then becomes fluctuant and eventually 'points' to the surface and discharges. Occasionally, in a non-lactating woman, a low-grade chronic breast abscess may develop and present as a tender lump without overt signs of infection. This may be a presentation of mammary duct ectasia, in which case the pus is sterile.

The early cellulitic phase is reversible if treated with appropriate antibiotics. Flucloxacillin is the antibiotic of choice on a 'best guess' basis. If antibiotics are started too late, or the wrong antibiotic is chosen, tissue damage and accumulation of polymorphs forms multiple loculi of pus. This can only be treated by surgical drainage. The need for surgical drainage has declined in recent years because of prompt and appropriate antibiotic treatment.

At operation, a skin incision is made over the most fluctuant area and the loculi are explored and broken down with a finger. If there is extensive damage, a drain may be inserted in the wound, and if there is significant residual cellulitis, antibiotics should be prescribed postoperatively.

MAMMARY DUCT ECTASIA

Mammary duct ectasia means dilatation of the larger breast ducts. These usually contain green fluid and sometimes sterile pus. If an ectatic duct ruptures, a chronic inflammatory response develops in the surrounding breast tissue. Plasma cells are a characteristic feature of the histology, which is described as *plasma cell mastitis*. Duct ectasia may occur because of obstruction by papillomata but the cause is more often obscure. A few ducts may be involved or the whole duct system.

Mammary duct ectasia is most common in the decade around the menopause. Patients typically present with a green nipple discharge and tender lumpiness beneath or close to the areola. Red tender areas may appear which simulate breast abscesses. Mammography sometimes shows diagnostic features. Management involves exclusion of carcinoma and surgical excision of the affected tissue if necessary. If mammary duct ectasia is extensive, sub-areolar excision of all the major ducts usually cures the condition.

Note that the term *plasma cell mastitis* describes a histopathological appearance seen in different conditions such as fat necrosis or ruptured ectatic duct. These evoke an inflammatory response in which plasma cells predominate. Like any intense inflammatory response, this produces a hard irregular mass. The term plasma cell mastitis should be reserved for histological description.

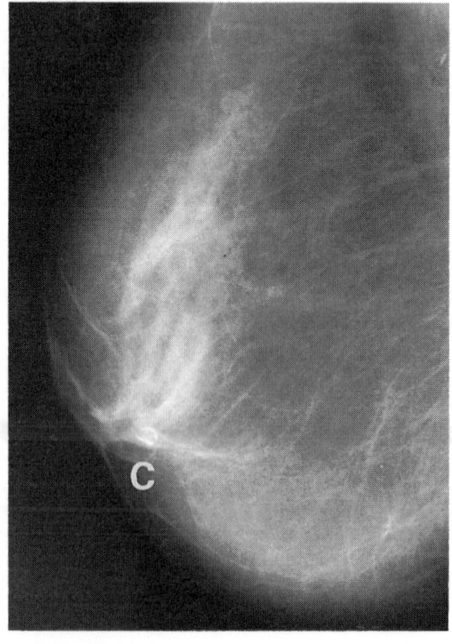

Fig. 27.26 Mammary duct ectasia

Radiopaque mass of dilated ducts with no features of malignancy. Large duct calcification **C** is also seen. Note the skin identation caused by fibrosis. Clinically, this condition can be mistaken for carcinoma

MALE BREAST DISORDERS

Any condition which occurs in the female breast can occur in the male. Only two conditions are clinically important: carcinoma and gynaecomastia. Any suspicious lumps should be removed. *Carcinoma* of the male breast is similar to that seen in women and is managed in the same way.

Gynaecomastia is benign hypertrophy of the breast disc and has a hormonal basis. Clinically, one or both breasts become abnormally enlarged. Gynaecomastia may be present at birth in response to maternal oestrogens crossing the placenta; the condition resolves spontaneously over several weeks. Likewise, in pubertal males, the changing hormonal environment may cause temporary but distressing breast enlargement which may require surgery. In older males, gynaecomastia may result from excess circulating oestrogens due to liver disease, drugs such as cimetidine and spironolactone, or exogenous oestrogens prescribed for the treatment of prostatic carcinoma.

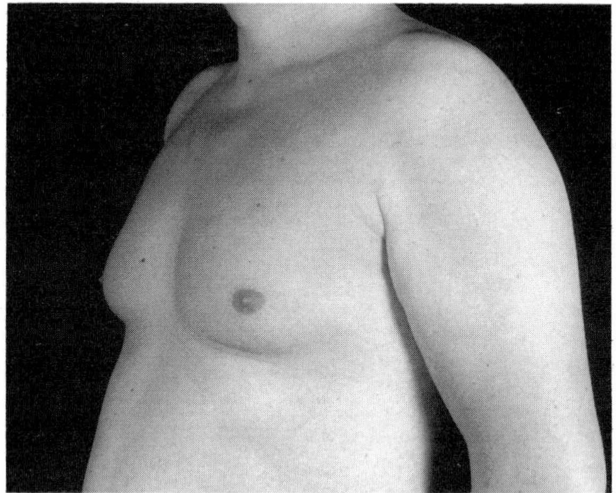

Fig. 27.27 Gynaecomastia

Pubertal gynaecomastia in a boy of 14 years. This will regress spontaneously if the cosmetic appearance can be tolerated

28 DISORDERS OF THE SKIN

Introduction

Only a small proportion of the enormous variety of skin disorders are surgically important. Unsightly lumps and possible malignant lesions fall into this category. Ulcers of the lower limb are common and usually of vascular or diabetic origin. Many venous ulcers are managed by dermatologists, but most of the remainder are managed by surgeons; these are discussed in Chapter 26. Ulceration also characterises many important, often malignant skin lesions.

Skin disorders comprise about 15% of new outpatient surgical referrals. Many only require excision biopsy under local anaesthetic. A small proportion of skin lesions have a potentially sinister course, particularly malignant melanoma. These must be accurately diagnosed and treated. Suspected malignant skin lesions are often managed jointly by dermatologists and surgeons. In general, the initial diagnostic referral should be made to the dermatologist, who sees many more skin conditions than the general surgeon.

Malignant melanomas comprise only 2% of all skin cancers in Northern Europe but, like basal cell and squamous cell carcinomas, their incidence closely correlates with sun exposure and fair skin. The incidence of all skin cancers is rising with the increase in foreign travel. Skin malignancies and their premalignant stages are much more common in sunny countries, like Australia, where they are reaching epidemic proportions.

Finally, the nails, which are specialised skin appendages, pose surgical problems in the form of infected ingrowing toenails and onychogryphosis. The rare subungual melanoma is an important diagnosis which should not be missed.

STRUCTURE OF NORMAL SKIN

The skin is made up of three main layers, the *epidermis*, the *dermis* and the *hypodermis*:

- The epidermis consists of four main layers — the basal layer, the prickle cell layer, the granular layer and the keratin layer. Cell division normally occurs only in the basal layer
- The underlying dermis consists of dense, tough interlacing collagen fibres; their orientation determines the lines of tension in the skin known as *Langer's lines*. These are surgically important because incisions parallel to them heal with minimal scarring

- The deepest layer of the skin is the hypodermis, which consists of loose fibro-fatty tissue. The hypodermis contains the skin appendages — sweat glands, hair follicles and their associated sebaceous glands. The hypodermis is only loosely connected to the *superficial fascia*, which makes the skin mobile over the deeper structures. The exceptions are the palms of the hands, the soles of the feet and the scalp, where the skin is tightly bound to the fascial layer

A working classification of surgically important skin lesions based on site of origin is given in Figure 28.1.

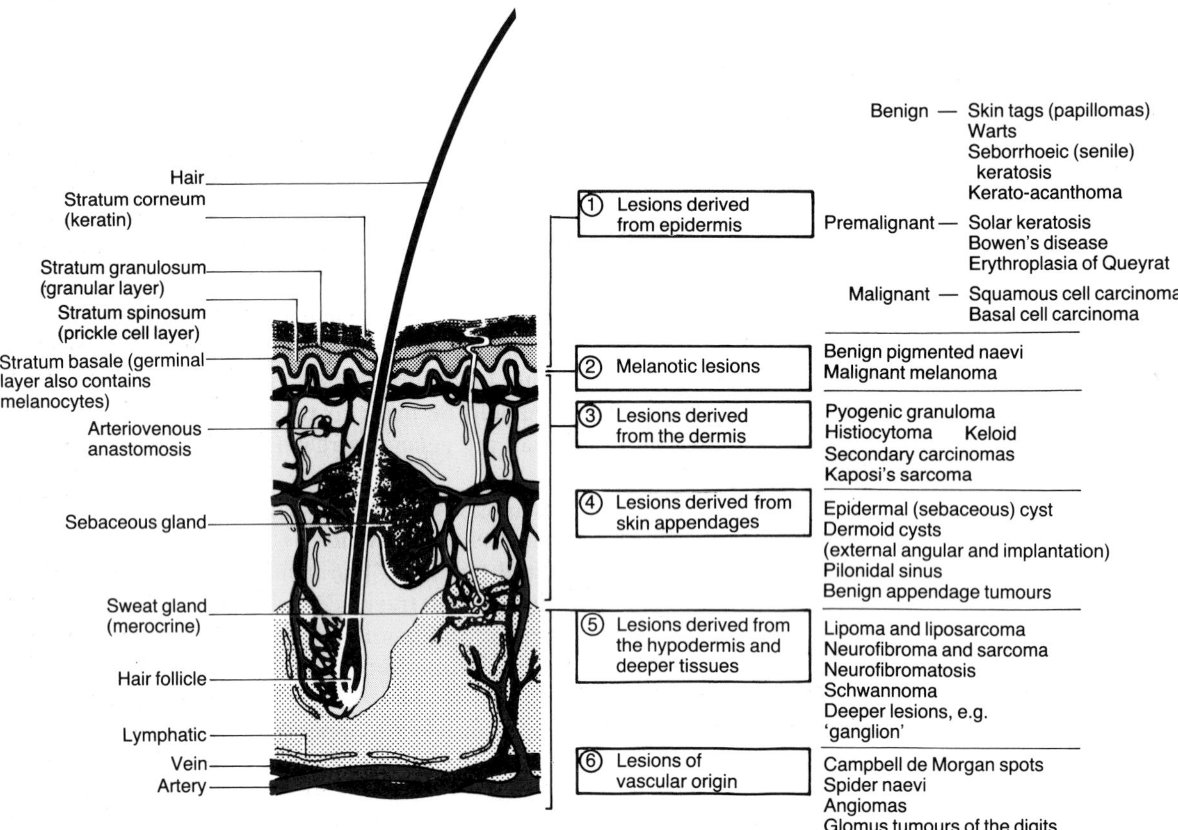

Fig. 28.1 Structure of the skin and lesions of surgical importance

SYMPTOMS AND SIGNS OF SKIN DISORDERS

The most common surgical skin complaint is a lump. This may be tender or painful, and it may have begun to bleed, discharge or ulcerate. The lesion may be pigmented or have changed colour. It may have appeared suddenly or enlarged rapidly, or there may have been some change in a long standing lesion.

Any one of these symptoms may prompt the patient to seek medical advice, but the most frequent seem to be the ugliness or inconvenience of a lesion to the patient. Elderly patients may only come reluctantly, and at the insistence of younger relatives. Some patients do not present until a lesion is huge, while others present with trivial lesions. Both types of patient may be worried by the thought of malignancy.

In practice (and in clinical exams!), the diagnosis of skin lesions rarely follows the conventional pattern of history taking, physical examination and investigations. Rather, the lesion is thrust before the doctor's eyes and a 'spot' diagnosis or differential diagnosis is made. History and examination are then used to see if they either confirm the diagnosis or narrow the differential possibilities. Figure 28.2 summarises the important clinical features of skin lesions and their diagnostic significance.

History taking and examination

As the patient describes the problem, the lesion is usually offered for examination. The clinician then has the questionable advantage of having seen the lesion; this may then guide the direction and emphasis of history taking. The patient should be questioned about other similar lesions or any regional lumps. Detailed inspection and palpation follow and by this time, a definite diagnosis or narrow differential diagnosis should have been established.

A general history must be taken at some point to establish whether there are any relevant systemic symptoms (e.g. weight loss suggests malignant cachexia), concurrent disorders (e.g. diabetes predisposes to infection and may influence surgical management), any history of previous similar lesions, surgical treatment or trauma to the affected area. For example, a history of previous rodent ulcers (basal cell carcinoma) makes this diagnosis more likely another time. Previous surgery or trauma can cause implantation dermoids or a chronic inflammatory response to a foreign body.

Family history is occasionally valuable in rare genetic disorders such as neurofibromatosis. *Social history* should include occupational details as these may be relevant. For example, natal cleft pilonidal sinus is more common in truck drivers. Exposure to carcinogens such as lubricating oils persistently spilt on the same area of clothing may result in squamous carcinoma. Outdoor workers, especially those from the tropics, are predisposed to all types of skin cancer. Chronic ulcers may be contracted during *foreign travel*, e.g. tropical ulcers, Madura foot, tuberculous or atypical mycobacterial ulcers. Occasionally, patients deliberately injure themselves, producing mysterious chronic lesions; a *psychiatric history* is valuable here, though rarely forthcoming.

Drug history is rarely relevant to 'surgical' skin lesions, apart from agents applied topically. Silver nitrate stick, caustic agents, and mechanical interference with wounds or lesions can distort the clinical picture.

The lesion is examined in detail, looking for the points described in Figure 28.2. In addition, general clinical examination should search for other similar lesions, regional lymphadenopathy or a primary malignancy arising elsewhere and metastasising to skin. For example, if inguinal lymph nodes are enlarged, rectal and genital examination should be carried out to exclude concealed carcinoma. The lower limbs, including the soles of the feet, should also be examined, looking especially for malignant melanoma.

Fig. 28.2 Symptoms and signs of skin disorders

SYMPTOMS AND SIGNS	DIAGNOSTIC SIGNIFICANCE
1. LUMP IN THE SKIN	
SIZE, SHAPE AND SURFACE FEATURES: Revealed by inspection —is the lesion smooth–surfaced, irregular, exophytic (i.e. projecting out of the surface)?	Epidermal lesions, such as warts, usually have a surface abnormality, but deeper lesions are usually covered by normal epidermis. A punctum suggests the abnormality arises from an epidermal appendage, e.g. epidermal (sebaceous) cyst
DEPTH WITHIN THE SKIN: Superficial and deep attachments. Which tissue is the swelling derived from?	Tends to reflect the layer from which lesion is derived (i.e. epidermis, dermis, hypodermis or deeper)
CHARACTER OF THE MARGIN: Discreteness, tethering to surrounding tissues, three-dimensional shape	A regular shaped, discrete lesion is most likely cystic or encapsulated (e.g. benign tumour). Deep tethering implies origin from deeper structures (e.g. ganglion). Immobility of overlying epidermis suggests a lesion derived from skin appendages (e.g. epidermal cyst)
CONSISTENCY: Soft, firm, hard, 'indurated', rubbery	Soft lesions are usually lipomas or fluid-filled cysts. Most cysts are fluctuant unless filled by semi-solid material (e.g. epidermal cysts), or the cyst is tense (e.g. small ganglion). Malignant lesions tend to be hard and irregular with an ill–defined margin (i.e. 'indurated') due to invasion of surrounding tissue. Bony-hard lesions are either mineralised (e.g. gouty tophi) or consist of bone (e.g. exostoses)
PULSATILITY	Pulsatility is usually transmitted from an underlying artery which may be abnormal (e.g. aneurysm or arteriovenous fistula)
EMPTYING AND REFILLING	Vascular lesions (e.g. venous malformations or haemangiomas) empty or blanch on pressure and then refill
TRANSILLUMINABILITY	Lesions filled with clear fluid such as cysts 'light up' when transilluminated
TEMPERATURE	Excessive warmth implies acute inflammation (e.g. pilonidal abscess)
2. PAIN, TENDERNESS AND DISCOMFORT	These most often imply acute inflammation. Pain also develops if a non–inflammatory lesion becomes inflamed or infected (e.g. inflamed epidermal cyst). Malignant lesions are usually painless
3. ULCERATION (i.e. loss of epidermal integrity, the inflamed base being formed by dermis or deeper tissues)	Tumours and kerato–acanthoma tend to ulcerate due to central necrosis. Surface breakdown also occurs in arterial or venous insufficiency (e.g. ischaemic leg ulcers), chronic infection (e.g. TB or tropical ulcers) or trauma

Fig. 28.2 (cont.)

SYMPTOMS AND SIGNS	DIAGNOSTIC SIGNIFICANCE
CHARACTER OF THE ULCER MARGIN	In benign ulcers, the margin is only slightly raised by inflammatory oedema. The base lies below the level of normal skin. Malignant ulcers begin as a solid mass of proliferating epidermal cells, the centre of which eventually becomes necrotic. The margin is typically elevated, 'rolled' and indurated by tumour growth and invasion
BEHAVIOUR OF THE ULCER	Malignant ulcers expand inexorably (though often slowly), but may go through cycles of breakdown and healing (often with bleeding)
4. COLOUR AND PIGMENTATION	
NORMAL COLOUR	If a lesion is covered by normal coloured skin then it must lie deep in the skin (e.g. epidermal cyst) or deep to the skin (e.g. ganglion)
RED OR PURPLE	Redness implies increased arterial vascularity, which is most common in inflammatory conditions like furuncles. Vascular abnormalities which contain a high proportion of arterial blood, such as Campbell de Morgan spots or strawberry naevi, are also red, whereas venous disorders such as port–wine stain are darker. Vascular lesions blanch on pressure
DEEPLY PIGMENTED	Benign naevi (moles) and their malignant counterpart, malignant melanomas, are nearly always pigmented. Other lesions such as warts, papillomas or seborrhoeic keratoses, may become pigmented later. Hairy pigmented moles are almost never malignant. Rarely, malignant melanoma may be non-pigmented (amelanotic). Darkening of a pigmented lesion should be viewed with suspicion as it may indicate malignant change
5. RAPIDLY DEVELOPING LESION	Kerato–acanthoma, warts and pyogenic granuloma may all develop rapidly and regress spontaneously. When fully developed, these conditions may be difficult to distinguish from malignancy. Spontaneous regression marks the lesion as benign
6. MULTIPLE, RECURRENT AND SPREADING LESIONS	In certain rare syndromes, multiple similar lesions develop over a period. Examples include neurofibromatosis and recurrent lipomata in Dercum's disease. Heavy sun exposure predisposes a large area of skin to malignant change. Viral warts may appear in crops. Malignant melanoma may spread diffusely (superficial spreading melanoma), or produce satellite lesions via dermal lymphatics
7. SITE OF THE LESION	Some skin lesions arise much more commonly in certain areas of the body. The reason may be anatomical (e.g. pilonidal sinus, external angular dermoid, or multiple pilar cysts of the scalp) or because of exposure to sun (e.g. solar keratoses or basal cell carcinomas of hands and face)
8. AGE WHEN LESION NOTICED	Congenital vascular abnormalities such as strawberry naevus or port–wine stain may be present at birth. Benign pigmented naevi (moles) may be detectable at birth, but only begin to enlarge and darken after the age of two

PRINCIPLES OF MANAGEMENT OF SKIN LESIONS

Many skin lesions can be diagnosed on the history and clinical examination, but wherever there is doubt, some form of *biopsy* is necessary. This is particularly true if there is any risk of malignancy. Biopsy is usually performed as part of the treatment process. Incision and excision biopsy techniques are illustrated in Chapter 3. Figure 28.3 summarises the options in the surgical management of skin conditions.

Fig. 28.3 Principles of management of 'surgical' skin disorders

Simple excision or other physical methods, e.g. electrocautery, laser therapy or cryotherapy — for small, obviously innocent lesions

Excision biopsy — if there is any risk of malignancy or the clinical diagnosis is doubtful (only for small lesions)

Biopsy — for large lesions. Definitive therapy is then planned according to the histology

Wide local excision with or without skin grafting — for malignant melanomas and sometimes for other large malignant lesions

Radiotherapy — an alternative to excision for basal cell carcinoma and primary squamous cell lesions. Also sometimes used in squamous cell carcinoma if regional lymph nodes are involved

Lymph node clearance — if nodes are involved by malignant melanoma or squamous carcinoma

BENIGN LESIONS DERIVED FROM THE EPIDERMIS

SKIN TAGS (SQUAMOUS CELL PAPILLOMAS)

Skin tags are small benign polypoid lesions up to about 5 mm in diameter. They consist of a loose connective tissue core covered by normal, often excessively pigmented, keratinised epithelium. They are common in adults and may occur on any part of the body, particularly the trunk, neck, axillae and groins. In these locations, they may be irritated by clothing and bleed. Unsightly or inconvenient lesions may be easily removed by cautery or excision (under local anaesthetic), or by tying a fine thread around the stalk (also under local anaesthetic) which leads to ischaemic atrophy.

WARTS

Warts are small, virus-induced epidermal tumours. They are characterised pathologically by irregular thickening of the epidermis with grossly excessive keratinisation and exaggerated dermal papillae. The morphology of the lesion depends on its location on the skin.

The *common wart* (verruca vulgaris), a papilliferous lesion up to 1 cm in diameter, is most common on the fingers and back of the hands. In children, warts are often multiple, and commonly occur on the face. Facial lesions are often less keratotic with a smoother, more dome-like shape. They are often called *juvenile warts* (verruca plana juvenilis). Lesions on the sole of the foot, *plantar warts* (verruca plantaris), become extremely keratotic and involuted due to pressure. They may extend deeply into the foot, causing considerable pain.

Warts may also occur on the genitalia, perineum and perianal area, in many cases, spread by sexual contact. Sometimes genital warts grow to a large size; these are known as *condylomata accuminata*.

Warts grow and then regress spontaneously over several months. They often, however, require treatment to relieve pain, irritation or inconvenience. Many are treated for aesthetic reasons. Keratolytic applications are the first choice of treatment. These include salicylic acid and podophyllin resin preparations. If this is unsuccessful, cryosurgery or cautery (with or without curettage) is used.

SEBORRHOEIC KERATOSIS

Seborrhoeic keratoses (*seborrhoeic warts*) are extremely common skin lesions in elderly patients; they sometimes occur in younger people. They are most often seen on the chest, face, neck and arms. Often, there are many lesions of different sizes with different intensities of pigmentation. They may be up to several centimetres in diameter. The lesions are slightly raised, sharply demarcated and plaque-like; they look and feel irregular and waxy. Sometimes they are so darkly pigmented that they cannot be distinguished clinically from superficial spreading malignant melanomas.

Histologically, a seborrhoeic keratosis is a localised proliferation of the basal layer of the epidermis. There is often hyperkeratosis in the surface crypts, resulting in round keratin nests. Seborrhoeic keratoses are sometimes called *basal cell papillomas* because of their origin, but they are not true neoplasms and are unrelated to basal cell carcinoma.

Treatment is only required for unsightly or easily traumatised lesions. As they are so superficial, they can be 'scraped off' with a scalpel or curette under local anaesthetic.

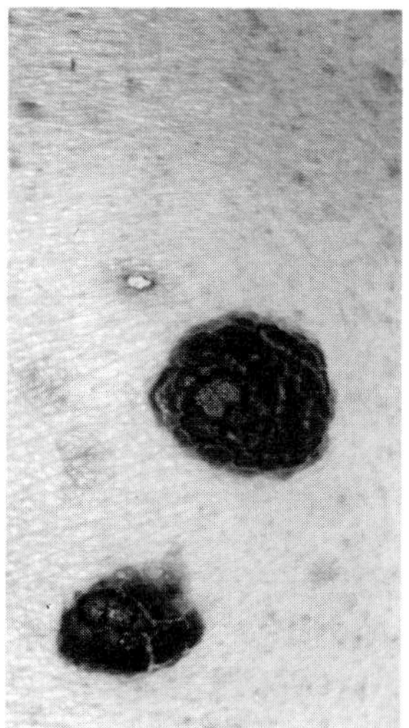

Fig. 28.4 Seborrhoeic keratoses

KERATO-ACANTHOMA

A keratoacanthoma is a nodular, usually single skin lesion, up to 2 cm in diameter. It has an irregular central crater containing keratotic debris. As its name implies, the histological lesion consists of localised tumour-like epidermal proliferation, with a thick prickle cell layer (*acanthosis*) and marked

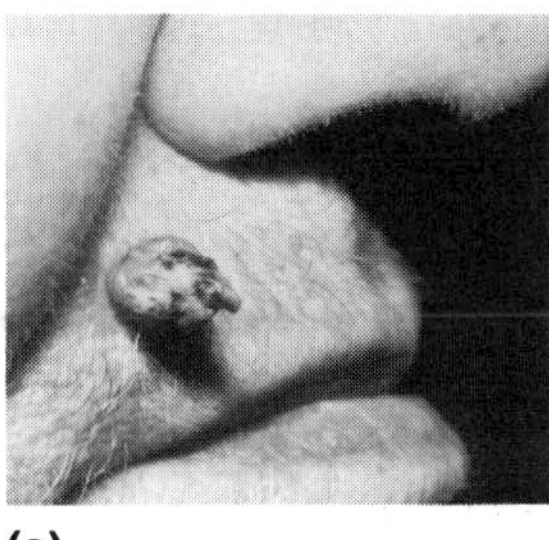

(a)

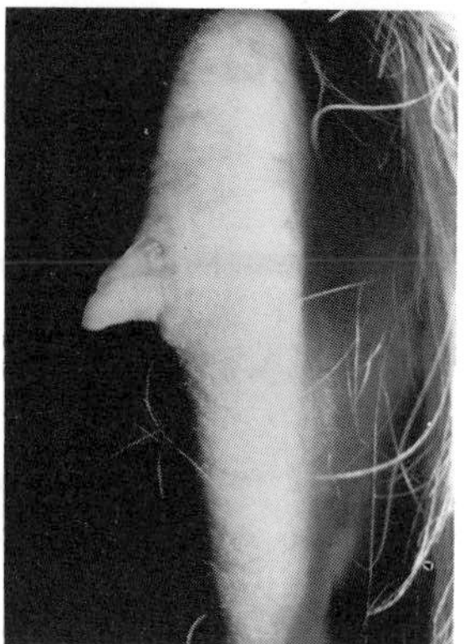

(b)

Fig. 28.5 Kerato-acanthoma and keratin horn

(a) This alarming looking lesion is a benign keratoacanthoma. The central keratin plug is characteristic. Resolution is spontaneous after a few weeks. **(b)** Keratin horn on pinna of an elderly man. If left, these can grow very large

keratinisation. Some epithelial cells are large and have atypical nuclei; the underlying dermis exhibits marked chronic inflammatory cell infiltration.

The importance of this benign lesion is that it can be difficult to distinguish clinically, and even histologically, from squamous carcinoma. Keratoacanthomas, however, tend to have a short life-cycle of 1–3 months and regress spontaneously, whereas squamous cell carcinomas continue to enlarge. Keratin horns may also look similar, but rarely regress. The cause of keratoacanthoma is unknown but its behaviour suggests a viral origin.

Diagnosis and treatment is by local excision unless the lesion is obviously regressing. If there is still diagnostic doubt, they should be followed up as for squamous carcinoma.

PRE-MALIGNANT EPIDERMAL CONDITIONS

SOLAR (SENILE) KERATOSIS AND INTRA-EPIDERMAL CARCINOMA

Pathology and clinical features

Solar keratoses are flat, well-demarcated, brown, scaly or crusty lesions with an erythematous base. They bleed easily if traumatised or scratched. Solar keratoses are often multiple, and are most common in middle-aged or elderly patients on sun-exposed parts, i.e. face, neck, arms and hands. The incidence is higher in farm workers, fishermen and other outdoor workers. Solar keratoses are especially common in fair-skinned people living in tropical or subtropical regions such as Australia or the southern USA.

The characteristic histological features are marked thickening of the keratin layer (*hyperkeratosis*) and the prickle cell layer (*acanthosis*). Deep in the epidermis, there is a variable degree of dysplastic change and abnormal mitotic activity. These features suggest malignant transformation, but most importantly, the basal layer remains intact.

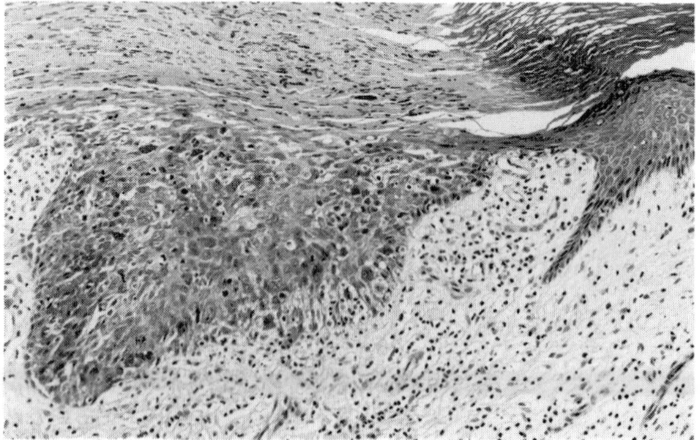

Fig. 28.6 Solar keratosis — histopathology

Photomicrograph showing severe dysplastic changes in a flat scaly lesion taken from the forearm of an elderly Australian farmer; the epidermis at the extreme right is normal. In this lesion the cells show severe nuclear and cytoplasmic atypia which extends through all layers to the surface, thus defining the lesion pathologically as carcinoma-in-situ

The epidemiology and pathology of solar keratosis suggest that it is a pre-malignant condition which predisposes to squamous carcinoma. Lesions in which the dysplastic changes extend from the basal layers to the surface are considered to be malignant. They are termed *carcinoma-in-situ* or *intra-epidermal carcinoma*. Clinically, these are more erythematous than the pre-malignant type, and are sometimes described as *Bowen's disease*. When Bowen's disease occurs on the glans penis, it is known as *erythroplasia of Queyrat*.

Management

Management of solar keratosis depends on the number, size and distribution of the lesions, the age of the patient, and whether the skin type predisposes to cancer. Isolated lesions are best excised. For multiple keratoses, excision biopsy of representative lesions should be initially performed to confirm the diagnosis. This is followed by excision biopsy, curettage or cryocautery of suspicious lesions. Patients should be advised repeatedly to minimise exposure to ultraviolet rays by wearing protective clothing and hats and applying total sunscreen creams. These patients should also be regularly examined for squamous cell carcinomas, basal cell carcinomas and melanomas, which are all more common in patients with marked sunshine exposure.

MALIGNANT EPIDERMAL LESIONS

SQUAMOUS CELL CARCINOMA

Pathology

Squamous cell carcinomas may occur anywhere on the skin, or on stratified squamous epithelium of the mouth, tongue, oesophagus, anal canal, glans penis or uterine cervix. Squamous cell carcinoma also occurs in metaplastic squamous epithelium in the bronchus or bladder.

Squamous cell carcinoma usually occurs in older age groups, in skin exposed repeatedly to ultraviolet light. Often, carcinoma develops from a pre-existing *solar (senile) keratosis*.

Much less commonly, squamous carcinoma develops in skin areas chronically exposed to *industrial carcinogens* such as ionising radiation, arsenic or chromium compounds, soot, tar, pitch or mineral oils. For example, carcinoma of the scrotum was once common in chimney sweeps; the recognition of soot as the predisposing factor was a milestone in understanding carcinogenesis.

Chronic inflammation also predisposes to squamous carcinoma, which may develop at the margins of osteomyelitic sinuses or long-standing ulcers. These are common in undeveloped countries where burns are poorly treated. An ulcer in which carcinoma arises is known as a *Marjolin's ulcer*.

Histologically, squamous cell carcinomas of the skin are usually well-differentiated, and the tumour cells resemble normal prickle cells. Keratin pearls and individual cell keratinisation are common features.

Clinical presentation

Squamous cell carcinoma usually presents as an enlarging painless ulcer with a rolled, indurated margin. Other lesions have an exophytic (outward growing,

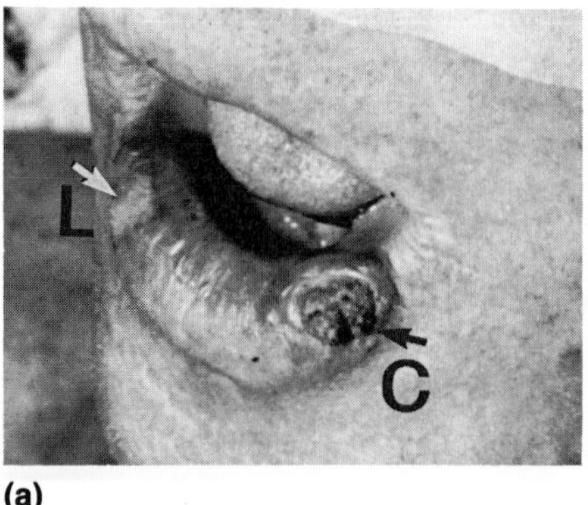

(a)

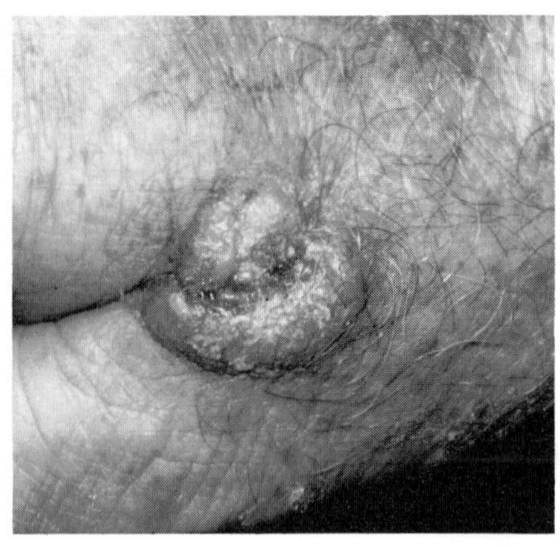

(b)

Fig. 28.7 Squamous carcinoma

(a) This 70-year-old man had been a pipe smoker for many years. The lesion on the left of his lower lip **C** is a well differentiated squamous cell carcinoma and was removed by wedge resection of the lip. The white lesion on the right of his lower lip **L** is *leukoplakia* (see Ch. 29) which, on histology, proved to be a carcinoma-in-situ. Pipe smoking predisposed to both lesions.
(b) Squamous carcinoma of the dorsum of the hand in an agricultural worker

proliferative) cauliflower-like appearance with areas of ulceration, bleeding or serous exudation. Squamous cell carcinomas invade the dermis and deeper tissues such as bone or cartilage; further spread is usually to regional lymph nodes. Distant metastases are uncommon.

Management of squamous cell carcinomas

Management involves first confirming the diagnosis by biopsy. This is followed by local radiotherapy or sometimes by excision of the carcinoma with a margin of normal tissue. Infiltrated lymph nodes are treated with *radiotherapy* or sometimes *block dissection* (i.e. removing all the regional lymph nodes in a single block of tissue). In general, these tumours respond favourably to radiotherapy and recurrence is unusual. Patients are usually reviewed annually for about five years after successful treatment.

BASAL CELL CARCINOMA

Pathology and clinical features

Basal cell carcinomas are common, and nearly always result from exposure to excess ultraviolet sunlight. Caucasians in tropical and sub-tropical regions have an extremely high incidence. Up to 50% of this group are affected at some time, often with multiple lesions. As for squamous cell carcinomas, basal cell carcinomas usually develop from middle age onwards, but their incidence is rising in younger 'sun-worshipers'. Males are affected at least twice as often as females, reflecting their greater occupational and recreational exposure to the sun.

Although any part of the skin can be involved, most arise on the upper part of the face, as shown in Figure 28.8. Because the lesions are so prominent, most patients present early rather than late.

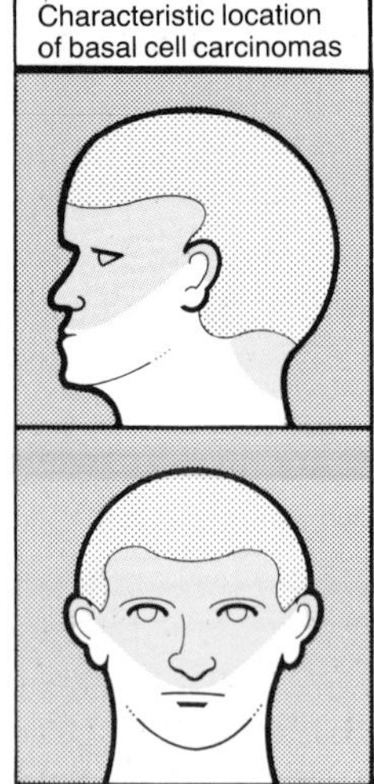

Fig. 28.8

Basal cell carcinomas begin as small pearly-white nodules with visible telangiectatic blood vessels. Early lesions may ulcerate, bleed and then heal again, but as they grow larger they form irregular ulcers (*rodent ulcers*) with a pearly rolled margin. Although basal cell carcinomas almost never metastasise they are definitely malignant, invading underlying bone and cartilage. Neglected lesions on the scalp or neck may even invade the brain or spinal cord.

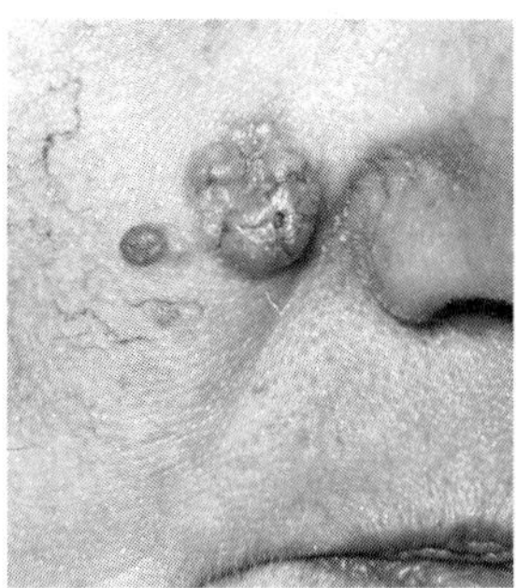

Fig. 28.9 Basal cell carcinoma (BCC)

The larger nodular lesion on the cheek of this woman aged 77 is a typical BCC. Note the pearly appearance of the lesion which is beginning to ulcerate. In this position, treatment with radiotherapy avoids distortion of the nasolabial fold. The smaller lesion lateral to the BCC is a benign naevus

Histologically, the tumour cells have strongly basophilic nuclei and little cytoplasm. The cells at the periphery are arranged in a palisade pattern reminiscent of normal basal cells.

Management of basal cell carcinomas

Small lesions are usually treated by radiotherapy, cryotherapy or curettage, although excision biopsy may be appropriate for isolated or suspicious lesions. Radiotherapy should be avoided on the nose or ear where cartilage is susceptible to radiotherapy and may undergo necrosis. Larger destructive lesions may require reconstructive plastic surgery and skin grafting.

MELANOTIC LESIONS

BENIGN NAEVI

The deeper layers of the epidermis contain scattered melanocytes which synthesise melanin. This pigment is then transferred to nearby epidermal cells where it is responsible for skin colour. The concentration of melanocytes in the skin is similar in all races, but the degree of skin pigmentation depends on the amount of melanin produced. Although colour is mainly determined by genetic factors, it is enhanced by exposure to the ultraviolet rays of sunlight (tanning).

Melanocytes originate from the neural crest and migrate to the ectoderm during embryological development. Hamartomatous accumulations of melanocytes may appear in the epidermis or dermis, or both, to form raised, variably pigmented lesions known as naevi or moles.

Lesions range in diameter from about 3–30 mm. The surface may be smooth or irregular and may contain hairs. According to clinical and histological features, naevi can be subdivided into five types: *junctional*, *intradermal*, *compound*, *blue* and *juvenile naevi*. The first three are closely related pathologically.

Junctional, intradermal and compound naevi

Junctional and intradermal naevi

Junctional naevi develop at or before puberty by accumulation of small clumps of melanocytes deep in the epidermis. These appear as small papules, slightly raised above the surface, but deeply pigmented because the melanocytes are close to the skin surface. After puberty, the junctional naevus cells are thought to proliferate and migrate into the dermis to form a larger mass of cells, an

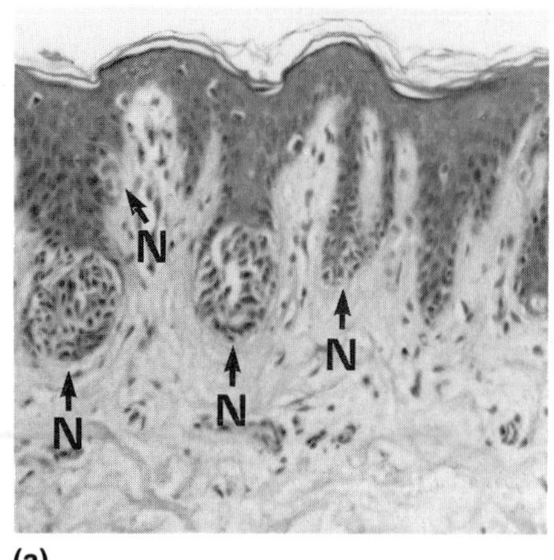

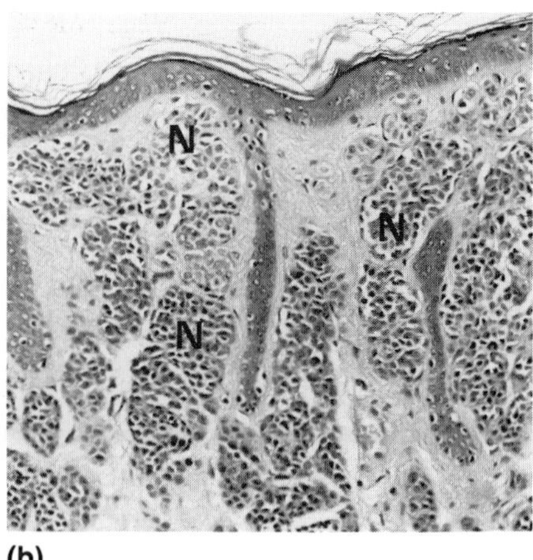

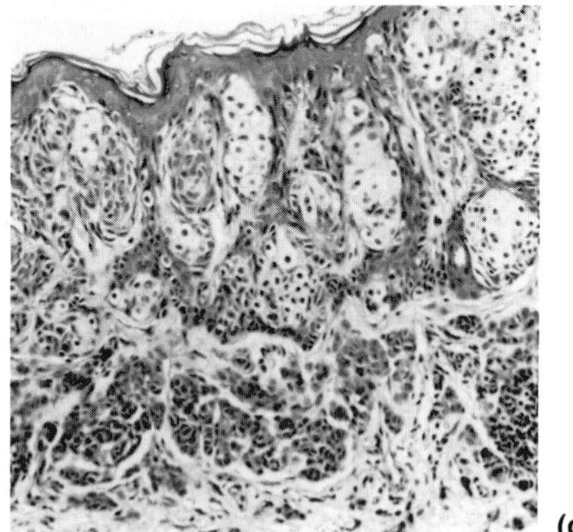

Fig. 28.10 Junctional, intradermal and compound naevi — histopathology

(a) *Junctional naevus*: aggregations of pale-stained naevus cells **N** (melanocytes) are located in the basal layer of the epidermis (i.e. at the junction of epidermis and dermis);
(b) *Intradermal naevus*: the naevus cells **N** form clumps in the upper dermis and are not found in the epidermis;
(c) *Compound naevus*: clumps of naevus cells are present in both the basal epidermis and upper dermis and are believed to represent a transitional type between junctional and intradermal naevi

intradermal naevus. These are usually found in adults as raised papules. They are larger than junctional naevi and paler, as the melanin is masked by the thickness of overlying skin.

Some intradermal naevi continue to enlarge; pilo-sebaceous elements become exaggerated to produce fleshy, dome-shaped or polypoid skin nodules often with protruding hairs. These slightly pigmented naevi are probably the most common skin lumps occurring on the face and are particularly seen in the elderly and in women.

Compound naevi

These contain junctional and intradermal components and look like something between the two, i.e. slightly raised, moderately pigmented papules. Compound naevi are probably a late transition from junctional to intradermal naevi occurring in early adulthood. Compound naevi are believed to be susceptible to transformation into aggressive malignant melanomas.

Blue naevi

Blue naevi are dark, blue-black, flat nodules formed by clumps of heavily pigmented melanocytes located deep in the dermis. The blue colour is an effect of the thick layer of overlying skin. Blue naevi occur at any age but are commoner in the young. Because of their dark colour they may be mistaken for malignant melanomas.

Juvenile naevi

Juvenile naevi are most common in the young but may occur at any age. Histologically, they are compound naevi. The cells are large and pleomorphic which would normally suggest malignancy. Despite this, the lesions are benign.

Lentigo

Lentigenes (the plural of lentigo) are benign pigmented lesions which may need to be considered in the differential diagnosis of potentially malignant melanotic lesions. They are large, heavily pigmented plaques, which develop on the face and hands of the elderly. Melanocytes are more numerous, and melanin production excessive but there is no accumulation of naevus cells. Lentigenes are benign but predispose to the superficial spreading variety of malignant melanoma.

Management of pigmented lesions

It is not particularly easy to distinguish clinically between the different types of benign naevi. Nor is it always easy to be sure that a pigmented lesion is not malignant. Excision biopsy is mandatory if there has been any recent change in a pigmented lesion or if there is any doubt about its nature. People are becoming increasingly aware that pigmented lesions can be malignant and so large numbers now seek medical advice. Fortunately, few will have malignant melanomas. If there is any suspicion of malignancy, specialist opinion should be sought. A dermatologist will usually be the first choice, but a surgeon will be involved if more than simple excision or biopsy is necessary.

In practice, if the patient or doctor is worried about a pigmented lesion, no matter how benign it looks, it is usually removed. Lesions subject to chronic irritation (e.g. at the waist, neck or palm) or in a site that is difficult to observe (e.g. sole of foot or genitalia) should certainly be removed. An elliptical incision removes the lesion together with a narrow margin of normal tissue (2–3 mm), enabling the skin edges to be readily apposed. All excised pigmented lesions should be examined histologically because a few benign looking lesions will turn out to be malignant.

MALIGNANT MELANOMA

Pathology

Malignant melanoma is a highly malignant tumour derived from melanocytes. The majority probably arise from pigmented naevi but some occur on normal skin. Although all skin is vulnerable, the most commonly affected sites are the lower extremities, including the soles of the feet, and the head and neck.

Malignant melanomas occasionally arise in the nail bed, the choroid of the eye or the oral mucosa. Most malignant melanomas are deeply pigmented but a few have no pigment at all and are thus known as *amelanotic melanomas*. These can only be diagnosed on histology.

The epidemiology of malignant melanoma is fascinating. They are rare in dark-skinned races, occurring mainly in fair-skinned people of northern European (Celtic) origin. The disease is extremely common in albinos of all races. Until recent times, malignant melanoma was quite rare in northern Europeans, but the incidence has dramatically risen over the last two decades. The highest incidence in the world is in northern and western Australia.

Ultraviolet radiation appears to be the essential aetiological factor. For other skin malignancies, a cumulative effect is most important, but for malignant melanoma, short periods of intense sun exposure, for example on a two week holiday, appear to be more carcinogenic. Prolonged but less intense exposure and tanning of the skin seem to offer some protection. There is evidence that unaccustomed exposure to strong sunlight, causing sunburn, suppresses general immunological responses and, by implication, immunological tumour surveillance. This might explain malignant melanomas on parts of the skin not generally exposed to the sun, e.g. soles of the feet.

Clinical features of malignant melanoma

Most malignant melanomas are black or dark brown, nodular lesions, which may bleed or ulcerate. Tumour cells rapidly invade the dermis and may spread laterally in dermal lymphatics. Lateral spread may produce *satellite lesions* around the primary nodule. If a pre-existing mole enlarges, darkens, bleeds, becomes inflamed, ulcerated or itchy, it should be regarded with great suspicion.

Malignant melanoma presents in two different forms, nodular and *superficial spreading*. The more common *nodular form*, which tends to invade deeply and metastasise early, has a much poorer prognosis than the *superficial spreading variety* which grows slowly and metastasises late. Elements of both may be present in the same lesion. Superficial spreading melanoma may arise in a lentigo, and can easily be mistaken for seborrhoeic keratosis.

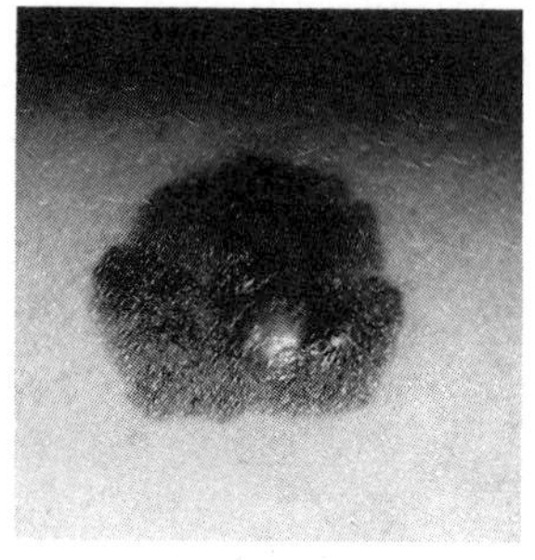

Fig. 28.11 Malignant melanoma

Pigmented lesion on the forearm in a 33-year-old woman. A small black lesion had been present for many years before starting to spread to reach its present diameter of 2.5 cm. Histologically, this proved to be the 'superficial spreading' type of malignant melanoma, usually associated with a better prognosis

In general, spread to regional lymph nodes occurs early. In the process, secondary lesions often appear along the course of the lymphatics between the primary and the draining nodes. Haematogenous spread also occurs later, to involve liver, bone, brain and other tissues. The behaviour of malignant melanoma is unpredictable, although lesions arising before puberty and in the elderly tend to be less aggressive. Rarely, disseminated lesions undergo complete spontaneous regression; indeed, a proportion of malignant melanomas show histological evidence of regression. Melanomas which exhibit marked lymphocytic infiltration have a better prognosis.

Management of malignant melanoma

The first objective in managing a pigmented lesion is to establish whether it is malignant. Unless malignancy is clinically obvious, small lesions are removed by excision biopsy, and more extensive lesions are sampled by incision biopsy.

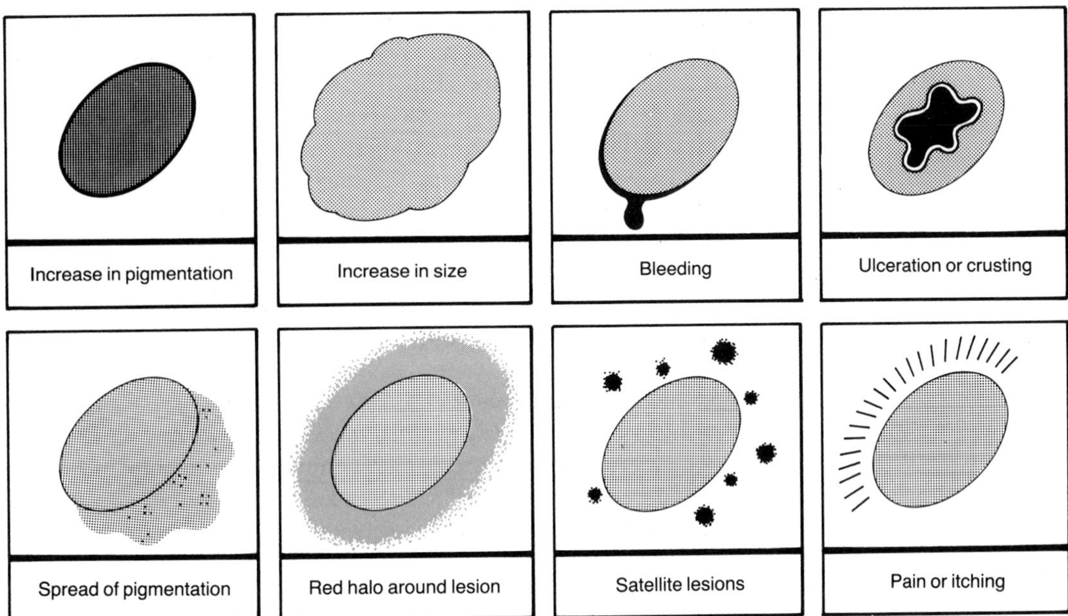

Fig. 28.12 Clinical features suggestive of malignant melanoma

Histologically, malignant melanomas are usually poorly differentiated with numerous mitotic figures. The presence of melanin is diagnostic, but amelanotic lesions can occur; these must be diagnosed by histochemical tests.

The *depth of invasion*, as determined by histological examination, is the most useful guide to prognosis. *Clark's levels* have traditionally been used for this purpose, as described in Figure 28.13. Many laboratories now prefer to use the measured depth of invasion of tumour cells. If this exceeds 0.76 mm from the granular layer, metastasis is deemed likely to have occurred to regional nodes. Some surgeons believe that in these circumstances, regional nodes must be removed if there is to be a chance of cure. In reality, tumour thickness is only one clue to possible tumour spread; the extent of lateral spread of the primary lesion, the extent of local lymphatic invasion and immunological and regressive features may be better indicators of tumour aggressiveness.

Malignant melanomas require wide local excision with a margin of at least five centimetres all round the lesion; the excision should extend down to the

Fig. 28.13 Depth of skin invasion as a prognostic indicator in malignant melanoma (Clark's classification)

CLARK'S LEVEL		5-year survival
I	Melanoma does not penetrate basement membrane	100%
II	Extends into papillary dermis	90–100%
III	Reaches junction between papillary and reticular dermis	80–90%
IV	Extends into reticular dermis	60–70%
V	Extends into subcutaneous fat	15–30%

deep fascia. Such an extensive wound usually requires skin grafting and leaves a cosmetically unattractive result. If involvement of regional lymph nodes is suspected or clinically apparent, these should be removed en bloc. Ideally, a corridor containing the lymphatic vessels which extend to the primary lesion should also be removed. This is often not practical. For example, a malignant melanoma near the middle of the back would, on this basis, require block dissection of axillary and groin nodes on both sides.

For suspected *superficial spreading melanomas*, incision biopsies are usually taken before complete excision. Less radical surgery is necessary than for nodular melanomas, as superficial spreading melanomas run a less aggressive course.

In practice, the decision to perform radical regional lymph node excision is first made on the basis of the site of the lesion. The second consideration is the thickness of the lesion, with more than 0.76 mm thick, or Clark's level III or deeper, as the critical level. Ideally all the histological evidence should be considered together and the treatment decided in consultation with the pathologist and perhaps dermatologist. Some surgeons defer regional node dissection for several weeks after local excision to allow tumour cells in the drainage area to be captured in regional nodes.

Adjuvant therapy in the form of intralymphatic radio-iodine ^{131}I may have some prophylactic value where nodes do not appear to be involved, or may be used about four weeks prior to regional node dissection. Cytotoxic agents have given disappointing results so far. Local treatment with BCG vaccine has been tried in an attempt to stimulate immunological defences but any response is temporary.

LESIONS DERIVED FROM THE DERMIS

PYOGENIC GRANULOMA

Pyogenic granuloma is a common inflammatory lesion of the skin which arises in response to minor penetrating foreign bodies such as splinters or thorns. Lesions are most common on the hands and feet but may also occur on the lips and gums. Pathologically, a pyogenic granuloma consists of a mass of exuberant granulation tissue containing numerous polymorphs. It usually develops over a period of about a week but does not often regress spontaneously.

Clinically, pyogenic granulomas are solitary, reddish-blue fleshy nodules which may be polypoid. The surface may be ulcerated, in which case the lesion may be clinically indistinguishable from amelanotic malignant melanoma. Pyogenic granuloma should be excised and the base curetted or cauterised to prevent recurrence.

KELOID SCARS

Keloids are formed by excessive deposition of collagen in the dermis during wound healing. The result is a bulging tumour-like mass covered by normal epidermis. The chest and neck are particularly susceptible. The problem appears to have a genetic basis as it is much more common in negroid people.

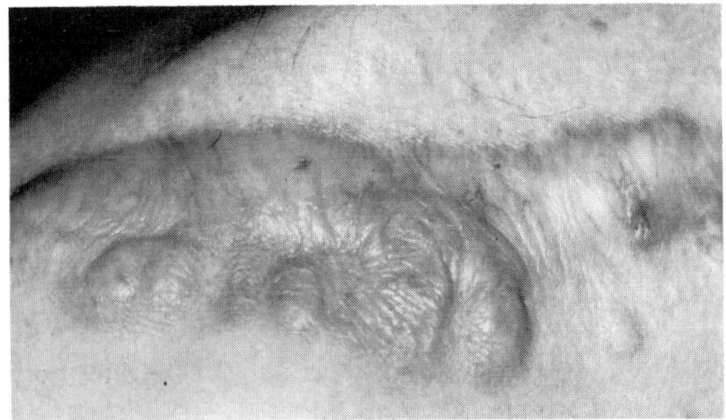

Fig. 28.14 Keloid scars

Keloid thickening of an abdominal wound. There were no known predisposing factors

Keloid formation may cause poor cosmetic results after injury, minor surgery, or even ear-piercing. Excising the lesion often makes scarring worse. Radiotherapy or local injection of corticosteroids may suppress keloid formation.

HISTIOCYTOMA

Histiocytomas, (also known as *dermatofibromas*), are common asymptomatic skin lesions occurring particularly on the limbs. They are firm nodules, about 5 mm in diameter and deep reddish-brown in colour. They are clinically important because they may be mistaken for malignant melanoma. Histologically, they contain numerous lipid-filled macrophages (*histiocytes*). One histological variant contains prominent vascular elements, and has given rise to the confusing term *sclerosing angioma*.

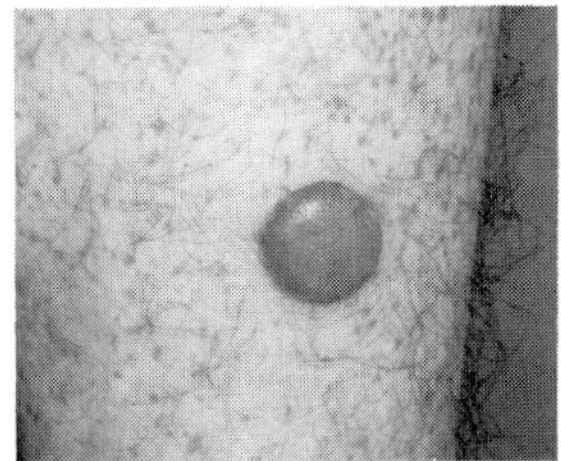

Fig. 28.15 Histiocytoma on lower leg

SECONDARY (METASTATIC) CARCINOMA

Metastatic tumour deposits may present as small hard painless skin nodules. They are usually located in the dermis and covered by normal epidermis. Breast carcinomas are the most common cause, but carcinomas of stomach, uterus, lungs, large bowel and kidneys also behave in this manner. In most patients, the primary lesion or other metastases will already have presented. Occasionally, biopsy of a mysterious skin lesion leads to the diagnosis.

Management of skin secondaries depends on the primary diagnosis but the prognosis is usually poor. Treatment is by local excision, radiotherapy or chemotherapy, depending on the severity of symptoms and the size, number and location of secondaries.

True skin metastases are a different entity from local spread of tumour or local implantation of cells during surgery, which are a particular feature of carcinoma of the breast.

KAPOSI'S SARCOMA

This once rare condition has leapt to prominence as one of the most frequent presentations of *acquired immune deficiency syndrome* (AIDS). The condition appears as multiple bluish-red to brown nodules or plaques, all of which are primary tumours. They most commonly occur on the limbs. The tumours are characterised by proliferating dysplastic fibroblasts, accompanied by chronic inflammation, endothelial proliferation and haemorrhage. Treatment of individual lesions is by excision biopsy.

LESIONS DERIVED FROM SKIN APPENDAGES

FURUNCLE (BOIL) AND CARBUNCLE

A furuncle is a staphylococcal abscess which develops in a hair follicle in the dermis. Diabetes mellitus can be a predisposing factor. The lesion rapidly enlarges and eventually 'points' at the surface, spontaneously discharging pus. The centre often contains a core of necrotic tissue. Once the pus has discharged and the necrotic tissue shed, the lesion heals spontaneously. Drainage may be encouraged with poultices or dressings, such as magnesium sulphate paste, which are said to draw the pus to the surface by osmosis. Antibiotics should be avoided if pus is present, as they inhibit spontaneous drainage and may lead to the formation of a chronic abscess.

Furuncles are most common in young men with acne, especially on the back of the trunk and lower limbs. Axillary furuncles are common in middle-aged females, and tend to recur. Surgical drainage is necessary only if a chronic abscess develops.

A furuncle may be the source of *septicaemia*, especially in uncontrolled diabetes. *Cavernous sinus thrombosis* is a rare but very serious (and often fatal) complication of a furuncle on the lateral aspect of the nose or infra-orbital area. This area drains into the cavernous sinus via the facial vein and inferior ophthalmic veins.

A *carbuncle*, also staphylococcal in origin, is larger than a furuncle and consists of a honeycomb of abscesses, often draining (inadequately) via multiple sinuses. The back of the neck is the usual site; here the skin is tightly bound by interlacing bundles of fibrous tissue. Treatment is with anti-staphylococcal antibiotics such as flucloxacillin as early as possible. The aim is to minimise pus formation and necrosis that would lead to skin loss and delay healing. If pus has formed, thorough desloughing and drainage of the abscesses is required. Carbuncles are more common in diabetic patients, and may bring the diabetes to light.

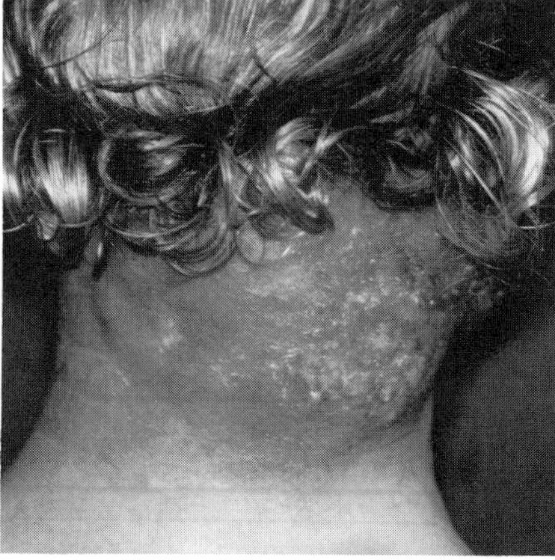

Fig. 28.16 Carbuncle on back of neck

CYSTS

Cysts are common skin lesions and by definition consist of an epithelial-lined cavity; this is filled with viscous or semi-solid epithelial degradation products. Most skin cysts probably arise from elements of hair follicles, possibly secondary to obstruction (*epidermal cysts* and *pilar cysts*). Occasionally, cysts also arise from developmental epithelial remnants (*dermoid cysts*) or by traumatic implantation of epithelial fragments (*implantation dermoids*).

Epidermal cysts

These are by far the most common skin cysts, and are often incorrectly described as '*sebaceous cysts*'. They are usually solitary and may be found anywhere on the body (except the palms or soles), most commonly on the trunk, face and neck. They range up to several centimetres in diameter. Epidermal cysts are smooth and rounded, and covered by normal epidermis in which a blocked duct (*punctum*) may be visible. On palpation, they have a doughy, fluctuant consistency and are usually not tender. They originate in the skin and are attached to it, but are mobile over deeper tissues. Multiple small epidermal cysts sometimes develop on the scrotal skin and cause considerable embarrassment.

Histologically, an epidermal cyst has a stratified squamous lining epithelium and is filled with keratin; this is consistent with its derivation from a hair follicle. The cyst contents are thick and waxy, and were originally thought to be sebaceous material. This gave rise to the erroneous name of sebaceous cyst.

Surgical removal (see Chapter 3)

Epidermal cysts are mainly removed for cosmetic reasons, but sometimes because they interfere with clothing or combing the hair.

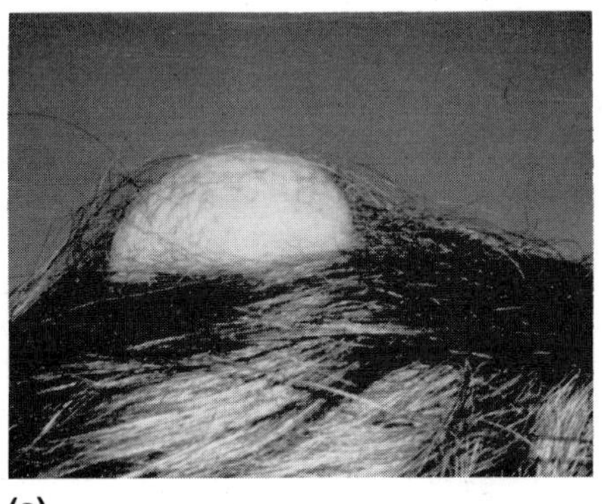

(a)

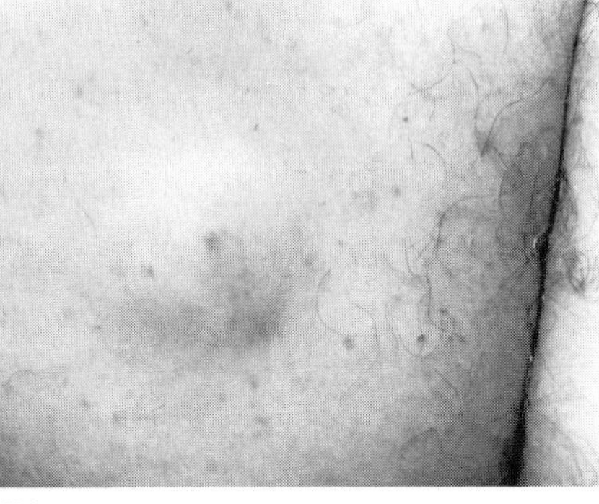

(b)

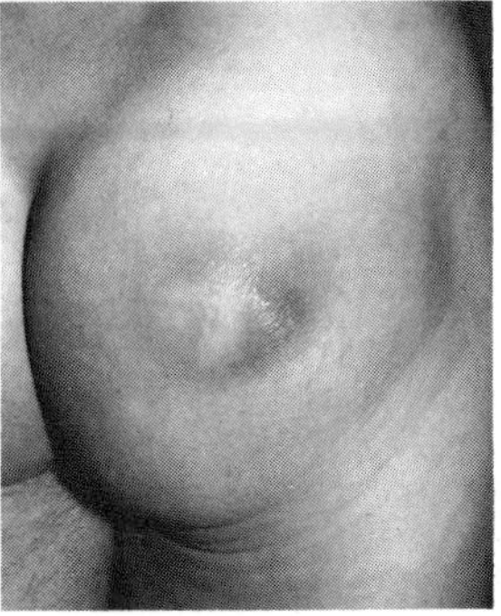

(c)

Fig. 28.17 Epidermal cysts
(a) This large epidermal (pilar) cyst of the scalp was clearly visible but several more were also palpable in the scalp hair of this 55-year-old man.
(b) Non-inflamed epidermal cyst in the skin of the buttock.
(c) Inflamed epidermal cyst of buttock

An incision is made over the cyst, taking care not to puncture the cavity. The cyst is then enucleated by blunt dissection and delivered from the wound in its entirety. This ensures all the epithelium is removed and will avoid recurrence.

Inflamed epidermal cysts

Trauma to epidermal cysts (often unnoticed), may cause some of the contents to escape into the surrounding tissues, exciting an intense foreign-body inflammatory response. The patient may complain of pain, swelling, redness and even spontaneous discharge of liquefied cyst contents; this looks like pus but is in fact sterile. These inflamed epidermal cysts are often described as 'infected' but this is rarely the case.

It is unwise to attempt removal of an acutely inflamed epidermal cyst because the tissue planes cannot be recognised and some of the epithelial lining is likely to be left. If pain is severe, liquefied cyst contents should just be drained. Culture of this material rarely yields any growth and so antibiotics are usually unhelpful. The cyst can be excised later in the usual way.

Pilar cysts

Some individuals develop multiple cysts on the scalp or less commonly on the face or neck. These range from a few millimetres to many centimetres in diameter, but grow very slowly. They can easily be excised under local anaesthesia.

Dermoid cysts

Dermoid cysts are pathologically similar to epidermal cysts in that they are lined by stratified squamous epithelium. As well as keratin, however, they contain hair, sebaceous glands and other ectodermal structures. Dermoids arise from cystic change in epithelial remnants left behind at lines of embryological fusion. They are usually found in the midline of the scalp, neck and lower jaw and at the outer angle of the eyebrow (*external angular dermoid*). Treatment is by excision.

Implantation dermoids

These small keratin-filled cysts arise from epidermal fragments implanted in the dermis by minor penetrating injuries. Though not derived from epidermal appendages, they are pathologically similar to epidermal cysts, but may contain small foreign bodies. Implantation dermoids are most often seen on the fingers, often under the scar of a previous laceration.

PILONIDAL SINUS AND ABSCESS

As the name implies, pilonidal sinuses, cysts and abscesses contain 'a nest of hairs'. They are common in young adults, particularly hirsute men, and are found at the upper end of the natal cleft. Here, between the buttocks, there is often a congenital dimple or pit. Fragments of hair falling from the back or the head accumulate in this nidus. The hairs slowly work their way into the dermis, with the cuticular scales on the hairs acting like barbs of an arrow. The process is encouraged by the massaging effect of sitting for long periods driving motor vehicles. Pilonidal sinus is thus common in truck and tractor drivers.

Pilonidal abscess

The mass of hairs and other skin debris in a pilonidal sinus excites a foreign-body inflammatory reaction, often merely resulting in a mildly or intermittently discharging sinus. If however the cavity becomes secondarily infected, an abscess develops and causes marked pain and swelling. Pilonidal abscesses are often multilocular. They sometimes drain spontaneously but rarely heal completely. Many require surgical drainage because of pain.

Pilonidal sinuses tend to run a long indolent course with chronic or intermittent purulent discharge via one or more sinuses to the skin surface. Periodic acute exacerbations may develop into abscesses which require urgent hospital admission for drainage.

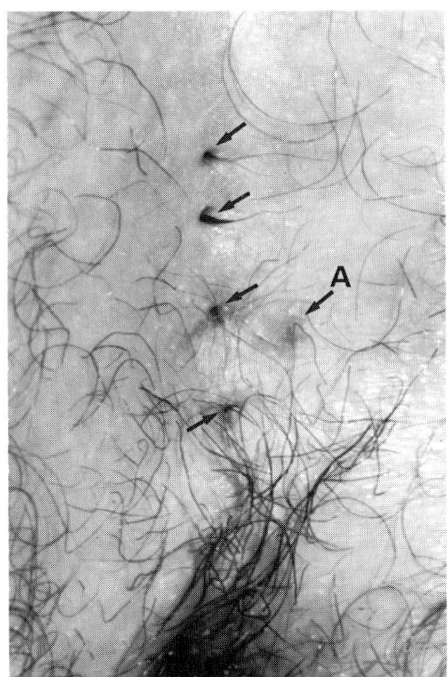

Fig. 28.18 Pilonidal sinus

The natal cleft of a young, hairy male, with several pilonidal sinuses visible (arrowed). There is obvious hair protruding from two of them. Note also the scar caused by drainage of a previous pilonidal abscess **A**

Treatment of pilonidal sinus

Definitive treatment aims to eliminate the nidus of hairs and associated cystic cavities, chronic abscesses and sinuses. At operation, obvious plugs of hair are first removed and then the sinus network is explored with probes, often aided by injecting blue dye into the sinuses. An elliptical wedge of tissue, incorporating the mass of sinuses, cysts and overlying skin is then excised. The

Fig. 28.19

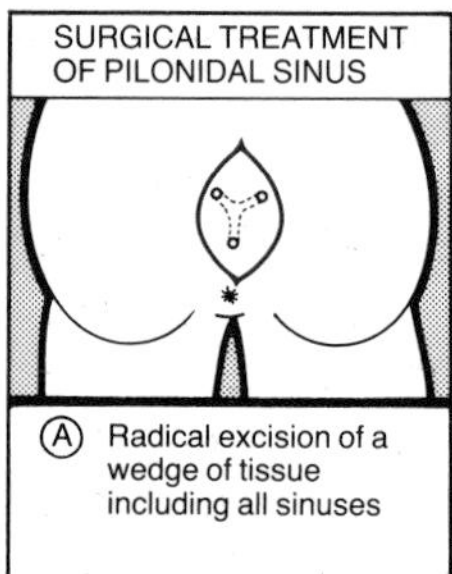

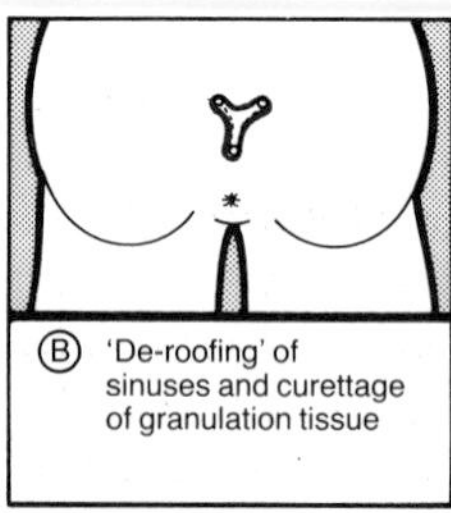

In either case the cavity is packed open to allow the wound to granulate up from the base and prevent healing over which would leave residual infection

incision often extends down to the sacral fascia. The resulting large defect bounded by healthy tissue is then packed and allowed to granulate from the base upwards. Healing takes several weeks but the patient can return home after a few days.

A less extensive surgical method known as *de-roofing*, shown in Figure 28.19, may be preferred. Another alternative treatment is *phenolisation*. In this, the sinus network is thoroughly curetted under general anaesthesia, and then filled with liquefied phenol for a minute or two. Phenol encourages fibrosis and may eliminate the cavity.

Despite surgery, pilonidal lesions commonly recur but this may be reduced by careful attention to hygiene. Daily baths and regular shaving of the area are recommended.

Occupational pilonidal sinuses

Pilonidal sinuses occasionally develop in the web spaces between the fingers in hairdressers. These are caused by implanted hairs from customers. A similar condition occurs in farmers, with hairs implanted from farm animals.

SEBACEOUS HYPERPLASIA

Localised hyperplasia of sebaceous glands on the nose and in nearby skin creases is common in both men and women. Sebaceous glands are plentiful in this area. The condition probably reflects a mildly abnormal response to sex hormones.

Apart from their unsightly appearance, these small nodular lesions may on occasion be clinically indistinguishable from basal cell carcinomas; the diagnosis is made on histology after excision biopsy.

In *rhinophyma*, an extreme manifestation of sebaceous hyperplasia, the nose becomes enlarged and lumpy. It is mainly seen in older men, and is said to occur in heavy drinkers.

BENIGN APPENDAGE TUMOURS

A variety of benign tumours arise from skin appendages. The most common is the *cylindroma*, which is derived from sweat glands. Diagnosis is usually made unexpectedly on histological examination of an excised nondescript skin lump.

LESIONS IN THE HYPODERMIS AND DEEPER TISSUES

CELLULITIS

Cellulitis is a diffuse spreading infection of the subcutaneous tissues and deeper layers of the skin. Beta haemolytic streptococci, usually Lancefield group A, are commonly responsible. These bacteria produce fibrinolysins and hyaluronidase which break down the protective intercellular barriers and promote spread of infection through the tissue planes. Although an intense neutrophil inflammatory response develops, pus rarely accumulates. Rather, the tissues become red and oedematous. If the skin surface is broken, a serous exudate is released.

Any part of the skin may develop cellulitis, the organisms usually gaining entry via a traumatic or surgical wound, although a wound is not always found. Clinically, the skin is greatly thickened, tense, hot, red and painful; the margins are fairly clearly demarcated from adjacent normal skin. Lymphatics draining the affected area become inflamed and *lymphangitis* develops. The inflamed lymphatics are visible as red streaks passing towards the regional lymph nodes which are also swollen and tender (*lymphadenitis*). Systemic features such as fever and tachycardia indicate bacteraemia or even septicaemia.

Cellulitis was a serious infection in earlier times, not least as a complication of surgery. It is now readily treated with antibiotics.

Cellulitis in the lower limb

Low-grade cellulitis may occur in the lower limb without evidence of any wound. This form of cellulitis is usually found in older women, and presents as a localised, but not clearly demarcated, brawny inflammation of the leg, usually without regional lymph node involvement or systemic features of infection. Predisposing factors are lymphatic obstruction or oedema from any cause. These infections often recur and are difficult to document bacteriologically because there is no wound and no infected exudate. Nevertheless, they usually respond to antibiotics (such as tetracycline), rest, elevation of the limb and compression stockings when the inflammation has settled. Recurrence is common at intervals of months or years.

A similar low-grade cellulitis may occur in the upper limb or chest wall as a result of lymphatic obstruction following radiotherapy for breast cancer.

Erysipelas

Erysipelas is an uncommon skin infection also caused by group A streptococci. In this condition, the infection is more superficial, involving only the dermis. The spreading inflamed area is very well demarcated, with the margin raised above the normal skin.

LIPOMA AND LIPOSARCOMA

Lipomas are benign tumours of fat. They may occur anywhere that fat is normally present, most often in the hypodermis of the trunk and limbs. Typically, they present in the supraclavicular fossa or over the deltoid muscle. Lipomas can also be found within the peritoneal cavity, including the bowel

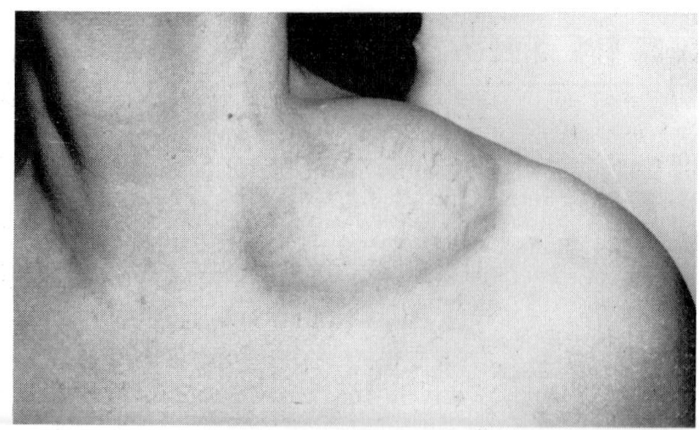

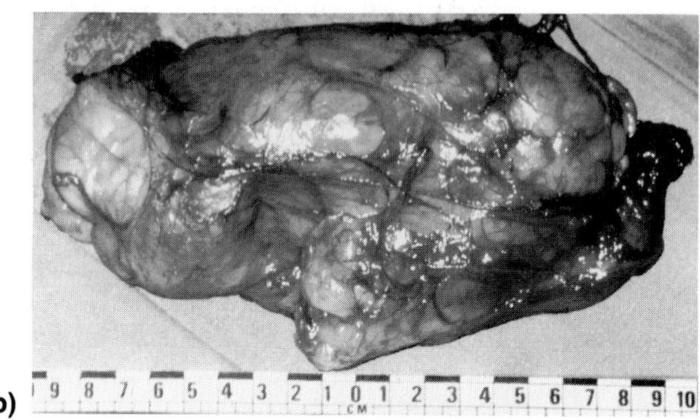

Fig. 28.20 Lipoma

(a) Large soft lipoma overlying the supraclavicular fossa in a 46-year-old woman. This is a common site for lipomas. It had been present for many years, but had recently started to enlarge. **(b)** The surgical specimen. Note that it is larger than its clinical appearance would suggest

submucosa, and within muscles or joints. They may also sometimes arise beneath periosteum.

Pathologically, lipomas consist of a multilobular mass of fatty tissue with thin fibrous septa. A thin fibrous capsule usually defines the lesion clearly from the surrounding tissue. Lipoma cells are histologically indistinguishable from normal adipocytes.

Lipomas vary in size from about 2–20 cm and are shaped like a flattened dome. The overlying skin is normal. Their consistency is soft and almost fluctuant. Lipomas are removed if they are inconvenient or unsightly. If the margin is poorly defined, recurrence is likely.

Liposarcoma is a rare malignant variant. It tends to occur in the retroperitoneal area and mediastinum rather than in the skin.

NEUROFIBROMA, NEUROFIBROMATOSIS AND SCHWANNOMA

Neurofibromas are benign tumours arising from the supporting fibroblasts of peripheral nerves. The tumour cells are loosely arranged in a gelatinous (myxomatous) intercellular material which often makes the lesion soft and pulpy to palpation. In the skin, neurofibromas may present as solitary sessile or pedunculated lesions in the vicinity of peripheral nerves.

The autosomal dominant inherited syndrome called *neurofibromatosis* (von Recklinghausen's disease) is characterised by multiple neurofibromas and cafe-au-lait spots; the latter are coffee-coloured skin patches. Sometimes, the neurofibromas are extremely numerous, and occasionally there is gross hypertrophy of subcutaneous tissues and skin folds. This extreme variation

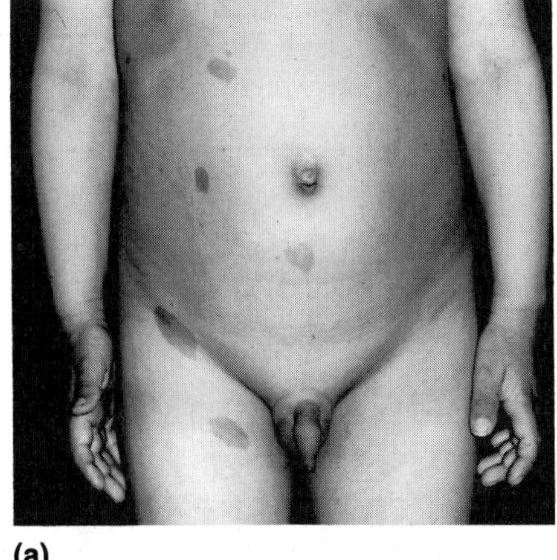

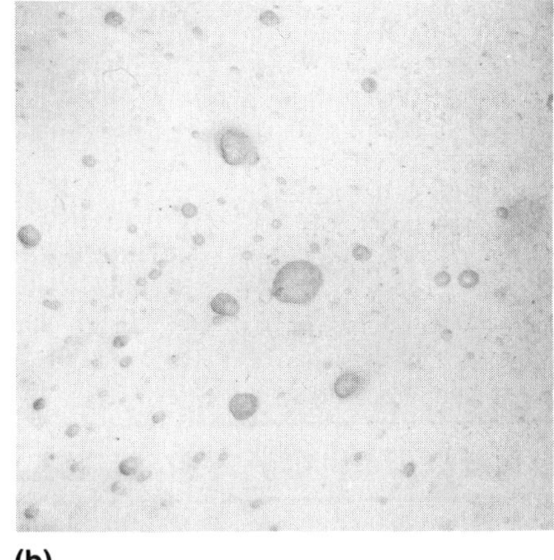

(a) (b)

Fig. 28.21 Von Recklinghausen's syndrome

(a) Cafe-au-lait patches. **(b)** Cutaneous neurofibromas

was immortalised by the famous 'elephant man' of Sir Frederick Treves. A small proportion of neurofibromas undergo malignant change into sarcomas.

Schwannomas are benign tumours arising from the Schwann cells supporting peripheral nerves. They present as firm, nodular lesions tethered to a nerve, and pressure on the tumour may cause pain in the area of distribution of the nerve. Treatment is by careful excision, attempting to preserve the affected nerve. This usually requires an operating microscope and microsurgical manipulation.

GANGLION

This extremely common and inappropriately-named condition is a cyst-like lesion derived from the lining of a synovial joint, tendon sheath or embryological remnants of synovial tissue. The 'cystic' space does not usually communicate with the associated joint or tendon sheath, and like synovial joint cavities, is not lined by epithelium. It contains a colourless, gelatinous fluid.

Ganglia present as skin lumps, usually about 1–2 cm in diameter, though sometimes larger. They are most common on the dorsum of the forearm and hand and around the ankle. They are rarely painful but sometimes cause

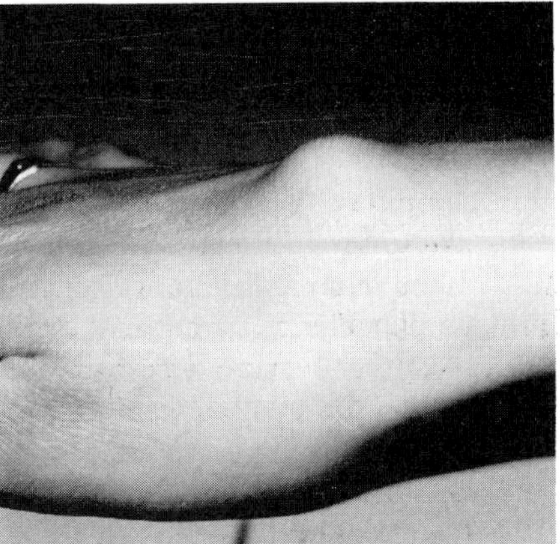

Fig. 28.22 Ganglion

This ganglion is in a common site, the dorsum of the hand

mechanical problems or interference with footwear. Ganglia are easily recognised by their smooth, hemispherical surface, and firm but slightly fluctuant 'cyst-like' consistency. The overlying skin is normal and mobile and the ganglion weakly transilluminable.

The age-old treatment for a ganglion was a sharp blow with a family bible, which dissipated the cyst contents into the tissues. Recurrence almost inevitably followed. Surgical excision is the accepted method of treatment now, but recurrence still often occurs.

LESIONS OF VASCULAR ORIGIN

CAMPBELL DE MORGAN SPOTS

Campbell de Morgan spots are small, bright-red spots which appear on the trunk, usually in the elderly. They represent highly localised capillary proliferation and have no clinical significance except for the titillation of bored examiners! Like other vascular lesions they blanch when compressed and then refill when pressure is removed.

SPIDER NAEVI

Spider naevi or telangiectases are small red lesions consisting of a central arteriole from which radiate dilated capillaries. This appearance explains their name. Isolated spider naevi may be found in normal individuals on the trunk, neck and face. Their numbers markedly increase in chronic liver disease, especially cirrhosis, and occasionally in pregnancy. Treatment is rarely required.

ANGIOMAS

Despite their name, angiomas are not true neoplasms but rather congenital hamartomas. They arise from localised excessive development of thin-walled blood vessels which may be of small diameter (*capillary haemangiomas*) or hugely dilated (*cavernous haemangiomas*). The histological appearance is often ambiguous, with most angiomas containing capillary and cavernous elements, as well as arteriovenous or even lymphatic components.

'Port-wine stains'

The most common haemangiomas are port-wine stains. These can occur anywhere on the body, but especially the face, neck and scalp, and cause considerable cosmetic distress. They are present from birth and remain unchanged throughout life. Lesions are flat or slightly elevated and reddish-blue. They have an asymmetrical outline and range up to many centimetres in diameter. Trauma may cause bleeding or ulceration.

Surgical treatment, often urged by anguished patients, is rarely successful except for small lesions. Sclerosing agents can be injected to promote thrombosis, organisation and progressive devascularisation, but results are disappointing. Argon lasers tuned to the colour frequency of haemoglobin are an encouraging innovation and give promising results in some patients. Regrettably, the use of covering cosmetic preparations remains the best advice for most.

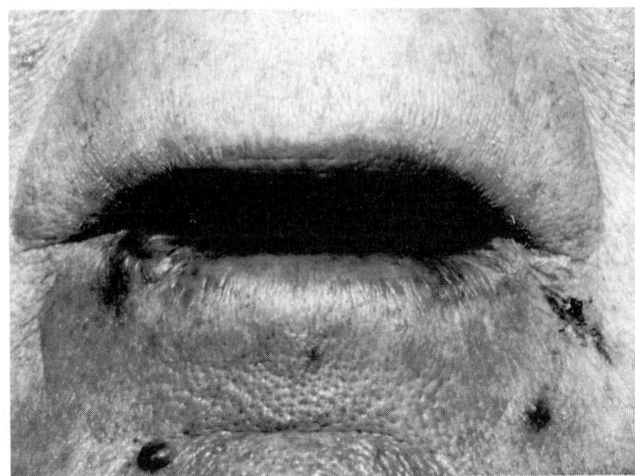

Fig. 28.23 Haemangiomas

Small haemangiomas of the lip and chin in an elderly man. These had been present since childhood. There were similar lesions inside the mouth

Strawberry naevi

The strawberry naevus is a distinct type of angioma. These occur in early childhood as bright-red fleshy lesions and grow for a few years before involuting spontaneously. Although they disappear and leave no scar, parents often insist on excision for cosmetic reasons. In the long term, surgical excision is not good management as it leaves an unnecessary scar.

Cystic hygroma

Cystic hygroma is a lymphangioma that presents as a lump in the neck usually during childhood; it is described in more detail in Chapter 29. Characteristically, the lesion is highly transilluminable.

Congenital syndromes

Gross vascular malformations form part of a number of rare congenital syndromes. These include *Sturge-Weber syndrome* (angiomas of the face and intracranial contents) and *Klippel-Trynawnay syndrome*. The latter syndrome usually affects one lower limb and the primary abnormality is multiple arteriovenous fistulae. These lead to hypertrophy of the limb (gigantism), gross varicose veins with venous ulceration, and cutaneous capillary naevi.

GLOMUS TUMOUR

This is a benign tumour derived from the glomus body, a small arteriovenous communication normally found in the peripheries. The glomus bodies are thought to play a part in controlling local blood flow. Glomus tumours occur

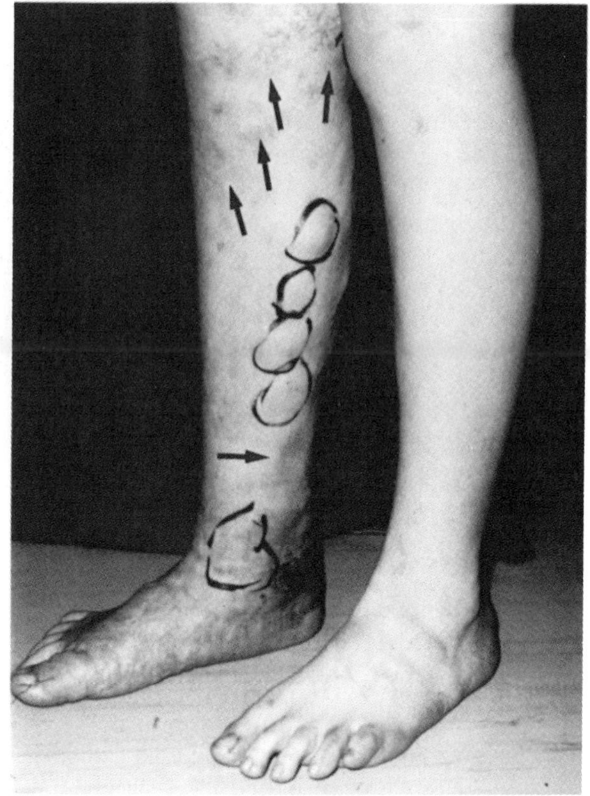

Fig. 28.24 Klippel-Trynawnay syndrome

Klippel-Trynawnay syndrome affecting the right leg in a male aged 19. The three characteristic features are gigantism due to multiple congenital arterio-venous fistulae, gross varicose veins (outlined in marking pen on the skin) and cutaneous capillary naevi (arrowed). In addition, this patient had a varicose ulcer, seen below the medial malleolus

singly, usually in the fingers and often beneath the nail. They are tiny (1–3 mm) red flat lesions which are exquisitely tender to the touch. Treatment is by surgical excision.

DISORDERS OF THE NAILS

INGROWING TOENAIL

Pathophysiology

Ingrowing toe nail occurs when the distal edge of the nail persistently cuts into the adjacent nail fold. The problem almost exclusively affects the great toe. In effect there is a laceration which cannot heal because of the presence of a foreign body (the toenail). Superimposed infection by a mixture of local bacterial and fungal flora complicates the picture. The combination of acute inflammation and attempts at tissue repair result in the formation of exuberant granulation tissue around the laceration and surrounding inflammatory swelling. Swelling aggravates trauma caused by the nail edge.

Ingrowing toe nail is mainly confined to teenagers and young adults, particularly males. It probably results from a combination of factors, including inadequate hygiene, unsuitable footwear, cutting the nails too short at the corners, and the macerating effect of sweat on the skin. High levels of

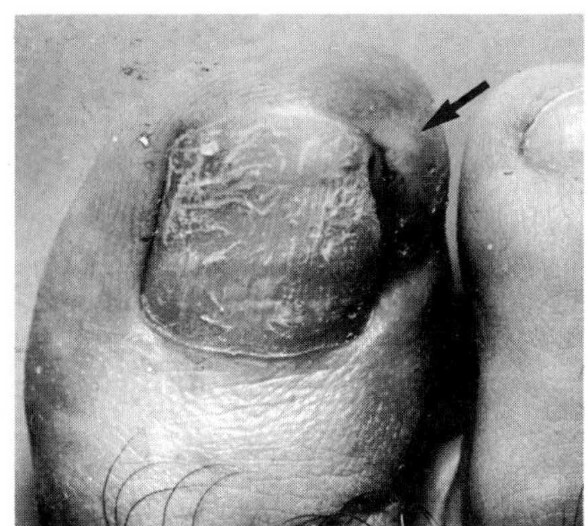

Fig. 28.25 Ingrowing toenail

Mild ingrowing toenail affecting the lateral edge of the right first toe. The patient has cut the corner from the nail to obtain relief. Note the ulcer near the cut edge of nail and the hypertrophy of nearby tissues (arrowed). This case responded to conservative treatment

circulating testosterone, as found in adolescence, may be an important aetiological factor.

Management

The main objective of treatment is to prevent persistent trauma by the nail edge. Surgical operations result in a week or more of pain and immobility, so conservative treatment should be tried first.

Conservative treatment

Simple conservative measures for all cases include regular bathing, frequent changes of socks (which should be made of cotton), avoiding tight or narrow shoes and avoiding trauma to the toe when inflamed, for example from kicking a football.

For an inflamed ingrowing toenail, foot soaks in warm saline should be carried out twice daily for at least ten minutes. Surgical spirit applied twice daily may also help.

A useful further measure, once inflammation is settling, is to pack a small pledget of cotton wool beneath the corner of the nail to lift the nail out of the laceration. At the same time, the nail fold can be pushed away by packing a small elongated pledget between the nailfold and the nail edge. These tiny packs can be left in place for days but need to be increased in size as the corner of the nail rises away from its bed.

These conservative measures, all undertaken by the patient, are often successful in even severe cases but require perseverence. Systemic antibiotics should only be used if infection is spreading, and topical antibiotics are of little use.

Surgical treatment

Surgical treatment involves avulsion of the whole nail, or one side of the nail. This immediately removes the 'foreign body' and permits rapid resolution. For recurrent ingrowing toenails, particularly if abnormal nail morphology is a contributory factor, part or all of the nail bed is best removed. The more

Fig. 28.26

OPERATIONS FOR INGROWING TOENAIL

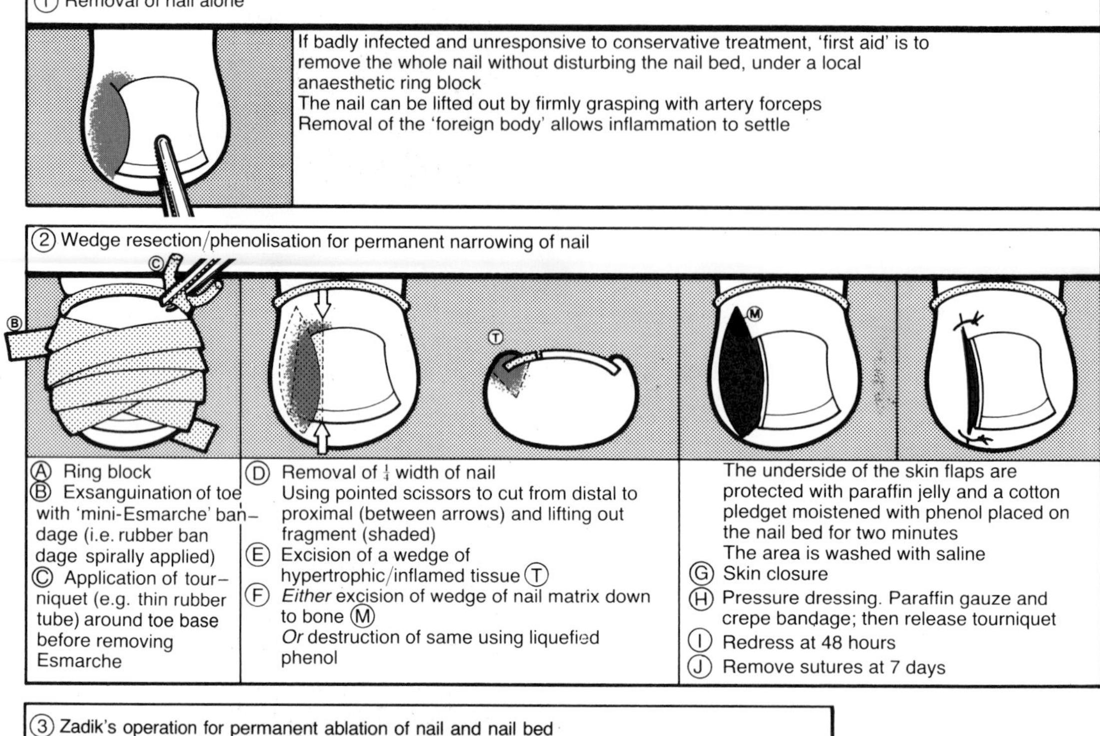

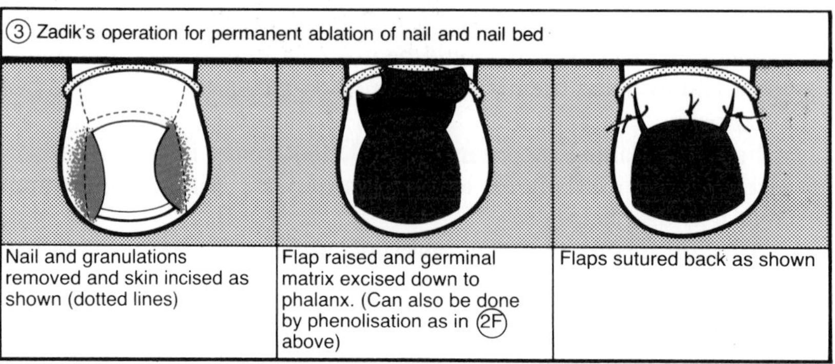

popular procedures are illustrated in Figure 28.26. The operations are usually performed under local anaesthesia using a ring block and tourniquet. Local anaesthetic incorporating a vasoconstrictor such as adrenaline must never be used in the digits because of the risk of ischaemic necrosis.

ONYCHOGRYPHOSIS

Onychogryphosis ('ram's horn nail') is a gross abnormality of nail growth. It most commonly affects the great toe nail, which becomes greatly thickened and distorted. Nail cutting with ordinary nail scissors then becomes impossible. Onychogryphosis is usually seen only in elderly patients, and probably results from previous trauma to the nail bed. The condition usually presents when it interferes with wearing shoes. A chiropodist can treat onychogryphosis by using grinding instruments at regular intervals. Surgical removal of the nail and ablation of the bed is sometimes performed.

Fig. 28.27 Onychogryphosis

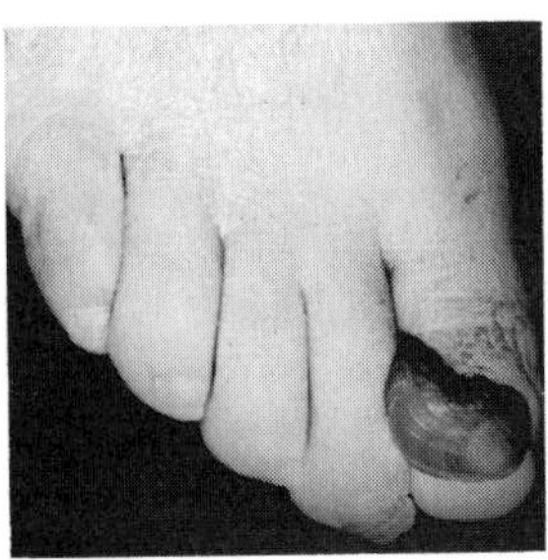

SUBUNGUAL MELANOMA

Malignant melanomas sometimes develop beneath finger or toe nails. Because of their location, they are difficult to diagnose. Pigmented melanomas are easily mistaken for old subungual haematomas, and amelanotic melanomas appear even more innocuous. Any lesion under the nail should therefore be biopsied to avoid the disaster of missing a potentially curable malignant melanoma.

Fig. 28.28 Subungual malignant melanoma

Aggressive malignant melanoma arising from beneath the nail of the first toe. Note the large main lesion and the satellite lesions nearby. This patient died of melanomatosis a year after this picture was taken

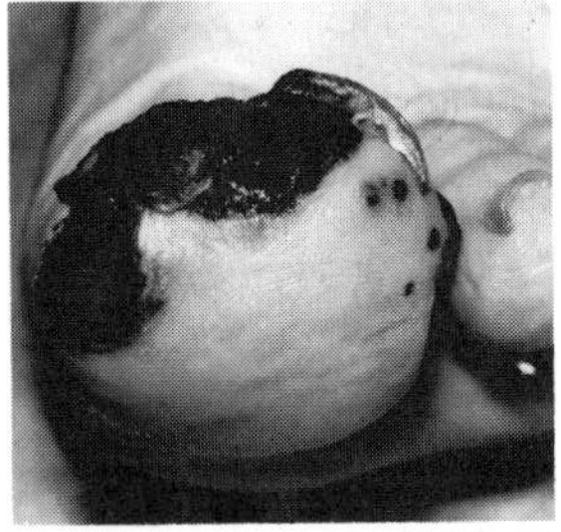

29 DISORDERS OF THE HEAD AND NECK

Introduction

The majority of head and neck disorders that reach the general surgeon are lumps of one sort or another. The main reasons for referral are either the need to exclude malignancy or for surgical treatment of a metabolic disorder such as thyrotoxicosis or hyperparathyroidism. There is a large overlap with other specialties, particularly ENT, dental and oral surgery, and dermatology.

Swellings of the thyroid gland may be confused with other swellings in the front of the neck. Thus, a complete examination of the head and neck should include the thyroid area.

Although problems in the mouth are usually managed by dental or oral surgeons, patients will often seek advice from another clinician. For this reason, most doctors should understand the essentials of oral and dental disease and their management.

LUMPS IN THE HEAD AND NECK

The concentration of so many different tissues in and around the head and neck is responsible for the profusion of conditions causing lumps in this area. Figure 29.1 provides a simple classification.

Fig. 29.1 Causes of a lump in the head or neck

1. **Thyroid disorders** (classified in Figure 30.1)
2. **Lymph node enlargement —**
   Lymphomas
   Secondary tumour deposits
   Local inflammatory lymphadenopathy from acute infections of the head and neck
   Local inflammatory lymphadenopathy from chronic infections such as tuberculosis
   Inflammatory lymphadenopathy as part of a generalised lymphadenopathy, e.g glandular fever or AIDS-related lymphadenopathy
3. **Congenital cysts** — thyroglossal, branchial and preauricular cysts, cystic hygroma and external angular dermoids
4. **Salivary gland disorders** — tumours, stones, rare autoimmune disorders such as Sjogren's syndrome
5. **Lumps in the skin** — any skin lesion may occur in the head and neck but the main problem is one of differential diagnosis e.g. lipomas and epidermal cysts
6. **Rare tumours** — carotid body tumours, carcinoma of the maxillary sinus, tumours and cysts of the jaw
7. **Actinomycosis** (very rare)

Special points in the history and examination

As always, the history will provide important clues to the diagnosis. The patient's age, the rate of growth of the lump and any associated symptoms such as pain, discharge, or swelling related to meals may lead quickly to the diagnosis.

Fig. 29.2 Characteristics of a lump

Site
Size
Shape
Surface characteristics
Fixation (superficial and deep)
Anatomical origin
Consistency
Fluctuance
Pulsatility
Temperature
Transilluminability
Bruit
Local lymphadenopathy

Fig. 29.3 Simple technique for palpating head and neck lymph nodes

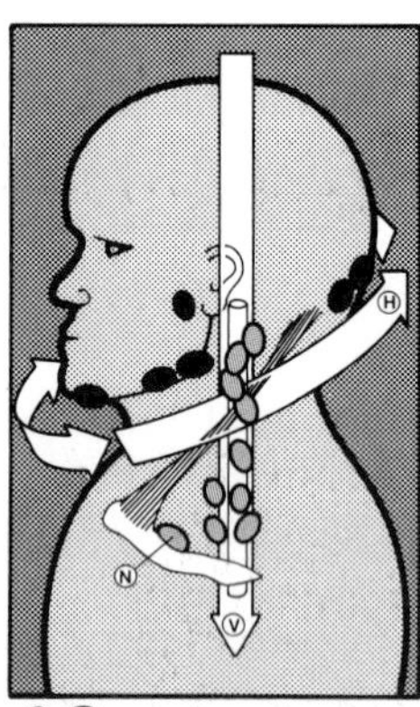

● (H) 'Horizontal' group of nodes

Palpate from behind patient, both sides simultaneously from submental, submandibular, jugulo-digastric, parotid to occipital

○ (V) 'Vertical' (internal jugular) nodes

Crossed obliquely by sternomastoid muscle and include anterior and posterior triangle nodes.

Search for enlarged Virchow's node **N** suggesting intra-abdominal malignancy

Most lumps in the head and neck are best examined with the patient sitting in a chair. This allows the examiner to palpate the lump from in front and behind. The examiner should establish the characteristics of the lump as summarised in Figure 29.2. At the same time, he or she should try to visualise the relationship of the lump to underlying anatomical structures. For example, a lump in the cheek may lie in the skin, the superficial part of the parotid, the buccinator muscle, the oral mucosa or the parotid duct. In clinical examinations, it is often useful to try to describe the characteristics of the lesion as if to a blind person.

The whole of the scalp, the back of the neck and the skin behind and in the ears, should be examined carefully. It is important to exclude primary tumours or infected lesions which may be producing lymph node enlargement. The lymph nodes of the head and neck must also be palpated. A simple method is to think of them as lying in two planes, the horizontal and the vertical, as shown in Figure 29.3. The nodes in each plane can then be examined with two or three simple manouvres. For any lump in the lower half of the face or submandibular region, the oral cavity should be examined to exclude salivary gland lesions, oral malignancies or sources of infection such as a dental abscess. For any lump in the parotid region, the integrity of the facial nerve should be formally tested.

DISORDERS OF THE ORAL CAVITY

The main disorders of the oral cavity are dental caries (decay) and its sequelae, inflammations of the gums and supporting bone (periodontal disease), tumours and premalignant conditions of the oral mucosa (leukoplakia and squamous carcinoma) and disorders of the accessory salivary glands such as retention cysts. The main symptoms and signs of oral disease are summarised in Figure 29.4.

Fig. 29.4 Symptoms and signs of oral disease and their main causes

Pain — dental caries and its sequelae, acute gingival inflammation such as pericoronitis and Vincent's infection

Bleeding — chronic gingival inflammation

Halitosis — dental caries and chronic periodontal disease

White lesions — epithelial dysplasia (leukoplakia), lichen planus and candidal infection

Oral ulceration — aphthous ulcers, squamous carcinoma, retained tooth roots, chronic tooth or denture trauma, and rare epidermal disorders (e.g. lichen planus or Behçets syndrome)

Discharging sinuses — periapical tooth abscess ('gum boil')

Bony lumps in the jaws — fibrous dysplasia, tumours, cysts, ectopic teeth

Salivary gland and duct-related lumps — retention cysts, submandibular duct stones, tumours

Examination of the oral cavity

For many doctors, asking the patient to open his mouth represents the entire oral examination. The following simple technique, illustrated in Figure 29.5, will enable most significant lesions to be seen without any special instruments or lighting.

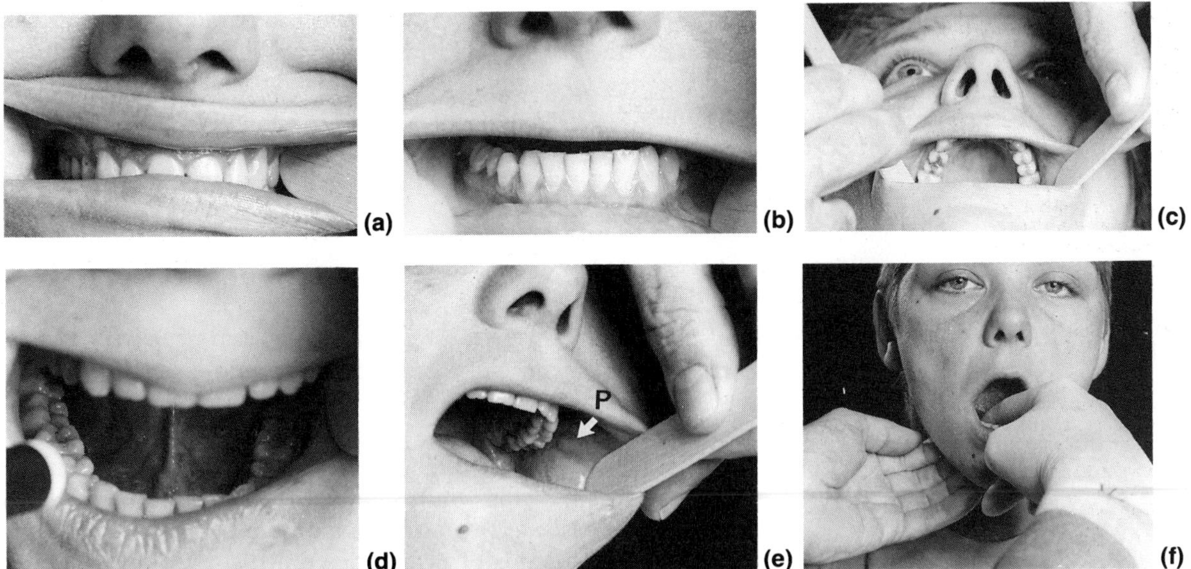

Fig. 29.5 Technique of oral examination

Teeth, gums and buccal sulci can be inspected by retracting the lips with wooden spatulae or fingers **(a)** and **(b)**. The palate is inspected by tilting the patient's head back and retracting the lips **(c)**, and the floor of the mouth and movements of the tongue examined as shown in **(d)**. The parotid papilla (arrowed) is demonstrated in **(e)**. Finally, bimanual palpation of the submandibular area, including the course of the submandibular duct, is performed with a gloved finger inside the mouth, as shown in **(f)**.

First, the patient should remove his dentures! The lips and their mucosal lining, and the lining of the cheeks and gums are then inspected. To do this, the lips are retracted by the examiner's fingers. At the same time, the teeth are inspected for gross decay and gingival inflammation. Painful inflammation is commonly related to a flap of gum over a partially erupted lower wisdom tooth.

If there is any suspicion of parotid disease, then the orifice of the parotiduct should be identified and palpated. This lies opposite the upper second molar tooth. The palate is examined easily if the patient tilts his head backwards. Finally, the tongue and floor of the mouth are inspected for mucosal lesions. To assist the examination, the patient first protrudes, then elevates, the tongue inside the mouth.

Lumps in the floor of the mouth, submandibular area and cheeks should be palpated bimanually as shown in Figure 29.5. Lumps in these areas are usually mobile and tend to move away from an examining finger.

DISORDERS OF THE SALIVARY GLANDS

Introduction

There are three pairs of major salivary glands, the *parotid*, *submandibular* and *sublingual* glands. The parotid produces serous saliva, the submandibular produces a mixed sero-mucous saliva and the sublingual produces a mucous secretion. The parotid and submandibular glands each drain into the mouth via a single long duct, whereas the sublingual glands drain via many small ducts.

The surgical disorders of the major salivary glands are benign and malignant tumours, stones, bacterial infections and rare autoimmune disorders, all of which present as salivary gland lumps. The oral mucosa also contains numerous small 'minor' salivary glands. Their main disorders are tumours and retention cysts.

SALIVARY GLAND TUMOURS

Pleomorphic adenoma

Pleomorphic adenoma is by far the most common neoplasm of salivary glands. It is also the most common cause of a lump in the parotid or submandibular gland. Most pleomorphic adenomas present in middle age or later, and both sexes are equally affected.

Pleomorphic adenomas are derived from salivary gland epithelium and are regarded as benign. Despite this, they show varying degrees of differentiation. The name *pleomorphic adenoma* was acquired from the varied histological appearance. Columns and islands of neoplastic epithelial cells are separated by a myxomatous connective tissue stroma which may contain areas resembling immature cartilage. This led early pathologists to believe that the tumour contained neoplastic tissue of both epithelial and connective tissue origin, thus generating the misleading name of *mixed salivary tumour*. Some tumours have no myxomatous tissue, and are described as *monomorphic* variants.

Although they do not metastasise, pleomorphic adenomas are often poorly circumscribed. Even when there appears to be a well-defined capsule, this is usually infiltrated with tumour, an important point when attempting removal. True malignant transformation occasionally takes place, usually to squamous cell carcinoma, with metastasis occurring to cervical nodes and sometimes the lungs.

Clinically, the tumour presents as a slowly growing, painless lump (see Figure 29.6). Most are in the parotid, some in the submandibular gland, and a few in minor salivary glands.

Parotid gland tumours usually occur in the superficial part of the gland, external to the plane of the facial nerve branches. Occasionally, they occur in the deep part of the gland, in more intimate association with the facial nerve. As the tumour is benign, it does not invade the nerve to cause a facial palsy. Facial nerve damage is, however, a risk during surgical excision, especially of deeper lesions. Patients should be warned of this possibility before operation.

If an older patient has a slowly growing parotid lump without a facial palsy, it is best to assume it is a pleomorphic adenoma. Definitive diagnosis can only be made histologically after excision.

Treatment of pleomorphic adenoma is by excision. For superficial lesions, this is by the operation of *superficial parotidectomy*, which involves excising all glandular tissue superficial to the plane of the facial nerve. Recurrence is uncommon. For deeper lesions, an attempt should be made to excise the entire lesion with a margin of normal gland, carefully identifying and preserving the branches of the facial nerve. When there is doubt about whether excision has been complete, postoperative radiotherapy is advisable.

The main complication of parotidectomy is damage to branches of the facial nerve. Damage to the temporal or upper zygomatic branches may prevent complete closure of the eye, leading to corneal drying and damage. Division

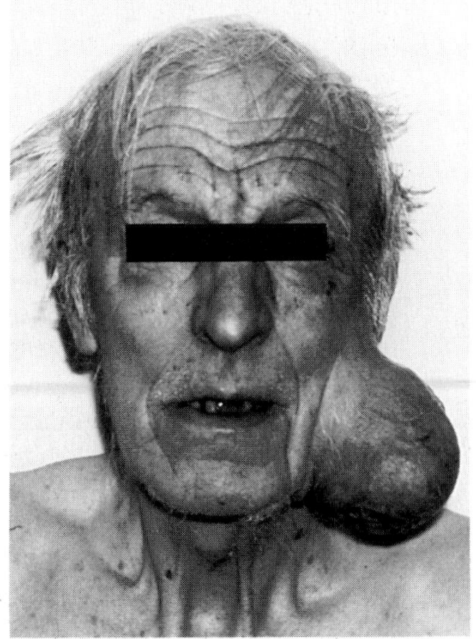

Fig. 29.6 Pleomorphic adenoma of parotid

Unusually large and very slow growing pleomorphic adenoma in an elderly man. These tumours usually present when much smaller

of the mandibular branch causes drooping of the angle of the mouth and embarrassing salivary dribbling. This may also complicate submandibular gland excision if the incision is incorrectly sited.

Salivary fistula is an occasional complication following parotid surgery, causing saliva to leak onto the face at meal times. The fistula usually resolves spontaneously after several months.

Frey's syndrome is a late complication of parotidectomy in as many as 25% of patients. It results from divided parasympathetic secretomotor fibres, originally innervating the gland, which then regenerate in the skin where they assume control of sweat gland activity. Facial sweating then occurs in response to salivatory stimuli, and is known as *gustatory sweating*.

Adenolymphoma (Warthin's tumour)

This unusual benign tumour constitutes less than 10% of salivary neoplasms. It occurs almost exclusively in the parotid glands. These tumours usually arise after middle age and there is a strong male predominance. They are sometimes bilateral.

Histologically, the tumour is composed of large glandular acini. The epithelium, similar to large salivary ducts, is embedded in dense lymphoid tissue in which lymphoid follicles may be seen. The histogenesis is not understood, but the glandular part may be hamartomatous salivary duct tissue within a normal parotid lymph node. A strong association with cigarette smoking has recently been demonstrated.

Adenolymphomas are invariably benign. They present as a parotid lump, indistinguishable from pleomorphic adenoma. The diagnosis can sometimes be made by fine-needle aspiration cytology, in which case, simple enucleation can be performed to remove the tumour. The standard treatment is, however, superficial parotidectomy. Adenolymphomas do not recur, but a satellite lesion may enlarge and present as another tumour.

Malignant primary salivary tumours

Malignant tumours comprise only a small proportion of neoplasms of major salivary glands, but form the major proportion of tumours in the minor (accessory) salivary glands scattered throughout the oral mucosa. Facial nerve weakness is diagnostic of parotid malignancy. The majority of malignant tumours are *adenocystic carcinomas* (also known as adenoid cystic carcinomas, and less accurately as cylindromas). The remainder include rare epithelial tumours such as *acinic cell carcinoma*.

Adenocystic carcinomas have a characteristic cribriform (sieve-like) microscopic appearance due to numerous small spaces in the tightly-packed tumour cell mass. These tumours are highly invasive, with early regional and systemic metastasis. Treatment involves wide mutilating surgery which usually destroys the facial nerve. Recurrence is unfortunately very common, and may occur as long as 5 years after apparently successful eradication. The tumours are unresponsive to radiotherapy and prognosis is almost uniformly poor.

Secondary tumours in salivary glands

The superficial part of the parotid gland contains lymph nodes which may become involved by secondary deposits from tumours of the face or scalp. In the same way, lymph node secondaries from the mouth may develop in the submandibular gland. The finding of a parotid or submandibular lump should therefore prompt a search for a primary tumour locally.

SALIVARY GLAND STONE DISEASE (SIALOLITHIASIS)

Pathophysiology

The submandibular gland and duct are prone to formation of calcified stones (calculi), which obstruct salivary outflow and predispose to infection. Calculi may occur in the parotid duct but this is much less common. The aetiology of salivary calculi is not known, but the submandibular gland may be vulnerable because of its more viscid secretion and elongated duct.

Stones are not the only cause of salivary gland damage. For both the parotid and submandibular gland, trauma to the duct orifice may result in stenosis and salivary stasis.

Submandibular stones may be found anywhere along Warthin's duct, including its course within the gland. Stones vary from several millimetres to centimetres in diameter. Those in the distal part of the duct tend to have an elongated 'date stone' shape

Clinical features

Salivary calculi rarely cause complete obstruction, but the patient usually experiences intermittent swelling or pain at meal times, when salivary flow is high. The swelling subsides over the next hour. Acidic foods such as lemon juice stimulate rapid salivary flow, and can be used as a test in clinic. Pain is not a prominent feature, rather, patients describe a sensation of fullness. Salivary calculi occasionally present with acute or chronic bacterial infection (*sialadenitis*).

Most of the submandibular gland lies deep to the mandible and so there is little to see on external examination. Palpation of the submandibular area confirms that the gland is moderately enlarged and firm. On intraoral examination, the tip of a stone impacted at the orifice of Warthin's duct may be visible (Figure 29.7). Bimanual palpation is the only way to assess the size of the gland and will also confirm the presence of a stone in the duct. Palpation is performed from the back towards the front of the mouth to avoid displacing a mobile stone into the gland.

Management of salivary calculi

Plain X-rays (occlusal and lateral-oblique views) will demonstrate most calculi. Contrast radiography of the duct system (*sialography*) is sometimes indicated if the history suggests stone disease, yet no stone is palpable or visible on plain X-ray. Sialography requires cannulation of the submandibular duct which may

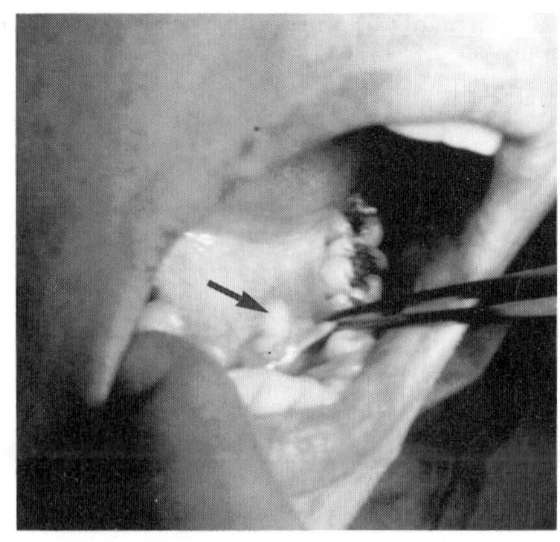

Fig. 29.7 Submandibular duct stone

This photograph shows a stone (arrowed) visible in the anterior part of Wharton's duct; it was removed under local anaesthesia via a longitudinal incision in the duct

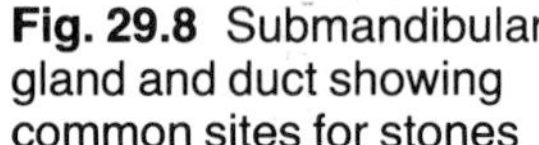

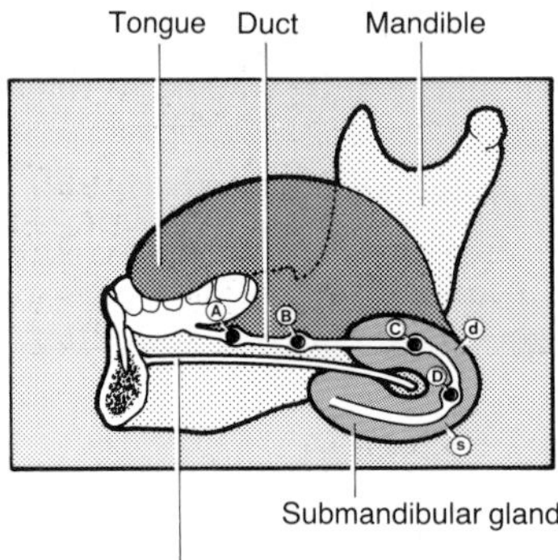

Note how the submandibular duct slopes downwards as it passes posteriorly. Thus the more posteriorly placed stones are increasingly difficult to remove from inside the mouth (Ⓐ → Ⓑ). Ⓒ and Ⓓ within the gland can only be removed by approaching the gland from the skin surface. Note also how the gland is in two parts, superficial and deep (ⓢ and ⓓ), wrapped around the posterior border of mylohyoid

Fig. 29.8 Submandibular gland and duct showing common sites for stones

reveal a stenosis of the duct orifice. Stenosis alone may produce symptoms similar to obstruction by a salivary calculus.

Calculi in the anterior two-thirds of the duct in the floor of the mouth are removed via an oral approach. A suture is first placed around the duct behind the palpable stone. This allows the duct to be lifted upwards and prevents the

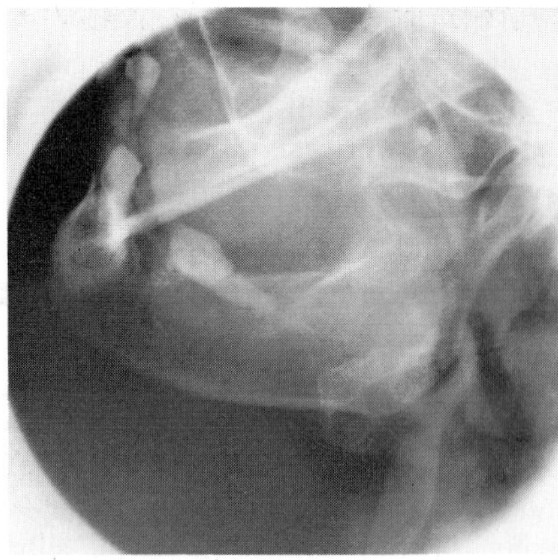

(a)

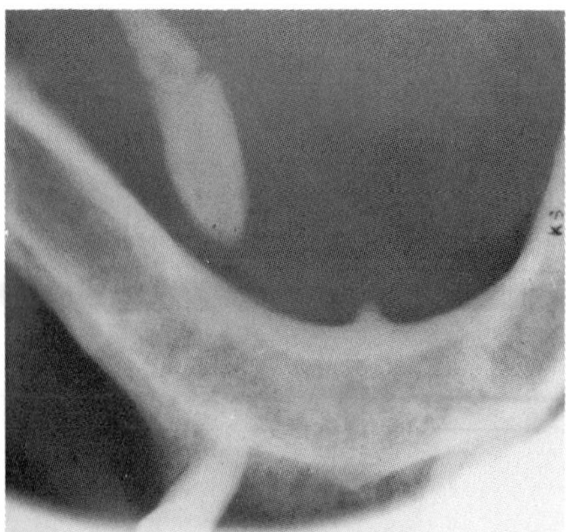

(b)

Fig. 29.9 Submandibular gland and duct calculi

(a) Lateral oblique plain X-ray, and **(b)** occlusal X-ray showing large 'date-stone' calculus in the right submandibular duct. These were easily palpable bimanually in the floor of the mouth and were removed via the oral route

stone from sliding back out of reach. A longitudinal incision is then made in the duct over the stone and the stone lifted out. The incision is not sutured but left open to improve salivary drainage. For small stones located at the duct orifice, a lacrimal probe is inserted into the duct and the orifice laid open.

Less commonly, calculi lie within the gland, where they are often multiple. The only way to remove the obstruction is to excise the entire submandibular gland through an incision below the mandible, carefully placed to avoid damaging the mandibular branch of the facial nerve.

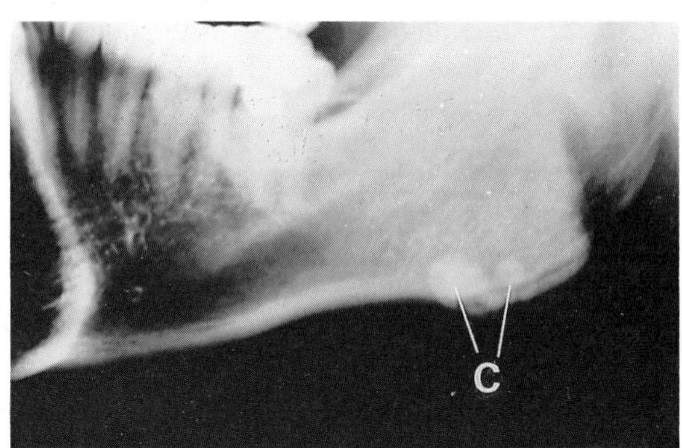

(a)

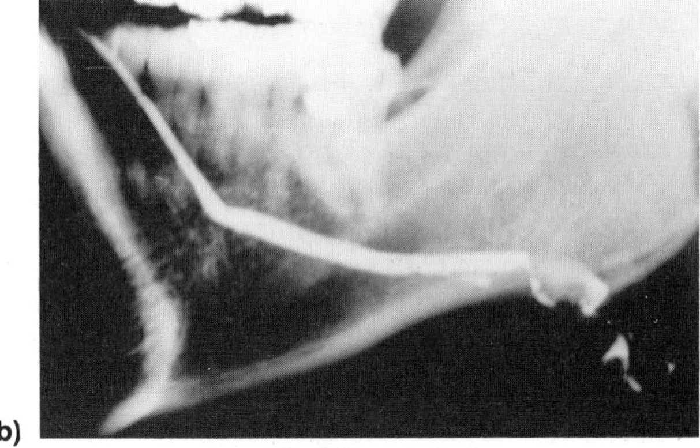

(b)

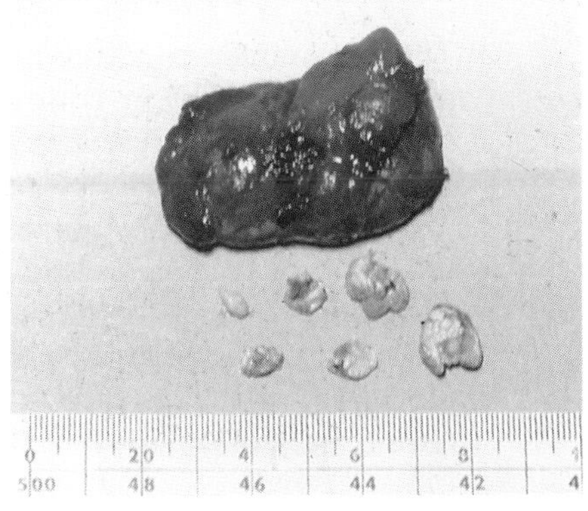

(c)

Fig. 29.10 Submandibular gland with stones

This 43-year-old man suffered chronic swelling and intermittent infection of the right submandibular gland: **(a)** Lateral plain X-ray showing calculi **C** within the gland. **(b)** Sialogram showing a normal Wharton's duct (note how rapidly it descends from the floor of the mouth). The stones within the gland are represented by filling defects in the contrast material. **(c)** The only means of dealing with the problem was excision of the gland via an extra-oral (submandibular) approach. The gland contained six calculi

INFLAMMATORY DISORDERS OF THE SALIVARY GLANDS

The salivary glands are subject to infection by both viruses (such as mumps) and bacteria. The glands may also be affected by rare, apparently autoimmune phenomena such as *Mikulicz's* and *Sjogren's syndromes*. Mumps is rare outside childhood and young adulthood, usually bilateral, and resolves spontaneously. It is rarely a surgical problem unless secondary bacterial infection supervenes.

Acute bacterial sialadenitis

This condition is now uncommon, almost always occurring in elderly or debilitated patients with poor oral hygiene. Dehydration and reduced salivary flow encourage ascending infection with oral flora, usually Strep. viridans or pneumococci.

The parotid gland is usually involved. The result is a painful, unilateral swelling accompanied by trismus, pyrexia and tachycardia. On examination, the parotid gland is tender and diffusely enlarged and a purulent discharge can be seen oozing (or can be 'milked') from the parotid duct orifice.

Bacterial sialadenitis should be treated promptly with parenteral antibiotics. If a parotid abscess has already formed, surgical drainage should be performed. *Acute parotitis* was once common in postoperative surgical patients due to dehydration and poor oral hygiene. Intravenous fluids and close nursing attention to mouth care have now made the condition rare.

Chronic sialadenitis

Prolonged obstruction of a major salivary gland by a ductal calculus causes chronic inflammation of the gland. The glandular secretory elements progressively atrophy, and are replaced by fibrous and adipose tissue. The duct system becomes dilated, fibrotic and infiltrated by chronic inflammatory cells. Chronic sialadenitis and salivary calculi usually involve the submandibular gland. The submandibular gland is swollen and there may be purulent discharge from the duct. The swelling is made worse by taking food.

Treatment is by removing the duct obstruction. In addition, antibiotics may be necessary. Glandular function may be irreversibly damaged if the process has been prolonged.

Recurrent sialadenitis

This uncommon condition, which may occur at any age, usually affects the parotid gland. One or both glands are subject to recurrent attacks of painful swelling. This is caused by low-grade bacterial infection, although no duct obstruction can usually be demonstrated.

Recurrent attacks cause swelling of the affected gland. Sialography shows dilatation of the duct system with terminal sacculation; this is described as *sialectasis*.

Treatment includes antibiotics, as indicated by culture of parotid duct discharge, as well as careful attention to oral hygiene. Intractable cases may require surgical removal of the gland.

Autoimmune salivary gland disorders

The salivary glands occasionally become involved in a chronic inflammatory process characterised by diffuse lymphoid infiltration and fibrosis. This is part of a poorly-understood autoimmune disorder which also involves lacrimal glands and mucous glands of the mouth and upper respiratory tract. The parotid and submandibular glands become diffusely and symmetrically enlarged, and salivary production is curtailed. The resulting dry mouth (*xerostomia*) not only causes distress and dysphagia, but predisposes to rampant dental caries. Diminished lacrymal secretions results in *kerato-conjunctivitis sicca*.

In isolation, the condition is known as *Mikulicz's syndrome*, but it may also occur in rheumatoid arthritis and other connective tissue disorders. In these cases, it is known as *Sjogren's syndrome*.

SALIVARY RETENTION CYSTS

Large retention cysts sometimes develop in the floor of the mouth. They reach several centimetres in diameter and are known as *ranulae*. The ranula typically appears as a blue-grey dome-like swelling beneath the tongue. It may burst spontaneously, discharging its contents and collapsing, but it almost invariably recurs. They are painless but occupy space in the mouth and treatment is often requested. Excision is difficult because of the tenous lining, and because of the proximity to vital structures in the floor of the mouth; incomplete removal leads to recurrence. The usual treatment, therefore, is marsupialisation i.e. de-roofing the cyst so that it opens into the floor of the mouth (see Figure 29.11).

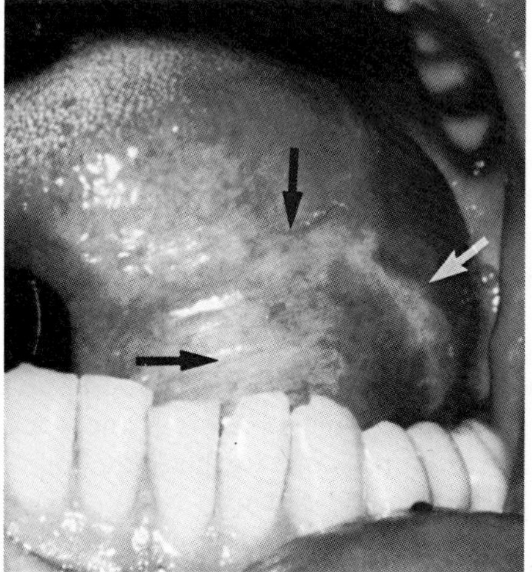
(a)

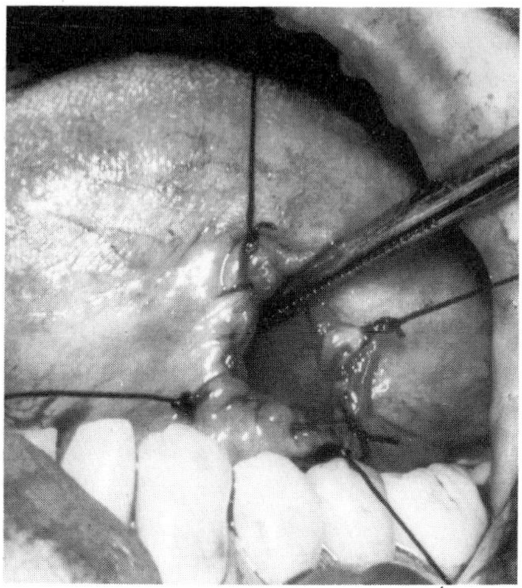
(b)

Fig. 29.11 Marsupialisation of ranula

(a) Large salivary retention cyst in the floor of the mouth displacing the tongue towards the opposite side. **(b)** Operative photograph showing the 'deroofed' cyst and the edges being sutured to the oral mucosa. The cavity rapidly 'filled in' from the base, obliterating the defect

LYMPH NODE DISORDERS OF THE HEAD AND NECK

Introduction

Patients are often referred to a surgeon for biopsy of an enlarged lymph node in the cervical region. Often there are no other symptoms or signs. *Isolated lymph node enlargement* may be caused by local disease within its field of drainage. Examples include tonsillitis or dental infection, tonsillar tuberculosis or a malignant oropharyngeal tumour. Nodes draining a bacterial infection may themselves suppurate, sometimes after the primary disorder has disappeared (see Figure 29.12).

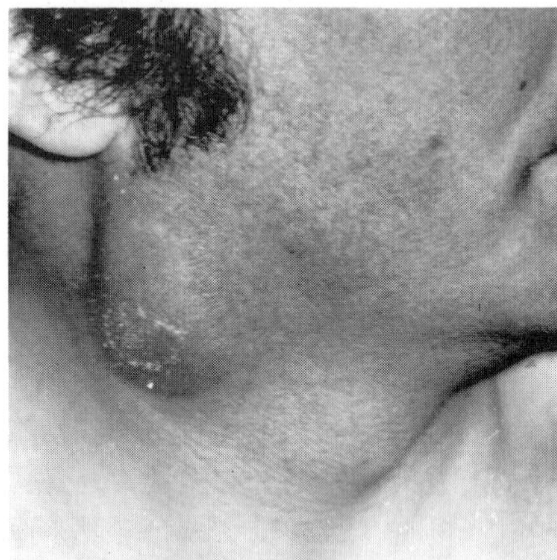

Fig. 29.12 Suppurating lymph node in the neck
This patient presented with a suppurating node in the neck which required external drainage. The primary site of sepsis was a dental abscess on a lower molar tooth

Alternatively, an enlarged cervical lymph node may be part of a *systemic lymphadenopathy* caused by glandular fever or lymphoma. Thus, any patient presenting with an enlarged lymph node requires careful examination of the head, neck and mouth. This includes thorough endoscopy of the whole pharyngeal area, usually by a specialist ENT surgeon. In addition, general examination should pay particular attention to axillary and inguinal lymph nodes, liver and spleen. If cervical lymph node biopsy is necessary, it should always be performed under general anaesthesia since the operation may be unexpectedly difficult. This is because lymph nodes are intimately related to so many vital structures, and furthermore, preoperative palpation tends to underestimate the size and extent of lymph node involvement.

CERVICAL TUBERCULOSIS

Tuberculosis involving the cervical glands (*scrofula*) was once common, the infection being acquired by drinking milk from cattle infected with bovine tuberculosis. Cervical tuberculosis is now extremely rare in developed countries, but may be seen in recent Third World immigrants. The primary infection occurs in the tonsils, but the condition presents with secondary involvement of the cervical nodes, which become progressively enlarged and matted together. In advanced cases, liquefaction of the caseous material forms *cold abscesses*. If untreated, these eventually drain onto the neck, and leave disfiguring scars.

In the past, surgery was often required to drain and remove the affected glands. With chemotherapy, this is now rarely necessary and surgery is mostly confined to excision biopsy for diagnosis.

LYMPHOMAS

An enlarged cervical lymph node is a common presentation of Hodgkin's disease or one of the other lymphomas. The disease is often at an early stage and there may be no other symptoms or clinical signs. The diagnosis is then made by histological examination of a biopsy specimen.

SECONDARY TUMOURS

Cervical lymph node metastases may originate from primary tumours in the head and neck, chest or abdomen. An enlarged lymph node may be the first indication of a tumour or a recurrence following treatment.

Tumours of the head and neck usually metastasise to nodes in the submandibular region and upper part of the anterior triangle. In contrast, tumours from the chest and abdomen usually metastasise to the lower part of the posterior triangle, particularly to *Virchow's node* which lies deep in the angle between the sternomastoid and the clavicle.

The following head and neck tumours metastasise to cervical lymph nodes:

- Squamous carcinoma and melanoma of the skin of neck, face, scalp and ear
- Squamous carcinoma of the mouth and tongue
- Squamous carcinoma of the nasopharynx, oropharynx, larynx and paranasal sinuses. The primary tumour may be exceedingly small
- Adenocystic carcinoma of the major or accessory salivary glands
- Papillary (and occasionally medullary) carcinomas of the thyroid

MISCELLANEOUS CAUSES OF A LUMP IN THE NECK

CONGENITAL CYSTS AND SINUSES

A variety of cystic lesions of congenital origin occur in the head and neck, and some of them may be associated with sinuses. All are uncommon except in clinical 'short-case' examinations! They can be subdivided into thyroglossal cysts, branchial cysts, fusion-line dermoid cysts, preauricular cysts and sinuses and cystic hygromas. All are true epithelial cysts except for cystic hygroma, which is a hamartomatous lymphatic malformation.

Branchial cysts, sinuses and fistulae

The exact embryological origin of these cysts is in dispute but they probably arise from remnants of the second pharyngeal pouch or branchial cleft. Branchial cysts usually present in late adolescence or early adulthood but sometimes even later. This late presentation is unusual for congenital lesions. Typically, the patient complains of a painless swelling in the side of the neck which may vary in size from time to time. Some patients present with a painful red swelling due to inflammation of a previously unnoticed cyst.

The lump lies deep to the sternomastoid, at the junction of its upper third and lower two-thirds. It protrudes forwards into the anterior triangle of the neck. On palpation the lump is soft and fluctuant. Provided it is not inflamed, the cyst usually transilluminates. Treatment is by surgical excision, although inflamed cysts may require initial drainage.

Branchial sinus and fistula presents as a discharging sinus near the lower end of the anterior border of the sternomastoid muscle. A sinus ends blindly on the lateral pharyngeal wall whereas a fistula communicates with the oropharynx near the tonsillar fossa. Surgical excision may be required.

Fusion-line dermoid cysts

Dermoid cysts of congenital origin may arise from epithelial remnants along lines of embryological fusion in the head and neck.

The most common are *external angular dermoids*, which are cystic swellings at the outer aspect of the supraorbital ridge. They are usually noticed soon after birth. On palpation these cysts are tense and firm, and do not transilluminate because of their thick keratinous contents. They are deeply fixed and therefore immobile. External angular dermoids are usually surgically removed during childhood for cosmetic reasons.

Midline dermoid cysts are described as teratoid cysts because they contain a mixture of ectodermal, mesodermal and endodermal elements (e.g. nails and teeth, glands, blood vessels). A rare phenomenon, dermoid cysts arise in the midline of the head or neck, usually during the first year of life. They should be removed surgically.

Preauricular cysts and sinuses

Small cysts and sinuses may arise from developmental abnormalities of the first and second branchial arches, which are involved in forming the external ear. The lesion becomes apparent in early childhood. They lie anterior to the tragus and present either as small lumps or as minute discharging sinuses which occasionally become infected. There may be an obvious associated abnormality of the auricle. Treatment is usually by surgical excision.

Cystic hygromas

Cystic hygromas are not true cysts but rather lymphatic hamartomas which form multilocular cyst-like spaces. Cystic hygromas may be huge and disfiguring lesions present at birth. Smaller lesions may present in older children or adolescents as a painless lump in the neck, just below the angle of the mandible. Cystic hygromas are soft and fluctuant and highly transilluminable.

Surgical excision may be difficult as these lesions often extend deeply into cervical and oro-facial tissues.

ACTINOMYCOSIS

Actinomycosis is a rare infection of the cervico-facial region. It is caused by *Actinomyces israelii*, an anaerobic gram-positive bacterium with an unusual filamentous growth pattern similar to fungal mycelia. Actinomycosis is a chronic

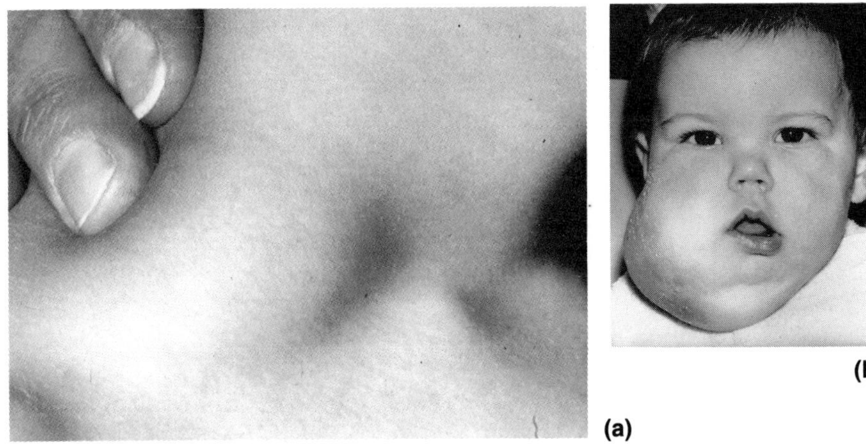

Fig. 29.13 Branchial cyst and cystic hygroma
(a) This 16-year-old girl was found to have a soft asymptomatic swelling, a branchial cyst, which is being displaced from beneath sternomastoid for this photograph.
(b) Very large cystic hygroma (lymphangioma) in a 12-month-old child which was present at birth

granulomatous infection with multilocular abscesses which drain to the overlying skin via multiple sinuses. The pus exuding from the sinuses contains characteristic yellow clumps of organisms known as '*sulphur granules*'. The infection stimulates much fibrosis.

The organism is an oro-pharyngeal commensal but gains access to the tissues via carious teeth, tooth extraction sockets or traumatic wounds. Initially, there is a painful intraoral swelling. Inflammation then spreads slowly into the tissues, causing firm swelling of the cheek, mandible and submandibular region ('lumpy jaw'). The infection eventually erodes into the salivary glands, jaws and adjacent structures. Suppurative foci drain onto the surface of the face forming chronic discharging sinuses.

Actinomycosis is treated with a prolonged course (four to six weeks) of high dose penicillin. If necessary, the abscess network is surgically explored and drained.

Cervico-facial actinomycosis was once common and its decline in developed countries is probably due to better oral hygiene and dental care. Actinomycosis may also occur in the ileo-caecal area, gaining access from an appendiceal perforation. Actinomycosis is now most often encountered in the pelvis as a complication of an intrauterine contraceptive device, although this is rare.

DISORDERS OF THE ORAL CAVITY

DENTAL CARIES

Pathophysiology and clinical features

Dental caries (dental decay) is the most common bacterial disorder in developed countries. The process begins when the protective enamel surface of the tooth is breached by the demineralising action of lactic acid. This is generated by commensal oral bacteria as a by-product of carbohydrate metabolism, particularly of refined sugar products. The most vulnerable sites for decay are the areas just below the contact points of adjacent tooth crowns, and the deep pits and fissures on the biting surface of molars and premolars. These sites are inaccessible to the natural oral cleansing mechanisms and to tooth brushing.

Once the enamel is breached, proteolytic bacteria gain entry to the less densely calcified dentine beneath, and cause its progressive destruction. The enamel remains intact until the supporting dentine is grossly undermined and the enamel fractures. Thus, dental caries may be well advanced before it is visible, even with a dental mirror and probe. In the meantime, the decay

Fig. 29.14
Pathophysiology and symptoms of dental caries and its sequelae

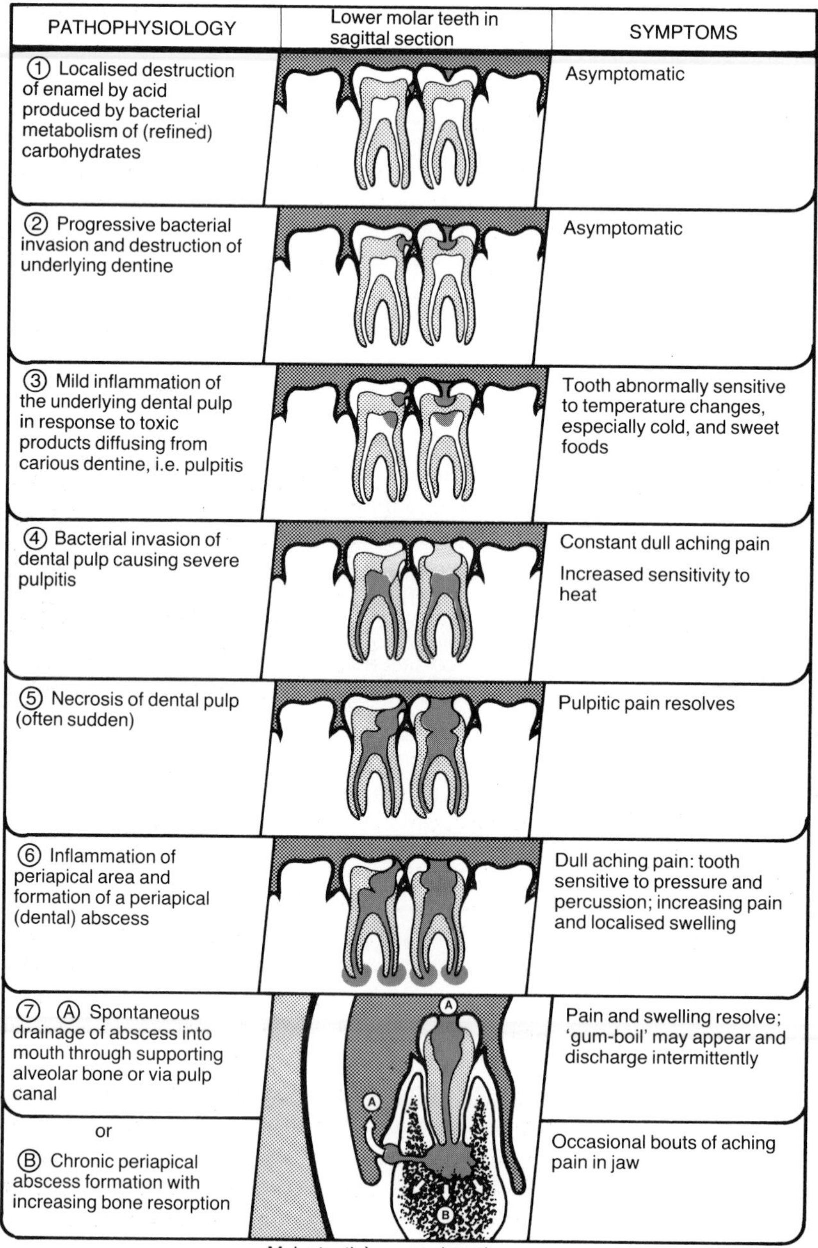

process is asymptomatic until close enough to the dental pulp to cause chemical inflammation and, eventually, bacterial invasion. The usual pathological process and corresponding symptoms are outlined in Figure 29.14.

Inflammation and bacterial invasion usually destroy the dental pulp and then spread to the periapical region where an abscess develops. This eventually drains into the mouth but causes painful oral and facial swelling beforehand.

The pain of dental caries is usually well localised and recognised as a 'toothache' by the patient. Dental pain may, however, be poorly localised and cause non-specific facial pain. Dental caries should always be considered before rarer diagnoses are accepted. Overall, however, a suprising amount of dental caries, even with periapical infection, is asymptomatic.

Management of dental caries

Provided the dental pulp has not been invaded by infection (i.e. become 'exposed'), a dentist can usually remove the carious enamel and dentine and restore it with a filling of silver amalgam, synthetic resin or gold. This is usually placed over a sedative and insulating lining. Once bacteria have invaded the pulp, this necrotic tissue must be removed by *endodontic treatment*, and the pulp cavity filled; this is known as 'root filling'. In this way, the tooth can often be saved.

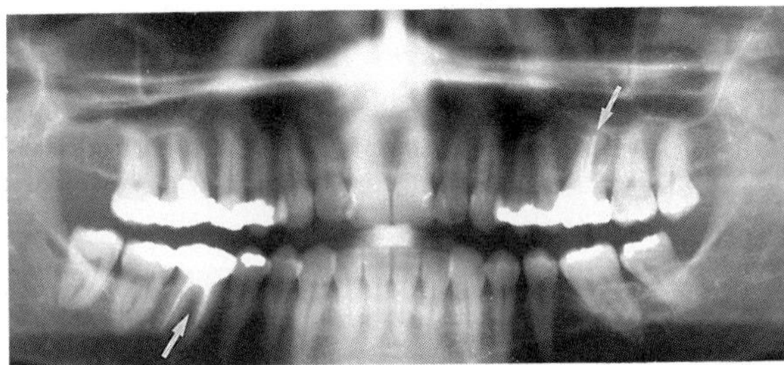

Fig. 29.15 Dental restorations and root fillings

This oral pantomograph (OPG) film shows silver amalgam restorations for caries in posterior teeth (shown as white radio-pacities) and 'silicate' restorations in front teeth (shown as relative radiolucencies in the upper incisors). In addition, the upper left first molar and the lower right first molar (arrowed) have radiopaque root canal fillings, necessitated by dental caries invading the pulp

Management of dental abscesses

A periapical abscess is the most common presentation of caries seen by the general medical practitioner or casualty officer. Primary treatment is drainage of pus as for other abscesses. Extracting the offending tooth is the most effective method, but if there is a chance of preserving the tooth, it can be drained via the root canal after drilling into the tooth. Wherever possible, patients with periapical abscesses should be referred to a dentist for treatment.

Large acute abscesses which are 'pointing', can be drained by incising the oral mucosa at the site of greatest fluctuation. Oral or intramuscular penicillin should be prescribed if there is spreading infection. Without swelling and other signs of an acute abscess, antibiotics have no part in the management of toothache. A dental abscess occasionally presents on the face (Figure 29.16) but will usually settle with extraction of the offending tooth. Dental abscesses are very rarely complicated by osteomyelitis.

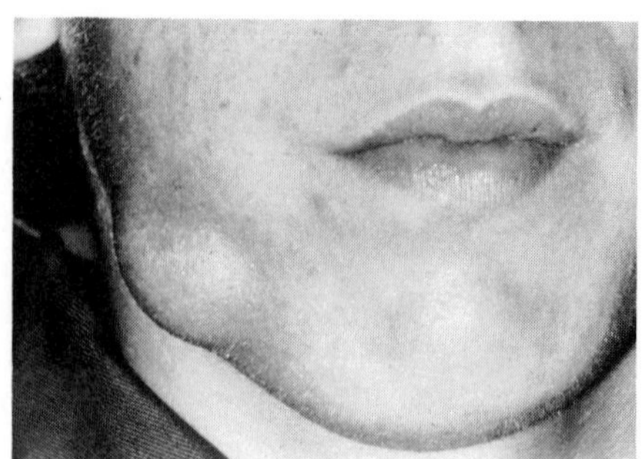

Fig. 29.16 Dental abscess pointing on the face

This young man presented to his doctor with an obvious abscess on the face; he was unaware that it arose from a tooth affected by dental caries. Once the tooth was removed, the abscess drained and the swelling settled

Tooth extraction and post-extraction problems

Medical practitioners are rarely required to extract teeth except in geographically isolated places. Caries prevention and modern restorative and endodontic techniques have made the need for extraction much less common. Patients, however, often attend general practitioners or accident and emergency departments following tooth extraction or surgical tooth removal, with problems of bleeding, pain and swelling.

a. Bleeding tooth socket

A small amount of blood mixed with saliva may appear to be a severe haemorrhage! The extraction site should be inspected for evidence of arterial bleeding, which produces blood clots in the mouth. The normal extraction socket should be filled with firm clot but there may be an ooze from the gingival margin. This is made worse if the anxious patient continually disturbs the clot by rinsing the mouth or 'exploring' the socket with the tongue. Aspirin as an analgesic may also promote bleeding by interfering with platelet activity.

Fig. 29.17

SUTURE TECHNIQUE FOR BLEEDING TOOTH SOCKET

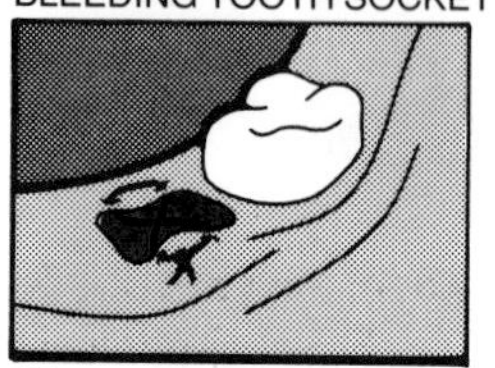

'Figure of eight' suture occludes bleeding gum edge on alveolar bone. Patient should bite for at least 10 minutes on a folded swab after suture to encourage clotting

Oozing or minor bleeding is easily controlled by the patient biting on a small dry pack such as a folded gauze swab. Pressure should be maintained for 10–15 minutes. More persistent bleeding is usually controlled by inserting several sutures through the gingival margins across the socket, partially closing the defect. This is illustrated in Figure 29.17. Afterwards, the patient should bite upon a small dry gauze pad. Suturing is performed under local anaesthetic, a small amount of which is infiltrated into the gingiva on each side of the socket. Silk or catgut sutures are preferred as they do not leave irritating sharp ends. Silk sutures are removed after 5–7 days, catgut sutures dissolve in about the same period.

If bleeding continues after these simple measures, then the patient should be investigated for a coagulation or platelet abnormality.

b. Pain after tooth extraction

Forceps extraction or surgical tooth removal may lead to a great deal of pain soon afterwards. Removal of lower molar teeth may cause trismus (masseteric spasm) making jaw movements painful and restricted. If there is no sign of infection, treatment is with analgesia, not antibiotics. Pain appearing several days after extraction is usually due to a superficial osteitis of exposed bone within the socket caused by failure of the socket to fill with organised clot. This condition, known as *dry socket*, is intensely painful and requires dental treatment. Antibiotic therapy is not helpful.

c. *Swelling after tooth extraction*

Soft tissue swelling is not common after tooth extraction with the exception of surgically removed lower third molars ('wisdom teeth'). Extraction of these teeth often causes marked swelling around the angle of the mandible (Figure 29.18), with trismus and pain. This swelling represents a normal inflammatory response and some interstitial haemorrhage rather than infection. The swelling subsides within a week or so postoperatively and again does not warrant antibiotic therapy.

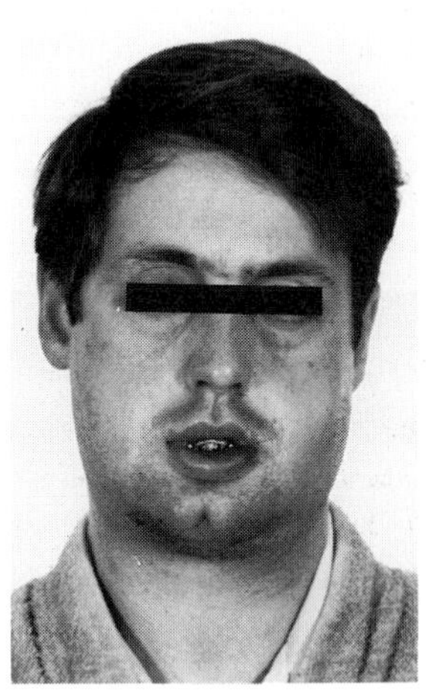

Fig. 29.18 Typical swelling following third molar removal

This patient presented to an accident and emergency department, believing he had postoperative infection. Swelling like this is to be anticipated after third molar surgery and, unless there are systemic features, does not usually represent infection

INFLAMMATION OF THE PERIODONTAL TISSUES

Gingivitis and periodontitis

Teeth are embedded in bony *alveolar ridges* in both upper and lower jaws. A thin layer of *cementum* (a bone-like material) on the root surface is joined to the bone of the socket by a tough collagenous tissue known as *periodontal membrane*. The oral mucosa bound to the alveolar bone (the *gingiva* or gums) normally forms a tight cuff around the tooth neck, protecting alveolar bone from bacteria and foreign material. A potential space between the gingival cuff and the enamel of the crown, known as the *gingival crevice* extends down to the cemento-enamel junction. At the free margin of the gingiva, the tough stratified oral epithelium becomes a thin vulnerable layer lining the gingival crevice.

If oral hygiene is inadequate, commensal bacteria colonise the gingival margin and form a white gelatinous *plaque* on the enamel. If allowed to persist, plaque becomes adherent to the tooth surface and becomes mineralised. This is known as *calculus*, and cannot be removed by tooth brushing. Bacterial toxins then cause inflammation of the gingiva, known as *marginal gingivitis*. This appears as swelling and redness of the gums and slight bleeding during tooth brushing.

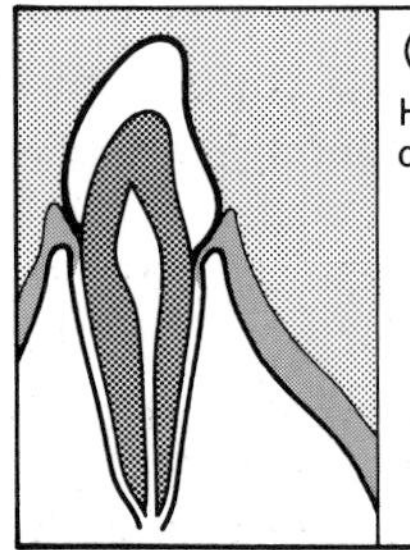

Ⓐ NORMAL GINGIVA

Healthy pink gingiva forming tight cuff around base of crown

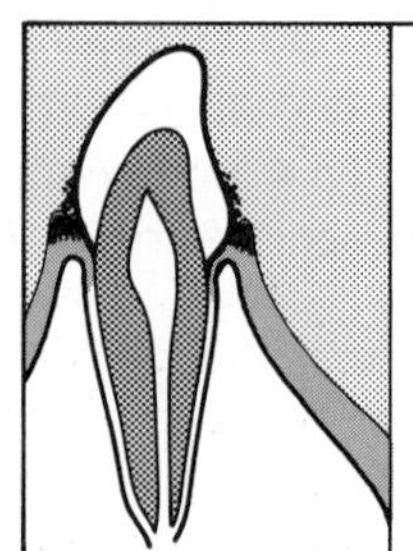

Ⓑ MARGINAL GINGIVITIS

Plaque accumulates around gingival margins

Toxins produced by bacteria cause marginal inflammation

Marginal gingiva becomes red, slightly swollen and bleeds easily

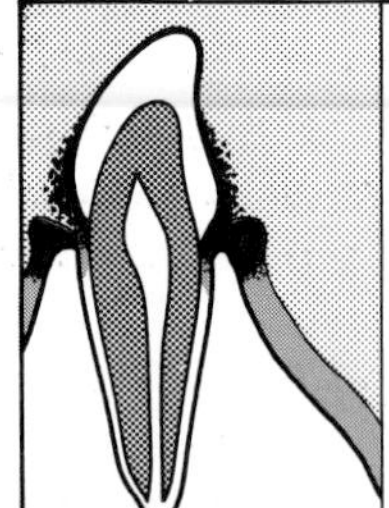

Ⓒ MODERATE GINGIVITIS

Loss of tight protective cuff of gingiva allowing accumulation of bacterial plaque and calculus in gingival crevice

More severe gingival inflammation

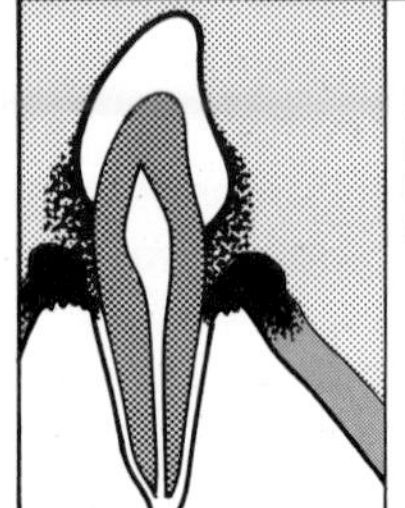

Ⓓ PERIODONTITIS

Inflammation involves supporting alveolar bone which is progressively resorbed so that adequate tooth support is eventually lost

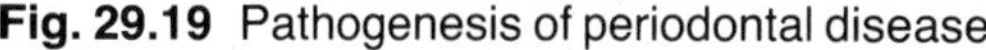

Fig. 29.19 Pathogenesis of periodontal disease

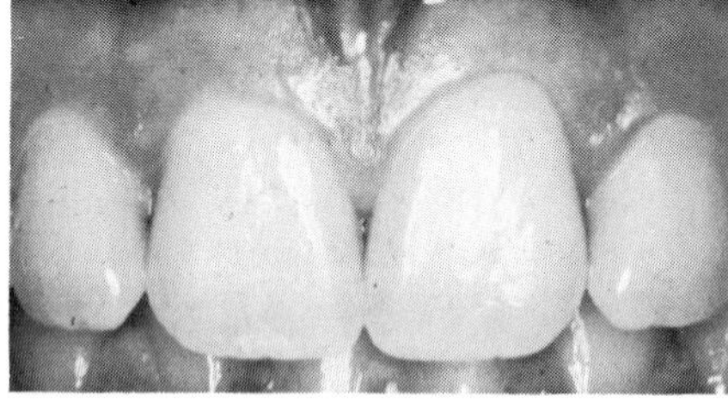

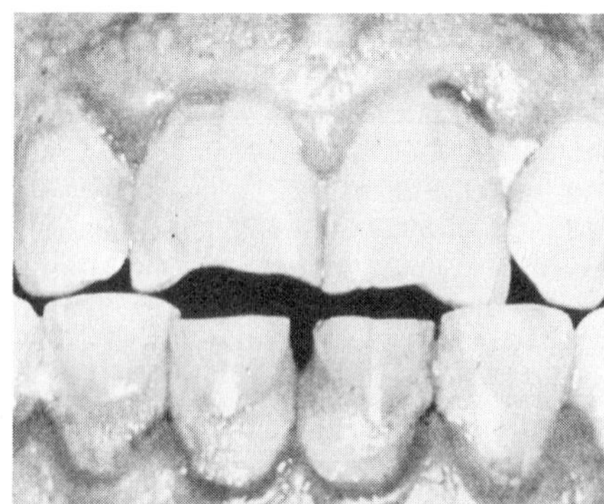

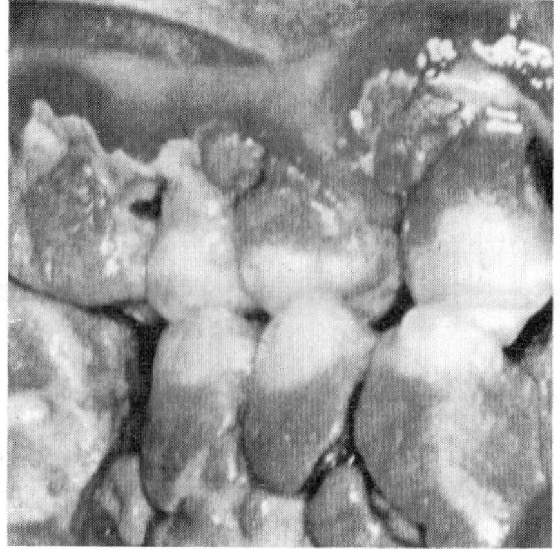

Fig. 29.20 Gingivitis and periodontitis

(a) Normal healthy gingivae. **(b)** Chronic gingivitis showing accumulated plaque and calculus around the gingival margins. At this stage, there has been no alveolar bone destruction and the inflammatory process is potentially reversible. **(c)** Gross chronic periodontitis with enormous accumulation of bacterial plaque and calculus, gross periodontal inflammation and loss of gingiva and supporting bone. These teeth were all loose and had to be extracted

As seen in Figure 29.20, gingivitis causes eversion of the gingival margin. This encourages more bacterial plaque and calculus to form in the gingival crevice and also results in greater gingival trauma from food. These both lead to more extensive gingival inflammation.

If untreated, inflammation gradually extends to involve the deeper supporting tissues. This causes progressive resorption of alveolar bone and destruction of the periodontal membrane, known as *periodontitis*. By this stage, the gingiva is thickened and inflamed with a purulent discharge from the gums. This explains the old term 'pyorrhoea'. Despite this, the patient is remarkably pain free, although halitosis is obvious to others!

As periodontal inflammation progresses, more alveolar bone is destroyed and the gums recede. The root surface becomes exposed to view, giving rise to the expression 'long in the tooth', once thought to be inevitable with advancing age. Teeth become increasingly mobile until they fall out or can be extracted with the fingers!

An acute *periodontal abscess* may develop at some point in the process. On the whole, however, periodontal disease is an insidious process from early adulthood, but it is almost entirely preventable. In adults, periodontitis (not dental decay, as is commonly supposed) is responsible for most lost teeth. The destruction of alveolar bone makes it difficult to construct satisfactory dentures for many of these patients, for lack of a retaining alveolar ridge.

Management of gingivitis and periodontitis

Gingivitis and periodontitis is almost entirely preventable by thorough and regular tooth brushing and use of dental floss, plus periodic dental scaling to remove inaccessible plaque and calculus.

Initial dental scaling, and careful oral hygiene instruction and supervision will cure gingivitis, which is a reversible condition. During the early stages of improved oral hygiene, bleeding will increase through brushing inflamed tissues. This soon subsides unless further periodontal treatment is needed.

Periodontitis also requires meticulous oral hygiene once the teeth have been thoroughly cleaned of plaque and calculus. Lost bone is never replaced, however, and the gingival contour remains abnormal, making effective oral hygiene difficult. Surgical recontouring of the gingiva and underlying bone (*gingivoplasty*) may sometimes be appropriate. It must be emphasised that antibiotics play no part in the treatment of chronic gingivitis and periodontitis. Antibiotics may, however, be useful for acute gingival conditions such as pericoronitis and Vincent's infection, described below.

Pericoronitis

This condition occurs when a lower third molar (wisdom tooth) is impacted against the second molar or the ramus of the mandible, so that its normal eruption into the mouth is prevented (see Figure 29.21). A flap of gingival tissue partly overlies the impacted tooth, creating a space around the buried tooth crown. Food and bacterial plaque collect here and lead to acute infection, which may extend into surrounding tissues, and even into the parapharyngeal area.

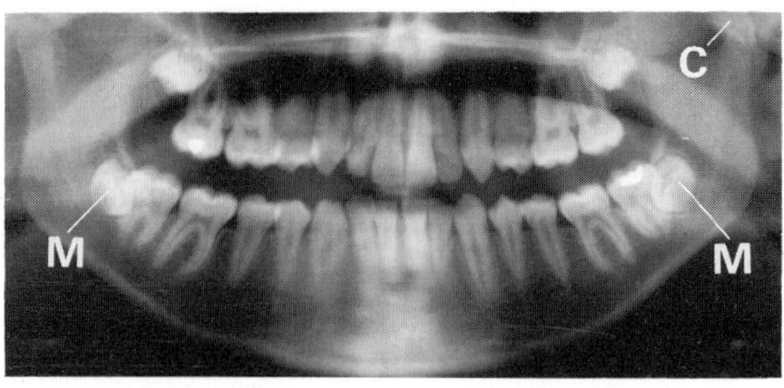

Fig. 29.21 Impacted lower third molars and pericoronitis

This OPG from a 16-year-old girl shows the whole lower jaw 'opened out'. Both lower third molars **M** are seen to be angled towards the second molars and impacted against them. The roots are not fully formed and there is little chance of these teeth erupting normally. These were an incidental finding, the X-rays having been taken to demonstrate a fracture of the left mandibular condyle **C**

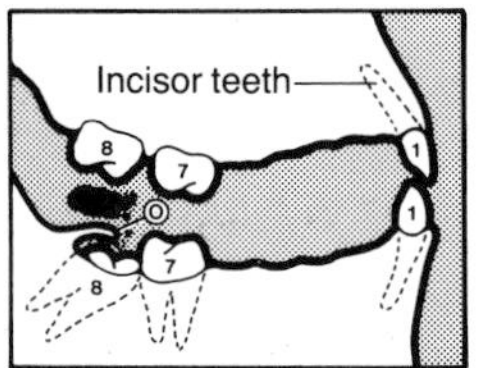

Lower wisdom tooth (8) unable to erupt because of inadequate length of alveolus
Example shown is the common variety, which tilts forwards (mesio-angular)
There is a flap of gum, or operculum (O) over the crown and the upper wisdom forces food under it leading to inflammation. 'First aid' treatment is to remove the upper 8.

The patient complains of severe, poorly localised pain near the angle of the mandible. Pain is aggravated by closing the jaw because the opposing tooth bites on the swollen gingival flap. On examination, the pericoronal tissues of the affected tooth are red and swollen with a purulent discharge exuding from beneath the gingival flap. Oral examination may be difficult because of trismus. Externally, the submandibular lymph nodes are enlarged and tender.

Management of pericoronitis

Pericoronitis is a cellulitis with incipient abscess formation. It is caused by a mixture of organisms which are usually sensitive to penicillin. It is treated locally by irrigating beneath the flap with hydrogen peroxide and the patient is advised to rinse the mouth several times daily with warm salty water. Rapid relief can be obtained by removing the upper wisdom tooth which impinges on the flap over the lower wisdom tooth. Oral penicillin is required if the patient is systemically unwell. Once the acute infection is over, the lower wisdom tooth should be removed surgically, especially if attacks are recurrent.

Acute ulcerative gingivitis (Vincent's infection)

This is an acute inflammatory condition with necrotising ulceration of the gingival margin. It is caused by a mixture of gram negative organisms, which are normal oral commensals. The most prominent bacteria are *Fuso-bacterium fusiformis, Borrelia vincenti* and *Bacteroides melaninogenicus*. Acute ulcerative gingivitis most commonly occurs in young adults who 'burn the candle at both ends' and become generally run down. Poor oral hygiene, pericoronitis and smoking may contribute. Acute ulcerative gingivitis is now uncommon, but was widespread among soldiers in the First World War when it gained the name 'trench mouth'.

There is an abrupt onset of gingival pain and bleeding, accompanied by a foul, often metallic taste, and marked halitosis. Cervical lymph nodes are enlarged and tender, and there may be fever, malaise and anorexia. Oral examination reveals characteristic ragged, punched-out ulceration of the gingival margin, especially between the teeth (see Figure 29.22). Ulceration elsewhere in the mouth is rare, except in severe cases where the pharyngeal mucosa becomes inflamed and ulcerated (*Vincent's angina*). Acute ulcerative gingivitis is easily distinguished from *herpetic gingivostomatitis*, the other acute ulcerative condition with systemic symptoms, being confined to the gingival margin, whereas herpetic ulcers are scattered all over the oral mucosa.

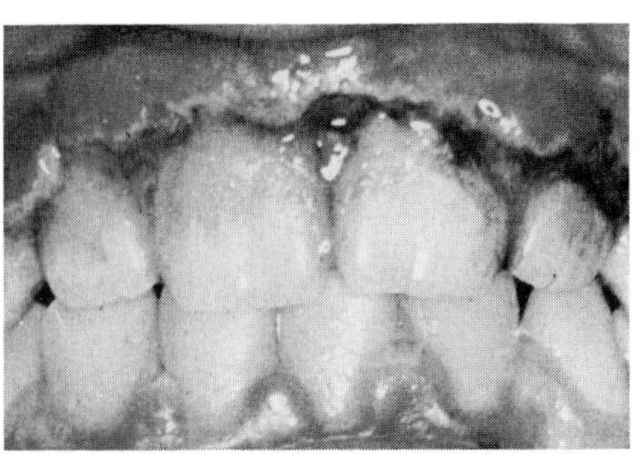

Fig. 29.22 Acute ulcerative gingivitis

This shows the typical appearance of acute ulcerative gingivitis ('Vincent's infection'); there is ulceration of the whole gingival margin with destruction of the interdental papillae, giving a ragged but almost straight gum margin (compare this with Figure 29.20b)

Management of acute (necrotising) ulcerative gingivitis

Vincent's infection rapidly responds to metronidazole tablets, usually with full recovery of gingival morphology; penicillin is also effective. Tooth brushing is extremely painful during an attack and the mouth should be frequently rinsed with warm water or weak hydrogen peroxide to keep it clean. Afterwards, careful attention to oral hygiene will usually prevent recurrence.

Epulis

An epulis is a benign, localised gingival swelling. Two types are recognised, fibrous epulis and giant cell epulis.

The *fibrous epulis* is simply a benign fibrous tissue tumour arising from the periodontal membrane or nearby periosteum. It forms a smooth, firm, slowly-growing lump, covered with normal gingiva. A fibrous epulis usually emerges between two teeth, which may be slightly pushed apart by pressure. Treatment is by local excision with curettage of the origin. Otherwise, the lesion may recur.

The *giant cell epulis* arises in a similar location but grows much faster. It forms an irregular red fleshy mass which ulcerates and bleeds. The lesion consists of numerous giant cells in a highly vascular stroma, which may invade local bone. Treatment involves extracting associated teeth and excising and curetting bone. This is the only way to avoid recurrence.

Pyogenic granulomas may occur on the gums or oral mucosa of the lips. They have a similar appearance to pyogenic granulomas of the skin (see Chapter 28).

TUMOURS OF THE ORAL MUCOSA

Pathophysiology and aetiology

The whole oral cavity, including the tongue, is invested by stratified squamous epithelium. Squamous cell carcinomas of the mouth account for about 3% of all malignancies. Like their counterparts on the skin, squamous carcinomas in the mouth usually occur in older patients. Men are affected twice as often as women.

Smoking is the usual cause in developed countries. Pipe and cigar smokers appear to be at greatest risk. The tongue and lower lip are the common sites of oral cancer, each accounting for about 25% of cases. Chronic irritation by

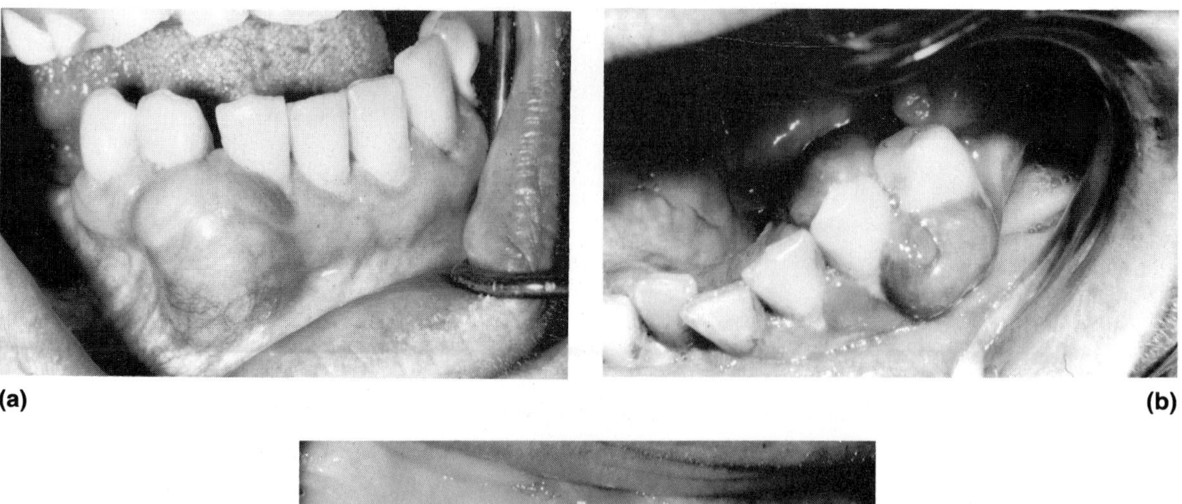

(a) (b)

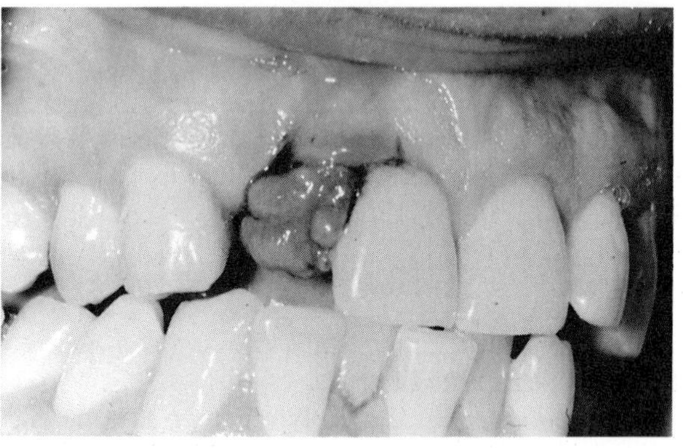

(c)

Fig. 29.23 Fibrous epulis, giant cell epulis and pyogenic granuloma of the gingiva
(a) Fibrous epulis and **(b)** giant cell epulis, both in typical interdental location. The fibrous epulis is the same colour as the gum, whilst the giant cell epulis is deeper red. **(c)** Pyogenic granuloma arising from the gum margin following extraction of an upper lateral incisor

ill-fitting dentures, jagged tooth restorations or alcohol abuse may contribute to the aetiology.

In India and Papua-New Guinea, the habit of chewing a small package of betel leaf, tobacco and lime, causes a very high incidence of carcinoma of the buccal mucosa.

Leukoplakia is a pre-malignant dysplastic condition found in 50% of patients with oral carcinoma.

Clinical features of oral cancer

Oral cancer usually presents as a chronic indurated ulcer, which slowly enlarges and fails to heal. Early lesions may present as a non-ulcerated mucosal swelling. Lesions are usually painless, unless they become secondarily infected, although advanced lesions may cause pain as they invade deeply. Carcinoma of the tongue, for example, may cause pain referred to the ear or pharynx.

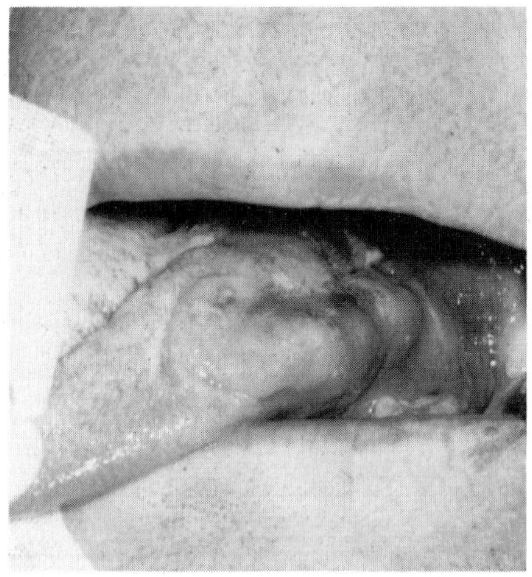

Fig. 29.24 Carcinoma of the tongue

Large ulcerating squamous cell carcinoma of tongue. By the time of presentation, cervical lymph nodes were already involved. This patient smoked 40 cigarettes per day

Oral squamous carcinomas are generally well differentiated. They invade locally but only metastasise to submandibular and cervical lymph nodes at a late stage. Spreading tumours of the posterior floor of mouth and tongue inhibit speech, mastication and swallowing. These are particularly distressing symptoms.

Management of oral cancer

A chronic oral ulcer which fails to heal after possible aggravating factors such as ill-fitting dentures have been removed, should undergo incision biopsy to exclude cancer.

Oral cancers are excised with a margin of normal tissue. This may not be possible anatomically or cosmetically, and often necessitates a major plastic surgical operation. Involved regional lymph nodes are removed by block dissection.

If excision is impractical, most of these tumours respond to radiotherapy. This may employ external beam treatment or radioactive implants. A disadvantage of radiotherapy, however, is that it damages salivary glands resulting in xerostomia (dry mouth). Apart from the discomfort, this predisposes to salivary gland infection.

Carcinoma of the lip has the best prognosis. The 5-year survival rate is over 60%, but for tumours of the tongue and floor of the mouth, this falls to only about 25%.

Leukoplakia

Leukoplakia means 'white plaque', and the term is used to describe white patches on the oral mucosa which cannot readily be scraped off. This distinguishes them from candidal infections. White plaques may be caused by oral lichen planus or lupus erythematosus, but the main importance of leukoplakia is that it may represent epithelial dysplasia or even carcinoma-in-situ.

The cheeks and tongue are most often affected, although dysplastic patches may develop anywhere in the oral mucosa. An innocent white line is often seen along the inside of the cheek; this corresponds to the line of biting surfaces of the teeth, and is caused by frictional hyperplasia.

Severe or extensive leukoplakia should be referred for specialist oral surgical opinion and biopsy. Areas of severe dysplasia require surgical removal, which may necessitate grafting.

MISCELLANEOUS DISORDERS CAUSING INTRAORAL SWELLING

RETENTION CYSTS OF THE ACCESSORY SALIVARY GLANDS

The oral mucosa contains numerous accessory mucous and serous salivary glands. Small retention cysts probably develop as a result of minor trauma to the duct. Most retention cysts are smaller than one centimetre in diameter. They commonly occur in the lower lip mucosa where they cause annoyance and are readily traumatised during speech or chewing. Retention cysts are blue-grey and are extremely soft to palpation. They often rupture spontaneously but usually reform. Small retention cysts can usually be completely enucleated under local anaesthesia; larger ones may need marsupialisation.

TUMOURS OF ACCESSORY SALIVARY GLANDS

Tumours occasionally arise in the accessory salivary glands. These are often malignant *adenocystic carcinomas*. They present as small, firm lumps in the oral mucosa or posterior palate, and are often noticed before invading deeply or metastasising. Treatment is by wide excision.

BONY EXOSTOSES

Local outgrowths of the jaw bones are common and may produce an intraoral lump. To the uninitiated doctor, this may be suspicious of neoplasia. The most common site is the centre of the hard palate, where it is known as a *torus palatinus*. A similar exostosis, usually bilateral, occurs inside the mandible, opposite the premolar teeth (*torus mandibularis*).

These lesions are extremely hard and covered by normal oral mucosa. Excision is rarely needed unless there are problems in wearing a removable denture.

CYSTS AND TUMOURS OF THE JAWS

Various cystic lesions and tumours arise in the jaws. Many are abnormalities of tooth-forming epithelium, either developmental or acquired. Most are rare and can usually be diagnosed radiologically. The jaws are occasionally the site of benign or malignant bone tumours, as found elsewhere. Examples are osteosarcomas and osteoclastomas.

Growth disorders of bone such as fibrous dysplasia and Paget's disease of bone may also affect the jaw.

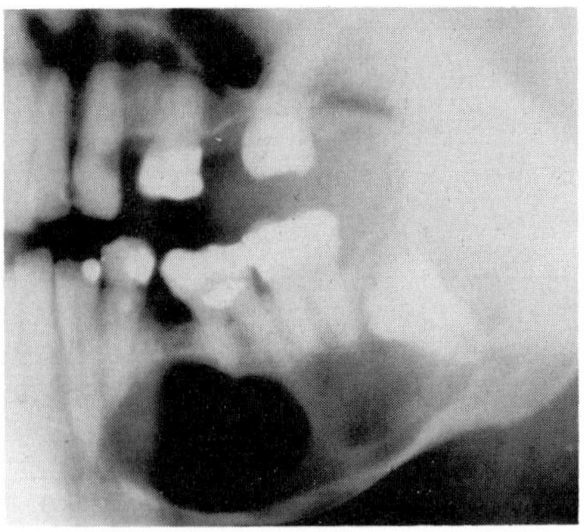

(a)

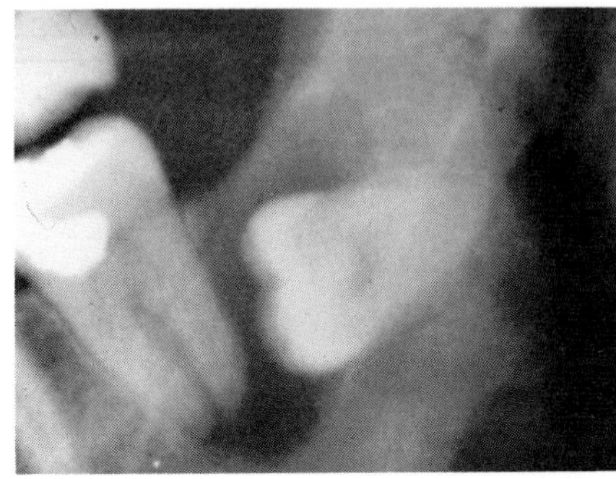

(b)

Fig. 29.25 Dental cyst and dentigerous cyst

(a) Large dental cyst in the mandible. This arose from tooth-forming epithelial remnants in the apical area of the lower left first molar tooth which was extracted several months beforehand due to chronic periapical infection.
(b) Dentigerous cyst associated with the crown of an unerupted lower third molar. These cysts originate from epithelial remnants of the tooth bud

30 DISORDERS OF THE THYROID AND PARATHYROID GLANDS

Introduction

Patients with disorders of the thyroid gland usually present to the surgeon in one of two ways, a mass in the neck or hyperthyroidism. In the first group with a thyroid mass, malignancy may be suspected or the mass may be causing cosmetic deformity or pressure symptoms. There may be a discrete thyroid lump or the whole gland may be enlarged (goitre). In most cases, the patient is clinically euthyroid (i.e. with normal thyroid activity) and biochemical tests of thyroid function are normal. In contrast, the second group of patients have usually been investigated and found to be hyperthyroid. They are then referred for thyroidectomy after unsatisfactory 'medical' treatment.

Parathyroid disorders usually reach the surgeon because of hypercalcaemia from excess parathormone secretion. This can only be successfully treated by surgical removal of the cause, which is usually parathyroid hyperplasia or adenoma, or very rarely, carcinoma.

DISORDERS OF THE THYROID

Diseases of the thyroid can be divided into four broad pathological categories:

- Developmental abnormalities
- Inflammatory and autoimmune disorders
- Hyperplastic and metabolic disorders
- Neoplasms

The main pathophysiological and clinical features are summarised in Figure 30.1.

Main clinical presentations of thyroid disease in surgical practice

a. Diffuse or generalised enlargement of the thyroid

The term *goitre* is often used to describe any generalised enlargement of the thyroid but it is imprecise descriptively and pathologically. Most generalised large thyroid swellings seen in developed countries are due to simple, non-toxic *colloid goitre* i.e. idiopathic diffuse hyperplasia or multinodular hyperplasia.

Where the condition is *endemic* (isolated, mountainous and underdeveloped regions such as Nepal), iodine deficiency is the usual cause. These goitres are often a symmetrical and soft to palpation. They are composed of many large hyperplastic nodules and can reach enormous sizes (see Figure 30.2). Although

Fig. 30.1 Diseases of the thyroid

CONDITION *(relative frequency in developed countries)*	**PATHOPHYSIOLOGY**	**CLINICAL FEATURES**
1. Developmental abnormalities		
a. Thyroglossal cyst *(uncommon)*	Cyst formation anywhere along the midline thyroglossal tract. This marks the line of embryological descent of the thyroid from the foramen caecum, via the hyoid bone, to the normal position in the neck.	Smooth, rounded swelling in midline of neck anywhere between the submental area and isthmus of thyroid. Usually found in children
b. Thyroglossal fistula *(rare)*	Incision into or incomplete removal of a thyroglossal cyst can cause a fistula	Fistulous opening near midline of neck. Becomes intermittently infected and discharges clear fluid or pus
c. Ectopic thyroid *(rare)*	Part or all of the thyroid lying anywhere along the thyroglossal tract	Usually symptomless but may present as an unusual swelling near foramen caecum at junction of anterior two–thirds and posterior third of tongue.
2. Inflammatory and autoimmune disorders		
a. Hashimoto's thyroiditis *(common)*	Diffuse lymphocytic infiltration of thyroid gland with progressive destruction of thyroid follicles. Over a period of years, leads to progressive atrophy and fibrosis. Various anti-thyroid antibodies usually present in serum in high titres. Polygenic inherited disorder which may be associated with other autoimmune disorders, e.g pernicious anaemia. Focal lymphocytic thyroiditis is probably a less severe variant of the same condition	Presents in adulthood with mild, diffuse, sometimes tender thyroid enlargement. Often the thyroid is not enlarged. Patient usually euthyroid at outset (sometimes mildly hyperthyroid) but later becomes insidiously hypothyroid. Affects females much more frequently
b. Graves' disease *(fairly common)*	Diffuse thyroid hyperplasia due to the action of a circulating immunoglobulin 'long acting thyroid stimulator' (LATS). This binds to thyroid acinar cells mimicking the effects of TSH and producing excess thyroid hormone	Diffuse thyroid enlargement, sometimes with bruit, but main feature is marked hyperthyroidism (thyrotoxicosis) causing weight loss, heat intolerance, tachycardia, hyperreflexia, tremor and sometimes exophthalmos

CONDITION	PATHOPHYSIOLOGY	CLINICAL FEATURES
c. De Quervain's acute thyroiditis *(uncommon)*	Diffuse inflammation of thyroid gland, probably viral in origin. Neutrophilic and later lymphocytic and histiocytic infiltration of gland occurs	Very tender, diffuse moderate thyroid enlargement, with or without systemic symptoms. Episodes last weeks to months and are often recurrent. Patient usually euthyroid but may be hyperthyroid in acute phase
d. Riedl's thyroiditis *(very rare)*	Dense fibrosis of thyroid gland. Possibly an autoimmune process	Extremely hard ('woody goitre') often asymmetrical thyroid mass suspicious of tumour. Sometimes produces symptoms from compression
3. Hyperplastic and metabolic disorders		
a. Simple non-toxic colloid goitre *(very common)*	Benign, diffuse or multi-nodular hyperplasia of thyroid follicles. Cause unknown but possibly minor abnormality of thyroid hormone synthesis	Diffuse or sporadic multinodular thyroid enlargement or single 'adenomatous' nodule or cyst. Patient clinically euthyroid and all thyroid function tests normal. Affects females much more than males
b. Endemic goitre *(very rare)*	Diffuse hyperplasia of thyroid follicles due to dietary iodine deficiency, or goitrogenic foods. Endemic in inland, underdeveloped countries, especially in mountainous areas.	Diffuse, often massive thyroid enlargement which may later become nodular. T4 is low or normal and TSH tends to be elevated
c. Drug induced goitre *(uncommon)*	Diffuse thyroid hyperplasia secondary to interference with thyroid hormone synthesis. Drugs causing this are antithyroid drugs used in therapy (e.g. carbimazole) or others like lithium and aminoglutethimide	Diffuse thyroid enlargement. Patient usually euthyroid. Can be prevented by using replacement dose of T4 concurrently with blocking drugs
d. Dyshormonogenesis *(very uncommon)*	Diffuse thyroid hyperplasia caused by a variety of uncommon genetic (recessive) defects affecting thyroid hormone synthesis	Presents at birth or in childhood with thyroid enlargement and severe hypothyroidism (cretinism). In developed countries, these defects are usually diagnosed at birth by neonatal screening tests before any goitre has developed
e. Physiological *(common)*	Diffuse thyroid hyperplasia often associated with pregnancy and puberty	Mild diffuse thyroid enlargement. Patient euthyroid

Fig. 30.1 (cont.)

CONDITION	PATHOPHYSIOLOGY	CLINICAL FEATURES
4. Neoplasms of the thyroid		
a. Thyroid adeno-carcinomas		
i) Papillary carcinoma *(relatively common)*	Papillary adenocarcinoma forms a complex branching structure with a fibrous stroma (papillary pattern). Variable degree of dysplasia. Commonly metastasises to cervical nodes but distant metastases rare	Slowly–growing firm thyroid lump or cervical lymph nodes or both. Occurs in adults and sometimes children. Excellent prognosis
ii) Follicular carcinoma *(relatively uncommon)*	Tumour forms a well-developed follicular pattern reminiscent of normal thyroid. Generally well differentiated but if metastasis occurs, it is usually distant, e.g. lungs and bone.	Similar presentation to follicular carcinoma but does not involve cervical nodes. Affects slightly older age group than papillary carcinoma
iii) Anaplastic carcinoma *(relatively uncommon)*	Aggressive tumour rapidly spreading beyond the confines of the gland	Diffuse, hard thyroid enlargement, often with symptoms of recurrent laryngeal or tracheal involvement. Affects elderly patients. Very poor prognosis
b. Medullary carcinoma of thyroid *(very uncommon)*	Well differentiated tumour derived from calcitonin secreting cells. Tumour contains extensive deposits of amyloid	Stony hard thyroid lump, possibly with secondaries in cervical nodes
c. Thyroid lymphoma *(rare)*	Diffuse lymphoid infiltration of thyroid gland	Diffuse thyroid enlargement. Patient euthyroid

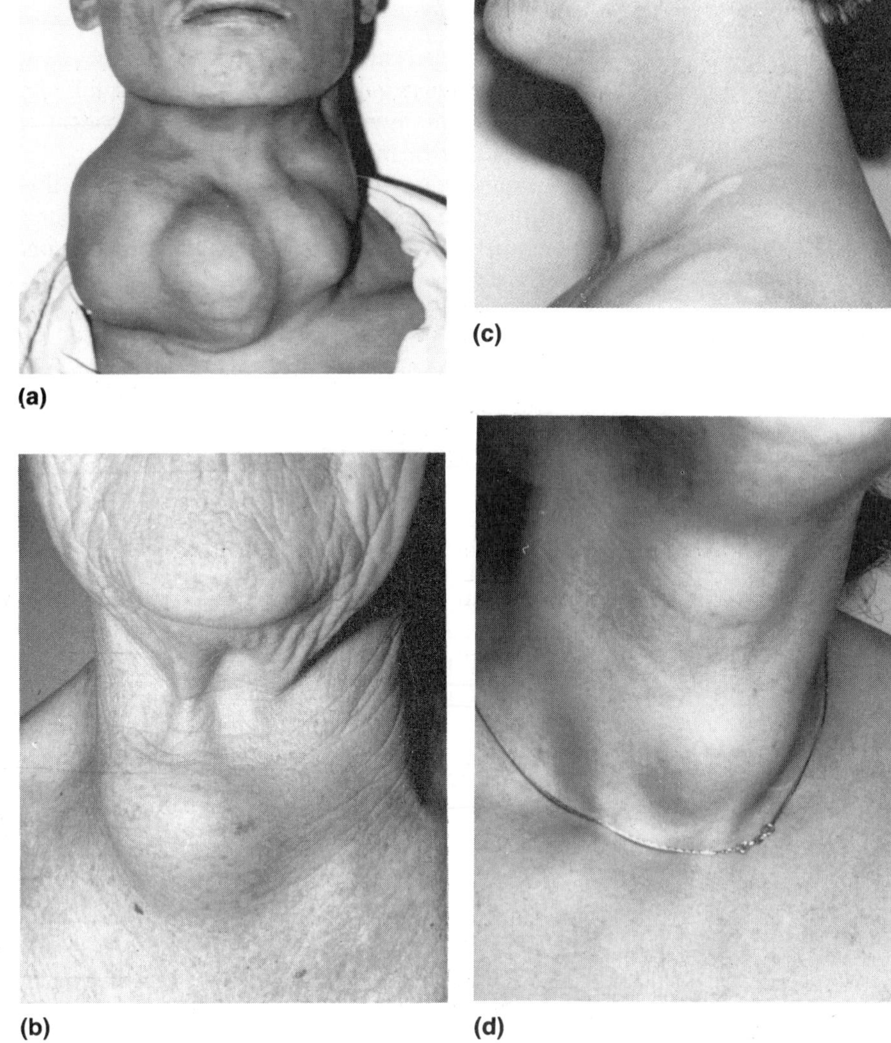

Fig. 30.2 Examples of thyroid swellings

(a) Endemic goitre. This condition, caused by iodine deficiency, is extremely common in isolated mountain regions. The thyroid can reach an enormous size, yet the patient suffers only minimal symptoms and is usually euthyroid. This typical example in a Nepalese man is only of moderate size by local standards! **(b)** Anaplastic carcinoma. Rapidly enlarging hard thyroid mass in an elderly woman; the mass was firmly tethered to strap muscles and deeper structures. **(c)** Graves' disease. Moderate diffuse enlargement of the whole thyroid in a thyrotoxic woman of 35. Note the area of depigmentation (vitilligo) which occasionally accompanies autoimmune thyroid disorders. This was treated by subtotal thyroidectomy after failure of medical treatment. **(d)** Solitary thyroid nodule. This asymptomatic nodule had been present for several years. It proved histologically to be a thyroid adenoma

unsightly, endemic goitres cause suprisingly few symptoms and the patient is usually euthyroid.

Anaplastic carcinomas may also cause large thyroid swellings in elderly patients (see Figure 30.2). There are usually symptoms of invasion into nearby structures. These include hoarseness, if there is recurrent laryngeal nerve involvement, and stridor if there is tracheal displacement or compression. The gland is hard on palpation. The uncommon *lymphomas* of the thyroid also present with diffuse thyroid enlargement.

In *Graves' disease*, there is usually a degree of smooth thyroid enlargement (see Figure 30.2), often increased by drug treatment. This is almost never the main presenting feature, however. Similarly, in *Hashimoto's* thyroiditis, the thyroid may be modestly enlarged but firmer and finely nodular on palpation.

b. 'Solitary' thyroid nodule

A common presentation of thyroid disease is a *solitary thyroid nodule*, an apparently isolated lump within the thyroid. These lumps are not usually obvious and are found incidentally by the patient or his doctor. They may first be noticed when the patient swallows.

A true solitary nodule may be a malignant thyroid tumour and this diagnosis must be excluded. Alternatively, an isolated lesion may be a nodule of idiopathic hyperplasia or a thyroid cyst. Both conditions fall within the spectrum of the pathological entity 'simple colloid goitre'. Hyperplastic nodules may be so discrete as to be described as *thyroid adenomas*.

An apparent solitary nodule may prove to be a focal accentuation of a generalised thyroid enlargement such as simple multinodular hyperplasia (colloid goitre), and less often, Hashimoto's thyroiditis.

c. Other features associated with thyroid enlargement

A new area of enlargement in a goitre may be due to haemorrhage into a cyst, an enlarging hyperplastic nodule or a carcinoma. If the thyroid grows behind the sternum into the anterior mediastinum, the trachea may be compressed or displaced and cause stridor. Stridor may only become obvious when the neck is in certain positions. Hoarseness or stridor may also result from invasion by an anaplastic carcinoma.

Pain and tenderness are uncommon presenting features in thyroid disease, but characterise the rare de Quervain's thyroiditis. Sometimes, in Hashimoto's thyroiditis, the thyroid is painful and tender.

d. Hyperthyroidism

The clinical manifestations of hyperthyroidism are summarised in Figure 30.3. Excessive thyroid hormone production is a feature of Graves' disease, when it is often desribed as *thyrotoxicosis*. Hyperthyroidism also occurs in the early stages of Hashimoto's thyroiditis. A solitary hyperplastic (adenomatous) nodule may produce so much thyroid hormone that it causes hyperthyroidism. This is known as a *toxic nodule*.

In general, thyroid adenocarcinomas are non-secreting but occasionally, a well differentiated carcinoma may cause thyrotoxicosis.

Fig. 30.3 Clinical manifestations of thyrotoxicosis

Metabolic — heat intolerance, increased appetite with weight loss, diarrhoea, menorrhagia

Cardiovascular — palpitations, tachycardia even while asleep, atrial fibrillation

Neuropsychiatric — hyperkinesis, insomnia, emotional instability, tremor, proximal myopathy

Ocular — exophthalmos including proptosis, lid retraction and eventually ophthalmoplegia

Cutaneous — pretibial myxoedema

e. Hypothyroidism

Hypothyroidism is usually the result of either late Hashimoto's thyroiditis or primary thyroid atrophy. In either case, the gland is small and fibrous and as such does not present to the surgeon. Hypothyroidism is a late complication in up to 25% of patients after subtotal thyroidectomy for thyrotoxicosis, and is inevitable after total thyroidectomy for carcinoma.

Special points in examining a thyroid swelling

Examining for a suspected thyroid swelling should begin with observing the front of the neck while the patient swallows. The characteristic rise and fall of the lump results from the thyroid gland's investment of pretracheal fascia which is attached to the larynx above. The normal thyroid is not visible, even on swallowing, and not normally palpable.

The thyroid area is next palpated from behind with the patient seated. This position is best for examining the size, shape and consistency of the gland. It also allows the lower edge of the swelling to be palpated to identify any retrosternal extension. The lobes of the thyroid lie deep to the sternomastoids and the strap muscles, and these tend to conceal thyroid enlargement and make it difficult to examine the whole gland.

The jugular chain of lymph nodes should be palpated for evidence of lymph node metastases, since this may be the sole presenting feature of papillary carcinoma. In thyrotoxicosis, auscultation of the thyroid may reveal a bruit because of the increased vascularity.

If there is suspicion of recurrent laryngeal nerve palsy because of hoarseness, tests of vocal cord function should be performed. The patient is asked to cough and to pronounce the sound 'ee', both of which will be abnormal if there is nerve damage.

General examination should look for signs of hyperthyroidism (tachycardia, atrial fibrillation, fine tremor and hypereflexia) and for signs specific to Graves' disease (exophthalmos and ophthalmoplegia).

Approach to investigation of a thyroid mass

The questions to be answered in investigating a thyroid mass are summarised in Figure 30.4 and described in detail below.

Fig. 30.4 Principles of investigation of a thyroid mass

General thyroid status — thyroid function tests and thyroid autoantibodies

Morphology of the gland, i.e. size, shape and physical consistency, effects upon surrounding structures — ultrasound, plain X-rays of thoracic outlet

Functional activity of glandular tissue — radioiodine tests of uptake and distribution

Tissue diagnosis — fine needle aspiration cytology, incision or excision biopsy

a. General thyroid status

First, it must be established whether the patient is *euthyroid*, *hyperthyroid* or *hypothyroid*. Serum thyroxine (T4) estimation is performed in all cases. Interpretation may be difficult during pregnancy and puberty because of elevated thyroid binding globulin, in which case free thyroxine, or free thyroxine index, is estimated. *Tri-iodothyronine* (T3) levels are occasionally measured if the patient is clinically hyperthyroid but serum thyroxine is normal. *Thyroid stimulating hormone* (TSH) is usually elevated in hypothyroidism, and should be measured if this is suspected.

Thyroid autoantibodies are assayed if autoimmune disease is a possibility. The presence of long acting thyroid stimulating factor (LATS) is diagnostic of Graves' disease. Hashimoto's thyroiditis is characterised by elevation of other thyroid antibodies such as anti-thyroglobulin or anti-mitochondrial antibodies.

b. Morphology of the gland

Ultrasound provides a simple, accurate and non-invasive method of establishing the size and shape of the gland. It can also determine whether there is displacement or compression of the trachea. Variation in tissue density such as cysts, localised areas of nodularity or invasion by anaplastic carcinoma are also demonstrated. Plain X-rays of the thoracic outlet are taken if there is suspicion of tracheal displacement or compression.

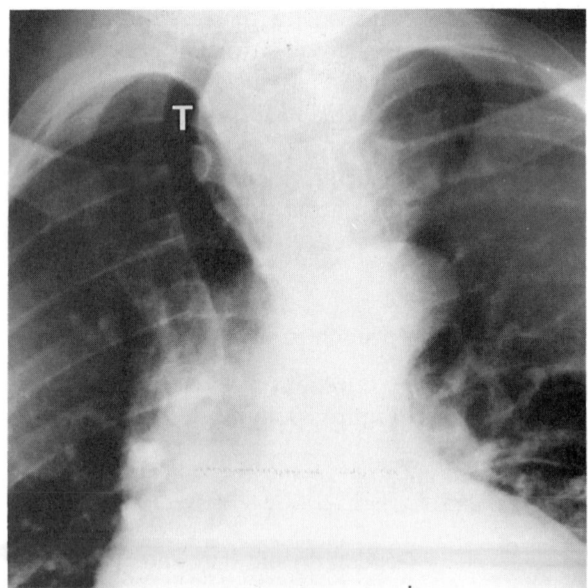

Fig. 30.5 Tracheal displacement by a goitre

This chest X-ray shows gross displacement of the trachea **T** to the right by a large retrosternal goitre. The patient presented with nocturnal stridor when she lay on her left side

c. Functional activity of glandular tissue

Injected radioactive isotopes of iodine are taken up by thyroid tissue in proportion to the rate of hormone synthesis. The gland is scanned after isotope

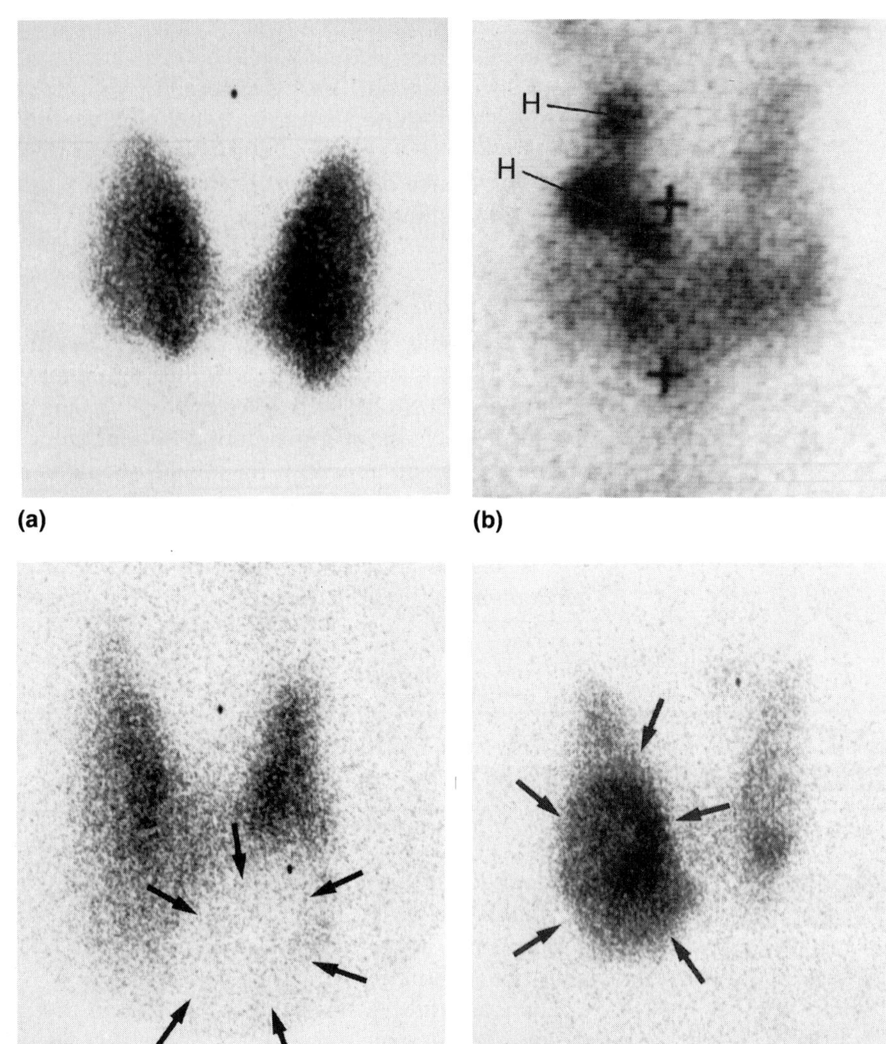

Fig. 30.6 Radioisotope thyroid scans

(a) This enlarged thyroid shows homogeneous tracer uptake typical of a simple colloid goitre.
(b) Heterogenous tracer uptake in a multinodular colloid goitre. The dark areas **H** are 'hot nodules'; to maintain the euthyroid state, the rest of the gland exhibits diminished uptake. The + signs indicate the positions of the thyroid cartilage and the suprasternal notch.
(c) Solitary 'cold' thyroid nodule. The area of low uptake (outline arrowed) at the lower left pole of the thyroid corresponds with a palpable nodule. In the case of a solid lesion (as confirmed by ultrasound) a cold nodule may indicate malignancy.
(d) Solitary 'hot' thyroid nodule. The area of high uptake (outline arrowed) in the lower part of the right lobe corresponds to a palpable mass. This patient was hyperthyroid and the lesion could be described as a 'toxic nodule'. Activity of the rest of the gland is suppressed by pituitary-mediated negative feedback from the high serum thyroxine level

injection to identify the distribution of isotope activity. This may fall into one of four patterns:

- *Diffuse, homogeneous uptake* — this is found in the normal gland or where there is diffuse hyperactivity, e.g. Graves' disease
- *Generalised but patchy uptake* — this occurs in multinodular goitre where the hyperplastic nodules are less active than the surrounding normal tissue
- *The cold nodule* — an isolated area devoid of isotope uptake indicates non-secreting tissue, i.e. tumour, inactive adenomatous nodule or cyst
- *The hot nodule* — this represents an autonomous focus of excess T4 secretion. The secretory activity of the surrounding normal thyroid tissue is suppressed. The patient is usually euthyroid but sometimes thyrotoxic ('toxic nodule')

An area where uptake is absent (or 'cold') is suspicious of carcinoma, especially if it is well demarcated, and solid on ultrasound examination. In this case, tissue diagnosis is essential. Very occasionally, thyroid malignancies secrete thyroid hormone and show as warm or hot nodules on isotope scanning. Isotope scanning can also identify and localise ectopic thyroid tissue (in the tongue or along the course of the thyroglossal duct) as well as retrosternal extension of a thyroid swelling.

d. Tissue diagnosis

Tissue diagnosis is usually only required for cold nodules. Fine needle aspiration cytology is used by some surgeons, but remains controversial; it is difficult to distinguish between well-differentiated tumours and benign lesions, and there is a theoretical risk of implantating tumour along the needle track.

The traditional approach for a cold nodule is complete excision by lobectomy. If papillary carcinoma is suspected, frozen section histology may be undertaken at the same time, because the treatment of choice for this condition is total thyroidectomy. Incision biopsy is occasionally used for diagnosing generalised thyroid enlargement where the chances of malignancy are low.

SPECIFIC CLINICAL PROBLEMS OF THE THYROID AND THEIR MANAGEMENT

THYRO-TOXICOSIS

Thyrotoxicosis most commonly results from Graves' disease. Hashimoto's thyroiditis is a much rarer cause. Occasionally, thyrotoxicosis is caused by a multinodular goitre which has become 'toxic', or an autonomous adenomatous 'hot' nodule.

There are three main treatment options in thyrotoxicosis: antithyroid drugs, radioisotope destruction of functioning thyroid tissue and partial thyroidectomy.

Carcinoma, a very rare cause of thyrotoxicosis, is occasionally diagnosed unexpectedly when a hot nodule is examined histologically.

Antithyroid drugs

Most cases of thyrotoxicosis are initially managed with antithyroid drugs which block synthesis of thyroid hormone. *Carbimazole* is the most popular, and restores serum hormone levels to normal over 4–8 weeks. A lower maintenance dose is then prescribed for one to two years. After this, more than half the patients remain euthyroid without further treatment. The remainder relapse in the succeeding months, necessitating further courses of carbimazole or a different form of therapy. In some patients, stable control cannot be achieved, and hypothyroidism alternates with hyperthyroidism.

Carbimazole occasionally causes a potentially fatal but reversible neutropenia. The white blood count should therefore be monitored about every three months during treatment. A sore throat or other infection in a patient on carbimazole should alert the patient and the doctor. Rashes, nausea, headache and arthralgia are also common side-effects of carbimazole, and if they occur, an alternative antithyroid drug such as *propylthiouracil* may be substituted. Poor control, frequent relapse, side effects and non-compliance lead to eventual surgical referral in up to 40% of patients.

Beta adrenergic blocking drugs such as *propranolol* rapidly control the distressing and dangerous effects of thyrotoxicosis. They may be used initially in extremely toxic patients until antithyroid drugs take effect, or if a patient urgently needs to be stabilised before thyroidectomy.

Radioactive iodide therapy

Radioactive iodide (^{131}I or ^{125}I), administered orally in doses 100 times higher than used for diagnostic scanning, may be used to treat thyrotoxicosis. This is especially appropriate for middle aged or elderly patients. Iodide is avidly taken up by the gland, after which emission of radiation destroys the most active thyroid tissue. The treatment is simple but the results are slow to take effect and unpredictable. Often late hypothyroidism occurs, requiring replacement therapy. There is also a small theoretical risk of inducing malignancy, and so the treatment is not advisable in the young. Radioactive iodide therapy is absolutely contraindicated in pregnancy because of the risk of genetic damage to the fetus.

Surgical removal of hyperactive thyroid tissue

Surgery for thyrotoxicosis may be indicated as follows:

- When a quick and effective cure is desired which avoids long term drug therapy and its drawbacks. It is often the best treatment for Graves' disease, particularly in younger patients, where the disease is not expected to burn itself out for many years
- When antithyroid drugs have proved unsatisfactory and radioiodide treatment is unsuitable
- Surgery is usually the most appropriate treatment for toxic multinodular goitre. Response to drug treatment in this condition is unreliable and surgery also deals with the cosmetic deformity
- Toxic solitary nodules ('hot nodules') are best excised to allow the suppressed normal thyroid to recover

Preoperative assessment and management of thyrotoxicosis

For all thyroid operations, preoperative assessment must include indirect *laryngoscopy* to demonstrate vocal cord function. This evaluates recurrent laryngeal nerve function should there later be a question of operative damage. Even without demonstrable cord damage, there is often a subtle change in voice quality after thyroidectomy. Patients should be warned of this before operation, especially if they are singers or politicians!

Wherever possible, thyroid function should be brought into the normal range before operation. The thyrotoxic state carries significant anaesthetic risks, especially of cardiac arrhythmias. Furthermore, manipulation of the gland may provoke massive release of thyroid hormone precipitating a potentially lethal 'thyrotoxic crisis'. Control of thyroid function is usually achieved with antithyroid drugs in the weeks preceding operation. If this fails, or if operation is very urgent, then beta adrenergic blocking drugs such as propranolol are used.

Antithyroid drugs cause increased vascularity of the gland which may add to surgical difficulty in toxic enlargement. It was formerly standard practice to administer *Lugol's iodine* solution orally for two weeks before operation, at the same time discontinuing antithyroid therapy. It was believed that this reduced vascularity and made the operation easier. Some surgeons still use Lugol's iodine, although its efficacy is unproven.

Partial thyroidectomy

Surgery for hyperthyroidism aims to remove enough thyroid tissue to render the patient euthyroid whilst preserving enough of the gland to prevent hypothyroidism. For Graves' disease or toxic multinodular goitre, about 10 gm of the gland is left intact. The technique of *sub-total thyroidectomy* leaves the posterior rim of each lobe in situ, thus minimising the risk of parathyroid or recurrent laryngeal damage. A low transverse collar incision along a skin crease gives the best cosmetic result. Meticulous care is required in ligating the *inferior thyroid artery* (after the recurrent laryngeal nerve is identified) and the *upper pole vessels*. Primary or reactionary haemorrhage is a serious complication causing major blood loss and laryngeal compression. To avoid suffocation from a postoperative bleed, instruments for emergency reopening of the wound should be kept at the patient's bedside after operation. The complications of thyroidectomy are summarised in Figure 30.8.

THYROID MALIGNANCIES

Thyroid malignancies are uncommon, comprising less than 1% of all malignant tumours. Nearly all originate from thyroid follicular cells and these form three distinct pathological entities. These are *papillary*, *follicular* and *anaplastic carcinomas*. Each has a characteristic pattern of behaviour and prognosis. With rare exceptions, these tumours do not secrete thyroid hormones.

About 7% of thyroid carcinomas arise from APUD C-cells which normally secrete calcitonin. These tumours are known as *medullary carcinomas* of the thyroid. *Lymphomas* occasionally involve the thyroid gland, causing diffuse thyroid enlargement.

Exposure to ionising radiation during childhood predisposes to thyroid carcinoma. This includes radiotherapy (once popular for treating 'status thymolymphaticus') and radioactive fallout. Many people exposed at the Hiroshima and Nagasaki bombings and the Bikini atoll nuclear tests developed thyroid tumours. In most cases, however, no aetiological factor can be identified.

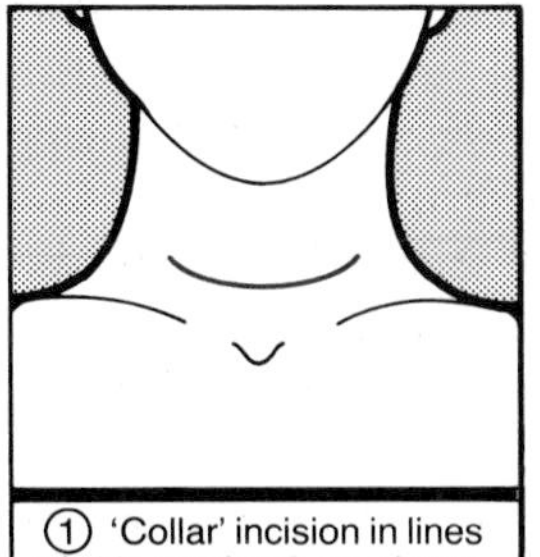

① 'Collar' incision in lines of skin tension 2 cm above suprasternal notch
Platysma divided in same line

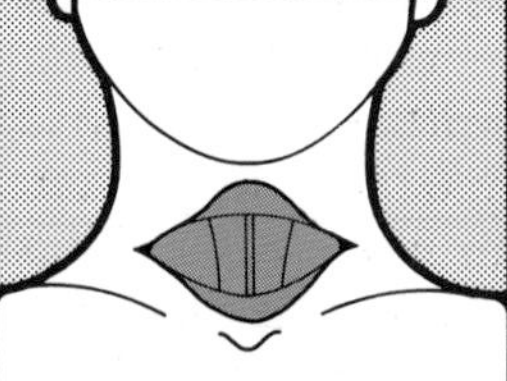

② Flaps mobilised *beneath* platysma down to suprasternal notch and up to thyroid cartilage

③ Incision made vertically in midline between strap muscles which are retracted laterally on side of interest (left side is shown here)

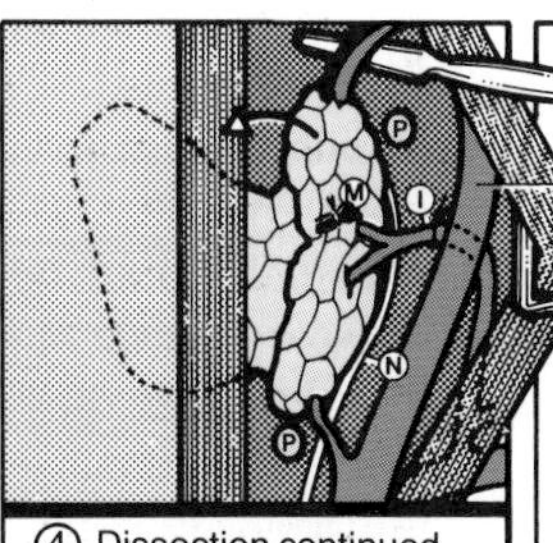

④ Dissection continued deep to strap muscles. Middle thyroid vein Ⓜ ligated and divided

⑤ Lateral lobe displaced anteriorly and inferior thyroid artery Ⓘ located and recurrent laryngeal nerve identified in groove between trachea and oesophagus Ⓝ. Inferior thyroid artery ligated lateral to nerve
Parathyroids identified Ⓟ

⑥ Upper pole vessels identified and ligated close to gland

⑦ Lower pole vessels ligated

⑧ a) *If partial thyroidectomy* approx 4 g gland left in situ and remainder dissected out, arresting bleeding from many small vessels entering gland from tracheal surface. Process repeated with other side

⑧ b) *If lobectomy or total thyroidectomy* whole lobe(s) excised, preserving recurrent laryngeal nerve and parathyroids

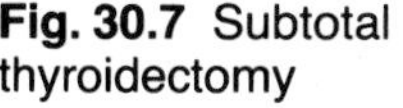

Fig. 30.7 Subtotal thyroidectomy

(a) This photograph shows the operation site after subtotal thyroidectomy for thyrotoxicosis. The collar incision is shown and the platysma muscle can be seen in the upper skin flap. A small thyroid remnant is sutured to the larynx and trachea on each side. A suction drainage tube has been placed in the wound.
(b) The resected specimen of thyroid

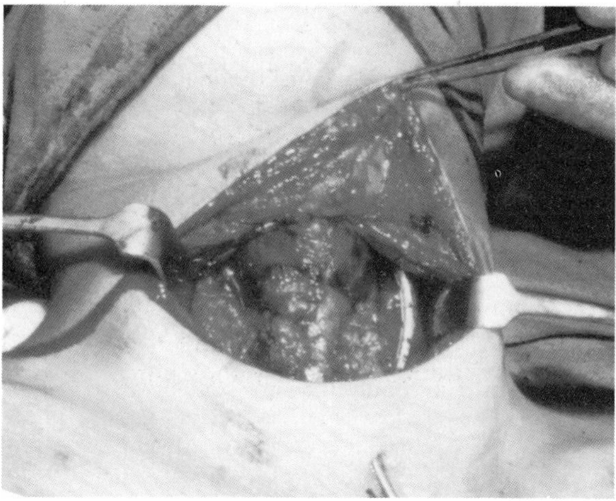

(a)

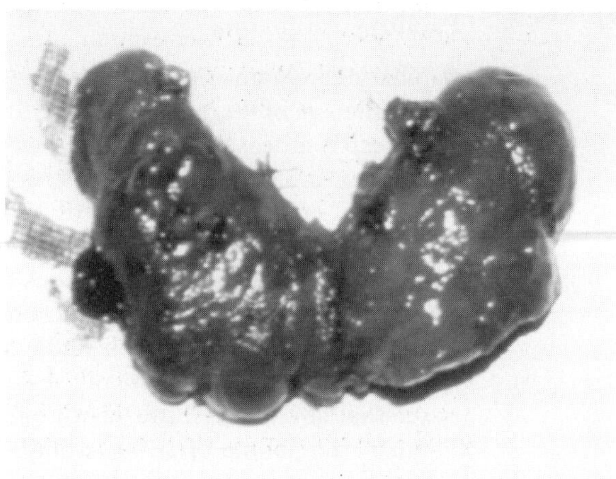

(b)

Fig. 30.8 Complications of thyroidectomy

PEROPERATIVE COMPLICATIONS

Uncontrollable haemorrhage — uncommon, usually results from a slipped ligature on the upper pole vessels which then retract

Unilateral or bilateral recurrent laryngeal nerve damage — bilateral nerve damage presents as laryngeal obstruction after tracheal extubation and necessitates immediate tracheostomy

Inadvertent damage to other structures — tracheal or oesophageal perforation, or damage to laryngeal muscles or nerves

IMMEDIATE POSTOPERATIVE COMPLICATIONS (within the first 12 hours)

Major haemorrhage — presents as rapid swelling of the neck, or a large volume of blood loss via the wound drain. This requires emergency surgical exploration of wound to achieve haemostasis

Mediastinal haemorrhage — presents with hypovolaemic shock

Laryngeal oedema — presents as stridor, rapidly progressing to respiratory obstruction. This requires endotracheal intubation

Thyrotoxic crisis — presents with abrupt onset of extreme agitation and confusion, hyperpyrexia, profuse sweating and rapid tachycardia or other arrhythmia. This requires emergency beta-adrenergic blockade, intravenous hydrocortisone and potassium iodide therapy. The mortality of thyrotoxic crisis is 10% from coma, pulmonary oedema or circulatory collapse

LATE POSTOPERATIVE COMPLICATIONS

Hypoparathyroidism — presents with muscle cramps, paraesthesiae and tetany within 36 hours of operation

Unilateral recurrent laryngeal nerve damage — presents with hoarseness of voice and defective cough

Superior laryngeal nerve damage — changes the quality of the voice

LONG TERM COMPLICATIONS

Hypothyroidism — often overlooked because it develops insidiously. Features are loss of energy, weight gain, depression and intellectual deterioration and intolerance of cold weather

Papillary carcinoma

Papillary carcinomas constitute about 80% of thyroid malignancies in adults below the age of 40, and nearly all thyroid malignancies in children. Females are affected at least twice as often as males. Histologically, the tumour forms a complex branching papillary structure with a fibrovascular stroma. There is a wide range of epithelial dysplasia from apparently benign to overtly malignant. Whatever the dysplasia, the tumours grow very slowly. They metastasise to cervical lymph nodes but rarely to more distant sites. Indeed, by the time of presentation, lymph nodes are involved in about 40% of patients (90% in children) and lymph node enlargement is of ten the sole presenting feature. The histology of involved lymph nodes is so close to normal thyroid tissue that at one time, this condition was known as 'lateral aberrant thyroid'. Papillary carcinoma often has a multicentric origin within the gland which is

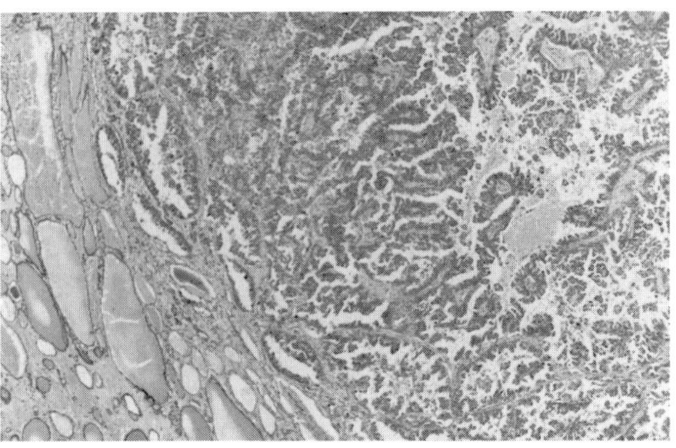

Fig. 30.9 Papillary carcinoma of the thyroid — histopathology

Part of a papillary carcinoma of the thyroid showing the typically papilliferous growth pattern of the tumour cells. Note, on the left, the compressed normal thyroid follicles at the margin of the tumour

important in treatment. The prognosis of papillary carcinoma is particularly good and it is remarkable that survival is not prejudiced by the presence of metastases.

Clinically, papillary carcinoma presents as a slow growing solitary thyroid nodule, or an enlarged cervical lymph node lateral to the gland. The patient is euthyroid. Thyroid isotope scanning usually shows no uptake in the palpable nodule. Sometimes, other tumour foci in the gland are large enough to appear as cold nodules. A patient presenting with just an enlarged cervical lymph node may be unexpectedly diagnosed as papillary carcinoma of the thyroid on histology of the node. Overall, the diagnosis of papillary carcinoma is usually made on investigation of a cold thyroid nodule.

The standard management of papillary carcinoma is *total thyroidectomy* because of the risk of other foci within the gland. Palpable cervical nodes are removed at the same operation. Technically, the operation is no more difficult than subtotal thyroidectomy. Hormone replacement with oral thyroxine is always necessary afterwards but rarely causes problems. Life expectancy after surgery approaches the normal span except in the unusual case of remote metastases. Tumour recurrence in the cervical nodes has little effect on prognosis, and is treated by excision.

Since papillary carcinomas progress so slowly, some surgeons prefer to retain one thyroid lobe, provided there are no palpable or isotope-detectable nodules. Their reasoning is that further tumours can be removed later without reducing life expectancy.

Follicular carcinoma

Follicular carcinoma is another well differentiated thyroid malignancy. Histologically, the neoplastic cells form a well developed *follicular pattern* which may be difficult to distinguish from benign adenomatous hyperplasia unless there is vascular invasion. The peak incidence of follicular carcinoma is between 40 and 50 years of age, an older group than papillary carcinoma. Generally, follicular carcinoma grows slowly and metastasises at a late stage. In contrast to papillary carcinoma, metastasis tends to occur via the blood stream, to the lungs, bone and other remote sites rather than to local lymph nodes.

Management usually involves removing the thyroid lobe containing the tumour. Follicular carcinoma is rarely multicentric, so total thyroidectomy is generally unnecessary to treat the local tumour. If however, distant metastases are present, total thyroidectomy is performed. This is to enhance iodine uptake by metastatic lesions, which can then be demonstrated by radio-iodine scanning and treated by high dose radioiodine.

Prognosis depends on the degree of invasion of blood vessels by the primary lesion and can be predicted from the histology. If there is no vessel invasion, 10-year survival is near 100%; this falls to about 30% if there is extensive local vascular involvement.

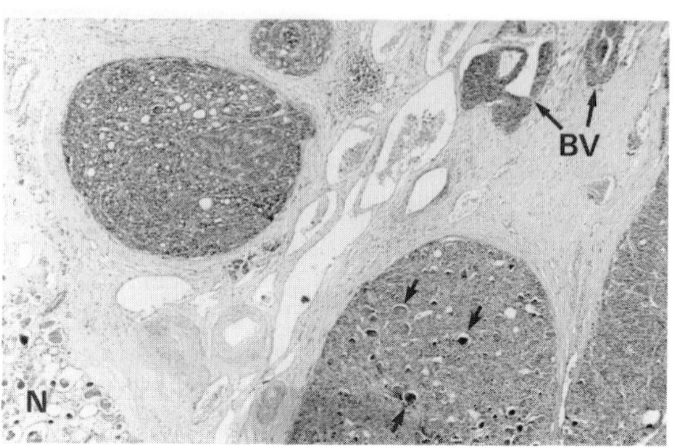

Fig. 30.10 Follicular carcinoma — histopathology

Margin of a follicular carcinoma showing masses of tumour cells exhibiting some follicular areas containing colloid (arrowed). Note the normal thyroid tissue **N** at the lower left of the field. Invasion of blood vessels **BV** by tumour provides evidence of malignancy

Anaplastic carcinoma

Anaplastic carcinomas are extremely aggressive tumours with an appalling prognosis. Most patients die within a year of diagnosis. The tumours are found almost exclusively in the elderly. In general, carcinomas in this age group are less aggressive than in the young; thyroid carcinomas are, however, more aggressive in the elderly.

Anaplastic carcinoma consists of sheets of very poorly differentiated cells which proliferate rapidly. The result is a diffuse, hard thyroid enlargement. The tumour soon invades surrounding structures, causing symptoms of tracheal and oesophageal obstruction and recurrent laryngeal nerve damage. There is also early dissemination to regional lymph nodes and haematogenous spread to the lungs, skeleton and brain.

Anaplastic carcinomas respond poorly to both radiotherapy and chemotherapy. Surgical treatment is directed at palliation of obstructive symptoms by removing tumour near the larynx and trachea.

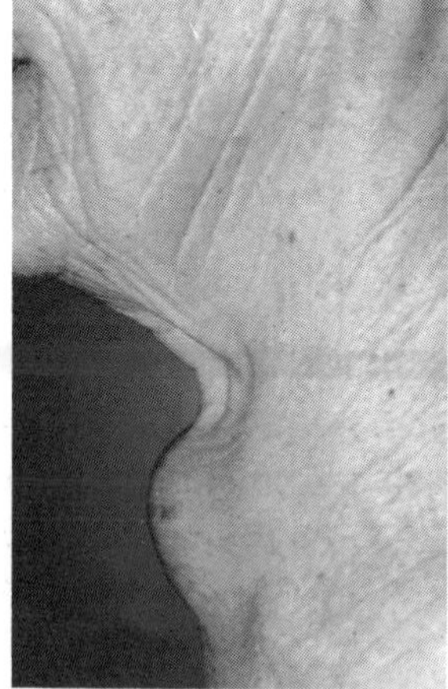

Fig. 30.11 Anaplastic carcinoma

This woman of 75 had noticed a swelling in her neck for more than a year which had enlarged rapidly over the three months before presentation. She presented because of stridor at night when lying on her left side. The thyroid enlargement was hard on palpation and did not rise fully on swallowing, appearing tethered to nearby structures. She underwent total thyroidectomy, but died of metastatic disease eight months later

Medullary carcinoma

This uncommon malignancy arises from parafollicular thyroid cells. The tumour often secretes abnormal quantities of *calcitonin*, which can be used as a measure of tumour recurrence after excision. The tumour may arise alone or with other APUD cell tumours. Medullary carcinoma is especially associated with *phaeochromocytoma*, as part of the *multiple endocrine neoplasia syndrome type II (M.E.N. II)*.

The tumour is of particular pathological interest because the stroma contains extensive deposits of amyloid. These make the tumour mass stony hard to palpation. The tumour grows relatively slowly, metastasising to regional lymph nodes.

The standard treatment is total thyroidectomy and clearance of anterior cervical and superior mediastinal lymph nodes. Without metastases, operation is often curative but when nodes are involved, 10-year survival falls to about 50%.

Thyroid lymphoma

Primary lymphomas of the thyroid are rare and possibly arise from pre-existing autoimmune (Hashimoto's) thyroiditis. Diagnosis can only be made on histology. The tumour is sensitive to radiotherapy.

GOITRES AND THYROID NODULES

As indicated earlier in Figure 30.1, several hyperplastic and metabolic disorders cause diffuse or nodular thyroid enlargement.

Idiopathic non-toxic thyroid hyperplasia

Most goitres referred to surgeons in developed countries are caused by simple, idiopathic hyperplasia of thyroid follicles. The condition probably begins with diffuse micronodular enlargement, and the nodules later become heterogeneously enlarged to form a *multinodular colloid goitre*. Within the same spectrum of disease are *solitary hyperplastic nodules* (which may actually be benign thyroid adenomas) and *thyroid cysts*, which are simply huge colloid-filled follicles.

The aetiology of simple thyroid hyperplasia is unknown, but is probably related to disordered sensitivity to TSH. In this sense, the condition may be analagous to fibroadenosis of the breast. The patient is usually clinically euthyroid and thyroid function tests are normal. Sometimes, thyroid hormone secretion escapes from hypothalamic control so the patient becomes hyperthyroid and occasionally thyrotoxic.

Within the gland, secretory activity is heterogeneous, explaining the patchy distribution of radio-iodine uptake on thyroid scans. Focal hormone secretion from 'hot' adenomatous nodules may be so great as to completely suppress the rest of the gland. The overall hormone secretion may still be within the euthyroid range; this may be considered the most extreme form of secretory heterogeneity.

Diffuse or multinodular idiopathic goitres develop slowly and cause little trouble until they have been present for many years.

The reasons patients present to surgeons with thyroid enlargement are:

- A goitre has become so large as to be cosmetically unacceptable
- A localised lump has appeared in the thyroid region. This may be a solitary adenomatous nodule or a solitary cyst. Alternatively, the apparent solitary lump may be part of an asymmetrical multinodular or multicystic enlargement
- A pre-existing multinodular goitre has undergone rapid asymmetric change. There are several possible causes, i.e. haemorrhage into a cyst or degenerate area of hyperplasia, or malignant change
- The patient has become hyperthyroid
- The patient has developed stridor from tracheal compression due to enlargement of a retrosternal extension of the thyroid.

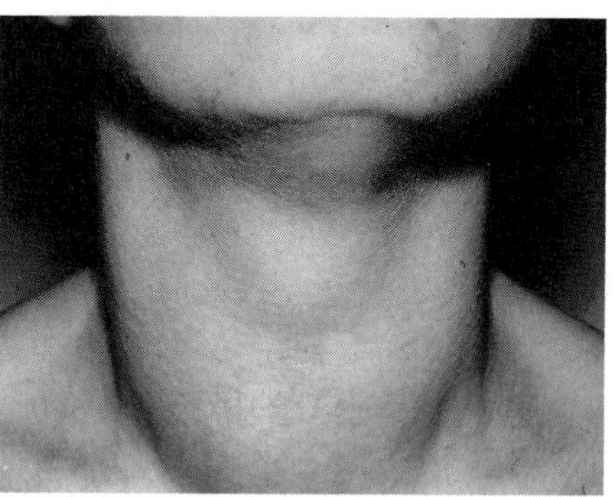

Fig. 30.12 Cosmetically unacceptable idiopathic goitre

This 25-year-old woman requested thyroidectomy for cosmetic reasons. This multinodular goitre had been present and slowly enlarging for several years. There was a strong family history of 'thyroid trouble'

Surgical management of goitre

The indications for surgery in idiopathic goitre are:

- Correction of cosmetic deformity
- Excision of a solitary toxic nodule
- Excision of a toxic multinodular goitre
- Excision of a lump suspicious of malignancy
- Excision of a compressive retrosternal thyroid

In principle, only enough thyroid tissue is removed to achieve the objective. The minimum amount of tissue remaining must be about 10 g.

Patients presenting for cosmetic reasons whose thyroids are only moderately enlarged may be treated with thyroxine. By suppressing TSH, thyroxine may shrink the gland to an acceptable size. Antithyroid drugs are ineffective for treating hypersecretion caused by idiopathic thyroid hyperplasia.

Thyroid cysts are diagnosed as fluid-filled lesions by ultrasound. Aspiration will confirm the diagnosis and cytology will exclude malignancy. Large or recurrent cysts are best treated surgically.

CONGENITAL THYROID DISORDERS

Introduction

The thyroid originates as a diverticulum in the midline between the first two pharyngeal pouches. Its origin is represented in the adult by the *foramen caecum*, which lies at the junction of the anterior two-thirds and the posterior third of the tongue. The calcitonin-secreting *parafollicular* cells originate from the *ultimobranchial body* of the fifth pouch. The thyroid diverticulum between the first two branchial pouches forms the *thyroglossal duct* which extends caudally through the developing tongue musculature. It passes down in relation to the hyoid bone (in front of, through or behind it) to reach its normal position below the larynx. By this time, it has become a bilobed structure, the lobes connected by a narrow central isthmus. The thyroglossal duct later degenerates.

Thyroglossal cyst and fistula

Part of the thyroglossal duct may persist and become cystic. Thyroglossal cysts present in young children, and occasionally adolescents, as a smooth, rounded, midline swelling at the front of the neck. Most thyroglossal cysts occur below the hyoid, although rarely, they are found in the submental region. A diagnostic feature is that the cyst rises when the patient swallows or protrudes the tongue. Most thyroglossal cysts are asymptomatic but they are prone to inflammation which causes pain and increased swelling. If an inflamed cyst is surgically drained, it may become an intermittently discharging *sinus*, often incorrectly described as a *thyroglossal fistula*.

Thyroglossal cysts are usually excised along with the thyroglossal tract up to the base of the tongue. This requires removing the middle third of the hyoid bone (*Sistrunk's operation*). Inflamed cysts are usually drained initially and later excised. A persistent sinus or a recurrent cyst will complicate incomplete excision.

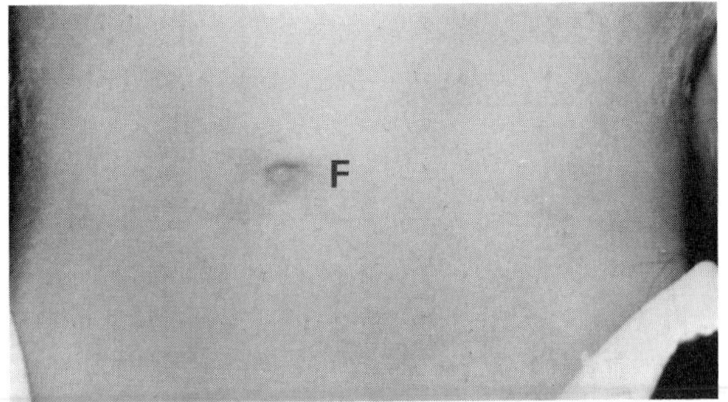

Fig. 30.13 Thyroglossal fistula

This photograph shows the anterior of the neck in a 14-year-old boy. An attempt had been made to remove a thyroglossal cyst several years previously. The inevitable result of incomplete surgical removal was an intermittently discharging fistula in the midline of the neck **F**

Ectopic thyroid gland

An ectopic thyroid gland is a rare congenital abnormality which results from interruption of normal descent. It may present in the same way as a thyroglossal cyst or as a lump in the tongue. As this may be the patient's only thyroid tissue, complete excision may not be appropriate.

DISORDERS OF PARATHYROID GLANDS

Introduction

Hyperparathyroidism is the most common clinical disorder of the parathyroid glands. Patients are usually referred to the surgeon after investigation of *recurrent urinary tract calculi*, or *hypercalcaemia*.

Mild hypercalcaemia is often found incidentally on biochemical screening. More severe hypercalcaemia presents with bone pain (with or without radiological changes), abdominal pain (caused by peptic ulcer or pancreatitis), constipation and dehydration. Mental changes include confusion, depression or even psychosis. Hypercalcaemia also occurs in chronic renal failure, associated with tertiary hyperparathyroidism. Note that hyperparathyroidism is only one cause of hypercalcaemia.

Control of serum calcium

Serum calcium level is normally maintained within a very narrow range by the combined effect of the hormones, parathormone and calcitonin. There must be an adequate dietary intake of calcium and vitamin D, which is essential for calcium absorption.

Fig. 30.14 Main control mechanisms for serum calcium

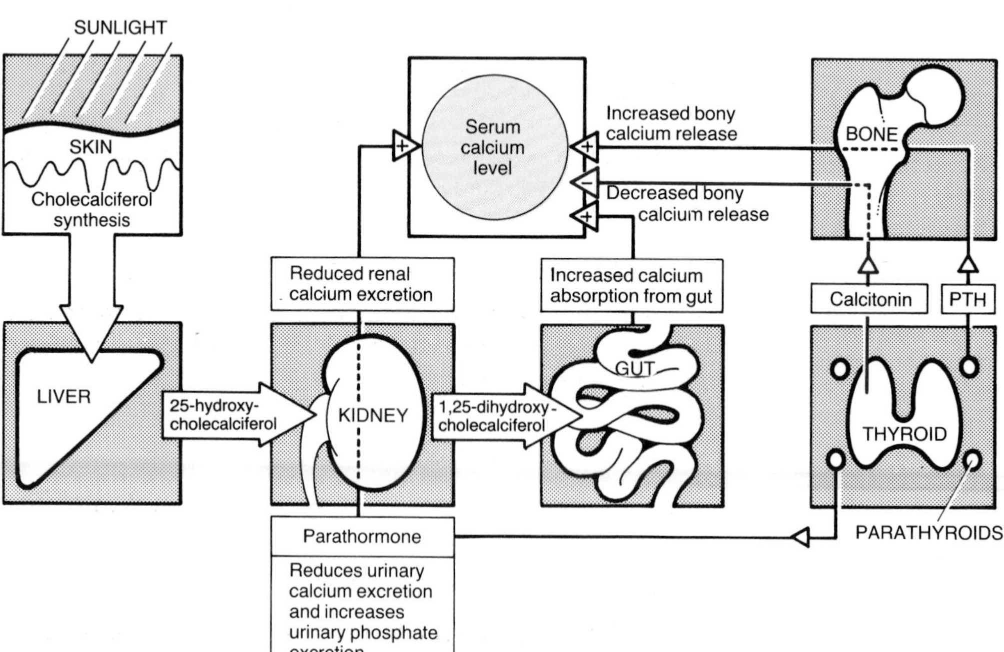

Parathormone raises serum calcium levels in the following ways:

- Increases osteoclastic activity and release of calcium from bone matrix. This liberates calcium into the circulation
- Enhances renal tubular reabsorption of calcium and diminishes reabsorption of phosphate
- Promotes calcium absorption from the small intestine; this involves vitamin D

Calcitonin, produced by the parafollicular C-cells of the thyroid gland, lowers serum calcium concentration by reducing osteoclastic activity and promoting osteoblastic activity. Calcitonin has a small influence on calcium metabolism compared with parathormone.

Vitamin D (as cholecalciferol) is produced by the action of sunlight on cholesterol derivatives in the skin. Cholecalciferol is then converted to 25-hydroxycholecalciferol in the liver, and further hydroxylated by the renal parenchyma to the active compound *1,25-dihydroxycholecalciferol*. This active compound is required for calcium absorption from the intestine.

Calcium homeostasis is thus dependent on normal functioning of parathyroids, liver and kidney, together with an adequate dietary intake of calcium, and suitable quantities of vitamin D from diet or exposure to sunlight.

HYPERPARATHYROIDISM

Hyperparathyroidism is classified as follows:

Primary hyperparathyroidism

a. Parathyroid adenoma

This is the most common cause of primary hyperparathyroidism. One of the four parathyroid glands becomes enlarged and replaced by a benign neoplasm which secretes parathormone in excessive amounts. Secretion by the other parathyroids is suppressed.

b. Diffuse parathyroid hyperplasia

This is an uncommon cause of primary hyperparathyroidism. The secretory cells of each of the glands undergoes idiopathic hyperplasia, resulting in excess hormone production.

c. Parathyroid carcinoma

This is extremely rare and involves only one of the parathyroid glands.

Secondary hyperparathyroidism

Secondary hyperparathyroidism occurs in response to reduced calcium absorption. It is mainly seen in *chronic renal failure* when there is defective absorption of calcium from the gut. This is primarily due to a failure of conversion of 25 hydroxycholecalciferol to 1,25 dihydroxy cholecalciferol in the diseased renal parenchyma. These patients are usually having regular renal dialysis. The parathyroid glands undergo *diffuse hyperplasia* in response to the reduced serum calcium. The output of parathormone increases, thereby mobilising bone calcium and reducing urinary excretion, in an attempt to maintain normal serum calcium levels.

Tertiary hyperparathyroidism

Tertiary hyperparathyroidism is a complication of prolonged secondary hyperparathyroidism. If the underlying cause of secondary hyperparathyroidism is corrected, e.g. by renal transplantation, serum calcium increases to normal levels yet parathyroid secretion remains abnormally high. The parathyroid glands remain hyperplastic, having become insensitive to the normal negative feedback from rising serum calcium levels.

Ectopic parathormone production

Some malignant tumours, such as oat cell carcinoma of the lung, secrete parathormone. The tumour is usually well advanced with widespread metastases.

Hyperparathyroidism is associated with raised serum calcium levels (and reduced serum phosphate levels) except in secondary hyperparathyroidism; in this disorder, serum calcium is normal or even depressed.

Raised serum calcium levels cannot be tolerated for long without causing serious systemic problems or damage to bone. From Figure 30.14, it might seem paradoxical that urinary tract calculi are a common presenting feature of hyperparathyroidism, since parathormone *reduces* urinary calcium excretion. The probable reason for stone formation is the excess phosphate excretion. This is associated with excessive urinary alkalinity, which predisposes to the formation of calcium salts.

Management of hyperparathyroidism

Diagnosis of hyperparathyroidism was difficult before the advent of radioimmunoassay for parathormone. Primary hyperparathyroidism is diagnosed if both serum calcium and parathormone levels are elevated, in the absence of renal failure or metastatic disease. In primary hyperparathyroidism, distinction between adenoma, diffuse hyperplasia and adenocarcinoma is not possible except by surgical exploration of the neck and examination of each parathyroid gland.

Surgical management

Surgery is the only treatment for primary and tertiary hyperparathyroidism. Secondary hyperparathyroidism is managed by giving oral vitamin D or calcium, however, if there is severe bone resorption, parathyroidectomy may sometimes be necessary. Hypercalcaemia due to ectopic parathormone

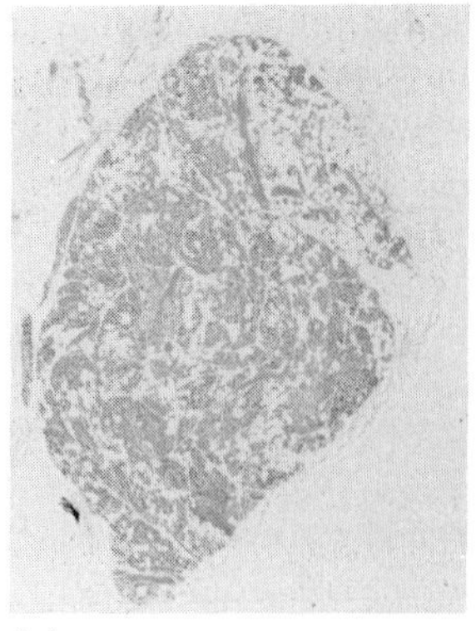

(a)

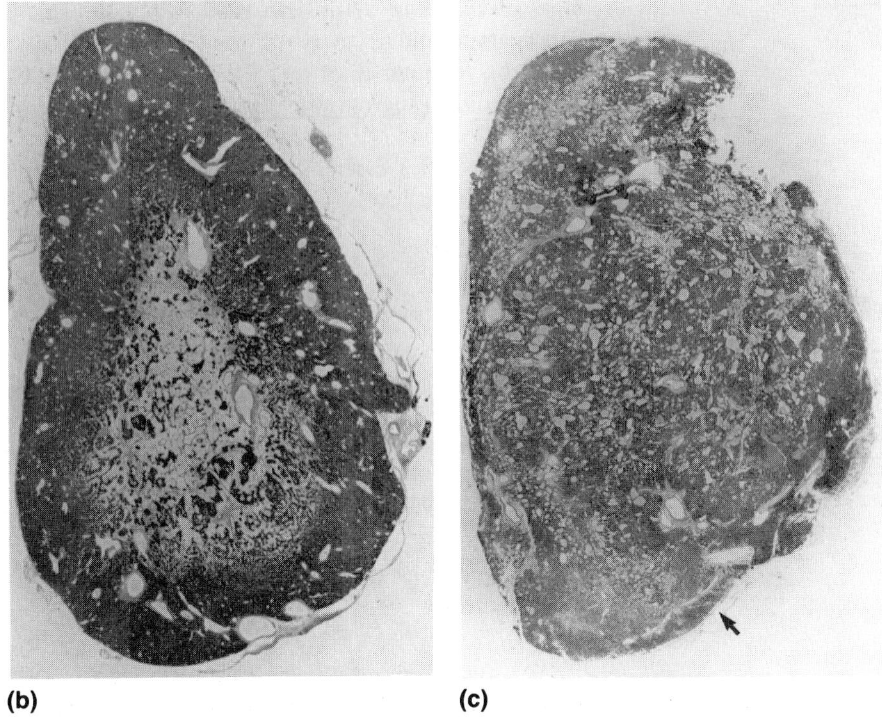

(b) (c)

Fig. 30.15 Parathyroid hyperplasia and adenoma — histopathology

These micrographs of parathyroid glands, all taken at the same magnification, show: **(a)** normal gland, **(b)** parathyroid hyperplasia and **(c)** a parathyroid adenoma. In (b), note the diffuse hyperplasia of the whole gland except for the central stroma. In (c), note that benign tumour cells occupy the whole gland except for a small rim of normal tissue (arrowed) at the periphery

production is managed medically as it is rarely possible to resect the parathormone secreting tumour.

There are normally two pairs of parathyroid glands, superior and inferior, lying close to the posterolateral aspect of the lateral lobes of the thyroid. The superior pair lie near the inferior thyroid artery at the middle of the gland. The inferior pair are usually located near the lower poles of the thyroid.

Parathyroid surgery is exacting and time-consuming, usually interrupted by histological examination of several frozen section biopsies during the course of the operation. The surgical access is the same as for thyroidectomy. The likely anatomical position of each parathyroid is then meticulously explored in the search for parathyroid tissue. Although the parathyroids have a characteristic yellow-brown colour, they are often extremely difficult to distinguish from thyroid tissue, especially if the tissues have been traumatised.

If one of the parathyroid glands is enlarged and the others are normal, the diagnosis is *parathyroid adenoma*, or rarely, *adenocarcinoma*. In either case, the abnormal gland is completely removed. If no individual gland is disproportionately enlarged, a diagnosis of *diffuse hyperplasia* can be made. In this case, enough parathyroid tissue must be removed to lower the parathormone level. At the same time, enough parathormone tissue must be retained to allow normal calcium homeostasis. The problem is that some parathyroid tissue may remain unidentified, however meticulous the surgery. Surgical practice varies in managing parathyroid hyperplasia. Some surgeons remove three and a half glands, while others remove all the parathyroid tissue and reimplant a small mass of tissue in a forearm muscle pouch. The advantage of this is that if hyperparathyroidism persists, then parathyroid tissue is more readily removed from the forearm than from the thyroid area. The disadvantage is that the parathyroid tissue may not become vascularised or may undergo atrophy.

Complications of parathyroidectomy are similar to those of thyroid surgery (see Figure 30.8 earlier). Hypoparathyroidism is more likely, however, and serum calcium levels must be carefully monitored in the early postoperative period.

HYPOPARATHYROIDISM

The most common cause of hypoparathyroidism is surgical removal or devascularisation of the parathyroid glands during thyroid or parathyroid surgery. It may also be a transient occurrence after excision of a parathyroid adenoma or subtotal parathyroidectomy, until the remaining suppressed parathyroid tissue recovers normal function. Autoimmune hypoparathyroidism may also occur occasionally.

Hypoparathyroidism presents clinically with the effects of hypocalcaemia. A fall in the serum calcium level increases neuromuscular excitability causing muscular cramps or even tetany in severe cases. An early symptom of hypocalcaemia is paraesthesia, especially around the lips. Post-operative patients should be routinely asked if they have experienced any tingling around the mouth.

Clinical tests for hypocalcaemia include tapping over the parotid gland which provokes transient contraction of the facial muscles (*Chvostek's sign*). A further test involves inflating a sphygmomanometer cuff on the upper arm to above systolic pressure. This induces carpal spasm within about three minutes (*'main d'accoucheur'*).

Early postoperative hypocalcaemia is treated with intravenous calcium gluconate. Persistent hypocalcaemia is controlled by oral administration of high doses of calcium and vitamin D.

31 PAEDIATRIC SURGERY

Introduction

Most surgery in children falls within the province of the general surgeon, although major congenital abnormalities and tumours are usually managed by regional paediatric surgical specialists and urologists. Not only does the range of conditions differ from those seen in adults, but the conditions themselves vary within different age groups. This is particularly true for conditions which present as acute emergencies. Reflecting this, paediatric emergencies may be considered under the headings of the *newborn* (the first few days of life), *infants and young children* (up to about two years) and *older children* (up to puberty). During puberty, the conditions merge with those of adulthood. The non-emergency and urogenital conditions tend to be less age-specific and are discussed separately later in the chapter.

ABDOMINAL EMERGENCIES IN THE NEWBORN

Introduction

The main abdominal emergencies in neonates are summarised in Figure 31.1. All except necrotising enterocolitis are congenital disorders. Diagnosis and management requires close cooperation between paediatricians and surgeons. Paediatricians play a particularly important role in both initial diagnosis and perioperative management of fluid and electrolyte balance and nutrition.

Intestinal obstruction is the underlying phenomenon in the majority of neonatal abdominal emergencies. Just as in adults, intestinal obstruction presents with vomiting, absolute constipation and, if the obstruction is in the distal bowel,

Fig. 31.1 Main abdominal emergencies occurring in the newborn

Gastrointestinal atresias and stenoses
Malrotation of the gut
Anorectal abnormalities
Meconium plugging
Meconium ileus
Hirschsprung's disease
Diaphragmatic hernia
Deficiencies in the abdominal wall (gastroschisis and exomphalos)
Necrotising enterocolitis

abdominal distension. Complete proximal obstruction such as oesophageal atresia, prevents the fetus from swallowing amniotic fluid as it does during the normal pregnancy, resulting in *polyhydramnios*. Indeed, if polyhydramnios is present at the time of delivery, gastrointestinal obstruction must be excluded before the baby is given its first feed.

The level of obstruction is indicated by the position of gas and fluid levels on plain abdominal radiography.

GASTRO-INTESTINAL ATRESIAS AND STENOSES

Atresia is defined as complete obliteration of a segment of the gastrointestinal tract which is thus completely obstructed, whereas a *stenosis* is an indistensible narrowing causing partial obstruction. These problems are most common in the oesophagus and small intestine.

Most atresias and some stenoses are acquired during late fetal life as a result of bowel wall ischaemia. The ischaemia may have been due to mechanical interference with the blood supply by bowel strangulation. Atresias and stenoses are rarely associated with other congenital malformations, although there is a higher incidence of duodenal abnormalities in Down's syndrome. This is probably due to incomplete canalisation of the bowel at the junction of foregut and midgut.

Oesophageal abnormalities

Fig. 31.2

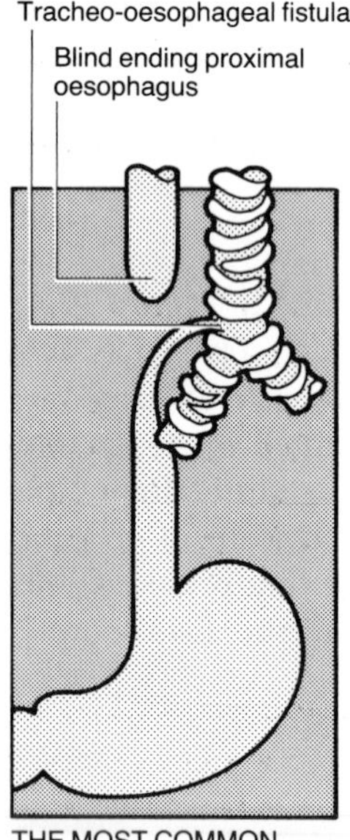

THE MOST COMMON VARIANT OF OESOPHAGEAL ATRESIA

Note: air enters GI tract via fistula and can be seen radiologically.
Gastric secretions may enter bronchial tree causing 'frothy' breathing

Potentially lethal oesophageal abnormalities occur in 1 in 3000 births. Oesophageal atresia may occur alone, but more commonly, it is associated with a fistulous communication between the trachea and either the proximal or the distal oesophageal segment (*tracheo-oesophageal fistula* or 'TOF'). In the most common variant, shown in Figure 31.2, acid reflux into the lungs occurs, and this is particularly destructive. Oesophageal abnormalities become apparent soon after birth; the baby cannot swallow milk or saliva, and persistently produces frothy mucus, chokes and becomes dyspnoeic.

Diagnosis is made by passing a nasogastric tube, which is arrested by the obstruction. The diagnosis is then confirmed by passing contrast material down the tube and taking a radiograph; the contrast will be arrested at the level of atresia. The presence of gas in the stomach indicates there must be a fistula between the distal oesophagus and the trachea.

Surgical treatment is required as soon as oesophageal atresia is diagnosed. The majority of cases are correctable by primary oesophageal anastomosis.

Duodenal atresia

The obstruction of duodenal atresia is usually below the entry of the common bile duct, resulting in *bile-stained vomiting*. Plain erect abdominal X-ray shows gas in the stomach and proximal duodenum; a gas bubble and fluid level are seen on each side of the upper abdomen (*'double bubble'*). Urgent surgery is needed to bypass the defect by creating a side-to-side anastomosis between proximal and distal duodenal segments.

Small intestinal atresias and stenoses are at least as common as oesophageal atresias. They may occur at any level and are sometimes multiple. Bile-stained

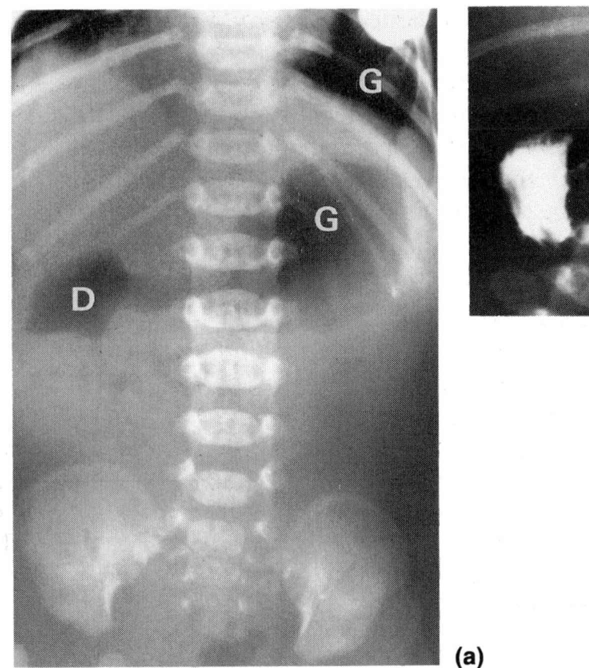

(a)

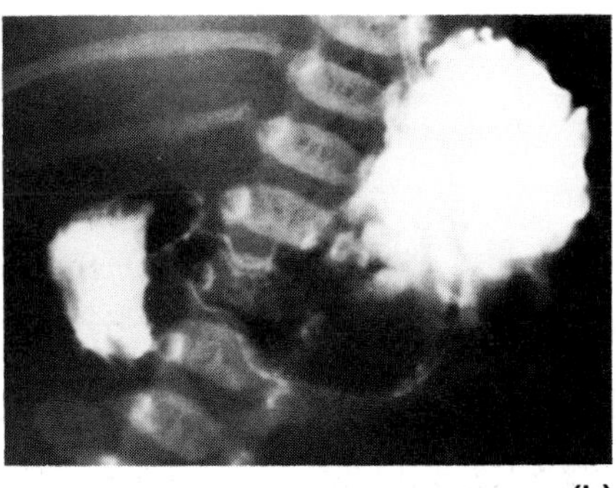

(b)

Fig. 31.3 Duodenal atresia

(a) Supine plain abdominal film in a neonate with duodenal obstruction. This film shows the typical 'double bubble' appearance of gas in the stomach **G** and the first part of the duodenum **D**. Fluid levels would be seen in an erect film. **(b)** A small amount of barium has been passed down the nasogastric tube and confirms that the obstruction is virtually complete

vomiting and abdominal distension are often associated with *visible peristalsis*. The baby may grimace and draw up its legs with pain. Plain radiography usually suggests the level of obstruction.

Treatment involves resection of the atretic or stenotic segment and end-to-end anastomosis.

MALROTATION OF THE GUT

During early embryological development, the midgut develops outside the abdominal cavity. By the end of the third month, the midgut has returned to the abdominal cavity, having rotated 270° anticlockwise in the process. Several rotational abnormalities may occur, and most cause obstruction just below the entry of the common bile duct (junction of foregut and midgut). The baby presents with bile stained vomiting, similar to duodenal atresia and the same 'double bubble' radiographic appearance is seen (see Figure 31.3 above).

ANORECTAL ABNORMALITIES

A variety of anatomical abnormalities occur in the anal region which obstruct the passage of faeces. These range from a simple low membranous obstruction in otherwise normal bowel, to higher obstructions where the rectum ends blindly above the pelvic diaphragm. The anal sphincter mechanism is usually intact. Anorectal abnormalities are often associated with urogenital abnormalities, and fistulas between bowel and genitourinary tract.

Diagnosis is made after the infant fails to pass meconium and then rectal examination reveals an 'imperforate anus'. The level of obstruction is established by taping a metal button over the anus and taking a plain abdominal X-ray with the baby turned upside down. The gap between rectal gas and the anal button indicates the extent of atresia. Low atresias can usually be corrected by a simple *cut-back operation*. High atresias are more complicated and require creation of a temporary colostomy followed later by sophisticated reconstruction in which the colon is 'pulled through' the sphincter to the anus. An intact sphincter mechanism allows normal continence to develop.

Failure to pass meconium soon after birth may also be caused by meconium plugging, meconium ileus or Hirschsprung's disease. Since meconium is formed by desquamation of bowel mucosal cells and is present throughout the bowel, the passage of meconium after birth does not exclude a proximal bowel obstruction.

OTHER CAUSES OF FAILURE TO PASS MECONIUM

Meconium plugging

Without any anatomical or functional abnormality of the bowel, the meconium in the rectum may sometimes form a viscous plug preventing normal defecation. The resulting distal bowel obstruction may be confused with a serious condition such as anorectal atresia. Meconium plugging is relieved by gentle digital examination of the rectum; the result is a satisfying gush of flatus and meconium.

Meconium ileus

Meconium ileus is the classic neonatal presentation of *cystic fibrosis*. The meconium is extremely viscous because insufficient bowel mucus is produced, and there is a deficiency of pancreatic enzymes which normally liquefy meconium. Thick putty-like meconium obstructs the ileum, producing gross abdominal distension, bile-stained vomiting and absolute constipation. Plain abdominal X-ray may show a mottled appearance due to lipid droplets within the meconium.

The obstruction may sometimes be relieved with enemas, but a temporary ileostomy is often required. Oral pancreatic enzyme supplements are needed to prevent recurrence.

Hirschsprung's disease

Hirschsprung's disease is a congenital abnormality in which there is failure of development of the parasympathetic plexuses in the submucosa and muscular layers of a segment of the large bowel. The disease may be confined to a very short segment of the distal rectum but more commonly involves a longer rectosigmoid segment. Sometimes the entire colon is involved. The affected segment is non-motile and obstructs faecal progress. The age of presentation and the severity of symptoms of obstruction are related to the length of the affected segment.

Some patients present with failure to pass meconium after birth, but the more common presentation is large bowel obstruction or extreme constipation during the first year. Uncommonly, Hirschsprung's disease presents in later childhood with chronic constipation. In these children, the defect involves only an *ultrashort segment*.

Diagnosis is suggested on barium enema by the finding of a narrowed rectal segment and dilated proximal bowel. Diagnosis is confirmed by deep rectal biopsy. Treatment involves resection of the affected segment and a procedure to restore continuity. A colostomy is required as a temporary procedure.

DIAPHRAGMATIC HERNIA

This common congenital disorder usually begins in early fetal life. A large hemidiaphragmatic defect allows herniation of a mass of gut into the chest on one side; the left side is usually affected. Normal development of the lung may be seriously impaired. Diaphragmatic hernia presents with gross respiratory distress at birth. Diagnosis is readily apparent on chest X-ray.

Surgery is required urgently and results are good unless there is irretrievable pulmonary hypoplasia.

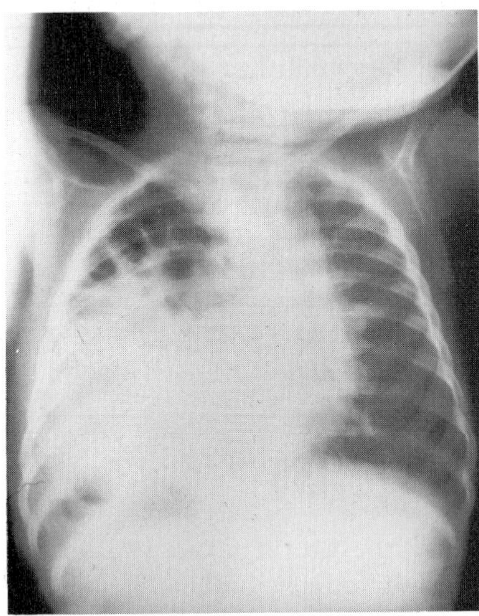

(a)

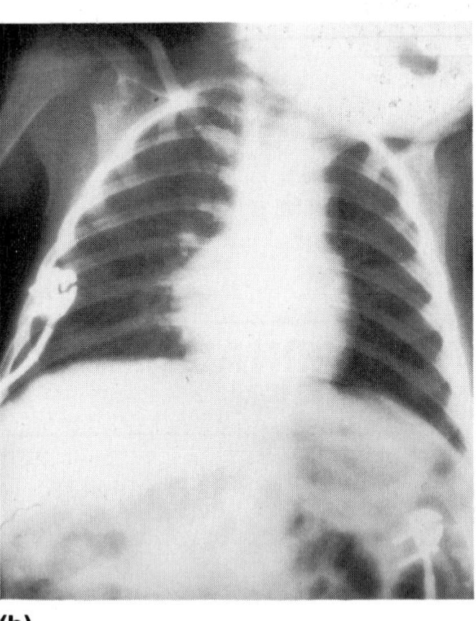

(b)

Fig. 31.4 Congenital diaphragmatic hernia

(a) Plain chest radiograph of a neonate with respiratory distress. This film shows a large opacity in the right lung field with obvious loops of bowel. This is a congenital diaphragmatic hernia, and is unusual on the right side as in the case. **(b)** Postoperative chest X-ray of the same infant showing complete lung expansion after repair of the diaphragmatic defect

DEFICIENCIES IN THE ABDOMINAL WALL

Major deficiencies in the anterior abdominal wall are an uncommon congenital abnormality, and are dramatically obvious at birth. They result from a midline defect in the abdominal wall so that much of the gut lies outside the abdominal cavity, with or without a membranous covering. In *gastroschisis*, coils of bare gut are exposed, whereas in *exomphalos*, the gut is invested by a thin layer of peritoneum.

Gastroschisis

In gastroschisis, the gut is oedematous, and the space within the abdominal cavity too small to allow the gut to be replaced without respiratory embarrassment. For this reason, the exposed gut is enclosed in a plastic bag which is sutured to the margin of the abdominal wall defect. Over the next few days, the gut is progressively eased back into the abdominal cavity, after which the defect can be repaired.

Exomphalos

Exomphalos presents in major and minor forms. In *exomphalos major*, most of the gut lies outside the abdominal cavity and is managed similarly to gastroschisis. In *exomphalos minor*, the bowel can be reduced and the defect repaired as a single procedure.

NECROTISING ENTERO-COLITIS

This often fatal disorder occurs in newborn babies, almost invariably the premature or seriously ill in special care baby units. The pathophysiology is poorly understood but probably involves ischaemia of the large bowel wall which then becomes invaded by gas-producing bacteria. Initially, there is adynamic bowel obtruction, presenting with abdominal distension, vomiting and diarrhoea with blood and mucus. If unrecognised, necrotising enterocolitis soon progresses to large bowel necrosis, perforation and generalised peritonitis.

Plain abdominal X-ray initially shows generalised gut dilatation with multiple fluid levels. Later, gas shadows may be seen in the bowel wall indicating bowel wall necrosis. Treatment includes vigorous resuscitative measures, broad spectrum antibiotics and surgical resection if incipient gangrene is suspected. Mortality remains high.

ABDOMINAL EMERGENCIES IN INFANTS AND YOUNG CHILDREN

Introduction

In children below the age of about two years, there are only four main abdominal causes for acute surgical admission; these are listed in Figure 31.5.

Fig. 31.5 Main abdominal emergencies occurring in infants and young children

Strangulated inguinal hernia
Hypertrophic pyloric stenosis
Intussuception
Swallowed foreign body

STRANGU-LATED INGUINAL HERNIA

Pathophysiology

Strangulated inguinal hernia is the most common cause of acute surgical admission in boys below the age of two. Strangulation follows incarceration of an indirect inguinal hernia. There is invariably a congenital patent processus vaginalis, although a frank hernia may not have been evident beforehand. Strangulated inguinal hernia may occur at any time from birth onwards and is most common during the first two years of life. The high incidence of strangulation in young children is a strong argument in favour of repairing any hernia in this age group as soon as it is discovered. There is a particularly high incidence of strangulation in premature babies.

Clinical features

Classically, a mother discovers a firm lump in the groin of her crying child. He may have vomited once or twice but the diagnosis is usually made before obstruction becomes established. On examination, the child is usually well. There is an obvious, irreducible lump in the groin which may extend into the scrotum.

Management

In a typical child presenting early, the hernia is not tender or red, and there is no risk that the strangulated bowel has yet become infarcted. An initial attempt is usually made to reduce the hernia in *gallows traction* using gravity, as shown in Figure 31.6, the child being sedated with a drug such as papaveretum. If this is successful, the child is kept in hospital and elective hernia repair performed at the earliest opportunity. If conservative management fails to reduce the hernia within about six hours, or if there is any clinical evidence of bowel infarction, then operation must be performed as an emergency procedure.

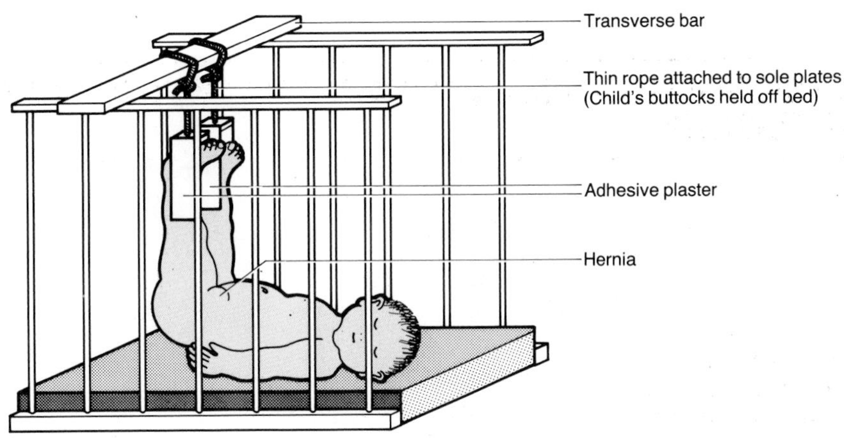

Fig. 31.6 Gallows traction for irreducible inguinal hernia

HYPERTROPHIC PYLORIC STENOSIS

Pathophysiology

This common condition of unknown aetiology nearly always presents between three and eight weeks of age. It presents with a sudden onset of complete *pyloric obstruction*. The underlying cause is marked hypertrophy of the circular muscle in the pyloric region of the stomach. The disorder occurs in about 1 in 400 normal babies and there is a male predominance of 4:1. Firstborn children are most commonly affected. Hereditary factors play a part since it is relatively common for siblings of affected children to develop the disease. It is also common for a parent or other close relative of an affected child to have had infantile pyloric stenosis.

Clinical features

Typically, the infant thrives for the first three or four weeks and then begins to vomit after every feed. The vomiting characteristically becomes *projectile*, i.e. large amounts of vomitus are hurled from the mouth rather than running down the baby's front. The vomitus is never bile-stained and this readily distinguishes pyloric stenosis from duodenal stenosis. Apart from the vomiting, the child appears well and is eager for further milk. With sustained vomiting, however, the child becomes progressively dehydrated and electrolyte depleted, and loses vigour. Examination often reveals no abdominal abnormality.

Diagnosis

The persistent vomiting leads to hospital admission, where the child's response to feeding is observed. At the same time, the abdomen is palpated. If pyloric stenosis is present, a mass about 2 cm in diameter is usually palpable deeply below the liver during the test feed. If gastric peristaltic waves are also visible through the abdominal wall, the diagnosis can be made with confidence. If the diagnosis remains in doubt, a barium meal examination will reveal complete pyloric obstruction.

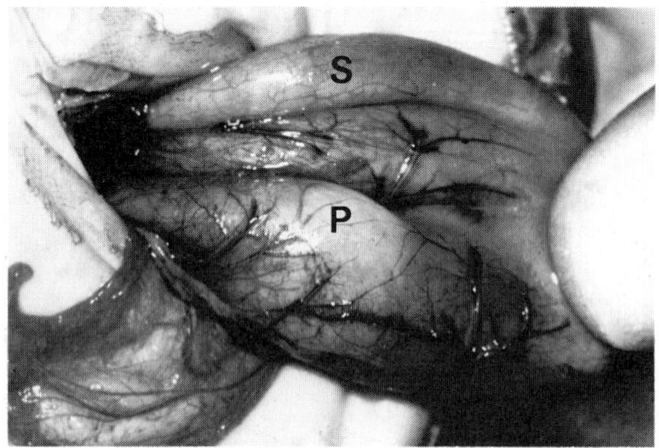

(a)

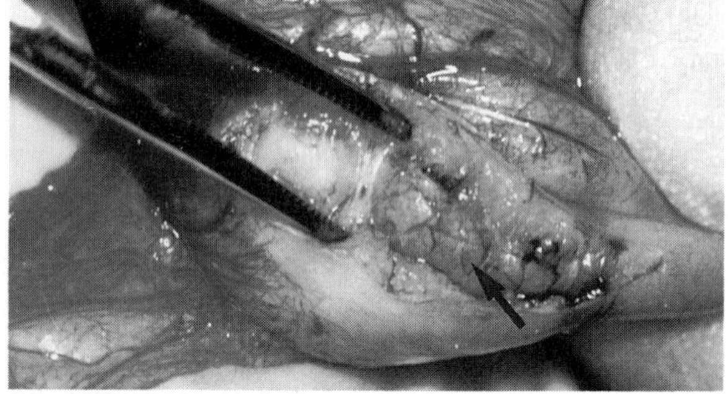

(b)

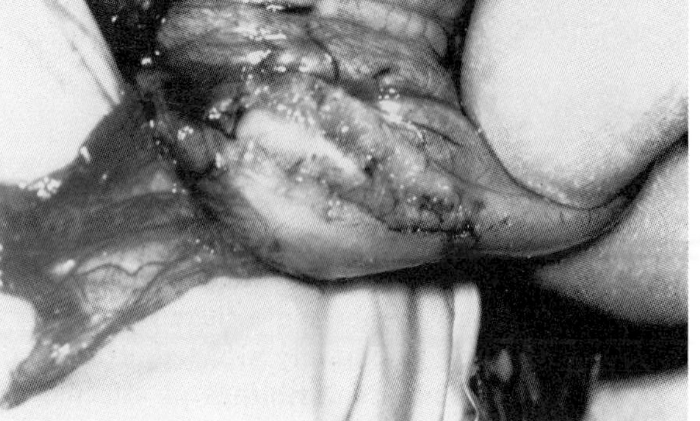

(c)

Fig. 31.7 Rammstedt's pyloromyotomy for hypertrophic pyloric stenosis

(a) A small transverse abdominal incision has been made and the stomach **S** and pyloric 'tumour' **P** delivered.
(b) The serosa over the tumour has been incised and the hypertrophic muscle split with forceps.
(c) The completed operation; the mucosa is seen bulging through the muscle split (arrowed)

Treatment is by *Rammstedt's pyloromyotomy* (see Figure 31.7). The muscle of the pylorus is split longitudinally down to but not including the mucosa; the mucosa bulges into the incision when the correct level is reached. Before operation, it is essential that any fluid and electrolyte abnormalities are corrected — the operation should only be performed on a well baby. The stomach is emptied by nasogastric aspiration and washed out with normal saline.

Postoperative recovery is rapid, and graded feeds are reintroduced over one to two days, beginning with a standard electrolyte solution.

INTUSSUSCEPTION

Pathophysiology

Intussusception is an acquired disorder most common between the ages of three months and two years. A segment of bowel becomes invaginated into the bowel immediately distal to it. The invaginated segment progressively elongates as it is propelled distally by peristalsis. *Ileo-caecal intussusception* is the most common variety. It is probably initiated by peristaltic action upon an enlarged Peyer's patch secondary to viral infection. The intussusception commonly extends well into the transverse colon and may even present at the anus.

Intussusception presents with bowel obstruction, but if untreated for more than about 10 hours, the affected segment undergoes venous infarction.

Intussusception sometimes occurs in adults, when the initiating factor is a bowel wall tumour or polyp.

Fig. 31.8

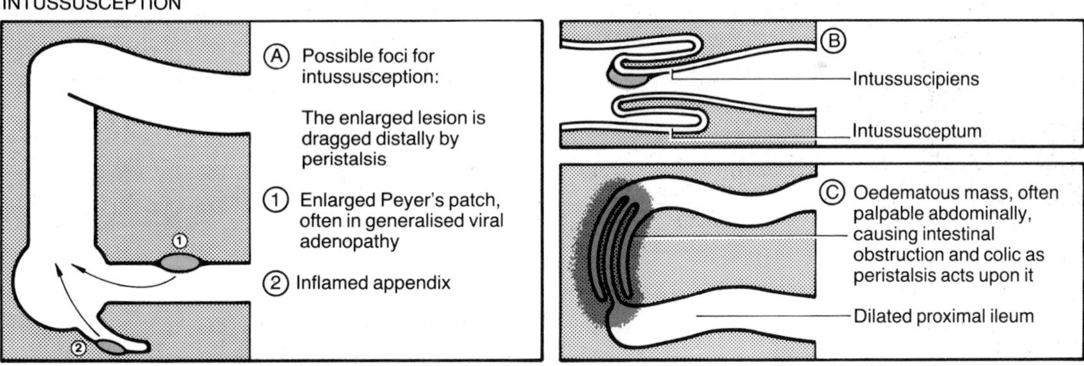

Clinical features

The classic presentation is bouts of severe colicky abdominal pain during which the child is doubled-up and screaming. These episodes are separated by periods of about an hour when the child appears entirely well. Within the first few hours, the child often passes a small amount of jelly-like blood described as *red-currant jelly stool* which is almost pathognomonic of intussusception. Vomiting begins later, consistent with the diagnosis of distal bowel obstruction.

On examination, a sausage-shaped mass is usually palpable, lying across the upper abdomen. The rectum is empty but may contain a little blood.

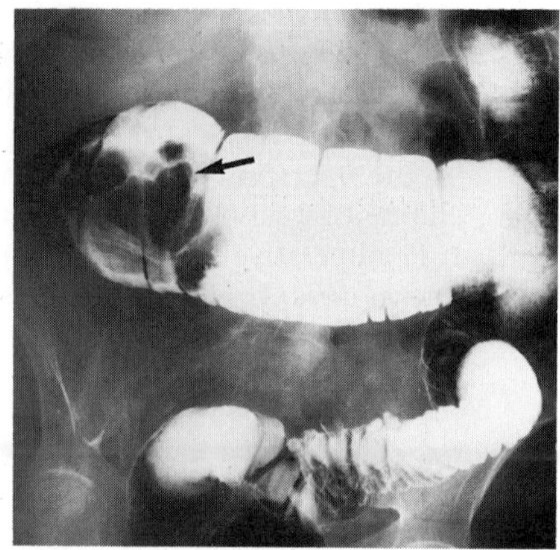

Fig. 31.9 Ileocolic-intussusception

This 2-year-old child presented as an emergency with spasms of abdominal pain, having passed 'red-currant jelly' rectally. This barium enema shows the typical appearance of large bowel obstruction by an intussusception of ileum (arrowed) which in this case has progressed to the transverse colon. The barium infusion pressure was increased, resulting in hydraulic reduction of the intussusception which did not recur

Management

If intussusception is suspected, barium enema should be performed urgently. Diagnosis is confirmed by the typical appearance shown in Figure 31.9. If gentle hydrostatic pressure is applied by elevating the bag containing barium, the intussusception may slowly reduce.

If this fails or infarction is suspected, laparotomy is performed urgently. The intussusception is reduced by gentle manipulation, and the appendix is usually removed. If the viability of the segment is in doubt, it must be resected.

SWALLOWED FOREIGN BODY

Young children examine their environment with their mouths and frequently swallow foreign bodies such as coins, safety pins, buttons or small plastic objects. The most dangerous swallowed foreign body is a small button-shaped mercury battery, because it is likely to disintegrate, releasing toxic mercury salts.

The narrowest part of the gastrointestinal tract is the cricopharyngeus sling at the upper end of the oesophagus. Foreign bodies (other than mercury batteries) that pass beyond this level are likely to pass all the way through the tract without incident. Only rarely does an object become arrested, usually in the terminal ileum or sometimes at the pylorus. Occasionally a sharp foreign body penetrates the bowel wall causing peritonitis.

Provided the child is well, management involves plain radiography which will show any metal-containing object and confirm that it is not in the bronchial tree. X-rays only need to be repeated if the foreign body has not passed spontaneously after 5 days. If the child develops abdominal pain, vomiting or bleeding, the object must be retrieved. If it is proximal to the pylorus, this may be by fibreoptic endoscopy, but if more distal, laparotomy is required. Swallowed mercury batteries are extremely dangerous and must be removed as soon as possible.

ABDOMINAL EMERGENCIES IN OLDER CHILDREN

THE ACUTE ABDOMEN

Differential diagnosis

From childhood to adolescence, acute abdominal pain is a common cause of surgical admission; usually, *appendicitis* is suspected. Appendicitis is described in detail in Chapter 14.

The major differential diagnosis is *constipation*, closely followed by *mesenteric adenitis*. The child with constipation is afebrile and systemically well. Mesenteric adenitis causes a higher fever than appendicitis, and the signs and symptoms settle quickly, usually within 24 hours. There is often a recent history of viral upper respiratory tract infection and enlarged cervical lymph nodes may be palpable.

Less commonly, acute abdominal pain in this age group is caused by a lower *urinary tract infection*, or occasionally a right lower lobe *pneumonia*. Both these diagnoses should be considered, and the urine tested. *Testicular torsion* (chapter 19) sometimes presents with just abdominal pain; the genitalia must always, therefore, be examined in boys with abdominal pain, although testicular torsion is uncommon before adolescence.

Fig. 31.10 Differential diagnosis of acute abdominal pain in pre–adolescent children

Acute appendicitis
Constipation
Mesenteric adenitis
Lower urinary tract infection
Right lower lobe pneumonia

Principles of management

If acute appendicitis is diagnosed when the child is first seen, operation should be performed without delay. More commonly, the diagnosis of appendicitis is uncertain. In these children, urinary tract infection should be excluded by urine microscopy. The child should be kept under close review, and re-examined at intervals of several hours. Soon, a worsening or improving trend will become apparent. This approach may be used both in general practice and after surgical admission. It reduces to a minimum psychological trauma and unnecessary operations, and also ensures that the diagnosis is not missed until peritonitis has become all too obvious.

NON-ACUTE ABDOMINAL PROBLEMS IN CHILDREN

Introduction

The main non-acute reasons for surgical referral in children are hernias and associated problems, abnormalities of testicular descent and foreskin problems, mainly phimosis. Less commonly, surgeons are asked to manage chronic or recurrent abdominal pain, chronic constipation, rectal bleeding, an abdominal mass or rectal prolapse. Many of these children present first to a paediatrician.

Unlike most of the acute conditions described earlier, non-acute conditions generally present across the whole age spectrum of childhood.

HERNIAS AND ASSOCIATED PROBLEMS

Persistence of the peritoneal sac associated with testicular descent causes three very common problems in boys: inguinal hernia, patent processus vaginalis and hydrocoele. These conditions all present as inguinal or scrotal swellings, usually in babies and preschool children. They are illustrated in Figure 31.11.

Inguinal hernia

Inguinal hernias in children arise because the processus vaginalis fails to close after testicular descent. They are therefore true congenital abnormalities. Anatomically, they are identical to indirect inguinal hernias in adults (see Chapter 19).

In childhood, an inguinal hernia usually presents as a lump at the external inguinal ring. The lump appears when the child cries but reduces spontaneously between times, so that when the child is seen by the surgeon, no abnormality may be detected. Most surgeons would accept a mother's history

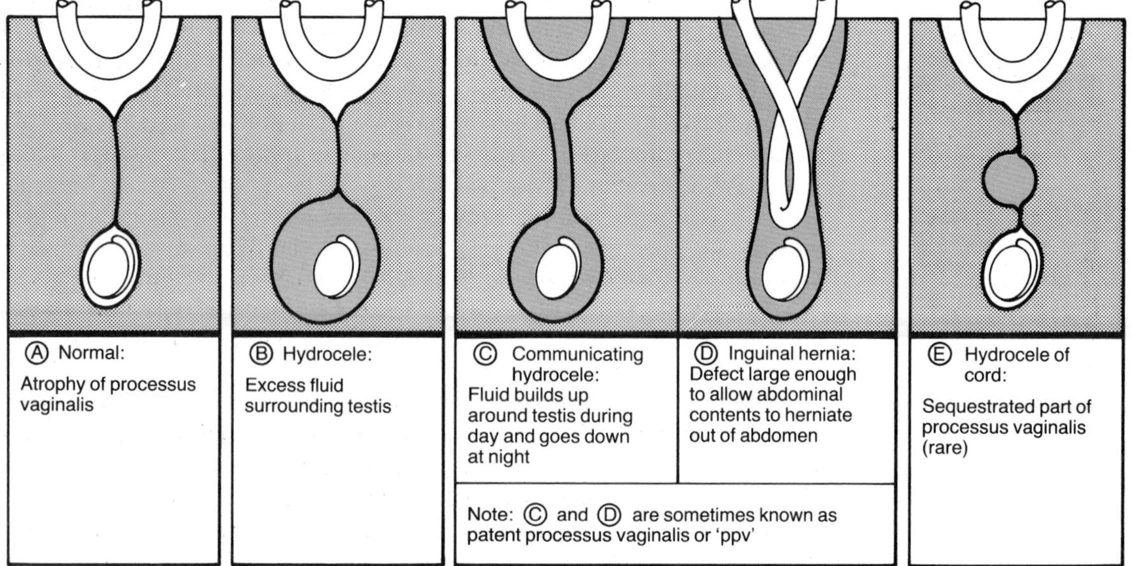

Fig. 31.11 Abnormalities associated with the processus vaginalis

of hernia even if no abnormality is found, and arrange surgical repair. Where the defect is larger, the lump is present all the time and simply expands during bouts of crying. Childhood inguinal hernias are prone to *strangulation*, when they present with pain and obstructive symptoms. Thus, inguinal hernias in children should be electively repaired without delay.

In adult inguinal hernias, a repair (*herniorrhaphy*) is necessary because an anatomical abdominal wall defect is important in the pathogenesis. In babies and children, there is no permanent abdominal wall defect and only the peritoneal sac needs to be removed (*inguinal herniotomy*).

Patent processus vaginalis

The term patent processus vaginalis should be reserved to describe a hydrocoele which communicates with the peritoneal cavity via a remnant too narrow to admit bowel. Children with these communicating hydrocoeles present with a history of scrotal swelling which increases during the day (as peritoneal fluid accumulates), and subsides during the night when the child lies flat. The condition is usually seen in toddlers up to the age of about three years.

Treatment is surgical excision of the peritoneal remnant as in herniotomy.

Infantile hydrocoele

Non-communicating hydrocoeles surrounding the testis are mostly seen in neonates and young babies. The hydrocoele results from incomplete reabsorption of fluid from within the tunica vaginalis after closure of the processus. The fluid will usually resorb slowly if untreated. Alternatively, it can be removed by needle aspiration, after which it does not recur.

Umbilical hernia

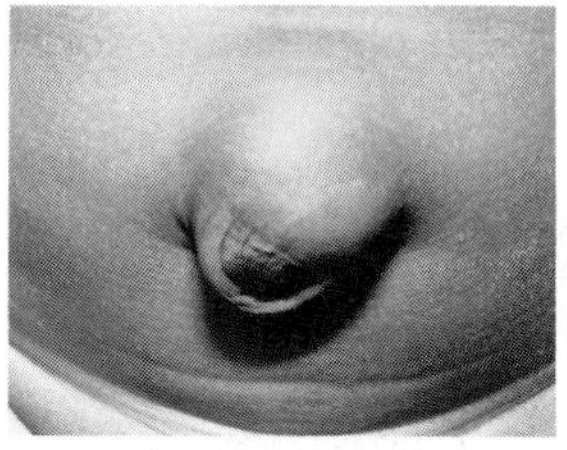

Fig. 31.12 Umbilical hernia

Many newborn babies have umbilical hernias, particularly if premature. Most will spontaneously shrink and disappear over the first year of life. Those that remain should be repaired as there is little chance of further improvement after that (see Figure 31.12). A small subumbilical incision allows emptying and ligation of the peritoneal sac and placement of a few non-absorbable repair sutures. The umbilicus is usually sutured to the repair to restore the normal recessed cosmetic appearance.

TESTICULAR MALDESCENT

In up to 4% of normal full-term newborn males, one or both testes has failed to reach the scrotum. This percentage is greatly increased with prematurity. By the age of one year, full descent will have occurred in most boys, leaving about 0.3% with maldescended testes.

Maldescent is associated with up to 30 times the normal risk of later testicular malignancy (although the risk is still small); surgical correction probably does not reduce this risk. In addition, maldescended testes tend to be subfertile and have an increased risk of traumatic injury or torsion. There is histological evidence that maldescent is often secondary to structural abnormalities of the testis.

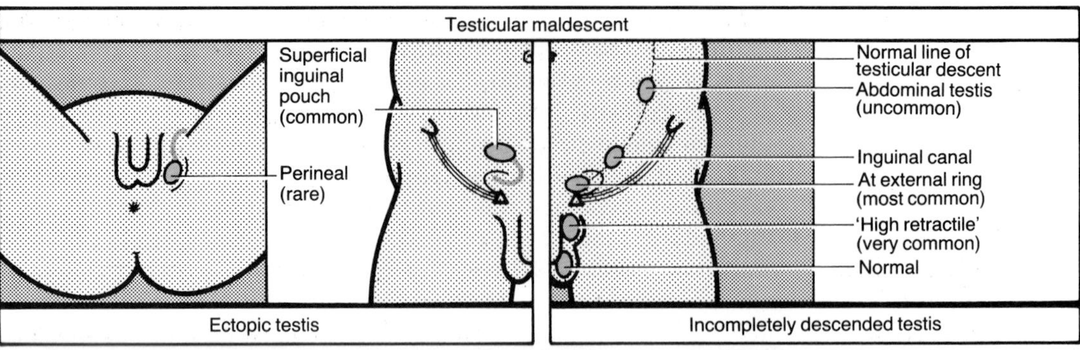

Fig. 31.13 Testicular maldescent

To minimise the risk of complications, boys are examined regularly from birth through school age to identify problems of maldescent and allow timely surgical correction (*orchidopexy*). Although orchidopexy has little influence on the predisposition to malignancy, a testicular tumour is more likely to be diagnosed early if the testis is in the scrotum. The influence of orchidopexy on fertility is probably marginal, except for any benefit gained from the cooler environment of the scrotum.

The maldescended testis may be arrested at any point on its path of descent from the posterior abdominal wall to the scrotum. Nearly all of them lie in the groin area, outside the external inguinal ring. In addition, the testis may be deflected from its normal path into the scrotum and come to lie in an ectopic position. The main sites of incomplete descent or ectopia are shown in Figure 31.13.

In most boys in whom the testis does not appear to be fully descended, the testis can be palpated in the scrotal neck and gently manipulated into its correct position. This is described as a *retractile testis* and requires no treatment; the testis become less retractile as the boy grows. Indeed, if the child is examined by the parents after a warm bath, the testis is usually fully descended.

In other boys, the testis can only be manipulated into the upper part of the scrotum. Although a small proportion of these will eventually descend completely (the 'high retractile' testis), the majority are truly incompletely descended and require surgical correction.

The optimum age for orchidopexy is debated, but the procedure is usually performed between the ages of three and eight years. The usual technique of orchidopexy involves mobilising the spermatic cord and placing the testis in a subcutaneous scrotal pouch outside the dartos muscle.

FORESKIN PROBLEMS

The foreskin is normally adherent to the glans until about the age of two years. For this reason, parents should be advised not to attempt to retract the foreskin before this age, as this may excite a fibrotic response. Some young boys develop stenos is of the preputial orifice (*phimosis*), probably due to a combination of recurrent low-grade balanoposthitis, chronic ammoniacal inflammation and ill-judged attempts at retraction by the parents.

Phimosis presents with chronic foreskin irritation or 'spraying' on micturition, often accompanied by 'ballooning' of the foreskin. There is often a recent history suggestive of acute balanoposthitis.

Most boys with phimosis require circumcision (described in Chapter 19). Attempts to dilate the phimosis are usually unsuccessful as this causes further scarring and rapid relapse.

Paraphimosis (see Chapter 19) sometimes occurs in children especially if there is a degree of phimosis. This causes the foreskin to become trapped in the coronal sulcus after the foreskin is retracted.

CHRONIC AND RECURRENT ABDOMINAL PAIN

Chronic or recurrent abdominal pain is a common problem in children of school age but in most, no cause is discovered and the problem gradually resolves; these children are often managed by paediatricians. The main organic causes are summarised in Figure 31.14, but psychological factors are fairly common and should not be overlooked (*periodic syndrome*).

Fig. 31.14 Organic causes of chronic or recurrent abdominal pain in children

Chronic constipation — common
Hydronephrosis — uncommon
Recurrent appendicitis — rare
Crohn's disease — rare
Gall stones — rare, sometimes associated with haemolytic anaemia
Peptic ulceration — rare

Chronic constipation

Chronic constipation is among the most common abdominal problems in children; it may present as *faecal soiling*, i.e. faecal overflow incontinence. In most children, the aetiology is unknown, but the condition usually responds to simple measures like a high fibre diet, regular attempts at defecation and, if necessary, a small daily dose of a laxative (lactulose or senna derivative). The problem should not be neglected as it may otherwise lead to lifelong problems. A tiny proportion of children with severe constipation have ultrashort segment Hirschsprung's disease as described earlier.

RECTAL BLEEDING

Rectal bleeding is a common problem in childhood, but is rarely caused by tumour or haemorrhoids. The usual causes in children are shown in Figure 31.15.

Fig. 31.15 Main causes of rectal bleeding in childhood

Anal fissure
Rectal polyps
Meckel's diverticulum

Anal fissure

Anal fissure occurs at any age during infancy and childhood and is probably initiated by straining to pass a large hard stool. The condition is readily diagnosed when digital rectal examination is found to be impossible because of extreme tenderness; the outer end of the fissure may sometimes be seen by parting the buttocks. Treatment involves gentle anal dilatation under general anaesthesia, followed by measures to prevent constipation.

Rectal polyps

Adenomatous polyps are a common cause of rectal bleeding in children. They may be single or multiple and usually occur in the rectum or sigmoid colon. They also occur elsewhere in the colon, and occasionally in the small intestine. Rectal polyps in children are almost never malignant.

Rectal bleeding is investigated as for adults, with digital examination followed by proctoscopy and sigmoidoscopy. If a polyp is seen, it is removed by diathermy snare. If no polyp is visible, barium enema is performed and any identified polyps removed later using fibreoptic colonoscopy.

Meckel's diverticulum

A Meckel's diverticulum is present in less than 2% of the population. It represents the embryological remnant of the *vitello-intestinal duct* which joined the fetal midgut and yolk sac. The diverticulum is situated on the anti-mesenteric border of the distal ileum about 60 cms from the ileocaecal junction. Meckel's diverticula are usually asymptomatic but may cause rectal bleeding or become inflamed and perforate.

Meckel's diverticula often contain a variety of gut-related tissues. These include *ectopic acid-secreting gastric mucosa*, which may cause peptic ulceration. In children below two years, this is an important cause of rectal bleeding. In older children, the ectopic gastric mucosa more often causes chronic occult bleeding, leading to iron deficiency anaemia. Much less commonly, peptic ulceration in a Meckel's diverticulum results in *perforation*.

If a Meckel's diverticulum is suspected as the cause of rectal bleeding, an attempt is made to confirm the diagnosis by radioisotope Meckel's scanning. An isotope is chosen which is concentrated in gastric mucosa. A negative scan does not, however, exclude the diagnosis, and laparotomy may have to be performed to examine the bowel directly.

If the neck is narrow, a Meckel's diverticulum may become inflamed in a manner identical to appendicitis, and cause similar symptoms and signs (see Figure 14.6). The diagnosis is only made at operation. As for appendicitis, the complications of gangrenous inflammation are perforation and peritonitis. Unlike the complications of peptic ulceration and bleeding, Meckel's diverticulitis is uncommon in children under ten years of age. The condition occurs in older children, adolescents and young adults.

RECTAL PROLAPSE

Transient rectal prolapse is a common and alarming childhood problem, usually occurring during the first two years of life. The most common cause is excessive straining during defecation, but it may be a presenting feature of cystic fibrosis. The majority of prolapses can be gently manipulated back into position without causing pain and will not recur if the stool is kept soft. If the problem is persistent or recurrent, proctoscopy and sigmoidoscopy are indicated. A rectal polyp is occasionally responsible, and can be removed by diathermy snare. If simple stool-softening measures fail to prevent recurrence, submucosal injections of phenol in oil are used to induce fibrosis. In the rare event of this failing, a perianal subcutaneous suture may be inserted.

ABDOMINAL MASS

An abdominal mass is an uncommon reason for surgical referral in children. It may be caused by a malignant embryonal tumour, most often a Wilm's tumour. Other causes include hydronephrosis and post-traumatic pancreatic pseudocyst.

Wilms' tumour

Wilms' tumour presents in early childhood, usually before the age of three years. The tumour arises in the kidney from embryonal renal tissue, hence the term *nephroblastoma*. The tumours are locally invasive and metastasise to the regional nodes, liver, lungs and bone. Often, a large abdominal mass is noticed by the mother as she bathes the child (see Figure 31.16). The mass is sometimes so large as to obscure its side of origin. Less common presenting features include haematuria, anorexia, weight loss, pyrexia and hypertension.

When surgery was the only treatment available, the cure rate was only about 10%. The modern combination of surgical resection, radiotherapy and chemotherapy, gives an excellent chance of complete cure even when distant metastases are present.

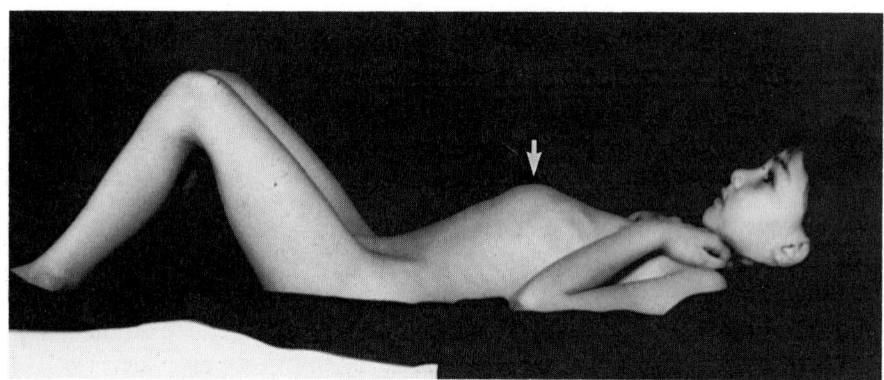

Fig. 31.16 Wilms' tumour
This 9-year-old girl presented with a large unilateral abdominal mass (arrowed), which was later confirmed to be arising from the left kidney (Wilms' tumour or nephroblastoma)

Neuroblastoma

Another embryonal tumour occurring in early childhood is the neuroblastoma. This is a highly malignant tumour arising from embryonal sympathetic nervous tissue in the adrenal gland or sympathetic chain. A less aggressive variant is the *ganglioneuroblastoma*. This tumour sometimes presents as an abdominal mass but the usual presentation is failure to thrive. The standard treatment is a combination of surgical resection, chemotherapy and radiotherapy, but the prognosis is poor.

UROLOGICAL DISORDERS IN CHILDREN

Introduction

All of the important urological disorders in children have a congenital origin, although not all congenital disorders of the urinary system present in childhood. The congenital urinary tract disorders and their clinical presentations are illustrated in Figure 31.17 and the important remediable disorders are described below.

Fig. 31.17 Congenital abnormalities of the urinary system (conditions presenting at birth or in childhood are highlighted)

NATURE OF ABNORMALITY	PRESENTATION
a) Kidney	
Bilateral agenesis (Potter's syndrome)	Oligohydramnios in pregnancy, still-born infant with characteristic appearance of face and ears
Unilateral agenesis, aplasia or hypoplasia	Usually an incidental finding at any age. There is often some abnormality on the other side
Multicystic kidney: usually unilateral dysplasia of kidney with multiple cysts	Usually presents in the neonate as an abdominal mass. Fatal if bilateral
Infantile polycystic disease: bilateral inherited disorder in which multiple small cysts replace renal parenchyma. Liver and pancreatic lesions also occur	Usually presents as gross abdominal distension in the neonate due to huge non–functioning kidneys; fatal
Medullary sponge kidney: cystic dilatation of collecting ducts of at least one medullary pyramid in one or both kidneys	May be found incidentally or as the cause of recurrent infection. Cysts usually become calcified and have a characteristic X–ray appearance.
Adult polycystic kidney: autosomal dominant disorder with multiple cysts throughout the renal parenchyma	Usually presents after age 30 with chronic renal failure, hypertension, haematuria or predisposition to infection
Solitary cysts: usually develop at one pole	Often incidental finding. May present with loin swelling or pain
Horseshoe kidney : fusion of lower poles of kidneys preventing their normal developmental ascent	Often found incidentally but may cause hydronephrosis due to pelvi–ureteric obstruction
Ectopic kidneys and rotational abnormalities due to failure of developmental ascent	Found incidentally or due to complications such as pelvi–ureteric obstruction

b) Pelvicalyceal system and ureters	
Pelvic hydronephrosis : dilatation of pelvicalyceal system due to congenital stenosis at pelvi–ureteric junction	Usually presents in childhood with loin pain or mass
Megaureter: abnormality of peristalsis of lower ureter resulting in gross proximal dilatation	Presents in young children with recurrent urinary tract infection to which it strongly predisposes
Ureterocoele: cystic dilatation of intravesical part of ureter due to stenosis of ureteric orifice	Often incidental finding. May cause infection or obstruction
Vesico–ureteric reflux : unilateral or bilateral abnormality of ureteric insertion into bladder	Presents in children as recurrent pyelonephritis which can severely damage the developing kidney
Duplex systems : partial or complete duplication of a ureter	Often incidental finding. May predispose to infection
Ectopic ureter : ureter does not open into the bladder but rather into some other part of the genital tract e.g. vagina	In females presents as dribbling incontinence but in males predisposition to infection
c) Bladder and urethra	
Agenesis of bladder : associated with other major abnormalities of genitourinary system	Present at birth and often fatal; very rare
Urachal abnormalities — cyst, sinus, patent urachus : due to persistence of urachal remnants	Patent urachus usually presents in childhood with urine dribbling from umbilicus. Cysts and sinuses may present in adulthood. Adenocarcinoma sometimes develops in urachal remnant in apex of bladder
Bladder diverticulum : forms by herniation of mucosa through defect in muscular wall. May be secondary to urethral valves	Usually presents as recurrent urinary tract infection
Bladder exstrophy : incomplete closure of lower abdominal wall in midline	Gross abnormality of genitourinary system obvious at birth
Urethral valves : usually occur in posterior urethra causing varying degrees of obstruction. Less obstructive valves may occur more distally	Severe cases present in the neonate with gross obstruction, renal failure and infection. Milder cases present later as recurrent urinary tract infection
Epispadias: urethral meatus located in abnormal position somewhere on dorsum of penis. Often associated with major abnormality of penis	Obvious at birth
Hypospadias : urethra opens in abnormal position on ventral aspect of penis due to defective fusion of urethral folds	Major cases obvious at birth. Minor cases have downward deviation of urinary stream and sometimes a degree of chordee

VESICO-URETERIC REFLUX

As described in detail in Chapter 24 and elsewhere, anatomical and functional abnormalities of the urinary tract strongly predispose to urinary tract infections. This is particularly true in children, where the commonest abnormality is *vesico-ureteric reflux*. For this reason, a single bacteriologically-proven urinary tract infection in a boy, and two or more in a girl, are indications for radiological or nuclear medicine investigation. Indeed, between 30 and 50% of children so investigated are found to have vesico-ureteric reflux.

Pathophysiology

In the normal, the distal ureter takes an oblique course through the muscular bladder wall, so that detrusor contraction during voiding acts as a sphincter, preventing reflux of urine from the bladder up the ureters (the *anti-reflux mechanism*). Vesico-ureteric reflux most commonly results from a minor congenital (often familial) abnormality of ureteric insertion, but may also be caused by other morphological abnormalities such as ectopic or duplex ureters, congenital megaureter (a peristaltic abnormality), bladder outlet obstruction, neuropathic bladder, and previous surgical procedures to the lower end of the ureter.

Reflux of sterile urine into the pelvicalyceal system during early childhood probably causes impairment of normal renal development and function. This is exacerbated by rises in back-pressure and greatly enhanced by bacterial infection, possibly even a single episode. Vesico-ureteric reflux of grade I and II (see Figure 31.18) appears to cause little damage but grades III and IV are associated with radiological 'clubbing' and distortion of calyces, and patchy loss of renal cortical substance; this is known as *reflux nephropathy*. Untreated reflux nephropathy may cause progressive irreversible renal damage, and if bilateral, may eventually result in renal failure.

Clinical presentation and investigation

Children of any age may present with isolated or recurrent upper urinary tract infections. Girls are more prone to infection than boys because of their short urethra and its proximity to the anus. Infants or young children with urinary tract infections may not exhibit symptoms and signs specific to the urinary tract and the diagnosis is often made on investigation of vomiting, fever or failure to thrive. Older children more typically suffer incontinence, frequency or dysuria or abdominal pain and tenderness.

Clinical examination seeks evidence of abnormal external genitalia, spina bifida and impaired perineal innervation (perineal sensation and anal sphincter tone).

Fig. 31.18 Grades of vesico-ureteric reflux on micturating cystography

Grade I — reflux into lower ureter only on micturition

Grade II — reflux into renal pelvis on micturition but no ureteric dilatation

Grade III — constant reflux into renal pelvis but no ureteric dilatation

Grade IV — constant reflux into renal pelvis with ureteric dilatation

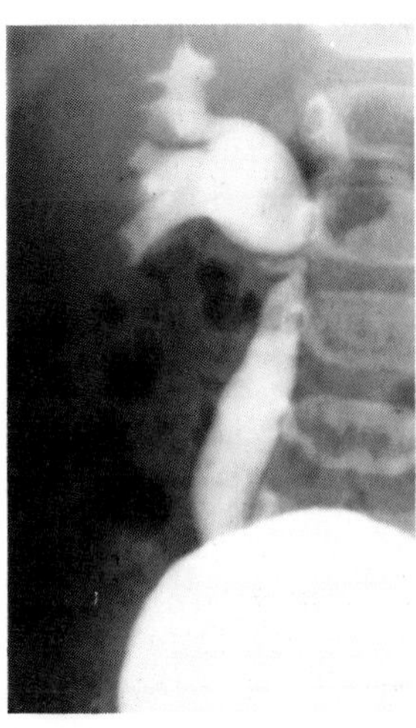

Fig. 31.19 Vesico-ureteric reflux

Micturating cysto-urethrogram (MCU) in a child with recurrent urinary tract infections. On voiding, the right ureter and pelvicalyceal system filled with contrast. This is defined as grade IV reflux

To demonstrate reflux, two methods can be used: micturating cystography or isotope cystography. *Micturating cystography* (Figure 31.19) is the standard investigation, and involves injecting contrast medium into the bladder via a urinary catheter. The catheter is then removed and X-rays are taken while the child voids urine. The radiological grades of reflux severity are shown in Figure 31.18 and provide a useful guide to the likelihood of future renal damage. More recently, static and dynamic *isotope studies* have been introduced, particularly for screening children suspected of reflux and for long term follow-up of children known to reflux. Isotope studies also provide additional information. DMSA, bound to renal tubules, demonstrates cortical scarring, whilst DTPA estimates glomerular filtration rate in each kidney (differential function) and reveals sites of urinary tract obstruction.

Management of vesico-ureteric reflux

If there are no other anatomical abnormalities and the ureter is not dilated (i.e. grades I and II), then there is an 85% chance of spontaneous resolution of vesico-ureteric reflux as the child grows. In the meantime, the urinary tract must be kept free of infection. This is done by encouraging regular voiding and a high fluid intake, avoiding constipation and maintaining perineal hygiene. At the same time, the child is maintained on continuous antibacterial chemotherapy (such as co-trimoxazole) until the danger of reflux is past. The child is followed up regularly, charting the progress of growth and development, blood pressure and serum creatinine. Radiography or isotope investigation of the urinary tract is repeated annually.

Surgical correction is required for more severe reflux and dilated ureters (i.e. grades III and IV) and for other obvious anatomical abnormalities. Surgery is also indicated for children who fail to progress on conservative management. The operations for simple reflux aim to re-implant the ureter in the bladder wall so that a length of it lies deep to the bladder mucosa; this is compressed flat by intraluminal pressure during voiding, thus restoring an anti-reflux mechanism.

If there is no renal scarring, the child can be discharged from follow up. If there is unilateral scarring, the blood pressure should be monitored long-term because of the risk of hypertension. If both kidneys are damaged, renal function must be monitored as well because of the risk of deterioration.

PELVI-URETERIC JUNCTION OBSTRUCTION

Pathophysiology

Obstruction at the pelvi-ureteric junction (PUJ) may present at any age from birth through to the end of the fourth decade. It presents with dilatation of the renal pelvis and calyces (*hydronephrosis*). The cause of obstruction may not be physical narrowing but instead a functional abnormality of the 'sphincter' mechanism. This normally prevents reflux of ureteric urine into the kidney when the ureters contract.

Obstruction at the PUJ increases the pressure in the collecting system and gradually causes deterioration in renal function. Stasis predisposes to infection.

Clinical presentation and diagnosis

Many patients with PUJ obstruction go undetected. Many others are discovered by chance on urography during investigation of an unrelated condition. Even in symptomatic patients, the condition may be intermittent. Some patients complain of aching pain in the renal area; others suffer bouts of severe abdominal or loin pain, sometimes with haematuria. The precipitating factor is often not identifiable, but symptoms are sometimes exacerbated by drinking large volumes of fluid, or by changes in posture.

In many patients, the diagnosis can be made on a standard IVU. The typical changes on the affected side are a prolonged nephrogram and a negative pyelogram (i.e. contrast persists in the renal cortex without opacifying the pelvis), delayed drainage of contrast from an often dilated renal pelvis, or a combination of these features. The only reliable sign, however, is spontaneous extravasation of contrast into parenchymal lymphatics. This is seen as 'contrast streaking' in the renal cortex.

A dilated renal pelvis on a standard urogram may just represent harmless stasis without obstruction, and diagnostic features of PUJ obtruction may become apparent only if a diuretic is given at the same time. A *radioisotope diuretic renogram* is a better way of distinguishing between simple stasis and stasis with obstruction: a characteristic isotope excretion curve is seen in about 80% of PUJ obstructions. The remainder are difficult to diagnose, requiring percutaneous intubation of the renal pelvis and sophisticated pressure and flow measurements (*the Whittaker test*).

Management

If PUJ obstruction is proved in symptomatic patients, particularly if renal function is impaired, operative treatment is required. The aim is to enlarge the pelvi-ureteric junction; this is known as *pyeloplasty*. Results are generally favourable but recovery of renal function may be incomplete.

HYPOSPADIAS AND EPISPADIAS

Hypospadias is a common congenital abnormality of the penis and urethra. It occurs in about 1 in 400 male births. The distal urethra fails to develop normally, so that the urethral meatus lies somewhere along the ventral surface of the penis from the glans to the perineum (see Figure 31.20). The remnant

Fig. 31.20 Hypospadias

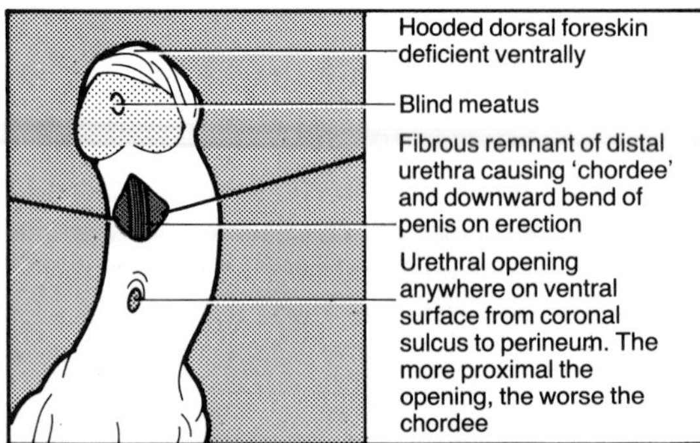

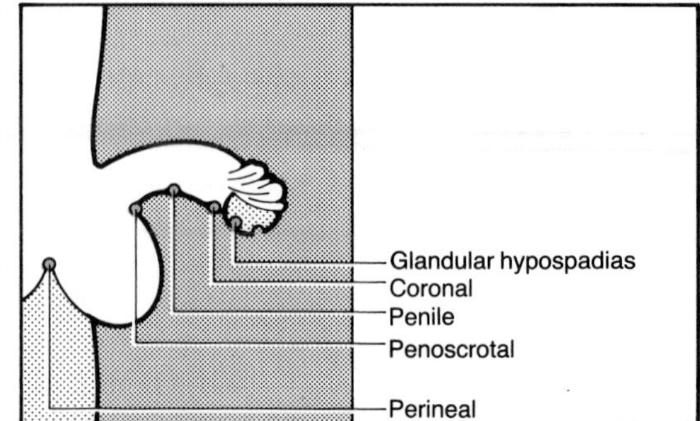

of urethral tissue distal to the meatus is fibrotic causing the penis to bend downwards on erection. This is known as *chordee*. The more proximal the urethral meatus, the worse the chordee. In addition, the ventral part of the foreskin is absent giving rise to a hooded appearance.

Repair is a highly specialised procedure and utilises the hood of foreskin. Thus circumcision should never be carried out without specialist advice.

Epispadias is much less common and may be associated with other major-genitourinary abnormalities. In epispadias, the urethral meatus is on the dorsal aspect of the penis.

URETHRAL VALVES

Urethral valves are congenital mucosal folds which may occur in the posterior male urethra. They impede or completely obstruct urinary flow. Complete obstruction becomes apparent soon after birth but partial obstruction may easily be overlooked. In either case, the back-pressure effects on the urinary tract soon lead to renal failure. Treatment is by endoscopic division of the valves as soon as possible.

PART IV
MANAGEMENT PROBLEMS OF SURGICAL IN-PATIENTS

32 MEDICAL PROBLEMS IN SURGICAL PATIENTS

Introduction

'Medical' disorders appear in surgical practice in four main ways:

- A pre-existing medical condition may cause a surgical admission because of progression, exacerbation or complications (e.g. foot problems in diabetics)
- A surgical condition may be complicated by an unrelated medical disorder. For example, a patient with rheumatoid arthritis on steroid therapy is vulnerable to impaired healing and recurrent infection
- A pre-existing medical condition can be exacerbated by operation. In chronic bronchitis, for example, general anaesthesia and postoperative sputum retention may precipitate a life-threatening chest infection
- An occult condition can become manifest under the stress of anaesthesia and operation. For example, postoperative myocardial infarction may result from coronary atherosclerosis

CARDIO-VASCULAR DISORDERS

Many surgical patients are elderly and are suffering with cardiovascular disorders. Together with respiratory disorders, cardiovascular disease accounts for the bulk of postoperative medical complications. Atherosclerosis is the commonest cause of cardiovascular diseases complicating surgery.

There are six main categories of cardiovascular disorder (although more than one may occur in the same patient):

- Ischaemic heart disease
- Cardiac failure
- Arrhythmias
- Hypertension
- Cerebrovascular disease
- Peripheral arterial disease

Emergency surgery in cardiac patients is about four times more likely to result in death than if the same operation is done electively. Thus, preoperative assessment and planning is vital for these patients.

1. Ischaemic heart disease

The most common manifestations of ischaemic heart disease are:

- Angina and previous myocardial infarction
- Cardiac failure
- Arrhythmias such as atrial fibrillation

Asymptomatic myocardial ischaemia may progress to infarction under the various stresses of anaesthesia and operation. These stresses include laryngoscopy and endotracheal intubation, excess pain, hypoxia, rapid blood loss, anaemia, hypotension, hypocarbia and fluid overload. For major operations, general anaesthesia and spinal anaesthesia carry similar risks; for minor procedures, local anaesthesia is far safer.

Clinical problems

a. Angina

Stable angina poses little increased risk during operation, but unstable angina is as dangerous as recent myocardial infarction. Nitrites, which dilate the coronary arteries and reduce preload and left ventricular work, protect the heart from hypoxia during general anaesthesia and should not be stopped in the perioperative period. A transdermal patch is a safe alternative to oral tablets. Beta adrenergic blockers, which reduce cardiac work and oxygen demand, should be continued unless cardiac failure develops.

b. Previous infarction

The risk of reinfarction associated with operation is about 6%. This is increased to about 30% if an operation is performed during the first three months of recovery. At six months the risk is 10–15 % which may be acceptable for important elective surgery. If reinfarction occurs in association with surgery, the risk of death is much greater than at other times. Thus, surgery after a heart attack should be postponed as long as possible.

Myocardial infarction associated with surgery usually occurs during the first postoperative week, not during the operation. Infarction may present with acute hypotension, cardiac failure, arrhythmia or cardiac arrest; pain is not always a feature. Diagnosis can usually be made by typical ECG changes, especially if a preoperative ECG is available. Serum enzyme levels are not always reliable because enzymes which rise after myocardial infarction, e.g. creatine kinase (CK) and lactate dehydrogenase (LDH), are also released by surgically damaged skeletal muscle. Measurement of cardiospecific isoenzymes (CK-MB and LD-1) will aid diagnosis.

Preoperative assessment of ischaemic heart disease

When taking a cardiac history, it is well worth asking specifically about previous myocardial infarction. Exercise tolerance should also be detailed, perhaps with the help of a physiotherapist, who can walk the patient around the hospital and up and down the stairs.

An ECG should be performed preoperatively on all patients over 60 years of age and on any patient with cardiac symptoms or signs. Preoperative ECGs may show arrhythmias, ischaemic changes, or evidence of previous infarction. They are also worth their weight in gold during the 3 a.m. assessment of a postoperative patient with chest pain!

2. Cardiac failure

The common causes of cardiac failure are ischaemic heart disease and hypertension. Less common causes include valvular disease, arrhythmias, thyrotoxicosis and severe anaemia (high output failure). Symptoms of cardiac failure include dyspnoea, tiredness and weakness, and loss of appetite. Signs include dependent oedema, raised venous pressure, tachycardia and peripheral cyanosis. Even if cardiac failure is stabilised preoperatively, there is still a mortality rate of 5%.

Clinical problems

a. Treated cardiac failure

Treatment is often inadequate and if so, must be corrected before operation. Plasma urea, electrolytes and creatinine should be measured preoperatively because patients taking diuretics may have abnormalities of fluid and electrolytes such as chronic dehydration or hypokalaemia.

Overtreatment with diuretics may cause:

- Thirst
- Postural hypotension
- Low plasma sodium concentration
- Raised plasma urea and creatinine
- Low plasma potassium (usually due to potassium-losing diuretics prescribed without potassium supplements)

b. Cardiac failure discovered preoperatively

Operation should be postponed until cardiac failure is treated and stabilised. Hasty preoperative diuretic therapy is dangerous because it may induce dehydration and electrolyte abnormalities. Vasodilatation caused by general anaesthesia reduces the plasma volume and lowers the blood pressure. This may precipitate acute myocardial infarction or a cerebrovascular accident.

c. Cardiac failure developing during or after operation

This problem most often results from poor tolerance of intravenous fluids, or unaccustomed supine posture. Prompt and vigorous diuretic therapy with intravenous frusemide is required to prevent worsening cardiac failure, hypoxia, chest infection, renal failure or other potentially lethal complications. Postoperative cardiac failure is best managed in an intensive care unit, using a CVP line to guide fluid replacement. In severe cases, a Swann-Ganz catheter should be used to monitor left atrial pressure. Perioperative cardiac failure may also be precipitated by myocardial infarction.

Preoperative assessment of cardiac failure

Chest X-ray will demonstrate cardiomegaly and may show signs of pulmonary oedema. These include upper lobe diversion, hilar congestion, septal Kerley B lines and pleural effusions. ECG may show evidence of arrhythmia, ischaemia or ventricular hypertrophy. If there is any doubt about the fitness of a patient for operation, a cardiological opinion should be sought.

3. Cardiac arrhythmias

Clinical problems

a. Atrial fibrillation

This is usually secondary to ischaemic heart disease but may be caused by mitral valve disease or thyrotoxicosis. Atrial fibrillation with a controlled ventricular rate (i.e. a normal pulse rate) causes minimal extra risk. Uncontrolled fibrillation may cause perioperative cardiac failure. It also increases the risk of arterial embolism from the left atrium. Adequate control should be achieved before operation with digoxin, occasionally supplemented with verapamil or beta-adrenergic blockers. Digoxin can be given intravenously if rapid control is necessary.

The therapeutic range of digoxin is narrow. Toxicity occurs if the dose is excessive or if renal excretion is impaired by chronic renal failure. The elderly are particularly prone to digoxin toxicity. Symptoms include anorexia, nausea and vomiting, which may be wrongly attributed to the operation. Assessment of patients on digoxin should include tests of renal function (plasma urea, electrolytes and creatinine), and if toxicity is suspected, digoxin levels.

b. Tachycardia

Postoperative sinus tachycardias are usually associated with hypotension, sepsis, cardiac failure, fluid overload, anxiety, or occasionally, thyrotoxicosis. Tachycardia may be the first sign of any of these problems. Primary cardiac abnormalities or phaeochromocytoma must be considered if the cause of tachycardia during operation is not apparent.

c. Bradycardia

Bradycardia is usually caused by heart block and the specific type can be determined by ECG. Single bundle branch block is usually innocent, but bifascicular block, in which conduction is impaired down two of the three main fascicles (right bundle plus anterior or posterior divisions of the left bundle) may progress to complete heart block (and low cardiac output) under anaesthesia. For these patients, a prophylactic temporary transvenous pacemaker should be inserted before operation.

Excessive digoxin may cause bradycardia. If the apex rate is below 60 beats per minute, that day's dose should be omitted and the regular dose reviewed.

A temporary or permanent cardiac pacemaker is not a problem for general anaesthesia. A surgical diathermy machine, if used too close to the control box, however, may induce a serious arrhythmia.

d. Arrhythmias developing during general anaesthesia

Significant arrhythmias develop under general anaesthesia in about 5% of patients. They can be precipitated by hypoxia, hypercapnia and hypo- or hyperkalaemia. Inadequately treated cardiac failure also predisposes to atrial arrhythmias. Preoperative investigations include ECG, full blood count, plasma electrolytes and digoxin level if appropriate.

4. Hypertension

About one in four patients coming to surgery are either hypertensive or receiving antihypertensive therapy. Most have essential hypertension, but other causes include oral contraceptives, renal parenchymal disease, renal artery stenosis or phaeochromocytoma.

Clinical problems

a. Mild to moderate essential hypertension

Patients with a systolic pressure less than 160–180 mm Hg and a diastolic less than 110 mm Hg are at minimal risk of cardiac complications unless there is some other cardiovascular disease. Sometimes, anxiety about the operation contributes to the hypertension and the blood pressure falls with preoperative bed rest. A labile blood pressure may, however, indicate widespread atherosclerosis. In younger patients with high blood pressure in this range, treatment is probably desirable, and non-urgent surgery should be postponed until the blood pressure can be stabilised at a lower level.

b. Treated hypertension

Diuretic therapy may cause fluid and electrolyte abnormalities. These should be corrected preoperatively. Most common antihypertensive drugs are cardioprotective and should not usually be stopped prior to general anaesthesia. These drugs include beta blockers, calcium antagonists, angiotensin converting enzyme inhibitors, vasodilators and methyl dopa. Postural hypotension may occur postoperatively, especially if there are associated problems of dehydration, fluid overload or anaemia.

Despite the patient being 'nil by mouth' in the immediate preoperative period, the normal dose of oral antihypertensive drugs should usually be given with a small amount of water. Sudden withdrawal of hypotensive drugs may cause dangerous rebound autonomic hyperactivity and lability of blood pressure for up to three days.

c. Severe or poorly controlled hypertension

These patients are at high risk of perioperative cardiac failure or stroke, particularly if there are swings of blood pressure. Unrecognised phaeochromocytoma may also cause uncontrollable cardiovascular abnormalities during anaesthesia and has a high mortality rate. Severely hypertensive or poorly controlled hypertensive patients should not undergo general anaesthesia and surgery until adequately treated.

Preoperative assessment of hypertensive patients

Chest X-ray may identify cardiomegaly or cardiac failure. An ECG may reveal signs of ventricular hypertrophy and ischaemia. Plasma urea and electrolytes should be measured in all patients on diuretics and in any patient with suspected chronic renal failure. It may be necessary to admit a severely hypertensive patient to hospital several days before operation to monitor the blood pressure before therapy and to establish the patient on a suitable antihypertensive regimen.

5. Cerebrovascular disease

Atherosclerosis of the cerebral vasculature may render the blood flow to the brain precarious. These patients have a high risk of stroke during the perioperative period from hypoxia, hypotension or increased blood viscosity secondary to dehydration. Cerebrovascular disease should be suspected if there is a history of stroke, transient ischaemic attacks (TIA) or senile dementia. Patients with ischaemic heart disease or peripheral vascular disease should also be assumed to have cerebrovascular disease.

The main surgical problems relate to patients who have had a previous stroke or who give a history of transient ischaemic attacks. An asymptomatic carotid bruit discovered on preoperative examination is a separate problem. In the UK, management is conservative, but in the USA, a prophylactic carotid endarterectomy is often performed.

If possible, operation should be avoided for at least two months after a stroke. Other than that, there are very few specific measures which will reduce cerebrovascular complications, although there are good theoretical reasons for prescribing low dose aspirin (75 mg daily) to inhibit platelet aggregation. The anaesthetist should be warned of any signs or symptoms suggestive of carotid artery disease so that special care can be taken to avoid hypotension during surgery.

6. Valvular disease

The common valvular abnormalities are listed here in decreasing order of frequency: mitral regurgitation, aortic stenosis, aortic regurgitation and mitral stenosis. Any may dangerously alter cardiovascular dynamics, but stenotic lesions are more serious than regurgitant ones.

Under perioperative stress, valvular disease may precipitate acute myocardial ischaemia, hypotension, cardiac failure, arrhythmias or thromboembolism. Valvular heart disease also predisposes to infective endocarditis. Thus certain operations need to be covered by antibiotic prophylaxis.

Aortic stenosis is the most serious valvular disease in a surgical patient because it limits cardiac output. The patient may already be functioning close to the limit with little reserve. Aortic stenosis usually occurs in the elderly and must be distinguished from the innocent flow murmur of aortic sclerosis, which is more common.

Clinical signs of aortic stenosis are:

- Slow rising upstroke of carotid pulse
- Hyperdynamic apex beat indicating left ventricular hypertrophy. (Note: the apex beat is only displaced laterally if aortic stenosis is complicated by cardiac failure)
- A systolic murmur radiating into the neck
- Left ventricular hypertrophy on ECG
- Valve calcification on chest X-ray (cardiac diameter is only increased if there is cardiac failure)

Clinical problems

a. History of rheumatic heart disease without significant symptoms or signs

The patient may or may not have a cardiac murmur, but when a murmur is present, this has often been assessed previously and any functional deficit documented. If not, specialist preoperative cardiological assessment is essential. In most patients, there is no special risk for general anaesthesia or surgery but antibiotic prophylaxis must be considered.

b. Murmur found at preoperative examination without a history of rheumatic fever, or symptoms or signs of rheumatic heart disease

This may be an innocent flow murmur, as in aortic sclerosis of the elderly, or may indicate a hyperdynamic circulation associated with anxiety or pregnancy. If there is doubt about the innocence of the murmur, a specialist opinion should be obtained. Operation may have to be deferred.

c. Symptomatic valvular disease

These conditions are potentially dangerous and require full preoperative assessment and treatment. Major valvular heart disease may be discovered in recent immigrants from undeveloped countries where rheumatic heart disease is prevalent. Patients with valvular heart disease undergoing general anaesthesia require monitoring of cardiac function during operation and probably intensive care afterwards.

d. Prosthetic valves

Replacement valves carry the greatest risk of infective endocarditis. For these patients, antibiotic prophylaxis is required for most invasive procedures.

Patients with some mechanical valves (such as the ball and cage type) are usually maintained on permanent oral warfarin anticoagulation. The more recent flap type of valve may not require anticoagulation but antiplatelet therapy is often used. Either treatment may predispose to operative bleeding but it is not usually advisable to stop treatment for the necessary two or three weeks before operation for fear of thrombotic valve complications.

Antiplatelet therapy is usually continued unaltered, but anticoagulation is often reduced; for many operations it is safe to continue warfarin therapy at a slightly lower level.

If much bleeding is anticipated, some surgeons stop warfarin two days preoperatively and substitute intravenous heparin. For patients with mitral valve prostheses, where the risk of thrombosis is high, full heparinisation is carefully maintained throughout the operative period. For other patients, heparin can be stopped twelve hours preoperatively and restarted once the danger of bleeding is over. The advantage of heparin over warfarin is that its effect can be reversed quickly with protamine if bleeding is excessive.

Infective endocarditis and indications for antibiotic prophylaxis

When blood is forced under pressure through a narrow orifice, laminar flow is disrupted, and eddy currents predispose to local thrombus formation. Thrombi may build up on damaged valve leaflets or the margins of a ventricular septal defect, for example, and then be colonised by circulating bacteria. This causes infective endocarditis. The left side of the heart is much more susceptible than the right because of the higher pressure and consequently greater potential for turbulence.

Gram positive cocci, especially *Strep. viridans*, are the most common causative organisms. Other bacteria such as coliforms, or fungi such as *Candida*, may also be responsible. Many types of operation and some invasive investigations cause a transient bacteraemia. Although the incidence of infective endocarditis following such procedures is small, the consequences may be catastrophic. The efficacy of prophylactic antibiotics is not absolutely proved, but it is all that is available. The relative risks associated with various cardiac and valvular lesions are summarised in Figure 32.1. The procedures most likely to cause bacteraemia are shown in Figure 32.2.

Fig. 32.1 Cardiovascular lesions at risk of infective endocarditis and indications for perioperative antibiotic prophylaxis

1. High risk conditions requiring prophylaxis
Prosthetic valve or other intracardiac surgery
Rheumatic valve disease
Congenital heart disease and aortic coarctation, whether or not corrected (Note: atrial septal defect is not a high risk)
Degenerative valve disease
Previous infective endocarditis

2. Low risk conditions — need for prophylaxis depends on likelihood of the operative procedure inducing a bacteraemia
Mitral valve prolapse
Haemodialysis shunts
Transvenous pacemakers
Ventriculo-atrial or ventriculo-peritoneal shunts for hydrocephalus

3. Minimal risk conditions not requiring antibiotic prophylaxis
Coronary bypass grafts
Closed patent ductus arteriosus
Closed atrial septal defect

Fig. 32.2 Procedures frequently associated with bacteraemia and requiring antibiotic cover in patients at risk of bacterial endocarditis

Surgical operations
Dental extractions and other procedures involving the gums
Tonsillectomy
Oesophageal dilatation
All gastrointestinal and biliary tract surgery
Most urological procedures including endoscopy, catheter insertion and removal, transrectal prostatic biopsy
Hysterectomy, dilatation and curettage, termination of pregnancy
Surgery of infected wounds and tissues
Cardiac surgery

Other procedures
Sigmoidoscopy, colonoscopy, barium enema and liver biopsy — prophylaxis is only required for patients with prosthetic heart valves

The choice of prophylactic antibiotics and the dose regimen depends on the anticipated organisms and the operative procedure. Recommendations vary between hospitals. Local bacteriology specialists may be consulted or a regimen from a national therapeutic publication such as the British National Formulary can be used.

RESPIRATORY DISEASES

Respiratory complications occur in up to 15% of surgical patients and are the leading cause of postoperative mortality in the elderly. The main postoperative complications are atelectasis, chest infection, aspiration pneumonitis and pneumonia. The risk of a respiratory complication is associated with the length of the anaesthetic. It is greatly increased by pre-existing respiratory disease like chronic airflow limitation, asthma or bronchiectasis. Other important factors include smoking, cardiac failure, obesity, old age and general debility.

Clinical problems

a. Chronic airflow limitation (chronic obstructive airways disease)

Chronic bronchitis and emphysema are common. They strongly predispose to postoperative chest complications, particularly bronchopneumonia, lobar collapse and pneumothorax. There is often a degree of reversible bronchoconstriction, and this can be assessed preoperatively by measuring expiratory peak flow before and after treatment with a bronchodilator.

Other chronic lung diseases include bronchiectasis, pneumoconiosis, pulmonary fibrosis, sarcoidosis and pulmonary tuberculosis.

The complication rate in chronic lung diseases can be greatly improved by careful preoperative assessment (including lung function tests) and treatment designed to bring the patient into optimum physical condition.

b. Cigarette smoking

Smokers have a five times greater risk of postoperative respiratory problems. This is partly due to pre-existing respiratory disease attributable to smoking. Smoking should be stopped at least four weeks before operation if any benefit is to be achieved. This gives time for recovery of respiratory functions such as bronchial ciliary activity. Stopping smoking just before surgery may actually be detrimental because of an increase in bronchial mucus production.

c. Current respiratory infections

Acute viral or bacterial upper respiratory tract infections are common in preoperative patients. The main question is whether the operation should be deferred. Patients with significant upper respiratory infections have reduced resistance to surgical trauma and infection. This alone may be grounds for cancelling an elective operation.

In children there is a particularly high risk of acute airways obstruction because of swelling of the bronchial mucosa in the narrow airways, and also because of increased secretions. This may result in lobar collapse or bronchopneumonia. There is also an element of bronchospasm in childhood infections which, when added to the already narrowed airways, leads to a difficult and dangerous anaesthetic. A 'wet' cough with a wheeze and a fever is an indication for cancelling the operation until normal function is recovered. Similar factors apply in adults but to a lesser extent.

Chronic conditions associated with infection such as bronchiectasis and cystic fibrosis are more difficult problems. Elective operations should be carried out during periods of remission, with intensive physiotherapy and prophylactic antibiotics perioperatively.

d. Asthma

Asthma is common in children and adolescents but may occur later in life as a component of chronic airflow limitation. The main elements of asthma are bronchoconstriction, bronchial wall oedema, excessive mucus production and airway plugging. All these factors predispose to atelectasis and infection.

Asthmatic problems can be exacerbated by the following factors associated with general anaesthesia and surgery:

- Endotracheal intubation
- Use of inhalational anaesthetic agents, e.g. nitrous oxide (halothane is less irritant)
- Dehydration (increases mucus viscosity)
- Limitation of movement and posture because of pain (inhibits clearance of secretions)
- The effects of certain drugs, e.g. beta blockers (may induce severe bronchospasm) or morphine (respiratory depressant)

In asthmatic patients, the usual medication should be continued in the perioperative period. Operation should be postponed during acute exacerbations.

e. *Previous chest problems*

A previous spontaneous pneumothorax may recur during anaesthesia or in the postoperative period. If respiratory function deteriorates postoperatively, the diagnosis of pneumothorax must be considered.

Previous chest surgery or radiotherapy increases the risk of postoperative infection. Physiotherapy before and after operation minimises the risk and should be arranged routinely for these patients.

f. *Previous pulmonary embolus or deep venous thrombosis*

These patients have a greatly increased risk of recurrent thromboembolism. Prophylactic measures are mandatory for all but the most minor procedures.

Preoperative investigation of respiratory disease

A chest X-ray should be performed on any patient with symptoms or signs of chest disease or dysfunction. There is no need to take 'routine' chest X-rays on all preoperative patients. Studies have shown that undirected screening of asymptomatic patients has an extremely low yield of abnormalities which are likely to influence surgical outcome.

Appropriate lung function tests, such as exercise spirometry, should be performed in patients with chronic lung disease. Peak flow measurements are useful to determine the extent of airflow limitation. The reversible element of bronchospasm can be assessed using peak flows before and after bronchodilators. Blood gas measurements are indicated if hypoxaemia or carbon dioxide retention is likely.

Perioperative management of respiratory disease and high risk patients

The following measures will maximise respiratory function and reduce the risk of postoperative complications:

- *Preoperative physiotherapy* — helps to prevent postoperative chest complications. Physiotherapy should include teaching the patient breathing exercises and correct posture

- *Drug therapy* — may need to be adjusted to achieve the optimum respiratory function. Theophyllines may be added to the therapy of asthma patients, for example, and nebulised salbutamol may improve the reversible component of chronic bronchitis. Prophylactic antibiotics are not commonly used for patients with chronic airflow limitation, but their prophylactic use in abdominal surgery may have the additional benefit of reducing infective chest complications. Preoperative bronchodilators given by inhaler or nebuliser may help to prevent an exacerbation of asthma perioperatively. Adequate hydration reduces the risk of retained secretions which might cause airways obstruction

- *Smokers* — should be encouraged to stop smoking from the time of booking for elective surgery. Smoking should be stopped at least four weeks preoperatively to achieve the optimum beneficial effect

- *Alternative methods of anaesthesia* — local, regional or spinal anaesthesia should be considered for patients with chronic respiratory disorders, but they are not necessarily the best solution. Physiotherapy and other supportive measures should be the same as for general anaesthesia. With the use of newer anaesthetic drugs and techniques, these patients may be better off with endotracheal intubation and ventilation using short-acting muscle relaxants. These techniques allow good bronchial toilet at the end of operation. In some patients, the respiratory function is better after the operation than before! Certain operations, such as transurethral resection of the prostate, are made more difficult under spinal anaesthesia if a patient with chest trouble coughs persistently during the procedure. General anaesthesia avoids this.

- *Early postoperative physiotherapy* — aims to enhance deep breathing, coughing and general mobility, greatly reducing the incidence of respiratory complications

- *Patients on long-term steroid therapy for airways obstruction* — need perioperative administration of intravenous steroids

GASTRO-INTESTINAL DISORDERS

The main gastrointestinal conditions giving rise to complications in surgical patients are dental problems, peptic ulcer disease and inflammatory bowel diseases. Previous abdominal surgery may also complicate inpatient treatment.

1. Dental problems

Teeth and artificial fixed crowns and bridges are vulnerable to damage during intubation. This causes not only cosmetic and medicolegal problems, but also exposes the patient to the risk of aspirating foreign bodies into the bronchi. Similarly, infected material from carious (decayed) teeth or inflamed gums may be aspirated. This causes a particularly grave aspiration pneumonia. Dentures should routinely be removed before operation for the same reason. In unconscious accident victims, the possibility of aspiration, swallowing or pharyngeal obstruction by a dental prosthesis should always be considered.

2. Peptic ulcer disease

Peptic ulcer disease can be a surgical problem in its own right, but surgical patients admitted for other reasons may also have an active peptic ulcer. Whether the ulcer is causing symptoms or not, it may be exacerbated by the stresses of surgical admission. These stresses include serious illness and trauma, operations, and drugs such as aspirin, non-steroidal anti-inflammatory drugs (NSAIDs) and corticosteroids. The result may be a sudden catastrophic haemorrhage (presenting as haematemesis or melaena), or occasionally perforation. Bleeding or perforation may also result from *acute stress ulceration* in the seriously ill patient. Stress ulceration is independent of chronic peptic ulcer disease, but acid-pepsin does play a part in its pathogenesis (see Chapter 9).

Patients with known peptic ulcer disease or strongly suggestive symptoms, should receive perioperative prophylaxis with H_2 receptor antagonists. Irritant drugs should be avoided.

Previous gastrectomy is associated with a number of long-term side effects. These include anaemia (due to deficiency of iron, vitamin B_{12} and occasionally folate) and rarely, osteomalacia. A full blood count should be included in the preoperative assessment of these patients.

3. Inflammatory bowel disease

Patients with chronic inflammatory bowel disease may be anaemic or malnourished if the disease is active. Patients may also be steroid dependent because of adrenal suppression from long-term steroid therapy. Occasionally immunosuppressive drugs such as azathioprine are being taken by the patient and may predispose to infection.

4. Previous abdominal surgery

Previous abdominal surgery results in scarring and sometimes multiple adhesions in the peritoneal cavity. Further operations on the same area are more difficult and take longer. In addition, there is greater risk of damage to structures which are adherent to the operation site. These include gut, ureters and major vessels.

LIVER DISORDERS

Pre-existing liver disease may have important consequences in the surgical patient and generally increases the risk of postoperative morbidity and mortality. A history of jaundice must be evaluated as it may be a clue to serious risks for both patient and medical staff.

Clinical problems

a. History of jaundice

A past history of jaundice suggests that the patient may be a carrier of hepatitis. Hepatitis B, (and non-A non-B hepatitis), is easily transmitted to surgical, nursing and laboratory staff. The main danger is from needle-stick injuries. Vaccination against hepatitis B is now recommended for health workers at occupational risk of infection. Hepatitis carriers among patients must be identified and special precautions adopted.

Most previously jaundiced patients will have suffered infective hepatitis (hepatitis A). There is little risk to staff because the infective agent disappears. In contrast, hepatitis B or hepatitis non-A non-B, is often carried for life. These diseases should be suspected if the illness associated with the previous jaundice was prolonged or serious. Jaundice contracted in underdeveloped countries should be regarded with suspicion because hepatitis B is often endemic. Hepatitis B is also common among male homosexuals. Drug addicts, who often share injection syringes, are at particular risk. Dishevelled, unkempt patients are particularly likely to be hepatitis carriers. Examination of these patients should include searching for intravenous injection sites which are characteristic of drug abuse. In high risk patients, screening should be performed for the surface antigen of the virus (HbsAg) before any other blood test.

b. History of jaundice following anaesthesia

The anaesthetic agent halothane is believed to cause an idiosyncratic hepatotoxicity in about 1 in 30 000 patients. The existence of this condition is, however, disputed by many doctors. It remains prudent however, to record exposure to halothane when jaundice occurs days or weeks after operation. Suspicion of previous halothane induced jaundice should be reported to the anaesthetist so the drug can be avoided. Further exposure to halothane may produce a more serious and more rapidly developing response.

c. Presence of obstructive jaundice

Surgery in this situation is usually being performed to relieve the obstruction. This carries a number of special risks which are described in Chapter 6. They include cholangitis, clotting disorders, deep vein thrombosis and acute renal failure.

d. The patient with known hepatitis

Patients with any form of hepatitis, whether viral or alcoholic, tolerate general anaesthesia and surgery very badly. The mortality risk is at least 30%. Surgery should be avoided unless absolutely essential. Gamma glutaryl transferase level is a fairly good indicator of excessive alcohol intake. Mean corpuscular volume (MCV) may also be raised, and should alert the doctor to the possibility of concealed alcoholism.

e. The patient with known cirrhosis

Patients with cirrhosis have a very high risk of perioperative morbidity and mortality. The main factors are:

- Anaemia
- Portal hypertension
- Defective synthesis of clotting factors
- Malnutrition
- Electrolyte disturbances (particularly hyponatraemia, hypokalaemia and metabolic alkalosis)
- Defective energy metabolism (gluconeogenesis and glycogenolysis)
- Abnormal drug metabolism
- Ascites

The main postoperative complications of cirrhosis are excessive bleeding, defective wound healing and susceptibility to infection.

Excessive bleeding results from several factors:

- Defective synthesis of clotting factors (all but factor VIII are synthesised in the liver)
- Thrombocytopenia (due to hypersplenism and depressed platelet production)
- Abnormal polymerisation of fibrin
- Portal hypertension (greatly expanded intra-abdominal venous network under high pressure). This, together with numerous vascular adhesions, makes dissection tedious, difficult and bloody

Portal hypertension may initially be discovered because of ascites or an acute upper gastrointestinal haemorrhage. (Note that only about half of such bleeding episodes in patients with portal hypertension are due to oesophageal varices. The rest are largely caused by peptic ulcer disease). If a patient with known oesophageal varices requires an operation, preoperative endoscopic assessment and injection with sclerosants may be appropriate.

Preoperative assessment and management of liver disease

Patients with liver disease should initially be tested for HBsAg (hepatitis viral surface antigen). Further blood tests should include full blood count, clotting screen and platelet count, plasma urea and electrolytes, bilirubin, transaminases, calcium, phosphate and gamma glutaryl transferase.

If prothrombin time is prolonged, vitamin K injections are given for several days preoperatively. If this fails to correct the abnormal clotting (as in severe hepatic impairment), fresh frozen plasma is given during the operation. If the patient is thrombocytopenic, platelet transfusion is also required.

RENAL DISORDERS

Chronic renal failure (CRF) is commonly encountered in general surgical patients. It is characterised by impaired homeostasis of fluid and electrolytes and impaired excretion of nitrogenous compounds. The risk of perioperative complications increases with the degree of renal failure. Patients can be divided into two groups, i.e. mild chronic renal failure, and moderate-to-severe chronic renal failure. Acute renal failure is usually a postoperative complication and is therefore described in the next chapter. Patients with pre-existing renal disease are particularly vulnerable to acute renal failure.

Clinical problems

a. Mild chronic renal failure

This is common in the elderly and is often associated with hypertension. The main management problem in surgical patients is impaired metabolism or excretion of drugs. Such drugs must therefore be given in smaller doses, calculated from charts supplied by the manufacturer. In practice, digoxin and gentamicin pose the main problem. Digoxin dosage is adjusted according to blood levels, measured 6 or more hours after the last dose. Gentamicin dosage is titrated according to blood levels measured immediately pre-dose and then 15 minutes after intravenous administration (or one hour after intramuscular administration).

Fluid and electrolyte homeostasis need not be a special problem in mild chronic renal failure provided fluid balance is carefully monitored in the perioperative period. Monitoring should include regular checks of plasma urea, electrolytes and creatinine, especially if the patient is receiving diuretic therapy.

Even mild renal failure implies a drastic reduction in renal reserve. Major reconstructive surgery to the abdominal aorta may interfere with normal renal function because of aortic cross-clamping near the renal arteries. This is exacerbated by transient hypotension caused by blood loss. The lack of renal reserve in these patients may progress to acute renal failure. Thus, renal function must be properly assessed before these operations by measuring plasma urea and creatinine. If these are abnormal, renal arteriography may be needed to exclude renal artery stenosis. In addition, special precautions must be taken during anaesthesia and surgery to avoid precipitating acute renal failure.

b. Moderate-to-severe chronic renal failure (CRF)

These patients are usually under the care of specialist physicians who should be involved in perioperative management. Patients may be receiving regular haemodialysis or ambulatory peritoneal dialysis; in such patients, surgery is usually for renal transplantation.

The main perioperative problems of severe chronic renal failure are:

- *Fluid overload* — this is caused by impaired fluid homeostasis and may require correction with diuretics and fluid retention. Fluid requirements in the perioperative period may be difficult to assess. They are best controlled by monitoring central venous pressure in an intensive care unit

- *Regulation of serum tonicity* — this is disordered in patients with severe chronic renal failure who are particularly vulnerable to hypo- and hypernatraemia. Care must be taken that the sodium content of intravenous fluids is appropriate for the individual

- *Hyperkalaemia* — this is a particular risk of advanced CRF. Patients with lesser degrees of CRF are vulnerable to rapid potassium shifts (due to transfusion, tissue damage or hypoxia) or changes in glomerular filtration rate (caused by cardiac failure or hypotension). Hyperkalaemia increases cardiac irritability and the risk of fatal arrhythmias. To minimise this risk, the preoperative plasma potassium level should ideally be stabilised below 5.0 mmol/l

- *Metabolic acidosis* — this tends to develop in moderate or severe CRF but it is usually compensated by chronic hyperventilation. This compensation is easily disrupted by general anaesthesia. It may also be disrupted by additional metabolic acidosis due to tissue ischaemia or general hypoxia

- *Chronic normochromic normocytic anaemia* — results from decreased erythropoietin production in CRF. Cardiovascular function is usually well adapted to this anaemia and preoperative transfusion should be avoided. Transfusion adds the further risks of precipitating fluid and electrolyte problems, and complicating tissue typing for future kidney transplantation. (Nonetheless, there is evidence that multiple blood transfusions reduce the rejection rate of renal transplants.)

Preoperative assessment

Hydration should be assessed by looking for clinical evidence of dehydration or fluid overload (skin turgor and jugular venous pressure). Plasma urea, electrolytes, creatinine and bicarbonate should be checked for abnormalities. Full blood count is checked for anaemia.

DIABETES MELLITUS

Diabetic patients are at special risk from general anaesthesia and surgery. Firstly, diabetics are predisposed to many medical disorders associated with a higher risk of perioperative complications. These are summarised in Figure 32.3. Secondly, stress (including surgery, trauma and infections) causes

Fig. 32.3 Special perioperative problems in diabetic patients

1. **Predisposition to ischaemic heart disease** — greater risk of postoperative myocardial infarction which has higher mortality in diabetics (infarction may be 'silent' due to autonomic neuropathy)
2. **Predisposition to diabetic nephropathy** — tendency to chronic renal failure
3. **Predisposition to peripheral vascular disease** — greater risk of perioperative strokes and lower limb ischaemia
4. **Predisposition to heel pressure sores**, especially if there is peripheral neuropathy
5. **Increased incidence of postoperative infection** in the wound, chest or urinary tract
6. **Obesity** (particularly common in maturity onset diabetes) is associated with increased operative morbidity
7. **Increased danger of cardiac arrest** due to autonomic neuropathy

increased production of catabolic hormones which oppose the action of insulin (see Chapter 1). This makes diabetic control more difficult. Thirdly, general anaesthesia, surgery and postoperative vomiting disrupt the delicate balance between dietary intake, exercise (energy utilisation) and diabetic therapy. Fourthly, diabetic ketoacidosis may cause an elevated leucocyte count and increased amylase level, which may confuse the diagnosis of an acute abdomen. Indeed, hyperglycaemia may sometimes present with abdominal pain. Fifthly, infection may not cause a pyrexia in a diabetic patient; thus infection may go undetected as the cause of deterioration.

Clinical problems

For the purposes of perioperative management, diabetics fall into three groups according to their diabetic therapy: insulin dependent, taking oral hypoglycaemic medications, or diet-controlled. Preoperative assessment should include evaluation of current diabetic control by serial blood glucose measurements. Cardiovascular and renal complications should be routinely screened by ECG and plasma urea and electrolyte estimations.

Perioperative management should attempt to maintain blood glucose level somewhere between 4 and 10 mmol/l. It is particularly important to avoid rapid swings which might result in acute hypoglycaemia. Surgery should be deferred if the blood glucose cannot be stabilised below 13 mmol/l. Above this level, there is an unacceptable risk of ketoacidosis or a hyperosmolar non-ketotic state.

a. Insulin-dependent diabetics

There are no hard and fast rules for managing these diabetics perioperatively but the general principles are:

- Establish good diabetic control preoperatively
- Give insulin as a continuous intravenous infusion during the operative period
- Give an infusion of dextrose (glucose) throughout the operative period to balance the insulin given and to make up for loss of dietary intake
- Add potassium to the dextrose infusion
- Monitor blood glucose and electrolytes 2–4 hourly throughout the operative and early postoperative period

A typical management protocol is given in Figure 32.4 and a recommended insulin infusion regimen in Figure 32.5. The key to successful management of diabetes is titrating the dose of insulin against frequent measurement of blood glucose. Finger-prick tests on the ward are adequate provided they are performed correctly by properly trained staff. The insulin dose is adjusted hourly according to the blood sugar results.

b. Diabetics controlled on oral hypoglycaemic drugs

Many of these patients are receiving short acting sulphonylureas such as glipizide or tolbutamide. Patients on long-acting drugs such as clorpropamide or

Fig. 32.4 Perioperative management of insulin-dependent diabetes

Preoperatively
1. Admit to hospital two to three days before operation
2. Establish good preoperative control — a twice daily mixture of short- and intermediate-acting insulin is usually adequate. If not, extra doses of short-acting insulin can be added
3. Monitor blood glucose throughout the day, e.g. before and after meals and at bed time
4. Plan the operation for as early as possible on the appointed day

Operation day
1. Starve from midnight and omit first dose of insulin
2. Check blood glucose and electrolytes before operating list commences — postpone if glucose level greater than 13 mmol/l or electrolyte abnormalities are found
3. Commence intravenous dextrose and insulin infusions
4. Check blood glucose and electrolytes at conclusion of operation (or at one to two hour intervals in a long operation)
5. Adjust concentration of infusions and rate of administration as required

Postoperatively
1. Check glucose 2 to 4 hourly and electrolytes 6 to 12 hourly and adjust infusion as indicated
2. Continue infusion until full oral diet is established, then reintroduce subcutaneous insulin, following the preoperative regimen

Fig. 32.5 Perioperative management of diabetics using insulin infusion

1. Intravenous 5% or 10% glucose infusion at 125 ml per hour
2. Constant pump-controlled intravenous soluble insulin infusion. This is adjusted according to 2–4 hourly blood glucose estimations
3. If there is a need to limit fluids, use 20% dextrose solution and infuse at 50 ml per hour

metformin (or both), should be changed several days before operation to a short-acting sulphonylurea. If this fails to provide adequate control, an insulin regimen can be used as above.

On the morning of the operation, the patient is starved in the usual manner and the short-acting sulphonylurea omitted. These drugs are reintroduced when oral intake is resumed. Blood glucose should be monitored regularly as for insulin dependent patients because it may still reach unacceptable levels, despite the lack of carbohydrate intake. If glucose rises above 13 mmol/l, it can be controlled by small subcutaneous doses of short-acting insulin, e.g. 6 units of soluble insulin. If a major operation is planned or if postoperative 'nil-by-mouth' is likely to be prolonged, it is best to use insulin and glucose infusions as for insulin-dependent diabetics.

c. Diabetics controlled by diet alone

These patients require no special perioperative measures if preoperative control is adequate. These patients cannot become hypoglycaemic and blood glucose rarely drifts above acceptable levels. All postoperative urine specimens should be tested for glucose and ketones as a precaution.

d. Diabetics poorly controlled on emergency admission

Any diabetic patient may be out of control on admission, particularly if admitted as an emergency. Uncontrolled diabetes may be due to infection or vomiting. The diabetes must first be brought under control with infusions of insulin, glucose and potassium. Rehydration will also be required before operation can proceed.

e. Abdominal pain and vomiting in a diabetic child

This often indicates diabetic ketoacidosis rather than an acute abdomen. If so, symptoms resolve when diabetic control is re-established by rehydration and insulin therapy. As a general rule, the vomiting precedes the abdominal pain in diabetic ketoacidosis, whereas the opposite occurs in an acute abdomen. **It must be reiterated that emergency laparotomy in an uncontrolled diabetic is extremely dangerous and must be avoided at all costs**. Conversely, an acute abdomen may precipitate diabetic ketoacidosis. If the abdominal symptoms fail to respond to diabetic therapy, a diagnosis of acute abdomen must be reconsidered.

THYROID DISEASE

1. Thyrotoxicosis

Surgery in untreated thyrotoxicosis carries a risk of thyrotoxic crisis. This has a mortality of at least 40%! In surgery for thyrotoxicosis, the patient should be rendered euthyroid preoperatively using antithyroid drugs or beta-adrenoceptor blockers. Beta blockers rapidly control the cardiovascular effects of thyrotoxicosis and can be used for urgent preoperative preparation. A thyrotoxic crisis may also occur if an undiagnosed thyrotoxic patient has an operation for another reason. Any patient with symptoms or signs of thyrotoxicosis should have a serum thyroxine estimation included in the preoperative assessment. If the patient has recently commenced carbimazole, a leucocyte count should be performed to check for neutropenia.

2. Hypothyroidism

Untreated hypothyroid patients are at moderate risk when undergoing surgery. They are more sensitive to CNS depressants and have a decreased cardiovascular reserve. They are also susceptible to electrolyte disorders. Severe infection, especially accompanied by trauma, a cold environment or depressant drugs, may precipitate myxoedema coma which is often fatal.

Hypothyroidism is common, particularly in women, and increases with age. Many patients are maintained on replacement therapy and are at no special risk. Patients previously treated for thyrotoxicosis may become insidiously hypothyroid. Symptoms and signs of hypothyroidism include weight gain, bradycardia, psychomotor depression, thinning eyebrows, coarse hair and skin, chronic constipation and hoarse voice.

If there is clinical suspicion of hypothyroidism, operation should be postponed and thyroid function checked by measuring T4 and TSH levels. If hypothyroidism is diagnosed, oral replacement therapy is commenced. If surgery must be performed urgently, it is usually best to proceed with the operation and begin oral treatment later.

DISORDERS OF ADRENAL FUNCTION

1. Adrenal insufficiency

The most common cause of adrenal insufficiency is hypothalamo-pituitary-adrenal suppression by long-term steroid therapy. It is occasionally caused by primary adrenal failure (Addison's disease) or pituitary ablation (due to tumour or surgery). Very rarely, it results from previous adrenalectomy. This may have been carried out for palliation of breast cancer, treatment for a hypersecretion syndrome, or primary surgery for an adrenal tumour.

In primary or secondary adrenal failure, the patient is usually already on oral steroid replacement therapy. In any case, the adrenals are unable to respond to the stress of trauma, surgery or infection, which would normally lead to increased secretion of glucocorticoids. The lack of adrenal response in these patients may cause acute postoperative cardiovascular collapse with hypotension and shock (*Addisonian crisis*).

Perioperative 'steroid cover'

Patients with potential adrenal insufficiency must be given 'steroid cover' during the perioperative period. This is usually in the form of intravenous hydrocortisone e.g. 100–200 mg prior to the operation, and 100 mg daily until recovery. It is better to give prophylactic hydrocortisone in doubtful cases than risk acute hypo-adrenalism. For any steroid-dependent patient, a doctor should write clearly in the notes 'Treat any unexplained collapse with hydrocortisone'.

2. Cushing's syndrome

Cushing's syndrome results from excess secretion of cortisol. This may be in response to excess ACTH secretion by a pituitary tumour. Occasionally, it is due to ectopic ACTH secretion (usually by a malignant tumour) and rarely due to a primary tumour of the adrenal. Clinically the patient may be plethoric, moon-faced, hypertensive and obese with abdominal striae. There may be a characteristic 'buffalo hump'. The most common cause of Cushingoid features is long-term steroid therapy for conditions such as rheumatoid arthritis or asthma. The main surgical problems in Cushingoid patients are hypertension, poor wound healing, infection and peptic ulceration. If the condition is due to steroid therapy, there is an additional risk of secondary adrenal insufficiency.

3. Phaeochromocytoma

Phaeochromocytoma is rare, and is usually diagnosed during investigation of paroxysmal hypertension. Sometimes, a phaeochromocytoma is discovered after wild swings of blood pressure are encountered during an operation. Phaeochromocytomas are usually located in the adrenal medulla but can occur retroperitoneally in embryological remnants of the organ of Zuckercandl. Diagnosis is made by finding high levels of catecholamine metabolites such as *vanillyl mandelic acid (VMA)* in the urine. Nowadays, the tumour is usually localised by CT scanning.

In the surgical management of phaeochromocytoma, there are two main problems: to control dangerous rises in blood pressure during operation, and to prevent hypotension afterwards. The former is caused by handling the tumour which increases catecholamine release, while the latter is the effect of chronic hypovolaemia. Hypovolaemia results from the high levels of circulating catecholamines before operation, which rapidly fall once the tumour is removed. Management involves gradual preoperative control of hypertension with alpha-adrenergic blocking drugs (e.g. phenoxybenzamine). As alpha blockade is increased, chronic hypovolaemia corrects, and this minimises postoperative hypotension. During operation, short-acting alpha- and beta-adrenergic drugs are used and a range of other drugs is kept ready to control swings in blood pressure. These patients are best managed by doctors with previous experience of the condition.

DIABETES INSIPIDUS

Diabetes insipidus results from inadequate secretion of vasopressin (anti-diuretic hormone) from the neurohypophysis (posterior pituitary). It is usually caused by ablation of the pituitary gland by tumour or surgery. The condition is uncommon. Most patients receive replacement therapy in the form of vasopressin or desmopressin by nasal insufflation. Patients with diabetes insipidus are prone to abnormalities of plasma electrolytes, which should be checked preoperatively. If ACTH production is impaired by anterior pituitary damage, these patients will also require steroid cover.

MUSCULOSKELETAL AND NEUROLOGICAL DISORDERS

Musculoskeletal and neurological disorders influence the outcome of surgery in two main ways. Firstly, any condition which hinders mobility predisposes to chest infection, deep venous thrombosis and pulmonary embolism, aspiration pneumonitis and pressure sores. The last is even more likely if there is also sensory impairment due to a stroke or diabetic peripheral neuropathy. Secondly, specific aspects of these disorders must be considered in relation to general anaesthesia, positioning on the operating table and the use of drugs.

1. Rheumatoid arthritis

Rheumatoid arthritis poses special problems related to chronic anaemia, drug therapy and spinal complications. (Some of these problems are shared by other collagen disorders):

- Normochromic normocytic anaemia is common in chronic inflammatory disorders, including rheumatoid arthritis. The anaemia is refractory to iron therapy and there is no benefit from preoperative transfusion unless haemoglobin concentration is extremely low
- Most rheumatoid patients are taking aspirin or other non-steroidal anti-inflammatory drugs, all of which strongly predispose to peptic ulceration.

Long-term steroid therapy may contribute to peptic ulceration. Chronic low-grade bleeding from the upper gastrointestinal tract may exacerbate the existing anaemia in these patients. Operative stress may also precipitate acute gastrointestinal haemorrhage

- Long-term steroid therapy may result in adrenal insufficiency under stress. Gold and penicillamine cause renal parenchymal damage, and bone marrow depression; NSAIDs may exacerbate chronic renal failure
- If rheumatoid arthritis involves the atlanto-axial joint, the transverse ligament may be destroyed, allowing the odontoid process to sublux. During general anaesthesia, the protective reflexes are lost. If the neck is hyperextended during intubation, there is a serious risk of injury to the spinal cord by the unrestrained odontoid

Preoperative assessment of the rheumatoid patient

Full blood count is essential to check for non-specific anaemia or iron deficiency anaemia. Plasma urea, electrolytes and creatinine are measured if there is any suspicion of chronic or drug-induced disturbance of renal function. Preoperative assessment must include examination of neck movements and cervical spine X-rays (Figure 32.6).

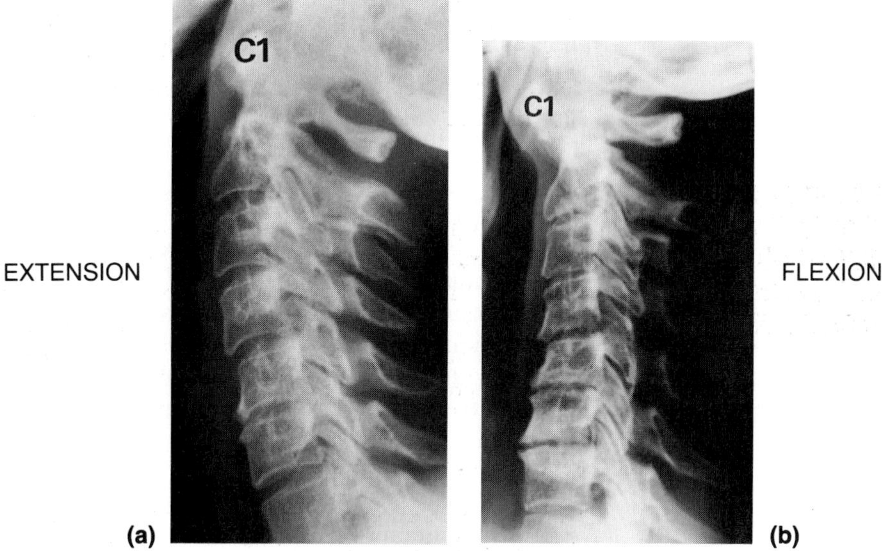

Fig. 32.6 Subluxation of the atlanto-axial joint in rheumatoid arthritis

This 62-year-old woman with long-standing severe rheumatoid arthritis required a major abdominal operation. Preoperative cervical films were taken to anticipate problems during anaesthesia. **(a)** Cervical spine in extension. **(b)** The same patient in flexion. Anterior subluxation is most apparent when the anterior border of the body of the atlas C1 is compared with that of the axis in the two pictures. This mobility is caused by destruction of the transverse axial ligament of the odontoid by pannus from the synovial joint. Under general anaesthesia, muscle relaxation may allow exaggeration of the subluxation, resulting in damage to the cervical cord

2. Epilepsy

Epilepsy is common and many routine surgical patients will therefore be taking anticonvulsive therapy. Fortunately, there is no particular risk from general anaesthesia or surgery. Indeed, the central depressive effect of general anaesthetic drugs is a powerful anticonvulsant!

HAEMATOLOGICAL DISORDERS

1. Anaemias

Severe anaemias are associated with increased perioperative morbidity and mortality. General anaesthesia poses the greatest single problem. Moderate anaemia, in which the haemoglobin concentration is more than 10 gm/dl, appears to impose no excess risk. For elective surgery, the haemoglobin concentration should be above this level before operation.

Management of anaemic patients depends on the cause of the anaemia. For patients on renal dialysis, there is no point in trying to raise the haemoglobin level as it rapidly falls again.

The cause of the anaemia may be the reason for the operation. Whether or not to transfuse before operation depends on the level of anaemia and the opinion of the anaesthetist. It may be preferable to avoid transfusion in young, fit patients but to transfuse the elderly or very ill patients who have less cardiorespiratory reserve. Transfusions should be given at least 24 hours before operation to minimise the risk of fluid overload and to ensure optimal red cell function. For iron deficiency anaemias, treatment with iron, vitamin B_{12} or folate may be all that is necessary before operation.

2. Haemoglobinopathies

Patients with *sickle cell disease* and *beta thalassaemia* have a high operative mortality and morbidity. They require intensive perioperative management with particular avoidance of hypoxia, infection, acidosis, dehydration and hypothermia. Patients with *sickle cell trait* are at much lower risk, and develop complications only if they become severely hypoxic. Sickle cell trait and disease occur amongst people of negroid origin, who should always be asked specifically about sickle cell disease. A sickle cell test must be performed preoperatively on any patient of negroid origin so that the anaesthetist can be prepared.

3. Polycythaemia

Polycythaemia may be caused by a primary myeloproliferative disorder such as *polycythaemia rubra vera (PRV)*. More commonly it is secondary to chronic cardiac or pulmonary disease. Heavy cigarette smoking also causes polycythaemia. There is an increased red cell mass in both primary and secondary polycythaemia, which causes a high haematocrit, hypervolaemia and increased blood viscosity. In PRV, there are often also excess platelets. Paradoxically, this is associated with defective haemostasis.

Some patients found to be polycythaemic do not have an increased red cell mass but rather a reduced plasma volume. This condition, known as *stress polycythaemia* is of unknown aetiology but is often associated with athero-sclerosis. Increased blood viscosity may lead to thromboembolic problems.

The main complications of polycythaemia rubra vera are haemorrhage, and arterial or venous thrombosis. The risk increases greatly once the haematocrit rises above 50%. In general, operation should be postponed to allow treatment by venesection or myelosuppression. If possible, the cardiovascular system should be allowed to stabilise for about a month after treatment. In an emergency, haematocrit may be reduced by preoperative venesection, making up the volume with 4.2% human albumin solution, gelatin infusion or normal saline.

4. Leukaemia, leucopenia and thrombocytopenia

Patients with these haematological disorders may need surgery for unrelated conditions. Complications, such as infection and haemorrhage, can be minimised by transfusing appropriate blood products such as white cell or platelet concentrates. In leukaemias and leucopenias, prophylactic antibiotics are often used.

5. Bleeding disorders

Bleeding diatheses such as *thrombocytopenia*, *von Willebrand's disease* (abnormal platelet function and factor VIII deficiency) and *haemophilia* are occasionally encountered in general surgical practice. Most surgical bleeding problems, however, are caused by uncontrolled anticoagulant therapy, liver disease, aspirin therapy and sometimes vitamin K malabsorption. The last occurs in obstructive jaundice and malabsorption syndromes.

A history of abnormal bleeding or factors which may predispose to abnormal bleeding are the most important pointers to a likely bleeding problem at operation. They should be sought from every surgical patient as follows:

- Excessive bleeding from simple cuts, previous surgery, dental extractions or childbirth
- Current use of anticoagulant drugs or aspirin
- A family history of bleeding disorders
- Intercurrent haematological or liver disease, cystic fibrosis or other malabsorption syndromes
- Recent jaundice
- Previous intestinal resection or bypass surgery

Any bleeding abnormality may lead to excessive bleeding at operation or recurrent bleeding in the early postoperative period. This may simply require additional care during surgical haemostasis but may well lead to runaway haemorrhage when clotting factors become exhausted. If this occurs, bleeding cannot be stopped by any means. Preoperative diagnosis and treatment is thus vital.

If a bleeding disorder is suspected, a *platelet count* and a *clotting screen* must be performed. A clotting screen includes *prothrombin time or ratio* and *activated partial thromboplastin time*. If an abnormality is revealed, further special investigations such as assay of individual clotting factors may be necessary. Operation should be deferred until the problem is overcome.

Clotting abnormalities (where platelet function is unaffected) are often responsible for recurrent bleeding after initial haemostasis has been achieved. In contrast, abnormal platelet numbers or function tends to cause excessive bleeding at operation and postoperative oozing. Other complications of clotting disorders include retroperitoneal or muscle haematomas and bleeding into joint cavities (haemarthroses). In contrast, platelet abnormalities tend to cause spontaneous bruising.

Clinical problems of bleeding disorders

a. Inherited clotting disorders

Haemophilia occurs in males. The disorder is a X-linked deficiency of factor VIII, or less commonly, factor IX. Cryoprecipitate or the appropriate anti-haemophilic factor is administered preoperatively and for up to two weeks after operation until the danger of secondary haemorrhage is over. Von Willebrand's disease is an autosomal dominant condition with abnormalities of both factor VIII and platelet function. It is managed perioperatively with fresh frozen plasma or cryoprecipitate.

b. Anticoagulant therapy

Long-term anticoagulant therapy with warfarin is commonly used in venous thromboembolism and for patients with mechanical heart valve prostheses. Patients on anticoagulants have a small extra risk of perioperative haemorrhage, particularly if control is poor. For most patients, some form of anticoagulation needs to be continued, particularly if a mechanical heart valve is in situ. Many doctors prefer to continue oral warfarin, reducing the prothrombin ratio slightly during the perioperative period. An alternative approach is to discontinue warfarin about four days before operation and convert to an intravenous heparin infusion. This can be closely adjusted or even reversed.

If anticoagulation has been prescribed for treatment of venous thromboembolism, some doctors prefer to discontinue warfarin two or three days before operation. The perioperative period is then covered with prophylactic subcutaneous low-dose heparin (see Chapter 33).

c. Liver disease

Bleeding disorders in cirrhosis are described earlier in this chapter and in the jaundiced patient are described in detail in Chapter 6.

d. Aspirin therapy

Aspirin has an irreversible inhibitory effect on platelet aggregation which persists for at least ten days. The effect is only reversed when the platelets have been replaced by new ones. Most non-steroidal anti-inflammatory drugs act on platelets in the same way. A similar but short-lived effect is also produced by high doses of intravenous penicillin. Aspirin ingestion, even in low doses, tends to result in oozing during and after operation, although this is rarely serious. Bleeding following dental extraction is a common manifestation of aspirin ingestion and can usually be controlled by sutures and pressure.

e. Malabsorption of fat-soluble vitamins

Vitamin K absorption may be impaired in pancreatic dysfunction, after resection of the distal ileum or in malabsorption syndromes. The problem is readily overcome by preoperative injections of vitamin K.

PSYCHIATRIC DISORDERS

1. Mental illness and mental handicap

Behavioural problems associated with mental illness and mental handicap can be minimised by a sympathetic and consistent approach from medical and nursing staff. Any procedure or investigation must be carefully explained to the patient in terms which can be understood. Patients should not be moved from bed to bed around the ward as this produces disorientation.

The patient's usual oral medication should be continued whenever possible. A parenteral substitute may be required if oral intake is restricted and behaviour is known to be unstable. Side effects and drug interactions are common with psychoactive drugs and these should be anticipated by checking with a formulary. *Monoamine oxidase inhibitors* (used as antidepressants) interact with sympathomimetic amines and narcotic analgesics causing severe hypertension. They should be discontinued at least two weeks preoperatively. *Tricyclic antidepressants* and *phenothiazines* also have a wide range of interactions. Plasma urea and electrolytes should be checked in all patients taking *lithium*, which may cause renal parenchymal damage.

2. Alcoholism and drug addiction

Alcoholics are prone to cirrhosis, malnutrition and peripheral neuropathies. Drug addicts are at risk of hepatitis, AIDS and other infections.

Alcohol potentiates general anaesthetic agents, and the inebriated patient needs smaller doses. In contrast, chronic alcohol abuse induces liver enzymes which break down anaesthetic agents and also increase tolerance to CNS depressants. Higher doses of anaesthetic agents will therefore be required. Similarly, larger doses of intravenous sedatives are required for procedures such as gastrointestinal endoscopy.

Opiate addiction leads to similar dosage problems. Doctors must be aware of feigned illness as a means of obtaining restricted drugs.

Problems of drug withdrawal

Withdrawal symptoms may develop unexpectedly during the postoperative period if drug or alcohol addiction has been concealed.

Alcohol withdrawal is characterised initially by irritability and tremors. Convulsions may develop after 24–48 hours. Full scale delirium tremens may appear as long as ten days after alcohol withdrawal. Delirium tremens is marked by mental confusion and hallucinations accompanied by fever, tachycardia, pallor, vomiting and sweats. Such signs also occur in other post-operative complications and alcohol withdrawal is an easily overlooked cause.

Alcoholic liver disease may result in episodes of hypoglycaemia. The symptoms of hypoglycaemia may be confused with those of delirium tremens. Hypoglycaemia should be excluded by measuring blood glucose.

Mild withdrawal states may be managed with regular oral doses of chlormethiazole or benzodiazepines. Parenteral B vitamins are usually given daily. If symptoms become pronounced, chlormethiazole can be administered by continuous intravenous infusion. A bolus dose is used initially, and the subsequent rate of administration is adjusted according to response. Oral drugs can usually be substituted after 48–72 hours. If the patient has a history of convulsions, phenytoin should also be given.

Opiate withdrawal symptoms are broadly similar to those of alcohol but generally less severe. Treatment is usually with a substitute drug such as methadone.

3. Senile dementia

Patients with senile dementia become even more confused when subjected to the strange and ever-changing environment of the surgical ward. They tolerate the stress of general anaesthesia and operation poorly. The potential benefit of any elective procedure must be carefully weighed against the possible adverse effects. Unfortunately, these patients often fail to become rehabilitated in their own homes after operation.

Sudden deterioration in mental state or increasing confusion may be provoked by infection, dehydration, electrolyte disturbances or overdose of drugs such as digoxin, hypnotics and sedatives. All these causes should be considered in any patient who undergoes mental deterioration in the perioperative period.

OBESITY

Gross obesity carries two to three times the normal risk of perioperative death or morbidity, as outlined in Figure 32.7. Whenever possible, weight should be reduced before operation, particularly if the operation is not urgent. Referral to a dietician may be helpful although self-help groups often provide stronger motivation. Preoperative screening procedures for obese patients include blood glucose estimation and ECG, even if the patient is asymptomatic.

Fig. 32.7 Surgical complications of obesity

Cardiopulmonary complications such as cardiac failure and chest infections — predisposing factors are atherosclerosis, increased demands on the cardiovascular system, decreased chest wall compliance, inefficient respiratory muscles and shallow breathing

Wound complications, e.g. infection, dehiscence — poor quality abdominal wall musculature with fat infiltration. Large 'dead space' in thick fat predisposes to haematoma formation

Deep venous thrombosis and pulmonary embolism — possibly due to general inertia

Complications with general anaesthesia
— physiological problems, e.g. intubation may be required because of the increased risk of aspiration and high pressure required for ventilation
— technical problems, e.g. intravenous cannulae are difficult to insert and intubation is more difficult. Clinical signs of dehydration and hypovolaemia are more difficult to elicit
— metabolic problems, e.g. altered distribution of drugs

Predisposition to various medical disorders — hypertension, ischaemic heart disease, diabetes, gall stones, gout

Operative difficulties — operations take longer to perform because of difficult access and vital structures obscured by fat

INTER-CURRENT DRUG THERAPY

Many drugs prescribed for 'medical' conditions have ramifications in the surgical patient. The most important of these commonly encountered in practice are summarised in Figure 32.8.

Fig. 32.8 Potentially dangerous drugs in the surgical patient

Glucocorticoids — predispose to peptic ulceration, delayed wound healing and infection. May lead to acute adrenal insufficiency causing cardiovascular collapse

Antihypertensive drugs — abrupt cessation may cause sympathetic overactivity resulting in rebound hypertension (a special problem with clonidine), or angina

Antidepressants — monoamine oxidase inhibitors (MAOIs) interact with tyramine-containing foods (such as cheese and yeast extracts), as well as sympathomimetic amines and narcotic analgesics. This interaction may cause a hypertensive crisis and potentiate narcotic effects

Oral contraceptives, stilboestrol and other sex hormones — increased risk of deep venous thrombosis and pulmonary embolism

Anticoagulants — predispose to haemorrhage

Diuretics — may cause electrolyte abnormalities and chronic dehydration

33 COMPLICATIONS OF SURGERY AND TRAUMA AND THEIR PREVENTION

Introduction

Any operation, major trauma or other surgical admission may be attended by a variety of complications. These not only cause additional pain and suffering to the patient but may put the patient's life at risk. Furthermore, complications place extra demands upon medical and nursing time and impose additional costs on already overstretched budgets. For example, a pelvic abscess or incisional hernia can nearly double the cost of a routine colonic resection.

While some complications are to an extent inherent in the condition being treated (e.g. deep venous thrombosis following multiple lower limb fractures), others arise from inexperience or errors of judgement (e.g. misdiagnosis), poor management practices (e.g. allowing pressure sores to develop) or even frank negligence (e.g. operation on the wrong side).

A large proportion of complications can be prevented or minimised by appropriate prophylactic measures, careful attention to detail and by early recognition of problems as they develop. Early diagnosis and treatment is essential as delay often leads to catastrophic 'snowballing' multisystem complications. Once three or more body systems become involved, mortality is extremely high, e.g chest infection and renal failure, complicating an operation for obstructive jaundice.

In respect of operative surgery, complications can be divided into the *general* complications of any operation, and the *specific* complications of individual operations. Both groups of complications can be subdivided into *immediate* (during operation or within the next 24 hours), *early postoperative* (during the first postoperative week or so), and *long-term*.

The complications of surgery can be divided into five broad categories as shown in Figure 33.1. This chapter covers categories 2, 3, 4 and the compli-

Fig. 33.1 Principle categories of surgical complications

1. **Complications predisposed to by intercurrent 'medical' disorders**, whether symptomatic or occult, e.g. ischaemic heart disease, chronic respiratory disease or diabetes mellitus (see Chapter 32)
2. **Complications of anaesthesia**
3. **Complications of any surgical condition**, e.g. pulmonary embolus, chest or urinary tract infection
4. **General operative complications**, e.g. haemorrhage or wound infection
5. **Complications of specific disorders and operations**

cations of abdominal surgery from category 5; 'medical' complications are discussed in Chapter 32. The complications associated with specific operations are discussed in the appropriate Chapters 8–31.

COMPLICATIONS OF ANAESTHESIA

General principles

Complications of anaesthesia are essentially the responsibility of the anaesthetist. The exception is local anaesthesia which is usually administered by the surgeon. Much of the preoperative assessment for an anaesthetic, whether spinal, epidural or general, falls to the junior members of the surgical team, who by anticipating complications, can prevent many of them. The main complications of anaesthesia are summarised in Figure 33.2.

COMPLICATIONS COMMON TO MOST OPERATIONS

RESPIRATORY COMPLICATIONS

Up to 15% of patients suffer from respiratory complications associated with general anaesthesia and major operations. The most common of these are *atelectasis*, *chest infection*, *aspiration pneumonitis* and *aspiration pneumonia*. Pre-existing lung disease greatly increases the risk of complications. Severely ill patients and burns or trauma victims are susceptible to the development of *adult respiratory distress syndrome*.

Effects of anaesthesia and surgery on respiratory function

Anaesthesia and surgery predispose to postoperative complications by altering lung function and compromising normal defence mechanisms as follows:

- Lung tidal volume may be reduced by as much as 50%, depending on the incision site. Thoracic, upper abdominal and lower abdominal incisions (in decreasing order of effect) particularly reduce lung volume
- Lung expansion is reduced by the *supine posture* during and after operation, *pain*, abdominal *distension*, abdominal *constriction* by bandages and the effects of *sedative drugs*
- Ventilation rate usually increases and there is loss of normal periodic hyperinflation
- Diminished ventilation and pulmonary perfusion result in reduced gaseous exchange
- Airway defences are compromised by loss of the cough reflex and diminished ciliary activity, which both lead to accumulation of secretions

Fig. 33.2 Common complications of anaesthesia

1. Local anaesthesia

Injection site — pain, haematoma, delayed recovery of sensation (direct nerve trauma), infection

Vasoconstrictors — ischaemic necrosis (if used in digits or penis)

Systemic effects of local anaesthetic agent

— idiosyncratic or allergic reactions (very rare)

— toxicity due to either excess dosage, or inadvertent intravenous injection. The same effect is produced by premature release of a Bier's block cuff. Toxic effects include: dizziness, tinnitus, nausea and vomiting, fits, CNS depression, bradycardia and asystole

2. Spinal, epidural and caudal anaesthesia

Failure of anaesthetic — anatomical difficulties or technical failure

Headache — loss of CSF or minor intrathecal haemorrhage

Intrathecal bleeding (especially if the patient is on anticoagulants)

Unintentionally wide field of anaesthesia

— in epidural anaesthesia, injection of local anaesthetic into the wrong tissue plane may give a spinal anaesthetic
— in spinal anaesthesia, if the anaesthetic agent flows too far proximally, respiratory paralysis may occur

Permanent nerve or spinal cord damage — injection of incorrect drug

Paraspinal infection — introduced by the needle

Systemic complications — severe hypotension or postural hypotension

3. General anaesthesia

Direct trauma to mouth or pharynx, e.g. teeth, artificial crowns and bridges

Inherited disorders
— malignant hyperpyrexia (any potent inhalational anaesthetic may be responsible)
— pseudocholinesterase deficiency (prolonged apnoea after succinylcholine)

Idiosyncratic or allergic reactions to anaesthetic agents
— minor effects e.g. postoperative nausea and vomiting
— major effects e.g. cardiovascular collapse, respiratory depression, halothane jaundice

Slow recovery from anaesthetic
— drug interactions
— inappropriate choice of drugs or dosage in relation to age or the requirements of day-case surgery

'Awareness' during anaesthetic — effective paralysis but ineffective anaesthesia

Disorders of fluid balance — inadequate or excessive replacement of fluids

Hypothermia
— long operations with extensive fluid loss
— large volume transfusions of cold blood

(Note : small neonates and infants are especially vulnerable to hypothermia)

Inadvertent trauma
— initiation of pressure sores
— pressure injury to nerves (especially ulnar and lateral popliteal)
— diathermy-pad burns
— corneal abrasions

Atelectasis

Pathophysiology and clinical features

Atelectasis or alveolar collapse occurs when airways become obstructed and air is absorbed from the air spaces distal to the obstruction. Bronchial secretions are the main cause of this obstruction. Predisposing factors include shallow ventilation, loss of periodic hyperinflation, inhibition of coughing and pooling of mucus. All of these are particular problems after thoracic and upper abdominal surgery. The resulting *ventilation-perfusion mismatch* produces a degree of right-to-left shunting, and tends to cause a fall in PaO_2. If the obstructed airways are small, there is only minor segmental collapse, in which case localising signs are minimal and X-ray appearance is unremarkable. Despite this, the overall extent of collapse may be large and cause significant hypoxaemia.

Obstruction of a major airway causes collapse and consolidation of a whole lobe, resulting in the typical clinical signs of dullness to percussion and reduced breath sounds or *bronchial breathing*. Chest X-ray will show the lobe to be contracted and opacified with mediastinal shift and compensatory expansion of other lobes.

Most cases of atelectasis are relatively mild and pass undiagnosed, although the patient may be slow to recover from operation. The patient may have a poor colour resulting from mild hypoxia, mild tachypnoea, tachycardia and low-grade pyrexia, which all resolve spontaneously within a few days. Sputum culture (if any is produced) is usually negative but infection may complicate severe cases.

Prevention of atelectasis

Atelectasis is best prevented by preoperative and postoperative physiotherapy. This includes deep breathing exercises, regular adjustments of posture and vigorous coughing. During postoperative physiotherapy, the wound should be supported by the patient's hand. Effective postoperative pain relief facilitates physiotherapy and mobility. For the initial recovery period, infiltration of the wound with local anaesthetic or epidural analgesia may be helpful. Nebulised bronchodilators such as salbutamol may assist the patient to cough up secretions. Severe cases of diffuse atelectasis may require endotracheal intubation and positive pressure ventilation. Lobar or whole lung collapse requires bronchoscopy to aspirate occluding mucus plugs.

Chest infections

Bronchopneumonia is the usual form of chest infection seen in surgical patients. It occurs secondarily to chronic lung disease, or following atelectasis or aspiration. *Haemophilus* and *Strep. pyogenes* are the common infecting organisms but coliforms may be responsible in elderly, debilitated or seriously ill patients. *Pseudomonas* bronchopneumonia occurs in patients on ventilators or with bronchiectasis.

Infection is manifest by pyrexia, tachypnoea, tachycardia and sometimes cyanosis. The mucopurulent sputum is thick, copious and green. Antibiotics, usually ampicillin or co-trimoxazole, are given on a 'best-guess' basis until sputum culture and sensitivities are available. Physiotherapy and encouragement to cough are equally important for recovery.

Aspiration pneumonitis

Aspiration pneumonitis (Mendelson's syndrome) is a sterile, chemical inflammation of the lungs resulting from inhalation of acidic gastric contents. There is often a clear history of vomiting or regurgitation, followed by a rapid onset of breathlessness and wheezing. This may later become complicated by infection, i.e. bronchopneumonia, with its typical symptoms and signs. Chest X-ray shows characteristic 'fluffy' opacities, particularly in the lower lobes, which are most affected for anatomical and postural reasons.

Aspiration occurs when protective laryngeal reflexes are suppressed. This may be due to impairment of consciousness (e.g. during recovery from general anaesthetic) or loss of consciousness as often occurs with head injuries. Aspiration may also result from local factors such as tracheostomy or nasogastric intubation.

Emergency anaesthesia in the unstarved patient poses special risks. Whenever possible, anaesthesia should be postponed for 4–6 hours after the last food or drink. In accident victims, it is important to note the time of last eating with respect to the time of the accident, as stress and anxiety may greatly delay gastric emptying. If general anaesthesia must be performed on the unstarved patient, a *crash induction* technique is employed: the supine patient is tilted head up and an endotracheal tube is inserted to protect the airway. At the same time, an assistant applies cricoid pressure to flatten the pharynx against the cervical spine, preventing reflux. Oral antacids may be given beforehand to neutralise gastric acidity. Metoclopramide, given by injection, may be used to hasten gastric emptying.

The patient with *bowel obstruction* is similarly at risk of aspiration. This is overcome by emptying the stomach preoperatively via a nasogastric tube and by using a crash induction anaesthetic technique.

The mortality from aspiration pneumonitis approaches 50% and urgent treatment must be started should it occur. This involves thorough bronchial suction via an endotracheal tube (or bronchoscope if necessary), followed by positive pressure ventilation and prophylactic antibiotics. Intravenous steroids are usually given to try to limit the inflammatory process, but their efficacy is unproven.

Aspiration pneumonia

Aspiration pneumonia may complicate aspiration pneumonitis, but more often it develops insidiously, following chronic aspiration of infected food and oropharyngeal secretions. In the surgical context, debilitated, confused or elderly patients are the usual victims, but aspiration pneumonia is also seen in alcoholics, drug addicts and stroke patients. The clinical features are of infection and lobar consolidation (usually of the lower lobe) progressing to *lung abscess* formation. The organisms are usually mixed oral anaerobes sensitive to penicillin, but prognosis depends more on the patient's general condition, and is usually poor.

Adult respiratory distress syndrome ('shock lung')

This syndrome of acute respiratory failure is characterised by rapid, shallow breathing, severe hypoxaemia, stiff lungs and diffuse pulmonary opacification on X-ray. It may develop in response to a variety of systemic and direct insults to the pulmonary alveoli and microvasculature.

Acute respiratory failure has long been known to occur in many disparate conditions and has been given many different names such as shock lung, wet lung, post-traumatic respiratory insufficiency, Da Nang lung (Vietnam war) and white lung. In 1976, it was finally realised that the underlying pathological phenomena were similar, and were directly related to the well-recogised respiratory distress syndrome of new-born babies. The main conditions with which adult respiratory distress syndrome (ARDS) is associated are summarised in Figure 33.3.

Fig. 33.3 Conditions associated with adult respiratory distress syndrome

Direct insults to the lung:
Lung contusion
Near drowning
Aspiration of gastric acid
Inhalation of smoke and corrosive chemicals, e.g chlorine, phosgene, nitrogen dioxide or ammonia
Radiation pneumonitis

Systemic insults to the lung:
Multiple trauma with shock
Septicaemic shock
Severe acute pancreatitis
Major head injuries ('neurogenic pulmonary oedema')
Fat, air and amniotic fluid embolism
Major blood transfusion reaction or massive blood transfusion
Disseminated intravascular coagulation
Cardiopulmonary bypass
Eclampsia
Severe allergic reactions
Drug overdose or sensitivity, e.g. heroin, barbiturates, paraquat, bleomycin

Pathophysiology of ARDS

The causative insults to the lung all have the effect of increasing the permeability of pulmonary capillaries, leading to leakage of protein-rich fluid into the alveolar interstitium. This causes interstitial oedema which *reduces lung compliance* and causes 'stiff lungs' and reduced alveolar ventilation.

The alveolar lining cells (type I pneumocytes) are also damaged in some way. The damage, combined with increased interstitial hydrostatic pressure, causes leakage of fluid into the alveolar spaces until they are filled. The result is disruption of the ratio of lung ventilation to perfusion (V/Q ratio), causing effective right-to-left shunting of blood. The intra-alveolar fluid later condenses to form a *hyaline membrane* which lines the alveoli. This is similar to the neonatal form of the disease.

The full clinical syndrome often only develops 24–48 hours after the initial insult. If the patient eventually recovers, the interstitial damage may result in diffuse *interstitial fibrosis*. It is important to note that cardiac failure plays no part in the development of ARDS, although cardiac failure may later complicate the condition.

Clinical features of ARDS

The main clinical finding is rapid shallow respiration with only scattered crepitations heard on auscultation. There is usually no cough, chest pain or haemoptysis. Blood gas analysis reveals low PaO_2 but the $PaCO_2$ remains normal, except in the most severe cases. Chest X-ray may be normal in the early stages, progressing rapidly through increased interstitial markings to complete 'white out' (see Figure 33.4). ARDS may be difficult to distinguish from cardiac failure except that cardiac diameter is normal in ARDS, and cardiac failure usually responds to diuretic therapy.

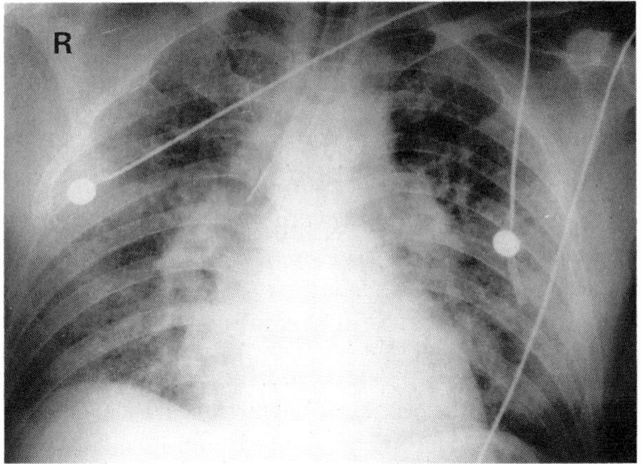

Fig. 33.4 Adult respiratory distress syndrome

Chest X-ray from a 62-year-old man admitted to intensive care with severe head injuries and multiple fractures. There is diffuse bilateral pulmonary shadowing typical of 'shock lung'. Note inadvertent placement of the endotracheal tube (identified by its radio-paque line) into the right main bronchus!

Treatment of ARDS

The overall objective is maintenance of respiratory function and cardiovascular stability while the underlying cause (e.g. septicaemia) is brought under control. This should be carried out under intensive care conditions. The sooner the treatment is begun, the greater the chance of recovery.

Most patients require mechanical *ventilation* with *positive end-expiratory pressure* (PEEP) to achieve adequate oxygenation and to try to reverse alveolar oedema and collapse. Fluid balance is complex in these patients and usually requires monitoring of both *right and left atrial pressures*; a central venous line is used to measure right atrial pressure, but left atrial pressure is measured indirectly as *pulmonary wedge pressure* via a *Swann-Ganz catheter*. Cardiac output can also be measured using the Swann-Ganz catheter. In these patients, diuretics do not control pulmonary oedema, but instead aggravate the hypovolaemia and shock associated with the underlying cause.

Renal failure is a common complication sometimes prevented by early use of drugs such as dopamine. The mortality rate for complicated cases of ARDS approaches 90%.

THROMBO-EMBOLISM

Pathophysiology

Venous thromboembolism is a major cause of complications and death after surgery or trauma. Venous blood is normally prevented from clotting within the veins by a complex series of mechanisms which include local inhibition of the clotting cascade, prompt lysis of small clots that do form, and continuous flow of blood. This subtle balance can be disturbed by several local and systemic factors, many poorly understood. Imbalance results in thrombus formation within the venous sinuses of the calf muscles and sometimes primarily in the pelvic veins. More often, distal thrombi form first, then propagate proximally to involve the femoral and pelvic veins. If thrombi in the larger vessels become detached, they circulate proximally to impact in the pulmonary arteries as *pulmonary emboli*.

The main predisposing factors to venous thromboembolism are summarised in Figure 33.5, but thromboembolism can also occur in healthy individuals with no apparent predisposing factors.

The risk of thromboembolism increases incrementally as the number and severity of local and systemic risk factor increases; this is neatly illustrated in Figure 33.6. The impact of many of the predisposing factors can be minimised by early mobilisation and prevention of local venous stasis. A number of specific preventive measures for high risk groups are described later.

Deep vein thrombosis

Deep vein thrombosis in the lower limbs (DVT) is often silent. Furthermore, the classic clinical features are found in only half the cases. These include swelling of the leg, tenderness of the calf muscles, increased warmth of the leg, and calf pain on passive dorsiflexion of the foot (*Homan's sign*). The presence of these features indicates that venous occlusion has extended at least as far as the popliteal veins.

Occlusion of the ilio-femoral veins tends to produce diffuse and sometimes massive swelling of the whole lower limb. In addition, there is tenderness over the femoral vein in the groin. In severe cases, the leg becomes painful and white, and boggy with oedema; this is known as *phlegmasia alba dolens*. In extreme cases, the limb becomes more painful and blue, with incipient venous infarction (*phlegmasia caerulea dolens*).

Despite the foregoing, up to 50% of substantial deep venous thromboses (DVTs) are *asymptomatic*, but these have the same potential for causing both pulmonary embolism and long term chronic venous insufficiency as sympto-

Fig. 33.5 Predisposing factors for deep vein thrombosis and pulmonary embolism

Trauma and surgery (complex systemic effects)
Direct trauma to the pelvis and lower limbs, especially fractures
Previous venous thromboembolism
Pre-existing lower limb venous disorders causing stasis
Venous stasis during general or regional anaesthesia (loss of calf muscle pump and postural pressure on the calves)
Malignant disease
Immobility, e.g. bedbound patients after operation or stroke
Cardiac failure
High-oestrogen oral contraceptive pill, oestrogen treatment
Pregnancy
Pelvic masses
Obesity
Dehydration
Blood disorders, e.g. polycythaemia and thrombocythaemia

Fig. 33.6 Varying risk of deep vein thrombosis

Age	Grade of surgery	Other risk factors	Risk of DVT
20	minor		1%
40	minor		3%
60	minor		10%
60	major		20%
60	major	previous DVT	50%
80	major		40%
80	major	previous DVT + infection or malignancy	96%

matic venous thromboses. To complicate the problem, as many as half the patients who develop swelling and pain in the calf after operation do not have deep vein thrombosis.

Diagnostic tests for DVT

Venography (phlebography) is the best diagnostic technique when deep venous thrombosis is suspected. It involves cannulating a small vein in the foot and injecting contrast material. Before the procedure, tourniquets are applied at the ankle and below the knee to direct superficial venous blood into the deep system. A typical venogram showing obstructed deep venous architecture is shown in Figure 33.7. Other techniques include detection of thrombi using radioisotopically-labelled fibrinogen (mainly used for research purposes) and Doppler ultrasound detection of flow in the femoral vein in response to squeezing the calf (sluggish or absent in deep vein thrombosis).

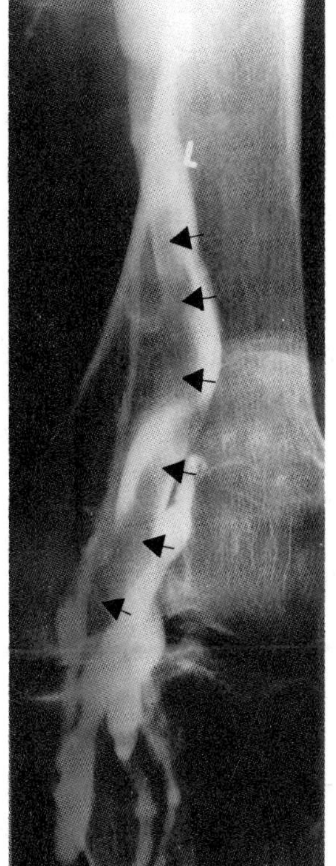

Fig. 33.7 Deep vein thrombosis

Venogram showing the popliteal veins in a patient who complained of calf pain five days after a laparotomy for obstructive jaundice. There is extensive thrombus in the deep veins (arrowed) which is only loosely attached to the vein wall and therefore in danger of embolisation to the lung

Pulmonary embolism

The classic picture of pulmonary embolism ('PE') is sudden dyspnoea and cardiovascular collapse, followed by pleuritic chest pain, development of a pleural rub and haemoptysis. ECG may show evidence of right heart strain (S wave in lead I, Q wave and inverted T wave in lead III). This clinical presentation, however, is uncommon and occurs only when 50% or more of the pulmonary arterial system is occluded. More extensive occlusion usually results in sudden death.

Smaller pulmonary emboli are more common and are often 'silent', presenting as non-specific episodes of general deterioration, confusion, breathlessness or chest pain. The patient often has a tachycardia and low-grade fever, and there are no diagnostic changes on ECG. The condition may be attributed to chest infection, atelectasis or cardiac failure unless a diagnosis of pulmonary embolism is considered. More specific diagnostic symptoms may occur with small pulmonary emboli, including localised *pleuritic chest pain* and small *haemoptyses* in the form of blood-streaked sputum. A small pulmonary embolus may herald a massive or fatal embolus, and must therefore always be treated seriously.

Venous thromboembolism is most common from about the fourth to the seventh postoperative day, but may present at any time during the first postoperative month.

Diagnostic tests for pulmonary embolism

Chest X-ray rarely shows specific changes. The best method of confirming the diagnosis is radioisotope *ventilation-perfusion scanning* (V/Q scanning) as shown in Figure 33.8. This involves two separate imaging procedures designed to demonstrate ventilation-perfusion mismatch. First, the patient inhales radioactive xenon gas and a gamma camera is used to detect the distribution of radioactivity within the air spaces of the lungs. The *ventilation scan* is followed by the *perfusion scan* in which an intravenous injection of radioisotopically labelled albumen microspheres is given. These lodge evenly throughout the pulmonary bed except where the pulmonary arteries are occluded by thrombus. This is again detected by gamma camera. In pulmonary embolism, distribution of isotope in the ventilation scan is normal, but areas of pulmonary underperfusion (emboli) show as defects in the perfusion scan. In areas of infection or atelectasis (which are underventilated), the ventilation scan is deficient but the perfusion scan is normal.

Pulmonary angiography is a more precise anatomical demonstration of the occluded vessels, and should be performed if embolism is strongly suspected but cannot be proved by other means. Pulmonary angiography is mandatory if an embolus is to be removed surgically or by less invasive means.

Management of venous thromboembolism

For most patients, removal of lower limb thrombus or pulmonary embolus is impractical. The main objective, therefore, in managing deep vein thrombosis and pulmonary embolism is to halt the coagulation process to prevent established thrombi propagating and new thrombi forming.

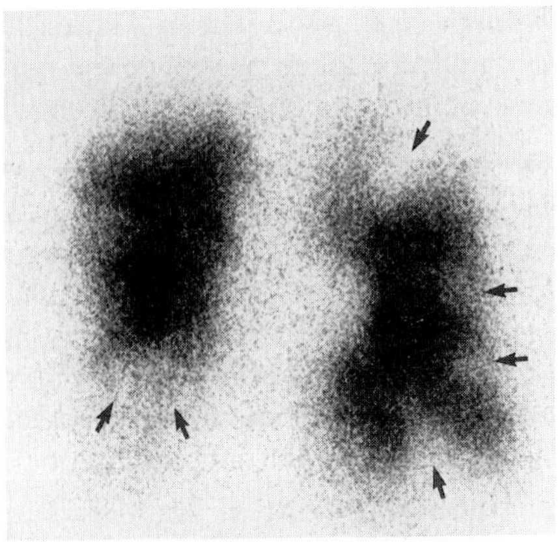

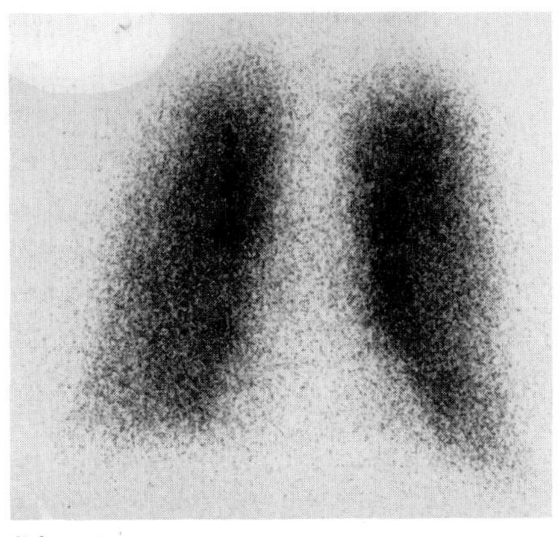

(a) (b)

Fig. 33.8 Ventilation–perfusion scan showing multiple pulmonary emboli

(a) Perfusion scan showing multiple filling defects (arrowed) typical of pulmonary emboli. **(b)** Normal ventilation scan from the same patient. Normal ventilation with impaired perfusion is typical of pulmonary embolism

Removal of thrombus is left to the normal body processes. In the lower limbs, venous thrombi eventually become organised and firmly attached to the vessel wall, posing no further risk of embolisation. The thrombus is later invaded by granulation tissue and the veins eventually become recanalised, thus restoring venous flow. In the process, the valves are often destroyed, leading to *chronic venous insufficiency* (Chapter 26). After pulmonary embolism, if the patient survives the initial embolic episode, the emboli are efficiently removed by local thrombolysis, leaving little functional deficit.

Initially, anticoagulation is achieved with *intravenous heparin*, commencing with a bolus dose of ten thousand units. This is followed by a continuous infusion of twenty to forty thousand units over each 24 hour period. Heparin anticoagulation takes effect immediately and is continued for about five days, by which time acute symptoms have usually subsided. In the meantime, oral *warfarin therapy* (which takes several days to become fully effective) is begun. Warfarin therapy is continued for three to six months, the period of highest risk of recurrent thromboembolism. Patients who suffer repeated thromboembolic episodes may have to be maintained on warfarin for life.

In the rare case of massive but non-fatal pulmonary embolism, surgical *embolectomy* may be appropriate. This is performed under total cardiopulmonary bypass and is therefore no small undertaking. Systemic thrombolytic therapy with *streptokinase* has been employed in this situation, but the high rate of serious bleeding in surgical patients precludes its use. The newer technique of manipulating a pulmonary artery catheter into the embolus and instilling high doses of local thrombolytic drugs is more promising. Note that thrombolytic therapy works slowly.

Prevention of venous thromboembolism

The importance of general measures in the prevention of venous thrombosis cannot be overemphasised. These include early *postoperative mobilisation*, *adequate hydration* and *avoiding calf pressure*. In addition, patients on oral contraceptives should stop taking them at least six weeks before operation.

For patients at high risk, as shown in Figure 33.5 earlier, specific prophylactic measures should be taken to reduce the risk of deep venous thrombosis (and consequent pulmonary embolism). Prophylactic measures include the following:

- *Low-dose subcutaneous heparin* — 5000 units of heparin given twice or three times a day subcutaneously provides the best prophylaxis against deep vein thrombosis short of full anticoagulation. It reduces the rate of postoperative deep venous thrombosis by about 70%. The intravascular antithrombotic effect is not due to anticoagulation, but results from stimulation of platelet factor *antithrombin III*; there should be no detectable in vitro anticoagulant effect or any clinically significant effects on haemostasis during or after operation
- *Calf compression devices* — several pneumatic and electrical devices are available for intraoperative calf compression to simulate normal muscle pump activity. These have the advantage of being non-invasive and easily applied to all patients, even those at low risk, but their efficacy is less than subcutaneous heparin
- *Graded-compression stockings* — the use of these stockings is simple and widely practised. Provided the stockings are full length and correctly fitted, graded-compression stockings offer a suitable level of prophylaxis for patients at low or moderate risk. The stockings must be worn during operation as well as during the early postoperative period
- *Intravenous dextran* — dextrans are high molecular weight polysaccharides, which are sometimes used as plasma substitutes. Intravenous dextran 70 has been shown to provide prophylaxis against deep venous thrombosis almost as effectively as low-dose heparin; 500 ml of a standard solution are given daily from the time of operation until the third postoperative day. The main disadvantages are the intravenous route, the large volume to be given and the occasional hypersensitivity reactions. All these have limited its more general use
- *Warfarin anticoagulation* — this is perhaps the best method of prophylaxis for elective operations, and is widely used for major elective surgery in the Netherlands. It is considered impractical by many surgeons, not least because of the supposed risk of incidental and operative haemorrhage. In addition, the logistics of establishing preoperative anticoagulation and continuing dose monitoring postoperatively, require a great deal of resources

FLUID AND ELECTROLYTE DISTURBANCES

Fluid and electrolyte disturbances such as *dehydration* or *fluid overload*, *hyponatraemia*, *hypokalaemia* and *hyperkalaemia* frequently develop in the postoperative period. Fluid and electrolyte abnormalities are particularly common after major surgery of the gut, especially if there have been massive fluid losses through vomiting, diarrhoea or sequestration in obstructed or adynamic bowel. These problems are fully discussed in Chapter 36.

TRANSFUSION COMPLICATIONS

The management of blood transfusion and its complications is described in detail in Chapter 3.

URINARY RETENTION

Acute retention of urine is common in the immediate postoperative period. The usual problem is that the patient has been unable to pass any urine following operation. The anuria is often drawn to the doctor's attention by a nurse several hours after operation, before the patient becomes distressed. If the diagnostic dilemma between acute retention and oliguria from poor renal perfusion or acute renal failure cannot be resolved clinically, ultrasound will show whether the bladder is full of urine.

Pathophysiology

Postoperative retention is much more common in men, particularly when there is a degree of prostatic hypertrophy. Patients with symptoms of bladder outflow obstruction ('prostatism') are at high risk of developing acute retention, although young male patients can also be affected.

All cases of acute postoperative urinary retention seem to result from a combination of the following factors:

- Difficulty in passing urine in the supine position
- Embarrassment at passing urine without sufficient privacy
- Accumulation of a large volume of urine during the operation and recovery from anaesthetic, causing overfilling of the bladder
- Transient disturbance of the neurological control of voiding by general or spinal anaesthesia
- Pain from an abdominal or inguinal wound inhibiting normal contraction of the abdominal musculature and relaxation of the bladder neck
- Certain operations predispose to acute retention, e.g. abdomino-perineal resection of rectum or bilateral inguinal hernia repair
- Constipation may interfere with voiding

Management of postoperative urinary retention

Conservative measures

Most cases of postoperative acute retention can be managed conservatively, bearing in mind the precipitating factors mentioned above. The earlier the problem is dealt with, the less likely is the patient to require catheterisation, which should be avoided if possible. The first step is to ensure there is adequate postoperative analgesia; this may be all that is required to enable the patient to pass urine. The next step is to help the patient out of bed in order to use a commode at the bedside or use a urine bottle standing at the bedside.

The patient will often need continuous support to stand if still 'groggy' from the anaesthetic or analgesia. For young male patients, a male assistant should be at hand if possible, as the presence of a young female can have a marked inhibitory effect!

If these measures fail, the patient should be wheeled into a bathroom for privacy and left alone for a while, if he is fit enough. The familiar sound of a tap left running often encourages micturition. If the patient still does not pass urine, it may be appropriate to encourage a bowel movement by means of a lubricant glycerine suppository. Defecation is usually accompanied by bladder neck relaxation and micturition, so this may help. In women, where the risk of bladder neck obstruction or urethral stricture is small, a single injection of *carbachol* is worth trying and may initiate micturition.

Catheterisation

If conservative measures fail, catheterisation will usually be necessary. In females, bladder drainage and immediate removal of the catheter is often all that is required. In males, the catheter is usually left in situ until the following morning or until the patient is well. Recurrent problems of retention are usually caused by bladder outlet obstruction and are managed as described in Chapter 21.

Gross faecal loading is common in the elderly in hospital and is probably the most frequent cause of acute retention (and faecal incontinence).

URINARY TRACT INFECTIONS

Urinary tract infections are extremely common in the postoperative period especially in women. The most obvious predisposing factor is catheterisation, although urinary tract infections commonly arise without urethral instrumentation. The cause is probably a combination of reduced urinary output, reducing 'flushing' of the bladder, incomplete bladder emptying in the supine posture, bacteraemia induced by operation or infection, and finally inadequate perineal hygiene.

Typical symptoms of dysuria and frequency may be less apparent or absent altogether. The diagnosis of urinary tract infection is often made on investigation of an unexplained pyrexia or septicaemia. Treatment is by ensuring adequate fluid input and prescription of appropriate antibiotics such as trimethoprim.

ACUTE RENAL FAILURE

Acute renal failure is defined clinically as the abrupt onset of oliguria or anuria, associated with a steep rise in blood urea concentration. This is caused by failure to excrete nitrogenous waste products. The usual cause is *acute tubular necrosis*, but acute renal failure is sometimes caused by nephrotoxins. These include the aminoglycoside antibiotics gentamicin and tobramycin, myoglobin (in the crush syndrome) and the hepatorenal syndrome associated with obstructive jaundice. Acute renal failure is also a particular complication of surgery of the abdominal aorta, in which the renal arteries may be occluded by inadvertent damage or occult embolism.

Pathophysiology of acute tubular necrosis

The renal tubules are acutely sensitive to a variety of metabolic insults, particularly hypoxia and certain toxins. Hypoxia readily occurs if renal perfusion falls significantly. The usual surgical cause is an episode of severe or prolonged hypotension. This may be the result of hypovolaemic shock (via haemorrhage or dehydration), cardiovascular collapse (caused by post-operative cardiac failure or myocardial infarction) or septicaemic shock. In the last, endotoxic tubular damage is probably an important factor. Pre-existing chronic renal disease increases a patient's susceptibility to acute renal failure.

Provided the insult to the renal tubules is not overwhelming, the damage to the tubular cells is confined to disruption of cellular metabolism rather than tissue necrosis. This is potentially reversible, provided the patient can be maintained in good general condition while tubular recovery takes place. Oliguria usually persists for about seven to ten days and is then followed by a spontaneous diuresis of unconcentrated urine. Urinary concentrating power then slowly improves as the tubules recover normal metabolic function.

Management of acute tubular necrosis

When *oliguria* or *anuria* occurs, the diagnostic problem is to differentiate acute tubular necrosis from less serious causes such as *reduced glomerular filtration* or *urinary retention*. Retention of urine can usually be diagnosed by abdominal examination, but if this is equivocal, bladder ultrasound will provide the answer. If the rate of urine production is in doubt, a catheter should be inserted to monitor hourly urine output. Low urine output is often caused simply by diminished glomerular filtration with enhanced tubular reabsorption. The primary cause is a modest reduction in renal perfusion, secondary to relative hypovolaemia. This usually arises if a perioperative fluid deficit is inadequately replaced; in this case, urine output may fall to as little as a few ml per hour. If fluid balance is not corrected, tubular necrosis may supervene.

If acute renal failure is mild, conservative measures, including fluid restriction, may sustain the patient until tubular function recovers. However, if complete renal failure develops, the plasma urea, creatinine and potassium concentrations rise in exorably and the patient usually requires dialysis. Haemodialysis is the usual method, although peritoneal dialysis may be appropriate if the patient has not undergone abdominal surgery.

Prevention of acute renal failure

Acute renal failure is largely preventable by careful attention to preoperative assessment, fluid balance, the prevention and prompt management of hypotension and septicaemia, and dose monitoring of potentially nephrotoxic drugs. In high risk patients (with pre-existing renal disease or obstructive jaundice, and those undergoing cardiopulmonary bypass or aortic surgery), intravenous mannitol given peroperatively may protect renal function by promoting an osmotic diuresis.

PRESSURE SORES

Pathophysiology

The elderly, debilitated and other bed-bound patients are extremely susceptible to developing pressure sores ('bed sores'), particularly over bony prominences such as the sacrum and heels (see Figure 33.9). Pressure sores

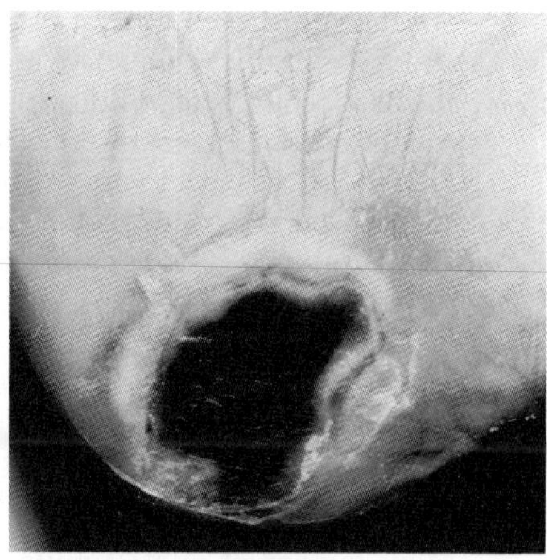

Fig. 33.9 Typical heel pressure sore

This elderly woman presented with peritonitis and had a stormy postoperative course. At some stage, this heel was allowed to remain too long in one position, resulting in deep necrosis. She had no evidence of peripheral arterial disease

occur because the frequent adjustment of position that normally occurs is lost through immobility. Diminished protective pain response probably plays some part. Tissue necrosis and subsequent failure to heal result from a combination of factors, including recurrent pressure ischaemia, poor tissue perfusion (from cardiac or peripheral vascular disease) and malnutrition.

Prevention and management of pressure sores

Pressure sores, once established, are difficult to eradicate and thus prevention must be given high priority in patients at risk. Relatively hard surfaces such as accident and emergency department trollies and operating theatre tables may initiate pressure sores in susceptible patients in less than an hour. Likewise, pressure sores can develop in a remarkably short time in a hospital bed, particularly if the patient is incontinent of urine or faeces. Prevention of pressure sores on the ward is mainly a nursing responsibility; indeed the incidence of pressure sores is a good indicator of the quality of nursing care.

Prevention of pressure sores involves the following procedures:

- Relieving pressure on the heels — use of ankle rests while on the operating table; use of heel pads, sheepskin rugs and 'bean-bags' on return to the ward
- Regular change of posture — for most patients, this involves encouragement to get out of bed, at least into a bedside chair, and to mobilise beyond this as much as possible. The bedbound patient requires regular turning so that the same skin area is not subjected to constant pressure
- Special bed surfaces to spread the load — these include simple sheepskin mattress covers, padded over-mattresses and electric ripple mattresses, water beds, sophisticated vibrating mattresses and suspended net beds
- Regular checking of pressure areas and local massage
- Management of incontinence

Treatment of established pressure sores is unsatisfactory unless the causative factors can be eliminated. This is often impossible in the permanently disabled patient. Avoiding pressure is the mainstay of treatment, supplemented by local cleansing and dressings designed to remove necrotic tissue and control secondary infection. Occasionally, major plastic surgery involving a rotational flap is justified for a sacral sore.

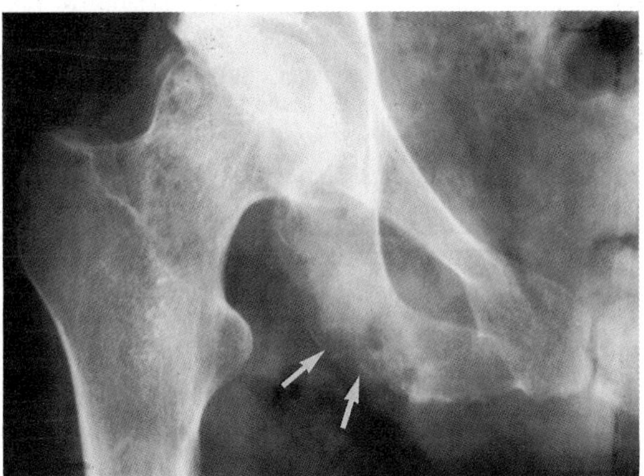

Fig. 33.10 Osteomyelitis of the ischial tuberosity secondary to pressure ulceration

X-ray of the pelvis in an elderly immobile woman showing osteomyelitis of the ischial tuberosity (arrowed) underlying a deep long-standing sacral pressure ulcer

GENERAL OPERATIVE COMPLICATIONS

The main complications of any operation are haemorrhage, infection, delayed wound healing, surgical damage to related structures and inadvertent trauma to the patient in theatre.

HAEMORRHAGE

Peroperative haemorrhage

Haemorrhage occurring during an operation (*primary haemorrhage*) should be controlled by the surgeon before the operation is completed; the methods have been described in Chapter 3.

Early postoperative haemorrhage

Haemorrhage during the immediate postoperative period usually indicates inadequate operative haemostasis or a technical mishap such as a slipped ligature or unrecognised trauma to a blood vessel.

After major blood loss requiring transfusion of stored blood, postoperative haemorrhage may be perpetuated by *consumption coagulopathy*, in which platelets and coagulation factors have been 'consumed' in a vain attempt at haemostasis. Occasionally bleeding results from a pre-existing but unrecognised bleeding diathesis or the use of aspirin-like drugs preoperatively.

Operations at particular risk of early postoperative haemorrhage include the following: major operations involving highly vascular tissues such as the liver or spleen, arterial surgery (in which the patient is usually heparinised) or operations which leave a large raw surface such as abdominoperineal resection of the rectum. This type of postoperative haemorrhage has been traditionally described as reactionary haemorrhage in the belief that it was a 'reaction' to the recovery of normal blood pressure and cardiac output. This concept is misleading and should now be discarded, especially since it may hinder the decision to re-explore a wound as a matter of urgency.

Management of early postoperative haemorrhage

It should be remembered that early postoperative haemorrhage is really a form of primary haemorrhage and if substantial, the patient must be surgically re-explored and the source of haemorrhage treated as at the original operation. It is wise to perform a clotting screen (including platelet count) and cross match an appropriate amount of bank blood as a preliminary measure. Good intravenous access should be ensured and a central venous pressure catheter inserted for monitoring. If heparin has been used at the original operation, protamine can be given to reverse any residual activity. If the clotting screen is abnormal, specific clotting factors such as fresh frozen plasma or platelet concentrates should be given. Many of these patients will stop bleeding with supportive measures and blood transfusion, but re-exploration must be considered at every stage.

Later postoperative haemorrhage

Haemorrhage occurring several days after operation is usually related to infection which erodes vessels at the operation site; this is known as *secondary haemorrhage*. Treatment involves managing the infection but exploratory operation may be required to ligate bleeding vessels.

INFECTION RELATED TO THE OPERATION SITE

Minor wound infections

The most common operative infection is the superficial wound infection occurring within the first postoperative week. This relatively trivial infection presents as localised pain, redness and a slight discharge. The organisms are usually staphylococci or streptococci derived from the skin. The infection usually settles without treatment. The exception is the patient in whom a prosthesis has been inserted, such as an arterial graft or artificial joint. For these patients, antibiotics must be given to prevent the devastating consequences of infection around the prosthesis.

Wound cellulitis and abscess

More severe wound infections occur most commonly after bowel-related surgery, when faecal organisms are usually incriminated. The majority present in the first postoperative week but they may occur as late as the third postoperative week, often after the patient has left hospital. These infections commonly present first with a pyrexia; examination of the wound reveals either a spreading *cellulitis* or localised *abscess formation*.

Cellulitis is treated with appropriate antibiotics after taking a wound swab for culture and sensitivity, whereas a wound abscess is treated by surgical drainage. This may simply involve suture removal and probing of the wound, but deeper abscesses may require re-exploration under general anaesthesia. In either case, the wound is left open to heal by secondary intention.

Intra-abdominal infection is discussed under complications of abdominal and bowel surgery later in this chapter.

Gas gangrene

Gas gangrene is an uncommon, acute, life-threatening wound infection, in which the anaerobic organisms multiply in necrotic tissue, particularly muscle (see Chapter 1).

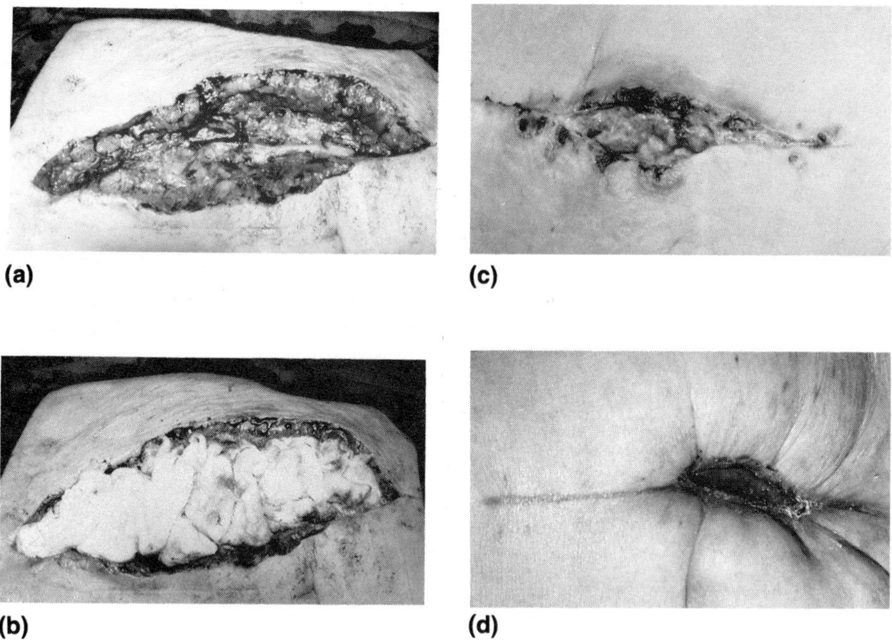

(a) (c)

(b) (d)

Fig. 33.11 Deep wound infection healed by secondary intention

This 80-year-old diabetic woman underwent laparotomy and the wound became infected with *Staphylococcus aureus*. This resulted in a wound abscess and necrosis of the wound edge. **(a)** The wound after all necrotic tissue has been excised. It was then packed with dry gauze, as shown in **(b)** and allowed to heal by secondary intention. The wound at three weeks **(c)** and eight weeks **(d)**. It was completely healed after two further weeks. Note the degree of wound contraction, which plays a major part in overcoming the tissue defect

Late infective complications

A late infective complication of surgery is a chronically discharging *wound sinus* which emanates from a deep chronic abscess. It usually relates to foreign material such as a non-absorbable suture or sometimes necrotic fascia or tendon. These sinuses commonly follow wound infections where healing is delayed and incomplete. Wound sinuses occasionally appear after apparent normal healing, particularly after insertion of a prosthesis.

Sinuses rarely heal spontaneously unless the foreign material is discharged, and the usual treatment is therefore re-exploration of the wound and removal of the offending substance.

IMPAIRED HEALING

Factors retarding wound healing

The vast majority of wounds heal without complication. It is a popular misconception that wounds heal slowly in the elderly; this is not so unless there are specific adverse factors. Wound healing in general is retarded if blood supply is poor (as in arterial insufficiency), or if the wound is under excess suture tension. Other factors which may retard wound healing are long-term steroid therapy, severe rheumatoid disease, malnutrition and vitamin deficiency, especially of vitamin C.

Wound dehiscence ('burst abdomen')

Wound dehiscence, i.e. total wound breakdown, is an uncommon problem. It affects about 1% of abdominal wounds and usually occurs about one week after operation. The sudden bursting open of the abdomen revealing coils of bowel is alarming to nurses and junior doctors but is remarkably pain-free for the patient! Infection and other factors already described may play a part but the usual cause is inadequate abdominal wall repair. This may be compounded by mechanical disruption caused by coughing or abdominal distension.

The wound should initially be covered with sterile swabs soaked in saline and the patient returned to the operating theatre within a few hours for repair. This usually involves placement of tension sutures which incorporate large 'bites' of the whole thickness of the abdominal wall.

Incisional hernia

Incisional hernia is a late complication of abdominal surgery. These hernias usually becoming apparent within the first postoperative year but sometimes develop as long as five years later; the overall incidence is about 10–15% of abdominal wounds. The hernia is caused by breakdown of the repair to the abdominal wall muscle and fascia. Predisposing factors are abdominal obesity, distension and poor muscle quality, inadequate closure technique, postoperative wound infection and multiple operations through the same incision.

An incisional hernia usually presents as a bulge in the abdominal wall near a previous wound. The condition is usually asymptomatic but occasionally a narrow-necked hernia presents with pain or strangulation. Once an

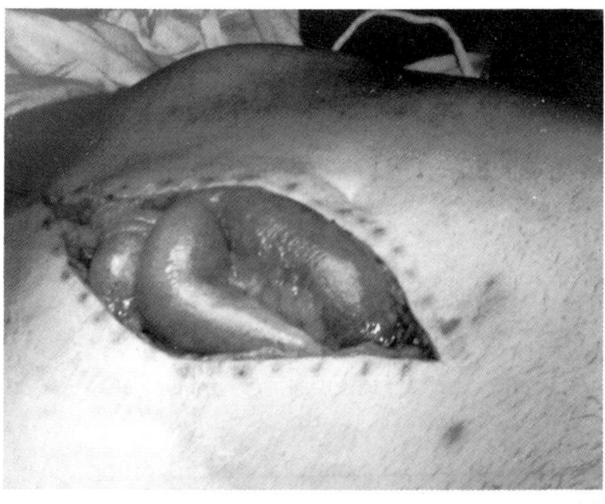

(a)

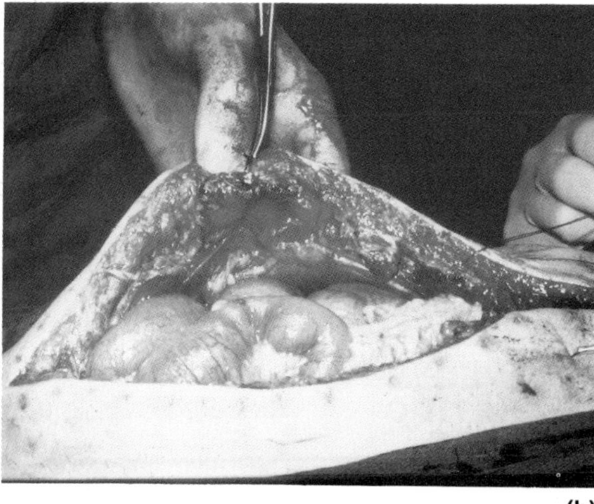

(b)

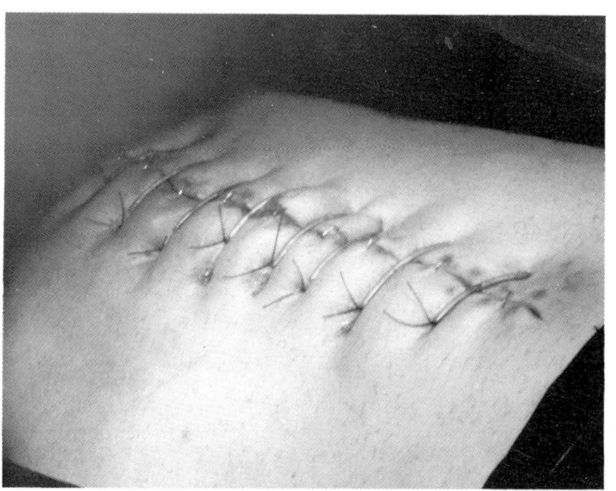

(c)

Fig. 33.12 Burst abdomen and repair with tension sutures

(a) Complete wound dehiscence six days after laparotomy for peritonitis. Note the exposed bowel spilling out of the wound. **(b)** Operative photograph showing insertion of 'tension sutures' through the whole thickness of the abdominal wall. **(c)** The completed wound repair

incisional hernia has appeared, it tends to enlarge progressively and may become a nuisance cosmetically or for dressing. Repair is indicated for strangulation, pain or inconvenience.

SURGICAL INJURY

Unavoidable tissue damage

Anatomical structures, particularly nerves, blood vessels and lymphatics, may be unavoidably damaged during operation. This is particularly true in cancer surgery, illustrated by facial nerve damage during total parotidectomy. This must be accepted as part of the operative risk and if possible, discussed with the patient beforehand. Sometimes the integrity or location of vulnerable structures can be established preoperatively, thus allowing better planning of the operation. For example, an IVU may be done to identify the course of the ureters in patients with colonic cancer, or indirect laryngoscopy may be done to assess vocal cord integrity prior to thyroid surgery.

Inadvertent tissue damage

Structures may be inadvertently damaged during operation. Examples include recurrent laryngeal nerve damage during thyroidectomy and trauma to the common bile duct during cholecystectomy. The main factors are inexperience, anatomical anomalies, attempts at arresting precipitous haemorrhage and tissue planes obscured by inflammation or malignancy. Signs of damage to structures at risk for specific operations should be sought in the postoperative period; for example, hoarseness after thyroidectomy or jaundice after cholecystectomy.

INADVERTENT OPERATING THEATRE TRAUMA

Apart from surgical trauma, patients are at risk of injury when anaesthetised. Special precautions are taken in the operating theatre to minimise these risks.

The most common complications caused by trauma in the operating theatre are:

- Ulnar and lateral popliteal nerve palsies
- Electrical burns from wet diathermy pads
- Excess pressure on the calf causing deep venous thrombosis
- Excess heel pressure causing pressure sores
- Cardiac pacemaker disruption by diathermy equipment
- Injury to diseased bones and joints from manipulation or positioning. These include dislocation of a rheumatoid atlanto-axial joint and dislocation of a prosthetic hip joint

COMPLICATIONS OF OPERATIONS INVOLVING BOWEL

DELAYED RETURN OF BOWEL FUNCTION

Temporary interruption of peristalsis

Any abdominal operation may temporarily disrupt peristalsis. This is particularly true where the operation is for peritonitis or obstruction, or if the operation involves extensive handling of the bowel. Operations involving the retroperitoneal area, such as aortic surgery, may also disrupt peristalsis. The mechanism is probably disturbance of parasympathetic activity. The problem is usually minor, mostly affecting the small intestine, and may cause nausea, anorexia and vomiting. This becomes obvious after oral fluids are reintroduced in the early postoperative period. This condition is often loosely described as *ileus* and is the reason for gradual reintroduction of fluids, followed by solids, after abdominal operations.

Complete adynamic obstruction

Occasionally, a much more prolonged and extensive form of adynamic bowel obstruction occurs. This presents with vomiting and protracted intolerance to oral intake. *Adynamic obstruction* must be distinguished from true mechanical obstruction, which may require reoperation (see Chapter 7).

Acute gastric dilatation

Occasionally, adynamic obstruction involves the stomach causing acute gastric dilatation, and a large volume of gastric and duodenal reflux secretions accumulate. The warning feature is when the patient suddenly vomits a large volume of fluid, which may result in fatal aspiration. Prevention of acute gastric dilatation is the main reason for nasogastric tubes being used after operations such as vagotomy and pyloroplasty, relief of mechanical bowel obstruction and aortic surgery. If acute gastric dilatation is suspected in any patient in whom recovery is unexpectedly slow, the abdomen should be examined daily for a succussion splash and a nasogastric tube passed if the result is positive.

'Pseudo-obstruction'

Adynamic obstruction involving the large bowel is conventionally described as pseudo-obstruction. It may follow any abdominal operation, especially if the retroperitoneal area has been disturbed as in nephrectomy or aortic surgery. Pseudo-obstruction is also a recognised complication of *non-abdominal operations* such as fractured neck of femur, especially in debilitated patients. Pseudo-obstruction may even occur without operation as a complication of severe hypokalaemia, trauma involving the lower spine and retroperitoneal area, or anti-Parkinsonian drugs.

MECHANICAL BOWEL OBSTRUCTION

Early postoperative mechanical obstruction

Postoperative mechanical obstruction of the bowel is uncommon. It may be caused by a loop of bowel becoming twisted or trapped in a peritoneal defect, unwittingly created at operation. *Fibrinous adhesions* may also cause obstruction, and these usually develop about one week postoperatively. In both cases, the obstruction may be transient and settle with conservative measures (nasogastric aspiration and intravenous fluids), or may progress to full-blown intestinal obstruction requiring laparotomy. Obstruction occurring after gastrectomy or gastroenterostomy may be due to oedema of the mucosa surrounding the anastomosis; this will usually settle eventually with conservative measures.

Late postoperative mechanical obstruction

Fibrinous adhesions may organise and persist as broad *fibrous adhesions* between adjacent loops of bowel or as isolated *fibrous bands* traversing the peritoneal cavity. These fibrous adhesions are a common cause of an isolated episode of small bowel obstruction or even strangulation. Adhesions may also cause recurrent bouts of bowel obstruction months or years after abdominal operations. Most cases will resolve spontaneously with conservative treatment, but failure to resolve or signs of strangulation will necessitate laparotomy.

ANASTOMOTIC FAILURE

Anastomotic leakage or breakdown is a major cause of postoperative morbidity after bowel surgery. Inadequate diagnosis and surgical intervention may lead to snowballing complications including septicaemia, fistulae and multi-organ failure.

Small anastomotic leaks are relatively common, and lead to small localised abscesses which are walled off by surrounding gut and omentum. Small leaks are clinically manifest by delayed recovery of bowel function due to local peristaltic dysfunction. Usually, the problem settles eventually with continued intravenous fluids and delayed reintroduction of oral intake. Reoperation is rarely necessary.

Major anastomotic breakdown results in large abdominal abscesses, septicaemia, generalised peritonitis or fistula formation. These are described below.

INTRA-ABDOMINAL ABSCESS

Abscess associated with bowel anastomosis

A large anastomotic leak from any part of the bowel may be walled off by small bowel and omentum as a vigorous intraperitoneal response (see Figure 33.13). This results in formation of an abscess near the anastomosis. The patient will either be non-specifically unwell with delayed recovery, a swinging pyrexia and signs of local peritonitis, or more seriously ill with septicaemia. A detailed description of the clinical features is given in Chapter 7.

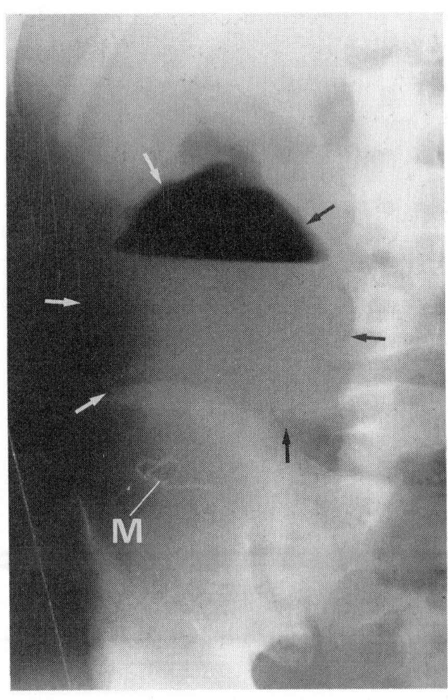

(a)

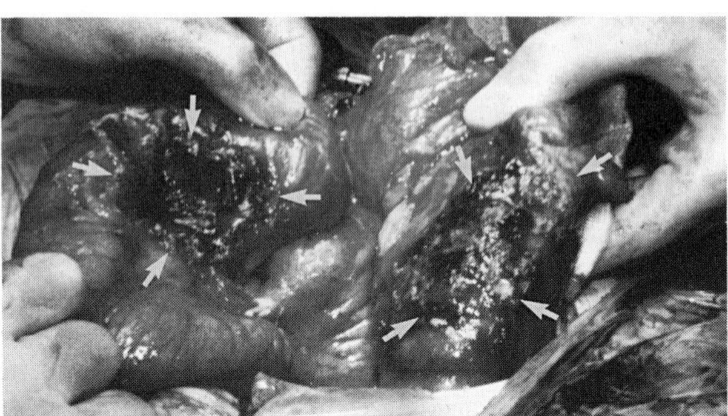
(b)

Fig. 33.13 Intra-abdominal abscess

(a) Intraperitoneal abscess following appendicectomy. Erect abdominal X-ray from a 16-year-old boy one week after removal of a perforated gangrenous appendix. He remained ill with anorexia and intermittent vomiting, general malaise and a swinging pyrexia. A large mass was palpable in the right side of the abdomen. The X-ray shows a huge abscess cavity (outline arrowed) with a gas bubble above a fluid (pus) level. Note the radiopaque marker **M** in a gauze swab packed into the open wound. **(b)** This 64-year-old woman had a right hemicolectomy for caecal carcinoma. The anastomosis performed between terminal ileum and transverse colon leaked and the patient developed symptoms and signs of an intra-abdominal abscess. At laparotomy, a localised abscess (arrowed) was found, walled off by loops of bowel

Reoperation is usually necessary to drain the abscess and prevent continued contamination of the peritoneal cavity. Where the anastomosis has broken down, both ends of the bowel should be brought out to form temporary stomas, since reanastomosis will almost certainly fail. The bowel can be rejoined once the local infection and metabolic upset have resolved.

Other intra-abdominal abscesses

Intra-abdominal abscesses may also develop at sites remote from an anastomosis, for example in the pelvis (*pelvic abscess*) or beneath the diaphragm (*subphrenic abscess*). These abscesses occur most commonly as a complication of treated peritonitis. They may also develop because of contamination of the operative site by faeces or other infected material, or by 'tracking' of an anastomotic abscess within the abdomen. Abscesses of this type usually produce a less severe illness than do those in direct communication with the bowel, described in the preceding section.

If an abscess is suspected, ultrasound or CT scanning may help to identify its location and guide needle aspiration, if appropriate. Surgical exploration may, however, be necessary.

PERITONITIS

Peritonitis in the postoperative period usually results from a major anastomotic breakdown causing widespread peritoneal contamination. Sometimes the cause of peritonitis is perforation of obstructed or ischaemic bowel or perforation of an incidental peptic ulcer. The clinical picture may develop rapidly over a few hours, or more insidiously over a few days if infection spreads from an intraperitoneal abscess. The patient is systemically ill with severe, generalised abdominal pain; the abdomen is tender and rigid to palpation (see Chapter 7 for more details). Generalised peritonitis progresses to septicaemic shock unless promptly treated.

The patient is resuscitated and commenced on intravenous antibiotics and then returned to theatre for laparotomy. The abdomen is explored, the underlying cause is treated and peritoneal toilet is carried out. Early and vigorous treatment will usually save the patient's life.

BOWEL FISTULA

Fistula formation usually results from an anastomotic leak, when its surrounding abscess discharges to the surface via the wound or along the track of an abdominal drain. The problem is compounded if there is distal bowel obstruction because the effluent is preferentially diverted via the fistula. Proximal small bowel fistulae result in the loss of large volumes of intestinal secretions containing digestive enzymes. This rapidly leads to dehydration and major electrolyte disturbances, and causes gross intra-abdominal inflammation and surface skin destruction. The more distal the origin of the fistula, the less destructive its consequences.

The general state of the patient with a fistula depends on the extent of intra-abdominal sepsis. If this is minimal and there is no distal obstruction, the fistula will close spontaneously within weeks or months, provided the patient can be sustained in the interim. Proximal small bowel fistulae require *total bowel rest*, with full *parenteral fluid replacement and nutrition*. Distal small bowel or large bowel fistulae may be managed with *enteral feeding* using low-residue elemental or semi-elemental fluid diets. These are often given via a fine-bore nasogastric tube.

When a fistula is associated with intra-abdominal sepsis, the patient is desperately ill, septicaemic and hypercatabolic. These patients need intensive care management. Laparotomy is required to bring the disrupted bowel ends to the surface as stomas and to drain the gross foci of infection; further laparotomies, even daily, may still be required before the intra-abdominal sepsis is brought under control. Mortality from such complicated fistulae is extremely high.

ACUTE BOWEL ISCHAEMIA

Acute bowel ischaemia is an uncommon postoperative complication, usually occurring after abdominal aortic surgery. Infarction of the sigmoid colon follows inferior mesenteric artery ligation (usually a necessary part of the operation) if the collateral supply is compromised by obliterative atherosclerosis of the remaining mesenteric arteries.

The patient has usually progressed satisfactorily at first, and then several days after operation, deteriorates unexpectedly. Finally, the patient collapses with peritonitis due to massive colonic necrosis and perforation. Clinical signs are non-specific, but plain abdominal X-ray may show the typical appearance of gas in the bowel wall. If acute bowel ischaemia is suspected, laparotomy must be performed immediately, as perforation is nearly always fatal. Even with timely surgery, the prognosis is bleak.

34 PREOPERATIVE ASSESSMENT AND PREPARATION

Introduction

When a patient is admitted to hospital for surgical investigation or treatment, a detailed history and examination (*clerking*) is undertaken by a junior hospital doctor. This procedure is not mainly concerned with diagnosing the primary disorder, but with anticipating complications and taking avoiding action.

PRINCIPLES OF ASSESSMENT

In preparing a patient for operation, the doctor needs to answer a series of questions, summarised in Figure 34.1. Answers from the history and examination may reveal the need for tests or some other action.

The majority of surgical cases are straightforward but preventable disasters can occur unless a thorough and systematic approach is used.

Patients at high risk of complications

The history and examination will reveal certain groups of patients who are at greater risk of occult illness or specific problems related to surgery. They need special investigations to identify hidden problems and to provide base-line information against which later changes can be measured. The common problems of high-risk groups of patients are summarised in Figure 34.2.

ESSENTIALS OF PRE-OPERATIVE ASSESSMENT

Although procedures vary in different hospitals, certain basic steps must be taken to ensure maximum safety of a patient before operation. These steps depend on the operation and the condition of the patient. The *need for an operation* must be reviewed on admission to hospital since circumstances can change significantly between booking and the time of operation. *Overt and occult illnesses* must also be considered in every patient.

Explanations to the patient and informed consent

The surgeon must carefully explain the diagnosis and the proposed operation to the patient beforehand. Patients, however, often absorb very little of what has been said, and fail to understand the full ramifications. This is because they are often anxious and disorientated when admitted, and most have little understanding of how their bodies work. This means the doctor must adopt a sympathetic and unhurried approach, and often must explain things more than once. By this means, the junior surgical doctor can ensure that the patient is giving genuine informed consent.

Fig. 34.1 Preoperative assessment and planning

1. DIAGNOSIS

What is the **(provisional) diagnosis**?

How **confident** is the diagnosis?

What are the **important facets of the history**?

What are the **findings on examination**?

What are the **results of investigations** already performed?

Have **tissue diagnoses** been obtained before admission to hospital?

Are any **further investigations** needed to confirm the primary diagnosis?

2. OPERATION

What **operation or procedure is planned**?

Have any **circumstances changed** relating to the planned operation —
Has the patient got better or worse?
Has any new diagnostic information appeared? (e.g. pulmonary metastases on a chest X-ray)
Is the planned operation still appropriate?

Are there any **special risks attending this particular operation**, i.e. intraoperative or postoperative? (e.g. risk of DVT after pelvic surgery)

Are there any **'routine' procedures** that need to be performed in relation to the operation ? (e.g. cross-matching blood if heavy blood loss is anticipated)

Are there **operation-specific actions** that need to be performed ? (e.g. examining vocal cord movement before thyroid surgery, arranging peroperative cholangiogram for cholecystectomy)

3. ANAESTHETIC

What **type of anaesthetic** is to be employed?

Can any **anaesthetic complications** be anticipated? (e.g. risk of postoperative chest infection after thoracotomy or upper abdominal surgery, risk of a patient with bowel obstruction inhaling vomitus during anaesthetic induction)

4. FITNESS FOR OPERATION

Is the **patient fit for the planned anaesthetic and operation**?

Are there any **intercurrent diseases** which are inadequately treated, or which might pose special problems? (e.g. insulin dependent diabetes, rheumatoid arthritis with cervical spine involvement)

Are any **preoperative investigations or treatments** needed for intercurrent disease ? (e.g. physiotherapy for chronic bronchitis, cervical spine radiology for rheumatoid arthritis)

Does the **surgical condition itself pose special problems**? (e.g. fluid or electrolyte disturbances as a result of vomiting)

Is the patient taking any **drugs which might cause problems** with anaesthesia or operation ? (e.g. MAOIs or steroids)

5. HIGH RISK

Is this patient, by virtue of the illness, **particularly predisposed to anaesthetic or surgical complications**?

6. AFTER THE OPERATION

Can any **special problems be anticipated** for this patient during the postoperative period and after discharge from hospital? (e.g. elderly patients living alone)

Are there any **problems specific to this anaesthetic or operation** with respect to recovery and rehabilitation ? (e.g. prostheses after mastectomy, limb fitting and rehabilitation following amputation)

Is any planning **required for operation-specific problems**?

Fig. 34.2 High risk groups for perioperative complications

Group	Particular risks	Management
Premature or tiny babies, neonates and infants	Fluid and electrolyte loss	Careful measurement and replacement
	Heat loss in operating theatre	Warming blanket, temperature monitoring
Patients over 60	Cardiovascular disease	ECG preoperatively & monitoring during operation; chest X–ray preoperatively
Elderly patients	Confusion	Multifactorial — see Chapter 35
	Hyponatraemia	Preoperative electrolyte estimations and correction
	Immobility	Good nursing and rehabilitation
Smokers	Postop chest infection and atelectasis	Stop smoking at least four weeks before operation. Preoperative chest X–ray. Preoperative and postoperative physiotherapy
	Increased risk of myocardial infarction	Preoperative ECG
Obese patients	Increased risk of DVT Reduced mobility	Prophylaxis (see Chapter 33)
Patients with intercurrent medical disease	Depends on medical condition	Problems discussed in Chapter 32

If the immediate postoperative period is likely to be unpleasant, and require admission to an intensive care unit, for example, it is kind to forewarn the patient and arrange a visit to the unit beforehand. Mentally handicapped and elderly patients have particular difficulty in adapting to changing circumstances, and care should be taken to familiarise them with facilities and staff.

At the time of obtaining consent, the *operation site should be marked* on the patient's skin with an indelible pen. This is particularly important if the operation could be performed on either side of the body, for example an inguinal hernia or limb amputation. This marking procedure also gives the patient an opportunity to agree which operation is to be done and on which side!

Liaison with anaesthetist

The anaesthetist should be informed in advance of the proposed operation and the condition of the patient; anaesthetists usually see patients themselves preoperatively to anticipate problems and prescribe premedication. The anaesthetist is ultimately responsible for ensuring that the patient is fit for operation.

Operating theatre arrangements

The house surgeon is responsible for informing the operating theatre nurses about the operation and making any special arrangements. If more than one patient is for operation, then a formal *operating list* should be prepared, giving full details of the name, age, sex, ward, and proposed operation for each patient. The side of the body to be operated on should be clearly indicated. In addition, any special requirements for instruments, intraoperative radiography or patient positioning must be noted on the list. In some hospitals, the amount of blood cross-matched for any patient is also recorded on the list.

Fig. 34.3 Essential steps in preoperative assessment and preparation

History taking

Physical examination

Collating pre-admission information about diagnosis

Arranging any further diagnostic investigations

Making special preparations for the particular operation

Investigating any intercurrent or occult illness suggested by clinical clerking

Discussing the operation with the patient and obtaining signed consent

Marking the operation site

Making arrangements for the operation with the operating theatre staff

Arranging and informing the anaesthetist

Prescribing premedication, prophylactic antibiotics and treatment to prevent venous thrombosis, as appropriate

Planning rehabilitation and convalescence

Planning the recovery period

Plans for rehabilitation and convalescence should be discussed with the patient and relatives in advance. The patient should be advised about the likely rate of recovery and the level of activity possible on discharge. In this way, social, business and domestic arrangements can be made in good time. If necessary, domestic or home nursing help can be arranged. Uncertainty about these matters often causes anxiety and hampers recovery.

CASE HISTORY

This case history illustrates the way a patient might be prepared for a major operation and the considerations which guide the preoperative management:

History

James Brown, a 70-year-old retired farmer, is admitted electively for the operation of anterior resection of the rectum for presumed carcinoma at the rectosigmoid junction.

Present complaint

He was seen urgently in an outpatient clinic three weeks beforehand, with a 5 week history of loose stools 3–5 times a day, without blood or mucus. He had lost about 4 kg in weight over the preceding three months, but remarked that he had been trying to lose weight anyway.

Outpatient investigation gave the following results:
Sigmoidoscopic examination — normal
Three stool specimens — positive for occult blood
Barium enema — 'apple-core' lesion at rectosigmoid junction
Ultrasound examination of liver — no metastases
Full blood count — haemoglobin 11.6 g/l, otherwise normal

Systems enquiry

He claimed to be generally well, but on systematic enquiry revealed that he became short of breath after walking 200 yards on the flat and had had occasional fast palpitations during the past few weeks. There were no other cardiovascular or respiratory symptoms. The only other symptom was a poor stream on micturition.

Past Medical History

He had undergone appendicectomy at the age of 14 with no anaesthetic complications, and he had a serious farming injury to his left elbow at the age of 20 years. He had been jaundiced without hospitalisation while in Asia during the Second World War. For about ten years he had been hypertensive and on drug treatment for five years. Three years before, maturity onset diabetes was discovered on routine urine testing and this was controlled by diet.

Family History

Mr Brown's mother had been obese, dying at the age of 55 from complications of diabetes. His brother had a major stroke at the age of 64. There was no family history of bowel disorder.

Social History

Mr Brown had been widowed for two years, his wife having died of breast cancer. He has a son and daughter, both married with young children, but living far away. He lives in a house with an upstairs lavatory, on a smallholding where he keeps a few animals. He is completely independent, and uses his car for shopping. He has smoked 20 cigarettes a day for many years, and drinks alcohol occasionally.

Drug history

He takes a beta-adrenergic blocker and a thiazide diuretic with potassium supplement each morning for hypertension, and he takes two aspirin tablets three times a day for pain in his left hip. He has been told in the past not to have penicillin, but he cannot recall why; he does not remember when he last had penicillin. He is not allergic to iodine.

Examination

General. Mr Brown is a fit looking man of 70, who does not appear to be anxious. He is tanned, with no apparent anaemia, cyanosis, jaundice, lymphadenopathy or clubbing, and there is no thyroid enlargement. His fingers are tobacco stained. He is not febrile.

Cardiovascular and respiratory system. Pulse is 68 beats per minute and regular, and blood pressure 150/110 mmHg. A soft systolic murmer is heard at the left sternal edge. There is no ankle swelling and jugular venous pressure is not elevated. Chest examination is unremarkable apart from odd crepitations which do not clear after coughing.

Abdomen. The abdomen is moderately obese and an appendicectomy scar is noted. The abdomen is soft with no apparent organomegaly but there is a suggestion of a mass in the left iliac fossa which is not indentable. External genitalia are normal. Rectal examination reveals a moderately enlarged smooth prostate and normal coloured stool.

Central nervous system and locomotor system. This is normal apart from a fixed flexion deformity of the left elbow at 90°.

Summary

A 70-year old man with probable rectosigmoid carcinoma without obvious dissemination, admitted for resection of the rectosigmoid area.

A problem list was constructed from this information, which led to further investigations and a management plan. The reasoning is shown in Figure 34.4.

Fig. 34.4 Example of preoperative assessment of a patient admitted for a major operation (case history given above)

Problem	Surgical significance	Plan of action for each problem
1. Mild diabetes mellitus	Is it under good control ?	All urine samples to be tested for glucose Random blood glucose estimation
2. Obesity	May make access difficult at operation	May necessitate insertion of wound drain at operation Predisposes to wound infection
	Increased risk of deep vein thrombosis or pulmonary embolism	Prophylaxis, eg low dose heparin, intravenous dextran or compression stockings
3. Hypertension (BP150/110)	How well is hypertension controlled on present medication?	Monitor blood pressure 4–hourly on admission and then decide about drug therapy
	Is elevated BP on admission just due to anxiety?	Check pulse rate and BP several times
	Are there other complications of hypertension such as ventricular hypertrophy or dilatation ?	Perform ECG and chest X–ray
4. Shortness of breath on exertion, recent palpitations	Are these merely symptoms of anxiety about the diagnosis or do they represent significant cardiac or respiratory disease ?	ECG and chest X–ray Possibly needs lung function tests
5. Poor urinary stream and large prostate	Possible carcinoma of prostate	Prostate should be palpated and possibly biopsied
	Possible difficulty of catheterisation at operation	Anticipate
	Risk of postoperative urinary retention when catheter removed	Anticipate

Fig. 34.4 (cont.)

Problem	Surgical significance	Plan of action for each problem
6. Jaundice in the past	History suggestive of Hepatitis A	Serological tests for hepatitis antigen ?
7. Smoker	Possible occult lung cancer	Chest X–ray
	Increased risk of postoperative chest infections	Preoperative physiotherapy and breathing exercises
	Increased risk of myocardial infarction	Anticipate
8. Left elbow injury	May be in the way during operation	Inform theatre staff about need for careful positioning on the operating table
9. Diuretic therapy	Are electrolytes and renal function normal?	Plasma urea, electrolytes and creatinine estimations
10. Aspirin therapy	Could gastric irritation partly account for the low haemoglobin ?	Use non–gastric irritant analgesics
11. Possible penicillin allergy	A penicillin is often used for prophylaxis or treatment of post-operative infections	Indicate penicillin allergy; alternative drugs must be used
12. Cardiac murmur	Is this clinically significant ? Is antibiotic prophylaxis necessary ?	Consult anaesthetist or cardiologist
13. Lives alone, looks after animals	Who will look after his animals while he is in hospital ? Who will look after him when he returns home ?	Discuss domestic arrangements and convalescence plans
14. Low haemoglobin	Not low enough to need preoperative transfusion but there is less reserve for the operation	Cross match at least two units of blood for operation
	Potentially extensive operation — may have large blood loss	Cross match extra blood, i.e. at least 4 units in all
15. May need temporary or even permanent colostomy	Will he be able to cope? What does he understand about stomas ?	Needs counselling and possible preoperative 'trial' of colostomy appliance (see Chapter 15)

Fig. 34.4 (cont.)

Problem	Surgical significance	Plan of action for each problem
16. Bowel will be opened during operation	Potential for faecal contamination of abdominal cavity and wound	Needs preoperative bowel preparation and prophylactic antibiotics
17. Lesion at pelvic brim	Does it involve the ureter?	Perform intravenous urogram ?

35 POSTOPERATIVE MANAGEMENT PROBLEMS

Introduction

Despite the best endeavours at diagnosis, preoperative assessment and surgical technique, unexpected symptoms and signs arise in the postoperative period which may herald a postoperative complication. Complications can be minimised by close postoperative patient observation. For example, daily auscultation of the chest may reveal a chest infection before symptoms appear.

Managing the common problems of fever, pain and collapse requires accurate diagnosis and early treatment if the complication is not to get out of hand. Making the diagnosis is often difficult as the postoperative patient may be anxious, in pain or not fully recovered from an anaesthetic. It is vital to conduct a thorough and systematic clinical assessment and if necessary, investigation, whatever the hour, of these potentially serious but often remediable complications.

COMMON POSTOPERATIVE PROBLEMS – DIAGNOSIS AND MANAGEMENT

The following problems commonly develop in the postoperative period, often 'after hours', and are the immediate responsibility of junior surgical doctors.

PAIN

Pain can be expected from most surgical wounds but, in most cases, gradually subsides over the first few days after operation. Some types of wound are more painful than others, for example vertical abdominal incisions, skin graft donor sites and inguinal hernia repairs. Postoperative analgesia is achieved with analgesic drugs or local or regional analgesia.

Analgesic drugs

Most patients require analgesic drugs in the postoperative period and for major operations, these are usually commenced in the operating theatre or in the recovery ward. Parenteral opiates such as *papaveretum*, *diamorphine*, *morphine* or *pethidine* are usually necessary.

Further postoperative analgesia will usually be required. The choice of drug, dose, frequency and route of administration depends on the operation. Analgesics commonly used for postoperative pain relief are summarised in Figure 35.1. Patients vary greatly in their tolerance of pain and their need for analgesics. Thus, the amount of analgesia must be tailored to individual need. Anxiety, exhaustion and sleep deprivation may greatly reduce pain tolerance; these should be considered in any patient who fails to respond to a reasonable amount of analgesia.

The dose of an analgesic must be sufficient to eliminate the pain without dangerous side-effects, and the drug should be given frequently enough to maintain continuous pain relief. This is best achieved by prescribing a particular dose at defined intervals. The alternative, prescribing a range of doses which can be given 'as required' at the discretion of nursing staff is not ideal, as the the drug tends to be given only on routine drug rounds or when the patient requests it. By that time the pain may have built up to an unnecessarily high level and require a larger dose to overcome it. Pain can be much more effectively controlled if it is never allowed to reach a high level. To achieve this, some hospitals are using devices which allow patients to give themselves small intravenous increments of opiates whenever they are needed. Continuous pain relief is thus easily achieved, and paradoxically, the total dose of drug used is less than with the conventional method. Alternatively, a continuous low-dose infusion of opiates may be used, controlling the dose with an infusion pump. This technique causes minimal sedation and respiratory depression whilst maintaining excellent continuous analgesia.

Local and regional analgesia

Another approach to postoperative pain relief is local or regional analgesia. This may reduce or eliminate the need for analgesic drugs. This is particularly important in patients with poor respiratory function in whom pain or opiates might precipitate respiratory failure.

Local analgesia can be achieved by infiltrating the wound edges at the end of the operation with long-acting local anaesthetic such as *bupivacaine*.

Regional analgesia can provide effective pain relief. *Intercostal nerve blocks* with local anaesthetics are useful for upper abdominal operations and *epidural anaesthesia*, using drugs such as morphine, is invaluable for lower abdominal and perineal operations. An epidural cannula is often left in-situ to allow 'top-ups' for prolonged postoperative analgesia.

Excessive postoperative pain

If the pain is not being controlled by what appears to be an adequate dose and frequency of analgesia, complications should be suspected. First, the dose should be reviewed in relation to the expected severity of pain and the weight of the patient. Next, local postoperative complications should be considered. Wound pain may be due to pressure from a *haematoma*. In limb trauma, bleeding into a fascial compartment must be diagnosed before ischaemia ensues ('*compartment syndrome*'). Wound pain increasing after the first 48 hours may

Fig. 35.1 Postoperative analgesics and their indications (approximate ascending order of analgesic strength)

Mild to moderate pain:

Paracetamol

Compounds of paracetamol and codeine, e.g. codydramol

Aspirin

Moderate pain:

Non-steroidal anti-inflammatory drugs, e.g. ibuprofen, indomethacin (also available as suppositories)

Paracetamol plus dextropropoxyphene (coproxamol)

Codeine or dihydrocodeine

Moderate to severe pain:

Buprenorphine (usually sublingual)

Morphine slow release tablets

Pethidine (usually intramuscular)

Morphine, diamorphine or papaveretum (intramuscular or sometimes intravenous)

be caused by *infection*. The wound will be unusually tender even before redness and induration develop. There is usually a pyrexia. Lastly, major complications may be the cause of pain.

Abdominal pain

After an abdominal operation, excessive pain may be caused by major intra-abdominal complications. These include haemorrhage, anastomotic leakage, abscess formation, gaseous distension due to ileus or air swallowing, urinary retention and bowel ischaemia. Constipation may also cause late postoperative pain. These complications are all described in Chapter 33.

As a general rule, serious complications cause deterioration in the patient's general condition, whereas the patient remains well with less serious complications like urinary retention or constipation.

FEVER

Fever is a common postoperative observation which is not always caused by infection. Nonetheless, a search should always be made for a focus of infection. The common ones are *superficial* or *deep wound infection, chest infection, urinary tract infection* and infection of an *intravenous cannula site*. If there is a central venous line, infection of this should always be suspected in a patient with unexplained pyrexia. Unfortunately, this can only be diagnosed by removing the line and culturing the tip for organisms. Blood cultures are often positive but do not reveal the source of infection.

Unrelated infections such as *viral upper respiratory tract infections* are easily overlooked. *Malaria* should be considered in a recent immigrant.

Common non-infective causes of pyrexia include *transfusion reactions, wound haematoma, deep venous thrombosis* and *pulmonary embolism*. Pyrexia is sometimes the only sign of an idiosyncratic or allergic *drug reaction*. Other rare causes of pyrexia include thyrotoxic crisis, phaeochromocytoma and malignant hyperpyrexia.

TACHYCARDIA

Tachycardia may simply indicate *pain* or *anxiety* but it is also a feature of *infection, circulatory disturbances* and *thyrotoxicosis*. Mild tachycardia may a sign of incipient *hypovolaemic shock* due to haemorrhage or dehydration. It may also herald *cardiac failure* which if missed, may progress to a life threatening complication. Tachycardia may be a sign of *atrial fibrillation*; this is confirmed by electrocardiography.

COUGH, SHORTNESS OF BREATH AND TACHYPNOEA

These symptoms are often associated with an overt respiratory problem such as *acute chest infection, aspiration of gastric contents, lobar collapse, pneumothorax* or an exacerbation of a pre-existing chronic lung disorder. Clinical examination and chest X-ray will rapidly diagnose most of them.

Shortness of breath and rapid shallow breathing are a feature of alveolar collapse (*atelectasis*) which may not be detected by clinical examination or chest X-ray. Atelectasis usually responds to chest physiotherapy. *Abdominal distension* may also cause rapid shallow breathing by inhibiting diaphragmatic movement. Shortness of breath and tachypnoea may be early features of *cardiac failure* or *fluid overload* but there are usually other clues such as tachycardia and basal crepitations.

A sudden onset of shortness of breath and tachypnoea may indicate *pulmonary embolism*, and this must be recognised and treated vigorously. *Adult respiratory distress syndrome* may occur in chest trauma, acute pancreatitis or septicaemia, and should be anticipated in these patients. Finally, respiratory symptoms may be due to *hyperventilation* induced by pain, anxiety or hysterical reaction to stress.

COLLAPSE OR RAPID DETERIORATION

The junior doctor on call is commonly asked to deal with a patient who has 'collapsed' or 'gone off' in a non-specific way. To make matters more difficult, the patient is often under the care of another surgical team and is not well known to the emergency doctor. An urgent diagnosis must be made. The more serious general possibilities are summarised in Figure 35.2.

In practice, the problem is tackled in the following order, which usually leads to a logical diagnosis:

- Brief history of the collapse and postoperative course to date
- Rapid clinical appraisal, i.e. general appearance, and changes in temperature, pulse, blood pressure and respiratory rate
- Review of:
  - Reason for admission and preoperative state
  - Other pre-existing diseases
  - The nature and extent of operation, including any particular operative problems

Fig. 35.2 Important causes of postoperative collapse or rapid deterioration

Hypovolaemic shock from acute blood loss or sudden decompensation in unrecognised hypovolaemia
Bowel strangulation or obstruction
Septicaemia
Severe local infection, e.g. chest or operation site
Myocardial infarction or other cause of rapid deterioration in cardiac function, e.g. gross fluid overload or sudden dysrhythmia
Pulmonary embolus
Hypoxia due to a respiratory disorder or respiratory depressant drugs
Cerebrovascular accident (may be without obvious limb paralysis)
Hypoglycaemia or hyperglycaemia associated with diabetes
Electrolyte disturbances, e.g. hyponatraemia
Drug reactions, e.g. anaphylaxis
Adrenal insufficiency, e.g. adrenal suppression by steroids

Extent of perioperative blood and other fluid losses (including sequestration in the gut)
Adequacy of fluid replacement
Drug therapy

- Detailed physical examination
- Special tests as suggested by clinical findings, e.g. ECG, chest X-ray, serum electrolyte estimation, full blood count

NAUSEA AND VOMITING

Drugs

Nausea and vomiting are common postoperative problems. The usual causes are side-effects from drugs used for premedication, general anaesthesia and postoperative analgesia. The major culprits are *opiates*. Antiemetics, such as prochlorperazine or metoclopramide, are usually given with opiates and are prescribed 'as required' for the early postoperative period. Nausea and sometimes vomiting later in the postoperative period may also be caused by drugs. The worst offenders are the sublingual analgesic *buprenorphine*, the *antibacterials* erythromycin and metronidazole, and *digoxin* overdosage (which should be anticipated in the elderly and in chronic renal failure).

Bowel obstruction

Serious or sustained vomiting 48 hours or more after operation is usually caused by failure of normal peristalsis of small bowel, stomach or large bowel. This may be caused either by *mechanical obstruction* or by *adynamic bowel*. Adynamic bowel problems may be a response to local factors such as bowel handling or a bowel wall haematoma, or to systemic abnormalities, particularly hypokalaemia. Adynamic bowel sometimes occurs in a debilitated patient with a severe non-abdominal illness, such as fractured neck of femur. Finally, faecal impaction is a common problem in the elderly or immobile patient. It may cause vomiting from what amounts to physical obstruction plus adynamic bowel.

Systemic disorders

Electrolyte disturbances, uraemia, hypercalcaemia and other systemic disorders may cause vomiting because of their central effects. Centrally mediated vomiting also occurs in *raised intracranial pressure*. This must be considered following head injuries, neurosurgical operations or in patients who may have cerebral metastases.

Haematemesis

Elderly postoperative patients sometimes produce a small quantity of 'coffee ground' vomit which is positive for blood on 'stick' testing. This rightly causes concern to nurses, but rarely indicates a major haematemesis. It probably results from trivial bleeding from mild, stress-related gastritis or reflux oesophagitis. No special treatment is usually required, but the patient should be closely observed for signs of internal bleeding.

Occasionally, a major upper gastrointestinal haemorrhage occurs in the postoperative patient. If there has been forceful vomiting, a Mallory-Weiss tear may be the cause. Major bleeding may also arise from exacerbation of a peptic ulcer or even oesophageal varices. Seriously ill patients and the victims of burns and head injuries are susceptible to *acute stress ulceration*, which may cause catastrophic gastrointestinal haemorrhage (see Chapter 9).

DISORDERS OF BOWEL FUNCTION

The main bowel function disorders which develop in the postoperative period are constipation, diarrhoea, adynamic bowel problems and intestinal obstruction.

Constipation

Constipation is common and becomes apparent several days after operation. It usually represents a failure to re-establish normal bowel function. The causes include restriction of oral fluids and fibre, difficulty or reluctance in using a bed pan, slow recovery of normal peristalsis and general lack of mobility. Anal pain is a powerful disincentive to defecation after surgery for anal conditions! Constipation causes great distress, especially in the elderly. It should be anticipated and prevented if possible by prescribing *bulk-forming agents* (ispaghula husk preparations), *osmotic laxatives* (e.g. lactulose) or *lubricant laxatives* (e.g. liquid paraffin). Irritant laxatives and bowel stimulants should be avoided.

For colonic surgery, large bowel cleansing procedures (enemas, osmotic laxatives and restriction of solid foods) are routinely carried out beforehand to prevent solid faecal matter disrupting the anastamosis. Bowel cleansing also reduces the risk of faecal contamination during operation. Impacted faeces may result in *overflow incontinence*, which must not be confused with diarrhoea from other causes. Thus any patient with abnormal bowel function should undergo rectal examination.

Diarrhoea

Transient diarrhoea frequently follows abdominal operations, and should be regarded as normal following bowel resections or operations to relieve intestinal obstruction. Persistent diarrhoea is an uncommon complication of *trunkal vagotomy*, presenting in the early postoperative period and continuing unabated.

Diarrhoea may also complicate *antibiotic therapy*. Several days after the onset of treatment, loose, frequent stools are passed, probably due to bacterial or fungal overgrowth. Less commonly, *antibiotic associated colitis* or *pseudomembranous colitis* may develop, and even become life-threatening. These are characterised by severe and persistent diarrhoea, sometimes containing blood (see Chapter 16).

After surgery of the abdominal aorta, blood-stained diarrhoea may sometimes occur several days postoperatively. This may indicate *large bowel ischaemia* due to surgical interference with its blood supply. This is a dangerous complication and requires urgent surgical exploration.

POOR URINE OUTPUT

Retention of urine

Abnormally low urinary output or complete failure to pass urine is a common postoperative problem. The most common cause is urinary retention, which usually occurs in males. It is readily diagnosed if there is a palpable suprapubic mass which is dull to percussion. Retention can readily be confirmed by ultrasound examination or, more invasively, by passing a urinary catheter.

Diminished urine production

Poor urine output commonly results from poor renal perfusion due to *hypotension* during the operation or *hypovolaemia* caused by inadequate fluid replacement. If untreated, this may progress to acute renal failure.

If hypovolaemia is suspected, then intravenous fluids should be increased ('fluid challenge'), while monitoring urine output. If the patient is hypotensive, the cause (cardiac failure or hypovolaemia, for example) must be identified and treated as so on as possible. If oliguria persists or worsens, then a urinary catheter should be inserted to ensure that the bladder is emptying and to measure hourly urine output. If urine output is still poor, many patients will respond to a small intravenous dose of a loop diuretic, e.g. 40 mg of frusemide. If these simple measures fail to improve urine output, then acute renal failure must be suspected.

Lastly, bilateral ureteric obstruction should be considered. This is extremely rare as a cause of postoperative low urine output. It can be diagnosed by renal ultrasound which will show bilateral hydronephrosis.

CHANGES IN MENTAL STATE

Marked mental changes may occur in the early postoperative period and are most common in the elderly. These changes are often loosely called 'confusion'. Common phenomena include clouding of consciousness, perceptual disturbances, incoherent speech and agitation or destructive behaviour, such as pulling out cannulas or catheters. Other features are loss of orientation, apathy and stupor, and stereotyped movements such as plucking at the bedclothes.

Elderly patients

The elderly are vulnerable to dementia or cerebrovascular insufficiency. There may thus be little tolerance of systemic insults which tip the balance against cerebral equilibrium.

Factors which predispose to postoperative mental changes in the elderly include:

- Dehydration
- Hyponatraemia
- Hypoxia (from chest infection or cardiac failure, for example)
- Infection (especially of the urinary tract)
- Drugs (particularly opiates and hypnotics)
- Uraemia
- Hypoglycaemia

In addition, pain, anxiety, sleep deprivation and disorientation caused by changes of environment (from ward to operating theatre and on to ITU, for example) may precipitate confusion.

Other causes of mental change

Marked alterations in behaviour in younger patients may indicate alcohol withdrawal or craving for drugs such as barbiturates or heroin. The history has usually been concealed at the time of admission.

JAUNDICE

General causes

Jaundice may develop several days postoperatively in a patient with no history of biliary disease. In these patients, the cause is usually a prehepatic or hepatic disorder. Causes of *prehepatic jaundice* include large blood transfusions, absorption of large haematomas or exacerbation of a haemolytic disorder such as thalassaemia or sickle cell trait (perhaps exacerbated by anaesthesia). *Hepatic* causes are less common. They include cholestasis (caused by infection near the liver, or drug idiosyncrasy), and liver cell toxicity from halothane idiosyncrasy.

Causes related to biliary or liver surgery

Patients subjected to biliary tract or liver surgery may become jaundiced after operation. The most likely cause is *obstruction* of the extrahepatic bile ducts due to retained stone, unrecognised surgical trauma or inadvertant duct ligation. Other causes include *infection* such as ascending cholangitis and systemic absorption of an intra-abdominal collection of bile.

36 FLUID, ELECTROLYTE, ACID–BASE AND NUTRITIONAL MANAGEMENT

Introduction

Most problems of fluid, electrolyte, acid-base and nutritional management are relatively simple and amenable to reason and common sense. Problems can be minimised if high risk patients are properly assessed preoperatively and their cardiovascular status and fluid balance monitored closely postoperatively. Plasma urea and electrolytes and haematocrit should be performed at least once daily.

Severely ill patients with abdominal sepsis and fistulae are most likely to suffer major fluid balance and nutritional problems. These are increasingly being managed with the help of experienced anaesthetists in intensive therapy units, where monitoring and therapy can be managed more precisely.

NORMAL FLUID AND ELECTROLYTE HOMEOSTASIS

Normally, the average adult loses between 2.5 and 3 litres of fluid in 24 hours. About one litre is lost insensibly from skin and lungs, 200 ml are lost in the faeces and the remaining 1300–1800 ml are passed as urine (about 60 ml/hour). Fluid is mainly derived by oral intake of fluids and food, but about 200 ml of water is produced as a by-product of metabolism. About 60–100 mmol of sodium ions and 60–100 mmol of potassium ions are lost each day in the urine, and this is balanced by a normal dietary intake.

When a patient is deprived of all oral intake (as occurs in the perioperative period or in coma) isotonic electrolyte solutions of different types are given intravenously as a substitute.

Fig. 36.1 Summary — normal daily fluid and electrolyte input and output

INTAKE	OUTPUT
Water Diet 2000 ml Metabolism 500 ml	Urine 1400 ml (minimum obligatory volume = 400 ml) Skin loss 500 ml (obligatory diffusion and vaporisation) *note:* sweating can cause loss of several extra litres Lung loss 500 ml (obligatory) Faecal loss 100 ml
Sodium Diet 150 mmol/ day (range 50–300 mmol)	Stool 5 mmol/day Skin transpiration 5 mmol/day (in the absence of sweating) Urine 140 mmol/day (can fall down to 15 mmol/day if required)
Potassium Diet 100 mmol/day (range 50–200 mmol)	Stool 10 mmol/day (obligatory) Skin <5 mmol/day Urine 85 mmol/day (rarely falls below 60 mmol/day)

Water and sodium

In an uncomplicated patient, the daily water and sodium requirements can be given as 2.5 to 3 litres of a standard *dextrose-saline* solution containing 4% dextrose and 0.18% sodium chloride (note: this has only one fifth the salt content of 'normal' or physiological saline). This fluid regimen is often, however, prescribed automatically, without considering special requirements of individual patients. For this reason, its general use should be discouraged. It can be used, however, when an intravenous infusion is required for a day or two, and there are no special fluid or electrolyte problems.

For most patients, the daily water and sodium requirements are best met by using appropriate quantities of *normal saline* solution (0.9% sodium chloride) and 5% *dextrose* (glucose) solution. Normal saline contains 154 mmol of sodium ions per litre. 500 ml will thus satisfy the daily sodium requirement of uncomplicated patients. 2–2.5 litres of 5% glucose make up the additional water requirement. The small amount of glucose present contributes little to nutrition but renders the solution isotonic.This prescription is altered for patients with electrolyte abnormalities or special requirements by varying the volume of physiological saline.

Potassium

Normal potassium requirements are met by infusing 60–80 mmol of potassium chloride in divided doses over each 24 hour period. Premixed intravenous fluids are now available with 20 mmol of potassium chloride per 500 ml container. If premixed containers are not available, potassium chloride can be added to intravenous solutions, but care must be taken to ensure thorough mixing. Concentrations of potassium chloride greater than 40 mmol in 500 ml should be avoided for general use, and bolus injections should never be given because rapid increases in plasma potassium may cause cardiac arrest.

Limits of compensatory mechanisms

Normally, the kidneys maintain fluid and electrolyte homeostasis despite large variations of fluid intake from hour to hour and day to day. The same also applies to fluid and electrolytes given intravenously. The kidneys' compensating ability, however, is reduced by renal parenchymal disease and chronic renal failure.

The total blood volume in the adult male is about 6 litres, of which about 55–60% is water (about 3.5 litres). Falls in blood volume which are not too rapid, can be compensated to a limited extent by fluid movement from the extracellular compartment. This compartment has a volume of more than 10 litres. If a deficit of more than 3 litres occurs in whole body fluid volume, this cannot be adequately sustained and intravascular volume becomes depleted. This is reflected in compensatory cardiovascular changes. Initially, there is a mild tachycardia but when the overall fluid deficit reaches 4 or 5 litres, the pulse rate becomes very rapid and hypotension develops. Note that patients on beta-adrenergic blocking drugs or with cardiac conduction defects may not

Fig. 36.2 Sample daily intravenous fluid regimens as a substitute for oral intake in uncomplicated cases

Prescription (1) for 24 hours (each bag to be given over 4 hours):

500 ml 0.9% sodium chloride + 20 mmol KCl
500 ml 5% dextrose
500 ml 5% dextrose + 20 mmol KCl
500 ml 5% dextrose
500 ml 5% dextrose + 20 mmol KCl
500 ml 5% dextrose

Prescription (2) for 24 hours (each bag to be given over 4 hours):

500 ml dextrose-saline (i.e. 4% dextrose + 0.18% NaCl) + 20 mmol KCl
500 ml dextrose-saline
500 ml dextrose-saline + 20 mmol KCl
500 ml dextrose-saline
500 ml dextrose-saline + 20 mmol KCl
500 ml dextrose-saline

be able to increase their heart rate and will therefore decompensate earlier. With 6 or more litres of fluid deficit, the limit of cardiovascular compensation is reached and the patient develops *hypovolaemic shock* (see Chapter 1).

In neonates, children, the elderly and the chronically ill, cardiovascular compensating ability is greatly reduced. A relatively small fluid and electrolyte imbalance may cause life-threatening complications.

PROBLEMS OF FLUID AND ELECTROLYTE DEPLETION

Surgical patients may suffer large losses of fluid and electrolytes as a result of disease, trauma, burns, surgical operations or surgical complications. These are summarised in Figure 36.3. In addition, many surgical patients are deliberately deprived of oral intake during the perioperative period.

Fig. 36.3 Sources of excess fluid loss in surgical patients

Blood loss — traumatic or surgical

Plasma loss — burns

Gastrointestinal fluid loss — vomiting, nasogastric aspiration, diarrhoea, sequestration in obstructed or adynamic bowel, loss through a fistula or an ileostomy

Inflammatory exudate into the peritoneal cavity — generalised peritonitis or acute pancreatitis

Septicaemia — massive peripheral vasodilatation causes relative hypovolaemia

Abnormal insensible loss — fever, excess sweating or hyperventilation

1. Loss of whole blood or plasma

Rapid and copious blood loss in traumatic injury or operative surgery primarily affects the intravascular compartment. Rapid loss of only 1 litre may cause hypotension or even hypovolaemic shock. When haemorrhage is less rapid, there is time for the extracellular compartment to replace the loss. Thus greater volumes can be lost before the cardiovascular system becomes compromised. The lost blood volume, though compensated by extracellular fluid shift, is still a loss to the system which must be restored either physiologically or by transfusion. If blood loss has ceased, the need for transfusion depends on the volume lost and on the previous haemoglobin concentration. Furthermore, the possibility of further blood loss must be anticipated by ensuring good venous access and cross matching bank blood. Acute blood loss of 500–1000 ml is usually treated by transfusion of plasma substitutes such as gelatin solutions. Larger volumes require whole blood (not packed cells!).

Slow chronic blood loss does not lead to fluid balance problems but may cause symptoms and signs of anaemia. Plasma loss from severe burns should be anticipated by using a standard formula to guide plasma replacement (see Chapter 5). This depends on the area burnt. Transfusion requirements are usually seriously underestimated unless an accepted formula is used.

2. Gastrointestinal fluid loss

Between 5 and 9 litres of electrolyte-rich fluid is normally secreted each day into the upper gastrointestinal tract as saliva, gastric juice, bile, pancreatic fluid and succus entericus (see Figure 36.4). The fluid is reabsorbed lower in the intestine.

Large volumes of water and electrolytes may be lost from the body by vomiting, nasogastric aspiration, diarrhoea, sequestration in obstructed or adynamic bowel, or drainage via a fistula or an ileostomy. If there is inflammation of the bowel, as in gastroenteritis or ulcerative colitis, inflammatory exudate may greatly increase the fluid lost as diarrhoea. Cholera may cause the loss of up to 10 litres of electrolyte-rich fluid in one day.

Abnormal fluid losses must be measured or estimated as accurately as possible. This enables intravenous replacement to be anticipated and so prevent symptoms of fluid and electrolyte depletion. From Figure 36.4, it can be deduced that vomitus and nasogastric aspirates usually contain about 120 mmol of sodium ions per litre and up to 10 mmol potassium ions per litre. Inflammatory diarrhoea contains a slightly lower concentration of sodium ions, but more than 40 mmol of potassium ions per litre. As a general rule, gastrointestinal fluid losses should be replaced by an equivalent volume of normal saline, with potassium chloride being added as necessary. In intestinal obstruction or adynamic ileus, fluid sequestrated in the bowel is replaced in a similar manner, although volume requirements cannot be measured accurately and have to be estimated. Fistulae and overactive ileostomies cause chronic fluid loss, which is high in chloride and bicarbonate.

Fig. 36.4 Daily gastrointestinal secretions and electrolyte composition

SECRETION	VOLUME (ml)	Na^+ (mmol/l)	K^+ (mmol/l)	Cl^- (mmol/l)	$HCO3^-$ (mmol/l)
Saliva	1000–1500	20–80	10–20	20–40	20–160
Gastric juice	1000–2500	20–100	5–10	120–160	nil
Bile	up to 1000	150–250	5–10	40–60	20–60
Pancreatic juice	1000–2000	120	5–10	10–60	80–120
Succus entericus	2000–3000	140	5	variable	variable

3. Intra-abdominal inflammatory fluid loss

Severe intra-abdominal inflammation, as in peritonitis or acute pancreatitis, may cause several litres of fluid, rich in plasma proteins and electrolytes, to be lost into the peritoneal cavity. This is best replaced, as well as can be estimated, by a combination of plasma or plasma substitutes and physiological saline.

4. Septicaemia

Septicaemia is associated with a large increase in capillary permeability. The result is extensive loss of protein and electrolyte-rich fluid from the circulation into the extracellular space, causing cardiovascular collapse and shock. In the same way as for fluid loss into the peritoneal cavity, this should be replaced with a combination of plasma, plasma substitutes and physiological saline.

The fluid volume required is difficult to estimate and so replacement is usually titrated to maintain cardiovascular stability (pulse rate and blood pressure) and urinary output (at least 30 ml per hour), whilst avoiding fluid overload and cardiac failure. In the severely ill patient, in whom the volume requirements are particularly difficult to judge, a central venous pressure line and perhaps a Swann-Ganz catheter make the task simpler and safer. These patients are best managed in intensive care units.

5. Abnormal insensible fluid loss

Abnormal insensible fluid loss can greatly increase overall fluid loss, particularly in the seriously ill patient. Insensible loss must be included in the fluid balance equation, especially if it is sustained for more than a short time. Fever increases insensible loss (mainly as exhaled water vapour) by approximately 20% for each degree C rise in body temperature. A pyrexia of 38.5° C for three days would therefore cause an extra litre of fluid loss. Similarly, prolonged hyperventilation, and also mechanical ventilation, cause large fluid losses. Sodium-rich fluid is lost in sweat. This is easily overlooked in fever and when the ward temperature rises in summer. The elderly, denied fluid preoperatively, are particularly vulnerable.

In summary, maintaining fluid balance in surgical patients depends on anticipating problems before they become irreversible; this includes estimating likely fluid losses to guide replacement, and infusing appropriate electrolyte solutions. Clinical signs of fluid imbalance should be sought (both dehydration and overload) and pulse rate, blood pressure and urine output monitored carefully in patients at risk. Regular measurements of plasma urea and electrolytes should be made. In patients with cardiac failure or shock, monitoring and treatment is best carried out in an intensive care unit, using central venous pressure and perhaps left atrial pressure to determine the volume of fluid replacement.

Physiological changes in fluids and electrolytes in response to surgery and trauma

The stresses of trauma or surgery cause a rise in the level of circulating catecholamines. Stress also stimulates the hypothalamo-pituitary-adrenal axis, which increases production of cortisol and aldosterone. This promotes renal conservation of sodium and water, so that both urine volume and urine sodium concentration fall.

Several factors may cause a fall in renal perfusion. These include haemorrhage, loss of oedema fluid into an area of trauma or operation, and cardiovascular changes in response to anaesthesia. The fall in renal perfusion activates the renin-angiotensin-aldosterone mechanism to sustain the blood pressure. This also promotes reabsorption of sodium and water from the renal tubules. By way of exchange, more potassium and hydrogen ions are lost in the urine. Postoperative urine output thus falls by several hundred ml per day, and the urine is low in sodium (less than 40 mmol/l), high in potassium (greater than 100 mmol/l) and acidic.

Water conservation is further enhanced by stress-mediated ADH secretion from the posterior pituitary. Normally, ADH release is mediated by a rise in plasma osmolality, i.e. a rising plasma sodium ion concentration.

At the site of trauma or operation, a volume of fluid is effectively, though temporarily, removed from the circulation as inflammatory oedema. The volume lost is balanced by that retained as a result of hormonal influences. More potassium is released by damaged tissues than the excess lost in the urine. Thus, postoperative plasma potassium level tends to rise in the first day or two. This is particularly true if stored blood has been transfused, which releases potassium from elderly stored red cells. For these reasons, potassium supplements are not usually needed for the first few postoperative days, provided the preoperative plasma potassium level is normal and potassium-losing diuretics are not being prescribed.

COMMON FLUID AND ELECTROLYTE PROBLEMS

1. Routine elective, and straightforward emergency operations

Most operations fall into this category. Most patients are fit before operation, although some have problems caused by diuretic therapy (for cardiac failure, hypertension or chronic renal failure). For these patients, plasma urea and electrolytes should be checked before operation. Loop and thiazide diuretics may cause *hypokalaemia* whilst potassium-sparing diuretics such as spironolactone, may result in *hyperkalaemia*. If abnormalities are found, operation should ideally be postponed until the problem is corrected. Hypokalaemia can usually be treated by oral potassium supplements or by adding a potassium-sparing diuretic. Hyperkalaemia is usually corrected by substituting a loop or thiazide diuretic.

Mild renal failure (plasma urea up to about 15 mmol/l and creatinine up to about 170 mmol/l) is not usually a contraindication to surgery. These patients tend to be mildly dehydrated however, and oral fluid intake should be strongly encouraged.

Management

For routine elective surgery, the patient is kept 'nil by mouth' for 6–12 hours preoperatively and will take very little oral fluid for up to 6 hours postoperatively. A fluid deficit of 1000–1500 ml is therefore common. This can usually be accommodated and is quickly made good once the patient is drinking normally. Intravenous fluids are therefore not required for many routine operations in adults. Some anaesthetists set up intravenous infusions for minor operations, mainly to ensure emergency venous access; these can be discontinued as soon as the patient is drinking satisfactorily. Occasionally, and despite the use of anti-emetics, patients vomit postoperatively. Intravenous fluids may be necessary if vomiting is prolonged.

Children, especially infants and neonates, are much more vulnerable to fluid deprivation because of their small total fluid content and disproportionate insensible losses. Even minor operations may cause dehydration. Intravenous fluids may therefore be necessary during operation, the volume and rate being calculated according to body weight.

As a rule, the sooner the body assumes control over fluid and electrolyte homeostasis the better. Intravenous fluids should be discontinued as soon as normal oral intake is resumed and urine output is satisfactory.

2. Major abdominal and other operations

Major operations, whether emergency or elective, and especially those involving the bowel, pose special fluid management problems. The principal reasons are:

- Patients are often elderly and are likely to have pre-existing fluid and electrolyte abnormalities and a diminished cardiovascular reserve
- Preoperative vomiting and restricted intake may result in dehydration and electrolyte abnormalities
- Blood loss during and after operation may be excessive
- Operations may take several hours
- The recovery period during which oral intake is nil or restricted may be long — several days after uncomplicated bowel surgery (e.g. hemicolectomy or gastrectomy), longer after peritonitis (e.g. perforated diverticulitis or an anastomotic leak)

It cannot be emphasised too much that careful pre- and postoperative assessment of patients having major surgery is essential. This should include clinical examination for evidence of dehydration (dry mouth and loss of normal skin turgor) or overhydration (elevated jugular venous pressure or cardiac failure). Plasma urea and electrolytes, creatinine and full blood count should also be measured. An elevated urea concentration with little elevation of creatinine is characteristic of dehydration. An abnormally high haematocrit (providing polycythaemia is not present) also indicates dehydration, especially if it was normal beforehand.

Management

If the patient is dehydrated, or has significant electrolyte abnormalities or has been vomiting, an intravenous infusion is set up to stabilise the patient before surgery. Dehydration should be corrected with normal saline. Blood loss from trauma or gastrointestinal bleeding is replaced with whole blood, although plasma or plasma substitutes can be used in an emergency as a holding measure.

Fluid management during the operation is the responsibility of the anaesthetist. An isotonic electrolyte infusion such as 500 ml Hartmann's solution is usually set up at the outset, often followed by a plasma substitute such as a gelatin solution. If operative blood loss exceeds about 750 ml, whole blood is usually given to make up the loss. If blood loss is less than 750 ml, the risks of transfusion usually outweigh the benefit. The exception is patients who were anaemic preoperatively (Hb about 10 g/dl).

A fluid regimen is planned for the postoperative 24 hours, taking into account lack of oral fluids and any further blood loss. For example, a further 500 ml blood loss may be expected from the drain after total hip replacement. In general, only 2 litres of intravenous fluids are required in the first 24 hours postoperatively. It is safer to err on the side of underhydration rather than overhydration, especially if there is a risk of cardiac failure from fluid overload. There is also a danger of precipitating acute urinary retention if an older man's bladder becomes overfilled before he has recovered enough to pass urine.

Intravenous fluids are continued postoperatively until bowel function has returned and free oral fluids resumed. The basic regimen shown in Figure 36.2 earlier is usually adequate. In the meantime, plasma urea and electrolytes should be checked daily. Potassium supplements will not usually be required until the third postoperative day.

3. Abnormalities of plasma sodium concentration

These abnormalities are usually discovered on routine measurement of electrolytes.

Hyponatraemia

The usual cause of hyponatraemia is insufficient sodium in intravenous fluids. This is especially common when replacing lost sodium-rich fluid from the gastrointestinal tract. Other causes include diuretic therapy and occasionally, inappropriate ADH production.

On the surgical ward, inappropriate ADH secretion is uncommon. It can occur in head injuries or neurosurgical patients, pneumonia, empyema, lung abscess and oat-cell carcinoma of the lung. Excess ADH increases renal tubular water reabsorption independently of sodium. This causes water overload and dilutional hyponatraemia. Inappropriate ADH secretion is the likely diagnosis if the urine osmolality is high and the plasma osmolality is low. Unless the hyponatraemia is caused by severe hyperglycaemia or a mannitol infusion, the plasma becomes hypotonic, resulting in cellular overhydration. In severe cases, cerebral oedema results. Mild hyponatraemia is asymptomatic but patients often become confused when the plasma sodium falls below about 120 mmol/l. Convulsions and coma occur below about 110 mmol/l.

Hyponatraemia can usually be treated simply by increasing the sodium content of intravenous fluids within the daily volume limit. Normal saline can be given continuously or, if the hyponatraemia is mild, alternate bags of 0.9% saline and 5% dextrose. If hyponatraemia is caused by inappropriate ADH secretion, this is managed by restricting fluid intake.

Hypernatraemia

This is an uncommon problem and, in the surgical patient, is usually iatrogenic. The usual cause is excess sodium administration in intravenous fluids. This is more likely to occur postoperatively, because aldosterone secretion is increased and sodium is conserved by the kidney. Hypernatraemia sometimes occur through excess water loss during prolonged mechanical ventilation. Very rarely, hypernatraemia is caused by *Conn's syndrome* (primary hyperaldosteronism).

Treatment involves encouraging the patient to drink more water or infusing fluids with a low sodium content.

4. Abnormalities of plasma potassium concentration

Plasma potassium abnormalities are often discovered on routine electrolyte estimation. A cause can usually be found and treatment is straightforward. Acid-base abnormalities can have a profound effect on plasma potassium concentration, but this may correct itself when the acid-base problem is treated.

Hypokalaemia

Preoperatively, hypokalaemia usually results from poor dietary intake, diuretic therapy, chronic diarrhoea, losses from a malfunctioning ileostomy or rarely, excess mucus secretion from a rectal villous adenoma. Rarely, hypokalaemia may be caused by primary hyperaldosteronism (Conn's syndrome).

Postoperative hypokalaemia is usually caused by inadequate potassium supplementation of intravenous infusions. The lack of intake is compounded by increased urinary losses from stress-induced secondary hyperaldosteronism.

Hypokalaemia causes skeletal muscle weakness and reduces gastrointestinal motility, with paralytic ileus in extreme cases. There is also a risk of sudden cardiac arrhythmias or even cardiac arrest. Hypokalaemia can usually be corrected with oral potassium supplements (effervescent or slow-release tablets). For postoperative patients with an intravenous infusion, potassium supplements are added as appropriate. The infusion rate should not exceed 15 mmol per hour.

Hyperkalaemia

This is less common in surgical patients than hypokalaemia. Preoperatively it is most commonly caused by chronic renal failure or high doses of potassium-sparing diuretics. Occasionally, non-steroidal anti-inflammatory drugs cause hyperkalaemia. Postoperatively, hyperkalaemia is usually iatrogenic, due to excessive intravenous potassium administration. It may also be associated with acute renal failure or large transfusions of old stored blood.

Hyperkalaemia is usually asymptomatic but when the plasma potassium concentration rises above 7.0 mmol/l, there is a high risk of sudden death from asystole. Potassium concentration at this level is a medical emergency and should be treated initially by intravenous infusion of insulin and glucose. This causes a shift of potassium from the extracellular to the intracellular fluid compartment. Lesser degrees of hyperkalaemia may be treated with cation exchange resins (e.g. calcium resonium) given orally or rectally. Severe renal failure may require dialysis treatment.

ACID–BASE DISTURBANCES

Significant acid-base abnormalities are uncommon in surgical patients and usually arise in seriously ill patients, many of whom will be managed in an intensive care unit.

1. Metabolic acidosis

Metabolic acidosis usually follows an episode of severe tissue hypoxia resulting from hypovolaemic shock, myocardial infarction or septicaemia. It is also seen in acute renal failure and uncontrolled diabetic ketoacidosis. Clinically, the patient has rapid, deep respirations (a respiratory compensatory mechanism). Arterial blood gas estimations show the characteristic picture of raised hydrogen ion concentration and low standard bicarbonate concentration with a low arterial pCO_2. Serum potassium concentration is elevated because of a shift from the intracellular compartment to the extracellular compartment.

Treatment is directed at the underlying cause. Bicarbonate infusion may be appropriate in severe cases.

2. Respiratory acidosis

This results from carbon dioxide retention in respiratory failure. The usual causes are severe postoperative chest complications or prolonged respiratory depression due to sedative, hypnotic or narcotic drugs. Serum hydrogen ion concentrations and pCO_2 are raised, but standard bicarbonate is normal. Treatment is directed at the underlying cause.

3. Metabolic alkalosis

Metabolic alkalosis is usually caused by severe and repeated vomiting or prolonged nasogastric aspiration in intestinal obstruction. This causes gross loss of gastric acid and classically occurs in pyloric stenosis. The patient becomes severely dehydrated and depleted of sodium and chloride ions; the condition is thus known as *hypochloraemic acidosis*. The kidney attempts to compensate by conserving hydrogen ions but this occurs at the expense of potassium ions. Patients become hypokalaemic not only from excess urinary loss, but also because potassium shifts into the cells in response to the alkalosis. Metabolic alkalosis also occurs with excessive intake of bicarbonate antacids to control dyspepsia (*milk-alkali syndrome*). With modern medical treatment of dyspepsia, and ready access to surgery, metabolic alkalosis of this type is now uncommon. Treatment of hypochloraemic acidosis involves rehydration with normal saline infusion and potassium supplements. Renal excretion of bicarbonate ions eventually corrects the alkalosis.

4. Respiratory alkalosis

This occurs when carbon dioxide is lost via excessive pulmonary ventilation. In surgical practice, the usual cause is prolonged mechanical ventilation during general anaesthesia or in the intensive care unit.

NUTRITIONAL MANAGEMENT IN THE SURGICAL PATIENT

Essential principles

Most surgical patients have no special nutritional requirements and easily withstand the short period of starvation associated with their illness and operation. A few patients need special nutritional support. This ranges from an easily prepared oral diet in diabetes to total parenteral nutrition for patients unable to absorb nutrients from the gastrointestinal tract. Figure 36.5 summarises the range of nutritional regimes and their main surgical indications.

Complete fluid diets and elemental diets were developed after research into the special requirements of manned space travel. They have proved valuable

Fig. 36.5 Special methods of nutrition and their indications

1. **Selective diets for specific indications,** e.g. diabetic, low protein (renal and liver failure), low fat (gall stones), high fibre (constipation, diverticular disease) or reducing (obesity)
2. **Liquidised normal diet** — for patients with partial oesophageal obstruction (e.g. stricture, tumour or Celestin tube) or teeth wired together for fractured mandible or gross obesity
3. **High protein, high calorie dietary supplements** — for chronically malnourished patients capable of a normal diet or debilitated convalescent patients
4. **Complete fluid diet,** i.e. 'semi-digested' minimal residue diets which can be administered orally or via fine-bore nasogastric tube — for nutritional support of the severely malnourished patient and the unconscious, ventilated and seriously ill patient in intensive care
5. **Elemental diet**, i.e. mixture of amino acids, glucose and triglycerides requiring no digestion and minimal absorptive capacity (usually given by fine-bore nasogastric tube) — for patients with minimal remaining bowel after massive resection and in the early stages of an exclusion diet for Crohn's disease
6. **Total parenteral nutrition (TPN)**, i.e. comprehensive intravenous nutrition — for patients with prolonged ileus or a very proximal fistula

for nutritional support of the severely malnourished patient and the patient with minimal bowel absorptive function. These *enteral diets* are available in a variety of proprietary formulae. They are about one fifth the cost of *parenteral nutrition* and intrinsically much safer. Parenteral nutrition should be reserved for conditions where it is specifically indicated. Similarly, the proprietary enteral diets should not be used if normal food can be given in some form.

Index